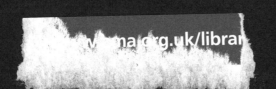

Meyler's Side Effects of Drugs

The International Encyclopedia of Adverse Drug Reactions and Interactions

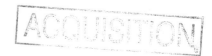

Complementary to this volume

Side Effects of Drugs Annuals 24–29 (1999–2006)
Edited by Jeffrey K. Aronson (Earlier annuals are no longer available in print)

Drugs During Pregnancy and Lactation, Second edition (2006)
Edited by Christof Schaefer et al.

The Law and Ethics of the Pharmaceutical Industry (2005)
By Graham Dukes

Introduction to Clinical Pharmacology, Fifth edition (2006)
By Marilyn Edmunds

Principles of Clinical Pharmacology, Second edition (2006)
Edited by Arthur Atkinson et al.

Writing Clinical Research Protocols (2006)
By E. De Renzo

A Pharmacology Primer (2003)
By Terry Kenakin

Publishing history of *Meyler's Side Effects of Drugs*

Volume*	Date of publication	Editors
First published in Dutch	1951	L Meyler
First published in English	1952	L Meyler
First updating volume	1957	L Meyler
Second volume	1958	L Meyler
Third volume	1960	L Meyler
Fourth volume	1964	L Meyler
Fifth volume	1966	L Meyler, C Dalderup, W Van Dijl, and HGG Bouma
Sixth volume	1968	L Meyler and A Herxheimer
Seventh volume	1972	L Meyler and A Herxheimer
Eighth volume	1975	MNG Dukes
Ninth edition	1980	MNG Dukes
Tenth edition	1984	MNG Dukes
Eleventh edition	1988	MNG Dukes
Twelfth edition	1992	MNG Dukes
Thirteenth edition	1996	MNG Dukes
Fourteenth edition	2000	MNG Dukes & JK Aronson
Fifteenth edition	2006	JK Aronson

*The first eight volumes were updates; the ninth edition was the first encyclopedic version, and updating continued with the Side Effects of Drugs Annual (SEDA) series.

At various times, full or shortened editions of volumes in the Side Effects series have appeared in French, Russian, Dutch, German, and Japanese.
The website of *Meyler's Side Effects of Drugs* can be viewed at:
   http://www.elsevier.com/locate/Meyler.

Meyler's Side Effects of Drugs

The International Encyclopedia of Adverse Drug Reactions and Interactions

Fifteenth edition

Editor

JK Aronson, MA, DPhil, MBChB, FRCP, FBPharmacol S
Oxford, United Kingdom

Honorary Editor

MNG Dukes, MA, DPhil, MB, FRCP
Oslo, Norway

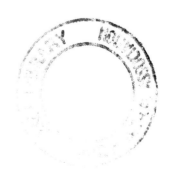

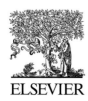

ELSEVIER

AMSTERDAM • BOSTON • HEIDELBERG • LONDON • NEW YORK • OXFORD
PARIS • SAN DIEGO • SAN FRANCISCO • SINGAPORE • SYDNEY • TOKYO

Elsevier
Radarweg 29, PO Box 211, 1000 AE Amsterdam, The Netherlands

Fifteenth edition 2006
Reprinted 2007

British Library Cataloguing in Publication Data
A catalogue record for this book is available from the British Library

Library of Congress Cataloging-in-Publication Data
A catalog record for this book is available from the Library of Congress

ISBN: 978-0-444-50998-7 (Set)
ISBN: 978-0-444-52251-1 (Volume 1)
ISBN: 978-0-444-52252-8 (Volume 2)
ISBN: 978-0-444-52253-5 (Volume 3)
ISBN: 978-0-444-52254-2 (Volume 4)
ISBN: 978-0-444-52255-9 (Volume 5)
ISBN: 978-0-444-52256-6 (Volume 6)

For information on all Elsevier publications
visit our website at books.elsevier.com

Printed and bound in *Great Britain*

07 08 09 10 10 9 8 7 6 5 4 3 2

Contents

Contributors

In this list the main contributors to the Encyclopedia are identified according to the original chapter material to which they made the most contribution. Most have contributed the relevant chapters in one or more editions of the *Side Effects of Drugs Annuals* 23-27 and/or the 14th edition of *Meyler's Side Effects of Drugs*. A few have contributed individual monographs to this edition.

M. Allwood
Derby, United Kingdom
Intravenous infusions—solutions and emulsions

M. Andersen
Odense, Denmark
Antihistamines

M. Andrejak
Amiens, France
Drugs affecting blood coagulation, fibrinolysis, and hemostasis

J.K. Aronson
Oxford, United Kingdom
Antiepileptic drugs
Antiviral drugs
Positive inotropic drugs and drugs used in dysrhythmias

S. Arroyo
Milwaukee, Wisconsin, USA
Antiepileptic drugs

I. Aursnes
Oslo, Norway
Drugs that affect lipid metabolism

H. Bagheri
Toulouse, France
Radiological contrast agents

A.M. Baldacchino
London, United Kingdom
Opioid analgesics and narcotic antagonists

D. Battino
Milan, Italy
Antiepileptic drugs

Z. Baudoin
Zagreb, Croatia
General anesthetics and therapeutic gases

A.G.C. Bauer
Rotterdam, The Netherlands
Antihelminthic drugs
Dermatological drugs, topical agents, and cosmetics

M. Behrend
Deggendorf, Germany
Drugs acting on the immune system

T. Bicanic
London, United Kingdom
Antiprotozoal drugs

L. Biscarini
Perugia, Italy
Anti-inflammatory and antipyretic analgesics and drugs used in gout

J. Blaser
Zurich, Switzerland
Various antibacterial drugs

C. Bokemeyer
Tübingen, Germany
Cytostatic drugs

S. Borg
Stockholm, Sweden
Antidepressant drugs

J. Bousquet
Montpellier, France
Antihistamines

P.J. Bown
Redhill, Surrey, United Kingdom
Opioid analgesics and narcotic antagonists

C.N. Bradfield
Auckland, New Zealand
General anesthetics and therapeutic gases

C.C.E. Brodie-Meijer
Amstelveen, The Netherlands
Metal antagonists

P.W.G. Brown
Sheffield, United Kingdom
Radiological contrast agents

A. Buitenhuis
Amsterdam, The Netherlands
Sex hormones and related compounds, including hormonal contraceptives

H. Cardwell
Auckland, New Zealand
Local anesthetics

A. Carvajal
Valladolid, Spain
Antipsychotic drugs

R. Cathomas
Zurich, Switzerland
Drugs acting on the respiratory tract

A. Cerny
Zurich, Switzerland
Various antibacterial drugs

G. Chevrel
Lyon, France
Drugs acting on the immune system

C.C. Chiou
Bethesda, Maryland, USA
Antifungal drugs

N.H. Choulis
Attika, Greece
Metals
Miscellaneous drugs and materials, medical devices,
and techniques not dealt with in other chapters

L.G. Cleland
Adelaide, Australia
Corticotrophins, corticosteroids, and prostaglandins

P. Coates
Adelaide, Australia
Miscellaneous hormones

J. Costa
Badalona, Spain
Corticotrophins, corticosteroids, and prostaglandins

P. Cottagnoud
Bern, Switzerland
Various antibacterial drugs

P.C. Cowen
Oxford, United Kingdom
Antidepressant drugs

S. Curran
Huddersfield, United Kingdom
Hypnosedatives and anxiolytics

H.C.S. Daly
Perth, Western Australia
Local anesthetics

A.C. De Groot
Hertogenbosch, The Netherlands
Dermatological drugs, topical agents, and cosmetics

M.D. De Jong
Amsterdam, The Netherlands
Antiviral drugs

A. Del Favero
Perugia, Italy
Anti-inflammatory and antipyretic analgesics and drugs
used in gout

P. Demoly
Montpellier, France
Antihistamines

J. Descotes
Lyon, France
Drugs acting on the immune system

A.J. De Silva
Ragama, Sri Lanka
Snakebite antivenom

H.J. De Silva
Ragama, Sri Lanka
Gastrointestinal drugs

F.A. De Wolff
Leiden, The Netherlands
Metals

S. Dittmann
Berlin, Germany
Vaccines

M.N.G. Dukes
Oslo, Norway
Antiepileptic drugs
Antiviral drugs
Metals
Sex hormones and related compounds, including
hormonal contraceptives

H.W. Eijkhout
Amsterdam, The Netherlands
Blood, blood components, plasma, and plasma products

E.H. Ellinwood
Durham, North Carolina, USA
Central nervous system stimulants and drugs that
suppress appetite

C.J. Ellis
Birmingham, United Kingdom
Drugs used in tuberculosis and leprosy

P. Elsner
Jena, Germany
Dermatological drugs, topical agents, and cosmetics

T. Erikkson
Lund, Sweden
Thalidomide

E. Ernst
Exeter, United Kingdom
Treatments used in complementary and alternative
medicine

M. Farré
Barcelona, Spain
Corticotrophins, corticosteroids, and prostaglandins

P.I. Folb
Cape Town, South Africa
Cytostatic drugs
Intravenous infusions—solutions and emulsions

J.A. Franklyn
Birmingham, United Kingdom
Thyroid hormones and antithyroid drugs

M.G. Franzosi
Milan, Italy
Beta-adrenoceptor antagonists and antianginal drugs

J. Fraser
Glasgow, Scotland
Cytostatic drugs

H.M.P. Freie
Maastricht, The Netherlands
Antipyretic analgesics

C. Fux
Bern, Switzerland
Various antibacterial drugs

P.J. Geerlings
Amsterdam, The Netherlands
Drugs of abuse

A.H. Ghodse
London, United Kingdom
Opioid analgesics and narcotic antagonists

P.L.F. Giangrande
Oxford, United Kingdom
Drugs affecting blood coagulation, fibrinolysis, and
hemostasis

G. Gillespie
Perth, Australia
Local anaesthetics

G. Girish
Sheffield, United Kingdom
Radiological contrast agents

V. Gras-Champel
Amiens, France
Drugs affecting blood coagulation, fibrinolysis, and
hemostasis

A.I. Green
Boston, Massachusetts, USA
Drugs of abuse

A.H. Groll
Münster, Germany
Antifungal drugs

H. Haak
Leiden, The Netherlands
Miscellaneous drugs and materials, medical devices, and
techniques not dealt with in other chapters

F. Hackenberger
Bonn, Germany
Antiseptic drugs and disinfectants

J.T. Hartmann
Tübingen, Germany
Cytostatic drugs

K. Hartmann
Bern, Switzerland
Drugs acting on the respiratory tract

A. Havryk
Sydney, Australia
Drugs acting on the respiratory tract

E. Hedayati
Auckland, New Zealand
General anesthetics and therapeutic gases

E. Helsing
Oslo, Norway
Vitamins

R. Hoigné
Wabern, Switzerland
Various antibacterial drugs

A. Imhof
Seattle, Washington, USA
Various antibacterial drugs

L.L. Iversen
Oxford, United Kingdom
Cannbinoids

J. W. Jefferson
Madison, Wisconsin, USA
Lithium

D.J. Jeffries
London, United Kingdom
Antiviral drugs

M. Joerger
St Gallen, Switzerland
Drugs acting on the respiratory tract

G.D. Johnston
Belfast, Northern Ireland
Positive inotropic drugs and drugs used in dysrhythmias

P. Joubert
Pretoria, South Africa
Antihypertensive drugs

A.A.M. Kaddu
Entebbe, Uganda
Antihelminthic drugs

C. Koch
Copenhagen, Denmark
Blood, blood components, plasma, and plasma products

H. Kolve
Münster, Germany
Antifungal drugs

H.M.J. Krans
Hoogmade, The Netherlands
Insulin, glucagon, and oral hypoglycemic drugs

M. Krause
Scherzingen, Switzerland
Various antibacterial drugs

S. Krishna
London, United Kingdom
Antiprotozoal drugs

M. Kuhn
Chur, Switzerland
Drugs acting on the respiratory tract

R. Latini
Milan, Italy
Beta-adrenoceptor antagonists and antianginal drugs

T.H. Lee
Durham, North Carolina, USA
Central nervous system stimulants and drugs that suppress appetite

P. Leuenberger
Lausanne, Switzerland
Drugs used in tuberculosis and leprosy

M. Leuwer
Liverpool, United Kingdom
Neuromuscular blocking agents and skeletal muscle relaxants

G. Liceaga Cundin
Guipuzcoa, Spain
Drugs that affect autonomic functions or the extrapyramidal system

P.O. Lim
Dundee, Scotland
Beta-adrenoceptor antagonists and antianginal drugs

H.-P. Lipp
Tübingen, Germany
Cytostatic drugs

C. Ludwig
Freiburg, Germany
Drugs acting on the immune system

T.M. MacDonald
Dundee, Scotland
Beta-adrenoceptor antagonists and antianginal drugs

G.T. McInnes
Glasgow, Scotland
Diuretics

I.R. McNicholl
San Francisco, California, USA
Antiviral drugs

P. Magee
Coventry, United Kingdom
Antiseptic drugs and disinfectants

A.P. Maggioni
Firenze, Italy
Beta-adrenoceptor antagonists and antianginal drugs

J.F. Martí Massó
Guipuzcoa, Spain
Drugs that affect autonomic functions or the extrapyramidal system

L.H. Martín Arias
Valladolid, Spain
Antipsychotic drugs

M.M.H.M. Meinardi
Amsterdam, The Netherlands
Dermatological drugs, topical agents, and cosmetics

D.B. Menkes
Wrexham, United Kingdom
Hypnosedatives and anxiolytics

R.H.B. Meyboom
Utrecht, The Netherlands
Metal antagonists

T. Midtvedt
Stockholm, Sweden
Various antibacterial drugs

G. Mignot
Saint Paul, France
Gastrointestinal drugs

S.K. Morcos
Sheffield, United Kingdom
Radiological contrast agents

W.M.C. Mulder
Amsterdam, The Netherlands
Dermatological drugs, topical agents, and cosmetics

S. Musa
Wakefield, United Kingdom
Hypnosedatives and anxiolytics

K.A. Neftel
Bern, Switzerland
Various antibacterial drugs

A.N. Nicholson
Petersfield, United Kingdom
Antihistamines

L. Nicholson
Auckland, New Zealand
General anesthetics and therapeutic gases

I. Öhman
Stockholm, Sweden
Antidepressant drugs

H. Olsen
Oslo, Norway
Opioid analgesics and narcotic antagonists

I. Palmlund
London, United Kingdom
Diethylstilbestrol

J.N. Pande
New Delhi, India
Drugs used in tuberculosis and leprosy

J.K. Patel
Boston, Massachusetts, USA
Drugs of abuse

J.W. Paterson
Perth, Australia
Drugs acting on the respiratory tract

K. Peerlinck
Leuven, Belgium
Drugs affection blood coagulation, fibrinolysis, and hemostasis

E. Perucca
Pavia, Italy
Antiepileptic drugs

E.H. Pi
Los Angeles, California, USA
Antipsychotic drugs

T. Planche
London, United Kingdom
Antiprotozoal drugs

B.C.P. Polak
Amsterdam, The Netherlands
Drugs used in ocular treatment

T.E. Ralston
Worcester, Massachusetts, USA
Drugs of abuse

P. Reiss
Amsterdam, The Netherlands
Antiviral drugs

H.D. Reuter
Köln, Germany
Vitamins

I. Ribeiro
London, United Kingdom
Antiprotozoal drugs

T.D. Robinson
Sydney, Australia
Drugs acting on the respiratory tract

Ch. Ruef
Zurich, Switzerland
Various antibacterial drugs

M. Schachter
London, United Kingdom
Drugs that affect autonomic functions or the
extrapyramidal system

A. Schaffner
Zurich, Switzerland
Various antibacterial drugs
Antifungal drugs

S. Schliemann-Willers
Jena, Germany
Dermatological drugs, topical agents, and cosmetics

M. Schneemann
Zürich, Switzerland
Antiprotozoal drugs

S.A. Schug
Perth, Australia
Local anesthetics

G. Screaton
Oxford, United Kingdom
Drugs acting on the immune system

J.P. Seale
Sydney, Australia
Drugs acting on the respiratory tract

R.P. Sequeira
Manama, Bahrain
Central nervous system stimulants and drugs that
suppress appetite

T.G. Short
Auckland, New Zealand
General anesthetics and therapeutic gases

D.A. Sica
Richmond, Virginia, USA
Diuretics

G.M. Simpson
Los Angeles, California, USA
Antipsychotic drugs

J.J. Sramek
Beverly Hills, California, USA
Antipsychotic drugs

A. Stanley
Birmingham, United Kingdom
Cytostatic drugs

K.J.D. Stannard
Perth, Australia
Local anesthetics

B. Sundaram
Sheffield, United Kingdom
Radiological contrast agents

J.A.M. Tafani
Toulouse, France
Radiological contrast agents

M.C. Thornton
Auckland, New Zealand
Local anesthetics

B.S. True
Campbelltown, South Australia
Corticotrophins, corticosteroids, and prostaglandins

C. Twelves
Glasgow, Scotland
Cytostatic drugs

W.G. Van Aken
Amsterdam, The Netherlands
Blood, blood components, plasma, and plasma products

C.J. Van Boxtel
Amsterdam, The Netherlands
Sex hormones and related compounds, including
hormonal contraceptives

G.B. Van der Voet
Leiden, The Netherlands
Metals

P.J.J. Van Genderen
Rotterdam, The Netherlands
Antihelminthic drugs

R. Verhaeghe
Leuven, Belgium
Drugs acting on the cerebral and peripheral circulations

J. Vermylen
Leuven, Belgium
Drugs affecting blood coagulation, fibrinolysis, and hemostasis

P. Vernazza
St Gallen, Switzerland
Antiviral drugs

T. Vial
Lyon, France
Drugs acting on the immune system

P. Vossebeld
Amsterdam, The Netherlands
Blood, blood components, plasma, and plasma products

G.M. Walsh
Aberdeen, United Kingdom
Antihistamines

T.J. Walsh
Bethesda, Maryland, USA
Antifungal drugs

R. Walter
Zurich, Switzerland
Antifungal drugs

D. Watson
Auckland, New Zealand
Local anesthetics

J. Weeke
Aarhus, Denmark
Thyroid hormones and antithyroid drugs

C.J.M. Whitty
London, United Kingdom
Antiprotozoal drugs

E.J. Wong
Boston, Massachusetts, USA
Drugs of abuse

C. Woodrow
London, United Kingdom
Antiprotozoal drugs

Y. Young
Auckland, New Zealand
General anesthetics and therapeutic gases

F. Zannad
Nancy, France
Antihypertensive drugs

J.-P. Zellweger
Lausanne, Switzerland
Drugs used in tuberculosis and leprosy

A. Zinkernagel
Zürich, Switzerland
Antiprotozoal drugs

M. Zoppi
Bern, Switzerland
Various antibacterial drugs

O. Zuzan
Hannover, Germany
Neuromuscular blocking agents and skeletal muscle relaxants

Foreword

My doctor is
A good doctor
He made me no
Iller than I was

Willem Hussem (The Netherlands) 1900–1974
Translation: Peter Raven

"*Primum non nocere*"—in the first place, do no harm—is often cited as one of the foundation stones of sound medical care, yet its origin is uncertain. Hippocrates? There are some who will tell you so;[1] but the phrase is not a part of the Hippocratic Oath, and the Father of Medicine wrote in any case in his native Greek.[2] It could be that the Latin phrase is from the Roman physician Galenius, while others attribute it to Scribonius Largus, physician to one of the later Caesars,[3] and there is a lot of reason to believe that it actually originated in 19th century England.[4] Hippocrates himself, in the first volume of his *Epidemics*, put it at all events better in context: "When dealing with diseases have two precepts in mind: to procure benefit and not to harm."[5] One must not become overly obsessed by the safety issue, but it is a necessary element in good medical care.

The ability to do good with the help of medicines has developed immensely within the last century, but with it has come the need to keep a watchful eye on the possibility of inflicting harm on the way. The challenge is to recognize at the earliest possible stage the adverse effects that a valuable drug may induce, and to find ways of containing them, so that risk never becomes disproportionate to benefit. The process of drug development will sometimes result in methods of treatment that are more specific to their purpose than were their predecessors and hence less likely to produce unwanted complications; yet the more novel a therapeutic advance the greater the possibility of its eliciting adverse effects of a type so unfamiliar that they are not specifically looked for and long remained unrecognized when they do occur. The entire process of keeping medicines safe today involves all those concerned with them, whether as researchers, manufacturers, regulators, prescribers, dispensers, or users, and it demands an effective and honest flow of information and thought between them.

For several decennia, concerned by its own errors in the past, the science of therapeutics put unbounded faith in the ability of well-planned clinical trials to arrive at the truth about the properties of medicines. Insofar as efficacy was concerned that was and remains a sound move, closing the door to charlatanism as well as to well-meant amateurism. Therapeutic trials with a new medicine were also able to delineate those adverse effects that occurred in a fair proportion of users. If serious, they would bar the drug from entry to the market altogether, while if transient and reasonably tolerable they would form the basis for warnings and precautions as well as the occasional contraindication. The problem lay with those adverse drug reactions that occurred rather less commonly or not at all in populations recruited for therapeutic trials, yet which could soon arise in the much broader spectrum of patients exposed to the drug once it was marketed across the world. The influence of race or climate might explain some of them; others might reflect interactions with foods, alcohol, or other drugs; yet others could only be explained, if at all, in terms of the particular susceptibility of certain individuals. Scattered across the globe, these effects might readily be overlooked, regarded as coincidental, or at worst dismissed contemptuously as "merely anecdotal".

The seriousness of the adverse effects issue became very apparent even as the reputation of controlled trials deservedly grew, and it touched on both newer and older drugs. The thalidomide calamity, involving several thousand cases of drug-induced phocomelia, was fortunately recognized by Widukind Lenz and others in the light of individual case reports within two years of the introduction of the product. On the other hand, generations elapsed between the patenting of aspirin in 1899 and the realization in 1965 that it might induce Reye's syndrome when used to treat fever in children. Such events, and many less spectacular, showed that, however vital well-controlled studies had become, there was good reason to remain alert for signals emerging from individual cases. Unanticipated events occurring during drug treatment might indeed reflect mere coincidence, but again they might not; and for many of the patients who suffered in consequence there was nothing in the least anecdotal about them.

Fortunately, the 1950s and 1960s of the 20th century saw the first positive reactions to the adverse reaction issue. Effective drug regulation emerged in one country after another. In 1952, Prof. Leo Meyler of The Netherlands produced his first "Side Effect of Drugs" to pull together data from the world literature. A number of national adverse reaction monitoring bureaux were established to gather data from the field and examine carefully reports of suspected side effects of medicines, creating the basis for the World Health Organization to establish its global reporting system. The pharmaceutical industry has increasingly realized its duty to collect and pass on the information that comes into its possession through its wide contacts with the health professions. Later years have seen the emergence, notably in Sweden and in Britain, of systems through which patients themselves can report possible adverse effects to the medicines they have taken. All these processes fit together in what the French language so appropriately terms "pharmacovigilance", with vigilance as the watchword for all concerned.

In this continuing development, the medical literature provides a resource with vast potential. The world is believed to have some 20 000 medical journals, of which a nuclear group of a thousand or so can be relied upon to publish reports and analyses of adverse effects—not only in the framework of formal investigations but also in letters, editorials, and reports of meetings large and small. Much of that information comprises not so much firm facts as emergent knowledge, based directly on experience in the field and calling urgently for attention. The book that Leo Meyler created has, in the course of fifteen editions and with the support of an ever-larger team of professionals, provided the means by which that attention can be mobilized. It has become the world's principal tool in bringing together, encyclopedically but critically, the evidence on the basis of which adverse drug effects and interactions can be recognized, discussed, and accommodated into medical practice. Together with its massive database and its complementary *Side Effects of Drugs Annuals*, it has evolved into a vital instrument in ensuring that drugs are used wisely and well and with due caution, in the light of all that is known about them.

There is nothing else like it, nor need there be; across the world, *Meyler* has become a pillar of responsible medical care.

M.N. Graham Dukes
Honorary Editor, *Meyler's Side Effects of Drugs*
Oslo, Norway

Notes

1. Lichtenhaeler C. Histoire de la Médicine, Fayard, Paris, 1978:117.
2. Smith CM. Origin and uses of *Primum non nocere*. J Clin Pharmacol 2005;45:371–7.
3. Albrecht H. Primum nil nocere. Die Zeit, 6 April, 2005.
4. Notably in a book by Inman T. *Foundation for a New Theory and Practice of Medicine*. London, 1860.
5. I am indebted to Jeffrey Aronson for his own translation of the Greek original from Hippocrates *Epidemics*, Book I, Section XI, which seems to convey the meaning of the original [ἀσκεῖν περὶ τὰ νοσημάτα δύο, ὠφελεῖν ἢ μὴ βλάπτειν] rather better than the published translations of his work.

Preface

This is a completely new edition of what has become the standard reference text in the field of adverse drug reactions and interactions since Leopold Meyler published his first review of the subject 55 years ago. Although we have retained the old title, *Meyler's Side Effects of Drugs*, the subtitle of this edition, *The Encyclopedia of Adverse Drug Reactions and Interactions*, reflects both modern terminology and the scope of the review. The structure of the book may have changed, but the *Encyclopedia* remains the most comprehensive reference source on adverse drug reactions and interactions and a major source of informed discussion about them.

Scope

The scope of the *Encyclopedia* remains wide. It covers not only the vast majority of prescription drugs, old and new, but also non-prescribed substances (such as anesthetics, antiseptics, lifestyle compounds, and drugs of abuse), herbal medicines, devices (such as blood glucose meters), and methods in alternative and complementary medicine. For this edition, entries on some substances that were regarded as obsolete, such as thalidomide and smallpox vaccine, have been rewritten and restored. Other compounds, such as diethylstilbestrol, although no longer in use, continue to cast their shadow and are included. Yet others, currently regarded as obsolete, have been retained, both for historical reasons and because one can never be sure when an old compound may once more become relevant or provide useful information in relation to another compound. Some drugs have been withdrawn from the market in some countries since the last edition of *Meyler* was published; rofecoxib, cisapride, phenylpropanolamine, and kava (see Piperaceae) are examples. Nevertheless, detailed monographs have been included on these substances because of the lessons that they can teach us and in some cases because of their relevance to other compounds in their classes that are still available; it is also not possible to predict whether these compounds will eventually reappear in some other form or for some new indication.

In the last 15 years there has been increasing emphasis on the use of high-quality evidence in therapeutic practice, principally as obtained from large, randomized clinical trials and from systematic reviews of the results of many such trials. However, while it has been possible to obtain useful information about the beneficial effects of interventions in this way, evidence about harms, including adverse drug reactions, has been more difficult to obtain. Even trials that yield good estimates of benefits are poor at providing evidence about harms for several reasons:

- benefits are usually single, whereas harms are usually multiple;
- the chance of any single form of harm is usually smaller than the chance of benefit and therefore more difficult to detect; however, multiple harms can accumulate and affect the benefit-to-harm balance;
- benefits are identifiable in advance, whereas harms are not or not always;

- the likely time-course of benefits can generally be predicted, while the time-course of harms often cannot and may be much delayed by comparison with the duration of a trial.

For all these reasons, larger and sometimes longer studies are needed to detect harms. In recent years attempts have been made to conduct systematic reviews of adverse reactions, but these have also been limited by several problems:

- harms are in general poorly collected in randomized trials and trials may not last long enough to detect them all;
- even when they are well collected, as is increasingly happening, they are often poorly reported;
- even when they are well reported in the body of a report, they may not be mentioned in titles and abstracts;
- even when they are well reported in the body of a report, they may be poorly indexed in large databases.

All this means that it is difficult to collect information on adverse drug reactions from randomized, controlled trials for systematic review. This can be seen from the evidence provided in Table 1, which shows the proportion of different types of information that have been used in the preparation of two volumes of the *Side Effects of Drugs Annual*, proportions that are likely be the same in this *Encyclopedia*.

Wherever possible, emphasis in this *Encyclopedia* has been placed on information that has come from systematic reviews and clinical trials of all kinds; this is reflected in new headings under which trial results are reported (observational studies, randomized studies, placebo-controlled studies). However, because many reports of adverse drug reactions (about 30%) are anecdotal, with evidence from one or just a few cases, many individual case studies (see below) have also been included. We need better methods to make use of the information that this large body of anecdotes provides.

Structure

The first major change that readers will notice is that the chapter structure of previous editions has given way to a monographic structure. That is because some of the information about individual drugs has previously been scattered over different chapters in the book; for example ciclosporin was previously covered in Chapter 37 and in scattered sections throughout Chapter 45; it is now dealt with in a single monograph. The monographs are arranged in alphabetical order, with cross-referencing as required. For example, if you turn to the monograph on cetirizine, you will be referred to the complementary general monograph on antihistamines, where much information that is relevant to cetirizine is given; the monograph on cetirizine itself contains information that is relevant only to cetirizine and not to other antihistamines. Within each monograph the material is arranged in the same way as in the *Side Effects of Drugs Annuals* (see "How to use this book").

Case Reports

A new feature, recognizable from the Annuals, but not incorporated into previous editions, is the inclusion of case reports of adverse effects. This feature reflects the fact that about 30% of all the literature that is reported and discussed in the Annuals derives from such reports (see Table 1). In some cases the only information about an adverse effect is contained in an anecdotal report; in other cases the report illustrates a variant form of the reaction. A case report also gives more immediacy to an adverse reaction, allowing the reader to appreciate more precisely the exact nature of the reported event.

Classification of Adverse Drug Reactions

Another new feature of this edition is the introduction of the DoTS method of classifying adverse drug reactions, based on the **Dose** at which they occur relative to the beneficial dose, the **Time-course** of the reaction, and individual **Susceptibility factors** (see "How to use this book"). This has been done for selected adverse effects, and I hope that as volumes of SEDA continue to be published and the *Encyclopedia's* electronic database is expanded, it will be possible to classify increasing numbers of adverse reactions in this way.

References

Because all the primary and secondary literature is thoroughly surveyed in the Annuals, the *Encyclopedia* has become increasingly compact relative to the amount of information available (even though it has increased in absolute size), with many unreferenced statements and cross-references to the Annuals, on the assumption that all the information would be readily available to the reader, although that may not always be the case. To restore all the reference material on which the *Encyclopedia* has been based as it has evolved over so many years would be a gargantuan task, but in this edition a major start has been made. Many references to original

material have been restored, and there is now hardly a statement that is not backed up by at least one reference to primary literature. In addition, almost all of the material that was published in Annuals 23 to 27 (SEDA-23 to SEDA-27) has been included, complete with citations. This has resulted in the inclusion of more than 40 000 references in this edition. Readers will still have to refer to earlier editions of the Annual (SEDA-1 to SEDA-22) and occasionally to earlier editions of *Meyler's Side Effects of Drugs* for more detailed descriptions, but now that the *Encyclopedia* is available electronically this will be repaired in future editions.

Methods and Contributors

I initially prepared the text of the *Encyclopedia* by combining text from the 14th edition of *Meyler's Side Effects of Drugs* and the five most recent annuals (SEDA-23 to SEDA-27). [Later literature is covered in SEDA-28 and the forthcoming SEDA-29.] I next restored missing references to the material and extended it where important information had not been included. The resulting monographs were then sent to experts for review, and their comments were incorporated into the finished monographs. I am grateful to all those, both authors of chapters in previous editions and Annuals and those who have reviewed the monographs for this edition, for their hard work and for making their expertise available.

Acknowledgements

This 15th edition of *Meyler's Side Effects of Drugs* was initiated and carefully planned with Joke Jaarsma at Elsevier, who has provided unstinting support during the production of several previous editions of *Meyler's Side Effects of Drugs* and the *Side Effects of Drugs Annuals*. Early discussions with Dieke van Wijnen at Elsevier about the structure of the text were invaluable. Professor Leufkens from the Faculty of Pharmacy at the University of Utrecht was instrumental in helping us to assemble the preliminary content for this edition; pharmacy students in his department entered the text

Table 1 Types of articles on adverse drug reactions published in 6576 papers in the world literature during 1999 and 2003 (as reviewed in SEDA-24 and SEDA-28)

Type of article	Number of descriptions* (%)
An anecdote or set of anecdotes (that is reported case histories)	2084 (29.9)
A major, randomized, controlled trial or observational study	1956 (28.1)
A minor, randomized, controlled trial or observational study or a non-randomized study (including case series)	1099 (15.8)
A major review, including non-systematic statistical analyses of published studies	951 (13.7)
A brief commentary (for example an editorial or a letter)	362 (5.19)
An experimental study (animal or in vitro)	263 (3.77)
A meta-analysis or other form of systematic review	172 (2.47)
Official statements (for example by Governmental organizations, the WHO, or manufacturers)	75 (1.07)
Total no. of descriptions*	6962
Total no. of articles	6576

* Some articles are described in more than one way

electronically into templates under the guidance of Joke Zwetsloot from Elsevier. Christine Ayorinde provided excellent assistance while I expanded and edited the material. The International Non-proprietary Names were checked by Renée Aronson. At Elsevier the references were then checked and collated by Liz Perill, who also copyedited the material, with Ed Stolting, and shepherded it through conversion to different electronic formats. Bill Todd created the indexes. Stephanie Diment oversaw the project and coordinated everyone's efforts.

The History of Meyler

The history of *Meyler's Side Effects of Drugs* goes back 55 years; a full account can be found at http://www.elsevier.com/locate/Meyler and the various volumes are listed before the title page of this set. When Leopold Meyler, a physician, experienced unwanted effects of drugs that were used to treat his tuberculosis, he discovered that there was no single text to which medical practitioners could turn for information about the adverse effects of drug therapy; Louis Lewin's text *Die Nebenwirkungen der Arzneimittel* ("The Untoward Effects of Drugs") of 1881 had long been out of print (SEDA-27, xxv–xxix). Meyler therefore surveyed the current literature, initially in Dutch as *Schadelijke Nevenwerkingen van Geneesmiddelen* (Van Gorcum, 1951), and then in English as *Side Effects of Drugs* (Elsevier, 1952). He followed up with what he called surveys of unwanted effects of drugs. Each survey covered a period of two to four years and culminated in Volume VIII (1976), edited by Graham Dukes (SEDA-23, xxiii–xxvi), Meyler having died in 1973. By then the published literature was too extensive to be comfortably encompassed in a four-yearly cycle, and an annual cycle was started instead; the first *Side Effects of Drugs Annual* (SEDA-1) was published in 1977. The four-yearly review was replaced by a complementary critical encyclopaedic survey of the entire field; the first encyclopaedic edition of *Meyler's Side Effects of Drugs*, which appeared in 1980, was labeled the ninth edition.

Since then, *Meyler's Side Effects of Drugs* has been published every four years, providing an encyclopaedic survey of the entire field. Had the cycle been adhered to, the 15th edition would have been published in 2004, but over successive editions the quantity and nature of the information available in the text has changed. In the new millennium it was clear that for this edition a revolutionary approach was needed, and that has taken a little longer to achieve, with a great deal of effort from many different individuals.

We have come a long way since Meyler published his first account in a book of 192 pages. I think that he would have approved of this new *Encyclopedia*.

J. K. Aronson
Oxford, October 2005

How to use this book

In a departure from its previous structure, this edition of *Meyler's Side Effects of Drugs* is presented as individual drug monographs in alphabetical order. In many cases a general monograph (for example Antihistamines) is complemented by monographs about specific drugs (for example acrivastine, antazoline, etc.); in that case a cross-reference is given from the latter to the former.

Monograph Structure

Within each monograph the information is presented in sections as follows:

GENERAL INFORMATION
Includes, when necessary, notes on nomenclature, information about the results of observational studies, comparative studies, and placebo-controlled studies in relation to reports of adverse drug reactions, and a general summary of the major adverse effects.

ORGANS AND SYSTEMS
Cardiovascular (includes heart and blood vessels)
Respiratory
Ear, nose, throat
Nervous system (includes central and peripheral nervous systems)
Neuromuscular function
Sensory systems (includes eyes, ears, taste)
Psychological, psychiatric
Endocrine (includes hypothalamus, pituitary, thyroid, parathyroid, adrenal, pancreas, sex hormones)
Metabolism
Nutrition (includes effects on amino acids, essential fatty acids, vitamins, micronutrients)
Electrolyte balance (includes sodium, potassium)
Mineral balance (includes calcium, phosphate)
Metal metabolism (includes copper, iron, magnesium, zinc)
Acid–base balance
Fluid balance
Hematologic (includes blood, spleen, and lymphatics)
Mouth and teeth
Salivary glands
Gastrointestinal (includes esophagus, stomach, small bowel, large bowel)
Liver
Biliary tract
Pancreas
Urinary tract (includes kidneys, ureters, bladder, urethra)
Skin
Hair
Nails
Sweat glands
Serosae (includes pleura, pericardium, peritoneum)
Musculoskeletal (includes muscles, bones, joints)
Sexual function
Reproductive system (includes uterus, ovaries, breasts)
Immunologic (includes effects on the immune system and hypersensitivity reactions)
Autacoids

Infection risk
Body temperature
Multiorgan failure
Trauma
Death

LONG-TERM EFFECTS
Drug abuse
Drug misuse
Drug tolerance
Drug resistance
Drug dependence
Drug withdrawal
Genotoxicity
Mutagenicity
Tumorigenicity

SECOND-GENERATION EFFECTS
Fertility
Pregnancy
Teratogenicity
Fetotoxicity
Lactation

SUSCEPTIBILITY FACTORS (relates to features of the patient)
Genetic factors
Age
Sex
Physiological factors
Cardiac disease
Renal disease
Hepatic disease
Thyroid disease
Other features of the patient

DRUG ADMINISTRATION
Drug formulations
Drug additives
Drug contamination (includes infective agents)
Drug adulteration
Drug dosage regimens (includes frequency and duration of administration)
Drug administration route
Drug overdose

DRUG–DRUG INTERACTIONS
FOOD–DRUG INTERACTIONS
SMOKING
OTHER ENVIRONMENTAL INTERACTIONS
INTERFERENCE WITH DIAGNOSTIC TESTS
DIAGNOSIS OF ADVERSE DRUG REACTIONS
MANAGEMENT OF ADVERSE DRUG REACTIONS
MONITORING THERAPY

Classification of Adverse Drug Reactions

Selected major reactions are classified according to the DoTS system (BMJ 2003;327:1222–5). In this system adverse reactions are classified according to the **Dose** at which they usually occur relative to the beneficial dose, the **Time-course** over which they occur, and the **Susceptibility factors** that make them more likely, as follows:

1 Relation to dose

- *Toxic reactions* (reactions that occur at supratherapeutic doses)
- *Collateral reactions* (reactions that occur at standard therapeutic doses)
- *Hypersusceptibility reactions* (reactions that occur at subtherapeutic doses in susceptible patients)

2 Time-course

- *Time-independent reactions* (reactions that occur at any time during a course of therapy)
- *Time-dependent reactions*
    - Immediate reactions (reactions that occur only when a drug is administered too rapidly)
    - First-dose reactions (reactions that occur after the first dose of a course of treatment and not necessarily thereafter)
    - Early reactions (reactions that occur early in treatment then abate with continuing treatment)
    - Intermediate reactions (reactions that occur after some delay but with less risk during longer- term therapy, owing to the "healthy survivor" effect)
    - Late reactions (reactions the risk of which increases with continued or repeated exposure), including withdrawal reactions (reactions that occur when, after prolonged treatment, a drug is withdrawn or its effective dose is reduced)
    - Delayed reactions (reactions that occur some time after exposure, even if the drug is withdrawn before the reaction appears)

3 Susceptibility factors

- *Genetic*
- *Age*
- *Sex*
- *Physiological variation*
- *Exogenous factors* (for example drug–drug or food–drug interactions, smoking)
- *Diseases*

Drug Names And Spelling

Drugs are usually designated by their recommended or proposed International Non-proprietary Names (rINN or pINN); when these are not available, chemical names have been used. If a fixed combination has a generic combination name (for example co-trimoxazole for trimethoprim + sulfamethoxazole) that name has been used; in some cases brand names have been used.

Spelling

Where necessary, for indexing purposes, American spelling has been used, for example anemia rather than anaemia, estrogen rather than oestrogen.

Cross-references

The various editions of *Meyler's Side Effects of Drugs* are cited in the text as SED-l3, SED-14, etc.; the *Side Effects of Drugs Annuals* 1-22 are cited as SEDA-1, SEDA-2, etc. This edition includes most of the contents of SEDA-23 to SEDA-27. SEDA-28 and SEDA-29 are separate publications, which were prepared in parallel with the preparation of this edition.

Indexes

Index of drug names

An index of drug names provides a complete listing of all references to a drug for which adverse effects and/or drug interactions are described. The monograph on herbal medicines contains tabulated cross-indexes to the plants that are covered in separate monographs.

Index of adverse effects

This index is necessarily selective, since a particular adverse effect may be caused by very large numbers of compounds; the index is therefore mainly directed to adverse effects that are particularly serious or frequent, or are discussed in special detail; before assuming that a given drug does not have a particular adverse effect, consult the relevant monograph.

Alphabetical list of drug monographs

The number in parentheses after each heading is the number of the corresponding chapter in the Side Effects of Drug Annuals (SEDA-28 and later) in which the item is usually covered.

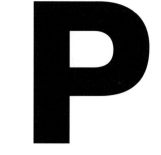

Paclitaxel

See also Cytostatic and immunosuppressant drugs

General Information

Paclitaxel is a complex plant product derived from the bark of the yew tree, *Taxus brevifolia*. It has been used for the treatment of metastatic carcinoma of the ovary and breast. It has also been investigated in the treatment of other carcinomas, including non-small-cell lung cancer, malignant melanoma, head and neck cancers, acute leukemias, and Kaposi's sarcoma. The recommended dosage for the treatment of ovarian and breast carcinoma is 175 mg/m^2 given intravenously over 3 hours every 3 weeks. However, various dosage and administration schedules have been investigated.

Mechanism of action

Paclitaxel acts by enhancing microtubule assembly and stabilizing microtubules (1,2). Microtubules consist of polymers of tubulin in dynamic equilibrium with tubulin heterodimers. Their principal function is the formation of the mitotic spindle during cell division, but they are also active in many interphase functions, such as cellular motility, intracellular transport, and signal transmission. Paclitaxel inhibits the depolymerization of tubulin, and the microtubules formed in the presence of paclitaxel are extremely stable and dysfunctional. This stabilization impairs the essential assembly and disassembly required for dynamic cellular processes, and death of the cell results through disruption of the normal microtubular dynamics required for interphase processes and cell division. In tumor cells, cytotoxicity is represented by the appearance of abnormal microtubular bundles, which accumulate during G2 and mitosis, blocking the cell cycle (3).

Pharmacokinetics

Paclitaxel has non-linear kinetics: peak plasma concentrations and drug exposure increase disproportionately with increasing doses and the pharmacokinetics depend on the schedule of administration. Saturation is reached with high-dose short infusions (4). Paclitaxel has been reported to follow both biphasic (5) and triphasic models (6). The half-life has been estimated at 6–13 hours after intravenous administration (7).

After intravenous administration, paclitaxel is extensively distributed, despite extensive binding to plasma proteins (89%), presumably albumin (2). Its routes of elimination have not been fully elucidated, but renal clearance accounts for an insignificant proportion of total systemic clearance, suggesting that metabolism, biliary excretion, or excretion via other routes are responsible for elimination (6). High concentrations of paclitaxel and its hydroxylated metabolites have been found in rat and human bile, suggesting hepatic metabolism (8). In all, 11 metabolites of paclitaxel have been identified, and paclitaxel metabolism to 6-α-hydroxypaclitaxel is an important detoxification pathway (6,9).

The effects of renal and hepatic dysfunction on paclitaxel elimination have not been studied extensively. Since renal clearance accounts for a small proportion of total clearance, dosage modifications are not considered necessary in patients with renal dysfunction.

One study has shown that patients with existing liver dysfunction have a reduced total body clearance of paclitaxel and require dosage reductions (10). A dosage reduction of 50% has been suggested in patients with moderate or severe hyperbilirubinemia or increased serum transaminases (4).

Paclitaxel is formulated in a mixture of ethanol and Cremophor EL (polyethoxylated castor oil). Cremophor reduced the electrophoretic mobility of serum lipoproteins along with the appearance of a lipoprotein dissociation product. After serum was exposed to Cremophor in vitro or in vivo there was substantial binding of paclitaxel to the lipoprotein dissociation product(s), and this could represent an important factor in the distribution of paclitaxel (11).

General adverse effects

A summary of the incidences of the adverse effects of paclitaxel in single-agent studies in 402 patients is given in Table 1 (12).

Organs and Systems

Cardiovascular

Paclitaxel causes disturbances in cardiac rhythm, but the relevance of these effects has not been fully elucidated. Originally, all patients in trials of paclitaxel were under continuous cardiac monitoring, owing to the risk of hypersensitivity reactions, and cardiac disturbances were therefore more likely to be detected. Many trials limited eligibility to patients without a history of cardiac abnormalities and to those who were not taking medications likely to alter cardiac conduction. The incidence of cardiac dysrhythmias in the population under study not treated with paclitaxel is unknown, and it is therefore not always possible to attribute dysrhythmias to paclitaxel in these patients. The Cremophor EL vehicle does not appear to be implicated in the incidence of dysrhythmias, although hypotension associated with hypersensitivity reactions may occur (13).

The most common effect of paclitaxel is asymptomatic bradycardia, which occurred in 29% of patients in one phase 2 trial (14) and in 9% of patients in a further assessment of 402 patients in phase 2 trials (15). One phase 1 trial showed no significant cardiac dysrhythmias (16), while another reported cardiac toxicity in 14% of patients, 74% of these being due to asymptomatic bradycardia (17). Bradycardia is not an indication for discontinuation of treatment, unless it is associated with atrioventricular conduction disturbances or clinically significant effects (for example symptomatic hypotension). More significant bradydysrhythmias and atrioventricular conduction disturbances have been reported during clinical trials, including Mobitz I (Wenckebach syndrome) and Mobitz II atrioventricular block (14,18).

Table 1 Incidences of adverse effects of paclitaxel

Adverse effect	Incidence (%)
Cardiovascular	
Bradycardia during infusion	10
Hypotension during infusion	23
Severe cardiovascular events	1
Abnormal electrocardiogram (all patients)	30
Abnormal electrocardiogram (patients with normal baseline)	19
Nervous system	
Peripheral neuropathy	
Any symptoms	62
Severe symptoms	4
Hematologic	
Neutropenia $<2 \times 10^9/l$	92
Neutropenia $<0.5 \times 10^9/l$	67
Leukopenia $<4 \times 10^9/l$	93
Leukopenia $<1 \times 10^9/l$	26
Thrombocytopenia $<100 \times 10^9/l$	27
Thrombocytopenia $<50 \times 10^9/l$	10
Anemia <11 g/dl	90
Anemia <8 g/dl	24
Liver	
Bilirubin raised	8
Alkaline phosphatase activity raised	23
Aspartate transaminase (AsT) activity raised	16
Gastrointestinal	
Nausea and vomiting	59
Diarrhea	43
Mucositis	39
Hair	
Alopecia	82
Musculoskeletal	
Myalgia/arthralgia	
Any symptoms	55
Severe symptoms	4
Immunologic reactions (with premedication)	
Any	41
Severe	2

One patient died in heart failure 7 days after receiving paclitaxel by infusion; this patient had no prior history of cardiac problems, apart from mild hypertension (19).

The authors of a review of the cardiac toxicity associated with paclitaxel in a number of studies concluded that the overall incidence of serious cardiac events is low (0.1%) (20). Heart block and conduction abnormalities occurred infrequently and were often asymptomatic. Sinus bradycardia was the most frequent, occurring in 30% of patients. The causal relation of paclitaxel to atrial and ventricular dysrhythmias and cardiac ischemia was not entirely clear. There did not appear to be any evidence of cumulative toxicity or augmentation of acute cardiac effects of the anthracyclines.

In an attempt to clarify further the cardiotoxicity of paclitaxel, its effect on cardiovascular autonomic regulation has been investigated in 14 women (21). The authors concluded that autonomic modulation of heart rate is impaired by paclitaxel, but they were unable to say whether it would return to normal on withdrawal. They also investigated the effect of docetaxel on neural cardiovascular regulation in women with breast cancer, previously treated with anthracyclines (22). They concluded that docetaxel did not impair vagal cardiac control. The changes that they observed in blood pressure suggest that docetaxel changes sympathetic vascular control, although these changes seemed to be related to altered cardiovascular homeostasis rather than peripheral sympathetic neuropathy.

Continuous cardiac monitoring is recommended for patients with serious conduction abnormalities; however, routine cardiac monitoring is considered unnecessary in patients without a history of cardiac conduction abnormalities (7). Further studies are needed to determine the risk in patients treated with paclitaxel with predisposing cardiac risk factors.

Respiratory

Effects of paclitaxel on the respiratory system are generally related to hypersensitivity reactions. One case of pneumonitis was possibly due to a hypersensitivity reaction to either paclitaxel or its vehicle Cremophor EL; treatment with corticosteroids resulted in improvement (23). One patient developed tachypnea and cyanosis and subsequently died of pulmonary edema 7 days after receiving an infusion of paclitaxel (19).

Nervous system

The most common nervous system effect is peripheral neuropathy, although one patient developed tonic-clonic seizures whilst receiving paclitaxel and required treatment with benzodiazepines and barbiturates (14). Motor weakness has occasionally been reported (24).

Neurotoxicity associated with paclitaxel is dose-dependent, cumulative, and characterized principally by a sensory and motor peripheral neuropathy. Neuropathy appears to be related to axonal degeneration and demyelination (25). Neurological toxicity is usually reversible after termination of therapy, and although it rarely requires withdrawal of therapy, it has been the dose-limiting adverse effect in some phase 1 trials (5,26). This effect became more apparent as higher doses of paclitaxel were used, particularly in combination with growth factors, which allow escalating doses of paclitaxel to be administered. A high-dose study has shown dose-related toxicity, with a dose-limiting ceiling at 775 mg/m^2, when paresthesia occurs (27). Patients with co-existing medical illnesses associated with peripheral neuropathy, such as diabetes mellitus and alcohol abuse, may be more prone to develop peripheral neuropathy.

Peripheral neuropathy presents as numbness, burning, and tingling in a glove-and-stocking distribution. Symptoms usually begin 24–72 hours after treatment with paclitaxel, with a symmetrical distal loss of sensation. Most cases occur at doses over 200 mg/m^2 and particularly after multiple courses (24–26). Mild to moderate sensory neuropathy has occurred in 52% of patients treated with doses of 175 mg/m^2, while only 36% experienced neuropathy at doses of at least 135 mg/m^2 (17,24,28,29). At the lower dose of 135 mg/m^2, the effects are usually limited to a mild sensory neuropathy (17,29).

The incidence of peripheral neuropathy increases substantially at doses above 250 mg/m^2 (14,16,18–20,

25,29–32). Neuropathy was the dose-limiting adverse effect in one phase 1 trial with doses of 275 mg/m^2, and patients experienced grade 2–3 neurotoxicity 1–3 days after treatment (5). The symptoms generally subsided within several weeks to months. A study of adverse effects in patients in phase 2 trials showed that peripheral neuropathy occurred in 62% of 402 patients (15). Of patients receiving higher doses (190 mg/m^2 or more), 80% had symptoms that were mild or moderate. In severe cases of peripheral neuropathy a dose reduction of 20% is recommended for subsequent courses (7).

Previous treatment with other neurotoxic agents may compound the problem. In one study symptoms of neurotoxicity were observed in one patient who received concomitant cisplatin with paclitaxel (33). However, signs and symptoms of neurotoxicity have been insignificant in combination treatments of cisplatin and paclitaxel in other trials (1). Pre-existing neuropathy as a result of previous therapy is not a contraindication to paclitaxel (7).

Tricyclic antidepressants, in particular amitriptyline, and venlafaxine are helpful in relieving symptoms of paclitaxel-induced peripheral neuropathy (1,26,33,34).

Sensory systems

Transient scintillating scotomata have been observed in the visual fields of both eyes in nine patients receiving paclitaxel infusions in doses of 175 and 225 mg/m^2 (35). Involvement of the optic nerve was confirmed, and this is likely to have been related to optic nerve conduction abnormalities associated with the neurological effects of paclitaxel. The abnormalities were not progressive and there was some degree of recovery, although one patient sustained a permanent reduction in vision.

Hematologic

Bone marrow suppression is a dose-limiting adverse effect often encountered with paclitaxel. Neutropenia occurs most commonly 8–10 days after treatment, and recovery usually occurs on days 15–21. Paclitaxel is relatively platelet-sparing, and thrombocytopenia and anemia are rare (26). There is no evidence that neutropenia is cumulative, suggesting that paclitaxel may not irreversibly damage hemopoietic stem cells (1).

Neutropenia is dose- and schedule-related and is less common with shorter infusion schedules. At doses of 110–250 mg/m^2 over 24 hours, neutropenia is usually severe, and grade 4 neutropenia develops in a large proportion of patients. Paclitaxel given as a 3-hour infusion causes less severe neutropenia (17,24,29). An analysis of patients receiving either a 3-hour or 24-hour infusion of 175 or 135 mg/m^2 showed that severe neutropenia was more common with the 24-hour infusions: 75% of patients developed severe neutropenia (absolute neutrophil count below 500×10^6/l) and episodes of fever (29). Doses of 200–250 mg/m^2 also cause severe neutropenia when paclitaxel was given as a 24-hour infusion, but recovery of neutrophil count was fairly rapid (13,14,26,33,36,37).

The duration of neutropenia is usually brief and treatment delays for unresolved adverse hematological effects at day 21 are rare. Paclitaxel-induced neutropenia does not always lead to infectious complications, and therefore a dosage reduction for neutropenia alone is not considered necessary (14,16,18–20,29,30).

Prior myelotoxic chemotherapy and/or radiotherapy appear to be major risk factors in determining the severity of neutropenia (1,13). Doses of 200 and 250 mg/m^2 over short infusion times induce minimal myelosuppression in patients who have had minimal prior therapy (26,30); however, seven patients (1.6%) died because of toxicity in another trial in patients with ovarian cancer who had received extensive previous chemotherapy; deaths were due to sepsis or severe neutropenia (13).

Other data suggest that neutropenia may be related to pharmacological exposure, and phase 1 studies have shown that the severity of paclitaxel-induced neutropenia correlates with the area under the paclitaxel concentration–time curve (36).

The incidence of neutropenia has also been investigated in combination schedules. Patients receiving paclitaxel in combination with cyclophosphamide have severe neutropenia more often than with single treatment (72% of patients). Paclitaxel given as a 24-hour infusion before cyclophosphamide is more likely to cause severe neutropenia compared with patients who receive cyclophosphamide first (31).

Attempts to overcome neutropenia include the use of human granulocyte colony stimulating factor (GCSF). The absolute neutrophil counts are generally higher and the duration of severe neutropenia is shorter when GCSF is given 24 hours after paclitaxel and continued until there is recovery of the neutrophil count. When paclitaxel is given in combination with GCSF, doses of 250 mg/m^2 given over 24 hours every 3 weeks are possible without inducing dose-limiting neutropenia (16). Three-hour infusion schedules have also been successful using doses of 250 mg/m^2 in combination with GCSF and doxorubicin (32). Other dose-limiting adverse effects tend to predominate when paclitaxel is given in higher doses in combination with GCSF.

Recommendations currently specify that patients should not be retreated with paclitaxel until the neutrophil count recovers to 2.5×10^9/l and the platelet count recovers to over 100×10^9/l (7).

Gastrointestinal

Severe nausea, vomiting, and diarrhea are uncommon with paclitaxel (1). Although about half of the patients in one study had vomiting or diarrhea, under 5% were severe events (15). In another phase 2 trial, there were 11 episodes of nausea and vomiting in 281 courses (14). Four patients developed diarrhea, but this was not clinically significant. Generally, symptoms of nausea, vomiting, and diarrhea associated with paclitaxel therapy are mild.

Mucositis and stomatitis have been reported with paclitaxel. Mucositis is characterized by ulceration of the lips, pharynx, and oral cavity, occurring 3–7 days after paclitaxel treatment (1,13,14,17,24,26,29,33,36–38). Mucositis appears to be more common during treatment of acute leukemias rather than solid tumors, when doses above 390 mg/m^2 are used (24). Severe mucositis occurred during second and third courses, suggesting a cumulative effect, and was more severe if treatment was given at 15 days or less after previous courses. Patients with hematological malignancies are more prone to breakdown of the mucosal barrier, and this may account for the increased incidence of mucositis. Narcotic analgesics are effective in controlling the pain associated with mucositis (1).

Severe abdominal pain occurred in 25 patients treated with intraperitoneal paclitaxel in doses over 175 mg/m^2 (39).

Transient paralytic ileus occurred in two patients in one study (29). Both patients were diabetic, and these symptoms may have been an additional manifestation of autonomic neuropathy.

Postmortem examinations of patients treated with paclitaxel have shown mucosal ulceration of the esophagus, stomach, small intestine, and colon (40). Changes associated with epithelial necrosis and mitotic arrest were most prominent in patients who had recently been treated with paclitaxel. These findings suggest that paclitaxel causes transient mitotic arrest associated with cell necrosis.

Urinary tract

Reversible renal insufficiency has been reported in one patient who was treated with paclitaxel by the intraperitoneal route (39).

Skin

Local venous effects, including erythema, tenderness, and discomfort, can occur at the injection site during paclitaxel infusion (13). Inflammation is evident within hours and usually resolves within 21 days. Inflammation occurs in areas of drug extravasation along with prolonged soft tissue injuries, and necrotic changes have been reported in one patient at the site of extravasation (41). Inflammation is most likely to be due to the drug, but the Cremophor EL vehicle may be implicated, as it produces mild inflammation in animals (41).

There is little information on the treatment of extravasation of paclitaxel, as it has not been common during clinical trials. However, a soft-tissue injury occurred in one patient at the site of previous extravasation after treatment with paclitaxel in a different limb (42). This resolved within 7 days.

Radiation dermatitis has been reported in a patient who received a single infusion of paclitaxel (43). This was attributed to the potentiation of radiation effects by paclitaxel because of the close time relation between the radiotherapy and paclitaxel therapy.

Hair

Alopecia occurs in nearly all patients who receive paclitaxel, but it has unique characteristics. Hair loss is sudden and complete, and many patients often experience loss of all body hair, including axillary and pubic hair, eyelashes, and eyebrows (28,44). The loss of body hair often occurs with cumulative therapy and is more severe after longer infusion times.

Nails

Onycholysis occurred in five of 21 patients who received more than six doses of paclitaxel 100 mg/m^2/week (45).

The authors also provided a useful review of onycholysis caused by other chemotherapy.

Musculoskeletal

An arthralgia/myalgia syndrome occurs 2–5 days after chemotherapy in about 20–30% of patients receiving paclitaxel and is possibly dose-related (1). It commonly occurs at doses above 170 mg/m^2 (29). Symptoms of myalgia usually involve the shoulder and paraspinal muscles, while arthralgia is common in the large joints of the arms and legs (1,13). Symptoms can be controlled by nonsteroidal anti-inflammatory drugs (13) and perhaps gabapentin (46). The incidence of arthralgia and myalgia is also increased in patients who receive GCSF, with symptoms occurring more frequently in 86% of patients compared with patients who receive similar doses without growth factor support (28%) (16).

The severity of myalgia and arthralgia correlated significantly with the total cumulative dose of paclitaxel 210 mg/m^2/cycle by 3-hour infusion in 247 patients with a median cumulative dose of 630 mg/m^2 (47).

Immunologic

Acute hypersensitivity reactions were common during phase 1 trials of paclitaxel, and this caused delays in the completion of many trials. Reactions were mild to severe and consisted of cutaneous flushing, bronchospasm, bradycardia, and hypotension; the reactions occurred after either the first or second dose (48). The mechanism of these reactions is uncertain, but they are thought to be non-immunologically mediated, and direct histamine release by mast cells is probably responsible. A large dose of Cremophor EL is used in the formulation of paclitaxel, and this may play an important part in these hypersensitivity reactions; Cremophor EL induces similar reactions in dogs by direct release of histamine (4).

In a study of 32 patients, 84% of those who received paclitaxel developed hypersensitivity reactions characterized by hypotension, respiratory distress, and urticaria (35). These symptoms further confirm that histamine is likely to be the cause of the reaction. The majority of reactions (53%) occurred within 2–3.minutes after the administration of paclitaxel and 78% within 10 minutes. There was one fatal reaction, characterized by hypotension and asystole. Most reactions to paclitaxel occurred after the first or second dose, and hypersensitivity reactions were more common with shorter infusion schedules. Since the duration of the infusion affected the incidence of hypersensitivity reactions, an extension of the infusion duration was investigated. Longer infusion schedules were associated with a reduced incidence of hypersensitivity reactions, the frequency of severe reactions being reduced from 12% or more to 5% with longer infusion times (5,15,49).

Premedication regimens of glucocorticoids and histamine H$_1$ and H$_2$ receptor antagonists have been used in an attempt to prevent hypersensitivity reactions in other phase 1 trials. These trials were successfully completed using infusion schedules of 1–120 hours and doses of 135–390 mg/m^2, with a lower incidence of hypersensitivity reactions (15,17,28,29,37,44,48). However, the use of premedication did not completely prevent such reactions.

There were incidences of 16, 13, and 7% with 3-hour, 6-hour, and 24-hour infusion schedules respectively, despite premedication (48), while only 1.5% of patients developed reactions in a trial with doses of 125–250 mg/m^2 over 24 hours with glucocorticoids and histamine receptor antagonists (29). Only one patient out of 26 developed a hypersensitivity reaction with doses of 150–250 mg/m^2 over 24 hours (26). The relative merits of longer infusion times and premedication are not entirely clear.

In one study of infusion of doses of 175–275 mg/m^2 over 6 hours without premedication, there was only one hypersensitivity reaction in 32 patients (49), while patients who received paclitaxel administered over 1 hour with premedication developed no serious hypersensitivity reactions (37). There were no hypersensitivity reactions in 40 patients who received fractionated doses of paclitaxel administered over 3–5 days, with cumulative doses of 120–250 mg/m^2 (36). In a randomized comparison of two doses of paclitaxel given by 3-hour or 24-hour infusions, premedication alone was sufficient to prevent hypersensitivity reactions with either infusion duration (29).

Premedication, consisting of dexamethasone 20 mg intravenously, 12 and 6 hours before the infusion, and diphenhydramine 50 mg and cimetidine 300 mg, intravenously 30 minutes before the infusion, are now routinely given before patients are treated with paclitaxel, and this, as well as a recommended infusion time of 3 hours, has reduced the incidence and severity of hypersensitivity reactions. A single dose of dexamethasone 16 mg given 30 minutes before paclitaxel was effective in preventing hypersensitivity reactions in 43 patients (38); however, whether a single dose of a glucocorticoid is sufficient for prophylaxis is controversial.

About 2% of all patients who receive paclitaxel with preventive premedication will develop a severe hypersensitivity reaction, characterized by dyspnea, hypotension, angioedema, and urticaria, and requiring treatment. Minor reactions occur in 39% of patients but do not require therapeutic intervention (7).

There was a 9% incidence of clinically important hypersensitivity reactions to paclitaxel in 450 women with gynecological malignancies treated with paclitaxel either alone or in combination regimens (50). There was a significant association between bee sting or animal allergy and paclitaxel hypersensitivity in 57 patients with a variety of tumors (51).

Drug–Drug Interactions

General

Drug interactions with paclitaxel have been reviewed (52). The most important of these are the pharmacodynamic interactions with other cytostatic drugs, but pharmacokinetic interactions have also been described.

Paclitaxel is metabolized by the cytochrome P$_{450}$ isoenzymes CYP2C and CYP3A4 (53), and drugs that inhibit or induce these isozymes would be expected to alter the metabolism of paclitaxel. In vitro ranitidine, diphenhydramine, vincristine, vinblastine, and doxorubicin had little or no effect on the metabolism of paclitaxel, but

barbiturates stimulated hydroxylation of the side-chain by induction of CYP3A isoforms (53).

Anthracyclines

The combination of doxorubicin plus paclitaxel is cardiotoxic. Various authors have suggested that after a median cumulative dose of 480 mg/m^2, 50% of patients will have a reduced left ventricular ejection fraction and 20% will develop congestive heart failure.

In 36 women with previously untreated metastatic breast cancer, paclitaxel dose-dependently increased the plasma concentrations of doxorubicin and its metabolite doxorubicinol; this was attributed to competition for biliary excretion of taxanes and anthracyclines mediated by P-glycoprotein (54).

Two studies of the combination of epirubicin plus paclitaxel have shown less reduction in left ventricular ejection fraction and no clinical evidence of cardiac failure (55,56).

Ketoconazole

In patients with ovarian cancer, ketoconazole, 100–1600 mg as a single oral dose 3 hours after paclitaxel 175 mg/m^2 as a 3-hour continuous intravenous infusion, did not alter plasma concentrations of paclitaxel or its principal metabolite, 6-alpha-hydroxypaclitaxel (57).

Platinum-containing cytotoxic drugs

In 21 patients with advanced non-small cell lung cancer carboplatin had no effect on the pharmacokinetics of paclitaxel 135–200 mg/m^2 as a 24-hour intravenous infusion (58). Peripheral neuropathy occurred in 13 of 37 patients treated with paclitaxel 175 mg/m^2 and carboplatin (59). The authors concluded that clinically important neurotoxicity increases with every cycle of chemotherapy. The peripheral neuropathy mainly affected sensory fibers without involving motor nerves. The same paclitaxel/carboplatin chemotherapy in 28 women caused no signs of acute central neurotoxicity or neuropsychological deterioration; however, 11 patients had a peripheral neuropathy (60).

References

1. Rowinsky EK, Cazenave LA, Donehower RC. Taxol: a novel investigational antimicrotubule agent. J Natl Cancer Inst 1990;82(15):1247–59.
2. Rowinsky EK, Onetto N, Canetta RM, Arbuck SG. Taxol: the first of the taxanes, an important new class of antitumor agents. Semin Oncol 1992;19(6):646–62.
3. Horwitz SB, Cohen D, Rao S, Ringel I, Shen HJ, Yang CP. Taxol: mechanisms of action and resistance. J Natl Cancer Inst Monogr 1993;(15):55–61.
4. Rowinsky EK, Donehower RC. Paclitaxel (taxol). N Engl J Med 1995;332(15):1004–14.
5. Wiernik PH, Schwartz EL, Strauman JJ, Dutcher JP, Lipton RB, Paietta E. Phase I clinical and pharmacokinetic study of taxol. Cancer Res 1987;47(9):2486–93.
6. Huizing MT, Keung AC, Rosing H, van der Kuij V, ten Bokkel Huinink WW, Mandjes IM, Dubbelman AC, Pinedo HM, Beijnen JH. Pharmacokinetics of paclitaxel and metabolites in a randomized comparative study in platinum-pretreated ovarian cancer patients. J Clin Oncol 1993;11(11):2127–35.

7. Bristol-Myers Squibb Pharmaceuticals. Taxol (paclitaxel). ABPI Data Sheet Compendium. 1995–1996.

8. Monsarrat B, Alvinerie P, Wright M, Dubois J, Gueritte-Voegelein F, Guenard D, Donehower RC, Rowinsky EK. Hepatic metabolism and biliary excretion of Taxol in rats and humans. J Natl Cancer Inst Monogr 1993;(15):39–46.

9. Gianni L, Kearns CM, Giani A, Capri G, Vigano L, Lacatelli A, Bonadonna G, Egorin MJ. Nonlinear pharmacokinetics and metabolism of paclitaxel and its pharmacokinetic/pharmacodynamic relationships in humans. J Clin Oncol 1995;13(1):180–90.

10. Wilson W, Berg S, Kang K. Phase I/II study of Taxol. 96 hour infusion in refractory lymphoma and breast cancer: pharmacodynamics and analysis of multi drug resistance (mdr-l). Proc Am Soc Clin Oncol 1993;335:134.

11. Sykes E, Woodburn K, Decker D, Kessel D. Effects of Cremophor EL on distribution of Taxol to serum lipoproteins. Br J Cancer 1994;70(3):401–4.

12. Abrams JS, Moore TD, Friedman M. New chemotherapeutic agents for breast cancer. Cancer 1994; 74(Suppl 3):1164–76.

13. Rowinsky EK, Eisenhauer EA, Chaudhry V, Arbuck SG, Donehower RC. Clinical toxicities encountered with paclitaxel (Taxol). Semin Oncol 1993;20(4 Suppl 3):1–15.

14. McGuire WP, Rowinsky EK, Rosenshein NB, Grumbine FC, Ettinger DS, Armstrong DK, Donehower RC. Taxol: a unique antineoplastic agent with significant activity in advanced ovarian epithelial neoplasms. Ann Intern Med 1989;111(4):273–9.

15. Onetto N, Canetta R, Winograd B, Catane R, Dougan M, Grechko J, Burroughs J, Rozencweig M. Overview of Taxol safety. J Natl Cancer Inst Monogr 1993;(15):131–9.

16. Schiller JH, Storer B, Tutsch K, Arzoomanian R, Alberti D, Feierabend C, Spriggs D. Phase I trial of 3-hour infusion of paclitaxel with or without granulocyte colony-stimulating factor in patients with advanced cancer. J Clin Oncol 1994;12(2):241–8.

17. Trimble EL, Adams JD, Vena D, Hawkins MJ, Friedman MA, Fisherman JS, Christian MC, Canetta R, Onetto N, Hayn R, Arbuck S. Paclitaxel for platinum-refractory ovarian cancer: results from the first 1,000 patients registered to National Cancer Institute Treatment Referral Center 9103. J Clin Oncol 1993;11(12):2405–10.

18. Rowinsky EK, McGuire WP, Guarnieri T, Fisherman JS, Christian MC, Donehower RC. Cardiac disturbances during the administration of taxol. J Clin Oncol 1991;9(9):1704–12.

19. Alagaratnam TT. Sudden death 7 days after paclitaxel infusion for breast cancer. Lancet 1993;342(8881):1232–3.

20. Arbuck SG, Strauss H, Rowinsky E, Christian M, Suffness M, Adams J, Oakes M, McGuire W, Reed E, Gibbs H, Greenfield R, Montello M. A reassessment of cardiac toxicity associated with Taxol. J Natl Cancer Inst Monogr 1993;(15):117–30.

21. Ekholm EM, Salminen EK, Huikuri HV, Jalonen J, Antila KJ, Salmi TA, Rantanen VT. Impairment of heart rate variability during paclitaxel therapy. Cancer 2000;88(9):2149–53.

22. Ekholm E, Rantanen V, Bergman M, Vesalainen R, Antila K, Salminen E. Docetaxel and autonomic cardiovascular control in anthracycline treated breast cancer patients. Anticancer Res 2000;20(3B):2045–8.

23. Goldberg HL, Vannice SB. Pneumonitis related to treatment with paclitaxel. J Clin Oncol 1995;13(2):534–5.

24. Rowinsky EK, Burke PJ, Karp JE, Tucker RW, Ettinger DS, Donehower RC. Phase I and pharmacodynamic study of taxol in refractory acute leukemias. Cancer Res 1989;49(16):4640–7.

25. Lipton RB, Apfel SC, Dutcher JP, Rosenberg R, Kaplan J, Berger A, Einzig AI, Wiernik P, Schaumburg HH. Taxol produces a predominantly sensory neuropathy. Neurology 1989;39(3):368–73.

26. Wiernik PH, Schwartz EL, Einzig A, Strauman JJ, Lipton RB, Dutcher JP. Phase I trial of taxol given as a 24-hour infusion every 21 days: responses observed in metastatic melanoma. J Clin Oncol 1987;5(8):1232–9.

27. Somlo G, Doroshow JH, Synold T, Longmate J, Reardon D, Chow W, Forman SJ, Leong LA, Margolin KA, Morgan RJ Jr, Raschko JW, Shibata SI, Tetef ML, Yen Y, Kogut N, Schriber J, Alvarnas J. High-dose paclitaxel in combination with doxorubicin, cyclophosphamide and peripheral blood progenitor cell rescue in patients with high-risk primary and responding metastatic breast carcinoma: toxicity profile, relationship to paclitaxel pharmacokinetics and short-term outcome. Br J Cancer 2001;84(12):1591–8.

28. Gore ME, Levy V, Rustin G, Perren T, Calvert AH, Earl H, Thompson JM. Paclitaxel (Taxol) in relapsed and refractory ovarian cancer: the UK and Eire experience. Br J Cancer 1995;72(4):1016–19.

29. Eisenhauer EA, ten Bokkel Huinink WW, Swenerton KD, Gianni L, Myles J, van der Burg ME, Kerr I, Vermorken JB, Buser K, Colombo N, Bacon M, Santabarbara P, Onetto N, Winograd B, Canetta R. European–Canadian randomized trial of paclitaxel in relapsed ovarian cancer: high-dose versus low-dose and long versus short infusion. J Clin Oncol 1994;12(12):2654–66.

30. Holmes FA, Walters RS, Theriault RL, Forman AD, Newton LK, Raber MN, Buzdar AU, Frye DK, Hortobagyi GN. Phase II trial of taxol, an active drug in the treatment of metastatic breast cancer. J Natl Cancer Inst 1991;83(24):1797–805.

31. Kennedy MJ, Donehower RC, Rowinsky EK. Treatment of metastatic breast cancer with combination paclitaxel/cyclophosphamide. Semin Oncol 1995;22(4 Suppl 8):23–7.

32. Fisherman JS, McCabe M, Noone M, Ognibene FP, Goldspiel B, Venzon DJ, Cowan KH, O'Shaughnessy JA. Phase I study of Taxol, doxorubicin, plus granulocyte-colony stimulating factor in patients with metastatic breast cancer. J Natl Cancer Inst Monogr 1993;(15):189–94.

33. Freilich RJ, Seidman AD. Pruritis caused by 3-hour infusion of high-dose paclitaxel and improvement with tricyclic antidepressants. J Natl Cancer Inst 1995;87(12):933–4.

34. Durand JP, Goldwasser F. Dramatic recovery of paclitaxel-disabling neurosensory toxicity following treatment with venlafaxine. Anticancer Drugs 2002;13(7):777–80.

35. Capri G, Munzone E, Tarenzi E, Fulfaro F, Gianni L, Caraceni A, Martini C, Scaioli V. Optic nerve disturbances: a new form of paclitaxel neurotoxicity. J Natl Cancer Inst 1994;86(14):1099–101.

36. Lokich J, Anderson N, Bern M, Coco F, Dow E, Moore C, Zipoli T, Gonzalves L. Multi-day fractionated administration schedule for paclitaxel. Ann Oncol 1995;6(9):883–5.

37. Hainsworth JD, Greco FA. Paclitaxel administered by 1-hour infusion. Preliminary results of a phase I/II trial comparing two schedules. Cancer 1994;74(4):1377–82.

38. Parikh B, Khanolkar S, Advani SH, Dhabhar B, Chandra M. Safety profile of single-dose dexamethasone premedication for paclitaxel. J Clin Oncol 1996;14(7):2189–90.

39. Markman M, Rowinsky E, Hakes T, Reichman B, Jones W, Lewis JL Jr, Rubin S, Curtin J, Barakat R, Phillips M, Hurowitz L, Almadrones L, Hoskins W. Phase I trial of intraperitoneal taxol: a Gynecoloic Oncology Group study. J Clin Oncol 1992;10(9):1485–91.

40. Hruban RH, Yardley JH, Donehower RC, Boitnott JK. Taxol toxicity. Epithelial necrosis in the gastrointestinal tract associated with polymerized microtubule accumulation and mitotic arrest. Cancer 1989;63(10):1944–50.

41. Ajani JA, Dodd LG, Daugherty K, Warkentin D, Ilson DH. Taxol-induced soft-tissue injury secondary to extravasation:

characterization by histopathology and clinical course. J Natl Cancer Inst 1994;86(1):51–3.

42. Shapiro J, Richardson GE. Paclitaxel-induced "recall" soft tissue injury occurring at the site of previous extravasation with subsequent intravenous treatment in a different limb. J Clin Oncol 1994;12(10):2237–8.

43. Raghavan VT, Bloomer WD, Merkel DE. Taxol and radiation recall dermatitis. Lancet 1993;341(8856):1354.

44. Peereboom DM, Donehower RC, Eisenhauer EA, McGuire WP, Onetto N, Hubbard JL, Piccart M, Gianni L, Rowinsky EK. Successful re-treatment with taxol after major hypersensitivity reactions. J Clin Oncol 1993;11(5):885–90.

45. Hussain S, Anderson DN, Salvatti ME, Adamson B, McManus M, Braverman AS. Onycholysis as a complication of systemic chemotherapy: report of five cases associated with prolonged weekly paclitaxel therapy and review of the literature. Cancer 2000;88(10):2367–71.

46. Nguyen VH, Lawrence HJ. Use of gabapentin in the prevention of taxane-induced arthralgias and myalgias. J Clin Oncol 2004;22(9):1767–9.

47. Kunitoh H, Saijo N, Furuse K, Noda K, Ogawa M. Neuromuscular toxicities of paclitaxel 210 mg m(-2) by 3-hour infusion. Br J Cancer 1998;77(10):1686–8.

48. Weiss RB, Donehower RC, Wiernik PH, Ohnuma T, Gralla RJ, Trump DL, Baker JR Jr, Van Echo DA, Von Hoff DD, Leyland-Jones B. Hypersensitivity reactions from taxol. J Clin Oncol 1990;8(7):1263–8.

49. Brown T, Havlin K, Weiss G, Cagnola J, Koeller J, Kuhn J, Rizzo J, Craig J, Phillips J, Von Hoff D. A phase I trial of taxol given by a 6-hour intravenous infusion. J Clin Oncol 1991;9(7):1261–7.

50. Markman M, Kennedy A, Webster K, Kulp B, Peterson G, Belinson J. Paclitaxel-associated hypersensitivity reactions: experience of the gynecologic oncology program of the Cleveland Clinic Cancer Center. J Clin Oncol 2000; 18(1):102–5.

51. Grosen E, Siitari E, Larrison E, Tiggelaar C, Roecker E. Paclitaxel hypersensitivity reactions related to bee-sting allergy. Lancet 2000;355(9200):288–9.

52. Baker SD. Drug interactions with the taxanes. Pharmacotherapy 1997;17(5 Pt 2):S126–32.

53. Monsarrat B, Royer I, Wright M, Cresteil T. Biotransformation of taxoids by human cytochromes P450: structure–activity relationship. Bull Cancer 1997;84(2):125–33.

54. Gianni L, Vigano L, Locatelli A, Capri G, Giani A, Tarenzi E, Bonadonna G. Human pharmacokinetic characterization and in vitro study of the interaction between doxorubicin and paclitaxel in patients with breast cancer. J Clin Oncol 1997;15(5):1906–15.

55. Rischin D, Smith J, Millward M, Lewis C, Boyer M, Richardson G, Toner G, Gurney H, McKendrick J. A phase II trial of paclitaxel and epirubicin in advanced breast cancer. Br J Cancer 2000;83(4):438–42.

56. Lalisang RI, Voest EE, Wils JA, Nortier JW, Erdkamp FL, Hillen HF, Wals J, Schouten HC, Blijham GH. Dose-dense epirubicin and paclitaxel with G-CSF: a study of decreasing intervals in metastatic breast cancer. Br J Cancer 2000;82(12):1914–19.

57. Jamis-Dow CA, Pearl ML, Watkins PB, Blake DS, Klecker RW, Collins JM. Predicting drug interactions in vivo from experiments in vitro. Human studies with paclitaxel and ketoconazole. Am J Clin Oncol 1997;20(6):592–9.

58. Kearns CM, Belani CP, Erkmen K, Zuhowski M, Hiponia D, Zacharski D, Engstrom C, Ramanathan R, Trenn MR, Aisner J, et al. Pharmacokinetics of paclitaxel and carboplatin in combination. Semin Oncol 1995; 22(5 Suppl 12):1–4; discussion 5–7.

59. Mayerhofer K, Bodner-Adler B, Bodner K, Leodolter S, Kainz C. Paclitaxel/carboplatin as first-line chemotherapy in advanced ovarian cancer: efficacy and adverse effects with special consideration of peripheral neurotoxicity. Anticancer Res 2000;20(5C):4047–50.

60. Mayerhofer K, Bodner-Adler B, Bodner K, Saletu B, Schindl M, Kaider A, Hefler L, Leodolter S, Kainz C. A paclitaxel-containing chemotherapy does not cause central nervous adverse effects: a prospective study in patients with ovarian cancer. Anticancer Res 2000;20(5C):4051–5.

Palivizumab

See also Monoclonal antibodies

General Information

Palivizumab is a humanized monoclonal antibody that inhibits an epitope at the A antigenic site of the F protein of respiratory syncytial virus subtypes A and B (1).

Palivizumab is generally well tolerated (2). Its most common adverse effects (over 5%) are rhinitis, cough, fever, pharyngitis, bronchiolitis, and diarrhea (3).

In 565 patients with respiratory syncytial virus infections palivizumab caused injection site reactions (2.3%), fever (1.5%), and nervousness/irritability (under 1%); no other adverse effects were reported (4).

Organs and Systems

Immunologic

The estimated risk of anaphylactic reactions to palivizumab is under one per 100 000 infants (5). No second-season subjects had a significant antipalivizumab antibody response (titer over 1:80) (6).

References

1. Scott LJ, Lamb HM. Palivizumab. Drugs 1999;58(2):305–11.

2. Mejias A, Chavez-Bueno S, Rios AM, Fonseca-Aten M, Gomez AM, Jafri HS, Ramilo O. Asma y virus respiratorio sincitial. Nuevas oportunidades de intervencion terapeutica. [Asthma and respiratory syncytial virus. New opportunities for therapeutic intervention.] An Pediatr (Barc) 2004;61(3):252–60.

3. Groothuis JR. Safety of palivizumab in preterm infants 29 to 32 weeks' gestational age without chronic lung disease to prevent serious respiratory syncytial virus infection. Eur J Clin Microbiol Infect Dis 2003;22(7):414–17.

4. Groothuis JR, Simpson SJ. Safety and tolerance of palivizumab administration in a large Northern Hemisphere trial. Northern Hemisphere Expanded Access Study Group. Pediatr Infect Dis J 2001;20(6):628–30.

5. Anonymous. Palivizumab: new indication. Moderate reduction in hospitalisation rate. Prescrire Int 2004; 13(74):213–16.

6. Lacaze-Masmonteil T, Seidenberg J, Mitchell I, Cossey V, Cihar M, Csader M, Baarsma R, Valido M, Pollack PF, Groothuis JR; Second Season Safety Study Group. Evaluation of the safety of palivizumab in the second season of exposure in young children at risk for severe respiratory syncytial virus infection. Drug Saf 2003;26(4):283–91.

Pancreatic enzymes

General Information

Pancreatic enzyme supplements are used to treat people who lack pancreatic secretions. Pancreatin, the British Pharmacopoeia standard, is an extract of pancreas, and contains enzymes with proteinase, amylase, and lipase activity; most commercial formulations are similar or identical (SEDA16, 358).

The effect of oral pancreatic enzyme supplementation (Creon 10 000 in a dose of 1000 units of lipase per gram of ingested dietary fat) on fat malabsorption has been evaluated in an open study in 24 patients with HIV infection (1). Pancreatic enzyme supplementation was highly effective in reducing fecal fat loss. There were no clinical adverse effects or changes in serum biochemistry attributable to the drug.

Organs and Systems

Metabolism

The effects of pancreatic exocrine supplements (four capsules with meals, two with snacks; each capsule containing lipase 10000 units, protease 37500 units, amylase 33200 units) on glucose metabolism have been studied in a 2-week parallel, randomized, placebo-controlled trial in 29 patients with chronic pancreatitis who had stool fat excretion of over 10 g/day, 18 of whom were diabetic and 15 of whom were malnourished (2). There were major problems with blood glucose control in 28 of the 29 patients.

Gastrointestinal

Colonic toxicity due to pancreatic enzyme supplements in children with cystic fibrosis has been reviewed (3). Since it was first reported in 1994, an increasing number of cases of fibrosing colonopathy due to pancreatic enzymes have been reported in children with cystic fibrosis in the UK, USA, and continental Europe. The disorder is not affected by age or sex, and the age at diagnosis is 9 months to 13 years.

- Fibrotic injury of the entire colon has been reported in an 8-year-old boy with cystic fibrosis who took pancreatic enzymes 12 000 IU/kg at each meal (SEDA23.36.65). He had earlier been taking 5000 IU/kg. The first colonic symptoms occurred 1 year after the increase in dose.

Evidence implicates high-strength formulations, which provide at least 22 000–25 000 IU of lipase per capsule (compared with low-strength and medium-strength formulations which provide up to 10 000 IU), and the association between pancreatic enzymes and colonopathy is clearly dose-related: the higher the dose greater the risk. There are several hypotheses about the pathogenesis of the condition. They include the following:

- toxicity due to the enteric coating (Eudragit L30D-55) used in high-strength pancreatic capsules;

- prolonged exposure of the colon to high-strength pancreatic enzymes because of the abnormally low small intestinal pH in cystic fibrosis, causing delay in dissolution of the enteric coating of the capsule (which occurs only above pH 5.5) until the enzymes reach the distal small intestine or even the large intestine;
- a colon-specific immune-mediated disorder or primary dysregulation of collagen synthesis in the colonic wall.

High-dose pancreatic enzyme formulations are no longer recommended for use in children because of the risk of fibrosing colonopathies (SEDA-19, 330) (SEDA-20, 322). A consensus meeting between the Cystic Fibrosis Foundation and the FDA in 1995 recommended that weight-based dosing should start at 1000 lipase units/kg per meal for children under 4 years and that the upper limit of the usual dosage should be 2500 lipase units/kg per meal and about half for snacks. This translates to a daily intake of 12 000–15 000 lipase units/kg, and the doses of other enzymes, such as protease, would be proportional (SEDA-21, 366).

Having reviewed the available epidemiological data, the UK's then Medicines Control Agency recommended that high-strength pancreatic enzymes coated with Eudragit L-30D-55 should be contraindicated in children under 15 years, that all high-strength formulations should be available only on prescription, and that no formulation should be used in a dosage over 10 000 IU/kg/day.

Pancreas

The effect of high-dose pancreatic enzymes on pancreatic function has been assessed in a double-blind study in 12 healthy volunteers, six of whom were given 18 capsules of Panzytrat (20 000 units of lipase, 18 000 units of amylase, and 1000 units of protease per capsule) daily for 4 weeks (4). There were no morphological or functional changes in the pancreas in those treated. None of the subjects had severe adverse effects. Two had transient mild nausea, epigastric pain, and heartburn. There were no abnormalities in liver function tests.

Drug Administration

Drug contamination

Pancreatic preparations can be bacterially contaminated (5).

Some formulations of pancreatic enzymes contain monohydroxy bile acids, which should not be administered to patients with liver disease (6).

References

1. Carroccio A, Guarino A, Zuin G, Verghi F, Canani RB, Fonatana M, Bruzzese E, Montalto G, Notarbartolo A. Efficacy of oral pancreatic enzyme therapy for the treatment of fat malabsorption in HIV-infected patients. Aliment Pharmacol Ther 2001;15:25(2).
2. O'Keefe SJD, Cariem AK, Levy M. The exacerbation of pancreatic endocrine dysfunction by potent pancreatic exocrine supplements in patients with chronic pancreatitis. J Clin Gastroenterol 2001;32:319–23.

3. Powell CJ. Colonic toxicity from pancreatins: a contemporary safety issue. Lancet 1999;353:911–15.
4. Friess H, Kleeff J, Malfertheiner P, Müller MW, Homuth K, Buchler MW. Influence of high-dose pancreatic enzyme treatment on pancreatic function in healthy volunteers. Int J Pancreatol 1998;23(2):115–23.
5. Lussi-Schlatter, Soliva, Speiser. Die antimikrobielle Behandlung von peroralen Enzympraparaten mit Gamma-Strahlen., Pharm Acta Helv, 1974;49(2):66–75.
6. Niessen, Konig, Molitor, Neef, Studies on the quality of pancreatic preparations: enzyme content, prospective bio-availability, bile acid pattern, and contamination with purines, Eur J Pediatr 1983;141(1):23–29.

Pancuronium bromide

See also Neuromuscular blocking drugs

General Information

Pancuronium bromide is a non-depolarizing muscle relaxant (1) with two quaternary ammonium groups on a steroid (androstane) skeleton. It is about 5–7 times as potent as D-tubocurarine. Protein binding occurs to both albumins and globulins, probably only to a relatively slight extent (10–20%), although reports vary from 10 to 90%. In contrast to most other non-depolarizing relaxants, pancuronium is metabolized at about 10–20%. Deacetylation in the liver probably accounts for the greater part of this biotransformation. The major metabolites are 3-monohydroxypancuronium, 17-monohydroxypancuronium, and (3,17)-dihydroxypancuronium; they are active pharmacologically, 3-monohydroxypancuronium being half as potent and the other two having 2% of the potency of pancuronium. About 40–50% of a dose is normally excreted in the urine and 5–10% in the bile over 24 hours as pancuronium plus its metabolites.

Pancuronium is reported to inhibit plasma cholinesterase (2) and this may be partly why the action of suxamethonium, given after a small dose of pancuronium, is prolonged. It also weakly inhibits acetylcholinesterase.

For tracheal intubation the usual dose is 0.1 mg/kg. When given after suxamethonium, 0.05 mg/kg is sufficient for good abdominal relaxation. Further doses of about one-quarter to one-third of the initial dose are given at intervals of 30–40 minutes to maintain relaxation. Reversal is easily achieved with neostigmine, provided there is some spontaneous return of neuromuscular transmission beforehand. If the evoked twitch height is less than 10% of the control value, there can be difficulty in reversing the blockade; this applies to all non-depolarizing relaxants, except perhaps vecuronium and atracurium.

The onset time for complete neuromuscular blockade is similar to that of D-tubocurarine and other non-depolarizing agents, namely 2–4 minutes. However, this is to some extent dose-dependent, and because of the relative lack of cardiovascular effects and histamine release, pancuronium can safely be given in higher dosages, thus producing good intubation conditions within 2 minutes. The dose of D-tubocurarine required to achieve similar conditions in 2 minutes would result in hypotension. As with D-tubocurarine, repeated doses can lead to accumulation and prolonged blockade.

In burned patients resistance to the neuromuscular blocking action of pancuronium may be encountered (3), as with other non-depolarizing relaxants.

Patients in whom pancuronium bromide is of value (4) include:

- patients with hypoxemia resisting mechanical ventilation and so cardiovascularly unstable that the use of sedatives is precluded;
- patients with bronchospasm unresponsive to conventional therapy;
- patients with severe tetanus or poisoning when muscle spasm prohibits adequate ventilation;
- patients with status epilepticus unable to maintain their own ventilation;
- shivering patients in whom metabolic demands for oxygen should be reduced;
- patients requiring tracheal intubation in whom suxamethonium is contraindicated.

Organs and Systems

Cardiovascular

Cardiovascular adverse effects are minimal with pancuronium. Ganglion blockade does not occur. Slight dose-dependent rises in heart rate, blood pressure, and cardiac output are common (5), but are often masked by the actions of other co-administered agents, such as fentanyl or halothane, which cause bradycardia or hypotension. These adverse effects of pancuronium are thus often beneficial and can be deliberately harnessed. Several mechanisms contribute: vagal blockade via selective blockade of cardiac muscarinic receptors (6), release of noradrenaline from adrenergic nerve endings (7), increased blood catecholamine concentrations (8), inhibition of neuronal catecholamine reuptake (9–11), and direct effects on myocardial contractility (12). These have been reviewed (13–15).

Occasionally nodal rhythm, atrioventricular dissociation, and tachydysrhythmias (such as ventricular extra beats or even bigeminy) develop, but these usually occur in association with halothane.

Supraventricular tachycardia has been reported after 8 mg pancuronium in a patient taking aminophylline (800 mg/day) (16).

Nodal rhythm can occur after injection of pancuronium. This dysrhythmia and bradycardia appear to be more common when neostigmine (plus atropine) is given for reversal of pancuronium-induced neuromuscular blockade than for reversal of D-tubocurarine or alcuronium (17); cholinesterase inhibition by pancuronium may contribute to the bradycardia in these circumstances.

Respiratory

Histamine release and bronchospasm are relatively rare with pancuronium but have been reported (SEDA-12, 117) (18–21).

Nervous system

Accidental injection into the cerebrospinal fluid of 4 mg of pancuronium resulted in generalized hypotonia, weakness, and hypoventilation (SEDA-15, 126) (22). Neostigmine given intravenously led to prompt recovery.

Sensory systems

Neonates with congenital diaphragmatic hernia often develop respiratory failure. To facilitate mechanical ventilation, neuromuscular blocking agents may be used. Sensorineural hearing loss can occur in survivors, with a reported incidence of up to 60%. It has been associated with the use of pancuronium. In a historical cohort study of 37 survivors of congenital diaphragmatic hernia, children with hearing loss had received significantly higher doses of pancuronium during respiratory failure than children without hearing loss (23). In addition, the cumulative dose of pancuronium correlated with the intensity of hearing loss in decibels. There were no differences with regard to oxygenation and ventilation parameters or to the cumulative dose of aminoglycosides, vancomycin, or furosemide, but children with hearing loss had received a higher cumulative dose of etacrynic acid. The authors admitted that the retrospective study design and the small sample size demanded cautious interpretation of their observations. For the time being, this report is not reason enough to avoid pancuronium if neuromuscular blockade is required. However, it should be remembered that the risk of severe neuromuscular disturbances associated with long-term administration of neuromuscular blocking agents militates against the routine use of these drugs in patients in intensive care, both children and adults. If muscle relaxants are given in this setting for more than a few hours, their effect should be monitored by a peripheral nerve stimulator to avoid overdose and drug accumulation. This may prove technically difficult in neonates.

Liver

Significant hyperbilirubinemia has been reported to occur more frequently in critically ill neonates given pancuronium than in a control group (24). The hyperbilirubinemia increased in the 4 days after withdrawal of pancuronium, whereas during the administration period the hyperbilirubinemia was less in the pancuronium group.

Body temperature

Malignant hyperthermia, possibly triggered by pancuronium, has been described (25), although pancuronium is generally considered to be safe in patients who are susceptible to the syndrome (26).

Second-Generation Effects

Fetotoxicity

There is placental transfer of pancuronium, but no untoward effects have been reported in neonates.

In a comparison of the onset and duration of paralysis produced by 0.2 mg/kg pancuronium ($n = 8$) or pipecuronium ($n = 8$) injected into the thighs of fetuses at 30–38 weeks gestational age, tachycardia occurred in four out of eight fetuses given pancuronium, and there was loss of beat-to-beat variability in two. No such changes were observed in any of the eight fetuses given pipecuronium (27).

Susceptibility Factors

Renal disease

Pancuronium appears to depend more on renal function for its elimination than D-tubocurarine does. Its action is, in most cases, significantly prolonged in renal insufficiency (28); in particular, spontaneous recovery is slow and adequate reversal of the block with neostigmine takes much longer than is generally expected (29). The response to pancuronium is much more unpredictable in renal insufficiency, with great interindividual variation in duration of blockade. Occasionally resistance to neuromuscular blockade with pancuronium is encountered (SEDA-13, 103) (28,30). This may be because of an increase in the volume of distribution. High plasma and tissue concentrations of 3-monohydroxypancuronium, sufficient to produce significant neuromuscular blockade, have also been measured in anuria (31). Monitoring of neuromuscular function is required in patients with appreciable renal dysfunction.

Hepatic disease

In hepatic disease, pancuronium seems to be more problematic than D-tubocurarine. Patients with cirrhosis have a prolonged half-life, a reduced clearance, and a markedly increased apparent volume of distribution (32). This is likely to result in the need for larger initial doses for adequate relaxation and prolongation of recovery of neuromuscular function.

Cholestasis can prolong the action of pancuronium, reducing its plasma clearance by 50%. This may be a result of raised bile salts, reducing the hepatic uptake of pancuronium (which is an important factor contributing to the total plasma clearance in normal patients) (SEDA-6, 130).

In patients undergoing liver transplantation, the dosage requirements for pancuronium and vecuronium by intravenous infusion were reduced by 57 and 50% respectively during the anhepatic phase (SEDA-17, 153), whereas atracurium requirements were not altered by exclusion of the liver from the circulation.

Other features of the patient

As with all muscle relaxants, abnormal reactions can occur in patients with neuromuscular diseases. In addition, muscle fibrillation has been reported, possibly due to pancuronium, in a patient with metachromatic leukodystrophy (33).

Pancuronium is relatively contraindicated, particularly in combination with halothane, in patients who may have raised catecholamine concentrations, or who are receiving drugs with sympathomimetic effects. Severe hypertension together with tachycardia can occur when pancuronium is given to a patient with a pheochromocytoma (34,35).

Caution should also be exercised in patients with thyrotoxicosis and with valvular stenosis, coronary artery insufficiency (36), or other conditions in which a tachycardia is hazardous.

Drug–Drug Interactions

Aminophylline

Aminophylline facilitates neuromuscular transmission, perhaps by increasing neurotransmitter release, through raising cyclic AMP concentrations at the neuromuscular junction via phosphodiesterase inhibition (37). This would account for the antagonism of pancuronium-induced blockade that has been reported in the presence of very high serum concentrations of theophylline (38).

Anticonvulsants

The long-term use of phenytoin has been associated with increased pancuronium requirements during neurosurgical operations (39), although the opposite effect might be expected from the quinine-like membrane-stabilizing activity of phenytoin.

Azathioprine

Azathioprine reduces sensitivity to pancuronium in experimental animals, possibly as a result of phosphodiesterase inhibition, increasing transmitter release (SEDA-4, 87) (40), (SEDA-13, 104).

Carbamazepine

Resistance to pancuronium, with a considerable shortening of recovery time, has been seen in patients taking long-term carbamazepine (SEDA-12, 118) (41); there was an inverse correlation between the daily dose and the recovery time.

Ciclosporin

Ciclosporin can cause considerable prolongation of the neuromuscular paralysis induced by pancuronium (42) in one patient (and also in another given vecuronium). Reversal required both neostigmine and edrophonium. Subsequently, recurarization occurred (SEDA-14, 116). Contributing factors could have been the solvent Cremophor EL in the ciclosporin formulation (Sandimmun) and minor renal dysfunction.

Corticosteroids

Corticosteroids have been reported to antagonize neuromuscular blockade due to pancuronium (43,44). In vitro studies in rats have shown a direct facilitating action of prednisolone on neuromuscular transmission (45), so that one would expect some antagonism of non-depolarizing relaxants in general.

Furosemide

Furosemide (1 mg/kg) shortened the recovery time from pancuronium blockade in neurosurgical patients with normal renal function (46). Phosphodiesterase inhibition and increased pancuronium excretion were suggested as possible explanations.

General anesthetics

Halothane anesthesia increases the risks of tachydysrhythmias when pancuronium is used (47).

Pancuronium lowers the MAC for halothane by 25% (48), although this has been disputed (SEDA-15, 124) (49).

Glyceryl trinitrate

Experiments in cats have demonstrated a significant prolongation and potentiation of the neuromuscular blockade induced by pancuronium during glyceryl trinitrate infusion (1 mg/kg/minute) started before the muscle relaxant was given. No prolongation was seen if suxamethonium, D-tubocurarine, or gallamine were used instead of pancuronium. Neostigmine reversal of the pancuronium block was not affected and neither was the plasma clearance of pancuronium changed over the 2 hours after the injection (50,51). The cause of this phenomenon, and whether it is applicable to humans, remains to be elucidated. However, more recent experiments (also in cats), using only moderate doses of pancuronium (and vecuronium), have failed to elicit any potentiation by glyceryl trinitrate (52).

Lithium carbonate

Prolonged neuromuscular blockade has been reported in patients taking long-term lithium given pancuronium (53). In animal experiments, lithium prolonged neuromuscular block due to pancuronium, suxamethonium, and decamethonium, but not that due to D-tubocurarine and gallamine (54); on the other hand, lithium was reported to have no or minimal effects on the blockade produced by pancuronium or D-tubocurarine (55). The mechanism of this interaction is not known, although possible mechanisms have been discussed (54). Caution, and monitoring are advisable.

Tricyclic antidepressants

The use of both halothane and pancuronium in patients taking tricyclic antidepressant has been reported as resulting in severe tachydysrhythmias. Experiments in dogs have shown that this combination can produce ventricular fibrillation and cardiac arrest (56). Enflurane also resulted in tachycardias in dogs given both imipramine and pancuronium acutely, but not when the imipramine was given chronically for 15 days beforehand. Pancuronium should not be used in patients taking tricyclic antidepressants.

Interference with Diagnostic Tests

Radiography

Complete relaxation in artificially ventilated neonates has resulted in apparent "gasless abdomens" on radiography and confusion in diagnosis. On discontinuation of paralysis, the normal appearance of gas-filled bowel was restored (57).

References

1. Roizen MF, Feeley TW. Pancuronium bromide. Ann Intern Med 1978;88(1):64–8.

2. Stovner J, Oftedal N, Holmboe J. The inhibition of cholinesterases by pancuronium Br J Anaesth 1975;47(9): 949–54.

3. Yamashita M, Shiga T, Matsuki A, Oyama T. Unusual resistance to pancuronium in severely burned patients: case reports. Can Anaesth Soc J 1982;29(6):630–1.

4. Speight TM, Avery GS. Pancuronium bromide: a review of its pharmacological properties and clinical application. Drugs 1972;4(3):163–226.

5. Coleman AJ, Downing JW, Leary WP, Moyes DG, Styles M. The immediate cardiovascular effects of pancuronium, alcuronium and tubocurarine in man. Anaesthesia 1972;27(4):415–22.

6. Saxena PR, Bonta IL. Mechanism of selective cardiac vagolytic action of pancuronium bromide. Specific blockade of cardiac muscarinic receptors. Eur J Pharmacol 1970; 11(3):332–41.

7. Domenech JS, Garcia RC, Sastain JM, Loyola AQ, Oroz JS. Pancuronium bromide: an indirect sympathomimetic agent. Br J Anaesth 1976;48(12):1143–8.

8. Cardan E, Nana A, Domokos M. Blood catecholamine changes after pancuronium bromide administration. Xth Congress of the Scandinavian Society of Anesthesiologists. Lund 1971;57.

9. Quintana A. Effect of pancuronium bromide on the adrenergic reactivity of the isolated rat vas deferens. Eur J Pharmacol 1977;46(3):275–7.

10. Docherty JR, McGrath JC. Potentiation of cardiac sympathetic nerve responses in vivo by pancuronium bromide. Br J Pharmacol 1977;61(3):P472–3.

11. Docherty JR, McGrath JC. Sympathomimetic effects of pancuronium bromide on the cardiovascular system of the pithed rat: a comparison with the effects of drugs blocking the neuronal uptake of noradrenaline. Br J Pharmacol 1978;64(4):589–99.

12. Seed RF, Chamberlain JH. Myocardial stimulation by pancuronium bromide. Br J Anaesth 1977;49(5):401–7.

13. Bowman WC. Pharmacology of Neuromuscular Function. 2nd ed. London/Boston/Singapore/Sydney/Toronto/Wellington: Wright, 1990.

14. Bowman WC. Non-relaxant properties of neuromuscular blocking drugs. Br J Anaesth 1982;54(2):147–60.

15. Marshall IG. Pharmacological effects of neuromuscular blocking agents: interaction with cholinoceptors other than nicotinic receptors of the neuromuscular junction. Anest Rianim 1986;27:19.

16. Belani KG, Anderson WW, Buckley JJ. Adverse drug interaction involving pancuronium and aminophylline. Anesth Analg 1982;61(5):473–4.

17. Heinonen J, Takkunen O. Bradycardia during antagonism of pancuronium-induced neuromuscular block. Br J Anaesth 1977;49(11):1109–15.

18. Heath ML. Bronchospasm in an asthmatic patient following pancuronium. Anaesthesia 1973;28(4):437–40.

19. Buckland RW, Avery AF. Histamine release following pancuronium. A case report. Br J Anaesth 1973;45(5):518–21.

20. Mishima S, Yamamura T. Anaphylactoid reaction to pancuronium. Anesth Analg 1984;63(9):865–6.

21. Bonnet MC, Julia JM, Chardon P, Kienlen J, du Cailar J. Àpropos d'un cas d'anaphylaxie au pancuronium. [Apropos a case of anaphylaxis caused by pancuronium.] Cah Anesthesiol 1986;34(3):253–5.

22. Peduto VA, Gungui P, Di Martino MR, Napoleone M. Accidental subarachnoid injection of pancuronium. Anesth Analg 1989;69(4):516–17.

23. Cheung PY, Tyebkhan JM, Peliowski A, Ainsworth W, Robertson CM. Prolonged use of pancuronium bromide and sensorineural hearing loss in childhood survivors of congenital diaphragmatic hernia. J Pediatr 1999;135(2 Pt 1):233–9.

24. Freeman J, Lesko SM, Mitchell AA, Epstein MF, Shapiro S. Hyperbilirubinemia following exposure to pancuronium bromide in newborns. Dev Pharmacol Ther 1990;14(4):209–15.

25. Waterman PM, Albin MS, Smith RB. Malignant hyperthermia: a case report. Anesth Analg 1980;59(3):220–1.

26. Gronert GA. Malignant hyperthermia. Anesthesiology 1980;53(5):395–423.

27. Fan SZ, Susetio L, Tsai MC. Neuromuscular blockade of the fetus with pancuronium or pipecuronium for intrauterine procedures. Anaesthesia 1994;49(4):284–6.

28. Somogyi AA, Shanks CA, Triggs EJ. The effect of renal failure on the disposition and neuromuscular blocking action of pancuronium bromide. Eur J Clin Pharmacol 1977;12(1):23–9.

29. Bevan DR, Archer D, Donati F, Ferguson A, Higgs BD. Antagonism of pancuronium in renal failure: no recurarization. Br J Anaesth 1982;54(1):63–8.

30. Gramstad L. Atracurium, vecuronium and pancuronium in end-stage renal failure. Dose-response properties and interactions with azathioprine. Br J Anaesth 1987;59(8): 995–1003.

31. Vandenbrom RH, Wierda JM. Pancuronium bromide in the intensive care unit: a case of overdose. Anesthesiology 1988;69(6):996–7.

32. Duvaldestin P, Agoston S, Henzel D, Kersten UW, Desmonts JM. Pancuronium pharmacokinetics in patients with liver cirrhosis. Br J Anaesth 1978;50(11):1131–6.

33. Quader MA, Healy TE. Muscle fibrillation following thiopentone and pancuronium bromide. An association with metachromatic leucodystrophy. Anaesthesia 1977; 32(7):644–6.

34. Hirano S, Ueki O, Misaki T, Hisazumi H, Hamatani K, Matsubara F, Miwa U. Severe hypertension and tachycardia associated with pancuronium bromide in a patient with asymptomatic pheochromocytoma. Hinyokika Kiyo 1984;30(5):709–13.

35. Jones RM, Hill AB. Severe hypertension associated with pancuronium in a patient with a phaeochromocytoma. Can Anaesth Soc J 1981;28(4):394–6.

36. Thomson IR, Putnins CL. Adverse effects of pancuronium during high-dose fentanyl anesthesia for coronary artery bypass grafting. Anesthesiology 1985;62(6):708–13.

37. Ono K, Nagano O, Ohta Y, Kosaka F. Neuromuscular effects of respiratory and metabolic acid–base changes in vitro with and without nondepolarizing muscle relaxants. Anesthesiology 1990;73(4):710–16.

38. Doll DC, Rosenberg H. Antagonism of neuromuscular blockage by theophylline. Anesth Analg 1979; 58(2):139–40.

39. Chen J, Kim YD, Dubois M, et al. The increased requirement of pancuronium in neurosurgical patients receiving dilantin chronically. Anesthesiology 1983;59:A288.

40. Dretchen KL, Morgenroth VH 3rd, Standaert FG, Walts LF. Azathioprine: effects on neuromuscular transmission. Anesthesiology 1976;45(6):604–9.

41. Roth S, Ebrahim ZY. Resistance to pancuronium in patients receiving carbamazepine. Anesthesiology 1987;66(5):691–3.

42. Crosby E, Robblee JA. Cyclosporine-pancuronium interaction in a patient with a renal allograft. Can J Anaesth 1988;35(3 Pt 1):300–2.

43. Meyers EF. Partial recovery from pancuronium neuromuscular blockade following hydrocortisone administration. Anesthesiology 1977;46(2):148–50.

44. Laflin MJ. Interaction of pancuronium and corticosteroids. Anesthesiology 1977;47(5):471–2.

45. Wilson RW, Ward MD, Johns TR. Corticosteroids: a direct effect at the neuromuscular junction. Neurology 1974; 24(11):1091–5.
46. Azar I, Cottrell J, Gupta B, Turndorf H. Furosemide facilitates recovery of evoked twitch response after pancuronium. Anesth Analg 1980;59(1):55–7.
47. Stirt JA, Sullivan SF. Aminophylline. Anesth Analg 1981;60(8):587–602.
48. Forbes AR, Cohen NH, Eger EI 2nd. Pancuronium reduces halothane requirement in man. Anesth Analg 1979; 58(6):497–9.
49. Fahey MR, Sessler DI, Cannon JE, Brady K, Stoen R, Miller RD. Atracurium, vecuronium, and pancuronium do not alter the minimum alveolar concentration of halothane in humans. Anesthesiology 1989;71(1):53–6.
50. Glisson SN, El-Etr AA, Lim R. Prolongation of pancuronium-induced neuromuscular blockade by intravenous infusion of nitroglycerin. Anesthesiology 1979;51(1):47–9.
51. Glisson SN, Sanchez MM, El-Etr AA, Lim RA. Nitroglycerin and the neuromuscular blockade produced by gallamine, succinylcholine, D-tubocurarine, and pancuronium. Anesth Analg 1980;59(2):117–22.
52. Schwarz S, Agoston S, Houwertjes MC. Does intravenous infusion of nitroglycerin potentiate pancuronium- and vecuronium-induced neuromuscular blockade? Anesth Analg 1986;65(2):156–60.
53. Borden H, Clarke MT, Katz H. The use of pancuronium bromide in patients receiving lithium carbonate. Can Anaesth Soc J 1974;21(1):79–82.
54. Hill GE, Wong KC, Hodges MR. Lithium carbonate and neuromuscular blocking agents. Anesthesiology 1977; 46(2):122–6.
55. Waud BE, Farrell L, Waud DR. Lithium and neuromuscular transmission. Anesth Analg 1982;61(5):399–402.
56. Edwards RP, Miller RD, Roizen MF, Ham J, Way WL, Lake CR, Roderick L. Cardiac responses to imipramine and pancuronium during anesthesia with halothane or enflurane. Anesthesiology 1979;50(5):421–5.
57. Siegle RL. Neonatal gasless abdomen: another cause. Am J Roentgenol 1979;133(3):522–3.

Pantoprazole

See also Proton pump inhibitors

General Information

Pantoprazole is a proton pump inhibitor.

Comparative studies

Pantoprazole 40 mg/day and ranitidine 150 mg bd for 8 weeks have been compared in the treatment of grades II and III reflux esophagitis in a randomized, double-blind trial in 256 patients (1). Symptom relief and healing rates were significantly better with pantoprazole. The incidences of adverse effects were similar in the two groups; the most commonly reported were diarrhea and somnolence with pantoprazole (2–3%) and headache, diarrhea, dizziness, increases in liver enzymes, and pruritus (2–4%) with ranitidine.

Pantoprazole 20 and 40 mg/day and nizatidine 150 mg bd for 8 weeks have been compared in the treatment of reflux esophagitis (grade II or worse) in a multicenter,

randomized, double-blind trial in 221 patients (2). Both doses of pantoprazole were more effective in relieving symptoms and healing erosive esophagitis than nizatidine. The incidences of adverse effects were similar in the three groups; the most commonly reported were diarrhea and headache.

Pantoprazole 20 mg/day and ranitidine 300 mg/day for 12 months have been compared in the relief of symptoms in a multicenter, randomized, double-blind trial in 307 patients with symptomatic gastro-esophageal reflux disease in primary care (3). Symptom control was significantly more effective and faster with pantoprazole than ranitidine. Adverse effects were similar in the two groups; the most common adverse effects were headache, diarrhea, nausea, constipation, and vomiting.

Pantoprazole 40 mg/day and pantoprazole 40 mg/day plus cisapride 20 mg bd for 8 weeks have been compared in the treatment of gastro-esophageal reflux disease in a multicenter, randomized, double-blind trial in 350 patients (4). The addition of cisapride did not significantly improve symptom control or healing rates. The frequency of adverse effects in the two groups was similar. Compliance was worse in the pantoprazole plus cisapride group.

References

1. Meneghelli UG, Boaventura S, Moraes-Filho JP, Leitao O, Ferrari AP, Almeida JR, Magalhaes AF, Castro LP, Haddad MT, Tolentino M, Jorge JL, Silva E, Maguilnik I, Fischer R. Efficacy and tolerability of pantoprazole versus ranitidine in the treatment of reflux esophagitis and the influence of *Helicobacter pylori* infection on healing rate. Dis Esophagus 2002;15(1):50–6.
2. Kovacs TO, Wilcox CM, DeVault K, Miska D, Bochenek W; Pantoprazole US Gerd Study Group B. Comparison of the efficacy of pantoprazole vs. nizatidine in the treatment of erosive oesophagitis: a randomized, active-controlled, double-blind study. Aliment Pharmacol Ther 2002;16(12): 2043–52.
3. Talley NJ, Moore MG, Sprogis A, Katelaris P. Randomised controlled trial of pantoprazole versus ranitidine for the treatment of uninvestigated heartburn in primary care. Med J Aust 2002;177(8):423–7.
4. van Rensburg CJ, Bardhan KD. No clinical benefit of adding cisapride to pantoprazole for treatment of gastro-oesophageal reflux disease. Eur J Gastroenterol Hepatol 2001;13(8):909–14.

Pantothenic acid derivatives

See also Vitamins

General Information

The pantothenic acid derivatives include pantothenic acid (BAN), pantothenol (BAN), dexpanthenol (rINN), and hopantenic acid (rINN).

Pantothenic acid (vitamin B_5) has been proposed as a treatment for hair loss. It has been used to treat pantothenic acid deficiency, acne, and rheumatoid arthritis. Over the past 30 years, only mild adverse reactions, such as rash and diarrhea, have been reported.

Hopantenate (calcium D-(+)-4-(2, 4-dihydroxy-3, 3-dimethylbutyramido)butyrate hemihydrate), or calcium hopantenate, is a homoanalog of l-pantothenate and has been used in Japan for the treatment of mental retardation with behavioral abnormalities. It represents one of the many attempts that have been made, so far unsuccessfully, to develop derivatives of substances belonging to the vitamin B group as agents for the treatment of brain or nervous disorders (SEDA-12, 328) (SEDA-13, 347).

Adverse effects, sometimes fatal, have been reported in patients taking calcium hopantenate, notably encephalopathy with metabolic acidosis and semicoma (1) and a Reye-like syndrome (2); this may be due to pantothenic acid deficiency, as hopantenate is a pantothenic acid antagonist. In elderly people, liver dysfunction and gastrointestinal upsets have been reported (3,4). In Japan, where the product was introduced in 1978, the control authorities in 1988 issued a series of warnings with respect to problems caused by hopantenate (5).

Organs and Systems

Cardiovascular

Eosinophilic pleural effusion with eosinophilic pericardial tamponade has been attributed to concomitant use of pantothenic acid and biotin (6).

- A 76-year-old woman developed chest pain and difficulty in breathing. She had no history of allergy and had been taking biotin 10 mg/day and pantothenic acid 300 mg/day for 2 months for alopecia. Chest X-rays showed pleural effusions and cardiac enlargement. Blood tests showed an inflammatory syndrome, with an erythrocyte sedimentation rate of 51 mm/hour and an eosinophil count of $1.2–1.5 \times 10^9$/l. Pericardiotomy showed an eosinophilic infiltrate. There was no evidence of vasculitis. Serological studies were negative for antinuclear antibodies, rheumatoid factor, viruses, bacteria, and Lyme disease. Stool examination and parasitological serologies were negative. A malignant tumor was excluded by mammography, thoracoscopy, and a CT scan. Myelography, a biopsy specimen of the iliac crest bone, and the concentrations of IgE, lysozyme, and vitamin B_{12} were also normal. A week after withdrawal of pantothenic acid and biotin she improved dramatically and her eosinophilia resolved.

Metabolism

As a pantothenic acid analogue, hopantenate can affect lactate generation, glucose metabolism, and ammonia disposal, and there have been two fatal cases in elderly people who developed disturbances of consciousness with lactic acidosis, hypoglycemia, and hyperammonemia (7).

Immunologic

Contact allergy to dexpanthenol is rare, but it occurs more often in some patients (for example those with eczema of the lower leg). Between 1992 and 1999, only 163 of 13 216 patients tested in the Information Network of Departments of Dermatology had a positive reaction to dexpanthenol. There have been no previous cases of occupational dexpanthenol sensitization caused by occupational exposure, but one has been reported in a junior nurse (8).

- Six weeks after starting training a 29-year-old nurse developed flushing and pruritus on the back of both hands and fingers, spreading to the forearms. Because of increased skin sensitivity she had been recommended to use skin protection measures; however, she did not use the skin protection cream that was available at the hospital but used a "Hand- und Hautsalbe" that had been designed for use especially in hairdressing salons. In addition to the lesions on her hands and arms she had periorbital shadowing, angular cheilitis, palmar hyperlinearity, and slightly generalized xerosis of the skin. She also reported seasonal rhinoconjunctivitis, intolerability of metals, and rhagades on the ears. After withdrawal of all supposed allergenic substances and local antieczematous therapy, the hand and arm lesions healed within a few days. Skin tests were positive for nickel-II-sulfate, imidazolidinyl urea, phenyl mercury acetate, and the hand cream, in which pantothenol (5% in vaseline) was identified as the allergen. She avoided the cream and the eczema did not recur.

References

1. Kimura A, Yoshida I, Ono E, Matsuishi T, Yoshino M, Yamashita F, Yamamoto M, Hashimoto T, Shinka T, Kuhara T, et al. Acute encephalopathy with hyperammonemia and dicarboxylic aciduria during calcium hopantenate therapy: a patient report. Brain Dev 1986;8(6):601–5.
2. Togashi K, Miura Y, Ishiyama S, et al. Two autopsied cases of sudden death associated with calcium hopantenate. Brain Devel 1984;6:230.
3. Noda S, Umezaki H, Yamamoto K, Araki T, Murakami T, Ishii N. Reye-like syndrome following treatment with the pantothenic acid antagonist, calcium hopantenate. J Neurol Neurosurg Psychiatry 1988;51(4):582–5.
4. Ohsuga S, Ohsuga H, Takeoka T, Ikeda A, Shinohara Y. [Metabolic acidosis and hypoglycemia during calcium hopantenate administration—report on 5 patients.] Rinsho Shinkeigaku 1989;29(6):741–6.
5. Anonymous. Calcium hopantenate. Information on Adverse Reactions to Drugs, 1988.
6. Debourdeau PM, Djezzar S, Estival JL, Zammit CM, Richard RC, Castot AC. Life-threatening eosinophilic pleuropericardial effusion related to vitamins B5 and H. Ann Pharmacother 2001;35(4):424–6.
7. Otsuka M, Akiba T, Okita Y, Tomita K, Yoshiyama N, Sasaoka T, Kanayama M, Marumo F. Lactic acidosis with hypoglycemia and hyperammonemia observed in two uremic patients during calcium hopantenate treatment. Jpn J Med 1990;29(3):324–8.
8. Scudlik C, Schnuch A, Uter W, Schwanitz HJ. Berufsbedingtes Kontaktekzem nach Anwenung einer Dexpanthenol-haltigen Salbe und Überblick über die IVDK-Daten zu Dexpanthenol (IVDK = Informationsverbund Dermatologischer Kliniken). Aktuel Dermatol 2002;28: 398–401.

Papaveraceae

See also Herbal medicines

General Information

The genera in the family of Papaveraceae (Table 1) include a variety of poppies and the greater celandine.

Chelidonium majus

Chelidonium majus (celandine, common celandine, greater celandine) contains a number of alkaloids, including chelidonine, chelerythrine, chelidocystatin, coptisine, sanguinarine, berberine, and sparteine.

Greater celandine was traditionally used to improve eyesight and in modern times has been used as a mild sedative, and antispasmodic in the treatment of bronchitis, whooping cough, asthma, jaundice, gallstones, and gall-bladder pain. The latex is used topically to treat warts, ringworm, and corns. A semisynthetic thiophosphate derivative of alkaloids from *C. majus*, called Ukrain, has cytotoxic and cytostatic effects on tumor cells (1).

Adverse effects
Hematologic
Hemolytic anemia has been reported after the oral use of a celandine extract; there was intravascular hemolysis, renal insufficiency, liver cytolysis, and thrombocytopenia; a direct antiglobulin test was positive (2).

Liver
Hepatitis has been attributed to celandine (3).

- A 42-year-old woman had been admitted twice to hospital with hepatitis (4). No toxic agent could be identified during the first episode, but detailed questioning during the second showed that in both cases she had self-prescribed a commercially available medication of common celandine. Withdrawal of this herbal remedy was followed by an unremarkable recovery.

Table 1 The genera of Papaveraceae

Arctomecon (bear poppy)
Argemone (prickly poppy)
Bocconia (bocconia)
Canbya (pygmy poppy)
Chelidonium (celandine)
Dendromecon (tree poppy)
Eschscholzia (California poppy)
Glaucium (horn poppy)
Hunnemannia (hunnemannia)
Macleaya (macleaya)
Meconella (fairy poppy)
Papaver (poppy)
Platystemon (cream cups)
Platystigma (queen poppy)
Roemeria (roemeria)
Romneya (Matilija poppy)
Sanguinaria (bloodroot)
Stylophorum (stylophorum)
Stylomecon (wind poppy)

- A 42-year-old woman developed acute hepatitis several weeks after taking a herbal formulation containing greater celandine and curcuma root for a skin complaint (5). After withdrawal recovery was rapid and hepatic function returned to normal within 2 months.

Ten cases of acute hepatitis induced by formulations of greater celandine were observed over 2 years in a German University hospital (6). Perhaps ironically, this product is popular in Germany for gastric and gall-bladder problems. In five cases there was marked cholestasis but no liver failure. After withdrawal of the product, the symptoms subsided and the liver enzymes normalized within 2–6 months. Unintentional rechallenge led to a further episode of acute hepatitis in one patient.

In addition to about 15 published cases, some 40 cases of liver damage from *C. majus* have been reported to the German regulatory authorities (7). The course of the hepatitis can be severe and can include cholestasis and fibrosis, but acute liver failure has not been observed. Based on these data, celandine has been banned for oral use in several countries.

Skin
Contact sensitivity has been attributed to *C. majus* (8).

Susceptibility factors
Some authors caution that the use of celandine in children should be discouraged because of an early fatal colitis in a 3-year-old boy (9); however, this report does not provide convincing evidence that the victim had indeed taken *C. majus*.

Papaver somniferum

Papaver somniferum (opium poppy) contains a variety of opioid and related alkaloids, including codeine, morphine, noscapine, papaverine, and thebaine. Crude opium is the air-dried latex obtained by incising the unripe capsules of *P. somniferum*. Paregoric is ammoniated tincture of opium (Scotch paregoric) or camphorated tincture of opium (English paregoric). The use of these formulations has largely been replaced by use of the purified compounds.

Adverse effects
The adverse effects of opium are generally the same as those of the pure compounds.

Respiratory
Of 28 workers in a pharmaceutical factory that produced morphine and other alkaloids extracted from the shells of *P. somniferum*, six had symptoms of sensitization and positive skin tests (10). A bronchial provocation test was positive in four of them, and in all six there was a specific IgE, detected by ELISA and RAST tests using an aqueous extract of *P. somniferum*.

Nervous system
- A young man dependent on "Kompot" or "Polish heroin", a domestic product produced from poppy straw or the juice of poppy heads (*P. somniferum*) and given intravenously, developed Guillain–Barré syndrome after severe intoxication induced by home-made heroin, barbiturates, and benzodiazepines (11).

"Kompot" contains variable amounts of morphine, heroin (diacetylmorphine), 3-monoacetylmorphine, 6-mono-acetylmorphine, acetylcodeine, and codeine, in addition to papaverine, thebaine, and narcotine.

References

1. Uglyanitsa KN, Nefyodov LI, Doroshenko YM, Nowicky JW, Volchek IV, Brzosko WJ, Hodysh YJ. Ukrain: a novel anti-tumor drug. Drugs Exp Clin Res 2000;26(5–6):341–56.
2. Pinto Garcia V, Vicente PR, Barez A, Soto I, Candas MA, Coma A. Anemia hemolitica inducida por *Chelidonium majus*. [Hemolytic anemia induced by *Chelidonium majus*. Clinical case.] Sangre (Barc) 1990;35(5):401–3.
3. Stickel F, Poschl G, Seitz HK, Waldherr R, Hahn EG, Schuppan D. Acute hepatitis induced by greater celandine (*Chelidonium majus*). Scand J Gastroenterol 2003;38(5):565–8.
4. Strahl S, Ehret V, Dahm HH, Maier KP. Nedrotisierende Hepatitis nach Einnahme pflanzlicher Heilmittel. [Necrotizing hepatitis after taking herbal remedies.] Dtsch Med Wochenschr 1998;123(47):1410–14.
5. Crijns AP, de Smet PA, van den Heuvel M, Schot BW, Haagsma EB. Acute hepatitis na gebruik van een plantaardig preparaat met stinkende gouwe (*Chelidonium majus*). [Acute hepatitis after use of a herbal preparation with greater celandine (*Chelidonium majus*).] Ned Tijdschr Geneeskd 2002;146(3):124–8.
6. Benninger J, Schneider HT, Schuppan D, Kirchner T, Hahn EG. Acute hepatitis induced by greater celandine (*Chelidonium majus*). Gastroenterology 1999;117(5):1234–7.
7. De Smet PA. Safety concerns about kava not unique. Lancet 2002;360(9342):1336.
8. Etxenagusia MA, Anda M, Gonzalez-Mahave I, Fernandez E, Fernandez de Corres L. Contact dermatitis from *Chelidonium majus* (greater celandine). Contact Dermatitis 2000;43(1):47.
9. Koopman H. Tödliche Schöllkraut-Vergiftung (*Chelidonium majus*). Vergiftungsf lle 1937;8:93–8.
10. Moneo I, Alday E, Ramos C, Curiel G. Occupational asthma caused by Papaver somniferum. Allergol Immunopathol (Madr) 1993;21(4):145–8.
11. Gawlikowski T, Winnik L. Zespol Guillain–Barré jako wynik zatrucia mieszanego "kompotem" i lekami. [Guillain–Barré syndrome as a result of poisoning with a mixture of "kompot" (Polish heroin) and drugs.] Przegl Lek 2001;58(4):357–8.

Papaveretum

See also Opioid analgesics

General Information

Papaveretum (Omnopon, Pantopon) is a mixture of several opium alkaloids.

Organs and Systems

Urinary tract

Renal insufficiency has been reported in a 60-year-old patient after the use of papaveretum for perioperative analgesia (SEDA-17, 83).

Second-Generation Effects

Teratogenicity

Because of possible teratogenicity, papaveretum is no longer recommended for women of child-bearing age (SEDA-17, 83).

Susceptibility Factors

Age

There was a 56% incidence of nausea and vomiting with papaveretum in 129 children 24 hours after circumcision with caudal epidural blockade (1).

Reference

1. Wilton NC, Burn JM. Delayed vomiting after papaveretum in paediatric outpatient surgery. Can Anaesth Soc J 1986; 33(6):741–4.

Papaverine

General Information

Papaverine is an alkaloid present in opium, although it is not related chemically or pharmacologically to other opium alkaloids. It has a direct relaxant effect on smooth muscle, partly attributable to inhibition of phosphodi-esterase.

Systemic adverse effects reported are hypotension and dizziness and, in rare cases, abnormal results of liver function tests (SEDA-15, 3).

Organs and Systems

Sexual function

Intracavernous administration of papaverine with phentolamine has been used in the diagnosis and treatment of erectile dysfunction. The major local adverse effect is prolonged erection, which usually occurs early during diagnostic testing and is reduced after dose adjustment; furthermore, local hematomas have been reported in a number of patients. It may be that patients most susceptible to priapism can be identified in advance by testing their erectile abilities in response to erotic stimulation (1). Long-term therapy can also cause intracavernous fibrosis but it can also lead to development of tolerance to the desired effect.

Reference

1. Fouda A, Hassouna M, Beddoe E, Kalogeropoulos D, Binik YM, Elhilali MM. Priapism: an avoidable complication of pharmacologically induced erection. J Urol 1989; 142(4):995–7.

Parabens

See also Disinfectants and antiseptics

General Information

Parabens (methyl, ethyl, propyl, and butyl esters of para-hydroxybenzoic acid) are used as preservatives in concentrations of 0.1–0.3% in pharmaceutical formulations and in concentrations of 0.01–0.1% in cosmetics and foods. In such concentrations they are devoid of systemic toxic effects, but allergic reactions have been reported.

Organs and Systems

Immunologic

Parabens can cause allergic contact dermatitis that can run an insidious course, especially when the parabens are in glucocorticoid ointments. In such cases, treatment leads to a protracted dermatitis without acute exacerbation, so that neither the patient nor the physician suspects parabens as a possible cause. A sensitization index of 0.8% was found in 273 patients with chronic dermatitis (1).

In 1973, in a multicenter study of 1200 individuals carried out by the North American Contact Dermatitis Group, there was a 3% incidence of delayed hypersensitivity reactions to parabens. General allergic reactions have also been reported after the injection of parabens-containing formulations of lidocaine and hydrocortisone and after oral use of barium sulfate contrast suspension, haloperidol syrup, and an antitussive syrup, all of which contained parabens (SEDA-11, 484).

Reference

1. Schorr WF. Paraben allergy. A cause of intractable dermatitis. JAMA 1968;204(10):859–62.

Paracetamol

General Information

A century after its introduction, acetylsalicylic acid (aspirin) is by far the most commonly used analgesic, sharing its leading position with the relative newcomer paracetamol (acetaminophen), and notwithstanding the fact that other widely used compounds, such as ibuprofen, have in recent years been introduced in over-the-counter versions. Both are also still being prescribed by physicians and are generally used for mild to moderate pain, fever associated with common everyday illnesses, and disorders ranging from head colds and influenza to toothache and headache. However, their greatest use is by consumers who obtain them directly from the pharmacy, and in many countries outside pharmacies as well.

Perhaps this wide availability and advertising via mass media leads to a lack of appreciation by the lay public that these are medicines with adverse effects. Both have at any rate been subject to misuse and excessive use, leading to such problems as chronic salicylate intoxication with aspirin and severe hepatic damage with paracetamol overdose. Both aspirin and paracetamol have also featured in accidental overdosage (particularly in children) as well as intentional overdosage.

In an investigation of Canadian donors who had not admitted to drug intake, 6–7% of the blood samples taken were found to have detectable concentrations of acetylsalicylic acid and paracetamol (1). Such drugs would be potentially capable of causing untoward reactions in the recipients.

To offer some protection against misuse of analgesics, many countries have insisted on the use of packs containing total quantities less than the minimum toxic dose (albeit usually the one obtained for healthy young volunteers and thus disregarding the majority of the population), and supplied in child-resistant packaging. Most important, however, is the need to provide education for the lay public to respect such medicines in general for the good they can do, but more especially for the harm that can arise, but can be avoided. There is a definite role for the prescribing physician, since informing the patient seems to prevent adverse events (2).

The sale of paracetamol or aspirin in dosage forms in which they are combined with other active ingredients offers considerable risk to the consumer, since the product as sold may not be clearly identified as containing either of these two analgesics. Brand names sometimes obscure the actual composition of older formulations that contain one or both of these analgesics in combination with, for example, a pyrazolone derivative and/or a potentially addictive substance. For instance, in Germany, with the EC harmonization of the Drug Law of 1990, the manufacturers of drugs already marketed before 1978 had the opportunity of exchanging even the active principles without being obliged to undergo a new approval procedure or to abandon their brand name. Combination formulations are still being promoted and sold, and not exclusively in developing countries. Consequently the patient who is so anxious to allay all his symptoms that he takes several medications concurrently may without knowing it take several doses of aspirin or paracetamol at the same time, perhaps sufficient to cause toxicity. It is essential that product labels clearly state their active ingredients by approved name, together with the quantity per dosage form (3).

The antipyretic analgesics share with the non-steroidal anti inflammatory drugs (NSAIDs) a common mechanism of action, namely the inhibition of prostaglandin synthesis from arachidonic acid and their release. More precisely their mode of action is thought to result from inhibition of both the constitutive and the inducible isoenzymes (COX-1 and COX-2) of the cyclo-oxygenase pathway (4). However, aspirin and paracetamol are distinguishable from most of the NSAIDs by their ability to inhibit prostaglandin synthesis in the nervous system, and thus the hypothalamic center for body temperature regulation, rather than acting mainly in the periphery.

Endogenous pyrogens (and exogenous pyrogens that have their effects through the endogenous group) induce the hypothalamic vascular endothelium to produce prostaglandins, which activate the thermoregulatory neurons by increasing AMP concentrations. The capacity of the antipyretic analgesics to inhibit hypothalamic prostaglandin synthesis appears to be the basis of their antipyretic action. Neither aspirin nor paracetamol affects the synthesis or release of endogenous pyrogens and neither will lower body temperature if it is normal.

While aspirin significantly inhibits peripheral prostaglandin and thromboxane synthesis, paracetamol is less potent as a synthetase inhibitor than the NSAIDs, except in the brain, and paracetamol has only a weak anti-inflammatory action. It is simple to ascribe the analgesic activity of aspirin to its capacity to inhibit prostaglandin synthesis, with a consequent reduction in inflammatory edema and vasodilatation, since aspirin is most effective in the pain associated with inflammation or injury. However, such a peripheral effect cannot account for the analgesic activity of paracetamol, which is less well understood.

The use of paracetamol as an antipyretic increased rapidly once phenacetin was no longer available and has received a boost more recently with wide acknowledgement of the role of aspirin as a causative agent in Reye's syndrome, resulting in the virtual disappearance of children's dosage forms of aspirin. While the incidence of adverse effects is reassuringly low, satisfaction must be tempered by appreciation of the relatively short duration of extensive clinical experience with paracetamol, its close relation to phenacetin, its low potency as an analgesic, and low public awareness of its potential adverse effects.

General adverse reactions

Although paracetamol is acceptably safe in usual dosages, there have been some reports that in patients with significant hepatic dysfunction or those taking substances that induce hepatic enzymes (for example ethanol, phenobarbital, isoniazid) even these doses may aggravate liver dysfunction, sometimes to the point of causing hepatic failure. The problem of overdosage is substantial. Allergic reactions, including urticaria, are seen occasionally. Anaphylactic shock has been reported.

Organs and Systems

Cardiovascular

Despite the high prevalence of the use of minor analgesics (aspirin and paracetamol) there is little information available on the association between the use of these analgesics and the risk of hypertension. A prospective cohort study in 80 020 women aged 31–50 years has provided some useful information (5). The women had participated in the Nurses' Health Study II and had no previous history of hypertension. The frequency of use of paracetamol, aspirin, and NSAIDs was collected by mailed questionnaires and cases of physician-diagnosed hypertension were identified by self-report. During 164 000 person-years of follow-up, 1650 incident cases of hypertension were identified. Overall, 73% of the cohort had used paracetamol at least 1–4 days/month, 51% had used aspirin, and 77% had used an NSAID. Compared with non-users of paracetamol the age-adjusted relative risk

(RR) of hypertension was significantly increased even in women who had used paracetamol for only 1–4 days/month (RR = 1.22; CI = 1.07, 1.39). There seemed to be a dose–response relation, as the RR of hypertension compared with non-users was 2.00 (CI = 1.52, 2.62) in women who had taken paracetamol for 29 days/month or more. For women using aspirin or NSAIDs at a frequency of 1–4 days/month the RRs were 1.18 (CI = 1.02, 1.35) and 1.17 (CI = 1.02, 1.36) respectively. However, after adjusting for age and other potential risk factors, only paracetamol and NSAIDs, but not aspirin, remained significantly associated with a risk of hypertension. In summary, the data from this study support the view that paracetamol and NSAIDs are strongly associated with an increased risk of hypertension in women, the risk increasing with increasing frequency of use. Aspirin did not seem to be associated with an increased risk. This conclusion contrasts with the results of some short-term studies that have shown no effect of paracetamol on blood pressure (6,7).

This study suggests that paracetamol can raise arterial blood pressure in a dose-related fashion, interfere with the actions of antihypertensive drugs, and prompt the need for new antihypertensive therapy. However, these results must be interpreted with caution, as there were some limitations: the assessments of analgesic use and hypertension were made using a self-reported questionnaire; relative risk can be influenced by many potentially confounding variables; the results are relevant only for young women and cannot be extrapolated to the general population.

Respiratory

Paracetamol can aggravate bronchospasm in patients who are sensitive to aspirin and other analgesics (8). In severe poisoning, paracetamol depresses respiratory function centrally through metabolic acidosis and coma (9).

An observational study, part of a population-based case-control study of dietary antioxidants and asthma, has shown an association between the regular use of paracetamol and the incidence of asthma and rhinitis in adults (10). After controlling for potential confounding factors the OR for asthma in daily users, compared with never users, was 2.38 (CI = 1.22, 4.64). Not unexpectedly, there was also an association in users and non-users of aspirin, strongest when cases with more severe disease were compared with controls. This adverse effect of paracetamol may be due to depletion of the antioxidant glutathione in the lungs. However, further studies are needed before paracetamol can be blamed for an increase in the prevalence and severity of asthma.

Nervous system

In patients who suffer from recurrent headaches, for example migraine, cluster headache, or tension headache, temporary relief for the constant or intermittent pains is obtained from each analgesic dose, but wears off after a few hours with the arrival of a new episode. The patient gets accustomed to this pattern and may use excessive doses of analgesics. This in turn can cause, worsen, and perpetuate headaches, leading to what is called analgesic-induced or rebound headache. Like migraine, analgesic-induced headache is more likely to occur in women and is associated with depression.

It is postulated that the mechanism by which analgesic abuse transforms a primary headache into a rebound headache involves serotonin: both platelet serotonin concentrations and uptake were lower in patients with analgesic-induced headache compared with migraine sufferers and non-headache sufferers. At the same time, there was upregulation of serotonin receptors on the platelet membrane (11,12). Extrapolating these findings to the nervous system, it has been suggested that excessive analgesic use suppresses serotonin pathways, contributing to aggravation of headaches. Paracetamol and codeine were the major culprits of the analgesics investigated.

Analgesic-induced headache has also been described in children. One report (13) described 12 children, aged 6–16 years, who gave a history of headaches on at least 4 days a week, for 3 months to 10 years. Eleven of the children had been taking paracetamol, six in combination with codeine, and one was taking ibuprofen alone. They were taking at least one dose of an analgesic for each headache and eight were taking analgesics every day. The headaches presented with increasing frequency and were related to overuse of analgesics, a typical finding in analgesic-induced headache. The analgesics were withdrawn; in six children the headaches resolved completely, another five children experienced a reduced frequency of headaches, and one resumed analgesic abuse.

A second report (14) was of a retrospective study of patients seen in a pediatric headache clinic. During 8 months, 98 patients were seen for headache; 46 of them suffered from daily or near daily headache and 30 were consuming analgesics daily. Follow-up information was available in 25. The average number of doses of analgesics per week they consumed was 26. The most commonly used medications were paracetamol and ibuprofen. In addition, a minority were taking combinations that contained aspirin, codeine, caffeine, propoxyphene, or butalbital, or other NSAIDs. Abrupt withdrawal of all analgesics concomitant with the use of amitriptyline 10 mg/day (in 22 patients) prompted a significant reduction in the frequency and severity of headache.

The data from these studies are comparable to previous observations reported in adults (SEDA-21, 95) and suggest that daily use of analgesics can cause daily or near daily headaches in children and adolescents. However, additional controlled prospective studies are needed to address the true frequency of analgesics rebound headache among children and to evaluate possible treatments.

Metabolism

Hypoglycemia has been recorded with paracetamol, particularly in children (15).

Hematologic

Agranulocytosis was recorded in a series in France (16), but does not appear to have been a significant clinical problem elsewhere.

Two patients developed immune thrombocytopenia attributed to metabolites of paracetamol (17).

- A 30-year-old man and a 66-year-old woman had taken paracetamol 1 g intermittently for headaches and other non-specific indications. Routine blood testing showed thrombocytopenia (50×10^9/l and 45×10^9/l respectively). They both stopped taking paracetamol, and their platelet counts rose to normal within 7–10 days. Their sera contained antibodies (IgG or IgA) that recognized normal platelets in the presence of the metabolite paracetamol sulfate.

This suggests that in patients with drug-induced immune thrombocytopenia, tests for metabolite-dependent antibodies can be helpful in identifying the responsible agent.

A hemolytic crisis has been recorded in a patient with glucose-6-phosphate dehydrogenase deficiency (18).

Gastrointestinal

In normal doses, paracetamol, in contradistinction to aspirin and the NSAIDs, is well tolerated by the gastrointestinal tract.

Liver

Paracetamol is directly hepatotoxic and can cause severe hepatic damage in dosages over 6–10 g (12–20 tablets).

Biliary tract

Acute biliary pain with cholestasis is an occasional complication (19,20).

Pancreas

Pancreatitis has been reported, but only in overdose (21).

Urinary tract

Apart from renal tubular necrosis, which is usually associated with hepatic toxicity, but is occasionally seen without hepatic damage, there have been reports of a nephropathy similar to that seen with phenacetin, after prolonged use of paracetamol alone or in combination with other NSAIDs (22–27).

Analgesic nephropathy
DoTS classification (BMJ 2003;327:1222–5)
Dose-relation: collateral effect
Time-course: delayed
Susceptibility factors: age (over 65); sex (women)
In a series of papers that appeared from 1950 onwards (28), Spüler and Zollinger in Switzerland recognized analgesic nephropathy as a condition resulting from prolonged excessive consumption of analgesic mixtures, usually containing phenacetin. The disease is characterized by renal papillary necrosis and interstitial nephritis. The prevalence is variable, being especially high when the use of minor analgesics is intensive. The evidence linking the disorder primarily to phenacetin has been reviewed extensively (SED-8, 169) (SED-8, 178) (SED-9, 123) (SED-10, 135) (SEDA-9, 75).

Over the last 50 years there has been a steady evolution in our knowledge of drug-related renal pathology, including the role of prostaglandins in the kidneys and the concept of two cyclo-oxygenase isozymes. In the 1960s a distinct clinical entity was identified, separate from

NSAID-induced renal toxicity, comprising interstitial nephritis and renal papillary necrosis. The condition, named analgesic nephropathy, was not uncommon and was serious. In a number of cases malignancies in the urinary tract also occurred.

The relation between long-term heavy exposure to analgesics and the risk of chronic renal disease has been the object of intensive toxicological and epidemiological research for many years (SEDA-24, 120) (29). Most of the earlier reports suggested that phenacetin-containing analgesics probably cause renal papillary necrosis and interstitial nephritis.

Nephropathy due to non-phenacetin-containing analgesics
There is no convincing epidemiological evidence that non-phenacetin-containing analgesics (including paracetamol, aspirin, mixtures of the two, and NSAIDs) cause chronic renal disease. Findings from epidemiological studies should be interpreted with caution, because of a number of inherent limitations and potential biases in study design (30). However, two methodologically sound studies have provided information on this topic.

The first was the largest cohort study conducted thus far to assess the risk of renal dysfunction associated with analgesic use (31). Details of analgesic use were obtained from 11 032 men without previous renal dysfunction participating in the Physicians' Health Study (PHS), which lasted 14 years. The main outcome measure was a raised creatinine concentration defined as 1.5 mg/dl (133 μmol/l) or higher and a reduced creatinine clearance of 55 ml/minute or less. In all, 460 men (4.2%) had a raised creatinine concentration and 1258 (11%) had a reduced creatinine clearance. Mean creatinine concentrations and creatinine clearances were similar among men who did not use analgesics and those who did. This was true for all categories of analgesics (paracetamol and paracetamol-containing mixtures, aspirin and aspirin-containing mixtures, and other NSAIDs) and for higher risk groups, such as those aged 60 years or over or those with hypertension or diabetes.

These data are convincing, because the large size of the PHS cohort should have made it possible to examine and detect even modest associations between analgesic use and a risk of renal disease. Furthermore, this study included more individuals who reported extensive use of analgesics than any prior case-control study. However, the study had some limitations, the most important being the fact that the cohort was composed of relatively healthy men, most of whom were white. These results cannot therefore be generalized to the entire population. However, the study clearly showed that there is not a strong association between chronic analgesic use and chronic renal dysfunction among a large cohort of men without a history of renal impairment.

The second study was a Swedish nationwide, population-based, case-control study of early-stage chronic renal insufficiency in men whose serum creatinine concentration exceeded 3.4 mg/dl (300 μmol/l) or women whose serum creatinine exceeded 250 μmol/l (2.8 mg/dl) (32). In all, 918 patients with newly diagnosed renal insufficiency and 980 controls were interviewed and completed questionnaires about their lifetime consumption of analgesics. Compared with controls, more patients with chronic renal insufficiency were regular users of aspirin (37 versus 19%) or paracetamol (25 versus 12%). Among subjects who did not use aspirin regularly, the regular use of paracetamol was associated with a risk of chronic renal insufficiency that was 2.5 times as high as that for non-users of paracetamol. The risk increased with increasing cumulative lifetime dose. Patients who took 500 g or more over a year (1.4 g/day) during periods of regular use had an increased odds ratio for chronic renal insufficiency (OR = 5.3; 95% CI = 1.8, 15). Among subjects who did not use paracetamol regularly, the regular use of aspirin was associated with a risk of chronic renal insufficiency that was 2.5 times as high as that for non-users of aspirin. The risk increased significantly with an increasing cumulative lifetime dose of aspirin. Among the patients with an average intake of 500 g or more of aspirin per year during periods of regular use, the risk of chronic renal insufficiency was increased about three-fold (OR = 3.3; CI = 1.4, 8.0). Among patients who used paracetamol in addition to aspirin, the risk of chronic renal insufficiency was increased about two-fold when regular aspirin users served as the reference group (OR = 2.2; CI = 1.4, 3.5) and non-significantly when regular paracetamol users were used as controls (OR = 1.6; CI = 0.9, 2.7). There was no relation between the use of other analgesics (propoxyphene, NSAIDs, codeine, and pyrazolones) and the risk of chronic renal insufficiency. Thus, the regular use of paracetamol, or aspirin, or both was associated dose-dependently with an increased risk of chronic renal insufficiency. The OR among regular users exceeded 1.0 for all types of chronic renal insufficiency, albeit not always significantly. These results are consistent with exacerbating effects of paracetamol and aspirin on chronic renal insufficiency, regardless of accompanying disease.

How can we explain the contrasting results of these two studies? A possible explanation lies in the different populations studied. In the PHS study, relatively healthy individuals were enrolled, while in the Swedish study all the patients had pre-existing severe renal or systemic disease, suggesting that such disease has an important role in causing analgesic-associated chronic renal insufficiency. People without pre-existing disease who use analgesics may have only a small risk of end-stage renal disease.

As up to 10% of about 42 000 dialysis patients have suffered from renal insufficiency due to analgesic nephropathy (in the postphenacetin era), German nephrologists have demanded the withdrawal from the market of medications that contain fixed combinations of analgesics (paracetamol, aspirin, or propyphenazone) plus caffeine, following the example of their American colleagues in the National Kidney Foundation (33).

Despite the fact that a careful evaluation of all epidemiological studies on non-narcotic analgesics showed no evidence that phenacetin-free combination drugs are more nephrotoxic than simple analgesics (29), the Belgian Public Health Authorities decided that combination analgesics are to become "prescription only" (34), as they have a "devastating" effect on the kidneys. However, contrasting opinions have been published (30,35).

The effect of the withdrawal of phenacetin in Germany in 1986 and its replacement with paracetamol in most analgesic mixtures resulted in a significant fall in the incidence of end-stage analgesic nephropathy from 30% in 1981–82 to 21% in 1991–92 and 12% in 1995–97 (36). However, whether this reduction can be taken as proof that only phenacetin and not paracetamol is nephrotoxic in compound analgesics is debatable (37). In fact, the German authors found that other factors, such as advanced age and an increasing prevalence of type II diabetes mellitus, affected the relative frequencies of primary renal disease in patients with end-stage renal disease to such a degree that the observed relative reduction in analgesic nephropathy may not have been related to a change from phenacetin to paracetamol. Thus, the relative reduction in the incidence of analgesic nephropathy cannot be used as an argument for the non-toxicity of compound analgesics that contain paracetamol.

Furthermore, despite withdrawal of phenacetin from the market, analgesic nephropathy has continued to occur. It has been estimated that analgesic-associated nephropathy still accounts for 20% of patients in the USA with interstitial nephritis. As recently as the mid-1990s, a German study showed that up to 10% of dialysis patients had suffered from renal insufficiency owing to analgesic nephropathy (SEDA-20, 89). There is evidence that paracetamol, which replaced phenacetin in analgesic combination formulations, is nephrotoxic as well (38,39). The withdrawal of combination analgesic products from over-the-counter sales in Sweden and Australia has markedly reduced analgesic nephropathy as a cause of end-stage renal disease in those countries (SEDA-21, 99). It is therefore not surprising that nephrologists on both sides of the Atlantic have suggested a ban on the advertising and over-the-counter sales of these medications.

Symptoms and signs
Clinical evidence suggestive of analgesic nephropathy includes nocturia, renal insufficiency with severe acidosis, persistent urinary tract infection with colic, hematuria, and hypertension (40,41). Nocturia resulting from failure to concentrate urine is usually the earliest functional defect, but like the other symptoms it is non-specific, rendering the diagnosis of analgesic nephropathy difficult. A CT scan showing bilateral small kidneys with bumpy contours, and papillary calcification is accepted to be of sufficient specificity (38,39).

Epidemiology
Analgesic nephropathy is mostly diagnosed between the ages of 30 and 70 years, with a peak in the fourth decade, and there is a familial predisposition (SEDA-6, 80).

The prevalence of analgesic nephropathy is particularly high when there is intensive use of analgesics. There is evidence from animal and clinical work to suggest that hypovolemia plays a part, and that the risk of nephropathy is greatest in women and the elderly. Because of the long latent period of over 10 years, the condition has continued to appear despite the withdrawal of phenacetin.

In Australia, where phenacetin was withdrawn from antipyretic analgesic formulations during 1962–75 (42),

analgesic nephropathy continued to be a major problem for a considerable time thereafter, reflecting the long latent period before the disorder develops; 22% of patients newly admitted to the Australian Kidney Foundation's dialysis and transplant registry in 1980 had analgesic nephropathy. The consumption of phenacetin-containing analgesics increased the risk of renal papillary necrosis in Australian women some 17-fold compared with non-consumers, while analgesics not containing phenacetin did not increase the risk of kidney damage (43).

In Belgium, the distribution of analgesic nephropathy in patients with terminal renal insufficiency was well correlated with the sale of drugs containing either aspirin + phenacetin or paracetamol + caffeine (SEDA-7, 75), and it is estimated that Belgium, after Australia, had the second highest incidence of analgesic nephropathy in the world.

Statistics published in 1981 from the European Dialysis and Transplant Association on the causes of chronic renal insufficiency suggested that in Europe about 3.1% of cases up to that time had been drug-induced; the figures cited varied from 0.4% in Spain to 17.5% in Switzerland. Some of the best-documented reports were those from Switzerland, where per capita consumption of phenacetin reached a peak of some 10 g annually between 1955 and 1968 (44). Between 1962 and 1978 the proportion of phenacetin users coming to autopsy increased from 1.8 to 3.1%.

In the USA only a very small proportion of phenacetin patients (in one series 2.8%) have a history of analgesic abuse (45).

True geographic differences cannot be proven from such figures, since the variation from country to country is largely due to inconsistent classification and differences in the selection of patients for dialysis and transplantation (46).

By the early 1980s, most countries had severely restricted or entirely prohibited the sale of phenacetin. Subsequent data from several of these countries suggested that the number of new patients with analgesic nephropathy fell as a result of the prohibition of phenacetin in analgesic mixtures.

Cause
It soon became clear that the major causative agent in analgesic nephropathy was phenacetin, improperly used long-term and especially in combinations with other analgesics, and this identification led to its virtual disappearance in the mid-1970s, following regulatory action.

In recent years it has become obvious that many of the NSAIDs are associated with renal disorders arising de novo or by aggravation of existent renal dysfunction. Inhibition of prostaglandin synthesis intrarenally leads to reduced vasodilator activity of PGE_1, which normally contributes to the maintenance of renal functional balance and protection against the vasoconstrictor effects of noradrenaline and angiotensin-II and the action of antidiuretic hormone. Some experimental work suggests a tendency for phenacetin and its metabolite paracetamol to concentrate in the renal medulla, possibly accounting for the papillary lesions most often associated with them.

There is no evidence that short-term use of cyclo-oxygenase inhibitors has any major deleterious effect on renal function in healthy individuals.

Although some authors have stressed the possible role of aspirin as a causal factor (SED-8, 169), a study of the safety of long-term ingestion of large cumulative doses did not confirm this (47). The patients in question, with seropositive rheumatoid arthritis, had taken aspirin continuously for 10 or more years (mean total dose per patient 36 kg, range 16–82 kg). Their normal creatinine and BUN concentrations, with maximum recorded specific gravities of urine greater than 1019 in 93% of patients, suggested that long-term salicylate ingestion does not cause renal damage or that the magnitude and long-term clinical significance of such damage is not significant. The fact remains, however, that the overwhelming sale of phenacetin was in the form of fixed combinations with aspirin (and sometimes with caffeine, codeine, and other components), and the possibility of some additive effect cannot retrospectively be excluded.

As the debate developed, the safety of paracetamol and its combination with aspirin, which had only come to the fore on a large scale as phenacetin disappeared, also came to be questioned. The difficulty in assigning specific roles to the various analgesics is partly related to the use of drug combinations but largely because of the prolonged time over which the disorder develops.

Susceptibility factors
The association between analgesic abuse and renal papillary necrosis is well established, but the existence of other unrecognized factors is highly probable (SEDA-6, 80). The female/male ratio of analgesic abusers as a whole in the Australian community is 2:1, but the ratio in analgesic nephropathy is about 6.5:1. Swiss data also point to a higher incidence than expected in women and in elderly subjects (28). Climatic factors and fluid intake have also been incriminated, since dehydration can aggravate the risk. Reports of an association between HLA genotype and analgesic nephropathy might explain why only a few of the many individuals who take large quantities of analgesics develop renal insufficiency (48).

Pathology
The primary renal lesions in phenacetin abusers are those involving the capillaries (49,50). In some 80% of cases there is capillary sclerosis, with reduplication of laminar transformation of the intima, due to reduplication of the basement membrane in the capillaries just below the urothelium in the papillae, renal pelvis, and lower urinary tract. It is these changes that make it possible to diagnose analgesic abuse from surgical or postmortem specimens, even when the clinical history is unknown. A morphological study of 21 transitional cell carcinomas in an Australian histopathology department disclosed 16 cases with papillary changes of the analgesic type. Of these patients, only two were known to be analgesic abusers (SEDA-6, 82).

The renal cortical and medullary tubules are similarly affected, since overuse of analgesic-containing formulations can affect the metabolism of the basement membranes of capillaries and tubules and result in thickening of the walls. In skin biopsy specimens from patients with a history of excessive intake of analgesics, thickening of dermal capillaries suggested that the microangiopathy

was not confined to the renal tract but also occurred in other organs (SEDA-6, 81).

Associated disorders
In the prospective Swiss Analgesic Study the risk of bacteriuria was about three times higher in those who abused analgesics heavily than in matched controls (51). The primary causes of mortality in this study were tumors and cardiovascular disease; only 7.5% died from primary renal disease due to pyelonephritis.

Renal papillary necrosis with retroperitoneal fibrosis secondary to analgesic abuse (involving aspirin, propoxyphene, and numerous other analgesics taken in large quantities for many years) has also incidentally been reported (SEDA-7, 94).

Patients with analgesic nephropathy have an increased risk of atherosclerosis. In a retrospective study their serum cholesterol and triglyceride concentrations were significantly higher than in a control group of similar age and with a similar degree of renal insufficiency due to other renal diseases (SEDA-6, 81). Some possible mechanisms of hyperlipidemia in analgesic nephropathy have been discussed, as this phenomenon is not sufficiently explained by end-stage renal insufficiency or by protein loss, as in the nephrotic syndrome (SEDA-7, 94).

Urinary tract tumors   Renal carcinoma has been associated with analgesic abuse an order of magnitude greater than in non-abusers (52–54), and the causal association has been recognized since 1965 (SEDA-6, 81) and repeatedly confirmed. In 1984 an authoritative consensus conference in the USA pointed to the evidence that very heavy and sustained use of some analgesic mixtures without phenacetin can also predispose to cancer of the urinary tract, particularly transitional cell carcinoma of the renal pelvis (55).

Of 422 inhabitants of Basel with malignant tumors of the lower urinary tract, 18.5% were users of phenacetin-containing analgesics, which means that carcinomas and sarcomas of the lower urinary tract were nearly 13 times as common in abusers as in non-abusers (54). Carcinoma of the renal pelvis was increased 77-fold, carcinoma of the ureter 89-fold, and carcinoma of the urinary bladder 7-fold. In Australia, in 274 urological patients who had abused phenacetin-containing products, renal symptoms appeared after an average latent period of 10 years; within the last decade of the period studied, 8% of this group (22 patients) had tumors of the urothelium.

In an Australian investigation of renal papillary carcinoma (SEDA-6, 81) the overall crude incidence rate was 1.6 per 100 000 population per year; 47% of the tumors were associated with analgesic abuse and analgesic nephropathy. The risk of renal papillary carcinoma among patients who regularly took analgesics was estimated to be 8 per 100 000 patients per year. Renal papillary carcinoma had a female-to-male ratio among analgesic abusers of 2.6:1, compared with 1:2 among those without analgesic-associated nephropathy. A similar epidemiological study from the USA (53) supported this association between analgesic nephropathy and tumors; 5.2% of patients with transitional carcinoma of the urinary tract diagnosed over 3 years had analgesic-associated nephropathy. The patients were predominantly younger women, who had renal pelvis tumors instead of bladder tumors and a higher mortality rate. In a historical prospective study of 146 patients with interstitial nephritis, 84 cases were associated with analgesics and in four patients transitional cell carcinoma developed. None of the 98 nephritic patients without analgesic-associated nephropathy developed transitional cell carcinoma. In 300 urological patients (75% women) in whom renal and extrarenal manifestations appeared after an average latency period of 20 years, 31 patients had a tumor of the urothelium.

Studies on the tumor-inducing effects of heavy use of analgesics, especially those that contain phenacetin, have given contrasting results (SEDA-21, 100) (56,57). Two case-control studies have been published on the role of habitual intake of analgesics on the occurrence of urothelial cancer and renal cell carcinoma.

In the first study, 647 cases of urothelial cancer (571 bladder, 25 ureter, and 51 renal pelvis) and an identical number of controls were enrolled (58). Exposure to compound analgesic (at least 1 kg of analgesic substances lifelong) showed a substance-specific association, with an increased risk ratio for renal pelvis cancer but not for cancers of the ureter or bladder. Among the different analgesics, anilide derivatives (intake over 1 kg) were associated with the highest risks of renal pelvis cancer, with respective odds ratios of 5.28 for phenacetin (CI = 0.34, 81) and 3.27 for paracetamol (CI = 0.25, 43); however, these odds ratios were not statistically significant. This lack of significance was due mainly to two factors, the high proportion of heavy analgesic use in controls and the low number of cases with renal pelvis cancer, which had the highest risk.

The second study (59) was aimed at clarifying the possible relation between analgesic use and renal cell carcinoma. In previous studies there was a consistent association between phenacetin and renal cell carcinoma, but inconclusive results with respect to non-phenacetin analgesics. In 1024 patients with renal cell carcinoma and an equal number of matched controls, regular use of analgesics was a significant risk factor for renal cell carcinoma (OR = 1.6; CI = 1.4, 1.9). The risk was significantly increased by all four major classes of analgesics (aspirin, NSAIDs, paracetamol, and phenacetin) and within each class of analgesic, the risk increased with increasing exposure. Individuals in the highest exposure categories had about a 2.5-fold increase in risk relative to non-users or irregular users of analgesics. However, exclusive users of aspirin who took aspirin 325 mg/day or less for cardiovascular problems were not at an increased risk of renal cell carcinoma (OR = 0.9; CI = 0.6, 1.4).

In contrast to these results, another large case-control study (60) in 1732 patients with renal cell carcinoma and 2039 controls showed no increase in the risk of renal cell carcinoma among regular users of phenacetin, paracetamol, and aspirin. There is no clear explanation of these disparate findings.

Conclusions
The history of analgesic nephropathy must not be dismissed as involving only a drug now obsolete.

Phenacetin, alone or in combination with other analgesics, was unwisely taken chronically by a large section of the public, and unless such misuse of analgesics can be avoided, there is much reason to fear that the story will be repeated with other agents and combinations.

If analgesics are discontinued in the early phases of nephropathy, there is a reasonable possibility of a return to normal renal function. It is wise to ensure that the dosage of aspirin or paracetamol, or of any NSAID, is kept as low as possible, that renal function is regularly assessed, and that prolonged use is avoided, especially in patients over 65 years of age, who seem to be at particular risk of analgesic nephropathy and who may also have pre-existing renal dysfunction, including marginally compensated asymptomatic renal insufficiency (40).

There is no evidence that short-term use of single cyclo-oxygenase inhibitors has any major deleterious effect on renal function in healthy, non-hypovolemic individuals, but even short-term use of a compound of this class is never a guarantee that nephropathy will not occur.

Skin

Rashes, usually erythematous, occur occasionally (61–63).

Paracetamol can rarely cause fixed drug eruptions (64,65), including an unusual non-pigmented fixed drug eruption (66).

Immunologic

Acute hypersensitivity reactions due to paracetamol are rare (SEDA-22, 114), but can be life-threatening (67).

Long-Term Effects

Mutagenicity

Animal studies have indicated a carcinogenic effect when paracetamol has been administered for prolonged periods in relatively high dosages. However, no clinical data are so far available to corroborate this. The matter cannot be dismissed entirely for the time being, in view of a report (68) of the development of chromosomal aberrations after prolonged use.

Second-Generation Effects

Fetotoxicity

Paracetamol crosses the placenta readily. However, there has been no published evidence of a teratogenic effect in the offspring of mothers who have taken paracetamol during pregnancy. A case of fetal death after a maternal overdose of paracetamol (30 g) has been described (SEDA-10, 73), but in another similar case, in which 22.5 g was taken in the 36th week, the fetus survived (SEDA-9, 96). Preliminary data from a longitudinal study have shown no adverse effects of therapeutic doses of paracetamol on either pregnancy or infant development (69).

Susceptibility Factors

Hepatic disease

It is generally considered inadvisable to use paracetamol in patients with active liver disease or severe liver dysfunction, patients with cachexia, or chronic alcoholics. Stable mild chronic liver disease does not seem to be a contraindication (70).

Drug Administration

Drug overdose

Paracetamol is one of the most commonly ingested medications in deliberate self-poisoning and accidental ingestion by children.

Fulminant hepatic failure occurs in 1–5% of cases of paracetamol overdosage 3–6 days after ingestion (71), with frequent deaths in people who take 20–25 g. There is only a narrow margin between the normal maximum 24-hour dosage and that which can cause liver damage and acute hepatic failure. Undoubtedly, some people are more susceptible than most to paracetamol toxicity, since although 6 g has been reported as toxic in some cases, most toxicity is seen with 12 g upwards (72,73). Nomograms have been developed to show the relation between plasma paracetamol concentrations over time and the risk of a serious outcome (SEDA-18, 94).

Epidemiology

Paracetamol is a widely-used, effective, and well-tolerated analgesic, but thanks also to its ready availability, it is the most commonly used substance in self-poisoning (SEDA-18, 94) (74) and a frequent cause of accidental overdose, especially in children (SEDA-22, 114), although children of 6 years and under are rarely subject to hepatotoxicity, even with accidental overdosage (75), possibly owing to age-dependent differences in paracetamol kinetics (76).

From prospective data (74,77), it has been estimated that around 58 000 people take paracetamol in overdose each year in England and Wales and that these episodes of poisoning prompted 3.3% of inquiries to US regional poisons centers (78), 10% of inquiries to the UK National Poisons Information Service (79), and up to 43% of all admissions to hospital with self-poisoning in the UK (80). Despite the availability of effective antidotes for patients who seek medical intervention early after an overdose, in the USA paracetamol alone accounted for 4.1% of deaths from poisoning reported to American poison centers in 1997 (78).

Paracetamol plus dextropropoxyphene, the combination known as co-proxamol, is available as a prescription-only analgesic in many countries. Self-poisoning can be lethal, as respiratory depression can occur from an excessive dose of dextropropoxyphene. In England and Wales, co-proxamol alone accounts for 5% of all suicides, and overdose is more likely to result in death than overdose with paracetamol alone or tricyclic antidepressants (81). Furthermore, although it is often prescribed, it is no more effective than paracetamol for short-term relief of pain. It should not be prescribed without good reason.

Symptoms and signs

While damage to the liver is effected within hours of ingestion, major clinical manifestations are seldom seen until some 24–48 hours. However, they can be prevented by early treatment. Thus, early history taking, a high index of suspicion, and prompt and repeated assays of plasma paracetamol concentrations are essential in emergency management. Primary signs, when they do appear, are those of liver failure, for example abdominal pain and tenderness, followed by jaundice, raised serum transaminases, and reduced concentrations of coagulation factors, resulting in a prolonged prothrombin time. It may be up to a week before severe liver failure ensues. Consciousness is not usually lost early on, but resistant cerebral edema can intervene in a few days secondary to hepatic failure.

Acute renal tubular damage occurs in association with the liver damage, together with muscle necrosis and hyperkalemia. The muscle necrosis, as demonstrated at autopsy in fatal cases (82), can itself exacerbate the severe electrolyte derangement, particularly marked hyperkalemia, that occurs in liver failure. The measurement of serum concentrations of coagulation factors V (below 10%) and VIII (VIII/V ratio over 30) can have predictive value and can thus be helpful in selecting patients who require liver transplantation (SEDA-17, 99).

- A 29-year-old woman with a psychiatric disorder took an overdose of paracetamol on nine separate occasions. On the last three occasions she developed a dose-dependent, late-onset, delayed hypersensitivity reaction, characterized by an erythematous rash over the entire body (83).

Risk factors
Alcohol

Alcohol abuse can predispose to paracetamol hepatotoxicity (84–91), even in moderate social drinkers who take therapeutic or modestly excessive doses (92), and there have been anecdotal reports of severe hepatotoxicity in chronic ethanol abusers after ingestion of 4 g/day (93). Alcoholics are more likely to exceed the recommended dosage of paracetamol and consequently may be at higher risk of hepatotoxicity than non-alcoholics (91,94).

The theory behind this effect involves induction by alcohol of CYP2E1, which metabolizes about 5% of a typical dose of paracetamol, producing the reactive hepatotoxic metabolite named N-acetylparabenzoquinone-imine (NAPQI), which is normally metabolized by glutathione (95). The rest of a therapeutic dose of paracetamol is conjugated to non-toxic forms of glucuronide and sulfate. Saturation of the detoxification pathway occurs with overdose of paracetamol (72), or sometimes in certain individuals who make long-term use of normal dosages (96), in patients with compromised hepatic function, with certain drug combinations, and in other conditions of glutathione deficiency. Ingestion of alcohol induces the activity of CYP2E1 and therefore predisposes the alcoholic patient to injury even at therapeutic doses of paracetamol (97).

Despite this theory, the evidence that therapeutic doses of paracetamol can produce liver injury in alcoholics is scanty (98,99). There has been only one study of the hepatotoxicity of paracetamol in therapeutic doses in alcoholic patients, a double-blind, randomized, placebo-controlled study in which 200 long-term alcoholic patients took placebo or paracetamol 1 g qds on two consecutive days (100). Paracetamol was not given until alcohol had been eliminated from the body. Liver injury, documented by increased serum transaminases, was not detected. Mean aspartate transaminase activity on day 4 was 38 U/l with paracetamol and 38 U/l with placebo. Only five patients who took placebo and four who took paracetamol had an increase in serum aspartate transaminase to greater than 120 U/l, and it did not exceed 200 U/l in any patient. Thus, repeated administration of the maximum recommended daily doses of paracetamol to alcoholic patients was not associated with liver damage. An older report also provided evidence that alcoholic patients are not at risk from therapeutic doses of paracetamol (70). The researchers concluded that the usual recommendations that alcoholic patients should use reduced doses of paracetamol or avoid it entirely are not based on firm evidence. However, the study had some limitations, as paracetamol was given for only 2 days in doses that did not exceed the maximum therapeutic daily dose. Moreover, the alcoholic patients enrolled in the study may not have been representative of those who would be at increased risk of paracetamol toxicity (101–103). It therefore seems wise to suggest that caution is still warranted with paracetamol in alcoholic patients.

Other drugs

Analgesic cocktails or the concurrent use of potentially hepatotoxic drugs increase the risk of paracetamol toxicity.

Drugs that induce liver microsomal enzymes, such as phenobarbital, phenytoin, carbamazepine, rifampicin, and isoniazid, can make paracetamol poisoning more severe (104,105). In patients taking such drugs the serum paracetamol concentration should be doubled before consulting the usual treatment nomogram.

Fasting

Potentiation of the toxic effects of paracetamol by fasting has been previously shown in animals. In 21 cases of paracetamol hepatotoxicity not due to intentional overdosage, fasting was significantly more common than recent alcohol use among patients who developed hepatotoxicity after a dosage of 4–10 g/day (SEDA-20, 96).

Prevention

Restricting supplies

The easy availability of paracetamol is reported to be the most common reason for its common use in overdose (106), and so reducing its availability might be an effective strategy. Therefore, in September 1998 legislation was introduced in the UK limiting the pack size of paracetamol to 20 units of 500 mg; at the same time nearly all formulations became available only in blister packs. The justification for this legislation was that analgesic self-poisoning is highly impulsive and is associated with both low suicidal intent and limited knowledge of the possible consequences; it was expected that the number of cases of

paracetamol overdose might be reduced by limiting its availability.

The impact of this legislation on mortality from paracetamol overdose has been assessed in a prospective study of mortality from paracetamol overdose before and after the new legislation (107). The evaluation included the number of patients referred to liver units or listed for liver transplantation, the number of episodes of overdose and tablets taken, the plasma concentration of paracetamol, and sales of paracetamol to pharmacies. In the years after the legislation the number of tablets of paracetamol formulations per packet fell markedly, as did the number of deaths from self-poisoning with paracetamol, the number of liver transplants and admissions to liver units with hepatic damage after paracetamol poisoning, and the number of episodes of overdose in which a large number of tablets was taken. On the basis of these results it seems that the legislation was relatively successful. The results suggested that the main factor was the reduction in the number of tablets per pack available for impulsive self-poisoning. However, the study had some limitations. The period assessed may have been too short for a full assessment of the impact of the legislation (108), and the effect of legislation on self-poisoning with other drugs was not examined (109).

It may be that limiting access to one type of drug simply increases the incidence of overdose with other potentially more dangerous medicines. If that is so, unless the availability of other medications is also controlled, the removal of one readily available medication, such as paracetamol, could lead to an increase in the use of other compounds with similar or even greater toxicity (for example aspirin, ibuprofen).

In Australia, paracetamol-containing medications were recalled during two periods in 2000, presenting a unique opportunity for a retrospective observational study of the effect of reduced availability of paracetamol on the incidence of deliberate self-poisoning and accidental pediatric poisoning with paracetamol and other over-the-counter analgesics (110). During the recall periods there was a significant increase in ibuprofen deliberate self-poisoning (RR = 1.86; 95% CI = 1.41, 2.44), while there was no statistically significant change in paracetamol and aspirin deliberate self-poisoning. In children there was a significant increase in the proportion of ibuprofen accidental poisoning but no significant change for aspirin and paracetamol.

These results suggest that reduced paracetamol availability increased poisoning with alternative analgesics (in particular ibuprofen) but had little effect on the incidence of paracetamol poisoning. Restriction of paracetamol-containing medications should be critically reconsidered as an effective strategy for preventing deliberate and accidental poisoning.

Adding antidotes to oral formulations

Because restricting the packet size cannot completely resolve the problem of paracetamol overdose, alternative measures have been proposed (SEDA-22, 114). Because of the beneficial effect of acetylcysteine in paracetamol overdose, it has been suggested that toxicity caused by paracetamol overdoses, whether intentional or not, could be prevented by formulating paracetamol with added acetylcysteine. It has been estimated that including 200 mg acetylcysteine for every 500 mg of paracetamol would prevent toxicity (111,112). Methionine has previously been added to oral paracetamol formulations for the same reason. For example, Paradote contains paracetamol 500 mg and methionine 100 mg, and the combination is called co-methiamol. However, adding methionine to every paracetamol tablet prompted contrasting opinions (SEDA-22, 114) (113,114). Pameton (paracetamol 500 mg + methionine 250 mg) was voluntarily withdrawn in the UK because of safety concerns, before any evaluation of its impact on overdose had been carried out (113). Paradote remains available in the UK, but similar formulations are not currently available in the rest of Europe or the USA.

Treatment

Gastric lavage, especially in the first hour after ingestion, is recommended.

Glutathione donors

Since the mechanism of damage appears to be the exhaustion or depletion of sulfhydryl groups, as available in glutathione, treatment consists of early replacement of those groups by administration of an alternative source of glutathione, either oral methionine or, better, N-acetylcysteine, either orally or intravenously. To be most effective, a glutathione donor should be given within 8–12 hours of ingestion of the overdosage, but even up to 24 hours administration can improve the outcome (115). Acetylcysteine is usually given intravenously, but a 20-hour treatment protocol for acute paracetamol overdose using oral acetylcysteine has also been proposed (116) and was effective in preventing hepatic injury after an acute overdose of paracetamol when therapy was begun within 8 hours after ingestion.

To reduce the chance of liver damage and death in cases of paracetamol overdosage, guidelines have been produced in many countries (74,117,118) to identify patients at high risk who need to be treated soon with acetylcysteine.

In general, such guidelines recommend that the antidote should be given to all patients with a serum paracetamol concentration over 200 µg/ml (1.32 mmol/l) 4 hours after ingestion. A nomogram, in which this value is joined to an end-point of 25 µg/ml (0.16 mmol/l) at 16 hours, allows identification over this period of the patients who must receive the antidote. If acetylcysteine is not administered, it has been calculated that over 60% of patients with serum concentration of paracetamol above the described treatment line develop serious liver damage and of these about 5% will die (119). No deaths have been reported in any of the major treatment trials, however high the initial serum paracetamol concentrations, provided acetylcysteine was given within 10 hours of paracetamol ingestion. These data support the hypothesis that serious liver damage and death should be very uncommon if treatment guidelines are followed and if the patient presents for medical advice within the critical time of 10 hours from poisoning.

However, a report (119) has described fatal overdose of paracetamol in four patients who presented within 10 hours with serum paracetamol concentrations below the treatment line who, in accord with the established guidelines, were not treated with the antidote and developed fatal acute liver failure. The report generated considerable debate by advocating changing the treatment line for the use of antidotes in patients at standard risk from paracetamol poisoning from that currently recommended to a lower line passing through 150 µg/ml at 4 hours and 30 µg/ml at 12 hours.

A second "high-risk patient" line, at about half the concentration of the conventional treatment line, has already been adopted in some guidelines for patients considered at adjunctive risk of liver damage, such as those taking long-term enzyme-inducing drugs, abusing alcohol chronically, or with poor nutrition and cachexia.

However, an absolute cut-off point between a non-toxic and a toxic paracetamol overdose does not exist. Many factors should be taken into consideration in correctly interpreting the measured serum concentrations. First, the timing of the blood sample in relation to the overdose is often uncertain, and when using treatment nomogram clinicians should assume the longest interval between poisoning and blood sampling that is consistent with the history. Secondly, the current treatment nomogram is useless when paracetamol overdosage has occurred over several hours or more rather than as a single episode. Thirdly, apart from the already mentioned known risk factors, some individual differences in susceptibility to paracetamol are not well understood.

Therefore, owing to these uncertainties, it seems wise to suggest that in judging whether or not to use an antidote, clinicians should always err on the side of caution: "If there is doubt about the timing or the need of treatment, treat" (74).

Other methods of treatment

The only alternatives to glutathione donors are charcoal hemoperfusion and hemodialysis, which can be effective up to 18 hours after dosage. However, the longer the time from ingestion to treatment, the less likely the condition is to be reversible and the more likely a fatal outcome.

Theoretically, inhibitors of cytochrome P450, like cimetidine, might be of value in the treatment of paracetamol overdosage, and preliminary animal data also suggest this (115).

Drug–Drug Interactions

Alcohol

The FDA has announced its intention to require alcohol warnings on all over-the-counter pain medications that contain acetylsalicylic acid, salicylates, paracetamol, ibuprofen, ketoprofen, or naproxen. The proposed warnings are aimed at alerting consumers to the specific risks incurred from heavy alcohol consumption and its interaction with analgesics. For products that contain paracetamol, the warning indicates the risks of liver damage in those who drink more than three alcoholic beverages a day. For formulations that contain salicylates or the mentioned NSAIDs three or more alcoholic beverages will increase the risk of stomach bleeding (120).

Argatroban

The thrombin inhibitor argatroban had no effect on the pharmacokinetics of five oral doses of paracetamol 1 g 6-hourly in 12 healthy volunteers; the argatroban was given as an intravenous infusion of 1.5 µg/kg/minute from hours 12 to 30 (121).

Oral contraceptives

Oral contraceptives accelerate the renal excretion of paracetamol, reducing its effect (SEDA-9, 90).

Phenytoin

Paracetamol is metabolized in part by CYP2E1, and inducers of CYP2E1 predispose patients to paracetamol hepatotoxicity. However, a possible interaction leading to hepatotoxicity with phenytoin has been reported in a 55–year-old woman taking paracetamol 1300–6200 mg/day over 10 days (122). Phenytoin induces CYP2C and CYP3A4 but not CYP2E1. As CYP3A4 may participate in paracetamol metabolism the induction of this isoform may also be responsible for paracetamol-induced hepatotoxicity.

Rifampicin

The addition of rifampicin in patients taking paracetamol can reportedly cause liver failure and encephalopathy (123).

- A 32-year-old woman, who had been taking paracetamol 2–4 g/day for several weeks, was given rifampicin 600 mg bd, and 2 days later developed agitation, confusion, and laboratory abnormalities indicative of severe liver injury. Both rifampicin and paracetamol were withdrawn and she was given acetylcysteine. Her liver dysfunction resolved.

The severe hepatotoxicity in this case was probably due to induction of CYP3A4 by rifampicin, but rifampicin-induced liver damage could not be excluded.

Warfarin

The anticoagulant effect of warfarin is potentiated by concomitant long-term paracetamol administration.

In an early, double-blind, placebo-controlled study of the interaction between coumarin anticoagulants and paracetamol, there was a statistically significant lengthening of the prothrombin time (124). The effect, although statistically significant, was very small and was considered to be clinically unimportant.

However, in a case-control study of the risk factors for excessive warfarin anticoagulation the investigators studied 289 patients prospectively, 93 with an International Normalized Ratio (INR) over 6.0 and 196 with an INR of 1.7–3.3 during warfarin therapy (125). Paracetamol intake was independently associated with a high INR and the effect was dose-related. At a dosage of about 2–4 g/week the adjusted odds ratio (OR) for having an INR over 6 was 3.5 (95% CI = 1.2, 10) compared with no intake of paracetamol. At an intake of 4–9 g/week the adjusted OR was 6.9 (95% CI = 2.2, 22), and at an intake over 10 g/week the OR was 10 (95% CI = 2.6, 38).

However, the results of this study must be interpreted with caution, for many reasons. First, despite these data and the widespread use of paracetamol as an analgesic in patients taking warfarin, only few reports from the literature have described serious hemorrhagic complications due to potentiation of anticoagulant effect of warfarin or acenocoumarol by paracetamol (126,127). Secondly, numerous factors in the Hylex study were independently associated with an increased likelihood of having an INR over 6.0 and it is therefore possible that overlap could have occurred between these factors and paracetamol intake. Thirdly, the biochemical mechanism by which paracetamol may interfere with warfarin is not well understood. The normal metabolism of warfarin, which occurs via hepatic cytochrome P450, is a complex mechanism that can be competitively and non-competitively inhibited by many drugs. The normal metabolism of paracetamol, particularly when large doses of paracetamol are ingested, also involves cytochrome P450. Thus, paracetamol can exhaust the capacity of cytochrome P450 and prevent the normal metabolism of warfarin. When the normal metabolism of warfarin is prevented by paracetamol, the amount of active, non-protein bound warfarin promptly increases and may double or triple in concentration in the blood. Some pharmacological data, however, makes this explanation uncertain. CYP2E1 and CYP1A2 partially metabolize paracetamol. CYP2E1 is not involved in warfarin metabolism, CYP1A2 partially metabolizes paracetamol and is responsible for metabolism of R-warfarin, the less potent anticoagulant of the two warfarin stereoisomers. While R-warfarin and paracetamol may compete for metabolism, it is unlikely that a drug that competes for or inhibits metabolism of the less potent R-warfarin would significantly increase the INR. Finally, despite sporadic case reports this potential interaction has been suggested to be clinically irrelevant on the basis of the extensive collective experience of many clinicians in managing patients who require anticoagulation (128,129).

Some pharmacokinetic studies have failed to show such an interaction (130). However, if this interaction happens in only a few individuals at risk, a formal pharmacokinetic study in a small number of subjects would probably fail to include enough of such individuals to detect an effect. A case-control study, on the other hand, would be the appropriate design for detecting this type of interaction.

Thus, the key message from this study is that in patients taking a stable warfarin regimen who begin to take repeated doses of paracetamol a possible interaction should be considered. The dose and duration of paracetamol therapy should be as low as possible and INR values should be monitored.

Zidovudine

Concomitant administration of paracetamol and zidovudine leads to inhibition of glucuronidation and to potentiation of the toxicity of each drug (131,132).

Interference with Diagnostic Tests

YSI glucose analyser

Paracetamol can cause false-positive reactions for glucose in serum and blood specimens examined using the YSI glucose analyser. The effect could be of considerable importance in patients admitted with suspected paracetamol overdosage.

References

1. MacIntyre A, Gray JD, Gorelick M, Renton K. Salicylate and acetaminophen in donated blood. CMAJ 1986;135(3):215–16.

2. Wynne HA, Long A. Patient awareness of the adverse effects of non-steroidal anti-inflammatory drugs (NSAIDs). Br J Clin Pharmacol 1996;42(2):253–6.

3. National Drugs Advisory Board. Availability of aspirin and paracetamol. Annual Report 1987;24.

4. Mitchell JA, Akarasereenont P, Thiemermann C, Flower RJ, Vane JR. Selectivity of nonsteroidal antiinflammatory drugs as inhibitors of constitutive and inducible cyclooxygenase. Proc Natl Acad Sci USA 1993;90(24):11693–7.

5. Curhan GC, Willett WC, Rosner B, Stampfer MJ. Frequency of analgesic use and risk of hypertension in younger women. Arch Intern Med 2002;162(19):2204–8.

6. Radack KL, Deck CC, Bloomfield SS. Ibuprofen interferes with the efficacy of antihypertensive drugs. A randomized, double-blind, placebo-controlled trial of ibuprofen compared with acetaminophen. Ann Intern Med 1987;107(5):628–35.

7. Chalmers JP, West MJ, Wing LM, Bune AJ, Graham JR. Effects of indomethacin, sulindac, naproxen, aspirin, and paracetamol in treated hypertensive patients. Clin Exp Hypertens A 1984;6(6):1077–93.

8. Schenck NL. Nasal polypectomy in the aspirin-sensitive asthmatic. Trans Am Acad Ophthalmol Otolaryngol 1973;77:30.

9. Roth B, Woo O, Blanc P. Early metabolic acidosis and coma after acetaminophen ingestion. Ann Emerg Med 1999;33(4):452–6.

10. Shaheen SO, Sterne JA, Songhurst CE, Burney PG. Frequent paracetamol use and asthma in adults. Thorax 2000;55(4):266–70.

11. Srikiatkhachorn A, Anthony M. Serotonin receptor adaptation in patients with analgesic-induced headache. Cephalalgia 1996;16(6):419–22.

12. Srikiatkhachorn A, Anthony M. Platelet serotonin in patients with analgesic-induced headache. Cephalalgia 1996;16(6):423–6.

13. Symon DN. Twelve cases of analgesic headache. Arch Dis Child 1998;78(6):555–6.

14. Vasconcellos E, Pina-Garza JE, Millan EJ, Warner JS. Analgesic rebound headache in children and adolescents. J Child Neurol 1998;13(9):443–7.

15. Ruvalcaba RH, Limbeck GA, Kelley VC. Acetaminophen and hypoglycemia. Am J Dis Child 1966;112(6):558–60.

16. Duhamel G, Najman A, Gorin NC, Stachowiak. Aspects actuels de l'agranulocytose (àpropos de 15 observations). [Current aspects of agranulocytosis (15 cases).] Ann Med Interne (Paris) 1977;128(3):303–6.

17. Bougie D, Aster R. Immune thrombocytopenia resulting from sensitivity to metabolites of naproxen and acetaminophen. Blood 2001;97(12):3846–50.

18. Heintz B, Bock TA, Kierdorf H, Maurin N. Haemolytic crisis after acetaminophen in glucose-(6)-phosphate dehydrogenase deficiency. Klin Wochenschr 1989;67(20):1068.

19. Waldum HL, Hamre T, Kleveland PM, Dybdahl JH, Petersen H. Can NSAIDs cause acute biliary pain with cholestasis? J Clin Gastroenterol 1992;14(4):328–30.

20. Wong V, Daly M, Boon A, Heatley V. Paracetamol and acute biliary pain with cholestasis. Lancet 1993;342(8875):869.

21. Gilmore IT, Tourvas E. Paracetamol-induced acute pancreatitis. BMJ 1977;1(6063):753–4.

22. Schwarz A, Kunzendorf U, Keller F, Offermann G. Progression of renal failure in analgesic-associated nephropathy. Nephron 1989;53(3):244–9.

23. McCredie M, Stewart JH. Does paracetamol cause urothelial cancer or renal papillary necrosis? Nephron 1988;49(4):296–300.

24. Walker RJ. Paracetamol, nonsteroidal antiinflammatory drugs and nephrotoxicity. NZ Med J 1991;104(911):182–3.

25. Pommer W, Bronder E, Greiser E, Helmert U, Jesdinsky HJ, Klimpel A, Borner K, Molzahn M. Regular analgesic intake and the risk of end-stage renal failure. Am J Nephrol 1989;9(5):403–12.

26. Sandler DP, Smith JC, Weinberg CR, Buckalew VM Jr, Dennis VW, Blythe WB, Burgess WP. Analgesic use and chronic renal disease. N Engl J Med 1989;320(19):1238–43.

27. Steenland NK, Thun MJ, Ferguson CW, Port FK. Occupational and other exposures associated with male end-stage renal disease: a case/control study. Am J Public Health 1990;80(2):153–7.

28. Spuhler O, Zollinger HU. Die chronische interstitielle Nephritis. [Chronic interstitial nephritis.] Helv Med Acta 1950;17(4–5):564–7.

29. Delzell E, Shapiro S. A review of epidemiologic studies of nonnarcotic analgesics and chronic renal disease. Medicine (Baltimore) 1998;77(2):102–21.

30. McLaughlin JK, Lipworth L, Chow WH, Blot WJ. Analgesic use and chronic renal failure: a critical review of the epidemiologic literature. Kidney Int 1998;54(3):679–86.

31. Rexrode KM, Buring JE, Glynn RJ, Stampfer MJ, Youngman LD, Gaziano JM. Analgesic use and renal function in men. JAMA 2001;286(3):315–21.

32. Fored CM, Ejerblad E, Lindblad P, Fryzek JP, Dickman PW, Signorello LB, Lipworth L, Elinder CG, Blot WJ, McLaughlin JK, Zack MM, Nyren O. Acetaminophen, aspirin, and chronic renal failure. N Engl J Med 2001;345(25):1801–8.

33. Tuffs A. German nephrologists demand painkiller ban. Lancet 1996;348:952.

34. Anonymous. Analgesics combos go Rx in Belgium. Scrip 1999;2424:4.

35. De Broe ME, Elseviers MM. Analgesic nephropathy. N Engl J Med 1998;338(7):446–52.

36. Schwarz A, Preuschof L, Zellner D. Incidence of analgesic nephropathy in Berlin since 1983. Nephrol Dial Transplant 1999;14(1):109–12.

37. Fox JM. Doubts about a particularly high nephrotoxicity of combination analgesics. Nephrol Dial Transplant 1999;14(12):2966–8.

38. Elseviers MM, Bosteels V, Cambier P, De Paepe M, Godon JP, Lins R, Lornoy W, Matthys E, Moeremans C, Roose R, et al. Diagnostic criteria of analgesic nephropathy in patients with end-stage renal failure: results of the Belgian study. Nephrol Dial Transplant 1992;7(6):479–86.

39. Elseviers MM, Waller I, Nenoy D, Levora J, Matousovic K, Tanquerel T, Pommer W, Schwarz A, Keller E, Thieler H, et al. Evaluation of diagnostic criteria for analgesic nephropathy in patients with end-stage renal failure: results of the ANNE study. Analgesic Nephropathy Network of Europe. Nephrol Dial Transplant 1995;10(6):808–14.

40. Prescott LF. Analgesic nephropathy: a reassessment of the role of phenacetin and other analgesics. Drugs 1982;23(1–2):75–149.

41. Cove-Smith JR, Knapp MS. Analgesic nephropathy: an important cause of chronic renal failure. Q J Med 1978;47(185):49–69.

42. Kincaid-Smith P. Analgesic nephropathy. BMJ (Clin Res Ed) 1981;282(6278):1790–1.

43. McCredie M, Stewart JH, Mahony JF. Is phenacetin responsible for analgesic nephropathy in New South Wales? Clin Nephrol 1982;17(3):134–40.

44. Murray RM. Analgesic nephropathy: removal of phenacetin from proprietary analgesics. BMJ 1972;4(833):131–2.

45. McAnally JF, Winchester JF, Schreiner GE. Analgesic nephropathy. An uncommon cause of end-stage renal disease. Arch Intern Med 1983;143(10):1897–9.

46. Schreiner GE, McAnally JF, Winchester JF. Clinical analgesic nephropathy. Arch Intern Med 1981;141(3 Spec No):349–57.

47. Emkey RD, Mills JA. Aspirin and analgesic nephropathy. JAMA 1982;247(1):55–7.

48. MacDonald IM, Dumble LJ, Doran T, et al. Increased frequency of HLA-B12 in analgesic nephropathy. Aust NZ J Med 1978;8:233.

49. Torhorst J. Nierenschädigung durch Analgetika: pathologische Anatomie und Morphogenese. Nephrol Klin Prax 1976;3:134.

50. Zollinger HU. 25 Jahre Phenacetinabusus. [25 years of phenacetin abuse.] Schweiz Med Wochenschr 1980;110(4):106–7.

51. Dubach UC. Die Bedeutung des Analgetikaabusus für chronische Harninfektionen. Therapiewoche 1981;31:7891.

52. Kung LG. Hypernephroides Karzinom und Karzinome der ableitenden Harnwege nach Phenacetinabusus. [Hypernephroid carcinoma and carcinoma of the urinary tract following phenacetin abuse.] Schweiz Med Wochenschr 1976;106(2):47–51.

53. Gonwa TA, Corbett WT, Schey HM, Buckalew VM Jr. Analgesic-associated nephropathy and transitional cell carcinoma of the urinary tract. Ann Intern Med 1980;93(2):249–52.

54. Mihatsch MJ, Manz T, Knusli C, Hofer HO, Rist M, Guetg R, Rutishauser G, Zollinger HU. [Phenacetin abuse III. Malignant urinary tract tumors in phenacetin abuse in Basle 1963–1977.] Schweiz Med Wochenschr 1980;110(7):255–64.

55. Consensus conference: Analgesic-associated kidney disease. JAMA 1984;251(23):3123–5.

56. Dubach UC, Rosner B, Pfister E. Epidemiologic study of abuse of analgesics containing phenacetin. Renal morbidity and mortality (1968–1979). N Engl J Med 1983;308(7):357–62.

57. Dubach UC, Rosner B, Sturmer T. An epidemiologic study of abuse of analgesic drugs. Effects of phenacetin and salicylate on mortality and cardiovascular morbidity (1968 to 1987). N Engl J Med 1991;324(3):155–60.

58. Pommer W, Bronder E, Klimpel A, Helmert U, Greiser E, Molzahn M. Urothelial cancer at different tumour sites: role of smoking and habitual intake of analgesics and laxatives. Results of the Berlin Urothelial Cancer Study. Nephrol Dial Transplant 1999;14(12):2892–7.

59. Gago-Dominguez M, Yuan JM, Castelao JE, Ross RK, Yu MC. Regular use of analgesics is a risk factor for renal cell carcinoma. Br J Cancer 1999;81(3):542–8.

60. McCredie M, Pommer W, McLaughlin JK, Stewart JH, Lindblad P, Mandel JS, Mellemgaard A, Schlehofer B, Niwa S. International renal-cell cancer study. II. Analgesics. Int J Cancer 1995;60(3):345–9.

61. Valsecchi R. Fixed drug eruption to paracetamol. Dermatologica 1989;179(1):51–2.

62. Thomas RH, Munro DD. Fixed drug eruption due to paracetamol. Br J Dermatol 1986;115(3):357–9.

63. Dussarat GV, Dalger J, Mafart B, Chagnon A. Purpura vasculaire au paracétamol: une observation. [Vascular purpura caused by paracetamol. A case.] Presse Méd 1988;17(31):1587.

64. Zemtsov A, Yanase DJ, Boyd AS, Shehata B. Fixed drug eruption to Tylenol: report of two cases and review of the literature. Cutis 1992;50(4):281–2.

65. Silva A, Proenca E, Carvalho C, Senra V, Rosario C. Fixed drug eruption induced by paracetamol. Pediatr Dermatol 2001;18(2):163–4.

66. Galindo PA, Borja J, Feo F, Gomez E, Encinas C, Garcia R. Nonpigmented fixed drug eruption caused by paracetamol. J Investig Allergol Clin Immunol 1999;9(6):399–400.

67. Ayonrinde OT, Saker BM. Anaphylactoid reactions to paracetamol. Postgrad Med J 2000;76(898):501–2.

68. Fyfe AI, Wright JM. Chronic acetaminophen ingestion associated with (1;7) (p11) translocation and immune deficiency syndrome. Am J Med 1990;88(4):443–4.

69. Anonymous. Paracetamol in pregnancy. Pharm J 1996;257:921.

70. Benson GD. Acetaminophen in chronic liver disease. Clin Pharmacol Ther 1983;33(1):95–101.

71. Brotodihardjo AE, Batey RG, Farrell GC, Byth K. Hepatotoxicity from paracetamol self-poisoning in western Sydney: a continuing challenge. Med J Aust 1992;157(6):382–5.

72. Meredith TJ, Prescott LF, Vale JA. Why do patients still die from paracetamol poisoning? BMJ (Clin Res Ed) 1986;293(6543):345–6.

73. Stricker BHC, Spoelstra P. Paracetamol (acetaminophen). In: Drug-Induced Hepatic Injury. Amsterdam: Elsevier, 1985:51–4.

74. Thomas SHL. Paracetamol (acetaminophen) poisoning. BMJ 1998;317:1609–10.

75. Penna A, Buchanan N. Paracetamol poisoning in children and hepatotoxicity. Br J Clin Pharmacol 1991;32(2):143–9.

76. Rumore MM, Blaiklock RG. Influence of age-dependent pharmacokinetics and metabolism on acetaminophen hepatotoxicity. J Pharm Sci 1992;81(3):203–7.

77. Thomas SH, Horner JE, Chew K, Connolly J, Dorani B, Bevan L, Bhattacharyya S, Bramble MG, Han KH, Rodgers A, Sen B, Tesfayohannes B, Wynne H, Bateman DN. Paracetamol poisoning in the north east of England: presentation, early management and outcome. Hum Exp Toxicol 1997;16(9):495–500.

78. Litovitz TL, Klein-Schwartz W, Dyer KS, Shannon M, Lee S, Powers M. 1997 Annual Report of the American Association of Poison Control Centers Toxic Exposure Surveillance System. Am J Emerg Med 1998;16(5): 443–97.

79. Vale JA, Proudfoot AT. Paracetamol (acetaminophen) poisoning. Lancet 1995;346(8974):547–52.

80. Bialas MC, Reid PG, Beck P, Lazarus JH, Smith PM, Scorer RC, Routledge PA. Changing patterns of self-poisoning in a UK health district. QJM 1996;89(12):893–901.

81. Hawton K, Simkin S, Deeks J. Co-proxamol and suicide: a study of national mortality statistics and local non-fatal self poisonings. BMJ 2003;326(7397):1006–8.

82. Ojeda VJ, Shilkin KB, Wright EA, Williams R. Massive hepatic necrosis and focal necrotising myopathy. Lancet 1982;1(8264):172–3.

83. Huitema AD, Soesan M, Meenhorst PL, Koks CH, Beijnen JH. A dose-dependent delayed hypersensitivity reaction to acetaminophen after repeated acetaminophen intoxications. Hum Exp Toxicol 1998;17(7):406–8.

84. Emby DJ, Fraser BN. Hepatotoxicity of paracetamol enhanced by ingestion of alcohol: report of two cases. S Afr Med J 1977;51(7):208–9.

85. Barker JD Jr, de Carle DJ, Anuras S. Chronic excessive acetaminophen use and liver damage. Ann Intern Med 1977;87(3):299–301.

86. Goldfinger R, Ahmed KS, Pitchumoni CS, Weseley SA. Concomitant alcohol and drug abuse enhancing acetaminophen toxicity. Report of a case. Am J Gastroenterol 1978;70(4):385–8.

87. McClain CJ, Kromhout JP, Peterson FJ, Holtzman JL. Potentiation of acetaminophen hepatotoxicity by alcohol. JAMA 1980;244(3):251–3.

88. Licht H, Seeff LB, Zimmerman HJ. Apparent potentiation of acetaminophen hepatotoxicity by alcohol. Ann Intern Med 1980;92(4):511.

89. Johnson MW, Friedman PA, Mitch WE. Alcoholism, non-prescription drug and hepatotoxicity. The risk from unknown acetaminophen ingestion. Am J Gastroenterol 1981;76(6):530–3.

90. Leist MH, Gluskin LE, Payne JA. Enhanced toxicity of acetaminophen in alcoholics: report of three cases. J Clin Gastroenterol 1985;7(1):55–9.

91. Seeff LB, Cuccherini BA, Zimmerman HJ, Adler E, Benjamin SB. Acetaminophen hepatotoxicity in alcoholics. A therapeutic misadventure. Ann Intern Med 1986;104(3):399–404.

92. Draganov P, Durrence H, Cox C, Reuben A. Alcohol–acetaminophen syndrome. Even moderate social drinkers are at risk. Postgrad Med 2000;107(1):189–95.

93. Zimmerman HJ, Maddrey WC. Acetaminophen (paracetamol) hepatotoxicity with regular intake of alcohol: analysis of instances of therapeutic misadventure. Hepatology 1995;22(3):767–73.

94. Seeff L, Zimmerman H. Acetaminophen hepatotoxicity in alcoholics. Ann Intern Med 1986;105(4):624–5.

95. Hinson JA, Pohl LR, Monks TJ, Gillette JR. Acetaminophen-induced hepatotoxicity. Life Sci 1981;29(2):107–16.

96. Itoh S, Matsuo S, Shiomi M, Ichinoe A. Cirrhosis following 12 years of treatment with acetaminophen. Hepato-Gastroenterology 1983;30:58.

97. Thummel KE, Slattery JT, Ro H, Chien JY, Nelson SD, Lown KE, Watkins PB. Ethanol and production of the hepatotoxic metabolite of acetaminophen in healthy adults. Clin Pharmacol Ther 2000;67(6):591–9.

98. Dart RC, Kuffner EK, Rumack BH. Treatment of pain or fever with paracetamol (acetaminophen) in the alcoholic patient: a systematic review. Am J Ther 2000;7(2):123–34.

99. Dart RC. The use and effect of analgesics in patients who regularly drink alcohol. Am J Manag Care 2001;7(Suppl 19):S597–601.

100. Kuffner EK, Dart RC, Bogdan GM, Hill RE, Casper E, Darton L. Effect of maximal daily doses of acetaminophen on the liver of alcoholic patients: a randomized, double-blind, placebo-controlled trial. Arch Intern Med 2001;161(18):2247–52.

101. Holtzman JL. The effect of alcohol on acetaminophen hepatotoxicity. Arch Intern Med 2002;162(10):1193.

102. Soll AH, Sees KL. Is acetaminophen really safe in alcoholic patients? Arch Intern Med 2002;162(10):1194.

103. Oviedo J, Wolfe MM. Alcohol, acetaminophen, and toxic effects on the liver. Arch Intern Med 2002;162(10):1194–5.

104. Marsepoils T, Mahassani B, Roudiak N, et al. Potentialisation de la toxicité hépatique et rénal du paracétamol par le phénobarbital. Jeur 1989;2:118.

105. Dossing M, Sonne J. Drug-induced hepatic disorders. Incidence, management and avoidance. Drug Saf 1993;9(6):441–9.

106. Hawton K, Ware C, Mistry H, Hewitt J, Kingsbury S, Roberts D, Weitzel H. Why patients choose paracetamol for self poisoning and their knowledge of its dangers. BMJ 1995;310(6973):164.

107. Hawton K, Townsend E, Deeks J, Appleby L, Gunnell D, Bennewith O, Cooper J. Effects of legislation restricting pack sizes of paracetamol and salicylate on self poisoning in the United Kingdom: before and after study. BMJ 2001;322(7296):1203–7.

108. Dargan P, Jones A. Effects of legislation restricting pack sizes of paracetamol on self poisoning. It's too early to tell yet. BMJ 2001;323(7313):633.

109. Isbister G, Balit C. Effects of legislation restricting pack sizes of paracetamol on self poisoning. Authors did not look at effects on all deliberate and accidental self poisoning. BMJ 2001;323(7313):633–4.

110. Balit CR, Isbister GK, Peat J, Dawson AH, Whyte IM. Paracetamol recall: a natural experiment influencing analgesic poisoning. Med J Aust 2002;176(4):162–5.

111. Andrus JP, Herzenberg LA, Herzenberg LA, DeRosa SC. Effects of legislation restricting pack sizes of paracetamol on self poisoning. Paracetamol should be packaged with its antidote. BMJ 2001;323(7313):634.

112. Law R. Severity of overdose after restriction of paracetamol availability. Why hasn't strategy for minimising paracetamol poisoning been enacted? BMJ 2001;322(7285):554.

113. Jones AL, Hayes PC, Proudfoot AT, Vale JA, Prescott LF. Should methionine be added to every paracetamol tablet? (No: the risks are not well enough known). BMJ 1997;315(7103):301–3.

114. Krenzelok EP. Should methionine be added to every paracetamol tablet? (Yes: but perhaps only in developing countries). BMJ 1997;315(7103):303–4.

115. Lewis RK, Paloucek FP. Assessment and treatment of acetaminophen overdose. Clin Pharm 1991;10(10):765–74.

116. Yip L, Dart RC. A 20-hour treatment for acute acetaminophen overdose. N Engl J Med 2003;348(24):2471–2.

117. UK National Poisons Information Service. National guidelines: management of acute paracetamol poisoning. Paracetamol Information Centre in collaboration with the British Association for Accident and Emergency Medicine. 1995.

118. Bialas MC, Evans RJ, Hutchings AD, Alldridge G, Routledge PA. The impact of nationally distributed guidelines on the management of paracetamol poisoning in accident and emergency departments. National Poison Information Service. J Accid Emerg Med 1998;15(1):13–17.

119. Bridger S, Henderson K, Glucksman E, Ellis AJ, Henry JA, Williams R. Deaths from low dose paracetamol poisoning. BMJ 1998;316(7146):1724–5.

120. Anonymous. Alcohol warning on over-the-counter pain medications. WHO Drug Inf 1998;12:16.

121. Inglis AM, Sheth SB, Hursting MJ, Tenero DM, Graham AM, DiCicco RA. Investigation of the interaction between argatroban and acetaminophen, lidocaine, or digoxin. Am J Health Syst Pharm 2002;59(13):1258–66.

122. Brackett CC, Bloch JD. Phenytoin as a possible cause of acetaminophen hepatotoxicity: case report and review of the literature. Pharmacotherapy 2000;20(2):229–33.

123. Stephenson I, Qualie M, Wiselka MJ. Hepatic failure and encephalopathy attributed to an interaction between acetaminophen and rifampicin. Am J Gastroenterol 2001;96(4):1310–11.

124. Boeijinga JK, Boerstra EE, Ris P, et al. De invloed van paracetamol op antistollingsbehandeling met coumarine-derivaten. Pharm Weekbl 1983;118:209.

125. Hylek EM, Heiman H, Skates SJ, Sheehan MA, Singer DE. Acetaminophen and other risk factors for excessive warfarin anticoagulation. JAMA 1998;279(9):657–62.

126. Bell WR. Acetaminophen and warfarin: undesirable synergy. JAMA 1998;279(9):702–3.

127. Bagheri H, Bernhard NB, Montastruc JL. Potentiation of the acenocoumarol anticoagulant effect by acetaminophen. Ann Pharmacother 1999;33(4):506.

128. Riser J, Gilroy C, Hudson P, McCay L, Willis TA. Acetaminophen and risk factors for excess anticoagulation with warfarin. JAMA 1998;280(8):696.

129. Amato MG, Bussey H, Farnett L, Lyons R. Acetaminophen and risk factors for excess anticoagulation with warfarin. JAMA 1998;280(8):695–6.
130. Kwan D, Bartle WR, Walker SE. The effects of acetaminophen on pharmacokinetics and pharmacodynamics of warfarin. J Clin Pharmacol 1999;39(1):68–75.
131. Shriner K, Goetz MB. Severe hepatotoxicity in a patient receiving both acetaminophen and zidovudine. Am J Med 1992;93(1):94–6.
132. Ameer B. Acetaminophen hepatotoxicity augmented by zidovudine. Am J Med 1993;95(3):342.

Paraffins

General Information

Paraffin is a name that is commonly used to denote a group of saturated alkane hydrocarbons with the general formula C_nH_{2n+2}, n being greater than 20. They take both solid and liquid forms. The solid form known as paraffin wax was discovered by Karl Reichenbach in 1830. Paraffins are mostly obtained from petroleum. Paraffin oil, used as a fuel, is also known as kerosene.

Hard paraffin

Hard paraffin is a mixture of solid hydrocarbons, also known as paraffin wax. It is used to stiffen ointments and creams and to coat capsules and tablets. At one time it was used for cosmetic enhancement, for example of the breasts, before silicone was introduced. It is also used in bismuth iodoform paraffin paste (BIPP) (see the monograph on bismuth).

Soft paraffins

White soft paraffin and yellow soft paraffin are mixtures of semi-solid hydrocarbons. They are used as bases for ointments, as emollients in skin diseases, and as lubricants in treating dry eyes. Soft paraffin is also known as petroleum jelly, petrolatum, and Vaseline.

Liquid paraffin

Liquid paraffin is a mixture of liquid hydrocarbons. Its main use has been as a lubricant laxative but it is not recommended, because of its adverse effects. Nevertheless, it continues to be used for this purpose and is reportedly as effective as lactulose (1). However, the erstwhile Committee on Safety of Medicines in the UK recommended the following precautions (2):

- pack sizes to be limited to 160 ml;
- liquid paraffin to be used only for the symptomatic relief of constipation;
- prolonged use to be avoided and the package label to state "repeated use is not recommended";
- to be contraindicated in children under 3 years of age.

Liquid paraffin has also been used in ointments, as an emollient in skin diseases, and as a lubricant in treating dry eyes. Injection of liquid paraffin into the pleural cavity (oleothorax) was a widely used treatment for pulmonary tuberculosis before effective antituberculosis drugs became available. Long-term complications continue to be reported (3–10).

Organs and Systems

Respiratory

Liquid paraffin can cause a lipoid pneumonia or pneumonitis if inhaled (11). This has been treated with bronchoalveolar lavage (12). Lipoid pneumonia in a 34-year-old fire-eater who inhaled liquid paraffin was treated with prednisolone, antibiotics, and urinastatin (13).

Nutrition

Liquid paraffin impairs the absorption of fat-soluble vitamins (A, D, E, and K). This has rarely been reported to be of clinical significance, although one case of rickets has been reported (14).

Hematologic

Reticulolymphoblastosarcomatosis with acquired hemolytic anemia and cryoglobulinemia complicated a paraffinoma after 50 years (15,16).

Gastrointestinal

Liquid paraffin leaks from the anus and can cause local irritation.

Immunologic

Although soft paraffin has been used to treat irritant contact dermatitis (17) and to protect the skin from other sensitizers (18), hypersensitivity reactions can occur, but are rare (19–26). Yellow soft paraffin is slightly more antigenic than white soft paraffin (24). Contact sensitization to a neat cutting oil containing chlorinated paraffin occurred in 12 men (27). Contact urticaria mimicking dermatitis has also been reported (28).

Sensitization to soft paraffins can cause false-positive drug patch tests (29).

- A 31-year-old woman with a long history of presumed atopic dermatitis actually had contact dermatitis due to the soft white paraffin that was present in the several medicaments (glucocorticoids, tacrolimus, pimecrolimus, and ciclosporin) that she had used to treat the skin (30).

Long-Term Effects

Tumorigenicity

There have been many reports of so-called paraffinomas, benign tumors due to granulomatous reactions, in patients using paraffin.

Paraffin used for breast enhancement can cause mammary paraffinomas, and there have been many such reports in men and women (31–51). The tumors can calcify but are benign; in one case there was no evidence of malignant transformation after 60 years (52), although in another case there was an associated malignancy (53). Lymphatic spread of paraffin has been described (54), as has sarcoid formation (55).

Paraffinomas have also been reported after the use of paraffin to enhance the male and female external genitalia (51,56–71).

When liquid paraffin is used as a laxative, paraffinomas can occur in the colon and rectum (72–75).

Paraffin used as packing after nasal surgery can cause nasal paraffinomas (76–81).

Other tissues in which paraffinomas have been reported include the orbit and eyelids (82–86), the lungs (87–94), the limbs (95–97), sometimes with subsequent calcification (98), the face (99–101), nose (102), and scalp (103), muscle (104), the bladder (105), and the ureter (106).

Although in most cases paraffinomas occur at the site of injection, remote deposition can occur, for example in the mediastinum (107–109).

- A 55-year-old woman, who had undergone intrapleural injection of paraffin for pulmonary tuberculosis 15 years before, developed a large left-sided chest wall mass and spinal paralysis (110). A paraffinoma had invaded the vertebral canal.

Paraffin deposition has also been reported in the retinal fundi, the liver, and the spleen, in addition to the lungs (111).

There is epidemiological evidence linking the use of liquid paraffin to gastrointestinal cancer (112). Malignant transformation of a paraffinoma has occasionally been suggested.

- An 82-year-old woman who had taken long-term liquid paraffin as a laxative, developed a lipoid pneumonia and a mesothelioma (113).

Susceptibility Factors

Age

Liquid paraffin is contraindicated in children under 3 years of age (2).

Drug–Drug Interactions

Anticoagulants

It is often stated that liquid paraffin should interact with oral anticoagulants because it inhibits the absorption of vitamin K. However, no evidence of such an interaction has been published.

References

1. Urganci N, Akyildiz B, Polat TB. A comparative study: the efficacy of liquid paraffin and lactulose in management of chronic functional constipation. Pediatr Int 2005; 47(1):15–19.

2. Committee on Safety of Medicines. Liquid paraffin—restricted indications and availability. Curr Probl 1990;(28):3.

3. Diukanova MIa. [Oleogranulomatosis of the lung as a late complication of oleothorax in a patient with pulmonary tuberculosis.] Arkh Patol 1979;41(6):49–52.

4. Haberkorn U, Layer G, Schmitteckert H, Marin-Grez M. Oleothorax nach 40 Jahren. [Oleothorax 40 years later.] Pneumologie 1989;43(12):715–18.

5. Halm H, Achatzy R, Macha HN, Wahlers B. Die Thrombose des linken Jugularis-Subclavia-Venenwinkels als seltene Spätkomplikation eines Oleothorax. [Thrombosis of the left jugular–subclavian vein junction as a rare late complication of oleothorax.] Pneumologie 1990;44(11):1264–6.

6. Kopka L, Friedrich M. Komplikation eines Oleothorax. [The complication of oleothorax.] Rofo 1992;157(2):190–1.

7. Kating WT, Müller M. Arrosion und pleurobronchiale Fistelung eines Oleothorax durch eine TBC-Kaverne. [Erosion and bronchopleural fistula of an oleothorax caused by a TBC cavern.] Rofo 1993;158(4):375–7.

8. Kirshenbaum KJ, Burke RC, Kirshenbaum MD, Cavallino RP. Pleurocutaneous fistula as a complication of oleothorax. CT findings in three patients. Clin Imaging 1995;19(2):125–8.

9. Kniehl E, Wenzler A, Joggerst B, Schorn T, Barcsay E. Rupture of therapeutic oleothorax leading to paraffin oil aspiration and dissemination of tuberculosis—a fatal late complication of tuberculosis therapy in the 1940s. Wien Klin Wochenschr 1998;110(20):725–8.

10. Freedman BJ, McCarthy DM, Feldman F, Feirt N. Fatty infiltration of osseous structures: a long-term complication of oleothorax—case report. Radiology 1999;210(2): 515–17.

11. Ohwada A, Yoshioka Y, Shimanuki Y, Mitani K, Kumasaka T, Dambara T, Fukuchi Y. Exogenous lipoid pneumonia following ingestion of liquid paraffin. Intern Med 2002;41(6):483–6.

12. Lauque D, Dongay G, Levade T, Caratero C, Carles P. Bronchoalveolar lavage in liquid paraffin pneumonitis. Chest 1990;98(5):1149–55.

13. Yokohori N, Taira M, Kameyama S, Kanemura T, Kondo M, Tamaoki J, Nagai A. [Acute form of exogenous lipoid pneumonia caused by inhalation of liquid paraffin in a fire-eater.] Nihon Kokyuki Gakkai Zasshi 2002; 40(7):588–93.

14. Sinclair L. Rickets from liquid paraffin. Lancet 1967 Apr 8;1(7493):792.

15. Colomb D, Croizat P, Morel P, Creyssel R, Jouvenceaux A, Desmonceaux H. [Reticulolymphoblastosarcomatosis with acquired hemolytic anemia caused by cold antibodies, and cryoglobulinemia having complicated a paraffinoma after 50 years' development.] Lyon Med 1962 18;94:635–44.

16. Colomb D. [The future of paraffinomas. Apropos of a case of reticulo-lymphoblasto-sarcomatosis with acquired hemolytic anemia caused by cold auto-antibodies and cryoglobulinemia, having complicated a paraffinoma having 50 years' development.] Ann Dermatol Syphiligr (Paris) 1962;89:36–46.

17. Odio MR, O'Connor RJ, Sarbaugh F, Baldwin S. Continuous topical administration of a petrolatum formulation by a novel disposable diaper. 2. Effect on skin condition. Dermatology 2000;200(3):238–43.

18. Shulakov NA, Novikov VE, Loseva VA, Makushkina VK, Kozlov NB, Iakushev PF, Bondarev DP. [Vaseline protection of the skin from the effects of the sealant Uniherm-6.] Gig Tr Prof Zabol 1990;(12):43–4.

19. Maibach H. Chronic dermatitis and hyperpigmentation from petrolatum. Contact Dermatitis 1978;4(1):62.

20. Dooms-Goossens A, Degreef H. Sensitization to yellow petrolatum used as a vehicle for patch testing. Contact Dermatitis 1980;6(2):146–7.

21. Lawrence CM, Smith AG. Ampliative medicament allergy: concomitant sensitivity to multiple medicaments including yellow soft paraffin, white soft paraffin, gentian violet and Span 20. Contact Dermatitis 1982;8(4):240–5.

22. Dooms-Goossens A, Dooms M. Contact allergy to petrolatums. (III). Allergenicity prediction and pharmacopoeial requirements. Contact Dermatitis 1983;9(5):352–9.

23. Dooms-Goossens A, Degreef H. Contact allergy to petrolatums. (II). Attempts to identify the nature of the allergens. Contact Dermatitis 1983;9(4):247–56.

24. Dooms-Goossens A, Degreef H. Contact allergy to petrolatums. (I). Sensitizing capacity of different brands of yellow and white petrolatums. Contact Dermatitis 1983;9(3):175–85.

25. Ayadi M, Martin P. Contact allergy to petrolatum. Contact Dermatitis 1987;16(1):51.

26. Kang H, Choi J, Lee AY. Allergic contact dermatitis to white petrolatum. J Dermatol 2004;31(5):428–30.

27. Scerri L, Dalziel KL. Occupational contact sensitization to the stabilized chlorinated paraffin fraction in neat cutting oil. Am J Contact Dermatitis 1996;7(1):35–7.

28. Grin R, Maibach HI. Long-lasting contact urticaria from petrolatum mimicking dermatitis. Contact Dermatitis 1999;40(2):110.

29. Ulrich G, Schmutz JL, Trechot P, Commun N, Barbaud A. Sensitization to petrolatum: an unusual cause of false-positive drug patch-tests. Allergy 2004;59(9):1006–9.

30. Kundu RV, Scheman AJ, Gutmanovich A, Hernandez C. Contact dermatitis to white petrolatum. Skinmed 2004;3(5):295–6.

31. Gumrich H. Die röntgenologische Darstellung eines Mammaparaffinoms. [Roentgenologic representation of mammary paraffinomas.] Medizinische 1955;14:500.

32. Tinckler LF, Stock FE. Paraffinoma of the breast. Aust NZ J Surg 1955;25(2):142–4.

33. Clarkson P. Local mastectomy and augmentation mammaplasty for bilateral paraffinoma of breasts. Nurs Mirror Midwives J 1965;121(152):13–16.

34. Munchow H. Paraffinolschaden im Gewebe am Beispiel verkalkter Paraffinome in den Mammae. [Paraffin-oil damage to tissue as in the example of calcified paraffinomas in mammae.] Radiol Diagn (Berl) 1966;7(6):743–7.

35. Bonvallet JM. Paraffinome des deux seins chez un homme. [Paraffinoma of both breasts in a man.] Chirurgie 1971;97(3):190–2.

36. Brombart JC. Un paraffinome du sein. Aspects radiologiques. [Breast paraffinoma. Radiological aspects.] J Belge Radiol 1972;55(5):585–7.

37. Alagaratnam TT, Ong GB. Paraffinomas of the breast. J R Coll Surg Edinb 1983;28(4):260–3.

38. Raven RW. Paraffinoma of the breast. Clin Oncol 1981;7(2):157–61.

39. Kay SP, Saad MN. Paraffinoma of the male breast: a case report. Br J Plast Surg 1983;36(4):522–3.

40. Tepavicharova P, Popmikhailova Kh, Videnov L. [Paraffinoma of the breasts.] Khirurgiia (Sofiia) 1988;41(4):90–3.

41. Czeti I, Siko PP. Removal of both breasts for paraffinoma and subsequent replacement. Acta Chir Plast 1988;30(2):122–4.

42. Yang WT, Suen M, Ho WS, Metreweli C. Paraffinomas of the breast: mammographic, ultrasonographic and radiographic appearances with clinical and histopathological correlation. Clin Radiol 1996;51(2):130–3.

43. Zekri A, Ho WS, King WW. Paraffinomes déstructifs des seins et de la paroi thoracique dus a l'injection de paraffine pour augmentation mammaire. A propos de trois cas et revue de la littérature. [Destructive paraffinoma of the breast and thoracic wall caused by paraffin injection for mammary increase. Apropos of 3 cases with review of the literature.] Ann Chir Plast Esthet 1996;41(1):90–3.

44. Alagaratnam TT, Ng WF. Paraffinomas of the breast: an oriental curiosity. Aust NZ J Surg 1996;66(3):138–40.

45. Sinclair DS, Freedy L, Spigos DG. Case 3. Altered breast: paraffin injection with development of paraffinomas. AJR Am J Roentgenol 2000;175(3):861;864–5.

46. Khong PL, Ho LW, Chan JH, Leong LL. MR imaging of breast paraffinomas. AJR Am J Roentgenol 1999;173(4):929–32.

47. Ho WS, Chan AC, Law BK. Management of paraffinoma of the breast: 10 years' experience. Br J Plast Surg 2001 Apr;54(3):232–4.

48. Wang J, Shih TT, Li YW, Chang KJ, Huang HY. Magnetic resonance imaging characteristics of paraffinomas and siliconomas after mammoplasty. J Formos Med Assoc 2002;101(2):117–23.

49. Peng NJ, Chang HT, Tsay DG, Liu RS. Technetium-99m-sestamibi scintimammography to detect breast cancer in patients with paraffinomas or siliconomas after breast augmentation. Cancer Biother Radiopharm 2003;18(4):573–80.

50. Chen JS, Liu WC, Yang KC, Chen LW, Huang JS, Chang HT. Reconstruction with bilateral pedicled TRAM flap for paraffinoma breast. Plast Reconstr Surg 2005;115(1):96–104.

51. Rintala A. Ulcerating paraffinoma. Ann Chir Gynaecol 1976;65(5):356–60.

52. Thiels C, Dumke K. Mammaverkalkung nach Paraffininjektion. [Breast calcinosis following paraffin injection.] Rofo 1977;126(2):173–4.

53. Pennisi VR. Obscure carcinoma encountered in subcutaneous mastectomy in silicone- and paraffin-injected breasts: two patients. Plast Reconstr Surg 1984;74(4):535–8.

54. Ooi GC, Peh WC, Ip M. Migration and lymphatic spread of calcified paraffinomas after breast augmentation. Australas Radiol 1996;40(4):404–7.

55. Montagnac R, Collet E, Schillinger F, Chapelon C. Sarcoidose secondaire a un paraffinome mammaire bilateral. [Sarcoidosis secondary to bilateral breast paraffinoma.] Presse Méd 1993;22(33):1707.

56. Bradley RH Jr, Ehrgott WA. Paraffinoma of the penis: case report. J Urol 1951;65(3):453–9.

57. May JA, Pickering PP. Paraffinoma of the penis. Calif Med 1956;85(1):42–4.

58. Masse R. Paraffinome peno-scrotal. [Paraffinoma of the penis and scrotum.] Ann Med Leg Criminol Police Sci Toxicol 1967;47(6):704–6.

59. Foucar E, Downing DT, Gerber WL. Sclerosing lipogranuloma of the male genitalia containing vitamin E: a comparison with classical "paraffinoma". J Am Acad Dermatol 1983;9(1):103–10.

60. Akkus E, Iscimen A, Tasli L, Hattat H. Paraffinoma and ulcer of the external genitalia after self-injection of Vaseline. J Sex Med 2006;3(1):170–2.

61. Podluzhnyi GA, Tigov AD, Braganets AM, Iakimenko VA. [The clinical picture, classification and surgical treatment of paraffinomas of the external genitalia.] Urol Nefrol (Mosk) 1991;(4):69–73.

62. Lee T, Choi HR, Lee YT, Lee YH. Paraffinoma of the penis. Yonsei Med J 1994;35(3):344–8.

63. Gfesser M, Worret WI. Paraffinome de pénis. [Paraffinoma of the penis.] Hautarzt 1996;47(9):705–7.

64. Jeong JH, Shin HJ, Woo SH, Seul JH. A new repair technique for penile paraffinoma: bilateral scrotal flaps. Ann Plast Surg 1996;37(4):386–93.

65. Muraro GB, Dami A, Farina U. Paraffinoma of the penis: one-stage repair. Arch Esp Urol 1996;49(6):648–50.

66. Steffens J, Kosharskyy B, Hiebl R, Schonberger B, Rottger P, Loening S. Paraffinoma of the external genitalia after autoinjection of Vaseline. Eur Urol 2000;38(6):778–81.

67. Cohen JL, Keoleian CM, Krull EA. Penile paraffinoma: self-injection with mineral oil. J Am Acad Dermatol 2001;45(6 Suppl):S222–4.

68. Cohen JL, Keoleian CM, Krull EA. Penile paraffinoma: self-injection with mineral oil. J Am Acad Dermatol 2002;47(5 Suppl):S251–3.

69. Moon du G, Yoo JW, Bae JH, Han CS, Kim YK, Kim JJ. Sexual function and psychological characteristics of penile paraffinoma. Asian J Androl 2003;5(3):191–4.

70. Santos P, Chaveiro A, Nunes G, Fonseca J, Cardoso J. Penile paraffinoma. J Eur Acad Dermatol Venereol 2003;17(5):583–4.

71. Eo SR, Kim KS, Kim DY, Lee SY, Cho BH. Paraffinoma of the labia. Plast Reconstr Surg 2004;113(6):1885–7.

72. Nairn RC, Woodruff MF. Paraffinoma of the rectum. Ann Surg 1955;141(4):536–40.

73. Bennett DH, Wade JS. Rectal paraffinoma. Proc R Soc Med 1969;62(8):818.

74. Nishio T, Sasai Y. [Paraffinoma.] Ryoikibetsu Shokogun Shirizu 1994;(4):268–70.

75. Yanagi H, Furukawa Y, Kusunoki M, Utsunomiya J. [Colorectal paraffinoma.] Ryoikibetsu Shokogun Shirizu 1994;(6):549–50.

76. Broadbent TR. Nasal paraffinoma following rhinoplasty. Northwest Med 1957;56(7):814–15.

77. Becker H. Paraffinoma as a complication of nasal packing. Plast Reconstr Surg 1983;72(5):735–6.

78. Montgomery PQ, Khan JI, Feakins R, Nield DV. Paraffinoma revisited: a post-operative condition following rhinoplasty nasal packing. J Laryngol Otol 1996;110(8):785–6.

79. Bachor E, Dost P, Unger A, Ruwe M. Paraffinome—eine seltene Komplikation nach endonasaler Chirurgie. [Paraffinoma—a rare complication following endonasal surgery.] Laryngorhinootologie 1999;78(6):307–12.

80. Mehendale FV, Sommerlad BC. Paraffinoma—a complication of Jelonet packs following rhinoplasty. Br J Plast Surg 2001;54(2):179–80.

81. Gryskiewicz JM. Paraffinoma or postrhinoplasty mucous cyst of the nose: which is it? Plast Reconstr Surg 2001;108(7):2160–1.

82. Mouly R, Dufourmentel C, Grupper C, Arouete J, Pailheret JP, Crehange JR. Huilome palpebral après injection intralacrymale. [Palpebral paraffinoma following intralacrimal injection.] Ann Chir Plast 1972;17(1):61–6.

83. Lieb W. Paraffingranulom des Unterlides. [Paraffin granuloma of the lower lid.] Klin Monatsbl Augenheilkd 1987;190(2):125–6.

84. Feldmann R, Harms M, Chavaz P, Salomon D, Saurat JH. Orbital and palpebral paraffinoma. J Am Acad Dermatol 1992;26(5 Pt 2):833–5.

85. Hintschich CR, Beyer-Machule CK, Stefani FH. Paraffinoma of the periorbit—a challenge for the oculoplastic surgeon. Ophthal Plast Reconstr Surg 1995;11(1):39–43.

86. Keefe MA, Bloom DC, Keefe KS, Killian PJ. Orbital paraffinoma as a complication of endoscopic sinus surgery. Otolaryngol Head Neck Surg 2002;127(6):575–7.

87. Berg R Jr, Burford TH. Pulmonary paraffinoma (lipoid pneumonia); a critical study. J Thorac Surg 1950;20(3):418–28.

88. McLetchie NG, De Profio FR, O'Rafferty FM. [Paraffinoma of the lung.] Treat Serv Bull 1952;7(9): 410–18.

89. Wood Ga, Mitchell SP. Pulmonary paraffinoma verified at thoracotomy; report of two cases. Calif Med 1953;79(6):452–4.

90. Nelson LM. Lipiodol swallow and paraffinoma of the lung. Br J Tuberc Dis Chest 1954;48(1):60–2.

91. Bordet F, Daumet P, Garnier C, Paillas J. [Pulmonary paraffinoma complicated by suppuration.] J Fr Med Chir Thorac 1959;13:547–53.

92. Vaidya MP. Oil granuloma (paraffinoma) of the lung. Postgrad Med J 1962;38:355–8.

93. Mouly R, Dufourmentel C. Les paraffinomes des membres. [Limb paraffinomas.] Ann Chir Plast 1964;16:210–18.

94. Borrie J, Gwynne JF. Paraffinoma of lung: lipoid pneumonia. Report of two cases. Thorax 1973;28(2):214–21.

95. Fasal P. Paraffinoma of the arms with granulomatous lesions over the elbows. AMA Arch Derm Syphilol 1950;62(6):928–9.

96. Rivas Diez B. Parafinomas ulcerados de ambas piernas; veinticinco anos de evolucion. [Ulcerating paraffinoma of both legs; 25 years of evolution.] Bol Tr Soc Argent Cir 1952 15;36(22):640.

97. Thiers H, Croisille M. Paraffinome des parties molles de la jambe (à propos d'un cas). [Paraffinoma of the soft parts of the leg (apropos of a case).] J Radiol Electrol Med Nucl 1969;50(1):83–4.

98. Galland MC, Cohen M, Aquaron R, Maurin R, Duick JP, Bouteiller JC, Sauget Y, Manez R, Pizzi-Anselme M, Pelissier JL, et al. Lipogranulome calcifie après injection d'huile gomenolée: un "paraffinome" 60 ans après. [Calcified lipogranuloma after gomenoleo oil injection: "paraffinoma" 60 years later.] Therapie 1990;45(1):27–32.

99. Duperrat B, Recht P, Lenoir JC. [Paraffinoma of the face caused by work accident.] Presse Méd 1960;68:691–2.

100. van der Waal I. Paraffinoma of the face: a diagnostic and therapeutic problem. Oral Surg Oral Med Oral Pathol 1974;38(5):675–80.

101. Vazquez-Martinez OT, Ocampo-Candiani J, Mendez-Olvera N, Sanchez Negron FA. Paraffinomas of the facial area: treatment with systemic and intralesional steroids. J Drugs Dermatol 2006;5(2):186–9.

102. Sinrachtanant C, Tantinikorn W, Warnnissorn M, Assanasen P. Sclerosing lipogranuloma of the nose: a new treatment using adipose tissue transplantation. Facial Plast Surg 2003;19(4):363–7.

103. Klein JA, Cole G, Barr RJ, Bartlow G, Fulwider C. Paraffinomas of the scalp. Arch Dermatol 1985;121(3):382–5.

104. Dumont-Fruytier M, Tennstedt D, Lachapelle JM. Paraffinomes multiples thoraco-abdominaux. [Multiple thoraco-abdominal paraffinomas.] Dermatologica 1980;160(3):208–14.

105. Moon WK, Kim SH, Lee SJ, Han MC. Paraffinoma in the urinary bladder: CT findings. J Comput Assist Tomogr 1992;16(2):308–10.

106. Kelleher J, Wilson S, Witherow RO. Paraffinoma of the ureter. Br J Urol 1987;59(1):92–3.

107. Kergin FG. Esophageal obstruction due to paraffinoma of mediastinum; reconstruction by intrathoracic colon graft. Ann Surg 1953;137(1):91–7.

108. Deck KA, Ruiz-Ayuso F, Steinbruck HG. Paraffinom im vorderen Mediastinum. [Paraffinoma in the anterior mediastinum.] Med Klin 1969;64(4):160–4.

109. Franks RE, Cleland WP. Mediastinal fibrosis from paraffin wax. Proc Thorac Cardiovasc Soc 1978;240:1515.
110. Shiiku C, Harada H, Yamamoto N, Ito T, Koizumi J, Matsui T, Abe T. [A case of paraffinoma after plombage with spinal paralysis.] Kyobu Geka 2002;55(2):178–80.
111. Lewis PD, Dayan AD. "Paraffinosis" secondary to bilateral oleothorax. Thorax 1965;20(5):436–40.
112. Boyd JT, Doll R. Gastro-intestinal cancer and the use of liquid paraffin. Br J Cancer 1954;8(2):231–7.
113. Meyniard O, Boissonnas A, Laisne MJ, Laroche C, Abelanet R. Pneumopathie chronique a l'huile de paraffine et modifications pleurales: hyperplasie mesothéliale et mésothéliome. [Chronic pneumonia caused by paraffin oil and pleural modifications: mesothelial hyperplasia and mesothelioma.] Rev Fr Mal Respir 1980;8(3):259–63.

Paraldehyde

General Information

Paraldehyde is the cyclic trimer of acetaldehyde, a colorless or slightly yellow-colored liquid. It has been used as an anticonvulsant, but because of its adverse effects and because it is difficult to use it has been replaced by more modern agents. However, it is still sometimes used to treat status epilepticus that is resistant to first-line drugs (1). The usual adult rectal dose is 10–20 ml.

Paraldehyde is a solvent for rubber, polystyrene, and styrene acrylonitrile co-polymer, and if parenteral administration is required it should ideally be given via a glass syringe (2). Plastic syringes start to break down after exposure of about 2 minutes (3). However, some plastic syringes are resistant to its effects for a few hours (4), and intravenous tubing is reportedly unaffected (5); in an emergency it has been given rapidly by plastic syringe.

Organs and Systems

Cardiovascular

Paraldehyde caused microembolization in a neonate immediately after the injection of 0.3 ml/kg (6). The skin below the waist became red, large purple vesicles formed, and there was loss of skin and sloughing of two toes.

Respiratory

Non-cardiac pulmonary edema has been reported with paraldehyde. In one case it followed the intravenous administration of 23 ml of paraldehyde over 10 hours (7) and in another 2 ml of undiluted paraldehyde followed 30 minutes later by 0.1 ml of a 10% solution (8).

Acid–base balance

Paraldehyde can cause a metabolic acidosis, due to inability of the renal tubules to acidify the urine; several cases have been described (9–15).

- A 35-year-old man who regularly took paraldehyde 15–20 ml/day took 200 ml and developed a metabolic acidosis (pH 7.12) and acute renal insufficiency (12). He was successfully treated with intravenous alkali and peritoneal dialysis.
- A 41-year-old woman took paraldehyde 20–50 g on three different occasions and developed a metabolic acidosis that mimicked diabetic ketoacidosis (13).
- A 49-year-old woman took paraldehyde 100 ml in 4 days; she became comatose and acidotic and required hemodialysis (14).
- A 30-year-old man taking anticonvulsants was given paraldehyde 40 ml intramuscularly; 6 hours later he collapsed and was found to have a lactic acidosis (15).

Drug Administration

Drug formulations

Paraldehyde easily oxidizes to acetic acid and acetaldehyde. It should be stored in an airtight container and protected from the light. It should not be used if it has a brown color or if it smells vinegary. It solidifies when cooled and may need to be warmed before use.

Drug administration route

Paraldehyde can be given orally, rectally, intramuscularly, or intravenously.

Oral and rectal administration can cause gastric and rectal irritation.

Intramuscular administration can cause sterile abscesses (16). Peripheral nerve injury has also been reported (17), but that is a hazard of any intramuscular injection (18).

Intra-arterial administration in one case caused generalized arterial and venous thrombosis (19).

Drug overdose

A 20-year-old man died after taking paraldehyde 16 g (20).

Drug–Drug Interactions

Alcohol

Paraldehyde has been used to treat delirium tremens, but eight patients with alcohol intoxication died unexpectedly after they were given paraldehyde 30–60 ml (21).

Disulfiram

Paraldehyde is metabolized in the liver to acetaldehyde (22), and the metabolism of aldehyde by aldehyde dehydrogenase is inhibited by disulfiram, causing aldehyde toxicity. The adverse effects of this have been shown in experimental animals (23) and there have been reports of confusional psychosis in patients given disulfiram and paraldehyde (24).

Intravenous fluids

About 10–16% of paraldehyde in 5% dextrose or 0.9% sodium chloride is lost when it is delivered from PVC bags through standard intravenous administration sets and burettes over 6 hours (25).

References

1. Armstrong DL, Battin MR. Pervasive seizures caused by hypoxic–ischemic encephalopathy: treatment with intravenous paraldehyde. J Child Neurol 2001;16(12):915–17.
2. Johnson CE, Vigoreaux JA. Compatibility of paraldehyde with plastic syringes and needle hubs. Am J Hosp Pharm 1984;41(2):306–8.
3. Addy DP, Alesbury P, Winter L. Paraldehyde and plastic syringes. BMJ 1978;2(6149):1434.
4. Lockman LA. Paraldehyde. In: Antiepileptic Drugs. Levy RH, Mattson RH, Meldrum BS, editors. New York: Raven Press, 1995:963–7.
5. Schallinger LE, Uden DL. The effect of paraldehyde on intravenous tubing sets. Pharmacotherapy 1989;9(6):381–5.
6. Wait RB, Greenhalgh D, Gamelli RL. Vascular injury in the neonate associated with intra-arterial injection of paraldehyde. Clin Pediatr (Phila) 1984;23(6):324.
7. Mountain R, Ferguson S, Fowler A, Hyers T. Noncardiac pulmonary edema following administration of parenteral paraldehyde. Chest 1982;82(3):371–2.
8. Sinai SH, Crowe JE. Cyanosis, cough, and hypotension following intravenous administration of paraldehyde. Pediatrics 1976;57(1):158–9.
9. Waterhouse C, Stern EA. Metabolic acidosis occurring during administration of paraldehyde. Am J Med 1957;23(6):987–9.
10. Elkinton JR, Huth EJ, Clark JK, Barker ES, Seligson D. Renal tubular acidosis with organic aciduria during paraldehyde ingestion; six year study of an unusual case. Am J Med 1957;23(6):977–86.
11. Hayward JN, Boshell BR. Paraldehyde intoxication with metabolic acidosis; report of two cases, experimental data and a critical review of the literature. Am J Med 1957;23(6):965–76.
12. Beier LS, Pitts WH, Gonick HC. Metabolic acidosis occurring during paraldehyde intoxication. Ann Intern Med 1963;58:155–8.
13. Hiemcke T. Metabole acidose door paraldehyde. [Metabolic acidosis due to paraldehyde.] Ned Tijdschr Geneeskd 1964;108:2165–7.
14. Gutman RA, Burnell JM. Paraldehyde acidosis. Am J Med 1967;42(3):435–40.
15. Linter CM, Linter SP. Severe lactic acidosis following paraldehyde administration. Br J Psychiatry 1986;149:650–1.
16. Adenipekun A, Soyannwo OA, Amanor-Boadu SD, Campbell OB, Oyesegun AR. Complications following sedation of paediatric oncology patients undergoing radiotherapy. West Afr J Med 1998;17(4):224–6.
17. Ohaegbulam SC. Peripheral nerve injuries from intramuscular injection of drugs. West Afr J Pharmacol Drug Res 1976;3(2):161–7.
18. Aronson JK. Routes of drug administration: 5. Intramuscular. Presc J 1995;35:32–6.
19. Gooch WM 3rd, Kennedy J, Banner W Jr, McGuire HJ. Generalized arterial and venous thrombosis following intra-arterial paraldehyde. Clin Toxicol 1979;15(1):39–44.
20. Hewer CL. In: Recent Advances in Anaesthesia and Analgesia. Churchill: London, 1948:35.
21. Kaye S, Haag HB. Study of death due to combined action of alcohol and paraldehyde in man. Toxicol Appl Pharmacol 1964;6:316–20.
22. Zaleska MM, Gessner PK. Metabolism of paraldehyde to acetaldehyde in liver microsomes. Evidence for the involvement of cytochrome P-450. Biochem Pharmacol 1983;32(24):3749–54.
23. Keplinger ML, Wells JA. The effect of disulfiram on the action and metabolism of paraldehyde. J Pharmacol Exp Ther 1957;119(1):19–25.
24. Christie GL. Three cases of transient confusional psychosis in patients receiving concurrent Antabuse and paraldehyde therapy. Med J Aust 1956;1(19):789–91.
25. Welty TE, Cloyd JC, Abdel-Monem MM. Delivery of paraldehyde in 5% dextrose and 0.9% sodium chloride injections through polyvinyl chloride i.v. sets and burettes Am J Hosp Pharm 1988;45(1):131–5.

Parathyroid hormone and analogues

General Information

Both intact parathyroid hormone and smaller N-terminal fragments are used. No adverse reactions have been reported with single infusions of up to 60 mg of synthetic human parathyroid hormone in diagnostic procedures (SEDA-13, 1307) (1,2). Although bone resorption increases if the hormone is given continuously or in high doses, it has an anabolic effect on bone when given intermittently. Synthetic parathyroid hormone fragments have therefore been used in the treatment of slow turnover osteoporosis. However, no improvement in fracture risk has been documented, and the anabolic effect may only be present in the first 12 months (3). The use of parathyroid hormone in the treatment of hypoparathyroidism is also under investigation, with the optimum dosage and target calcium concentrations yet to be determined.

The adverse effects of parathyroid hormone that have been reported in clinical trials are mild and include transient bone pain, nausea, and local irritation at the injection site (4).

Parathyroid hormone has potent anabolic effects on the skeleton if given intermittently; being used in clinical trials. Initial concerns about the development of osteosarcoma in rats after prolonged treatment with high doses of parathyroid hormone have not been confirmed in human trials, but surveillance continues (5). In one study there was a mild increase in creatinine, which was thought not to have clinical significance (6). Mild nausea (7) and arthralgia (7,8) have also been reported.

Nausea was reported in 18% and headache in 13% of 552 women who took parathyroid hormone 40 micrograms, compared with 8% of the 544 women who took placebo (9).

Organs and Systems

Cardiovascular

Parathyroid hormone lowers the blood pressure by a direct effect on vascular smooth muscle, and there are isolated instances of hypotension or tachycardia (10). Pre-injection blood pressure was normal in 1093 women randomized to parathyroid hormone (PTH_{1-34}), and dizziness was reported infrequently in 541 women taking 20 micrograms/day but not in 552 taking 40 micrograms/day (9).

Mineral balance

Mild asymptomatic hypercalcemia is common during treatment with parathyroid hormone (11). The hypercalcemia is persistent, and requires dosage reduction in 3% of patients using 20 micrograms/day and in 11% using 40 micrograms/day (12). Transient mild hypercalciuria and increased serum phosphate are common but do not usually limit therapy.

In a randomized study in premenopausal women also treated with nafarelin, four of 23 women randomized to PTH$_{1-34}$ 500 IU/day had a serum calcium concentration over 2.67 mmol/l 4 hours after the injection; the concentration normalized after the dose of parathyroid hormone was reduced and other treatment was continued (7).

In another study, two of 10 men who were randomized to receive subcutaneous PTH$_{1-34}$ 400 IU/day for 18 months had serum calcium concentrations over 2.6 mmol/l after 1 or 3 months; the concentrations normalized after reduction of the dose of parathyroid hormone (8).

Hypercalcemia was present in 11% of 541 women 4–6 hours after parathyroid hormone 20 micrograms/day and in 28% of 552 women after 40 micrograms/day (9). The dose was halved because of hypercalcemia in 3 and 11% of the women taking 20 and 40 micrograms/day respectively. Nine of the women taking 40 micrograms/day stopped treatment because hypercalcemia persisted after dosage reduction.

Combining parathyroid hormone with antiresorptive agents may prevent or minimize hypercalcemia. None of 27 women randomized to estrogen plus parathyroid hormone PTH$_{1-34}$ 25 micrograms/day became hypercalcemic during a 3-year study (13).

Skin

Local reactions at sites of subcutaneous injection are common but are usually limited to transitory redness (7,8).

Subcutaneous nodules at the injection site developed in two of 17 women after more than 2 years of administration in a clinical trial (14). Two of 27 women randomized to parathyroid hormone developed nodules at injection sites; however, this could have been due to a contaminant, as both women received parathyroid hormone from the same batch (13).

Immunologic

Dose-dependent antiparathyroid hormone antibodies developed in under 10% of 1093 women in one study; however, there was no reduction in efficacy (9).

Long-Term Effects

Tumorigenicity

The rate of osteosarcoma in animal and human trials of parathyroid hormone has been reviewed (15). Rats treated with parathyroid hormone for 2 years had a high dose-dependent rate of osteosarcoma, up to 48% in animals given 75 micrograms/kg; human trials were therefore interrupted (16). However, the anabolic effect of parathyroid hormone is much greater and occurs much earlier in rats than in humans, possibly because of fundamental differences in bone biology: moreover, osteosarcoma has never been associated with primary, secondary, or tertiary hyperparathyroidism in humans (15). There has been no evidence of osteosarcoma in several hundred patients involved in parathyroid hormone clinical trials lasting up to 3 years, after 5 years minimum follow-up (15).

Drug–Drug Interactions

Bisphosphonates

Alendronate significantly reduced the anabolic effect of parathyroid hormone when the two were used in combination, both in postmenopausal women (17) and in men (18). It seems likely that this interaction will also apply to other bisphosphonates, although the mechanism has not been determined.

References

1. Mallette LE. Synthetic human parathyroid hormone 1–34 fragment for diagnostic testing. Ann Intern Med 1988;109(10):800–4.
2. Mallette LE, Kirkland JL, Gagel RF, Law WM Jr, Heath H 3rd. Synthetic human parathyroid hormone-(1–34) for the study of pseudohypoparathyroidism. J Clin Endocrinol Metab 1988;67(5):964–72.
3. Dempster DW, Cosman F, Parisien M, Shen V, Lindsay R. Anabolic actions of parathyroid hormone on bone. Endocr Rev 1993;14(6):690–709.
4. Winer KK, Yanovski JA, Cutler GB Jr. Synthetic human parathyroid hormone 1-34 vs calcitriol and calcium in the treatment of hypoparathyroidism. JAMA 1996;276(8):631–6.
5. Whitfield J, Morley P, Willick G. The parathyroid hormone, its fragments and analogues—potent bone-builders for treating osteoporosis. Expert Opin Investig Drugs 2000;9(6):1293–315.
6. Hodsman AB, Fraher LJ, Watson PH, Ostbye T, Stitt LW, Adachi JD, Taves DH, Drost D. A randomized controlled trial to compare the efficacy of cyclical parathyroid hormone versus cyclical parathyroid hormone and sequential calcitonin to improve bone mass in postmenopausal women with osteoporosis. J Clin Endocrinol Metab 1997;82(2):620–8.
7. Finkelstein JS, Klibanski A, Arnold AL, Toth TL, Hornstein MD, Neer RM. Prevention of estrogen deficiency-related bone loss with human parathyroid hormone-(1–34): a randomized controlled trial. JAMA 1998;280(12):1067–73.
8. Kurland ES, Cosman F, McMahon DJ, Rosen CJ, Lindsay R, Bilezikian JP. Parathyroid hormone as a therapy for idiopathic osteoporosis in men: effects on bone mineral density and bone markers. J Clin Endocrinol Metab 2000;85(9):3069–76.
9. Neer RM, Arnaud CD, Zanchetta JR, Prince R, Gaich GA, Reginster JY, Hodsman AB, Eriksen EF, Ish-Shalom S, Genant HK, Wang O, Mitlak BH. Effect of parathyroid hormone (1–34) on fractures and bone mineral density in postmenopausal women with osteoporosis. N Engl J Med 2001;344(19):1434–41.
10. Morley P, Whitfield JF, Willick GE. Parathyroid hormone: an anabolic treatment for osteoporosis. Curr Pharm Des 2001;7(8):671–87.
11. Body JJ, Gaich GA, Scheele WH, Kulkarni PM, Miller PD, Peretz A, Dore RK, Correa-Rotter R, Papaioannou A,

Cumming DC, Hodsman AB. A randomized double-blind trial to compare the efficacy of teriparatide [recombinant human parathyroid hormone (1–34)] with alendronate in postmenopausal women with osteoporosis. J Clin Endocrinol Metab 2002;87(10):4528–35.

12. Rubin MR, Bilezikian JP. The potential of parathyroid hormone as a therapy for osteoporosis. Int J Fertil Womens Med 2002;47(3):103–15.

13. Cosman F, Nieves J, Woelfert L, Formica C, Gordon S, Shen V, Lindsay R. Parathyroid hormone added to established hormone therapy: effects on vertebral fracture and maintenance of bone mass after parathyroid hormone withdrawal. J Bone Miner Res 2001;16(5):925–31.

14. Lindsay R, Nieves J, Formica C, Henneman E, Woelfert L, Shen V, Dempster D, Cosman F. Randomised controlled study of effect of parathyroid hormone on vertebral-bone mass and fracture incidence among postmenopausal women on oestrogen with osteoporosis. Lancet 1997;350(9077):550–5.

15. Tashjian AH Jr, Chabner BA. Commentary on clinical safety of recombinant human parathyroid hormone 1–34 in the treatment of osteoporosis in men and postmenopausal women. J Bone Miner Res 2002;17(7):1151–61.

16. Vahle JL, Sato M, Long GG, Young JK, Francis PC, Engelhardt JA, Westmore MS, Linda Y, Nold JB. Skeletal changes in rats given daily subcutaneous injections of recombinant human parathyroid hormone (1–34) for 2 years and relevance to human safety. Toxicol Pathol 2002;30(3):312–21.

17. Black DM, Greenspan SL, Ensrud KE, Palermo L, McGowan JA, Lang TF, Garnero P, Bouxsein ML, Bilezikian JP, Rosen CJ; PaTH Study Investigators. The effects of parathyroid hormone and alendronate alone or in combination in postmenopausal osteoporosis. N Engl J Med 2003;349(13):1207–15.

18. Finkelstein JS, Hayes A, Hunzelman JL, Wyland JJ, Lee H, Neer RM. The effects of parathyroid hormone, alendronate, or both in men with osteoporosis. N Engl J Med 2003;349(13):1216–26.

Parecoxib

See also COX-2 inhibitors

General Information

Parecoxib sodium is an injectable COX-2 inhibitor developed for the treatment of acute pain. It is a prodrug of a sulfonamide-based COX-2 inhibitor, valdecoxib, a potent anti-inflammatory and analgesic drug. The published information on this compound is inadequate to draw any conclusion about its tolerability. Single-dose and multiple-dose studies have not shown any safety problems compared with placebo (1–4). In small short-term endoscopic studies parecoxib was much better tolerated than the non-selective NSAID ketorolac (5,6). However, it should be noted that valdecoxib was withdrawn in 2005 (7).

References

1. Sorbera LA, Leeson PA, Castaner J, Castaner RM. Valdecoxib and parecoxib sodium. Analgesic, antiarthritic, cyclooxygenase inhibitor. Drugs Future 2001;26:133–40.

2. Cheer SM, Goa KL. Parecoxib (parecoxib sodium). Drugs 2001;61(8):1133–41.

3. Karim A, Laurent A, Slater ME, Kuss ME, Qian J, Crosby-Sessoms SL, Hubbard RC. A pharmacokinetic study of intramuscular (i.m.) parecoxib sodium in normal subjects J Clin Pharmacol 2001;41(10):1111–19.

4. Daniels SE, Grossman EH, Kuss ME, Talwalker S, Hubbard RC. A double-blind, randomized comparison of intramuscularly and intravenously administered parecoxib sodium versus ketorolac and placebo in a post-oral surgery pain model. Clin Ther 2001;23(7):1018–31.

5. Stoltz RR, Harris SI, Kuss ME, LeComte D, Talwalker S, Dhadda S, Hubbard RC. Upper GI mucosal effects of parecoxib sodium in healthy elderly subjects. Am J Gastroenterol 2002;97(1):65–71.

6. Harris SI, Kuss M, Hubbard RC, Goldstein JL. Upper gastrointestinal safety evaluation of parecoxib sodium, a new parenteral cyclooxygenase-2-specific inhibitor, compared with ketorolac, naproxen, and placebo. Clin Ther 2001;23(9):1422–8.

7. Cotter J, Wooltorton E. New restriction on celecoxib (Celebrex) use and the withdrawal of valdecoxib (Bextra). CMAJ 2005;172(10):1299.

Parenteral nutrition

General Information

Parenteral nutrition should be tailored to the needs of the individual, but on average should provide about 25 kcal/kg/day. Solutions for long-term parenteral nutrition should contain:

- about 30% carbohydrate, usually in the form of glucose, providing 60% of the energy requirements
- 30–50% fat in the form of a lipid emulsion such as soya oil
- amino acids, 150–250 kcal/g of nitrogen
- sodium and potassium
- calcium, phosphate, and magnesium
- bicarbonate
- vitamins
- trace elements (chromium, cobalt, copper, fluoride, iodide, iron, manganese, molybdenum, selenium, zinc)

The benefits and safety of parenteral nutrition have been considerably improved in recent years by innovative strategies, such as supplementation with medium-chain triglycerides, glutamine, or branch-chain amino acids.

Observational studies

GAB-88 is an infusion solution containing amino acids (3%), dextrose (7.5%), and electrolytes in a dual-chamber plastic bag. It has been evaluated in 39 non-operative patients who were unable to tolerate oral feeding or to take adequate amounts by mouth (1). When it was given in a daily dose of 1.0–2.5 liters for 7–19 days, there was an improvement in nutritional status without obvious adverse effects. There was mild vascular pain in four patients, but no phlebitis. There were no other clinically significant adverse reactions.

In 28 Japanese institutions, GAB-88 was infused continuously via a peripheral vein at a rate of 30–45 ml/kg/day for 5 postoperative days after partial gastrectomy for gastric cancer in 92 patients and compared with a similar commercial formulation; no particular adverse events emerged (2,3).

No serious adverse effects were noted in a phase 1 clinical study of GAB-88 aimed at determining its safety and pharmacokinetics in eight healthy men who were given three different doses (0.15 g/kg/hour, 0.3 g/kg/hour, and 0.5 g/kg/hour) at 1-week intervals. Serum electrolytes did not change significantly, except for zinc (4).

General adverse effects

Many of the safety issues in parenteral nutrition relate to the fact that the process is inherently unphysiological (5). Instead of periodic ingestion of nutrients via the gastrointestinal tract resulting in gradual entry of nutrients into the blood, nutrients are infused directly at a constant rate. The gastrointestinal tract as a mediator of nutrient absorption, the periodicity of nutrient administration, and the natural biorhythms of hormone secretion are all lost.

Common problems in the past were fat overload syndrome, metabolic acidosis, hyperglycemia, and hypertriglyceridemia (6). These problems are now rare. Increasing efforts have been made to avoid adverse effects such as central venous catheter infection and hepatic dysfunction. Major developments in the future are likely to be achieved with the identification of nutrients, hormones, or other active compounds that can positively influence outcome beyond the safe provision of 40 essential nutrients in proper amounts, which is what principally has been achieved to date (7). Liver damage is still a major problem. The most common micronutrient deficiency is of thiamine.

In an assessment of the clinical use of nutrients, and the tendency that has been noted in the past to overfeed with carbohydrate, lipid, and micronutrients, attention has been drawn to the adverse effects of oversupply (8).

The emerging discipline of nutritional pharmacology and the related legislative and ethical issues require expert attention and analysis. Scientific study of the nutritional and pharmacological aspects of these substances will provide new and safer forms of therapy in a number of medical conditions.

Organs and Systems

Cardiovascular

Infusion phlebitis presents a problem in parenteral nutrition. Various alternative techniques of administration have been compared in order to identify means of countering this problem (9). Mechanical trauma appears to be a causative factor; it can be reduced by limiting the time of exposure of the vein wall to nutrient infusion and by minimizing the amount of prosthetic material within the vein (10). This is likely to be even more important in small veins. In one study the addition of heparin (500 U/l) and hydrocortisone (5 micrograms/ml) significantly reduced the risk of thrombophlebitis from 0.43 to 0.11

episodes per patient-day, and a reduction in osmolality of the solution resulted in a further ten-fold fall in the incidence of thrombophlebitis (11). Other work has concluded that the incidence of infusion phlebitis is minimized during parenteral nutrition by cyclic infusion of nutrient solutions and by rotation of venous access sites (12).

Respiratory

The clinical differentiation of chylothorax from leakage of parenteral nutrition fluid into the pleural space can be difficult. However, in one case the diagnosis of leakage of parenteral nutrition fluid was made by additional tests of electrolytes, showing very high concentrations of potassium (11.3 mmol/l) and glucose (128 mmol/l), ruling out chylothorax (13).

In an acute experiment, infusion of fat emulsion (Intralipid) for 60 minutes (mean dose 0.07–0.16 g/kg/hour) in neonates with lung disease was found to lead consistently to a 10% fall in transcutaneous PO_2 (transcutaneous oxygen tension). There was no change in PCO_2. This is evidence that Intralipid contributes to the hypoxia of respiratory distress in neonates; it should be used with caution in this group, and not at all in infants with pulmonary disease (14).

Nervous system

Two children developed neurological complications of fat emulsion therapy, including focal and generalized seizures, weakness, and altered mental status, before any systemic findings were in evidence (15). Biopsy and autopsy findings included cerebral endothelial and intravascular lipid deposition. These complications are potentially reversible with alteration of the parenteral nutrition content, highlighting the importance of their early recognition.

- Acute hemiplegia and seizure developed in a 24-year-old patient following accidental catheterization of the right common carotid artery for parenteral nutrition infusion (16). Magnetic resonance imaging of the brain showed lesions in the frontal lobe and putamen, consistent with an ischemic stroke.

Considerable interest has been stimulated in the pathogenesis of critical illness polyneuropathy during artificial nutrition (17). This condition (initially functional, but proceeding to an axonal polyneuropathy, demonstrable postmortem by histological evidence of axonal degeneration) is familiar to intensive care units, and it is an important cause of weaning failure. The neurological disability can last for some 6 months, but it is likely to be reversible if the cause is recognized early and treatment withdrawn before permanent axonal changes occur. There is a strong association with sepsis and multiple organ dysfunction syndrome, the nervous system being yet another focus of organ failure. The autonomic nervous system is commonly involved, and patients are likely to show early cardiovascular instability requiring antihypotensive medication. It seems that artificial feeding after starvation leads to reduced activity of the enzymes involved in glucose oxidation, with the result that nutrient glucose causes accumulation of phosphorylated glycolytic intermediates; this in turn causes a block in the energy cascade that is an essential element in the development of axonal polyneuropathies. Although the exact chain of events is not known, there is evidence that there are disturbances of the microcirculation and increased microvascular permeability, which can lead to endoneural edema with resulting primary axonal degeneration of peripheral nerves (18). A sensitive bioassay capable of identifying a low molecular weight fraction toxic to rat spinal motor neurons has been identified in the sera of these patients (19,20).

Cases of Wernicke's encephalopathy caused by thiamine deficiency during parenteral nutrition are reported (21).

- A 13-year-old girl with acute myeloid leukemia received parenteral nutrition and chemotherapy. After a second cycle of chemotherapy she developed persistent nausea and vomiting, nystagmus, ophthalmoplegia, and brisk deep tendon reflexes on the left. Her level of consciousness deteriorated progressively. A CT scan was normal, but an MRI scan showed caudate nucleus lesions, cortical involvement, and typical diencephalic and mesencephalic abnormalities. She was given mannitol and dexamethasone, but without improvement. However, after intravenous thiamine her symptoms gradually improved; she recovered within 1 month and the MRI abnormalities disappeared.

The authors suggested that this case showed how MRI can play a role in the diagnosis of Wernicke's encephalopathy, but that there was unusual involvement of the frontal and parietal cortex and the caudate nuclei.

Metabolism

Ammonium

Hyperammonemia has occurred during parenteral nutrition as a component of therapy for renal insufficiency (22). The hyperammonemia presented as a change in mental status, developing about 3 weeks after initiation of parenteral nutrition therapy; in most cases the episodes are of increasing duration and paroxysmal. In three of the patients, serum amino acid analysis in the acute phase showed reduced concentrations of ornithine and citrulline (the respective substrate and product of condensation with carbamyl phosphate at its entry into the urea cycle). Concentrations of arginine, the precursor to ornithine, were raised.

Carbohydrates

The effects of parenteral nutrition on endocrine and exocrine functions of the pancreas have been investigated in experimental rats (23). The conclusion was that after parenteral nutrition treatment the insulin secretory response to glucose is impaired, the exocrine pancreas is hypoplastic, and the storage pattern of pancreatic exocrine enzymes is altered.

Lipids have an adverse effect on carbohydrate metabolism under basal conditions. The infusion of 20% triglyceride emulsion with heparin during basal insulin and glucose turnover conditions resulted in a rise of plasma free fatty acids from 0.4 to 0.8 mmol/l at a low rate of infusion (0.5 ml/minute for 2 hours) to between 1.6 and

2.1 mmol/l at a high rate (1.5 ml/minute for 2 hours). There were similar increases in plasma concentrations of glycerol, acetoacetate, and hydroxybutyrate. The infusions resulted in significant increases in C-peptide concentrations, but had no effects on any of the other indices of carbohydrate metabolism that were examined (plasma glucose, lactate, and pyruvate concentrations), or on carbohydrate oxidation rates. By blocking the compensatory release of insulin by the intravenous administration of somatostatin and by simultaneous replacement of basal insulin and glucagon concentrations, these workers found that there was a significant increase in plasma glucose and in hepatic glucose output, and reduced glucose clearance. It was concluded that exogenous lipids may have adverse effects on carbohydrate metabolism under basal conditions, and that healthy individuals normally compensate for this by additional secretion of insulin (24).

Preoperative parenteral nutrition can be a major cause of hyperglycemia, which has been associated with an increased risk of postoperative infection. The frequency of hyperglycemia and infectious complications has been studied in a prospective, randomized, controlled, non-blind trial in 40 patients who required parenteral nutrition for at least 5 days (25). They were given either a hypocaloric regimen (1 liter containing nitrogen 70 g and dextrose 1000 kcal) or a standard weight-based regimen begun with similar amounts initially but with gradual increases in calorie and nitrogen contents to 25 kcal and 1.5 g nitrogen/kg, up to one-third of the calories being given as fat. There were no significant differences between the two groups with regard to hyperglycemia or infections. The higher calorie regimen provided significant nutritional benefit in terms of nitrogen balance compared with the hypocaloric regimen.

Some children receiving parenteral nutrition have abnormal glucose tolerance. When this was studied in 12 patients, aged 5.7–19 years, receiving cyclic nocturnal parenteral nutrition, patients with normal glucose tolerance had an insulin response to intravenous glucose tolerance testing similar to that of normal people of the same age (26). Two patients with abnormal glucose tolerance had a reduced capacity to release insulin, whereas insulin sensitivity was unchanged in one of them. Patients with a limited capacity to release insulin, either constitutional or acquired, may not be able to produce enough insulin in these conditions and they may develop glucose intolerance during parenteral nutrition. Insulin sensitivity was not a key factor in the alteration of glucose tolerance in this study.

In five patients with multiple trauma given sodium lactate as part of parenteral nutrition there was a 20% fall in glycemia, a 43% fall in insulinemia, a 34% reduction in net carbohydrate oxidation (assessed by indirect calorimetry), and a 54% fall in plasma glucose oxidation (assessed using $^{13}CO_2$). Respiratory oxygen exchange was increased by 3.7% owing to a 20% thermic effect of lactate, but respiratory CO_2 exchange was not altered. PaO_2 fell by 11.3 mmHg, suggesting that the increased oxygen consumption was matched by an appropriate increase in spontaneous ventilation. Arterial pH increased from 7.41 to 7.46. It appears that sodium lactate given in parenteral nutrition during short intravenous nutrition in critically ill patients as a metabolic substrate limits hyperglycemia but contributes to metabolic alkalosis and does not spare ventilatory demand (27).

Lipids

The fat overload syndrome, characterized by a sudden rise in serum triglycerides, hepatosplenomegaly, intravascular coagulopathy, and end-organ dysfunction, is today an uncommon complication of intravenous administration of fat emulsion. Its higher incidence in the past may have been due to the greater phospholipid content of intravenous solutions in use at the time. The syndrome is a consequence of fat sludging within the microvasculature in organs such as the spleen, liver, kidney, lungs, brain, and retina. Necrosis in these organs suggests that emboli are responsible for the clinical symptoms and functional impairment that results. Plasma exchange has been successfully used in a patient with this syndrome who had not responded adequately to conventional medical therapy (28).

Critically ill patients are at greatest risk of fat overload syndrome when they are given lipid emulsions intravenously. Some of these patients already have impaired lipid metabolism and they are at risk of developing fat intolerance. These are the very patients who are likely to be given parenteral nutrition, including fat emulsions. Patients with increased serum triglyceride concentrations (for example, in hypothyroidism, with inborn errors of lipid metabolism, renal insufficiency, and severe sepsis, especially gram-negative sepsis) are at greatest risk. There is impaired metabolism of fats in advanced liver disease. Continuous heparin infusion may also lead to a decreased elimination capacity (29).

Fatty acids

Patients undergoing home parenteral nutrition for severe malabsorption or reduced oral intake can exhaust their stores of essential fatty acids, causing clinical effects, mainly dermatitis. In a comparative study of fatty acid profiles in 37 healthy control subjects and 56 patients receiving home parenteral nutrition, reduced small bowel length was associated with aggravated biochemical signs of essential fatty acid deficiency (30). This applied to total n-6 fatty acids and not to n-3 fatty acids. There were skin problems in 25 of the 56 patients receiving home parenteral nutrition. Patients receiving home parenteral nutrition had biochemical signs of essential fatty acid deficiency. Parenteral fluids did not increase the concentration of essential fatty acids to values comparable with those of control subjects. However, 500 ml of 20% fat emulsion (Intralipid) once a week was sufficient to prevent an increase in the Holman index (an indicator that reflects optimum proportions of polyunsaturated fatty acids).

Linoleic acid and alpha-linoleic acid are essential fatty acids that are provided in any long-term parenteral nutrition by administering fat emulsions at least twice a week. Fatty acid deficiency is a common complication of severe end-stage liver disease. The ability of short-term intravenous lipid supplementation to reverse fatty acid deficiencies has been studied in patients with chronic liver disease and low plasma concentrations of fatty acids (31). Short-term supplementation failed to normalize triglycerides.

Phospholipids

Although choline is not regarded as an essential nutrient for humans, it has been described as being "conditionally essential" in patients receiving parenteral nutrition. Choline is a methyl-group donor, a component of phospholipids, and a precursor of acetylcholine and lecithin. In animal models and healthy human beings, choline deficiency impairs liver function. Studies in patients receiving long-term parenteral nutrition have shown that low levels of plasma choline are common and are associated with hepatic steatosis.

- Choline deficiency developed in a 41-year-old woman with advanced cervical cancer who underwent prolonged parenteral nutrition (32). Her liver function tests became abnormal and she became jaundiced and complained of nausea and vomiting. The serum choline concentration was 5.77 mmol/l and there was histological evidence of hepatic steatosis. There was steady improvement with oral choline supplementation, 3 g/day, and with oral glutamine 15 g/day. There was a 45% improvement in serum choline concentration over baseline.

Intravenous fat emulsions contain choline, but not in sufficient amounts to prevent choline deficiency (32,33).

Nutrition

Amino acids

Carnitine

In septicemic patients with multi-organ dysfunction syndrome serum carnitine concentrations are in the reference range, and they remain unchanged over treatment for 10 days with parenteral nutrition without carnitine supplementation. This has been established in 28 septicemic patients, mean age 53 years, whose mean APACHE II score on admission was 17. Of these patients, 10 had septicemia with multi-organ dysfunction syndrome and 18 had uncomplicated septicemia. There were no differences in patients given long-chain triglycerides (n = 16) and a 1:1 mixture of long-chain and medium-chain triglycerides (n = 12). It does not appear from these findings that carnitine deficiency plays a significant role in the pathogenesis of multi-organ dysfunction syndrome complicating septicemia, whether or not parenteral nutrition is given in the acute phase of the illness (34).

Deficiency of carnitine has been described in all of a series of surgical neonates receiving parenteral nutrition (35); carnitine intake was far below the recommended minimal need of 11 mmol/kg per day. Although only three of the infants had clinical symptoms suggestive of carnitine deficiency, the authors recommended carnitine supplementation for all neonates receiving parenteral nutrition for more than 2 weeks. It has been suggested that a deficiency of l-carnitine may be responsible for steatosis and steatohepatitis in patients on parenteral nutrition, but one experimental study in adult women throws much doubt on this theory (36). However, in another series of patients who had depletion of erythrocyte and plasma glutathione peroxidase activity during parenteral nutrition (37), supplementation with selenium resulted in normalization of glutathione peroxidase activity within 3–4 months, which is consistent with the time-course for bone marrow erythrocyte production.

Glutamine

Animal studies have shown that raised plasma glutamate concentrations increase cerebral edema whenever the blood–brain barrier is disturbed. In a prospective study of 23 neurosurgical patients requiring parenteral nutrition, glutamine-containing regimens were compared with parenteral nutrition regimens that excluded glutamine (38). The former doubled plasma glutamine concentrations compared with controls, and the authors concluded that glutamine-containing solutions cannot be recommended for patients with a disturbed blood–brain barrier.

In a study of the safety and efficacy of l-glutamine when added to parenteral nutrition solutions of patients being treated at home, glutamine was stable in home parenteral nutrition solutions for at least 22 days. Supplementation of home parenteral nutrition solutions with l-glutamine in a dose of 0.285 g/kg for 4 weeks in seven stable patients resulted in increases in hepatic enzymes in two patients, requiring withdrawal of the glutamine/parenteral nutrition mixtures at the end of weeks 2 and 3. A third patient's liver enzymes rose at the end of week 4. These abnormalities subsided after withdrawal. Plasma concentrations of glutamine rose during the first 3 weeks of supplementation, but these increases were not statistically significant. It appears that hepatic toxicity can be associated with supplementation of home parenteral nutrition solutions with l-glutamine, without a demonstrable beneficial effect on intestinal absorptive capacity, as measured by d-xylose absorption (39). Other work seems to confirm the lack of benefit from adding glutamine in the form of its dipeptide, though it proved harmless (40).

Thiamine

Thiamine deficiency has been reported (41).

- A young man developed marked deterioration in his vision and oscillating vision, despite normal optic fundi, during parenteral nutrition; he went on to develop a characteristic Wernicke's encephalopathy, confirmed by characteristic findings on MRI brain scan (42). The serum vitamin B_1 concentration was 110 pg/ml (reference range: 200–500). He responded fully to thiamine 300 mg/day in addition to betamethasone for 4 weeks.
- Parenteral nutrition was used to support a patient requiring autologous blood stem-cell transplantation, but vitamins were excluded (the reason was not identified). After about 28 days, the patient suddenly developed severe metabolic acidosis, heart failure, and deep coma. Thiamine was immediately infused, with rapid improvement.

In the second case, the authors were unsure if the associated graft failure was due to the acute metabolic acidosis or thiamine deficiency, since the absence of thiamine in the diet leads to poor glucose oxidation, resulting in accumulation of lactic acid and metabolic acidosis, which is refractory to any treatment except thiamine supplementation.

Vitamins

More than 40 cases of fulminant beriberi have been described in patients receiving parenteral nutrition (43). The condition becomes evident 4–40 days after the start of parenteral nutrition, and is more likely to develop in patients with malignancies, ulcerative colitis, and short bowel syndrome, and in those receiving chemotherapy. The severity of metabolic acidosis is very high and refractory to bicarbonate administration, but it responds quickly to intravenous thiamine. Rapid intravenous administration of thiamine is imperative, and the patient should be transferred urgently to an intensive care unit when parenteral nutrition-induced fulminant beriberi develops.

A further consequence of thiamine depletion during parenteral nutrition can be severe lactic acidosis (44). Six cases have been described from Japan with associated hypotension, Kussmaul's respiration, and clouding of consciousness, as well as abdominal pain not directly related to the underlying disease. During parenteral nutrition administration there was blockade of oxidative decarboxylation of alpha-keto acids such as pyruvate and alpha-ketoglutarate, resulting in pyruvate accumulation and massive lactate production. None of the patients responded to sodium bicarbonate or other conventional emergency treatments for shock and lactic acidosis. Thiamine replenishment with intravenous doses of 100 mg every 12 hours resolved the lactic acidosis and improved the clinical condition of three patients.

These various reports stress the need to supplement parenteral nutrition with thiamine-containing vitamins unless there is adequate dietary intake, and to monitor serum thiamine and erythrocyte transketolase activity so that supplementary thiamine can be given in good time, if necessary intravenously (45). Giving thiamine will not rectify the various disorders if hepatic function is severely disturbed, because then thiamine is not phosphorylated and hence remains physiologically inactive.

Electrolyte balance

Hyperkalemia in one published case was attributed to combined treatment with octreotide and heparin (enoxaparin) in parenteral nutrition (46). It was suggested that both enoxaparin and octreotide had contributed in this case to the development of hyperkalemia since they reduce urinary potassium excretion.

Mineral balance

Calcium

Calcium is normally considered to be safe in parenteral nutrition, and relatively high quantities are often included in neonatal and pediatric formulations. However, there is a risk of hypercalciuria. The pathogenesis of hypercalciuria is not readily explicable on the basis of endocrine or metabolic effects, but it has been postulated to be due to excessive calcium or vitamin D intake or aluminium overload.

- A 6-year-old girl with Hirschsprung's disease had jejunostomy at 1 month followed by parenteral nutrition (47). Her calcium intake was 1–1.5 mmol/kg/day. Her urinary calcium rose from 3 months of age; her serum calcium concentrations remained within the reference range but started to rise when she was 3–4 years old. At 5–6 years of age she showed growth retardation and deteriorating renal tubular function with bilateral nephrocalcinosis. The calcium content of the parenteral nutrition was reduced, her serum and urinary calcium concentrations stayed within the reference ranges, and her renal function and growth rate improved.

After persistent hypercalciuria, osteopenia can develop, causing "metabolic bone disease," pathological fractures, and immobilization. Hypercalciuria can also lead to nephrolithiasis and nephrocalcinosis, factors that can impair renal function. Intravenous chlorothiazide has been successfully used for its hypocalciuric effect, with remarkable effect over a period of 6 months in a 13-year-old child who had received parenteral nutrition for 6 years. Calcium excretion and tubular reabsorption of phosphate returned to normal (48). What is not clear from this study is whether the drug actually has a positive long-term beneficial effect on metabolic bone disease.

Increasing the inorganic phosphorus content of parenteral nutrition formulas reduces hypercalciuria due to parenteral nutrition in experimental animals and humans. Urinary calcium excretion is significantly lower when patients receive higher inorganic phosphorus formulae, without changing the load of ultrafilterable calcium or filtered calcium, but significantly reducing fractional calcium excretion. There were no differences in serum concentrations of ionized calcium, parathyroid hormone, 25-hydroxycolecalciferol, 1,25-dihydroxycolecalciferol, or urinary cyclic AMP between different treatments with inorganic phosphorus formulae. Thus, increasing the inorganic phosphorus content of the parenteral nutrition formula reduces urinary calcium content by increasing renal tubular calcium resorption. This effect is not due to alterations in the parathormone/1,25-dihydroxycolecalciferol axis, but more probably reflects a direct action of inorganic phosphorus on the renal tubules (49).

Phosphate

Since chronic renal insufficiency is frequently complicated by rises in serum potassium, phosphate, and magnesium, parenteral nutrition solutions used to treat malnourished patients with chronic renal insufficiency are usually prepared with little supplementation of these cations. Four patients with chronic renal insufficiency developed significant hypophosphatemia 3–5 days after starting parenteral nutrition. Other electrolyte abnormalities included hypomagnesaemia ($n = 1$) and hypokalemia ($n = 3$) (50). Hypophosphatemia may be the most significant of the electrolyte risks in this clinical setting, and the electrolytes of such patients should be monitored closely when nutritional support is begun.

Hypophosphatemia has received continued attention, resulting in the need to recognize the importance of maintaining awareness of the possibility of low phosphate concentrations, monitoring phosphate concentrations closely during the first week of therapy, and supplementing with phosphate cautiously while serum concentrations remain in the reference range (51,52).

Excess phosphate is only likely to be administered as a result of medical error.

- Hyperphosphatemia complicated by calcification of subcutaneous arteries and skin infarcts has been reported in a patient with sepsis who received an unintended excess

of phosphate in parenteral nutrition (53). The patient had unintentionally received total elemental phosphorus infused over a 7-week period in the daily amount of 1.8–4.2 g (median 3.1 g), over three times the normal daily requirement. Serum phosphorus increased to 3.02 mmol/l (reference range 0.76–1.46 mmol/l). Calcification of subcutaneous arteries was complicated by widespread infarcts of the anatomically related skin and subcutis, apparently the result of hypoperfusion of these vessels during an episode of septic shock. The infarcts were characterized by blotchy skin discoloration.

Metal metabolism

Aluminium

Over the years, problems have arisen as a result of the presence of significant amounts of aluminium in parenteral nutrition solutions; in particular they have been held responsible for hypercalciuria and its consequences (54). Parenterally administered aluminium bypasses the gastrointestinal tract, which normally serves as a protective barrier to aluminium entry into the blood. In the past, aluminium contamination of casein hydrolysate, which was used as a source of protein in parenteral nutrition solutions, was associated with low-turnover osteomalacia and with encephalopathy in uremic patients. Premature infants are still at risk of aluminium accumulation as a result of prolonged parenteral nutrition (as are patients receiving plasmapheresis with albumin contaminated in its preparation with aluminium). Metabolic bone disease can result (54).

Deposition of aluminium in bone seems to relate to the appearance of bone disorders (55), although it is probably not the only cause and some studies have failed to detect a clear relation. In one critical study the bone response to parenteral nutrition containing high amounts of aluminium and ergocalciferol (25 micrograms/day), administered for 6–72 months, was compared with that to parenteral nutrition containing amino acids with reduced amounts of aluminium and ergocalciferol (5 micrograms/day) for 9–58 months, and various other solutions. Bone formation varied inversely with both plasma aluminium and bone surface aluminium, suggesting that plasma or bone surface aluminium, acquired during parenteral nutrition, reduces bone formation and leads to patchy osteomalacia (56). One should add, however, that in this study the switch to amino acids rather than casein not only influenced aluminium intake but also that of protein and ergocalciferol, both of which could be relevant to bone responses.

No effective treatment has been established for aluminium-loaded patients other than identifying the primary source of aluminium contamination and reducing or eliminating it with an appropriate substitute constituent. Prospective studies of serum aluminium concentration and urinary aluminium excretion in children receiving long-term parenteral nutrition would allow better definition of the extent to which aluminium loading remains a problem (5).

Copper

Patients who develop cholestatic jaundice during chronic parenteral nutrition can develop significant hematological complications due to hypocupremia.

- A 36-year-old woman with short bowel syndrome developed progressive liver dysfunction 6 months after the start of parenteral nutrition (57). Trace elements had been omitted because of cholestasis and persistent hyperbilirubinemia. After 15 months she became dependent on erythrocyte transfusions and her neutrophil and platelet counts fell steadily. After 19 months her serum copper concentration was 4 ng/ml (reference range 11–24 ng/ml, 0.17–0.38 µmol/l). Provision of trace elements for 2 months was associated with increased serum copper concentration and neutrophil and platelet counts, independent of erythrocyte transfusions. When the serum copper concentration reached 30 µmol/l copper was discontinued. Over the next 3 months, the copper concentration fell to 1.6 µmol/l and neutrophil and platelet counts fell precipitously. Once again, the copper concentration and neutrophil and platelet counts recovered with copper supplementation.

Because copper is excreted primarily in the bile, some experts advocate reducing or curtailing copper supplementation in patients with chronic hyperbilirubinemia. The earliest signs of copper deficiency are peripheral blood cytopenias (typically anemia and neutropenia) and occasionally thrombocytopenia, caused by reduced bone marrow production. The authors recommended that serum copper should be monitored quarterly and that copper should be included in the parenteral nutrition mixture three times a week, adjusting the frequency in response to serum copper concentrations.

Three adult cases in which copper deficiency developed during long-term parenteral nutrition without copper supplementation have been described. All three patients were suffering from malabsorption when therapy was instituted, and overt symptoms of copper deficiency developed an average of 5.8 months after the start of parenteral nutrition. Leukopenia with neutropenia and low plasma concentrations of copper and ceruloplasmin were seen in all cases (58).

- Copper deficiency has been reported in a patient with Crohn's disease after removal of copper from the parenteral nutrition because of severe cholestasis (59). The patient developed pancytopenia with severely depressed serum copper concentrations after 8 weeks. Bone-marrow biopsy confirmed the cause as copper deficiency. Although intravenous replacement of copper improved the patient's anemia and other markers, he suddenly died of cardiac tamponade.

Manganese
The dangers of hypermanganesemia as a result of parenteral nutrition are well documented. They are mainly associated with neurological toxicity. The causes of hypermanganesemia are poorly understood, but cholestasis is suspected as a key factor. There has been an attempt to identify the main factors associated with increased plasma manganese in a prospective study in 21 subjects (60). Hypermanganesemia was not only related to increased quantities infused but also to persistent inflammation (which can alter manganese metabolism) and cholestasis (causing reduced manganese biliary excretion). Neurological complications appeared to be marginal, despite the fact that manganese brain deposition is frequent. The authors suggested that manganese status

must be regularly monitored during long-term parenteral nutrition.

When oral intake is precluded, the recommended daily parenteral supplementation of manganese is 0.15–0.8 mg. Manganese is mainly excreted in the bile; during cholestasis serum manganese levels may rise, and manganese toxicity can result. Hypermanganesemia after parenteral nutrition when first reported was linked to portosystemic encephalopathy. Patients with liver disease were particularly at risk.

- Manganese deposition in the brain has been reported after 28 days of parenteral nutrition including manganese 20 µmol/day (61). The serum manganese concentration was raised (4.9 µmol/l) 34 days postoperatively, 13 days after stopping parenteral nutrition. MRI scans showed symmetrical hyperintense lesions in the globus pallidus, which gradually improved as serum manganese concentrations fell to normal.

The authors concluded that even short-term perioperative parenteral nutrition can result in manganese deposition, especially if there is liver impairment.

Excess manganese can accumulate in the brain, resulting in toxic psychosis ("manganese madness") and parkinsonism. One striking report involves a middle-aged woman receiving parenteral nutrition supplemented with trace elements from the first postoperative day after a Whipple's procedure; she developed obstructive jaundice, and her serum bilirubin concentration peaked at 179 µmol/l on the ninth postoperative day (62). She simultaneously developed increasing confusion, aggression, and choreoathetoid movements. The serum manganese concentration was 26 ng/ml (reference range below 10 ng/ml). When supplementation of manganese was substantially reduced there was progressive improvement in her confusion and other neurological signs. On the basis of this experience the authors warned against the use of standard dosages of manganese in patients with obstructive jaundice.

In manganese madness, neuroleptic drugs may be ill-advisedly administered. However, they themselves can potentiate manganese toxicity and have serious adverse effects of their own. Trivalent manganese promotes oxidation of phenothiazines, increasing free-radical formation, and may increase a patient's susceptibility to haloperidol (63). MRI brain scans in 13 of 57 children aged 6 months to 10 years receiving long-term parenteral nutrition who were being investigated because of hypermanganesemia showed characteristic increased signal intensity on T1-weighted images in seven cases, with no abnormalities on T2-weighted images. All the patients had increased whole blood manganese concentrations, suggesting that the basis for the MRI abnormality was deposition of manganese within the basal ganglia and other cerebral tissues (64). In other studies these MRI changes disappeared or abated after withdrawal of manganese supplements or exposure, but the Parkinson-like neurological manifestations appear to be permanent.

Serum manganese concentrations are not a reliable indicator of the concentrations attained in the brain. However, in one reported case with neurological complications in which alterations in basal ganglia and cerebral signal intensity had been detected during life by magnetic resonance, postmortem showed raised concentrations of manganese in the radiologically abnormal areas (65).

The relation between dose and erythrocyte concentrations of manganese has been studied in patients receiving parenteral nutrition, including manganese 500 micromol/day, for periods varying from a few days to many months (66). While concentrations during short-term parenteral nutrition were normal, patients who had been receiving parenteral nutrition for up to 30 days had raised concentrations. Of 21 patients who had been receiving parenteral nutrition for over 1 month, 15 had raised erythrocyte manganese concentrations, although in this group there was no clear relation with liver test abnormalities or renal function. In three patients there was evidence of neurological damage. The authors recommended that all patients receiving parenteral nutrition for more than 30 days should be monitored for serum manganese concentrations, that the recommended dose of manganese should not exceed 100 micrograms/day, and that manganese should be eliminated from nutrition solutions when the serum concentration is raised. The authors also recommended that manganese should not be added to parenteral nutrition solutions for patients with chronic liver disease.

It is not known with certainty whether manganese accumulation is hepatotoxic in humans, but in rats it causes mild though reversible intrahepatic cholestasis. Manganese may prove to be an overlooked cause of hepatotoxicity, as it is excreted via bile. Of 53 children who had been given parenteral nutrition for over 6 weeks, 35 had biochemical evidence of cholestatic liver disease, and in all those cases the serum manganese concentration was over 360 nmol/l (67). The highest serum manganese concentrations were found in children under 2 years of age; it is possible that biliary excretion of manganese at this age is less efficient.

The possible link between hypermanganesemia and cholestasis has been investigated in patients receiving long-term parenteral nutrition (68). The authors concluded that cholestatic liver disease does not contribute to increased blood manganese concentrations in such patients, and that plasma concentrations reflect recent manganese exposure and impaired excretion when cholestasis is present. They also emphasized that serum concentrations are a poor marker and that erythrocyte manganese concentrations should be used instead.

Selenium

The signs of selenium deficiency include skeletal myopathy and cardiomyopathy, and selenium deficiency continues to be reported in cases in which this essential element has not been added to parenteral nutrition solutions during long-term administration (69).

In a report dating from 1987, low selenium concentrations were found in four children receiving long-term parenteral nutrition. There was erythrocyte macrocytosis ($n = 3$), loss of pigmentation of hair and skin ($n = 2$), raised transaminase and creatine kinase activities ($n = 2$), and profound muscle weakness ($n = 1$). Intravenous supplementation with selenium for 3–12 months resulted in progressive improvement in all these (70).

Selenium deficiency caused by parenteral nutrition can cause heart failure.

- A 38-year-old man with Crohn's disease had been receiving parenteral nutrition for 16 years, from the age of 22 years (71). After 6 years of parenteral nutrition he developed heart failure and ventricular extra beats associated with selenium deficiency. A serum concentration of 62 ng/ml was measured (reference range 80–230). Selenium supplements improved his condition but did not normalize left ventricular function. He was given selenium supplements and was free from heart failure for 11 years, but the echocardiographic findings gradually deteriorated and he died of congestive heart failure at the age of 38 years. At autopsy, his heart showed linear fibrosis in the interventricular septum, confined to the right side. The subendocardial region and the right ventricular free wall were relatively spared.

The authors proposed that the cardiac changes in this case were characteristic of the cardiomyopathy related to selenium deficiency. Once fully developed, left ventricular dysfunction may be irreversible, even after the use of selenium supplements.

Selenium deficiency has also been reported to have caused a myopathy.

- A 35-year-old man developed selenium deficiency after repeated administration of parenteral nutrition for 13 years (72). The deficiency syndrome manifested as muscle weakness but not pain in both arms and legs, especially the thighs. There was a dominant proximal muscle weakness and reduced deep tendon reflexes. There was a progressive rise in serum creatine kinase activity, mainly of the MM type. Serum aldolase and lactate dehydrogenase were significantly raised. Peripheral muscle electromyography showed a myogenic pattern of short duration and amplitude. Muscle biopsy showed myopathic changes, with mild variation in size, regeneration of muscle fibers and muscle cell necrosis. There was no infiltration of inflammatory cells. The serum concentration of selenium was very low (1 ng/ml, reference range 97–160). After treatment for 3 months with selenium infusions the muscle weakness began to resolve and the creatine kinase activity improved. The muscle weakness did not disappear completely and serum selenium concentrations did not return to normal for more than 4 months after treatment. Eventually, and after about 5 months, there was virtually complete resolution of the muscle weakness and serum creatine kinase abnormality.

Selenium is a constituent of glutathione peroxidase, an enzyme that catalyses the oxidation of reduced glutathione by hydrogen peroxide and other hydroperoxides to form oxidized glutathione and water. In addition, glutathione peroxidase reduces phospholipid hydroperoxide in cell membranes. Selenium deficiency, as well as glutathione depletion, reduces resistance against oxidative stress, resulting in lipid peroxidation. Selenium via glutathione peroxidase may be one of the key mediators in response to oxidative stress. Cardiomyopathy and hyperglycemia are additional possible complications of selenium deficiency, but they were not noted in this case.

Acid–base balance

Lactic acidosis can occur through thiamine deficiency during parenteral nutrition (73).

- A 13-year-old boy underwent bone marrow transplantation and received parenteral nutrition without vitamins. After 15 days he had acute life-threatening lactic acidosis refractory to bicarbonate and Tris. Intravenous thiamine 100 mg produced satisfactory clinical and biochemical responses.

The authors suggested that in any patient receiving parenteral nutrition without added vitamins who develops lactic acidosis, thiamine deficiency should be suspected.

Hematologic

Erythrocytes

The major cause of megaloblastic anemia in children is folate deficiency. The following case indicates the importance of including regular supplementation of parenteral nutrition with folate (74).

- A Japanese boy, born at 34 weeks with congenital microvillous atrophy, was given parenteral nutrition 7 days after birth. The mixture included trace elements and most vitamins, but not folate. At 3 months he became lethargic, with facial pallor and hepatosplenomegaly. He had a hemoglobin of 6.9 g/dl with thrombocytopenia and a normal white blood cell count. Bone marrow showed typical megaloblasts. The serum folate concentration was 0.6 (reference range 2.4–9.8) ng/ml and vitamin B_{12} was 290 (249–938) pg/ml. These findings indicated megaloblastic anemia due to folate deficiency. Daily intramuscular folate 30 micrograms/kg and vitamin B_{12} 40 micrograms/kg improved his anemia and thrombocytopenia and his serum folate concentration returned to normal after 14 days. Both vitamins were then added daily and there was no recurrence of anemia, but he died at 4 months because of sepsis.

It is estimated that the minimum daily requirement of folate is 5 micrograms/kg. Liver stores are about 160 micrograms in premature children, and 220 micrograms in full-term infants. Infants who require parenteral nutrition will rapidly become folate deficient unless folic acid is included in the regimen. Since many multivitamin supplements do not contain folic acid, its inclusion should be ensured by the addition of folic or folinic acid.

Iron deficiency anemia can also be an important adverse effect of long-term parenteral nutrition. It is usually caused by partial or complete absence of iron from the regimen, inadequate absorption if oral iron is substituted, or chronic iron loss from gastrointestinal lesions. In a retrospective study, the records of 55 patients on long-term parenteral nutrition (more than 6 months) were examined for evidence of iron deficiency anemia (75). All had received home parenteral nutrition, comprising amino acids, glucose, and fat emulsion, with appropriate electrolytes, vitamins, and trace elements, but without iron. All had taken substantial amounts of food despite malabsorption. Iron deficiency anemia was identified in patients whose hemoglobin concentration was less than 12 g/dl and who had at least one the following:

serum iron less than 600 ng/ml and TIBC less than 3500 ng/ml; iron to TIBC ratio (or transferrin saturation) 16% or less; or serum ferritin less than 15 ng/ml. Iron studies had been monitored at about 3-monthly intervals, reduced to yearly if no problems were found. In 30 patients there was evidence of iron deficiency anemia; ten of these were detected at the start of home parenteral nutrition, and the other 20 developed iron deficiency anemia during treatment. Many had evidence of acute blood loss, for example from the gastrointestinal or genitourinary tracts. The time between the start of parenteral nutrition and the development of anemia was 2–97 (mean 29) months. Mild iron loss from the gastrointestinal tract was identified as the predominant cause. Regular treatment with small amounts of iron (10–15 mg/day had been used in these patients) added to the parenteral nutrition regimen appeared to be safe and efficacious, with no reported adverse effects. In contrast, total dose infusion of iron (for example, iron dextran infusion) had adverse effects in 25% of patients.

Iron is an essential element in nutrition, and its inclusion in any long-term parenteral nutrition regimen should be mandatory. However, it is not included in all trace element formulations, although this varies from country to country; most European products include 20 µmol of iron in trace element formulations. While it might be considered unnecessary to include iron as a daily supplement, because of safety and pharmaceutical considerations, there is ample evidence that the use of iron-containing trace element formulations is both safe and efficacious, with no associated adverse effects.

Histiocytosis

Sea-blue histiocytes containing granulations and hemophagocytosis can be seen on bone marrow smears, and there can be bone marrow sequestration of radiolabeled autologous erythrocytes. The constellation of hematological abnormalities suggests an activation of the monocyte-macrophage system by the fat emulsion (76).

Sea-blue histiocytes have been reported in bone marrow secondary to parenteral nutrition including fat-emulsion sources in seven patients with severe thrombocytopenia undergoing long-term parenteral nutrition required by extensive small-bowel resection (77). All patients received intravenous fat emulsion (Intralipid 20%) for 3–18 months. Bone marrow biopsy showed sea-blue histiocytes dispersed amongst hemopoietic cells or arranged in aggregates adjacent to osseous lamellae and blood vessels or separated from bone trabeculae. The significance of these histological findings in association with parenteral nutrition and thrombocytopenia is not known.

When one young woman on chronic parenteral nutrition for short bowel syndrome presented with hepatosplenomegaly and pancytopenia (78), bone marrow examination showed the sea-blue histiocytes to be lipid-laden macrophages. The total amount of fat in the regimen was subsequently reduced, and there was partial hematological improvement. The condition observed in this patient is analogous to that which occurs in Gaucher's disease and Niemann-Pick disease.

Leukocytes

Septic complications associated with total parental nutrition may be partly due to neutrophil dysfunction, though this has not been demonstrated (79).

Platelets

Hematological abnormalities have been found to be associated with prolonged administration of intravenous fat emulsion in children on a program of long-term cyclic parenteral nutrition. Recurrent thrombocytopenia is common and platelet lifespan is reduced. In one study (80), thrombocytopenia occurred in 66% of patients, but most of these had taken drugs that might have interfered with platelet function. Hypercoagulability was not found in the majority of cases.

It seems clear that platelet counts should be performed on a regular basis in patients receiving prolonged parenteral nutrition with fat emulsion (Intralipid). If a low platelet count develops, reduction or termination of administration is indicated (76). Clinical findings further point to hyperactivity of the macrophage in the reticuloendothelial system related to long-term treatment with Intralipid.

Coagulation

The activation of coagulation that occurs during parenteral nutrition is thought to be aggravated by coincidental infection; experimental work in healthy humans provides evidence that in patients receiving parenteral nutrition bacterial infection may facilitate the occurrence of venous thrombosis by synergistic stimulation of the coagulation system. Warfarin resistance has been found to develop during high dose propofol infusion, which contains 10% soybean oil as an emulsified preparation (81). Despite increasing the daily dose of warfarin to 30 mg, anticoagulation was not achieved until propofol was withdrawn. Lipid emulsions interfere pharmacodynamically with warfarin activity by enhancing the production of clotting factors, facilitating platelet aggregation, or supplying vitamin K; they may also facilitate warfarin binding to albumin. It follows that where patients with intestinal absorptive deficiencies who receive high-dose lipid emulsions require reliable anticoagulation heparin rather than warfarin should be used. If warfarin is given, the response should be monitored daily.

To test the hypothesis that infection facilitates activation of coagulation during parenteral nutrition, healthy subjects were injected intravenously with endotoxin (2 ng/kg) after they had received either standard parenteral nutrition for 1 week ($n = 7$) or normal enteral feeding ($n = 8$) (82). Compared with enteral feeding, parenteral nutrition was associated with selectively enhanced activation of the coagulation system (plasma concentrations of thrombin-antithrombin III complexes) during endotoxemia. Activation of the fibrinolytic system (plasminogen activator activity, tissue-type plasminogen activator, plasminogen activator inhibitor type 1) proceeded similarly in both groups. Bacterial infection, a common complication in patients receiving parenteral nutrition, may aggravate the occurrence of another common complication (venous thrombosis) by synergistic stimulation of the coagulation system. Lipids were not included in the parenteral

nutrition in this study, and it is possible that the shift towards thrombogenesis may be even more pronounced in patients receiving parenteral nutrition containing lipids.

Gastrointestinal

The proportion of patients on parenteral nutrition in whom cholestasis is accompanied by necrotizing enterocolitis has increased markedly in the past ten years. Little is known about the nature of this association. In one study, directed primarily to cases of necrotizing enterocolitis and bowel necrosis or perforation who required surgical intervention, it was found that the incidence of accompanying cholestasis was much higher in those patients who had received parenteral nutrition; necrotizing enterocolitis may make the liver more susceptible to the hepatotoxic effects of parenteral nutrition (83). In an animal study using neonatal piglets (84) parenteral nutrition produced a significant reduction in weight and length of the gastrointestinal tract, particularly in the proximal small bowel. The proximal small-bowel weight was reduced by 67–72% compared with controls; similar, but less marked, differences were found in the distal small bowel. If these findings apply to man they mean that parenteral nutrition, while necessary for survival, is at least temporarily detrimental to intestinal growth and development and thus to enteral absorption of nutrients.

Normal enterally-administered nutrition prevents the development of gut barrier failure through several mechanisms which fail to come into play when nutrition is provided parenterally (85).

Liver

Both short-term parenteral nutrition and long-term parenteral nutrition can cause liver damage (86,87). Some adult patients develop cirrhosis (88), but there is a particularly high prevalence of hepatic complications of parenteral nutrition in children (89). The clinical spectrum includes cholestasis, cholelithiasis, hepatic fibrosis with progression to biliary cirrhosis, and the development of portal hypertension and liver failure in a significant number of children who are totally parenterally fed. The pathogenesis is multifactorial and is related to prematurity, low birth weight, and the duration of parenteral nutrition. The degree and severity of the liver disease is related to recurrent sepsis, including catheter sepsis, bacterial translocation, and cholangitis. Lack of enteral feeding leads to reduced gut hormone secretion, reduced bile flow, and biliary stasis, all of which may be important in the development of cholestasis. Even in the absence of frank gallstones, there is a high incidence of biliary tract sludge and microlithiasis in patients receiving parenteral nutrition, highlighting the necessity for preventive measures and for vigilance for acute pancreatitis (90). There is evidence in rats that hepatic steatosis may be an early marker of liver toxicity caused by parenteral nutrition, preceding biochemical disturbances (91). If so, reversal of early hepatic steatosis should spare the liver from further damage. There is an inverse relation between the incidence of parenteral nutrition-associated cholestasis and both gestational age and birth weight (92).

Intestinal transplantation is combined with liver transplantation in 46% of cases, because of terminal liver failure (93). Of 78 patients who had received parenteral nutrition for more than 2 years ($n = 66$) and/or had short bowel syndrome and could not be weaned from parenteral nutrition ($n = 12$), 58 developed chronic cholestasis and 37 developed one or more severe liver complication (serum bilirubin concentration 60 µmol/l, factor V (proaccelerin) 50%, portal hypertension, encephalopathy, ascites, bleeding from the gastrointestinal tract, or histological findings consisting of extensive fibrosis and cirrhosis) after 6 (3–132) months and 17 (2–155) months respectively. Liver disease was responsible for deaths in 6.5% of the patients (22% of deaths).

Patients treated with interleukin-2 (IL-2) develop profound anorexia, malaise, loss of energy, mucositis, nausea, and vomiting, which can contribute to poor nutrition. In 21 patients who took a normal diet (controls) and 16 who received parenteral nutrition during IL-2 treatment, parenteral nutrition improved serum calcium and potassium concentrations, particularly during spontaneous diuresis after completion of IL-2 treatment (94). Unexpectedly, parenteral nutrition reduced the frequency and severity of cholestatic jaundice caused by IL-2, the pathophysiological basis of which is unknown. A brief period of parenteral nutrition during IL-2 treatment was well tolerated and it corrected the calorie and protein malnutrition. Parenteral nutrition also improved control of serum electrolytes, particularly calcium, potassium, and magnesium concentrations, although there was more marked hypophosphatemia during IL-2 treatment. The reason for this change is not clear.

Frequency

In a prospective prevalence study of liver disease in 90 patients with permanent intestinal failure receiving parenteral nutrition liver biopsy was performed in 57 (95). Chronic cholestasis developed in 58 patients after a median of 6 (range 3–132) months, and 37 developed complicated liver disease after a median of 17 (range 2–155) months. Chronic cholestasis was significantly associated with a risk of liver disease independent of parenteral nutrition, a bowel remnant shorter than 50 cm, and a lipid intake of 1 g/kg/day or more; liver disease related to parenteral nutrition was significantly associated with chronic cholestasis and a parenteral lipid intake of 1 g/kg/day or more. The authors concluded that the prevalence of liver disease increased with the duration of parenteral nutrition and was one of the main causes of death in patients with permanent intestinal failure. Parenteral intake of long-chain lipid emulsion should be restricted to less than 1 g/kg/day.

Mechanisms and susceptibility factors

Several mechanisms have been proposed to explain the cholestasis that occurs during parenteral nutrition, but there is little direct evidence to support any of them. Nutrient deficiencies that may be critical for hepatic uptake, biotransformation, and secretion of bile may be involved. Deficiency of taurine, which is important for bile acid conjugation, may cause cholestasis in premature infants. Certain amino acids may act as toxins. Reduced

hormonal and neural stimulation of hepatic bile secretion may be a factor in patients who are not receiving nutrition enterally. Increased production by intestinal bacteria of lithocholate, which is a hepatotoxic bile acid, or retention of lithocholate in the liver, might account for the cholestasis. It is unclear whether it is the lipid or the carbohydrate component of parenteral nutrition solutions that determines the development of cholestasis during parenteral nutrition (96). In one study in neonates receiving parenteral nutrition the number of operations (amongst other factors) was significantly related to the development of cholestasis, possibly because of the stress of surgery itself or to the repeated administration of anesthetic agents or morphine (97). Some animal work suggests that gallbladder sludge and cholestasis during parenteral nutrition result from a reduction in both the bile salt-dependent and bile salt-independent fractions of canalicular bile flow (98). Another possible causal factor is an accumulation in the body of phytosterols derived from soya oil and/or soya lecithin used to make the intravenous lipid emulsion. There is a close association between phytosterolemia and cholestatic liver disease; animal work provides evidence that increasing the content of phytosterols in cell membranes can interfere with the function of important transport proteins involved in the secretion of bile (99,100). Phytosterol-induced changes in neutrophil function also lead to impaired phagocytosis of bacteria and an increased risk of sepsis; the latter is responsible for further damage to hepatocytes. Finally, in neonates who are at high risk of developing parenteral nutrition-associated cholestasis when receiving a prolonged course of parenteral nutrition lack of gastrointestinal hormone formation, including cholecystokinin, may be responsible. In a prospective controlled study, patients who received cholecystokinin prophylaxis had concentrations of direct bilirubin significantly lower than in the non-treated group (101).

Increased hepatic lipogenesis and reduced transport function are important in the fatty liver associated with parenteral nutrition. Providing ample quantities of essential amino acids mitigates but does not prevent this. This highlights the importance of total caloric intake. If insufficient amounts of amino acids are taken together with adequate non-protein calories, protein deficiency analogous to kwashiorkor can develop. Hepatic lipid accumulates, but lipoprotein synthesis is limited. Carnitine supplementation minimizes fatty infiltration of the liver in patients receiving dextrose-based parenteral nutrition, which supports the idea that carnitine deficiency plays a role in the development of this complication. However, carnitine can ordinarily be synthesized from the essential amino acids methionine and lysine, which are present in all commercially available parenteral nutrition formulae. Hepatic tissue requirements may be increased under conditions of stress, contributing to the development of a fatty liver by impairment of transport and oxidation of fatty acids by mitochondria.

Raised concentrations of lithocholate, portal bacteremia, and/or endotoxemia have all been suggested as contributing to hepatic triaditis in patients with inflammatory bowel disease receiving parenteral nutrition. Toxic amino acids or their metabolic products, excessive calorie administration and a disturbed carbohydrate/protein ratio may also influence the development of triaditis. Steatonecrosis is also known to occur when nutritional depletion develops. Inadequate administration of a critical nutrient or combination of nutrients might be involved in the pathogenicity of this lesion.

The high incidence of cholestatic liver disease associated with long-term parenteral nutrition in infants who have undergone major gut resection is linked to high plasma concentrations of phytosterols, compounds that resemble cholesterol but have an alkylated side-chain (99). The phytosterols that accumulate in patients receiving parenteral nutrition are derived from the soya oil and/or soya lecithin that is used to make the intravenous lipid emulsion. There is a strong association between phytosterolemia and cholestatic liver disease, which suggests a possible causative association. Experiments in neonatal piglets have suggested that phytosterols, given without any of the other components of parenteral nutrition, can reduce bile flow. The authors suggested that increasing the content of phytosterols in cell membranes may interfere with the function of important transport proteins involved in the secretion of bile. If a 20% lipid emulsion is infused at a rate of more than 50 ml/kg/week into a premature neonate who has had a major gut resection, and if this rate of infusion is continued for 2 months, the plasma phytosterol concentration is likely to rise to a value close to 25% of the total plasma sterols. The mechanism of the liver injury and effect on bile flow caused by parenteral nutrition is likely to be more complex than a simple sterol-induced change in membrane fluidity. Intravenous lipid emulsions that do not contain phytosterols may be safer.

The possible link between cholestasis and intravenous fat emulsions has been investigated in five patients (aged 2 months to 15 years) receiving parenteral nutrition, all of whom had signs of liver disease (102). In particular, the possible role of phytosterols, natural contaminants of fat emulsions, in causing liver disease was evaluated. Three developed steatosis with non-icteric hepatic dysfunction. High plant phytosterol concentrations in patients receiving parenteral nutrition were related to liver dysfunction and depended on the degree of cholestasis and the dosage of fat emulsion. However, this evidence does not prove that plant phytosterols contribute to the development of liver disease in susceptible individuals, and the authors concluded that in patients with steatosis associated with parenteral nutrition, lipid emulsions should not be withdrawn.

In a retrospective study of the incidence of cholestasis and liver failure in 42 patients with intestinal resection in the neonatal period who subsequently became dependent on parenteral nutrition support, the effect of various associated clinical factors on the incidence and severity of cholestasis was determined (103). Cholestasis developed in 28 while they were receiving parenteral nutrition. In 21 patients, the raised direct bilirubin concentration returned to normal while they continued to receive parenteral nutrition. Seven patients progressed to liver failure. Patients without cholestasis had been dependent on parenteral nutrition for longer than patients with cholestasis. It was clear from this study that cholestasis in neonates with intestinal resection is not simply a function of the duration of exposure to intravenous nutrition.

The results instead suggested that infection early in life, when the developing liver may be uniquely sensitive to cholestatic injury and additionally stressed by intravenous nutrition, may play an important role.

The role of lipid emulsions in cholestasis associated with long-term parenteral nutrition has been investigated retrospectively in 10 children with a total of 23 episodes of cholestasis, associated with thrombocytopenia in 13 cases (104). Changes in lipid delivery, associated with increased daily amounts, preceded complications in more than half the cases, while temporary reduction in lipid administration led to normalization of bilirubin in 17 episodes. The authors concluded that lipid supply is one of the risk factors for cholestasis associated with parenteral nutrition. They recommended that when cholestasis occurs, lipid should be temporarily withdrawn, especially if there is associated thrombocytopenia.

In a randomized, controlled study of 244 infants one group ($n = 123$) received lower concentrations of manganese (0.0182 micromol/kg/day as Peditrace 1 ml/kg/day) while the second ($n = 121$) received 1 micromol/kg/day (as Ped-el 4 ml/kg/day) (105). All other components of the parenteral nutrition regimen were standardized. Monitoring comprised whole-blood manganese and serum direct bilirubin concentrations, the indicator for the development of cholestasis being a peak bilirubin concentration over 50 micromol/l. Those who were given extra manganese had higher peak whole blood manganese concentrations and higher peak serum direct bilirubin concentrations, but the differences were not significant. The two groups did not differ in terms of the occurrence of cholestasis (63/121 versus 57/123), but more infants in the high manganese group developed a more severe degree of hyperbilirubinemia. The authors concluded that the pathogenesis of cholestasis during parenteral nutrition is probably multifactorial, and that a high manganese intake is a significant contributory factor.

The link between cholestasis during home parenteral nutrition and inflammatory markers has been investigated in 17 patients on long-term home parenteral nutrition and 10 age-matched and sex-matched controls (106). Liver enzyme concentrations were used as markers of liver disease. Circulating inflammatory and immune markers were determined as measures of inflammatory activity. There were abnormal liver function tests in 14 of the patients. Alkaline phosphatase was positively correlated with markers of persistent inflammation and immune activation. Liver enzyme activities were also related to the amounts of total intravenous calories and calories originating from carbohydrates, but not lipids, in contrast to other recent data. The authors suggested that these results confirm that the number of infused calories contributes to liver toxicity in patients receiving home parenteral nutrition and strongly imply that sustained inflammation is probably a key factor in worsening the associated cholestasis.

Management

There is no effective treatment of liver damage during parenteral nutrition, except for using enteral nutrition as soon as possible. However, the benefits of ursodeoxycholic acid, a naturally occurring non-toxic hydrophilic bile acid, have been evaluated in a retrospective chart review of six infants who received oral ursodeoxycholic acid 15–30 mg/kg/day for at least 1 month (107). Ursodeoxycholic acid was safe and led to some early reduction in bilirubin concentrations, although there was no improvement in other markers of liver function. Clearly, the possible benefits have yet to be firmly established. Ursodeoxycholic acid may prevent or reduce the hepatocyte damage and cholestasis caused by high concentrations of hydrophobic bile acids by increasing the concentrations of hydrophilic non-hepatotoxic bile acids in the bile, by reducing histocompatibility antigens displayed by hepatocytes, or by a direct cytoprotective effect (108).

One cause of deteriorating liver function resulting from long-term parenteral nutrition is attributable to excessive or persistent calorie intake. Cyclic parenteral nutrition is a procedure of intermittent delivery (either during the day or at night over 10–12 hours). During the non-infusion period the central venous catheter is heparin-locked. In a prospective study the effect of early use of cyclic parenteral nutrition on deterioration of liver function has been studied in 65 patients with impaired liver function (109). The patients were divided into three groups based on bilirubin concentrations (over 85 µmol/l, 170 µmol/l, and 340 µmol/l). Each of the subgroups was divided into control (continuous parenteral nutrition) or test (cyclic parenteral nutrition). Patients on non-cyclic parenteral nutrition had significantly increased bilirubin and alkaline phosphatase, but the difference between the control and test groups was not significant in those patients with the most severe liver failure before the study. The authors were therefore unable to confirm the possible value of cyclic parenteral nutrition in reducing deterioration in liver function, although the results suggested that, at least in mild or moderate liver failure, there may be some benefit in reducing hepatocellular damage and progressive jaundice.

Urinary tract

There was a profound reduction in renal function associated with very long-term parenteral nutrition (continuing for periods longer than 10 years) in 29 of 33 patients studied: a reduction in estimated creatinine clearance of 0.6–15.4% per year (110). Tubular function, as determined by the tubular reabsorption of phosphate, was impaired in 52%. Although nephrotoxic drug use, bacteremia, fungemia, age, and infection rate accounted for part of the decline in renal function, most of it was unexplained.

In some infants receiving parenteral nutrition nephrocalcinosis occurs. Parenteral nutrition solutions contain the oxalate precursors ascorbate and glycine, and in one study of very low birth weight infants (111) administration of parenteral nutrition protein of about 0.5 g/kg/day was associated with an increased urinary oxalate/creatinine ratio; the effect was dose-dependent. Raised urinary oxalate concentrations may be a factor in the pathogenesis of nephrocalcinosis in these infants.

Musculoskeletal

There is massive evidence that parenteral nutrition therapy itself can affect bone adversely, especially bone density (5,112,113). Depletion of bone mineral is common

in patients dependent on long-term parenteral nutrition (114). It is difficult to identify the role of a single nutrient in the development of bone disease during parenteral nutrition. The pathogenicity may be multifactorial and different in patients at different ages: in growing infants increased mineral requirement can be of particular importance, whereas other factors (such as aluminium toxicity) can occur in both adults and children. Since mineral status can be critical, particularly in small preterm infants, non-nutritional factors, including chronic use of potent loop diuretics and altered acid-base status, can affect urine mineral loss, cell metabolism, and consequently bone mineralization. Other factors that can play a role in the pathogenesis of bone disease associated with parenteral nutrition make reports confusing; they include lack of periodic enteral feeding, underlying intestinal disease including malabsorption and inflammation, neoplasm, and drug-induced alterations in calcium and bone metabolism.

In adults receiving long-term parenteral nutrition, despite its anabolic effects on other tissues, there is no improvement in bone density. Infants treated with parenteral nutrition from birth also develop low bone density for age, suggesting that parenteral nutrition treatment in some way contributes to the osteopenia (5). A 17% long-term increase in spinal bone mineral content has been shown in patients who have received parenteral nutrition solutions without vitamin D. However, this rise was nearly balanced by a 15% fall in hip bone mineral content (115). In a Danish study of bone mineral content in adults receiving home parenteral nutrition for short bowel syndrome, despite the fact that all were on free oral intake as a supplement to the parenteral nutrition, 47% had mandibular osteoporosis while 33% had osteoporosis in the forearm and radiographic changes of osteoporotic fractures in the vertebral column. Dental and periodontal tissues were normal (116).

In general, the question of whether parenteral nutrition adversely affects calcium regulation is unclear. Human studies are confounded by uncontrolled variables, including the degree to which food is taken orally; gut absorption; underlying disease; medications that adversely affect bones, including glucocorticoids; and aluminium contamination of parenteral nutrients. Calcium loss in the urine is often described, but the pattern is not consistent. Non-human primate work can provide some insight, but here too the findings are difficult to interpret. In one such study it was not possible to show a negative calcium balance with the use of parenteral nutrition in the absence of underlying disease (114). However, at higher rates of intravenous nutrition negative calcium balance has been demonstrated in such a model (117), while in other work evidence has been obtained that there is initial calciuria (and a negative calcium balance), which improves within 2 weeks (5). Some evidence seems to show that in premature infants receiving parenteral nutrition the mixture should contain higher calcium and phosphorus concentrations in prematurity than in childhood in order to avoid rickets and to promote improvement in existing rickets (118).

Cytokines such as interleukin-1, interleukin-6, and tumor necrosis factor alfa influence bone resorption and have been invoked as a cause of type 1 osteoporosis.

Parenteral nutrition in experimental rats enhances the catabolic effect of tumor necrosis factor alfa (119). The role of parenteral nutrition-induced cytokine release or activity, especially of IL-1, IL-6, and tumor necrosis factor alfa, in causing hypercalciuria and reduced mineralization in patients receiving parenteral nutrition needs to be clarified (119).

Metabolic bone disease in children receiving parenteral nutrition manifests primarily as osteopenia and, on occasion, fractures (5). The etiology is multifactorial: calcium and phosphate deficiency play a major role in the preterm infant but the part played by aluminium toxicity in this population is unknown. Lack of reference values of bone histomorphometry in the premature infant, as well as lack of reference data for biochemical markers of bone turnover in these patients, contributes to the uncertainty. Other factors that may play a role in the pathogenesis of bone disease associated with parenteral nutrition include lack of periodic enteral feeding; underlying intestinal disease, including malabsorption and inflammation; the presence of neoplasms; and drug-induced alterations in calcium and bone metabolism. However, the true incidence and prevalence of parenteral nutrition-associated bone abnormalities in pediatric patients are unknown.

Sexual function

Priapism has been reported as a complication of parenteral nutrition (160).

- A man developed a persistent painful penile erection 12 hours after the administration of a 12% fat emulsion (120). This was thought to have been caused by venous thrombosis in the corpora cavernosa, and the priapism was immediately relieved by bilateral corpora cavernosa spongiosa shunts, although the patient remained impotent.

Three different mechanisms have been postulated for this complication of parenteral nutrition:

1. an increase in blood coagulability
2. adverse effects on erythrocytes
3. fat embolism

In this case it was felt that the 20% fat emulsion had increased platelet activity, which was already increased before the start of therapy, and that this had predisposed to the development of priapism. The authors pointed out that a shunt procedure should be performed as soon as possible if erectile capacity is to be preserved.

Immunologic

Parenteral nutrition can adversely affect the immune system, thereby increasing the risk of infection and sepsis, for example by impairing neutrophil function, blocking the function of the reticuloendothelial system, and altering cell-mediated immunity. However, much of the evidence has been obtained in experiments using large bolus doses; the immunological effects of more conservative doses administered as continuous infusions over 12–24 hour/day are less clear. As the chylomicron-like lipid is metabolized, increased triglyceride concentrations may alter the function of macrophages by reducing chemotaxis and phagocytic capacity, although this has not been consistently demonstrated. Excessive parenteral administration of lipid may overload the mononuclear cells of the reticuloendothelial system, resulting in an inability to clear bacteria from the bloodstream. Studies of the alterations in cellular immunity associated with intravenous infusions of lipid emulsions have produced mixed results. Increases in B lymphocyte and T lymphocyte counts, increased lymphocyte mitogenesis, and increased production of interleukin-2 have been reported in patients receiving parenteral lipids. Others have reported no change or reductions in natural killer cell counts, helper-to-suppressor cell ratios, and antibody-dependent cellular cytotoxicity compared with patients not receiving intravenous lipids. No significant changes in serum immunoglobulin or complement concentrations have been observed secondary to intravenous lipid administration.

A growing area of interest is the use of intravenous medium-chain triglycerides, which have a different metabolic fate to long-chain triglycerides and may not have similar detrimental effects on the reticuloendothelial function, leukocyte activity, and eicosanoid production. Another focus of research is the differences observed between the various lipid components and fatty acids. The polyunsaturated fatty acid content of cell membranes, an important factor in the structural and functional integrity of the cell, can be altered by the provision of increased amounts of *n*-3 fatty acids in place of *n*-6 fatty acids. In a 1987 study, the effects of different parenteral nutrition solutions on in vitro lymphocyte reactivity and measured lymphocyte responsiveness were investigated in patients during treatment (121). In vitro lymphocyte responses were significantly depressed by a fat emulsion at concentrations similar to those achieved in clinical practice, but were unaffected by dextrose or amino acid solutions. These and similar finding by others indicate that careful consideration should be given before using fat emulsions in patients whose cell-mediated immunity is already impaired.

Immune function has been studied in ten surgical infants (aged under 6 months) requiring parenteral nutrition in two consecutive phases: (a) after 31 days with no enteral feeding (parenteral nutrition) and (b) after 4.7 days from the addition to parenteral nutrition of small volumes of enteral feeding. Host bactericidal activity against coagulase-negative staphylococci, measured by an in vitro whole blood model, was lowest in the patients who received parenteral nutrition, and it increased significantly after the addition of small enteral feeds, approaching the levels measured in controls. Production of tumor necrosis factor-alfa was low during parenteral nutrition and rose significantly after the addition of small enteral feeds in patients on parenteral nutrition. The increase in killing of coagulase-negative staphylococci after the addition of small enteral feeds correlated significantly with the duration of enteral feeding. The mechanism causing impaired immune function during parenteral nutrition is not known, and it is probably multifactorial. Neither is it understood how small additional enteral feeds affect host bactericidal activity (122).

Allergic reactions

Severe allergic reactions can occur to parenterally administered lipid solutions. Such reactions may be mistaken for symptoms of the underlying disease or adverse effects of cytostatic chemotherapy (123). There is some evidence that the presence of soya bean proteins is responsible.

In 1989 the Perioperative Anaphylactic Reactions Study Group began an epidemiological survey of anaphylactoid reactions during anesthesia. Details recorded about patients who have suffered an anaphylactic reaction include demographic information and the results of allergy testing. In the most recent survey 1750 patients were reported from 27 diagnostic centers during January 1992 to June 1994 (124). Plasma substitutes accounted for 5.0% of the reactions observed. Intravenous infusions carry a comparatively small risk of anaphylaxis in the perioperative period. Other surveys come to a similar conclusion (125).

Allergic reactions have been reported infrequently in children receiving parenteral nutrition. The length of exposure before the reaction, the severity of the response, and the component responsible are variable.

- Anaphylaxis has been reported in a 4-year-old child when parenteral nutrition was resumed after a 5-day interruption in therapy after prior treatment 16 days after surgery for Wilms' tumor.

The authors considered the reaction to have been a type 1 IgE-mediated allergic response, although the causative agent was not identified. It was considered unlikely that individual amino acids had stimulated the allergic response, although the possibility of aggregated amino acids acting as a potential sensitizing agent could not be excluded. A component of the multivitamin mixture was considered the more likely explanation; the substances administered were vitamin E, vitamin K_1, the preservatives butylated hydroxyanisole (BHA) and butylated hydroxytoluene (BHT), and polysorbate emulsifiers (126).

Anaphylaxis linked to vitamin B complex in a parenteral nutrition regimen has been reported (127).

- An 8-year-old girl had a diaphragmatic hernia repaired at 7 days of age and had two episodes of adhesion ileus at 8 months. After laparotomy she was given all-in-one parenteral nutrition and after 21 days developed a reddish rash on her face and chest. The rash was pruritic and resolved quickly after intravenous diphenhydramine. She was readmitted 15 days after discharge because of malnutrition. Parenteral nutrition was restarted and she rapidly became irritable and developed an itchy rash over her face and trunk and swelling of her lips and eyelids. Parenteral nutrition was discontinued, diphenhydramine was given, and her symptoms abated rapidly. The possibility of hypersensitivity to a component of the parenteral nutrition was considered, and by a process of elimination the cause of the reaction was identified as the vitamin product MVI No 1. This was further confirmed by a skin test 1 year after the anaphylactic episode, but using a vitamin B complex solution.

Previous reports of anaphylactic reactions to parenteral nutrition have been identified as being caused by fat emulsion, vitamin K, iron dextran, and in particular multivitamins. This appears to be the first report of a reaction to vitamin B complex injection. However, neither the source of the vitamin B complex test product nor its formulation was identified by the authors, and there is doubt about the specific allergens responsible for the allergic response in this case.

Infection risk

Infection has long been recognized as a risk of parenteral nutrition and it has proved impossible to eliminate it (SEDA-22, 379). Once established, sepsis can increase the risk of fat overload syndrome. In an extensive study in Taiwan there was sepsis with positive blood cultures in 56 of 378 children receiving parenteral nutrition; the risk factors were longer duration of parenteral nutrition, age under 3 months, the use of central venous catheters, gastrointestinal disease as an indication for parenteral nutrition, low birth weight, and short gestational age in prematurity (128).

Various explanations have been offered for the occurrence of sepsis during parenteral nutrition, quite apart from the fact that the solution itself may be contaminated. Phytosterols can cause changes in neutrophil function. Cholestasis may play a role and then be further aggravated by the sepsis, creating a vicious circle. And fat emulsion may reduce hepatic phagocytosis. In vitro evidence using material from preterm infants suggests that administration of Intralipid may interfere with the binding of IL-2 to the specific receptors on their activated lymphocytes, with suppression of the immune response (129).

However, the clinical significance of these various mechanisms has been questioned. Some experimental in vitro work on human white cells suggests that the effect is markedly dose-dependent; it has been suggested that very few inhibitory effects on phagocytic cells will be found if lipid emulsion rates are kept at around 0.08 g/kg/hour (20). It is also notable that in one large series of premature very low birth weight infants in whom the use and duration of treatment with parenteral nutrition were associated with short gestational age and low birth weight, children treated with parenteral nutrition had a higher risk of sepsis usually caused by *Staphylococcus epidermidis* or *Staphylococcus aureus* (130). Thus, although the risk of sepsis in this age group appears to be significantly increased by parenteral nutrition, the causative organisms were fairly benign. It was concluded that the advantages of parenteral nutrition outweighed the risk of sepsis in this group of infants.

The incidences of bacteremia and fungemia during the first month after bone marrow transplantation for hematological malignancies have been studied in a prospective comparison in 512 patients. The patients were randomly assigned to receive 6–8% (low dose) or 25–30% (standard dose) of total energy as a 20% lipid emulsion. An adaptive randomization scheme, stratified for various treatments and transplant type, ensured that confounding treatment variables did not differ between the groups. Of 482 evaluable patients, 55 in the standard-dose group developed bacteremia or fungemia compared with 54 in the low-dose group. There was no association between the incidence of bacteremia or fungemia and intravenous lipid. Similar results were obtained when the results were analysed according to intention to treat, when bacterial or fungal infections at all sites were included, and when the observation period was extended to 60 days. These results suggest that moderate amounts of intravenous lipid rich in linoleic acid are not associated with an increased incidence of bacterial or fungal infections in patients undergoing bone marrow transplantation and receiving parenteral nutrition (131).

In infants of very low birth weight, fungal colonization and the association between fungal colonization and systemic fungal diseases was significantly linked to prolonged administration of antibiotics, parenteral nutrition, and fat emulsion (Intralipid) (132). Of 116 infants with birth weights under 1500 g, fungal colonization was detected in 25, of whom 17 developed colonization by 2 weeks of life. *Candida albicans* (61%) and *Candida parapsilosis* (29%) were the two most common organisms. The rectum (76%) was the most frequent site of colonization. Cultures were taken from the oropharynx, rectum, skin (groin and axilla), urine, and endotracheal aspirates in the first 24 hours after birth and weekly thereafter. There was an association between colonization and subsequent fungemia in one infant, representing 4% of colonized infants. It was also noted that although fungal colonization represents a risk factor for invasive candidiasis in infants of very low birth weight, candidiasis in this population is not invariably associated with prior colonization. Factors other than fungal colonization can also contribute to the occurrence of invasive candidiasis.

In a study of the independent risk factors for nosocomial coagulase-negative staphylococcal bacteremia among neonates of very low birth weight, after adjusting for the severity of the underlying illness, there was a significant association between coagulase-negative staphylococcal bacteremia and exposure during hospitalization to intravenous lipids (133). The study was conducted in 590 consecutively admitted neonates with birth weights under 1500 g, in two neonatal intensive care units, with a case-control study of 74 cases of coagulase-negative staphylococcal bacteremia and 74 pairs of matched controls. The independent risk factors for bacteremia were intravenous lipids (odds ratio 9.4), mechanical ventilation (OR = 2.0), and short peripheral venous catheters (OR = 2.6). It would appear that exposure to intravenous lipids at any time during hospitalization remains, and has possibly become an increasingly important risk factor for coagulase-negative staphylococcal bacteremia. In neonates of very low birth weight 85% of these bacteremias are now attributable to lipid therapy. In contrast, the relative importance of intravenous catheters as an independent risk factor has declined. Mechanical ventilation in the week before bacteremia has emerged as a risk factor for bacteremia.

There is evidence that lipid emulsion, which is cleared by the Kupffer cells of the reticuloendothelial system, can adversely affect reticuloendothelial function by reducing its ability to remove blood-borne bacteria. In a study of the blood clearance and organ localization of viable ^{35}S-radiolabelled *Escherichia coli* after slow intraperitoneal and more rapid intravenous administration of 20% fat emulsion in Sprague-Dawley rats, although there was

rapid bacterial blood clearance in control and test animals, there was a significant change in the organ localization of bacteria as a result of the administration of lipid emulsion. There was a slight increase in lung localization of bacteria in rats that received intraperitoneal fat emulsion, and a significant increase in lung trapping of bacteria in rats that received intravenous fat emulsion. Liver localization of bacteria was reduced in all groups after fat emulsion. The data are understood to indicate that intravenous fat emulsion reduces hepatic phagocytosis and increases pulmonary localization of *E. coli*, and it is thought that this may produce greater susceptibility to infection. Patients with underlying sepsis are at greatest risk. The capacity of the lungs to kill sequestered bacteria is not known. Thus, increased bacterial lung localization may result in local inflammation and other pulmonary complications, and in the re-emergence into the blood of *E. coli*, with systemic sepsis as a result (134).

Second-Generation Effects

Teratogenicity

The developmental toxicity of a 20% lipid emulsion containing a 3:1 ratio of medium-chain to long-chain triglycerides has been examined in animals. Administration was once-daily intravenously to rats and rabbits during organogenesis. Maternal and embryo/fetal toxicity were also assessed. There were no adverse effects on fetal parameters for rats even in the presence of maternal toxicity. However, embryo and fetal toxicity (resorptions) and skeletal abnormalities were noted in rabbits (135). The adverse fetal effects were probably the result of dietary deprivation, maternal toxicity, or both rather than representing a direct teratogenic effect.

Susceptibility Factors

Age

Since lipoprotein lipase activity is reduced in premature babies and babies who are small for gestational age, and since bacterial and viral infections adversely affect lipoprotein lipase activity and can precipitate fat overload, it follows that fat emulsion should be administered with great caution, or even temporarily withheld, in small infants with proven or suspected sepsis (134).

Cholestatic liver disease is a frequent complication of prolonged parenteral nutrition, especially in preterm infants, with an occurrence rate that can approach 60% after 2 weeks of parenteral nutrition. In a retrospective survey of the incidence of liver dysfunction in 94 children (mean age 5 years) receiving parenteral nutrition over 2 years, liver disease was identified in over 50% of cases, with a nadir during the second week of parenteral nutrition (50). The most closely associated factors were length of parenteral nutrition and sepsis. In premature low birth weight infants hepatobiliary dysfunction with histological changes has been attributed to parenteral nutrition (48). Other risk factors include high baseline serum bile acids, reduced hepatic extraction, and an underdeveloped ileal transport system for conservation of bile acids. These lead to a reduced pool of bile acids and consequent exposure of the liver to toxic bile acids. The liver damage is aggravated by sepsis, ischemia, necrotizing enterocolitis, or surgery.

The pattern and prognosis of liver injury in children is distinct from that seen in adults, despite some overlap; liver disease develops in 40–60% of infants who require long-term parenteral nutrition for intestinal failure (89). The longer parenteral nutrition is used in neonates the greater is the risk of developing cholestasis, and the risk approaches 100% in neonates who receive parenteral nutrition for more than 8 weeks, especially if parenteral nutrition has been started very early in life (83,136). The particularly high risk in infants can be explained by factors that are specific to this age group; namely, immaturity of the enzyme systems responsible for hepatic conjugation, disturbance in the physiological patterns of enteral nutrition, and excessive secondary bile acid production and absorption from a contaminated small bowel. The bile of premature and newborn infants differs in its composition from that of adults, and this may account for the differences in solubility (137). Histologically one is likely to find cholestasis (intracellular or canalicular), periportal inflammation, fibrosis, and bile ductular proliferation (138). Sepsis can make cholestasis more severe. The clinical manifestations of cholestasis in infants include a progressively rising conjugated bilirubin concentration starting after 2 weeks of parenteral nutrition. Liver biopsy characteristically shows bile duct proliferation, bile plugs, and congestion. The clinical consequences include increased rates of sepsis, cirrhosis, liver failure, and death (139), though if parenteral nutrition can be withdrawn the condition is in principle reversible (138). Cholelithiasis is much less common in these children, but the administration of large amounts of amino acids and a high ratio of non-protein (kcal/ml) increased the risk of formation of gallstones and sludge. Conversely, these are prevented by the administration of appropriate amounts of fat (140). It has been recommended that ultrasound examination of the gallbladder be performed in children maintained on parenteral nutrition for longer than 30 days, and early elective cholecystectomy performed if parenteral nutrition-associated cholelithiasis develops (141).

A theory has been proposed regarding a possible mechanism by which parenteral lipid solutions injure preterm infants; namely, by free radical-induced lipid peroxidation in the lipid solution (142,143). How this happens is not explained. The result can be pulmonary damage and chronic lung disease. Premature infants are thought to be at particularly high risk. However, others (144,145) have suggested that Cooke's interpretation (142) was not based on solid clinical evidence, and that the data that he derived from his observations should be tested in controlled studies before parenteral nutrition is prescribed for infants of very low birth weights.

Other features of the patient

Thrombosis can occur, especially (for unclear reasons) in patients suffering from AIDS. The incidence of symptomatic central venous thrombosis in patients with AIDS receiving home parenteral nutrition has been estimated at 0.009 per patient-month (80). However, in one retrospective study of malnourished patients with AIDS, none of whom had had a previous venous thrombosis, and who were treated with parenteral nutrition for a long period, the rate of central venous thrombosis in patients taking warfarin was 0.016 thromboses per patient-month, both in those taking warfarin and in those not so treated; in this series no hypercoagulability was found.

In a prospective study of the effects of parenteral medium-chain and long-chain triglycerides on lymphocyte subpopulations and function in severely malnourished patients with acquired immunodeficiency syndrome (AIDS), long-chain triglycerides were compared with a balanced emulsion of long-chain and medium-chain triglycerides (146). Administration was over 6 days. With 2 g/kg/day of lipids, long-chain triglycerides caused significant abnormalities in lymphocyte function, expressed as a reduction in phytohemagglutinin A response. Such abnormalities were not observed with long-chain plus medium-chain triglycerides, which reduced IgM and increased the C3 fraction.

Drug Administration

Drug formulations

Precipitates can develop in parenteral nutrition admixtures because of a number of factors such as the concentration, pH, and phosphate content of the amino acid solutions, the calcium and phosphorus additives, the order of mixing, or the mixing process. The consequences can be serious. In one cohort study of hospitalized patients who received peripheral parenteral nutrition, a subgroup developed unexplained chest pain, dyspnea, cardiopulmonary arrest, or new interstitial infiltrates on chest radiograph. A change in the amino acid source of a parenteral nutrition mixture was associated with respiratory adverse events that ranged from interstitial infiltrates to sudden death. The events apparently resulted from infusion of calcium phosphate precipitate in an opaque admixture, and the deposition of the crystals in the pulmonary microvasculature (147).

The United States Food and Drug Administration issued a safety alert in 1994 regarding the potentially life-threatening formation of precipitates in parenteral nutrition admixtures (148). They had received reports of two deaths and at least two cases of respiratory distress during intravenous infusion of a three-in-one parenteral nutrition mixture (amino acids, carbohydrates, lipids). The mixture contained 10% FreAmine III (amino acids + magnesium acetate + phosphoric acid + potassium chloride + sodium acetate + sodium chloride), dextrose, calcium gluconate, potassium phosphate, other minerals, and a lipid emulsion. The solution may have contained a precipitate of calcium phosphate. Autopsies revealed diffuse microvascular pulmonary emboli containing calcium phosphate.

The FDA has recommended the following steps to decrease the hazard of injury through precipitation (149):

1. The amounts of phosphorus and calcium added to the admixture are critical. The solubility of the added calcium should be calculated from the volume at the time that the calcium is added. It should not be based on the

final volume. The line should be flushed between the addition of any potentially incompatible components.

2. A lipid emulsion in a three-in-one admixture obscures the presence of a precipitate. Therefore, if a lipid emulsion is needed, either use a two-in-one admixture with the lipid infused separately, or add the calcium before the lipid emulsion according to the recommendations in 1 above. If the amount of calcium or phosphate which must be added is likely to cause a precipitate, some or all of the calcium should be administered separately. Such separate infusions must be properly diluted and slowly infused to avoid serious adverse events related to the calcium.

3. During the mixing process, parenteral nutrition admixtures should be periodically agitated to check for precipitates. This check should be conducted both before and during the infusion. Patients and caregivers should be trained to inspect for signs of precipitation. They should also be trained to stop the infusion and seek medical assistance if precipitates are noted.

4. A filter should be used when infusing either central or peripheral parenteral nutrition admixtures. Data are not available to determine which size filter is most effective in trapping precipitates.

5. Parenteral nutrition mixtures should be administered within the following time frames: if stored at room temperature, the infusion should be started within 24 hours after mixing; if stored at refrigerated temperatures, the infusion should be started within 24 hours of rewarming. Because warming parenteral nutrition mixtures may contribute to the formation of precipitates, once administration begins, care should be taken to avoid excessive warming of the mixture.

Mirtallo has added to the FDA guidelines, stressing the need to ensure that an appropriate dose of calcium is prescribed, to follow appropriate procedures when mixing parenteral nutrition solutions and to use automatic mixing devices strictly in accordance with the manufacturer's instructions (150). He has stressed the fact that more information is needed to substantiate the usefulness of filters in preventing adverse effects caused by the infusion of particulate matter present in parenteral nutrition admixtures.

It has been pointed out that calcium phosphate precipitates more readily in warm than in cold solutions. Precipitation can occur in solution at room temperature, even if an identical cold solution is clear. A precipitate can also form when a clear solution, stored refrigerated or at room-temperature, is warmed to body temperature. Thus, visual inspection and even in-line filters, if they are distal to the side of precipitation, may not prevent infusion of the precipitate (151).

Drug contamination

Since the introduction of parenteral nutrition in hospital care the potential microbiological risks associated with the manufacture, preparation, and administration of these products have abated but not disappeared (133,152). Fatal infectious complications still occur. The parenteral nutrition mixture is a good growth medium for microorganisms, more conducive to microbial growth than glucose or amino acid solutions. Storage of mixtures allows time for microbial multiplication, often to counts of millions per ml. Commonly isolated organisms from parenteral nutrition solutions are coagulase-negative staphylococci, *S. aureus*, *Candida* species, *Serratia* species, and *Enterobacter* species. Infection with *Malassezia furfur* is a rare but serious complication strongly associated with parenteral nutrition in young children, now documented in some 50 reports (153). *Candida* infection is a particular problem in patients receiving parenteral nutrition. Even organisms such as *S. epidermidis* and *Bacillus* species, relatively non-pathogenic in normal circumstances, can multiply in the infusion to such large numbers as to have disastrous effects. Many of these commensal organisms tend to be insensitive to antibiotics. In an open-system aseptic process of preparation the estimated risk of contamination, according to the World Health Organization, is one in 3000. Microbiological and environmental quality control assurance needs to be continuous.

The average rate of episodes of catheter-related bacteremia in patients receiving parenteral nutrition is 3–5%. Higher rates are reported for long-term patients. Patients with a nosocomial infection have an 11-fold higher risk of acquiring an additional nosocomial infection compared with those with no infection. Prompt removal of the catheter and targeted antimicrobial treatment remains the standard approach for febrile episodes in these circumstances. However, many catheter-related infections caused by coagulase-negative staphylococci can successfully be treated with the catheter still in place (154).

Drug administration route

Local extravasation of parenteral nutrition fluid can occur. Two patients developed an intense inflammatory reaction that was successfully controlled with repeated local administration of the hyaluronidase analogue chondroitin sulfatase (155). Although the exact mechanism of tissue toxicity by extravasated parenteral nutrition is not understood, it seems likely to be related to osmolarity, pH, and ions. The area affected may become blistered, with darkening of the skin, or ischemic, depending on whether the skin thickness is partially or fully damaged. In children, extravasation can have devastating consequences, such as deep necrosis, amputation, severe sequelae in the affected limb, or other complications, such as subdural collection of fat emulsion, liporrhachis, and acute abdomen after intra-abdominal extravasation. Children are at special risk, because very young infants and children are unable to communicate the pain that results from the pressure of extravasated fluid. Other individuals in this situation are comatose patients, those under general anesthesia, and patients who are being resuscitated. Other risk factors that predispose to extravasation are related to venepuncture technique, state of the patient, and medication delivery. Special care should be taken when high-osmolarity (1000–1700 mosmol/l) peripheral parenteral nutrition is administered, as fluids of this osmolarity are likely to cause severe tissue damage if extravasated. Fluids should not generally exceed 600–900 mosmol/l in order to minimize the risk of this complication. The position of the catheter needs to be regularly checked. Fat emulsions are harmless to the tissues if extravasated.

After a preterm infant developed parenteral nutrition ascites after infusion through a low umbilical vein catheter, a follow-up study of eight patients, all of whom developed hypotension and ascites, showed that each had an umbilical vein catheter overlying the liver on plain X-ray (156). The catheters had been in place for a mean of 8.9 days before extravasation. Ultrasound in four patients showed hepatic parenchymal damage around the umbilical vein catheter tip. Parenteral nutrition given through abnormally placed umbilical vein catheters is not without risk, and correct placing of the catheter is paramount.

Drug–Drug Interactions

Glucocorticoids

Infants of very low birth weight have reduced tolerance to intravenous fat emulsions, with consequent hyperlipidemia. Since glucocorticoids are often used to prevent or treat chronic lung disease, and since they can cause hyperlipidemia, this potential drug interaction has been investigated in a randomized double-blind trial (157). The results supported the hypothesis that dexamethasone increases triglyceride serum concentrations, and the authors recommended that low birth weight infants who are receiving both dexamethasone and fat emulsion should be monitored carefully for signs of impairment of lipid tolerance.

Propofol

Drugs with a high lipid content, when given concurrently with lipid-containing parenteral nutrition, can aggravate the problems of lipid overload (29). The anesthetic, propofol, which is used for continuous sedation in a dose of 1–3 mg/kg/hour (an equivalent of 300–500 ml of a 10% fat emulsion), may aggravate the symptoms and pathological effects of fat overload (29).

Warfarin

Warfarin resistance has been described in a patient with short bowel syndrome receiving intravenous lipid (158). Up to 20 mg of warfarin was given daily without increase in the International Normalized Ratio (INR). Although intravenous lipid has been reported anecdotally to account for warfarin resistance, this report suggests that the more likely explanation was the reduced surface area for drug absorption secondary to total surgical removal of the patient's duodenum and gastrojejunostomy. However, several other reports have refuted a correlation between warfarin resistance and short bowel syndrome. Conversely, warfarin resistance has occurred secondary to intravenous lipid administration in a patient with only 12 cm of small bowel; the patient had been given oral warfarin while he received daily fat emulsion (Intralipid) to prevent fatty acid deficiency (159).

References

1. Shin S, Kamada T, Fusamoto H, Nakamura K, Kojima G, Mukuda T, Kimura K, Akeyama T, Yoneda S, Shimazu T, Sueyoshi K, Mikami H, Meren H, Nakano S. Clinical effects of GAB-88, an amino acid injection with dextrose and electrolytes, in nonoperative patients in internal medicine. Jpn Pharmacol Ther 1994;22(Suppl 4):149–59.

2. Saito Y, Ohyanagi H, Matsuno S, Tamakuma S, Ohara T, Mutoh T, Mori T, Sowa M, Hioki K, Kakegawa T, Yamakawa M, Usami M, Kido Y, Mizote H, Nakano S, Furuya K. Clinical effects of GAB-88, an amino acid injection with dextrose and electrolytes, in patients after partial gastrectomy. A comparative study with a commercial product. Jpn Pharmacol Ther 1994;22(Suppl 4):119–48.

3. Saito Y, Ohyanagi H, Matsuno S, Mashima Y, Ohara T, Tamakuma S, Mutoh T, Matsubara Y, Mori T, Sowa M, Hioki K, Kakegawa T, Mizote H, Furuya K, Nakano S, Yamakawa M, Kido Y. A phase II clinical study of GAB-88, an amino acid injection with dextrose and electrolytes, in patients after gastrointestinal surgery. Jpn Pharmacol Ther 1994;22(Suppl 4):97–118.

4. Shima K, Tahara Y, Matsuzaki S. A phase I clinical study of GAB-88, an amino acid injection with dextrose and electrolytes. Jpn Pharmacol Ther 1994;22(Suppl 4):75–95.

5. Klein GL. Metabolic bone disease of total parenteral nutrition. Nutrition 1998;14(1):149–52.

6. Barnoud D, Fontaine E, Leverve X. Complications métaboliques de la nutrition parenterale. Med Nutr 1995;31:158–67.

7. McCowen KC, Chan S, Bistrian BR. Total parenteral nutrition. Curr Opin Gastroenterol 1998;14:157–63.

8. Elia M. Changing concepts of nutrient requirements in disease: implications for artificial nutritional support. Lancet 1995;345(8960):1279–84.

9. Kane KF, Lowes JR. Peripheral parenteral nutrition and venous thrombophlebitis. Nutrition 1997;13(6):577–8.

10. May J, Murchan P, MacFie J, Sedman P, Donat R, Palmer D, Mitchell CJ. Prospective study of the aetiology of infusion phlebitis and line failure during peripheral parenteral nutrition. Br J Surg 1996;83(8):1091–4.

11. Madan M, Alexander DJ, Mellor E, Cooke J, et al. A randomised study of the effects of osmolality and heparin with hydrocortisone on thrombophlebitis in peripheral intravenous nutrition. Clin Nutr 1991;10:309–14.

12. Kerin MJ, Pickford IR, Jaeger H, Couse NF, et al. A prospective and randomised study comparing the incidence of infusion phlebitis during continuous and cyclic peripheral parenteral nutrition. Clin Nutr 1991;10:315.

13. Wolthuis A, Landewe RB, Theunissen PH, Westerhuis LW. Chylothorax or leakage of total parenteral nutrition? Eur Respir J 1998;12(5):1233–5.

14. Marks KH, Turner MJ, Rothberg AD. Effect of Intralipid infusion on transcutaneous oxygen and carbon dioxide tension in sick neonates. S Afr Med J 1987;72(6):389–91.

15. Schulz PE, Weiner SP, Haber LM, Armstrong DD, Fishman MA. Neurological complications from fat emulsion therapy. Ann Neurol 1994;35(5):628–30.

16. Bohlega S, McLean DR. Hemiplegia caused by inadvertent intra-carotid infusion of total parenteral nutrition. Clin Neurol Neurosurg 1997;99(3):217–19.

17. Waldhausen E, Mingers B, Lippers P, Keser G. Critical illness polyneuropathy due to parenteral nutrition. Intensive Care Med 1997;23(8):922–3.

18. Berek K, Margreiter J, Willeit J, Berek A, Schmutzhard E, Mutz N. Critical illness polyneuropathy—only due to parenteral nutrition? Intensive Care Med 1997;23(8):923–4.

19. Bolton CF, Young GB. Critical illness polyneuropathy due to parenteral nutrition. Intensive Care Med 1997;23(8):924–5.

20. Waitzberg DL, Bellinati-Pires R, Salgado MM, Hypolito IP, Colleto GM, Yagi O, Yamamuro EM, Gama-Rodrigues J, Pinotti HW. Effect of total parenteral nutrition with different lipid emulsions of human

monocyte and neutrophil functions. Nutrition 1997; 13(2):128–32.

21. D'Aprile P, Tarantino A, Santoro N, Carella A. Wernick e's encephalopathy induced by total parenteral nutrition in a patient with acute leukaemia: unusual involvement of caudate nuclei and cerebral cortex on MRI. Neuroradiology 2000;42(10):781–3.

22. Nakasaki H, Katayama T, Yokoyama S, Tajima T, Mitomi T, Tsuda M, Suga T, Fujii K. Complication of parenternal nutrition composed of essential amino acids and histidine in adults with renal failure. J Parenter Enteral Nutr 1993;17(1):86–90.

23. Fan BG, Salehi A, Sternby B, Axelson J, Lundquist I, Andren-Sandberg A, Ekelund M. Total parenteral nutrition influences both endocrine and exocrine function of rat pancreas. Pancreas 1997;15(2):147–53.

24. Boden G, Jadali F. Effects of lipid on basal carbohydrate metabolism in normal men. Diabetes 1991;40(6):686–92.

25. McCowen KC, Friel C, Sternberg J, Chan S, Forse RA, Burke PA, Bistrian BR. Hypocaloric total parenteral nutrition: effectiveness in prevention of hyperglycemia and infectious complications—a randomized clinical trial. Crit Care Med 2000;28(11):3606–11.

26. Lienhardt A, Rakotoambinina B, Colomb V, Souissi S, Sadoun E, Goulet O, Robert JJ, Ricour C. Insulin secretion and sensitivity in children on cyclic total parenteral nutrition. J Parenter Enteral Nutr 1998;22(6):382–6.

27. Chiolero R, Schneiter P, Cayeux C, Temler E, Jequier E, Schindler C, Tappy L. Metabolic and respiratory effects of sodium lactate during short i.v. nutrition in critically ill patients. J Parenter Enteral Nutr 1996;20(4):257–63.

28. Kollef MH, McCormack MT, Caras WE, Reddy VV, Bacon D. The fat overload syndrome: successful treatment with plasma exchange. Ann Intern Med 1990;112(7):545–6.

29. Lindholm M. The ability of critically ill patients to eliminate fat emulsions. J Drug Dev 1991;4(Suppl 3):40–2.

30. Jeppesen PB, Hoy CE, Mortensen PB. Essential fatty acid deficiency in patients receiving home parenteral nutrition. Am J Clin Nutr 1998;68(1):126–33.

31. Duerksen DR, Nehra V, Palombo JD, Ahmad A, Bistrian BR. Essential fatty acid deficiencies in patients with chronic liver disease are not reversed by short-term intravenous lipid supplementation. Dig Dis Sci 1999;44(7):1342–8.

32. Hager L. Choline deficiency and TPN associated liver dysfunction: a case report. Nutrition 1998;14(1):60–2.

33. Shronts EP. Essential nature of choline with implications for total parenteral nutrition. J Am Diet Assoc 1997;97(6):639–46, 649.

34. Garnacho Montero J, Ortiz Leyba C, Jimenez Jimenez F, Monterrubio Villar J, Fernandez Vega MD, Garcia Garmendia JL. Niveles de L-carnitina en pacientes criticos septicos con nutricion parenteral. [L-carnitine levels in critical septic patients receiving parenteral nutrition.] Nutr Hosp 1998;13(2):77–80.

35. Tibboel D, Delemarre FM, Przyrembel H, Bos AP, Affourtit MJ, Molenaar JC. Carnitine deficiency in surgical neonates receiving total parenteral nutrition. J Pediatr Surg 1990;25(4):418–21.

36. Bowyer BA, Miles JM, Haymond MW, Fleming CR. L-carnitine therapy in home parenteral nutrition patients with abnormal liver tests and low plasma carnitine concentrations. Gastroenterology 1988;94(2):434–8.

37. Cohen HJ, Brown MR, Hamilton D, Lyons-Patterson J, Avissar N, Liegey P. Glutathione peroxidase and selenium deficiency in patients receiving home parenteral nutrition: time course for development of deficiency and repletion of enzyme activity in plasma and blood cells. Am J Clin Nutr 1989;49(1):132–9.

38. Stover JF, Kempski OS. Glutamate-containing parenteral nutrition doubles plasma glutamate: a risk factor in neurosurgical patients with blood–brain barrier damage? Crit Care Med 1999;27(10):2252–6.

39. Hornsby-Lewis L, Shike M, Brown P, Klang M, Pearlstone D, Brennan MF. L-glutamine supplementation in home total parenteral nutrition patients: stability, safety, and effects on intestinal absorption. J Parenter Enteral Nutr 1994;18(3):268–73.

40. van Zaanen HC, van der Lelie H, Timmer JG, Furst P, Sauerwein HP. Parenteral glutamine dipeptide supplementation does not ameliorate chemotherapy-induced toxicity. Cancer 1994;74(10):2879–84.

41. Sawada M, Tsurumi H, Hara T, Goto H, Yamada T, Oyama M, Moriwaki H. Graft failure of autologous peripheral blood stem cell transplantation due to acute metabolic acidosis associated with total parenteral nutrition in a patient with relapsed breast cancer. Acta Haematol 2000;102(3):157–9.

42. Suzuki S, Kumanomido T, Nagata E, Inoue J, Niikawa O. Optic neuropathy from thiamine deficiency. Intern Med 1997;36(7):532.

43. Kitamura K, Yamaguchi T, Tanaka H, Hashimoto S, Yang M, Takahashi T. TPN-induced fulminant beriberi: a report on our experience and a review of the literature. Surg Today 1996;26(10):769–76.

44. Nakasaki H, Ohta M, Soeda J, Makuuchi H, Tsuda M, Tajima T, Mitomi T, Fujii K. Clinical and biochemical aspects of thiamine treatment for metabolic acidosis during total parenteral nutrition. Nutrition 1997;13(2):110–17.

45. Schiano TD, Klang MG, Quesada E, Scott F, Tao Y, Shike M. Thiamine status in patients receiving long-term home parenteral nutrition. Am J Gastroenterol 1996; 91(12):2555–9.

46. Brown RO, Hamrick KD, Dickerson RN, Lee N, Parnell DH Jr, Kudsk KA. Hyperkalemia secondary to concurrent pharmacotherapy in a patient receiving home parenteral nutrition. J Parenter Enteral Nutr 1996;20(6):429–32.

47. Ikema S, Horikawa R, Nakano M, Yokouchi K, Yamazaki H, Tanaka T, Tanae A. Growth and metabolic disturbances in a patient with total parenteral nutrition: a case of hypercalciuric hypercalcemia. Endocr J 2000; 47(Suppl):S137–40.

48. Muller D, Eggert P, Krawinkel M. Hypercalciuria and nephrocalcinosis in a patient receiving long-term parenteral nutrition: the effect of intravenous chlorothiazide. J Pediatr Gastroenterol Nutr 1998;27(1):106–10.

49. Berkelhammer C, Wood RJ, Sitrin MD. Inorganic phosphorus reduces hypercalciuria during total parenteral nutrition by enhancing renal tubular calcium absorption. J Parenter Enteral Nutr 1998;22(3):142–6.

50. Duerksen DR, Papineau N. Electrolyte abnormalities in patients with chronic renal failure receiving parenteral nutrition. J Parenter Enteral Nutr 1998;22(2):102–4.

51. Druml W, Kleinberger G. Hypophosphatemia in patients with chronic renal failure during total parenteral nutrition. J Parenter Enteral Nutr 1999;23(1):45–6.

52. Duerksen DR, Papineau N. Response to Drs Druml and Kleinberger. J Parenter Enter Nutr 1999;23:46.

53. Janigan DT, Perey B, Marrie TJ, Chiasson PM, Hirsch D. Skin necrosis: an unusual complication of hyperphosphatemia during total parenteral nutrition therapy. J Parenter Enteral Nutr 1997;21(1):50–2.

54. Klein GL. The aluminium content of parenteral solutions: current status. Nutr Rev 1991;49(3):74–9.

55. Lipkin EW, Ott SM, Klein GL. Heterogeneity of bone histology in parenteral nutrition patients. Am J Clin Nutr 1987;46(4):673–80.

56. Vargas JH, Klein GL, Ament ME, Ott SM, Sherrard DJ, Horst RL, Berquist WE, Alfrey AC, Slatopolsky E, Coburn JW. Metabolic bone disease of total parenteral nutrition: course after changing from casein to amino acids in parenteral solutions with reduced aluminium content. Am J Clin Nutr 1988;48(4):1070–8.

57. Fuhrman MP, Herrmann V, Masidonski P, Eby C. Pancytopenia after removal of copper from total parenteral nutrition. J Parenter Enteral Nutr 2000;24(6):361–6.

58. Fujita M, Itakura T, Takagi Y, Okada A. Copper deficiency during total parenteral nutrition: clinical analysis of three cases. J Parenter Enteral Nutr 1989; 13(4):421–5.

59. Spiegel JE, Willenbucher RF. Rapid development of severe copper deficiency in a patient with Crohn's disease receiving parenteral nutrition. J Parenter Enteral Nutr 1999;23(3):169–72.

60. Reimund JM, Dietemann JL, Warter JM, Baumann R, Duclos B. Factors associated to hypermanganesemia in patients receiving home parenteral nutrition. Clin Nutr 2000;19(5):343–8.

61. Kondoh H, Iwase K, Higaki J, Tanaka Y, Yoshikawa M, Hori S, Osuga K, Kamiike W. Manganese deposition in the brain following parenteral manganese administration in association with radical operation for esophageal cancer: report of a case. Surg Today 1999;29(8):773–6.

62. Taylor S, Manara AR. Manganese toxicity in a patient with cholestasis receiving total parenteral nutrition. Anaesthesia 1994;49(11):1013.

63. Mehta R, Reilly JJ. Manganese levels in a jaundiced long-term total parenteral nutrition patient: potentiation of haloperidol toxicity? Case report and literature review. J Parenter Enteral Nutr 1990;14(4):428–30.

64. Quaghebeur G, Taylor WJ, Kingsley DP, Fell JM, Reynolds AP, Milla PJ. MRI in children receiving total parenteral nutrition. Neuroradiology 1996;38(7):680–3.

65. Alves G, Thiebot J, Tracqui A, Delangre T, Guedon C, Lerebours E. Neurologic disorders due to brain manganese deposition in a jaundiced patient receiving long-term parenteral nutrition. J Parenter Enteral Nutr 1997;21(1):41–5.

66. Fitzgerald K, Mikalunas V, Rubin H, McCarthey R, Vanagunas A, Craig RM. Hypermanganesemia in patients receiving total parenteral nutrition. J Parenter Enteral Nutr 1999;23(6):333–6.

67. Reynolds AP, Kiely E, Meadows N. Manganese in long term paediatric parenteral nutrition. Arch Dis Child 1994;71(6):527–8.

68. Wardle CA, Forbes A, Roberts NB, Jawhari AV, Shenkin A. Hypermanganesemia in long-term intravenous nutrition and chronic liver disease. J Parenter Enteral Nutr 1999;23(6):350–5.

69. Ishihara H, Kanda F, Matsushita T, Chihara K, Itoh K. White muscle disease in humans: myopathy caused by selenium deficiency in anorexia nervosa under long term total parenteral nutrition. J Neurol Neurosurg Psychiatry 1999;67(6):829–30.

70. Vinton NE, Dahlstrom KA, Strobel CT, Ament ME. Macrocytosis and pseudoalbinism: manifestations of selenium deficiency. J Pediatr 1987;111(5):711–17.

71. Inoko M, Konishi T, Matsuse S, Kobashi Y. Midmural fibrosis of left ventricle due to selenium deficiency. Circulation 1998;98(23):2638–9.

72. Tsuda K, Yokoyama Y, Morita M, Nakazawa Y, Onishi S. Selenium and chromium deficiency during long-term home total parenteral nutrition in chronic idiopathic intestinal pseudoobstruction. Nutrition 1998; 14(3):291–5.

73. Vossbeck S, Lindner M, Schulz A, Lindner W. Lebensbedrohliche, durch thiaminmangel bedingte,

74. laktatazidose unter total parenteraler ernahrung ohne vitaminzufuhr. Monatsschr Kinderheilkd 2000;148:841–4.

74. Kaneko K, Shimizu T, Nagaoka R, Fujiwara S, Igarashi J, Ohtomo Y, Yamashiro Y. Megaloblastic anemia in an infant receiving total parenteral nutrition. Pediatr Int 2002;44(1):101–2.

75. Khaodhiar L, Keane-Ellison M, Tawa NE, Thibault A, Burke PA, Bistrian BR. Iron deficiency anemia in patients receiving home total parenteral nutrition. J Parenter Enteral Nutr 2002;26(2):114–19.

76. Goulet O, Girot R, Maier-Redelsperger M, Bougle D, Virelizier JL, Ricour C. Hematologic disorders following prolonged use of intravenous fat emulsions in children. J Parenter Enteral Nutr 1986;10(3):284–8.

77. Maier-Redelsperger M, Girot R. Sea-blue histiocytes in bone-marrow due to a long-term total parenteral nutrition including fat-emulsions. Br J Haematol 1997;97(3):689.

78. Meiklejohn DJ, Baden H, Greaves M. Sea-blue histiocytosis and pancytopaenia associated with chronic total parenteral nutrition administration. Clin Lab Haematol 1997;19(3):219–21.

79. Plusa SM, Webster N, Primrose JN. Neutrophil adhesion molecule expression and response to stimulation with bacterial wall products in humans is unaffected by parenteral nutrition. Clin Sci (Lond) 1996;91(3):371–4.

80. Duerksen DR, Ahmad A, Doweiko J, Bistrian BR, Mascioli EA. Risk of symptomatic central venous thrombotic complications in AIDS patients receiving home parenteral nutrition. J Parenter Enteral Nutr 1996;20(4):302–5.

81. MacLaren R, Wachsman BA, Swift DK, Kuhl DA. Warfarin resistance associated with intravenous lipid administration: discussion of propofol and review of the literature. Pharmacotherapy 1997;17(6):1331–7.

82. van der Poll T, Levi M, Braxton CC, Coyle SM, Roth M, ten Cate JW, Lowry SF. Parenteral nutrition facilitates activation of coagulation but not of fibrinolysis during human endotoxemia. J Infect Dis 1998;177(3):793–5.

83. Moss RL, Das JB, Raffensperger JG. Total parenteral nutrition-associated cholestasis: clinical and histopathologic correlation. J Pediatr Surg 1993;28(10):1270–4.

84. Morgan W 3rd, Yardley J, Luk G, Niemiec P, Dudgeon D. Total parenteral nutrition and intestinal development: a neonatal model. J Pediatr Surg 1987;22(6):541–5.

85. Qiu JG, Delany HM, Teh EL, Freundlich L, Gliedman ML, Steinberg JJ, Chang CJ, Levenson SM. Contrasting effects of identical nutrients given parenterally or enterally after 70% hepatectomy: bacterial translocation. Nutrition 1997;13(5):431–7.

86. Baker AL, Rosenberg IH. Hepatic complications of total parenteral nutrition. Am J Med 1987;82(3):489–97.

87. Burstyne M, Jensen GL. Abnormal liver functions as a result of total parenteral nutrition in a patient with short-bowel syndrome. Nutrition 2000;16(11–12):1090–2.

88. Ito Y, Shils ME. Liver dysfunction associated with long-term total parenteral nutrition in patients with massive bowel resection. J Parenter Enteral Nutr 1991;15(3):271–6.

89. Kelly DA. Liver complications of pediatric parenteral nutrition—epidemiology. Nutrition 1998;14(1):153–7.

90. Gafa M, Sarli L, Miselli A, Pietra N, Carreras F, Peracchia A. Sludge and microlithiasis of the biliary tract after total Gastrectomy and postoperative total parenteral nutrition. Surg Gynecol Obstet 1987; 165(5):413–18.

91. Nussbaum MS, Fischer JE. Pathogenesis of hepatic steatosis during total parenteral nutrition. Surg Annu 1991;23(Pt 2):1–11.

92. Teitelbaum DH. Parenteral nutrition-associated cholestasis. Curr Opin Pediatr 1997;9(3):270–5.

93. Cavicchi M, Crenn P, Beau P, Degott C, Boutron MC, Messing B. Severe liver complications associated with long-term parenteral nutrition are dependent on lipid parenteral input. Transplant Proc 1998;30(6):2547.

94. Samlowski WE, Wiebke G, McMurry M, Mori M, Ward JH. Effects of total parental nutrition (TPN) during high-dose interleukin-2 treatment for metastatic cancer. J Immunother 1998;21(1):65–74.

95. Cavicchi M, Beau P, Crenn P, Degott C, Messing B. Prevalence of liver disease and contributing factors in patients receiving home parenteral nutrition for permanent intestinal failure. Ann Intern Med 2000;132(7):525–32.

96. Craig RM, Coy D, Green R, Meersman R, Rubin H, Janssen I. Hepatotoxicity related to total parenteral nutrition: comparison of low-lipid and lipid-supplemented solutions. J Crit Care 1994;9(2):111–13.

97. Drongowski RA, Coran AG. An analysis of factors contributing to the development of total parenteral nutrition-induced cholestasis. J Parenter Enteral Nutr 1989;13(6):586–9.

98. Truskett PG, Shi EC, Rose M, Sharp PA, Ham JM. Model of TPN-associated hepatobiliary dysfunction in the young pig. Br J Surg 1987;74(7):639–42.

99. Clayton PT, Whitfield P, Iyer K. The role of phytosterols in the pathogenesis of liver complications of pediatric parenteral nutrition. Nutrition 1998;14(1):158–64.

100. Iyer KR, Spitz L, Clayton P. BAPS prize lecture: New insight into mechanisms of parenteral nutrition-associated cholestasis: role of plant sterols. British Association of Paediatric Surgeons. J Pediatr Surg 1998;33(1):1–6.

101. Teitelbaum DH, Han-Markey T, Drongowski RA, Coran AG, Bayar B, Geiger JD, Uitvlugt N, Schork MA. Use of cholecystokinin to prevent the development of parenteral nutrition-associated cholestasis. J Parenter Enteral Nutr 1997;21(2):100–3.

102. Bindl L, Lutjohann D, Buderus S, Lentze MJ, v Bergmann K. High plasma levels of phytosterols in patients on parenteral nutrition: a marker of liver dysfunction. J Pediatr Gastroenterol Nutr 2000;31(3):313–16.

103. Sondheimer JM, Asturias E, Cadnapaphornchai M. Infection and cholestasis in neonates with intestinal resection and long-term parenteral nutrition. J Pediatr Gastroenterol Nutr 1998;27(2):131–7.

104. Colomb V, Jobert-Giraud A, Lacaille F, Goulet O, Fournet JC, Ricour C. Role of lipid emulsions in cholestasis associated with long-term parenteral nutrition in children. J Parenter Enteral Nutr 2000;24(6):345–50.

105. Fok TF, Chui KK, Cheung R, Ng PC, Cheung KL, Hjelm M. Manganese intake and cholestatic jaundice in neonates receiving parenteral nutrition: a randomized controlled study. Acta Paediatr 2001;90(9):1009–15.

106. Reimund JM, Duclos B, Arondel Y, Baumann R. Persistent inflammation and immune activation contribute to cholestasis in patients receiving home parenteral nutrition. Nutrition 2001;17(4):300–4.

107. Levine A, Maayan A, Shamir R, Dinari G, Sulkes J, Sirotta L. Parenteral nutrition-associated cholestasis in preterm neonates: evaluation of ursodeoxycholic acid treatment. J Pediatr Endocrinol Metab 1999;12(4):549–53.

108. Spagnuolo MI, Iorio R, Vegnente A, Guarino A. Ursodeoxycholic acid for treatment of cholestasis in children on long-term total parenteral nutrition: a pilot study. Gastroenterology 1996;111(3):716–19.

109. Hwang TL, Lue MC, Chen LL. Early use of cyclic TPN prevents further deterioration of liver functions for the TPN patients with impaired liver function. Hepatogastroenterology 2000;47(35):1347–50.

110. Buchman AL, Moukarzel A, Ament ME, Gornbein J, Goodson B, Carlson C, Hawkins RA. Serious renal impairment is associated with long-term parenteral nutrition. J Parenter Enteral Nutr 1993;17(5):438–44.

111. Campfield T, Braden G. Urinary oxalate excretion by very low birth weight infants receiving parenteral nutrition. Pediatrics 1989;84(5):860–3.

112. Foldes J, Rimon B, Muggia-Sullam M, Gimmon Z, Leichter I, Steinberg R, Menczel J, Freund HR. Progressive bone loss during long-term home total parenteral nutrition. J Parenter Enteral Nutr 1990;14(2):139–42.

113. Koo WW. Parenteral nutrition-related bone disease. J Parenter Enteral Nutr 1992;16(4):386–94.

114. Lipkin EW. A longitudinal study of calcium regulation in a nonhuman primate model of parenteral nutrition. Am J Clin Nutr 1998;67(2):246–54.

115. Verhage AH, Cheong WK, Allard JP, Jeejeebhoy KN, Harry M. Vars Research Award. Increase in lumbar spine bone mineral content in patients on long-term parenteral nutrition without vitamin D supplementation. J Parenter Enteral Nutr 1995;19(6):431–6.

116. von Wowern SN, Klausen B, Moller EH. Knogletab of oral status hos patienter i parenteral ernaering i hjemmet. [Bone loss and oral health status in patients on home parenteral nutrition.] Ugeskr Laeger 1997;159(33):4982–5.

117. de Vernejoul MC, Messing B, Modrowski D, Bielakoff J, Buisine A, Miravet L. Multifactorial low remodeling bone disease during cyclic total parenteral nutrition. J Clin Endocrinol Metab 1985;60(1):109–13.

118. Tsai JR, Yang PH. Rickets of premature infants induced by calcium deficiency. A case report. Changgeng Yi Xue Za Zhi 1997;20(2):142–7.

119. Jeejeebhoy KN. Metabolic bone disease and total parenteral nutrition: a progress report. Am J Clin Nutr 1998;67(2):186–7.

120. Hebuterne X, Frere AM, Bayle J, Rampal P. Priapism in a patient treated with total parenteral nutrition. J Parenter Enteral Nutr 1992;16(2):171–4.

121. Francis DM, Shenton BK. Fat emulsion adversely affects lymphocyte reactivity. Aust NZ J Surg 1987;57(5):323–9.

122. Okada Y, Klein N, van Saene HK, Pierro A. Small volumes of enteral feedings normalise immune function in infants receiving parenteral nutrition. J Pediatr Surg 1998;33(1):16–19.

123. Weidmann B, Lepique C, Heider A, Schmitz A, Niederle N. Hypersensitivity reactions to parenteral lipid solutions. Support Care Cancer 1997;5(6):504–5.

124. Laxenaire MC, Cottineau C, Neidhardt M, Tunon De Lara M, Rakotoseheno JC, Bricard H, Vergnaud MC, Laroche D, Dubois F, Jacson F, Claussner-Poulignan M, Jacquot C, Zambelli P, Hautier MB, Facon A, Orsel I, Motin J, Dubost R, Courvoisier L, et al. Substances responsables des chocs anaphylactiques peranethesiques. Troisième enquête multicentrique française (1992–1994). [Substances responsible for peranesthetic anaphylactic shock. A third French multicenter study (1992–94).] Ann Fr Anesth Reanim 1996;15(8):1211–18.

125. Theissen JL, Zahn P, Theissen U, Brehler R. Allergische und pseudoallergische reaktionen in der anästhesie. Teil I: Pathogenese Risikofaktoren, substanzen. [Allergic and pseudo-allergic reactions in anesthesia. I: Pathogenesis, risk factors, substances.] Anasthesiol Intensivmed Notfallmed Schmerzther 1995;30(1):3–12.

126. Market AD, Lew DB, Schropp KP, Hak EB. Parenteral nutrition-associated anaphylaxis in a 4-year-old child. J Pediatr Gastroenterol Nutr 1998;26(2):229–31.

127. Wu SF, Chen W. Hypersensitivity to vitamin preparation in parenteral nutrition: report of one case. Acta Paediatr Taiwan 2002;43(5):285–7.

128. Yeung CY, Lee HC, Huang FY, Wang CS. Sepsis during total parenteral nutrition: exploration of risk factors and

determination of the effectiveness of peripherally inserted central venous catheters. Pediatr Infect Dis J 1998;17(2):135–42.

129. Sirota L, Straussberg R, Notti I, Bessler H. Effect of lipid emulsion on IL-2 production by mononuclear cells of newborn infants and adults. Acta Paediatr 1997;86(4):410–13.

130. Beganovic N, Verloove-Vanhorick SP, Brand R, Ruys JH. Total parenteral nutrition and sepsis. Arch Dis Child 1988;63(1):66–7.

131. Lenssen P, Bruemmer BA, Bowden RA, Gooley T, Aker SN, Mattson D. Intravenous lipid dose and incidence of bacteremia and fungemia in patients undergoing bone marrow transplantation. Am J Clin Nutr 1998;67(5):927–33.

132. Huang YC, Li CC, Lin TY, Lien RI, Chou YH, Wu JL, Hsueh C. Association of fungal colonization and invasive disease in very low birth weight infants. Pediatr Infect Dis J 1998;17(9):819–22.

133. Avila-Figueroa C, Goldmann DA, Richardson DK, Gray JE, Ferrari A, Freeman J. Intravenous lipid emulsions are the major determinant of coagulase-negative staphylococcal bacteremia in very low birth weight newborns. Pediatr Infect Dis J 1998;17(1):10–17.

134. Katz S, Plaisier BR, Folkening WJ, Grosfeld JL. Intralipid adversely affects reticuloendothelial bacterial clearance. J Pediatr Surg 1991;26(8):921–4.

135. Henwood S, Wilson D, White R, Trimbo S. Developmental toxicity study in rats and rabbits administered an emulsion containing medium chain triglycerides as an alternative caloric source. Fundam Appl Toxicol 1997;40(2):185–90.

136. Yip YY, Lim AK, R J, Tan KL. A multivariate analysis of factors predictive of parenteral nutrition-related cholestasis (TPN cholestasis) in VLBW infants. J Singapore Paediatr Soc 1990;32(3–4):144–8.

137. Mashako MNL, Cezard JP, Boige N, Chayvialle JA, et al. The effect of artificial feeding on cholestasis, gallbladder sludge and lithiasis in infants: correlation with plasma cholecystokinin levels. Clin Nutr 1991;10:320–7.

138. Chou YH, Yau KI, Hsu HC, Chang MH. Total parenteral nutrition-associated cholestasis in infants: clinical and liver histologic studies. Zhonghua Min Guo Xiao Er Ke Yi Xue Hui Za Zhi 1993;34(4):264–71.

139. Mullick FG, Moran CA, Ishak KG. Total parenteral nutrition: a histopathologic analysis of the liver changes in 20 children. Mod Pathol 1994;7(2):190–4.

140. Komura J, Yano H, Tanaka Y, Tsuru T. Increased incidence of cholestasis during total parenteral nutrition in children—factors affecting stone formation. Kurume Med J 1993;40(1):7–11.

141. King DR, Ginn-Pease ME, Lloyd TV, Hoffman J, Hohenbrink K. Parenteral nutrition with associated cholelithiasis: another iatrogenic disease of infants and children. J Pediatr Surg 1987;22(7):593–6.

142. Cooke RW. Factors associated with chronic lung disease in preterm infants. Arch Dis Child 1991;66(7 Spec No):776–9.

143. Andersson S, Pitkanen O, Hallman M. Parenteral lipids and free radicals in preterm infants. Arch Dis Child 1992;67(1):152.

144. Williams AF. Factors associated with chronic lung disease in preterm infants. Arch Dis Child 1992;67(3):351.

145. Wilson DC, McClure G, Halliday HL, Reid MM, Dodge JA. Nutrition and bronchopulmonary dysplasia. Arch Dis Child 1991;66(1 Spec No):37–8.

146. Gelas P, Cotte L, Poitevin-Later F, Pichard C, Leverve X, Barnoud D, Leclercq P, Touraine-Moulin F, Trepo C, Bouletreau P. Effect of parenteral medium- and long-chain triglycerides on lymphocytes subpopulations and functions in patients with acquired immunodeficiency syndrome: a prospective study. J Parenter Enteral Nutr 1998;22(2):67–71.

147. Shay DK, Fann LM, Jarvis WR. Respiratory distress and sudden death associated with receipt of a peripheral parenteral nutrition admixture. Infect Control Hosp Epidemiol 1997;18(12):814–17.

148. Nightingale SL. Safety alert on hazards of precipitation associated with parenteral nutrition. JAMA 1994;271:1472.

149. Lumpkin MM. Safety alert: hazards of precipitation associated with parenteral nutrition. Am J Hosp Pharm 1994;51(11):1427–8.

150. Mirtallo JM. The complexity of mixing calcium and phosphate. Am J Hosp Pharm 1994;51(12):1535–6.

151. Hasegawa GR. Caring about stability and compatibility. Am J Hosp Pharm 1994;51(12):1533–4.

152. Allwood MC. Microbiological risks in parenteral nutrition compounding. Nutrition 1997;13(1):60–1.

153. Jatoi A, Hanjosten K, Ross E, Mason JB. A prospective survey for central line skin-site colonization by the pathogen Malassezia furfur among hospitalized adults receiving total parenteral nutrition. J Parenter Enteral Nutr 1997;21(4):230–2.

154. Widmer AF. Management of catheter-related bacteremia and fungemia in patients on total parenteral nutrition. Nutrition 1997;13(Suppl 4):S18–25.

155. Gil ME, Mateu J. Treatment of extravasation from parenteral nutrition solution. Ann Pharmacother 1998;32(1):51–5.

156. Coley BD, Seguin J, Cordero L, Hogan MJ, Rosenberg E, Reber K. Neonatal total parenteral nutrition ascites from liver erosion by umbilical vein catheters. Pediatr Radiol 1998;28(12):923–7.

157. Sentipal-Walerius J, Dollberg S, Mimouni F, Doyle J, Gilmour C. Effect of pulsed dexamethasone therapy on tolerance of intravenously administered lipids in extremely low birth weight infants. J Pediatr 1999;134(2):229–32.

158. Brophy DF, Ford SL, Crouch MA. Warfarin resistance in a patient with short bowel syndrome. Pharmacotherapy 1998;18(3):646–9.

159. Lutomski DM, Palascak JE, Bower RH. Warfarin resistance associated with intravenous lipid administration. J Parenter Enteral Nutr 1987;11(3):316–18.

160. Douchain F, Hode E, Paul JC, Bakhache P, Pautard JC. Priapisme aigu après une perfusion d'émulsion lipidique à 10 p. 100 chez un enfant mucoviscidosique. [Acute priapism after infusion of 10% fat emulsion in a child with cystic fibrosis.] Presse Méd 1990;19(9):429.

Paroxetine

See also Selective serotonin re-uptake inhibitors (SSRIs)

General Information

Paroxetine is a phenylpiperidine derivative. Its half-life is about 17–22 hours and about 95% of it is bound to plasma proteins. Its metabolites have no more than 1/50 of the potency of the parent compound in inhibiting serotonin re-uptake. The metabolism of paroxetine is accomplished in part by CYP2D6, saturation of which at therapeutic doses appears to account for the non-linearity of paroxetine kinetics at higher doses and increasing durations of treatment. The adverse effects of paroxetine are those of the SSRIs in general. Commonly observed adverse events in placebo-controlled clinical trials were weakness, sweating, nausea, reduced appetite, somnolence, dizziness, insomnia, tremor, nervousness, ejaculatory disturbance, and other male genital disorders. Paroxetine seems to have a higher incidence of withdrawal symptoms than other SSRIs.

Organs and Systems

Cardiovascular

Electrocardiographic changes, with a prolonged QT_c interval and bradycardia, have been reported with paroxetine (1).

Nervous system

Serotonin syndrome

The serotonin syndrome is a recognized complication of SSRI treatment. Usually it occurs as part of a drug interaction, when the serotonergic effects of SSRIs are augmented by medications that also have serotonin-potentiating properties (SEDA-22, 14) (SEDA-25, 16). Occasionally, however, the serotonin syndrome can occur after SSRI monotherapy.

- A 23-year-old Japanese woman with major depression took a single dose of paroxetine (20 mg) and 1 hour later had agitation, myoclonus, mild hyperthermia (37.5 °C), sweating, and diarrhea, symptoms that meet the criteria for the serotonin syndrome; she recovered with supportive treatment over 3 days (2).

Blood concentrations of paroxetine were not obtained, but the authors reported that the patient was homozygous for the 10* form of the CYP2D6 allele, which is associated with low CYP2D6 activity in vivo. While this is an interesting observation, it is unlikely by itself to explain the patient's sensitivity to paroxetine, because this genotype is not uncommon in the Japanese population, and if a lot of Japanese have this genotype, the serotonin syndrome with SSRI monotherapy would be quite common, given the widespread prescription of SSRIs. However, it reinforces clinical advice that in patients new to SSRI treatment it is advisable to start therapy with half the standard dose.

Dystonias

Acute dystonia has been described during the first days of paroxetine treatment (SEDA-17, 19).

Paroxetine-induced akathisia has been described in an 81-year-old man with bipolar depression. The akathisia began one week after paroxetine treatment (20 mg/day) and remitted within 6 days of withdrawal (3).

The authors pointed out that it is important to recognize SSRI-induced akathisia, because increasing agitation and restlessness early in treatment can be mistaken for worsening depression. In addition, case reports have suggested that akathisia can be associated with suicidal impulses.

Sensory systems

Tricyclic antidepressants can precipitate acute glaucoma through their anticholinergic effects. There are also reports that paroxetine can cause acute glaucoma, presumably by pupillary dilatation.

- An 84-year-old woman developed acute closed-angle glaucoma after taking paroxetine for 6 days (SEDA-21, 13).
- A 70-year-old woman taking paroxetine developed acute closed-angle glaucoma (4).
- A 91-year-old developed bilateral acute closed-angle glaucoma after taking paroxetine (5).

Three patients taking paroxetine for interferon-alpha-induced depression developed retinal hemorrhages, including one with irreversible loss of vision (6).

Psychological, psychiatric

In three children (two aged 9 years and one aged 10 years) who took paroxetine 10–20 mg/day for the treatment of childhood obsessive-compulsive disorder, symptoms of mania, including overactivity, pressure of speech, irritability, and antisocial behavior, occurred within 3 weeks of starting paroxetine and remitted after paroxetine withdrawal or dosage reduction (7). Symptoms of mania are rare in childhood, suggesting that the elevated mood in these cases was a direct effect of the paroxetine.

Psychomotor retardation with semistupor has been reported in one patient taking paroxetine; however, she was also taking antipsychotic drugs, which may have contributed (SEDA-18, 20).

Endocrine

Serotonin pathways are involved in the regulation of prolactin secretion. Galactorrhea has been associated with paroxetine (8).

Serotonin pathways are involved in the regulation of prolactin secretion. Amenorrhea, galactorrhea, and hyperprolactinemia have been reported in a patient taking SSRIs.

- A 32-year-old woman taking paroxetine 40 mg/day had a raised prolactin concentration (46 ng/ml) and galactorrhea, both of which resolved a few days after paroxetine withdrawal (9).

Hematologic

Clozapine and SSRIs are often used together, because depressive syndromes are common in patients with schizophrenia. Clozapine carries a relatively high risk of agranulocytosis, but this adverse effect is very rarely seen with SSRIs, although a case of possible fluoxetine-induced neutropenia has been described (SEDA-22, 15). Two cases in which the addition of paroxetine to clozapine was associated with neutropenia have been reported (10). The patients had been taking stable doses of clozapine for 6–12 months and had previously tolerated other SSRIs without adverse hematological consequences. In both cases the white cell count recovered when clozapine was withdrawn, although paroxetine was continued.

Fluoxetine has infrequently been associated with abnormal bleeding, including ecchymoses, melena, and hematuria. Spontaneous ecchymoses have been reported in a woman taking paroxetine (11).

- A 47-year-old woman who had had bilateral mastectomies for breast cancer became depressed and was given paroxetine 20 mg/day. After 15 days she developed widespread multiple ecchymoses over the arms, legs, and abdomen. Her platelet count, prothrombin time, partial thromboplastin time, and bleeding time were normal. Paroxetine was withdrawn, and 5 days later, the bruising had markedly abated and no new lesions were identified. She was subsequently treated with a tricyclic antidepressant without recurrence of the ecchymoses.

The authors noted two earlier reports of ecchymoses with paroxetine, with normal laboratory values. They speculated that an indirect effect on platelet function through inhibition of platelet 5-HT uptake may be involved.

Paroxetine caused neutropenia in a patient whose white cell count fell to 2.9×10^9/l (neutrophils 1.37×10^9/l) (12). The white cell count gradually recovered over 6 weeks after paroxetine withdrawal.

Liver

Hepatotoxicity associated with paroxetine has been documented in two case reports (SEDA-21, 12). Severe hepatitis has been reported in two young women who took Atrium (febarbamate + difebarbamate + phenobarbital) and paroxetine (13). Liver biopsy showed lesions compatible with drug-related injury. Both recovered completely. The authors suggested that simultaneous treatment with Atrium and paroxetine increased each drug's hepatotoxicity.

Sexual function

Delayed ejaculation associated with paroxetine has been reported (SEDA-18, 21).

Immunologic

A skin reaction consistent with a vasculitis has been reported.

- A 20-year-old woman taking paroxetine 10 mg/day for obsessive-compulsive disorder developed multiple purple lesions on the fingers of both hands after 15 weeks (14). The lesions disappeared after 1 week but returned in 2 days after rechallenge with paroxetine.

Long-Term Effects

Drug withdrawal

Sudden withdrawal of paroxetine has been associated with nausea, dizziness, tremor, insomnia, irritation, and agitation (SEDA-17, 20). In three cases, a withdrawal reaction occurred with paroxetine, despite tapering of the dose for 7–14 days before discontinuation; the symptoms were the same as in earlier reports, but also included in one case myalgia, and in another rhinorrhea and visual phenomena similar to those associated with migraine (15). The authors suggested that cholinergic mechanisms and functional changes in 5-HT may play a role in the mediation of withdrawal symptoms.

Drug Administration

Drug overdose

There were gastrointestinal symptoms and CNS disturbances in patients who took overdoses of paroxetine, the largest amount being 850 mg (16).

Drug–Drug Interactions

Beta-blockers

Paroxetine can cause clinically important increases in plasma concentrations of metoprolol (17).

Clozapine

In a prospective study, paroxetine (20 mg/day), a potent inhibitor of CYP2D6, did not increase clozapine concentrations ($n = 14$), and the authors therefore suggested that CYP2D6 is not an important pathway of metabolism of clozapine (18). However, other studies (SEDA-21, 22) have shown that paroxetine can increase clozapine concentrations, suggesting that this combination should be used with caution.

Linezolid

SSRIs can also cause pharmacodynamic drug interactions for some time after withdrawal, through residual serotonin reuptake blocking activity.

- A 56-year-old woman with a postoperative wound infection developed the serotonin syndrome when she was given the antibiotic linezolid intravenously (19). The dose of paroxetine had been tapered and it had been withdrawn 5 days before.

Linezolid inhibits monoamine oxidase activity and has been reported to cause serotonin toxicity in combination with paroxetine. While some patients have apparently taken the combination of linezolid and an SSRI safely, this report suggests that patients taking combined treatment should be monitored for serotonin toxicity.

Methadone

Methadone-maintenance treatment is now established by controlled trials as effective in managing patients with opioid dependence. SSRIs are often co-prescribed for such patients, and there have been reports that SSRIs can increase methadone concentrations, presumably by inhibition of CYP2D6 (SEDA-25, 15). The effect of adding paroxetine (20 mg/day) to the treatment regimen has been studied in 10 opiate-dependent patients taking methadone maintenance (20). Methadone concentrations increased on an average by about one-third, although there was much individual variation. There were no obvious clinical consequences, presumably because the patients were fairly tolerant to the effects of methadone. However, the authors cautioned that sudden withdrawal of an SSRI in methadone users has the potential to trigger opioid-withdrawal symptoms.

Tricyclic antidepressants

Paroxetine can cause clinically important increases in plasma concentrations of tricyclic antidepressants (21).

Triptans

Treatment of 12 healthy volunteers with paroxetine (20 mg/day for 14 days) did not alter the pharmacokinetics or pharmacodynamic effects of an acute dose of rizatriptan (10 mg orally) (22). These data are reassuring, but (as with sumatriptan) it is possible that sporadic cases of 5-HT neurotoxicity could still occur when rizatriptan is combined with an SSRI.

Risperidone

The addition of paroxetine 20 mg/day to risperidone 4–8 mg/day in 10 patients with schizophrenia produced a 45% increase in plasma concentrations of risperidone and its active metabolite, 9-hydroxyrisperidone (23). One of the patients developed signs of drug-induced Parkinson's disease following the addition of paroxetine.

The serotonin syndrome occurred in a patient taking paroxetine plus an atypical antipsychotic drug, risperidone (24).

• A 53-year-old man took paroxetine 40 mg/day and risperidone 6 mg/day, having previously taken lower doses of both. Within 2 hours he developed ataxia, shivering, and tremor. He had profound sweating but was apyrexial, and was confused, with involuntary jerking movements of his limbs. He recovered without specific treatment over the next 2 days.

This was the first report of the serotonin syndrome in a patient taking an SSRI and an atypical antipsychotic drug. The reaction was unexpected because risperidone, in addition to being a potent dopamine receptor antagonist, is also a 5-HT$_2$-receptor antagonist. Subsequent animal studies suggested that 5-HT$_2$-receptor antagonists increase the firing of serotonergic neurons, perhaps through a postsynaptic feedback loop. This could account for potentiation of the effects of SSRIs by 5-HT$_2$-receptor antagonists, such as risperidone.

References

1. Erfurth A, Loew M, Dobmeier P, Wendler G. EKG – Veran derungen nach faroxetineo Drei Fallberichte. [ECG changes after paroxetine. 3 case reports.] Nervenarzt 1998;69(7):629–31.
2. Kaneda Y, Kawamura I, Fujii A, Ohmori T. Serotonin syndrome—"potential" role of the CYP2D6 genetic polymorphism in Asians. Int J Neuropsychopharmacol 2002;5(1):105–6.
3. Bonnet-Brilhault F, Thibaut F, Leprieur A, Petit M. A case of paroxetine-induced akathisia and a review of SSRI-induced akathisia. Eur Psychiatry 1998;13:109–11.
4. Lewis CF, DeQuardo JR, DuBose C, Tandon R. Acute angle-closure glaucoma and paroxetine. J Clin Psychiatry 1997;58(3):123–4.
5. Kirwan JF, Subak-Sharpe I, Teimory M. Bilateral acute angle closure glaucoma after administration of paroxetine. Br J Ophthalmol 1997;81(3):252.
6. Musselman DL, Lawson DH, Gumnick JF, Manatunga AK, Penna S, Goodkin RS, Greiner K, Nemeroff CB, Miller AH. Paroxetine for the prevention of depression induced by high-dose interferon alfa. N Engl J Med 2001; 344(13):961–6.
7. Diler RS, Avci A. SSRI-induced mania in obsessive-compulsive disorder. J Am Acad Child Adolesc Psychiatry 1999;38(1):6–7.
8. Bonin B, Vandel P, Sechter D, Bizouard P. Paroxetine and galactorrhea. Pharmacopsychiatry 1997;30(4):133–4.
9. Morrison J, Remick RA, Leung M, Wrixon KJ, Bebb RA. Galactorrhea induced by paroxetine. Can J Psychiatry 2001; 46(1):88–9.
10. George TP, Innamorato L, Sernyak MJ, Baldessarini RJ, Centorrino F. Leukopenia associated with addition of paroxetine to clozapine. J Clin Psychiatry 1998;59(1):31.
11. Cooper TA, Valcour VG, Gibbons RB, O'Brien-Falls K. Spontaneous ecchymoses due to paroxetine administration. Am J Med 1998;104(2):197–8.
12. Moselhy HF, Conlon W. Neutropenia associated with paroxetine. Ir J Psychol Med 1999;16:75.
13. Cadranel JF, Di Martino V, Cazier A, Pras V, Bachmeyer C, Olympio P, Gonzenbach A, Mofredj A, Coutarel P, Devergie B, Biour M. Atrium and paroxetine-related severe hepatitis. J Clin Gastroenterol 1999;28(1):52–5.
14. Margolese HC, Chouinard G, Beauclair L, Rubino M. Cutaneous vasculitis induced by paroxetine. Am J Psychiatry 2001;158(3):497.
15. Barr LC, Goodman WK, Price LH. Physical symptoms associated with paroxetine discontinuation. Am J Psychiatry 1994;151(2):289.
16. Grimsley SR, Jann MW. Paroxetine, sertraline, and fluvoxamine: new selective serotonin reuptake inhibitors. Clin Pharm 1992;11(11):930–57.
17. Hemeryck A, Lefebvre RA, De Vriendt C, Belpaire FM. Paroxetine affects metoprolol pharmacokinetics and pharmacodynamics in healthy volunteers. Clin Pharmacol Ther 2000;67(3):283–91.
18. Wetzel H, Anghelescu I, Szegedi A, Wiesner J, Weigmann H, Harter S, Hiemke C. Pharmacokinetic interactions of clozapine with selective serotonin reuptake inhibitors: differential effects of fluvoxamine and paroxetine in a prospective study. J Clin Psychopharmacol 1998;18(1):2–9.
19. Wigen CL, Goetz MB. Serotonin syndrome and linezolid. Clin Infect Dis 2002;34(12):1651–2.
20. Begre S, von Bardeleben U, Ladewig D, Jaquet-Rochat S, Cosendai-Savary L, Golay KP, Kosel M, Baumann P, Eap CB. Paroxetine increases steady-state concentrations of (R)-methadone in CYP2D6 extensive but not poor metabolizers. J Clin Psychopharmacol 2002;22(2):211–15.
21. Leucht S, Hackl HJ, Steimer W, Angersbach D, Zimmer R. Effect of adjunctive paroxetine on serum levels and side-effects of tricyclic antidepressants in depressive inpatients. Psychopharmacology (Berl) 2000;147(4):378–83.
22. Goldberg MR, Lowry RC, Musson DG, Birk KL, Fisher A, De Puy ME, Shadle CR. Lack of pharmacokinetic and pharmacodynamic interaction between rizatriptan and paroxetine. J Clin Pharmacol 1999;39(2):192–9.
23. Spina E, Avenoso A, Facciola G, Scordo MG, Ancione M, Madia A. Plasma concentrations of risperidone and 9-hydroxyrisperidone during combined treatment with paroxetine. Ther Drug Monit 2001;23(3):223–7.
24. Hamilton S, Malone K. Serotonin syndrome during treatment with paroxetine and risperidone. J Clin Psychopharmacol 2000;20(1):103–5.

Passifloraceae

See also Herbal medicines

General Information

The family of Passifloraceae contains the single genus *Passiflora*.

Passiflora incarnata

Passiflora incarnata (apricot vine, grenadille, passion flower, passion vine) is widely touted as a herbal sedative and anxiolytic (1). It contains harman alkaloids.

Adverse effects

Passion flower has reportedly caused prolongation of the QT interval (2).

- A 34-year-old woman developed nausea, vomiting, drowsiness, a prolonged QT interval, and episodes of non-sustained ventricular tachycardia after self-medication with passion flower for 1 day. She made a full recovery after withdrawal of the passion flower.

The authors suggested that the adverse event had been caused by harman alkaloids from *P. incarnata*.

Five patients developed altered consciousness after taking the herbal product Relaxir for insomnia and restlessness, produced mainly from the fruit of the passion flower (3).

References

1. Krenn L. Die Passionsblume (*Passiflora incarnata* L.)—ein bewahrtes pflanzliches Sedativum. [Passion Flower (*Passiflora incarnata* L.)—a reliable herbal sedative.] Wien Med Wochenschr 2002;152(15-16):404–6.
2. Fisher AA, Purcell P, Le Couteur DG. Toxicity of *Passiflora incarnata* L. J Toxicol Clin Toxicol 2000;38(1):63–6.
3. Solbakken AM, Rorbakken G, Gundersen T. Natur medisin som rusmiddel. [Nature medicine as intoxicant.] Tidsskr Nor Laegeforen 1997;117(8):1140–1.

Pazufloxacin

See also Fluoroquinolones

General Information

Pazufloxacin is an injectable quinolone antibiotic with bactericidal effect against cephalosporin-resistant, carbapenem-resistant, and aminoglycoside-resistant strains of bacteria.

Organs and Systems

Skin

In in vivo studies in animal models of phototoxicity, pazufloxacin was less potent than nalidixic acid, ofloxacin, ciprofloxacin, or sparfloxacin, and there was no photoallergenicity (1).

Drug–Drug Interactions

Theophylline

Co-administration of pazufloxacin and theophylline has been studied in rats (2). Pazufloxacin reduced the clearance of theophylline by about 25%. In seven healthy volunteers taking modified-release theophylline, intravenous pazufloxacin mesilate increased serum theophylline concentrations; analysis of the urinary excretion of theophylline and its metabolites suggested that CYP1A2 had been inhibited (2). Theophylline concentrations need to be monitored if pazufloxacin is co-administered.

References

1. Nagasawa M, Nakamura S, Miyazaki M, Nojima Y, Hayakawa H, Kawamura Y. [Phototoxicity studies of pazufloxacin mesilate, a novel parenteral quinolone antimicrobial agent—in vitro and in vivo studies.] Jpn J Antibiot 2002;55(3):259–69.
2. Niki Y, Watanabe S, Yoshida K, Miyashita N, Nakajima M, Matsushima T. Effect of pazufloxacin mesilate on the serum concentration of theophylline. J Infect Chemother 2002;8(1):33–6.

Pedaliaceae

See also Herbal medicines

General Information

The genera in the family of Pedaliaceae (Table 1) include sesame.

Harpagophytum species

Harpagophytum procumbens (devil's claw, grapple plant, wood spider) contains the iridoids harpagoside and procumbide. It is used to treat pain in the joints and lower back, although the quality of trials demonstrating efficacy is poor and there is variability from formulation to formulation (1).

Adverse effects

It is sometimes stated that *H. procumbens* should be avoided during pregnancy because of its supposed abortifacient effect, but the oxytoxic properties of the plant remain to be verified. There may be an interaction with warfarin (2).

Table 1 The genera of Pedaliaceae

Ceratotheca (ceratotheca)
Craniolaria (craniolaria)
Harpagophytum (devil's claw)
Ibicella (yellow unicorn plant)
Martynia (martynia)
Proboscidea (unicorn plant)
Sesamum (sesame)

References

1. Chrubasik S, Conradt C, Black A. The quality of clinical trials with *Harpagophytum procumbens*. Phytomedicine 2003;10(6–7):613–23.
2. Izzo AA, Di Carlo G, Borrelli F, Ernst E. Cardiovascular pharmacotherapy and herbal medicines: the risk of drug interaction. Int J Cardiol 2005;98(1):1–14.

Pefloxacin

See also Fluoroquinolones

General Information

Pefloxacin is a fluoroquinolone antibiotic that inhibits *Plasmodium falciparum* in vitro. It is effective against *Plasmodium yoelii* infections in mice.

Observational studies

In humans pefloxacin was tested in a dosage of 400 mg every 12 hours for 3 days against chloroquine-resistant *P. falciparum* infections in Madagascar, and proved successful in 9 out of 22 cases; seven further cases responded at first but recrudescence followed. The investigators suggested that pefloxacin should be used as a complementary drug rather than as a primary antimalarial drug.

There was a significant reduction in proteinuria in ten children with idiopathic nephrotic syndrome after pefloxacin therapy (mean dose 2–4.6 mg/kg/day for 4–8 weeks) (1). All had received a course of cyclophosphamide at least 6 months before. One patient discontinued pefloxacin within 2 weeks because of nausea and vomiting, one complained of arthralgia, and one developed nail discoloration.

The efficacy and safety of pefloxacin, 15–20 mg/kg bd for 14–28 days in combination with ceftazidime and amikacin, have been investigated in 21 children (aged 7–16 years) with mucoviscidosis or aplastic anemia (2). Combined therapy had good clinical efficacy. Arthropathy developed frequently and children at risk were over 10 years old and had a history of allergies.

General adverse effects

The adverse effects of pefloxacin are those of the fluoroquinolones, which are generally well tolerated. Gastrointestinal complaints occur in some 3–6%, and have included (in declining order of frequency) nausea, abdominal discomfort, vomiting, and diarrhea. Colitis due to *Clostridium difficile* infection has been reported infrequently. Nervous system effects have been less common, but headache, dizziness, agitation, sleep disturbances, and more rarely seizures, delirium, and hallucinations have been reported. Allergic reactions are infrequent. Photosensitivity reactions have been reported. The quinolones cause cartilage erosion in weight-bearing joints in young growing animals, and the long-term use of pefloxacin in growing children, such as would be required for prophylaxis, should be avoided. In bacteria that have developed resistance to fluoroquinolones, cross-resistance with chemically unrelated antibiotics, such as tetracycline and chloramphenicol, is possible.

Organs and Systems

Musculoskeletal

In vitro, pefloxacin was more toxic to tendons than ofloxacin, ciprofloxacin, or levofloxacin (3). In rodents, pefloxacin (400 mg/kg for several days) caused oxidative damage to the type I collagen in the Achilles tendon; these alterations were identical to those observed in experimental tendinous ischemia and a reperfusion model (4). Oxidative damage was prevented by the co-administration of *N*-acetylcysteine (150 mg/kg). Several cases of rupture of the Achilles tendon have been reported during or shortly after the use of fluoroquinolones, including five case in which pefloxacin was used (5).

The efficacy and safety of pefloxacin, 15–20 mg/kg bd for 14–28 days in combination with ceftazidime and amikacin, have been investigated in 21 children (aged 7–16 years) with mucoviscidosis or aplastic anemia (2). Combined therapy had good clinical efficacy. Arthropathy developed frequently and children at risk were over 10 years old and had a history of allergies.

In patients with mucoviscidosis treated with pefloxacin the most common adverse event was arthropathy, and the symptoms disappeared 3 days to 3 months after drug withdrawal (6).

Immunologic

Pefloxacin in suprabactericidal concentrations (2.0 mg/ml and 0.4 mg/ml) markedly suppressed T lymphocyte proliferation in blast transformation; 0.08 mg/ml did not (7). Pefloxacin in a maximal effective dose (200 mg/kg) suppressed delayed hypersensitivity skin reactions in mice.

Susceptibility Factors

Renal disease

In moderate impairment of renal function, prolongation of the dosage interval of pefloxacin should be considered; pefloxacin should be avoided in severe renal impairment (8).

Drug–Drug Interactions

Theophylline

Pefloxacin inhibits theophylline metabolism (9).

References

1. Sharma RK, Sahu KM, Gulati S, Gupta A. Pefloxacin in steroid dependent and resistant idiopathic nephrotic syndrome. J Nephrol 2000;13(4):271–4.
2. Postnikov SS, Semykin SIu, Kapranov NI, Perederko LV, Polikarpova SV, Khamidullina KF. [Evaluation of tolerance and efficacy of pefloxacin in the treatment and prevention of severe infections in children with mucoviscidosis and aplastic anemia.] Antibiot Khimioter 2000;45(8):25–30.
3. Pouzaud F, Rat P, Cambourieu C, Nourry H, Warnet JM. [Tenotoxic potential of fluoroquinolones in the choice of

surgical antibiotic prophylaxis in ophthalmology.] J Fr Ophtalmol 2002;25(9):921–6.

4. Simonin MA, Gegout-Pottie P, Minn A, Gillet P, Netter P, Terlain B. Pefloxacin-induced achilles tendon toxicity in rodents: biochemical changes in proteoglycan synthesis and oxidative damage to collagen. Antimicrob Agents Chemother 2000;44(4):867–72.
5. Ribard P, Audisio F, Kahn MF, De Bandt M, Jorgensen C, Hayem G, Meyer O, Palazzo E. Seven Achilles tendinitis including 3 complicated by rupture during fluoroquinolone therapy. J Rheumatol 1992;19(9):1479–81.
6. Postnikov SS, Semykin SIu, Polikarpova SV, Nazhimov VP. [Pefloxacin in the treatment of patients with mucoviscidosis.] Antibiot Khimioter 2002;47(4):13–15.
7. Artsimovich NG, Nastoiashchaia NN, Navashin PS. [Effect of pefloxacin on immune response.] Antibiot Khimioter 2001;46(4):11–12.
8. Ma L, Sun C, Wu J. [Study of pefloxacin concentration in blood and sputum in the aged pneumonia patients with impairment of renal function.] Zhonghua Jie He He Hu Xi Za Zhi 2001;24(10):596–8.
9. Brouwers JR. Drug interactions with quinolone antibacterials. Drug Saf 1992;7(4):268–81.

Pemirolast

General Information

Pemirolast is a mast-cell stabilizer, like cromoglicate, used in eye-drops for the treatment of allergic disorders (1). It has also been used to prevent coronary artery restenosis after the insertion of a stent (2).

In a 7-day, double-blind, single-dose, crossover, parallel-group study, 45 adults with asymptomatic eyes were randomized to bilateral pemirolast, cromoglicate, or ketorolac at each of three visits (1). Overall discomfort was significantly less with pemirolast than with cromoglicate or ketorolac. Burning/stinging and tearing were also significantly less with pemirolast than with cromoglicate.

In a 1-day, randomized, double-blind, single-dose study in which 48 subjects received pemirolast in one eye and nedocromil in the other, overall discomfort was significantly less with pemirolast than with nedocromil (1).

The most common adverse effects of pemirolast are headache, rhinitis, and mild cold- or flu-like symptoms. After ocular administration for 2 weeks, plasma concentrations were detectable, but with no significant accumulation (SEDA-24, 534).

References

1. Shulman DG, Amdahl L, Washington C, Graves A. A combined analysis of two studies assessing the ocular comfort of antiallergy ophthalmic agents. Clin Ther 2003;25(4):1096–1106.
2. Ohsawa H, Noike H, Kanai M, Hitsumoto T, Aoyagi K, Sakurai T, Sugiyama Y, Yoshinaga K, Kaku M, Matsumoto J, Iizuka T, Shimizu K, Takahashi M, Tomaru T, Sakuragawa H, Tokuhiro K. Preventive effect of an antiallergic drug, pemirolast potassium, on restenosis after stent placement: quantitative coronary angiography and intravascular ultrasound studies. J Cardiol 2003;42(1):13–22.

Pemoline

General Information

Pemoline has similar actions to dexamfetamine and is used in the management of hyperactivity disorders in children (1).

Organs and Systems

Liver

During the past two decades there have been many reports of liver failure resulting in death or transplantation in patients being treated for ADHD with pemoline. However, a descriptive meta-analysis of the existing scientific literature and drug reporting databases showed that current assumptions of the risk of acute hepatic failure posed by pemoline alone are overestimates.

- A 7-year-old boy with Duchenne muscular dystrophy and attention deficit hyperactivity disorder (ADHD) developed acute hepatic failure, with features of autoimmune hepatitis (2). The only medications he had taken were pemoline (56 mg/day) and cyproheptadine (2 mg/day). Pemoline was withdrawn after 8 months as the presumed cause of his raised transaminases. Two weeks later he developed an altered mental state, jaundice, and encephalopathy. The histological features of the liver and his autoimmune antibody panel were consistent with autoimmune hepatitis. He was treated with corticosteroids and azathioprine and recovered.
- A 9-year-old boy with ADHD taking pemoline developed signs and symptoms of liver failure requiring liver transplantation (3).

The evidence linking pemoline to life-threatening liver failure prompted the Food and Drugs Administration to require the manufacturer to add a black box warning to the package insert, whereas in the UK the Committee on Safety of Medicines withdrew marketing approval for pemoline, citing safety and a lack of adequate evidence of efficacy as the reason (4).

Drug Administration

Drug overdose

There has been a report of pemoline-induced acute movement disorders after presumed overdose (5).

- Two 3-year-old identical male twins were found playing with an empty bottle of pemoline that had originally contained 59 tablets. They had a history of attention deficit disorder previously unsuccessfully treated with methylphenidate, but no history or family history of movement disorders. Choreoathetoid movements began 45 minutes to 1 hour after ingestion. The children received gastrointestinal decontamination and high doses of intravenous benzodiazepines but continued to have choreoathetosis for about 24 hours and were discharged at 48 hours.

Five children who took excessive amounts of pemoline have been described (6). They had a relatively benign course and their symptoms appeared to be primarily accentuated pharmacological effects on the central nervous and cardiovascular systems. Sinus tachycardia, hypertension, hyperactivity, choreoathetoid movements, and hallucinations were most commonly observed, consistent with previous reports.

Possible rhabdomyolysis occurred after overdose, accompanied by raised serum creatine kinase activity in three of four patients in whom it was measured; this appears to be common in acute pemoline poisoning. After ingestion, symptoms occurred within 6 hours and lasted up to 48 hours in all cases.

Gastric lavage and activated charcoal are considered to be effective decontamination measures, whereas ipecac-induced emesis should be avoided after massive ingestion, because of the risk of seizures. Aggressive use of benzodiazepine is a reasonable first choice to treat associated involuntary movements, tremor, hyperactivity, and agitation. Chlorpromazine or haloperidol can also be used, especially for serious, life-threatening symptoms, including hypertensive crises and severe hyperthermia, and labetalol or sodium nitroprusside are reasonable choices for rapid stabilization of blood pressure.

References

1. Shevell M, Schreiber R. Pemoline-associated hepatic failure: a critical analysis of the literature. Pediatr Neurol 1997;16(1):14–16.
2. Hochman JA, Woodard SA, Cohen MB. Exacerbation of autoimmune hepatitis: another hepatotoxic effect of pemoline therapy. Pediatrics 1998;101(1 Pt 1):106–8.
3. Adcock KG, MacElroy DE, Wolford ET, Farrington EA. Pemoline therapy resulting in liver transplantation. Ann Pharmacother 1998;32(4):422–5.
4. Anonymous. Committee on safety of medicines. Volital (pemoline) has been withdrawn. Curr Probl Pharmacovig 1997;23:9–12.
5. Stork CM, Cantor R. Pemoline induced acute choreoathetosis: case report and review of the literature. J Toxicol Clin Toxicol 1997;35(1):105–8.
6. Nakamura H, Blumer JL, Reed MD. Pemoline ingestion in children: a report of five cases and review of the literature. J Clin Pharmacol 2002;42(3):275–82.

Penicillamine

General Information

Penicillamine is dimethylcysteine or 2-amino-3-mercapto-3-methylbutyric acid, a sulfur-containing amino acid. It has three functional groups: an alpha-amine, a carboxyl, and a sulfhydryl, which largely determine its pharmacological effects. Because the levorotatory isomer, L-penicillamine, is a pyridoxine antagonist and toxic, the racemic mixture has been replaced for medicinal purposes by purified D-penicillamine. Here "penicillamine" refers to the D-isomer unless otherwise specified.

Acetylpenicillamine is a weaker chelating agent than penicillamine, has no effect on collagen cross-links, and is not effective in rheumatoid arthritis. It has been used in the treatment of mercury poisoning (1).

As its name suggests, penicillamine is a degradation product of penicillin. There have been several reviews of the chemistry, pharmacokinetics, and pharmacology of penicillamine (SED-12, 537) (2). After oral administration about two-thirds (50–70%) of a dose of penicillamine is absorbed. As much as 33% can be degraded in the gut before absorption can take place. With a half-life of less than 1 hour, penicillamine is rapidly cleared after oral administration, largely by formation of disulfides with plasma albumin and with low-molecular weight thiols, such as cysteine and glutathione. Low-molecular weight disulfides constitute the major urinary metabolites. The penicillamine-albumin disulfide, on the other hand, has a long half-life. The consequence of this is slow accumulation: in healthy volunteers pseudo-steady-state plasma concentrations of penicillamine-albumin disulfide are not reached until the second week of daily administration. Peak plasma concentrations of penicillamine occur at 1.5–4 hours after ingestion and range from 5 μmol/l after 150 mg to 28 μmol/l after 800 mg (when conventional-release oral formulations are used). About 80% of penicillamine is protein-bound; about 7% occurs as L-cysteine-D-penicillamine disulfide, 5% as penicillamine disulfide, and 6% as free penicillamine. A large proportion is rapidly excreted in the urine, mainly as the disulfide or as the disulfide metabolite conjugated with cysteine; formation and excretion of the latter can cause cysteine depletion. Some penicillamine is converted to S-methyl-penicillamine and is either excreted by the kidneys or metabolized in the liver. Although S-methylation is a quantitatively minor elimination pathway, S-methyl-penicillamine is a potential substrate for sulfoxide formation, and patients with rheumatoid arthritis who form the sulfoxide at a reduced rate are at greater risk of adverse effects (3). The concentrations of penicillamine and its metabolites within cells and at the cell surface are largely unknown, but may be relevant to variability in response in regard to cellular sites of action.

Uses

Penicillamine is mainly used in the treatment of rheumatoid arthritis, Wilson's disease, and cystinuria. Although penicillamine and gold compounds were both originally used in rheumatoid arthritis on the basis of erroneous pharmacological hypotheses, they have been strongholds in the treatment of debilitating rheumatoid arthritis for more than a quarter of a century (4). Whereas they do not have much effect on the progression of joint damage, they have unexpectedly been found to be associated with a remarkable diversity of serious adverse reactions. In hindsight, they have played central roles in improvements in the understanding of the pathology of rheumatoid arthritis and of the methods of studying the benefits and harms of therapeutic strategies in rheumatoid arthritis and other chronic progressive diseases.

General trends in the treatment of rheumatoid arthritis in the past decade have been more aggressive treatment in early disease with disease-modulating antirheumatic drugs (DMARDs) (5) and the use of combinations of DMARDs (6). Strategies for improving the long-term outcome in rheumatoid arthritis include early specialist referral for DMARD treatment and the avoidance of NSAID-induced gastrointestinal and renal toxicity (7). However, a 28-year observational study in Austria of the patterns of use of DMARDs has illustrated how penicillamine has given way to other drugs, in particular methotrexate and sulfasalazine (8,9). The advent of novel drugs with different mechanisms of action, such as cytokine antagonists, has empowered rheumatologists with effective new instruments (10–12).

Some believe that early, aggressive, and continuous use of DMARDs and of combinations thereof slows joint destruction, modifies the natural course of the disease, and improves outcome (13,14). On closer inspection, however, the evidence still seems thin. Schemes for treatment and monitoring are variable and complex, and none is demonstrably superior to any other. It is in any case always important to tailor treatment to the needs of the individual patient rather than following rigid guidelines.

In other reviews, the conclusion has again been reached that the long-term use of DMARDs, including penicillamine, is limited by both frequent loss of response and serious adverse reactions, and that the advantages of combination DMARDs treatments remain controversial (15,16) (SEDA-19, 229) (SEDA-20, 219) (SEDA-25, 266). In particular, the treatment of juvenile rheumatoid arthritis is difficult, since DMARDs are often poorly active in children and some (gold compounds, sulfasalazine) cause special adverse reactions, such as the macrophage activation syndrome (which in turn can lead to severe infections) (17). There is still much to be achieved and improved. As Fries has put it (16): "Determining the most clinically useful DMARD combinations and the optimal sequence of DMARD use requires effectiveness studies, Bayesian approaches and analyses of long-term outcomes. Such approaches will allow optimization of multiple drug therapies in rheumatoid arthritis, and should substantially improve the long-term outcome for many patients." In the same paper it was emphasized that patients taking penicillamine should have blood cell counts and urine protein measurements every 2 weeks during drug titration and then about monthly for as long as treatment lasts.

Since the recognition of the superior effectiveness of methotrexate and the publications of the Pediatric Rheumatology Collaborative Study Group, penicillamine has been used infrequently in juvenile rheumatoid arthritis. The maximum daily dose is about 10 mg/kg (750 mg/day) (18). This dosage is reached in three equal steps, each of 6–8 weeks' duration. Perhaps more than gold, penicillamine acts slowly, taking 9 months to 3 years for maximum effectiveness.

In a small trial, penicillamine together with metacycline was not effective in progressive multiple sclerosis (19).

Observational studies

In an Austrian study, patients with rheumatoid arthritis were followed for a mean of 10 years (20). Of 27 courses of penicillamine, 13 were discontinued because of adverse effects, 12 because of lack of effectiveness, and two because of remission. Furthermore, an analysis of the reasons for DMARD withdrawal in patients in the Czech and Slovak Republics has underlined the fact that lack of effectiveness is, in addition to adverse effects, an important reason for stopping penicillamine (21).

General adverse effects

In clinical trials about 50% of patients experienced one or more adverse effects and withdrawal was necessary in about one-third (22–26). A mucocutaneous reaction (for example a rash or stomatitis) is the most frequent reason for discontinuing the drug (27). Long-term follow-up studies have shown that many patients (up to 80%) stop taking penicillamine, either because of adverse effects or lack of efficacy (27–31).

Adverse effects are less common when small doses are used, when increments are made only slowly, when patients are closely monitored, and when penicillamine has been tolerated for some years. However, in a meta-analysis of a large series of clinical trials, dose was not a strong determinant of the risk of adverse effects (dose range 500–1250 mg/day) (26). With regard to the safe use of penicillamine the words of Huskisson (1981) are still true (32): "Perhaps the most important aspect of the surveillance of patients receiving penicillamine is the need for the physician and patient to be able to contact each other. The physician must find the patient if his blood count changes. The patient must find the physician if he becomes ill. Disasters have occurred when patients consulted physicians who were unaware of the problems of penicillamine and instituted unwise therapy for them. Penicillamine can only be used by those who know how to use it and skilful management [of its adverse effects] is a most important aspect, perhaps the most important aspect of the treatment."

In patients with rheumatoid arthritis, delayed disease complications or serious intercurrent disorders can be mistaken for complications of treatment with penicillamine or other drugs (SEDA-21, 252). Anyone responsible for a patient taking penicillamine must bear in mind that serious adverse reactions can occur suddenly and at any time during treatment, even with very small doses (as low as 125 mg/day) and after many years. Penicillamine can be the unexpected cause of serious adverse reactions as an additive to Chinese herbs (33).

Early effects are gastrointestinal upsets and, more characteristically, loss of taste. Although a fall in the number of platelets is common, serious thrombocytopenia is less frequent. After long-term use of high doses, skin collagen and elastin are impaired, resulting in increased friability and sometimes in disorders such as perforating elastoma or cutis laxa; the latter has also been observed in neonates.

Hypersensitivity reactions are frequent early in a course of penicillamine, with urticarial or maculopapular rashes, fever, and lymphadenopathy. Cross-allergy to penicillin can occur. In addition, the use of penicillamine can be complicated by a unique variety of often serious autoimmune reactions, involving the skin, kidneys, liver, lungs, muscles, or other organs. Proteinuria is found in more than 10% of patients and sometimes develops into the nephrotic syndrome. Pemphigus, myasthenia gravis, polymyositis, or a lupus-like syndrome occur in smaller percentages.

Reactions such as aplastic anemia, Goodpasture's syndrome, or thrombotic thrombocytopenic purpura (Moschcowitz's syndrome) are rare but serious.

Although lymphatic malignancies have been described in a few patients using penicillamine (SEDA-11, 212) (SEDA-8, 237), a causal relation is considered unlikely.

Combinations with other drugs used in rheumatoid arthritis

Adding chloroquine or hydroxychloroquine to penicillamine in the management of rheumatoid arthritis probably offers no therapeutic advantages, produces more adverse effects, and may even be less effective (SEDA-10, 223) (34–37). A combination of penicillamine and sulfasalazine seems to be more effective, although the extent of the advantage is uncertain, and adverse effects may be more frequent (34). In one study penicillamine and intramuscular gold together produced much earlier improvement, but efficacy and adverse effects did not differ significantly compared with either drug alone. In an open, uncontrolled study, the combination of penicillamine and intramuscular gold yielded the highest proportion of remissions in patients with refractory rheumatoid arthritis (34). The possible consequences of previous intolerance to gold compounds in association with adverse reactions to penicillamine administration have been reviewed (SEDA-8, 236); at present no firm conclusions can be made. Penicillamine does not chelate gold stores in the body.

Comparisons with other drugs used in rheumatoid arthritis

In an outpatient study in New Zealand, the changing patterns were studied in the use of "slow-acting" antirheumatic drugs (38). There were increases in the use of methotrexate and of drugs in combination, whereas there was a marked reduction in the use of auranofin. Penicillamine had the highest "average toxicity" score. However, despite the increased popularity of sulfasalazine and immunosuppressive drugs, drugs such as penicillamine continue to be used worldwide. In a long-term follow-up study, the proportion of patients who continued to take their first DMARD or who were in remission at 5 years was 53% for penicillamine, compared with 34% for aurothiomalate, 31% for auranofin, and 30% for hydroxychloroquine (39). Of the 179 patients who used penicillamine, 36 stopped taking it because of adverse effects (see Table 1). In an open, randomized, follow-up study of patients with rheumatoid arthritis, 98 were allocated to penicillamine (median daily dose 750 mg, range 375–1000 mg) and 102 to sulfasalazine (40). Over follow-up for 12 years as many as 95 patients (48%) died, four from peptic ulcer disease complications, illustrating the prevalence of premature mortality in patients with rheumatoid arthritis. Only four of the 98 patients continued to take penicillamine. Major reasons for withdrawal of penicillamine, other than death, were adverse effects ($n = 47$) and lack or loss of effect ($n = 36$) (see Table 1). In neither study was any of the deaths thought to have been related to penicillamine. The picture given in Table 1 illustrates the remarkable diversity and seriousness of the adverse reactions pattern of penicillamine.

Table 1 Adverse effects leading to the withdrawal of penicillamine in two studies

Reference	(40)	(39)
Total number of patients	98	179
Patients with adverse effects	47 (48%)	37 (20%)
Proteinuria	17	8
Rash, pruritus, or mouth ulcers		16
Nausea/vomiting	7	2
Rash	9	
Abdominal pain/dyspepsia	2	4
Thrombocytopenia	4	1
Leukopenia	2	2
Mouth ulcers	4	
Malaise	1	1
Exacerbation of joint pains		1
Myasthenia gravis		1
Pemphigus		1
Lupus-like syndrome	1	

A diagnostic and monitoring database program called DIAMOND runs across a network of personal computers throughout the Staffordshire Rheumatology Centre (41). For about 10 years, drug histories, blood test results, and clinical correspondence files for about 2000 patients have been accessible, and the system is linked to the main hospital pathology database. The DIAMOND system has been used to study adverse reactions and durations of treatment for commonly prescribed DMARDs, including penicillamine (combination treatments excluded). With a median survival time of 34 months, penicillamine held an intermediate position, between methotrexate (<96 months) and azathioprine (13 months) at the extremes; 38% of the patients continued to take penicillamine after 5 years. There were strong associations between penicillamine and both proteinuria and thrombocytopenia, both well-established adverse effects of penicillamine. Myasthenia gravis occurred in eight of 582 penicillamine users (1.4%) and not in patients using other DMARDs.

Prevention

Some 15 years ago, a more aggressive "sawtooth" strategy (early continual serial use) for the treatment of rheumatoid with disease-modifying drugs (DMARDs) was advocated (SEDA-19, 229). There is now evidence that DMARDs, when carefully monitored, are both less toxic and less effective than previously thought (42). Apparently, the sawtooth strategy has not changed the balance of benefit and harm of these drugs. No single DMARD or combination of DMARDs stood out favorably with respect to efficacy, toxicity, or survival. Ineffectiveness, rather than toxicity, was the main reason for drug withdrawal. A Canadian study has added to the evidence that the long-term results of treatment with DMARDs, such as penicillamine and gold, are disappointing, as well as in patients treated early in the course of their disease (43). After 3 years, only 30% were still taking penicillamine. After 6 years only 20% of patients had not been withdrawn, and there were no substantial differences between the drugs.

The effect of a patient education program, taught by rheumatology nurse practitioners, on adherence of patients to treatment with penicillamine has been studied

(44). The program significantly and persistently increased adherence over a period of 6 months in 51 patients compared with 49 controls (who used penicillamine without the educational program). Most of the patients (in both groups) had adverse effects, including thrombocytopenia in two and myasthenia gravis in one. The number of patients who asked to have penicillamine withdrawn was far higher in the control group ($n = 12$) compared with the patient education group ($n = 2$). Taste disturbances, for example, led to self-withdrawal in four patients, all in the control group. On the other hand, the patients in the patient education group were much more reluctant to withdraw, even in the event of serious adverse effects.

Dose relation

In a comparison of high doses (750–1000 mg/day) and low doses (125 mg every other day) of penicillamine in the treatment of early diffuse systemic sclerosis, there were no differences in efficacy (45). However, 16 of the 20 adverse event-related withdrawals were in the high-dose group. Seven of the 34 patients in the high-dose group had proteinuria (over 1 g/day) compared with only one of the 32 patients in the low-dose group. On the other hand, and in accordance with previous experience (SED-14, 723), other recorded adverse reactions, including myasthenia gravis, flu-like illness, thrombocytopenia, stomatitis, and rash, were only slightly more common in the high-dose group.

Time-course

Certain adverse effects occur predominantly during the first few months of treatment, for example taste alterations and non-specific hypersensitivity reactions, whereas others are more frequent during the second half-year of treatment (thrombocytopenia, proteinuria) or become apparent even later (for example collagen insufficiency). However, almost the entire spectrum of possible adverse reactions can occur at any time and without warning throughout a course of treatment with penicillamine. Although different schemes may be used, the monitoring of penicillamine treatment usually includes regular testing of platelet and white cell counts, a blood smear, proteinuria, and hematuria.

Organs and Systems

Cardiovascular

Penicillamine has no direct effect on the cardiovascular system. However, penicillamine-associated polymyositis can involve cardiac muscle and cause dysrhythmias, Adams–Stokes attacks, and death. Necrotizing vasculitis can occur as an immunological reaction to penicillamine (46). The effect of penicillamine on collagen and elastin fibers, which causes characteristic skin lesions, also includes the vascular wall, but effects of vascular insufficiency have not been reported.

Respiratory

Although penicillamine has no direct effects on the lungs (47), its use is associated with a spectrum of pulmonary injury: interstitial and alveolar reactions, pulmonary fibrosis, bronchiolitis obliterans, and pulmonary/renal syndromes (48–52). However, the differentiation between drug reactions and pulmonary disorders secondary to rheumatic or other underlying diseases is often difficult. The clinical presentation of bronchiolitis obliterans is acute, with cough, shortness of breath, and other non-specific respiratory complaints. The prognosis is often poor. Two separable but overlapping groups have been described: acute and chronic cellular bronchiolitis with less conspicuous scarring, and constrictive bronchiolitis, with histology varying from fibrotic and inflammatory lesions to complete small airway obliteration (SED-12, 539) (51,53–55).

In addition, several autoimmune reactions to penicillamine can secondarily affect pulmonary function. Penicillamine-induced polymyositis (56) or myasthenia gravis can cause respiratory failure, even requiring ventilatory support (57). The diagnosis and management of lupus-induced pleurisy have been reviewed (58).

Alveolar hemorrhage can occur with penicillamine, usually as part of a life-threatening pulmonary-renal syndrome resembling Goodpasture's syndrome (59,60).

Rhinitis, bronchospasm, and asthma can occur as a manifestation of hypersensitivity to penicillamine (SEDA-5, 248) (61–63) and rarely of the Churg–Strauss syndrome (64). Rhinitis can also be a symptom of penicillamine-induced pemphigus (65). In one patient a large pulmonary cyst developed concomitantly with skin lesions characteristic of the use of large doses of penicillamine (66). Microscopic derangement of the elastic fibers predominated. Although the frequency is uncertain, penicillamine can be associated with recurrent respiratory tract infections, that is secondary to IgA deficiency (67,68) or as part of the "yellow nail syndrome" (SEDA-9, 223).

Nervous system

Penicillamine, both L-penicillamine and the racemic mixture, strongly inhibit pyridoxal-dependent enzymes, cause pyridoxine deficiency in animal experiments, and are neurotoxic. Although this effect is much weaker with D-penicillamine, a few case reports have shown that D-penicillamine can also occasionally cause a polyneuropathy, as either a toxic or an allergic reaction (69–72). Rarely, an optic neuropathy (73) or a polyradiculoneuropathy (Guillain–Barré syndrome) (74,75) can occur.

When penicillamine is started in patients with Wilson's disease, pre-existing neurological involvement can acutely worsen; convulsions, muscle spasms, and coma can occur and death can follow (76–81). Worsening of neurological symptoms after starting therapy with penicillamine can occur in up to 50% of neurologically affected patients with Wilson's disease (79,80) and penicillamine can precipitate serious neurological injury in previously asymptomatic patients (82,83). It is uncertain if this results from alterations of copper distribution at submolecular, subcellular, transcellular, or transorganic levels, or whether it results from some other property of penicillamine (for example its capacity to donate sulfhydryl groups). Since the initial damage may be caused by copper decompartmentalization, it has been suggested that pretreatment with lipid-soluble antioxidants, such as vitamin E, may be useful (77), whereas at least some of these effects may reflect secondary pyridoxine deficiency. Supplementary oral pyridoxine may be advisable (80).

Two patients have been described with the internuclear ophthalmoplegia syndrome, probably induced by penicillamine. In one it was secondary to serious progressive intracerebral necrotizing vasculitis (46), in the other the underlying condition was a myasthenic reaction (84). Isolated cases have been described of neuromyotonia (85) and diffuse fasciculations (86), attributed to penicillamine.

Myasthenia

Penicillamine can induce a myasthenia gravis-like reaction, indistinguishable from idiopathic myasthenia gravis (33,57,82,87–101). It develops in up to 4% of patients using penicillamine, is most often described in patients with rheumatoid arthritis, but can also occur with other indications (for example biliary cirrhosis (102) or eosinophilic fasciitis (103)). However, it reportedly does not occur in Wilson's disease (104). The reaction often starts with involvement of ocular muscles, but any striated muscle can become involved. In contrast to other drug causes, it is characteristic of penicillamine-related myasthenia that about 90% of patients have antiacetylcholine receptor antibodies (101). The antigenic properties of circulating acetylcholine receptor antibodies in penicillamine-induced and idiopathic myasthenia are similar to those in recent-onset cases of spontaneous myasthenia gravis (92,99). Antistriational and antinuclear antibodies (105) can be present, and a sensitive immunoassay for striational autoantibodies can be used to monitor patients taking penicillamine for the development of myasthenia (94). In one study, measurement of acetylcholine receptor antibodies was considered to be of little or no use in routine monitoring of patients using penicillamine, because in 20% of patients antibodies were detected at least on one occasion, although none of the patients had signs or symptoms of myasthenia, and the antibody tests returned to normal despite continuation of the drug (106). Others have advised annual monitoring of every patient taking penicillamine, to detect subclinical changes in neuromuscular transmission and by acetylcholine receptor antibody testing (107,108).

- A 68-year-old woman, with HLA type DR1+, had been taking penicillamine (dose not specified) for 9 months for erosive seropositive rheumatoid arthritis (109). T cell clones were highly specific for D-penicillamine, but not for L-penicillamine or D-cysteine, and were restricted to HLA DR1. They responded well to blood mononuclear cells prepulsed with D-penicillamine but not to autologous B cell lines pulsed with D-penicillamine.

Apparently, penicillamine can couple directly to distinctive peptides resident in surface DR1 molecules on circulating macrophages or dendritic cells. In another article, apparently concerning the same patient, the same group described the selection of T cell clones specific for the ϵ (rather than the α or γ) subunit, responding to peptide ϵ 201–219 (110). They were restricted to HLA-DR52a (a member of the strongly predisposing HLA A1-B8-DR3 haplotype). Since these T cells had a pathogenic Th1 phenotype with the potential to induce complement-activating antibodies, they could be important targets for selective immunotherapy. In another patient, penicillamine-related myasthenia gravis developed simultaneously with polymyositis and pemphigus (111).

In spite of the similarities, there are some differences between spontaneous and penicillamine-induced myasthenia in respect to genetics. Myasthenic reactions to penicillamine appear to occur in a special genetic subgroup of patients, in whom there is a higher prevalence of the HLA antigens DRI and Bw35, and a lower prevalence of the antigens DR3 (which is associated with idiopathic myasthenia) and DR4 (which is increased in rheumatoid arthritis) (112,113).

Myasthenia usually improves rapidly after withdrawal of penicillamine, but it may have a protracted course. Fatal cases have occurred. Unrecognized myasthenia can present with prolonged paralysis after general anesthesia. For this reason, for patients taking penicillamine undergoing anesthesia the same precautions are advisable as for patients known to have myasthenia gravis (114). Penicillamine unexpectedly caused myasthenia gravis when present as an unrecognized adulterant in Chinese herbs (33).

Sensory systems

Alteration or loss of taste is a characteristic adverse effect of penicillamine. Depending on the dose used, taste impairment (dysgeusia) occurs in 10–25% of patients and when daily doses in excess of 900 mg are used this increases to over 50% (SED-11, 466) (23,115). It usually develops in about the sixth week of treatment. Patients complain of requiring increasing amounts of sugar and spices. Food does not taste normal, but salty or metallic, or like cotton wool or blotting paper. Identification of certain foods becomes difficult. Absolute taste loss can ensue but the sense of smell is unaltered. Spontaneous recovery usually follows within 6–8 weeks, despite continuation of the drug. Dysgeusia can occur at any time and can be persistent (116).

In a review of drug-induced olfactory disorders, penicillamine was mentioned as a cause of abnormal smell (117). However, there may have been confusion with its effect on taste.

In patients with Wilson's disease, penicillamine is rapidly attached to copper and, although higher doses are used, taste disturbances develop in a lower frequency, about 4% (SED-8, 536). It has been suggested that dysgeusia is related to deficiency of copper or zinc, but a strong connection between taste impairment and urinary copper excretion has not been demonstrated (118). Serum copper concentrations remained within normal limits and copper supplements were not effective in prevention (119).

In another study, there was an association with reduced serum zinc concentrations, and taste recovered after zinc supplements were given, although it should be remembered that spontaneous recovery occurs in most patients (120).

Taste alterations have been reported with other sulfhydryl compounds, including pyritinol, captopril, and propylthiouracil (121), suggesting that the thiol moiety is involved. However, dysgeusia has not been observed in many studies on the use of penicillamine in children (SEDA-7, 258) (122).

Optic neuropathy has only rarely been reported in association with penicillamine (73). In one patient, blurred vision occurred as a result of the development of bilateral choroidal hemorrhage complicating penicillamine-induced thrombocytopenia (123).

Ocular pseudotumor has been described in one patient as part of an ANCA-positive vasculitis (124).

Endocrine

A few patients are on record with suspected penicillamine-induced thyroiditis, one case being associated with a myasthenic reaction (125,126).

Metabolism

Penicillamine had a small effect on urinary glucaric acid excretion in patients with rheumatoid arthritis (127). This effect was thought to be the result of an indirect effect on hepatic metabolism and not to be related to disease activity.

Anti-insulin antibodies and hypoglycemia
One of the remarkable autoimmune phenomena that penicillamine can cause is the induction of anti-insulin antibodies, with resultant hypoglycemia (autoimmune hypoglycemia) (128,129). In these patients, there are high concentrations of immunoreactive insulin, despite undetectable free insulin. When penicillamine is withdrawn antibody titers fall sharply. The occurrence of hypoglycemia rather than hyperglycemia is not fully understood (130).

In two previously well-controlled diabetic patients taking penicillamine who developed hypoglycaemia, no reference was made to anti-insulin antibodies (131).

In a study using a competitive radiobinding assay, as many as 43% of patients with rheumatoid arthritis using penicillamine had autoantibodies against insulin (132). These antibodies did not appear to affect pancreatic beta-cells, as the response to intravenous glucose was normal and there were no episodes of hypoglycemia. Other sulfhydryl compounds that have occasionally been reported to cause autoimmune hypoglycemia are tiopronin, pyritinol, and thiamazole (methimazole) (133).

Enzyme inhibition
In in vitro studies penicillamine inhibited angiotensin-converting enzyme (ACE) and carboxypeptidase (134). Penicillamine interferes with the functions of the copper-containing enzyme ceruloplasmin, and some of the penicillamine- and copper-containing complexes formed in vivo have a superoxide dismutase effect (2). In patients with scleroderma, penicillamine normalized collagen metabolism, by inhibiting beta-galactosidase activity (135).

Nutrition

L-penicillamine strongly inhibits pyridoxal-dependent enzymes and causes pyridoxine deficiency in animals. Although D-penicillamine is much less active in this respect, there is some reduction in pyridoxine, and in a report of penicillamine-associated polyneuropathy, pyridoxine supplements for patients receiving D-penicillamine were advised (69).

Metal metabolism

Penicillamine is a potent chelator of metals. The stability of complexes of metals with penicillamine varies in the following order (from highest to lowest): mercury, lead, nickel, copper, zinc, cadmium, cobalt, iron, manganese (136–138). Most human data refer to copper, lead, and mercury.

Because of the strong affinity of penicillamine for copper and other metals, it is used in the treatment of Wilson's disease and lead poisoning. In other patients, however, this effect may sometimes cause deficiencies (SED-8, 531), especially of copper (SEDA-10, 223). Copper deficiency has been thought to play a role in the occasionally reported alopecia and in the loss of taste that is often experienced by patients with rheumatoid arthritis taking penicillamine (but rarely in Wilson's disease), but this could not be confirmed (118).

Penicillamine-induced deficiency of both copper and iron has been held responsible for the development of anemia (139), but serum iron concentrations do not usually change in patients using penicillamine (SED-8, 535).

The influence on metals such as copper and zinc may be difficult to assess, since penicillamine not only increases the excretion but also the absorption of these metals (140). A zinc deficiency syndrome, with skin lesions, alopecia, granulocytopenia, and eye damage, has been described in association with penicillamine (141).

Hematologic

The pathogenesis of hematological reactions to penicillamine is uncertain, but the available evidence suggests that pharmacological as well as immunological processes may be involved (142–144).

In the ARAMIS PMS Program, hematological events regarded as adverse effects of penicillamine, calculated per 1000 person-years, were as follows: pancytopenia 10, low white blood cell count 8, low platelet count 18, and polycythemia 2 (145). Serious blood dyscrasias, although rare, are among the most important adverse effects of penicillamine (SED-12, 541) (146,147). The assessment of the frequency of penicillamine-related hematological reactions can be hindered by the use of other potentially hemotoxic drugs, such as analgesics or gold compounds.

Eosinophilia can occur in up to 25% of patients using penicillamine, but is of little value in predicting serious hypersensitivity reactions (148).

Thrombocytopenia occurs in about 10–16% of patients and requires withdrawal in up to 10% (22,23,115), but these percentages vary considerably, presumably reflecting the use of different doses of penicillamine and different definitions of thrombocytopenia. In a series of 309 spontaneous case reports of drug-related thrombocytopenia, penicillamine was the fifth most common cause (18 cases, 6%) (149). The fall in platelet count is usually transient, but it is occasionally a warning of impending profound and dangerous thrombocytopenia or other serious hematological reactions, such as aplastic anemia or thrombotic thrombocytopenic purpura. Thrombocytopenia mainly develops during the first 6 months of penicillamine administration and appears to be associated with certain HLA antigens (DRA4, A1, C4BQO). Platelet counts fall to some extent in about 75% of patients taking penicillamine and it can be difficult to decide when to withdraw it. Platelet counts are recommended initially at 2-weekly intervals and subsequently each month, in addition to clear instructions to the patient. Weekly checks are needed when counts fall to between 100 and 70×10^9/l, and daily checks when below 70. If the platelet count falls progressively or falls below 70×10^9/l penicillamine should be immediately withdrawn (150).

In all but one of 26 children with Wilson's disease who were treated with penicillamine 20 mg/kg/day, there were fewer adverse reactions than expected: two patients developed a rash, one patient had to stop taking the drug because of a lupus-like syndrome, and another had thrombocytopenia, which resolved after treatment with prednisone (151).

Concurrent thrombocytopenia and anemia have been attributed to penicillamine (152).

- A 66-year-old woman had taken penicillamine 200 mg/day for 8 months for long-standing systemic sclerosis, together with erythromycin (800 mg/day) for prophylaxis of pulmonary infection. Her platelet count was 39×10^9/l and her hemoglobin concentration 7.3 g/dl. The leukocyte count was 3×10^9/l with a normal differential count. There was no hemolysis. A bone marrow aspirate showed mild hypoplasia and reduced megakaryopoiesis. Incubation with penicillamine produced inhibition of erythroid and megakaryocyte burst-forming units, but not of granulocyte/macrophage colony-forming units, suggesting a selective effect of penicillamine on erythropoiesis and megakaryopoiesis. The blood cell counts recovered gradually on withdrawal of both penicillamine and erythromycin, treatment with corticosteroids, and a blood transfusion.

The authors did not make reference to the effects of incubating the bone marrow with erythromycin.

There have been several cases of thrombotic thrombocytopenic purpura or Moschcowitz's syndrome, characterized by intravascular coagulation, thrombocytopenia, and hemolysis, as a rare but life-threatening complication of penicillamine (153–156). There is one case report of Evans' syndrome, thrombocytopenic purpura in combination with autoimmune hemolytic anemia, in suspected association with penicillamine (157). In this patient antiplatelet antibodies as well as antibodies against erythrocytes were detected.

Penicillamine can cause other serious hematological reactions such as agranulocytosis and aplastic anemia (27,144,146,158–167).

- Pure red-cell aplasia developed in a 40-year-old woman as a rare idiosyncratic hematological reaction to penicillamine (105). Withdrawal of the drug, which had been taken in a daily dose of 500 mg for rheumatoid arthritis, and a short course of glucocorticoids was followed by permanent recovery.

Sideroblastic anemia has been attributed to penicillamine (168).

Because of its effect on ceruloplasmin and, in turn, the utilization of stored iron, penicillamine is considered to be able to cause iron deficiency anemia (139,169,170).

Penicillamine can also cause hemolytic anemia (SEDA-8, 535) (171), although good clinical evidence of this is lacking. A positive Coomb's test can occur as part of a lupus-like syndrome (172).

Polycythemia (145), leukocytosis, and thrombocytosis have been mentioned in association with penicillamine, but data are lacking.

Mouth and teeth

Stomatitis is a troublesome adverse effect of DMARDs. Ulcers of the oral mucosa are not uncommon in patients taking penicillamine (188,173) and lead to withdrawal in 3.1% of patients (174). However, stomatitis may be a consequence of multiple factors, including hematinic deficiency, virus or Candida infection, recurrent aphthous ulceration, or Sjögren's syndrome. Moreover, aphthous stomatitis often occurs in users of non-steroidal anti-inflammatory drugs (175).

When high doses are used, stomatitis may reflect impaired collagen synthesis. In one patient, mucosal ulcers were associated with leiomyomatosis in the peripheral serosa, which in turn caused intestinal obstruction (176). In another patient taking penicillamine for Wilson's disease, the removal of an impacted maxillary third molar was followed by the development of an oroantral fistula, presumably as a result of impaired collagen synthesis and disturbed wound healing (177). Furthermore, oral ulcers may be an important warning sign of penicillamine-induced agranulocytosis.

Cheilosis has also been reported (178). Oral lesions in patients using penicillamine may be due to pemphigus, cicatricial pemphigoid, or lichen planus, even in the absence of lesions outside the oral cavity. In 56 consecutive patients taking penicillamine, oral lichen planus was found in as many as seven (179). Penicillamine-induced cicatricial pemphigoid can be associated with oral ulcers as well as lesions of the esophagus, and stenosis can develop.

Gastrointestinal

Gastrointestinal complaints, including nausea, vomiting, heartburn, abdominal distress, and diarrhea, occur in up to one-third of patients starting penicillamine and may account for up to half of the withdrawals in the first 3 months of treatment (SED-12, 541) (22,23,173). However, penicillamine is not known to be ulcerogenic (SED-8, 535) (SEDA-2, 217) (180), and the nature of gastrointestinal effects is not clear. Gastrointestinal symptoms are less frequent with initially low doses that are slowly increased. Taking penicillamine with food improves tolerance but reduces its absorption.

- A woman taking penicillamine developed dysphagia, heartburn, and weight loss; numerous large aphthoid ulcers were found in the esophagus (181).

Sulfhydryl compounds can damage the gut mucosa, but examination of the mucosa of cysteinuric patients who reported gastrointestinal upsets while taking penicillamine showed no evidence of structural damage (182).

Although less well documented than with gold, penicillamine can also occasionally cause life-threatening colitis (183).

Liver

Several case reports have demonstrated that penicillamine can cause liver damage (SEDA-13, 199) (184), mainly cholestatic hepatitis, often associated with other signs of hypersensitivity such as fever, rash (185), and pulmonary (159,186) or hematological reactions (162). In two children with Wilson's disease, penicillamine was thought to have caused persistence of a pre-existing increase in aminotransferase activity (187).

- A 30-year-old Japanese man with polyarthritis, in whom sodium aurothiomalate for 3 years had been ineffective, was given penicillamine 200 mg/day (188). After 10 days he became febrile and 2 days later jaundiced. A lymphocyte stimulation test against penicillamine was positive, suggesting type IV hypersensitivity. Later on he had a good response to tiopronin, without further adverse reactions.

In 29 Chinese patients, there was evidence in one that DMARDs and chronic viral hepatitis have synergistic hepatotoxic effects (189). However, the relevance of this anecdotal observation is uncertain.

Copper and iron are both capable of electron exchange and play a complex role in oxygen utilization. Copper proteins are critical in the transfer and transport of iron (190). In four patients with Wilson's disease, the fall in serum ceruloplasmin concentrations after treatment with penicillamine was associated with increased hepatic iron content; in two of these patients serum ferritin was increased (191). In another patient a liver biopsy taken after 15 years of treatment with penicillamine and zinc showed iron-laden hepatocytes, whereas histochemically detectable iron had been absent from an initial biopsy (192). The copper-containing protein ceruloplasmin and its membrane-bound homolog hephaestin are pivotal in iron metabolism. In addition there are intracellular transfer proteins ("chaperones") that deliver copper to ferroxidase proteins. Intracellular ferroxidase proteins accelerate the efflux of iron through stimulating the conversion of Fe^{2+} to Fe^{3+} and subsequent binding to transferrin. Presumably, excess loss of copper due to penicillamine or penicillamine plus zinc can reduce ferroxidase activity and cause intracellular iron deposition and paradoxical deterioration in liver function. Therefore, during treatment of Wilson's disease when the non-ceruloplasmin-bound copper falls to within the reference range (<150 ng/ml), the maintenance dose of penicillamine should be reduced to the minimum needed; temporary withdrawal of penicillamine may even be indicated (190).

Pancreas

There have been three poorly documented cases of pancreatitis attributed to penicillamine (SED-8, 385) (SEDA-2, 217).

Urinary tract

Penicillamine is often associated with renal damage. Proteinuria occurs in about 10–25% of patients taking penicillamine (SED-11, 464) (22,23,115,145,193–196) and occurs in 50% of patients with cysteinuria (SEDA-8, 236).

However, microalbuminuria is common in patients with rheumatoid arthritis and may reflect either rheumatoid nephropathy or renal injury caused by penicillamine (or other drugs, such as gold compounds) (197). In about 5% of patients, proteinuria is the reason for withdrawing penicillamine. To avoid renal damage, response-dependent prescribing is recommended in rheumatoid arthritis, starting with a low dose and making increments at intervals of at least 1–2 months. Frequent urine testing is necessary, particularly during the first 18 months. Mild proteinuria (<1 g/day) occurs most frequently, is often transient, and may be coincidental. Moderate proteinuria may be penicillamine-induced but need not be progressive or clinically harmful; close monitoring is indicated in such cases, and a temporary reduction in dose is advisable, although withdrawal of penicillamine may not be needed. When proteinuria increases, nephrotic syndrome can develop, necessitating withdrawal (198). In cysteinuria it is advisable to withdraw penicillamine when proteinuria exceeds 5 g/day (199), but in rheumatoid arthritis a lower limit of 2 g/day has been proposed (200). Nephropathy mainly develops during the second 6 months of treatment with penicillamine (200). It is more frequent in patients with a low sulfoxidation capacity (3,201) and with the HLA antigens DR3 and B8 (SEDA-11, 212) (202). Although nephropathy is thought to be rare in Japanese people (SEDA-8, 235) (25), it has been encountered in Japan (203).

In a comparison of high doses (750–1000 mg/day) and low doses (125 mg every other day) of penicillamine in the treatment of early diffuse systemic sclerosis, seven of the 34 patients in the high-dose group had proteinuria (over 1 g/day) compared with only one of the 32 in the low-dose group (45). Rheumatoid arthritis is a risk factor for renal disease, and the distinction from adverse drug reactions can be difficult in these patients (SED-14, 729).

On the basis of experience in one patient and 10 published case histories, the "scleroderma-pulmonary-renal syndrome," a rare and usually fatal complication of systemic sclerosis, characterized by fulminant alveolar hemorrhage and rapidly progressive renal insufficiency, has been reviewed (204). In their patient penicillamine was continued, and the disease progressed. Five of the 11 patients in their review had been using penicillamine.

In a prospective study of renal disease in 235 patients with early rheumatoid arthritis, persistent proteinuria and a raised serum creatinine concentration were predominantly related to drugs, including penicillamine and other DMARDs, whereas isolated hematuria was more directly associated with the activity of the disease process (205). Risk factors for drug-induced proteinuria were raised C-reactive protein, raised erythrocyte sedimentation rate, and age over 50 years.

Of 44 patients with rheumatoid arthritis, 24 had proteinuria (206). Two of these had drug-related nephropathy (penicillamine and gold, respectively); both had non-selective tubuloglomerular proteinuria, type V.

The principal renal lesion associated with proteinuria is membranous glomerulopathy or minimal-change glomerulopathy (196,201,207,208), characterized by minor thickening of the basement membrane or no change on light microscopy, but striking disturbances of the glomerular structures on electron microscopy (fusion of epithelial cell foot processes, subepithelial electron-dense deposits, and mesangial cell hyperactivity). Immunofluorescence microscopy shows granular deposits that contain IgG and C3 (209). These immunoglobulin deposits are not the result of precipitation of circulating immune complexes, as was previously thought. The available evidence suggests that the nephritogenic antigen, although still not identified, is expressed in the glomerulus and the immune complexes are formed in situ (207,210). Although proteinuria may be profound, serum creatinine is usually unaltered and penicillamine glomerulopathy usually has a good prognosis. Proteinuria can nevertheless continue for longer than 12 months after withdrawal and microscopic lesions can persist for longer. Although penicillamine nephropathy is more frequent when high doses are taken, it can also occur with small doses (for example 125 mg/day). On rechallenge, nephropathy does not necessarily relapse (SEDA-10, 218), and a history of previous gold nephropathy is not thought to be a risk factor (203). In one study, titers of antigalactosyl antibodies were correlated with the prior development of penicillamine (or gold) nephropathy (211).

Occasionally, penicillamine-associated renal injury is proliferative and progressive, extending beyond the basement membrane, with crescent formation in the glomeruli, and encompassing other renal structures, for example in the case of renal vasculitis, IgM nephropathy (212), or as part of a more general reaction; persistent renal insufficiency can develop and death can follow (196,213–218).

Penicillamine-induced lupus-like syndrome can be associated with proliferating glomerulonephritis with mesangial involvement and interstitial infiltrates (213,219). In such cases antibodies to native DNA can be found.

A rare but life-threatening complication of penicillamine is the development of a Goodpasture's syndrome-like reaction, characterized by alveolar hemorrhage, crescentic glomerulonephritis, and fever (59,220–224). In contrast to genuine Goodpasture's syndrome, circulating antiglomerular basement membrane antibodies are not detected (222), perhaps because the antigen concerned is not present in the test extracts used (223). Patients who have taken immunosuppressive therapy have a comparatively good outcome, but plasmapheresis and hemodialysis may be needed (220).

Serious renal injury can develop as a late complication of pre-existing benign penicillamine nephropathy (220,225). Unfortunately, microscopic hematuria has limited predictive value for imminent serious renal injury, since in most patients who take penicillamine it is a transient or coincidental finding (SEDA-7, 260). The diagnosis of penicillamine-induced renal injury is often difficult because of the frequent association of rheumatoid arthritis with renal disorders (198,204,226–228), including spontaneous membranous glomerulopathy (229), or with injury caused by concomitant analgesics (230).

In a comprehensive study of 158 Japanese patients with rheumatoid arthritis, there was an obvious relation between membranous nephropathy and exposure to disease-modifying antirheumatic drugs (DMARDs) in 40 of 49 patients (231). In this study penicillamine (15%), bucillamine (67%), and gold compounds (17%) clearly predominated.

A patient with nephrotic syndrome that developed soon after the start of treatment with penicillamine has been described in detail (232).

- A 12-year-old boy with a history of a generalized pruritic rash after penicillin took penicillamine up to 500 mg/day for Wilson's disease. He had a rash after using penicillamine for 1 week. The penicillamine was stopped for 3 days. He developed nephrotic syndrome 2 weeks after restarting penicillamine. On electron microscopy, there was the typical picture of minimal change disease with extensive foot process effacement.

In rare cases penicillamine can cause extracapillary glomerulonephritis with more extensive and serious glomerular injury leading to progressive and persistent renal insufficiency. One such patient has been described with a review of 26 similar published cases (233).

- A 51-year-old woman, who used penicillamine, maximum dose 600 mg/day, for systemic sclerosis, developed microscopic hematuria after 11 months. The penicillamine was withdrawn. Three months later she had progressive renal insufficiency. A biopsy showed extracapillary glomerulonephritis, with central fibrinoid necrosis and segmental mesangial proliferation, and marked tubulointerstitial lesions. After treatment with glucocorticoids, cyclophosphamide, and 12 plasma exchanges her renal function improved slightly.

In half of the 26 patients renal damage was associated with alveolar hemorrhage (233). In eight patients plasma exchange treatment was performed. Seven patients died, including four with alveolar hemorrhage; 12 ended up with more or less chronic renal insufficiency. Only seven patients regained normal renal function; five of these had had plasma exchange.

- Acute renal insufficiency together with diffuse alveolar hemorrhage and bilateral pulmonary infiltrates was suspected to have been caused by penicillamine (500 mg/day for 6 months) in a 34-year-old white woman, who took penicillamine for progressive systemic sclerosis (234). Because of disseminated intravascular coagulation, a biopsy was not made and the role of penicillamine remained uncertain.

Hemolytic–uremic syndrome has been described in a patient with paradoxical rapid progression of systemic sclerosis (235).

- A 58-year-old man with a complex history of Hashimoto's thyroiditis and mixed cellularity Hodgkin's disease in complete remission developed systemic sclerosis involving the skin and the lungs but not the kidneys. He was given penicillamine 250 mg/day and prednisone 60 mg/day. After a few weeks there was rapidly progressive skin thickening, spreading from the hands to the trunk. However, his treatment was not altered, and 4 months later he developed hemolytic–uremic syndrome with microangiopathic hemolytic changes, thrombocytopenia, and acute renal insufficiency, with proteinuria, hematuria, and granular casts in the urine. The renal insufficiency persisted and he died with fulminant sepsis.

Three case reports from Belgium and France have illustrated the fact that rarely proliferative crescent-forming extracapillary glomerulonephritis and renal insufficiency can also occur (236,237). All three patients had taken penicillamine for systemic sclerosis. Antimyeloperoxidase antineutrophil cytoplasm antibodies were found in all three; one patient also had alveolar hemorrhage (that is Goodpasture's syndrome).

A clinical algorithm for the management of hematuria, for example in patients taking penicillamine or NSAIDs, has been published (238). It should be borne in mind that in such patients hematuria may be symptomatic of underlying pathology (for example a tumor of the urinary tract).

In one study in children with low-level lead poisoning, urinary incontinence was mentioned as a suspected adverse effect of penicillamine (239).

Skin

There is probably no other medicine that causes skin reactions with such a high frequency and of such striking diversity as penicillamine (see Table 2).

During the first few weeks of treatment, allergic reactions occur in about one patient in five (SED-11, 465) (25).

Maculopapular or urticarial rashes are frequent and can be associated with pruritus, edema, lymphadenopathy, arthralgia, fever, and eosinophilia. Patients with previous hypersensitivity to penicillin are more likely to experience a rash when taking penicillamine. Cross-allergy to penicillin can occur, but the risk of a severe allergic reaction to penicillamine in penicillin-allergic patients is thought to be low (240,241). Skin reactions may be more common in the presence of the HLA antigen DRw6 (242), and rashes and febrile reactions were more frequent in patients with anti-Ro(SSA) antibodies (243). Early allergic reactions do not usually necessitate permanent withdrawal of penicillamine, and can often be overcome by lowering the dose or by timely withdrawal of the drug and the use of a

Table 2 Penicillamine-associated skin disorders

Maculopapular or urticarial rashes
Seborrheic dermatitis
Lichen planus-like eruptions
Psoriasiform eruptions
Erythema annulare
Photosensitivity
Pemphigus (erythematosus, foliaceus, vulgaris)
Bullous pemphigoid
Cicatricial pemphigoid
Dermatomyositis
Graft-versus-host reactions
Systemic lupus-like syndrome
Discoid lupus; subacute cutaneous lupus
Erythema multiforme and toxic epidermal necrolysis
Tardive dermopathy (friability, miliary papules, hemorrhagic bullae)
Elastosis perforans serpiginosa
Pseudoxanthoma elasticum
Cutis laxa (hyperelastica)
Cutaneous pseudolymphoma
Acantholytic dermatosis (Grover's disease)

glucocorticoid. On the other hand, a non-specific eruption can be the first sign of a serious penicillamine-induced skin disorder, for example pemphigus.

There were no serious adverse reactions in 55 children who received 66 courses of low-dose penicillamine (about 15 mg/kg/day for a mean period of 77 days) for mild to moderate lead poisoning (244). However, in three children penicillamine was withdrawn because of a transient rash.

Paradoxically, penicillamine is occasionally involved in the development of rare diseases for which it is also sometimes used, such as systemic sclerosis-like lesions (245) and circumscribed scleroderma (or morphea) (246,247).

A rash or photosensitivity can also occur as part of the penicillamine-induced lupus-like syndrome (248–250). Type II bullous systemic lupus erythematosus (251) and necrotizing vasculitis (46) have been attributed to penicillamine. In one report, a hypersensitivity reaction to penicillamine with a skin rash and fever was associated with low back pain (252).

Erythema multiforme and toxic epidermal necrolysis are considered to occur as adverse reactions to penicillamine (SEDA-12, 465) (167).

Various other skin lesions have been described.

- In one inconclusive case report acantholytic dermatosis (Grover's disease) was described as a suspected adverse reaction to penicillamine (253). This is a papulovesicular eruption in elderly people, characterized histologically by focal acantholytic dyskeratosis.
- In a female patient acne and hirsutism developed in association with breast enlargement, probably induced by penicillamine (254).
- In a 31-year-old Korean woman with Wilson's disease, high doses (1–2 g/day) of penicillamine led to the development of a dermopathy, with mildly itchy, matchhead-sized, cream-colored papules on top of dark reddish plaques on both knees and elbows (255).

Penicillamine can cause localized scleroderma (also known as morphea), which has been reviewed (257). Bullous lesions can occur in scleroderma (localized, generalized, or systemic), and this highlights the diagnostic problems in such patients (258). In one of the four case histories presented in this paper, the bullous eruption, in a patient taking penicillamine for systemic sclerosis, was diagnosed as penicillamine-induced pemphigus foliaceus.

- A man with a history of penicillin allergy developed a hypersensitivity reaction of the penis when his wife was taking penicillamine (259).

Effects on collagen and elastin

When penicillamine is administered for a long time and in high doses (for example for Wilson's disease) it can cause a characteristic delayed skin eruption, with increased friability, hemorrhagic bullous lesions, and miliary papules (66,260–266). The lesions develop predominantly in those parts of the skin that are often exposed to trauma. This disorder is a manifestation of the effects of penicillamine on collagen and elastin. Occasionally, these eruptions imitate other rare dermatological diseases and take the shape of elastosis perforans serpiginosa, cutis hyperelastica (cutis laxa) (267), or pseudoxanthoma elasticum (268–270); however, the histological and ultrastructural characteristics of the penicillamine variants differ from those of the spontaneous disorders.

In delayed penicillamine skin disorders, abnormal elastic tissue also exists in non-lesional skin, and has occasionally been documented in other organs (lungs, blood vessels, ileum, visceral adventitia, joint tissue), but the clinical implications of these findings are uncertain. In one study, multiple lymphangiectases and bloodvessel-lymphatic anastomoses were observed (263). Clinically manifest impairment of collagen and elastin has been reported in association with much lower penicillamine doses than had previously been recognized (271–273). In five of eight patients receiving penicillamine for rheumatoid arthritis, there was elastic fiber damage in joint capsules, suggesting that penicillamine-associated collagen injury may be common (273), although in only one case there was also elastic fiber damage in a skin biopsy. The fact that the lesions in delayed penicillamine skin disorders concentrate in flexural areas (neck, axillae, antecubital fossae, and buttocks) may reflect the accelerated turnover rate of elastin in these areas, secondary to shearing stresses and stretching. Perhaps impairment of collagen interferes with wound healing.

Presumably, the mechanism underlying penicillamine dermopathy is inhibition by penicillamine of cross-linkage of collagen fibers. In addition, the enzyme lysyl oxidase, required for the cross-linking of collagen fibers, is copper-dependent and may be inhibited by copper chelation by penicillamine. Another argument for a possible role of copper deficiency is the fact that cutis laxa is common in Menke's disease, a rare genetically determined disturbance of copper metabolism. Perforating elastoma occurs when abnormal elastic fibers accumulate, cause a foreign body reaction, and are transepidermally eliminated. Although the patient was also thought to have elastolytic involvement of the lining of the upper respiratory tract, there was no objective evidence of this.

Elastosis perforans serpiginosa, cutis laxa, and pseudoxanthoma elasticum

In rare cases, penicillamine dermopathy mimics elastosis perforans serpiginosa, cutis laxa, or pseudoxanthoma elasticum.

Elastosis perforans serpiginosa

Elastosis perforans serpiginosa starts as red umbilicated papules that coalesce to form annular (serpiginous or arcuate) lesions with clear centres. There are microscopically thickened coarse elastic fibers, extruding through narrow epidermal channels.

- A 37-year-old Japanese woman, who was taking penicillamine (500 mg/day) for systemic sclerosis, developed papules distributed in characteristic arcuate patterns of the skin of her neck (274). Histologically there was transepidermal elimination of degenerative elastic particles.

Cutis laxa

Cutis laxa presents with loose redundant skin folds, reduced elasticity of the skin, and connective tissue involvement.

- An 84-year-old woman, who had been taking penicillamine 1.2 g/day for 50 years for Wilson's disease, developed generalized, rapidly progressive, acquired cutis laxa (275). Faulty production of collagen and elastin fibers lead to gross folding of the skin, giving it an appearance reminiscent of the folds of the cerebral cortex.

In one patient the characteristic features of both of elastosis perforans serpiginosa and cutis laxa developed (276).

- A 36-year-old man, who had had Wilson's disease since the age of 4 years, had used penicillamine for about 13 years in a dosage of 2–3 g/day. He developed an itching papular eruption, which initially resolved after withdrawal of the drug but recurred and progressed 6 months later. Generalized cutis laxa developed, with perforating elastolytic nodules on the neck and elastosis perforans serpiginosa over the shoulders. A biopsy showed perforating channels from the dermis through the epidermis, with a surrounding inflammatory infiltrate and horseshoe-shaped multinuclear giant cells phagocytosing abnormal elastic fibers. Van Giesen staining showed a lumpy-bumpy appearance of elastin fibers, typical of penicillamine dermopathy, as originally described by Bardach et al. (SED-14, 730).

Pseudoxanthoma elasticum

Pseudoxanthoma elasticum is characterized by coalescent yellow waxy papules with a "plucked chicken" appearance (because of the prominence of follicular orifices in the papules) and a marked laxity and wrinkling of the skin, resulting in redundant skin folds. In delayed penicillamine skin disorders gross abnormalities of elastic and collagen fibers are seen on electron microscopy. Elastic fibers have "moth-eaten," "saw-toothed," or "bramble bush thorns" appearances. Collagen fibers show large differences in thickness. Elastic tissue stains show an increase in the number of elastic fibers and irregular serrated fibers. The elastin content of lesional skin is three times greater than normal, whereas the number of elastin cross-links is only 15% of normal. In electron photomicrographs, dermal elastic fibers are studded with multiple perpendicular buds of different sizes and shapes, described as "lumpy-bumpy" and show varying degrees of fragmentation. Aggregations of granular elastinophilic material surround the central core of normal mature elastic tissue. In contrast to spontaneous pseudoxanthoma elasticum there is no calcium deposition in elastic fibers.

- A 47-year-old man had been using penicillamine 1.5 mg/day for 18 years for Wilson's disease. He developed pseudo-pseudoxanthoma combined with dysphagia and dyspnea. Biopsy specimens showed systemic involvement of elastic fibers, including skin, lung, esophageal muscle, gum, and pharyngeal and cervical connective tissue. All biopsies showed abnormal elastic fibers, consisting of a central core of uneven thickness with many lateral arborizations. There were branches at right angles to the main fibers, with perpendicular lateral arborizations off these, producing a stag-horn or fractal appearance. On the other hand, the adjacent collagen fibers were normal in structure.

Pseudo-pseudoxanthoma elasticum, caused by the use of high doses of penicillamine, has also been described (277).

Wound healing

In the past, penicillamine, because of its effects on collagen synthesis, has been suspected of interfering with normal wound healing. Experience of 217 operations in 150 patients did not show such effects, and consequently, there does not seem to be a need for stopping penicillamine before surgery (278). On the other hand, a few reports have suggested that penicillamine can, at least in some patients, have deleterious effects on wound healing (177,279).

Pemphigus

Pemphigus is a bullous autoimmune disorder of the skin, characteristically associated with antidesmoglein antibodies. Although many different drugs have been described as a cause of pemphigus, there is a remarkably strong predominance of penicillamine (and other sulfhydryl compounds) (280–283). Three groups of pemphigus-inducing drugs can be distinguished (284):

1. thiol drugs (for example penicillamine);
2. "masked thiol drugs" (sulfur-containing drugs that undergo metabolic changes to form thiol groups, for example piroxicam, beta-lactam compounds);
3. drugs with an active amide group (for example dipyrone, enalapril).

Thiol-related pemphigus usually presents as the foliaceus variant, with comparatively few immunofluorescence findings and a good prognosis, whereas drugs with an active amide group can provoke pemphigus vulgaris with a less favorable prognosis on drug withdrawal. A pemphigus-like eruption (284–297) develops in 1–2% of the users of penicillamine (SEDA-11, 213). Penicillamine is by far the most frequent cause of the drug-related variant.

- A 71-year-old woman taking penicillamine (dosage not specified) developed pemphigus vulgaris rather than pemphigus foliaceus, which is the usual form of pemphigus that penicillamine causes (298). She presented with pustular bullae (due to secondary infection with *Pseudomonas aeruginosa*), and the indication for penicillamine was not rheumatoid arthritis but systemic sclerosis.
- A 64-year-old woman, who had used penicillamine 500 mg/day for 3 years for rheumatoid arthritis, developed a bullous skin eruption affecting her neck and limbs (299). After treatment with prednisolone (dose not specified) she improved, but relapsed when the dose was reduced below 10 mg. Eleven months after the onset of blistering, penicillamine was discontinued and within 2 months the prednisolone was also stopped, with no recurrence of the eruption during 12 months follow-up. Direct immunofluorescence was positive for immunoglobulin G and complement component C3,

and indirect immunofluorescence was positive on the roof of the NaCl split skin preparation.

A consultation of the database of the Committee on Safety of Medicines in London showed that 41 cases of bullous pemphigoid have been reported in suspected connection with penicillamine, suggesting that this adverse reaction is less rare that the published literature suggests.

Pemphigus usually recedes when penicillamine is stopped, but can persist for many years (286,296), and recur on rechallenge (300); fatal cases have occurred (301,302). Pemphigus that continues after drug withdrawal is referred to as triggered pemphigus, whereas a reaction that clears soon after withdrawal is called induced pemphigus (285). Although it is usually rapidly reversible, penicillamine-induced pemphigus can run a protracted course (SED-14, 730). In a report from the Netherlands, penicillamine-related pemphigus foliaceus was highly resistant to treatment for 7 years (303). Eventually the intravenous administration of low doses of normal human immunoglobulin (40 mg/kg/day for 5 days in cycles of 3 weeks), together with dexamethasone pulse therapy, led to remission.

The entire clinical and pathological spectrum of pemphigus can occur in association with penicillamine, that is pemphigus erythematosus, pemphigus foliaceus, pemphigus vulgaris, and bullous pemphigoid (297). In this order of sequence the level of blister formation descends from the superficial layers to the deeper layers of the epidermis toward the basement membrane and subepidermal tissue. Penicillamine-induced pemphigus is predominantly of the foliaceus type. As in spontaneous pemphigus, antidesmoglein antibodies are present, although they may not be found in early stages. In pemphigus vulgaris antibodies react with desmoglein 3 and in pemphigus foliaceus with desmoglein 1, suggesting that different antigens are involved (304,305). The antibody reactivity of patients with idiopathic and penicillamine-related pemphigus appeared to be the same (284), which is suggestive of a similar basic molecular mechanism. Sometimes the characteristic lesions of different eruptions, for example pemphigus, bullous or cicatricial pemphigoid, lupus erythematosus, discoid lupus, or seborrheic dermatitis, can be seen in one and the same patient taking penicillamine (SEDA-11, 213) (SEDA-15, 239) (300). This suggests differences in the pathogenic process rather than the simultaneous occurrence of different reactions.

Penicillamine has epidermotropic properties and accumulates in the skin. There are several possible mechanisms involved in penicillamine-induced pemphigus (SED-12, 544):

- penicillamine may cause acantholysis by direct destruction of epidermal intercellular attachment (without pemphigus antibodies) (306–308);
- the drug may induce autoantigens through modification of epidermal differentiation or interaction with epidermal tissues;
- penicillamine may change immunological tolerance, influence T-suppressor cells, and elicit autoimmune responses (280,281).

There is still uncertainty about the precise underlying processes. Apart from a reduced frequency of the rheumatoid arthritis-associated antigen B15, penicillamine-induced pemphigus does not appear to be strongly associated with a characteristic HLA antigen pattern (309,310).

Penicillamine-induced pemphigus can pose diagnostic difficulties, for example because it can present as a non-specific rash, seborrheic dermatitis, erythema annulare (311), isolated stomatitis, or even rhinitis (65). Because of the friability of the superficial blisters, the bullous nature of pemphigus erythematosus and pemphigus folia-ceus may be overlooked.

Since beta-lactam antibiotics also appear to be asso-ciated with pemphigus, especially ampicillin and amoxi-cillin, an earlier hypothesis (SEDA-5, 244) that this (and perhaps other reactions) to beta-lactam antibiotics may in fact be induced by the hydrolytic metabolite penicilla-mine has received attention (280,283).

A rare but potentially serious skin reaction to penicil-lamine is cicatricial pemphigoid (312,313). These patients can have symblepharon and entropion of the eyes, ulcers in the mouth, and blistering lesions on the trunk, extre-mities, and perineum (314). Involvement of the esopha-geal or vaginal epithelium can cause stenosis.

Ulcerative lesions of the vagina can occur in patients taking penicillamine, as a manifestation of pemphigus or cicatricial pemphigoid, or following impaired collagen synthesis (SED-8, 533) (315).

Graft-versus-host-like eruptions

Although rarely described, skin reactions that mimic graft-versus-host disease are an established complication of penicillamine (SED-14, 731). The similarity of the pathology of these drug-induced eruptions to those that occur after bone marrow transplantation has been reviewed (316). The drug-related eruptions may have different manifestations and can, for example, resemble smallpox, lichen planus (317), eczema, or other eruptions (318). However, their histological features are similar to those seen in cutaneous graft-versus-host disease, in par-ticular eruptions in which liquefactive necrosis is seen at the interface between the epidermis and the cutis. One of the possible mechanisms involved in hypersensitivity reactions to sulfhydryl-containing drugs is based on the immune response of T cells to the sulfhydryl group, which arises when binding of IL-2 to the IL-2 receptor induces autoreactive T cells (319). The concentrations of IL-2 and IL-2 receptor were closely associated with the onset and severity of cutaneous graft-versus-host disease, suggesting an etiological similarity between the disease and skin eruptions induced by sulfhydryl-containing drugs. Proliferation of autoreactive T cells is induced by the binding of IL-2 to its receptor in these patients.

With seven cases in 56 consecutive patients taking peni-cillamine in one study, oral lichen planus may be fairly frequent (179). Most patients have erosive oral lichen planus, but bullous, plaque-like, or "classic" lichen planus can occur. Rarely a psoriasiform eruption has been reported with penicillamine (320).

Hair

Alopecia has occasionally been reported in association with penicillamine (145), but is ill-understood; hair loss can occur in association with polymyositis (321).

Nails

The peculiar yellow nail syndrome (SEDA-9, 223), char-acterized by dystrophy of the nails, lymphedema, pleural effusion, and bronchial involvement, has occasionally been reported in association with penicillamine and also with bucillamine (SEDA-9, 223) (SED-13, 612) (322–325). It has been suggested that penicillamine and bucillamine, because of their structural similarity to cysteine, might disturb nail growth by interfering with keratin synthesis. Although the nail changes and injury to other organs probably develop by different mechan-isms, in patients with nail changes a careful search for possible systemic disorders is needed.

Monosymptomatic nail changes, with longitudinal rid-ging, transverse or longitudinal defects of the nail plate, absence of lunulae, and a tendency toward onychoschizia, can also occur as adverse effects of penicillamine (326).

Musculoskeletal

Joint symptoms in patients taking penicillamine vary from "creaking" and subjective discomfort and worsening of joint pain to severe arthralgia (327–329). Paradoxical acute severe exacerbation of rheumatoid arthritis has been reported in three patients, probably induced by penicillamine (330). Arthritis can also be a manifestation of penicillamine-induced systemic lupus erythematosus.

Although rare, Wilson's disease may itself be asso-ciated with a polyarthritis resembling rheumatoid arthritis and when it develops during the use of penicillamine it can be mistaken for an adverse reaction to the drug (331). Demineralization osteopathy has been reported in a study on the use of D-penicillamine in Wilson's disease (SED-8, 536).

- Progressive eosinophilic fasciitis with muscular involve-ment in a 35-year-old Brazil woman has been attributed to penicillamine (250 mg/day) (332).

In a prospective analysis of 74 women with systemic sclerosis, low bone mineral density and densitometric osteoporosis were related to the menopause and not to the previous use of penicillamine or other drugs (333).

Reproductive system

Gigantism of the breasts (macromastia) can occur in patients using penicillamine (SEDA-8, 238) (255,334–338). It usually develops in women and very rarely as gynecomastia in men (337,339). There is resemblance to the pubertal form of massive breast enlargement. It can be painful and has been encountered in pre- and postmenopausal women, with normal and increased prolactin concentrations. Histological examina-tion mainly shows increased connective tissue and no changes in the glandular tissue.

- In one patient, the breasts were tender and grew pro-gressively larger during each menstrual period.
- A 55-year-old premenopausal woman took penicilla-mine 1 g/day for 2 years for localized scleroderma (340). She used no other drugs. She noticed a gradual enlargement of her breasts, from a size B to size D+ bra cup. There were no palpable masses or tenderness. The only abnormal laboratory test finding was a positive test

for homogeneous antinuclear antibodies (titer < 1:80), which is often found in patients with scleroderma. Serum prolactin was normal. Penicillamine was withdrawn and the breast enlargement regressed over 3 months; the bra cup size reverted to B.

- In a 25-year-old woman with Wilson's disease, treatment with penicillamine (1.5 g/day) was first followed by the development of hirsutism, mainly of the face (255). After she started to use an oral contraceptive, her breasts enlarged rapidly and she experienced cyclic mastodynia; in addition, gingival hyperplasia developed. All symptoms improved on withdrawal of penicillamine, but additional mammoplasty was needed.

The sequence of events in the last patient suggested that the use of the oral contraceptive contributed to the development of macromastia.

In one case breast enlargement was accompanied by systemic lupus erythematosus (341).

- A 37-year-old woman with a 7-year history of rheumatoid arthritis had taken penicillamine for about 1–2 years (dose not specified). When she presented at the Cambridge Breast Unit she had had rapidly increasing painful enlargement of the breasts for 7 months. The breasts were symmetrically enlarged (from an A cup to DD) and had thickened and erythematous skin. There were several palpable masses; mammography showed no evidence of malignancy and an ultrasound scan showed large hypo-echoic nodules with engorged vessels. Histology of a large lump in the left breast showed a fibroadenoma. Immunohistochemistry for estrogen receptors showed 50% nuclear staining. She had stopped taking penicillamine 2 months before because of a lupus-like syndrome with thrombocytopenia, lymphopenia, and positive ANA and DNA antibodies (whether single-stranded or double-stranded was not stated).

Although breast gigantism is a rare manifestation of idiopathic SLE, in this case autoimmune substances could have stimulated mammary duct proliferation or mimicked estrogen or other growth factors in the breast.

Immunologic

Several experimental studies in humoral and cell-mediated immune systems have demonstrated numerous effects of penicillamine on the immune system; these findings are in keeping with a reduction in the overactivity of helper T lymphocyte that is found in rheumatoid arthritis (2,342). There is a fall in the numbers of immunoglobulin-secreting cells, and cultured mononuclear cells produce less IgA, IgG, and IgM. There is suppression of the autologous mixed lymphocyte reaction (343) and reduced hydroxyl radical generation from polymorphonuclear leukocytes (344). Penicillamine reduces the clearance of immune complexes and inhibits the complement cascade (345).

Penicillamine is uniquely likely among therapeutic drugs to cause autoimmune reactions (see Table 3).

Clinically and pathologically these variants of autoimmune disorders are closely similar to or indistinguishable from the spontaneous diseases. A major difference is that the patients usually recover when penicillamine is withdrawn. Differences in HLA configurations also

Table 3 Autoimmune-like reactions reported in suspected association with penicillamine

Pemphigus (erythematosus, foliaceus, vulgaris)
Bullous pemphigoid, cicatricial pemphigoid
Graft-versus-host-like skin eruptions
Myasthenia gravis
Dermatomyositis/polymyositis
Glomerulonephritis
Lupus-like syndrome
Goodpasture's syndrome
Autoimmune hypoglycemia
Thyroiditis
Sjögren's syndrome
Aplastic anemia
Thrombocytopenia
Agranulocytosis
Thrombotic thrombocytopenic purpura (Moschcowitz's syndrome)
Evans' syndrome
Churg–Strauss syndrome
Necrotizing vasculitis
Guillain–Barré syndrome

suggest that penicillamine-induced and spontaneous autoimmune disorders occur in different populations.

During penicillamine treatment autoantibodies develop in a high proportion of patients without clinical disease (346). For example, penicillamine can be associated with the development of anticentromere antibodies (347,348). Although these are usually a marker of serious autoimmune diseases, in association with penicillamine, the phenomenon was not accompanied by clinical symptoms and disappeared after stopping the drug.

In the serum of three patients with acute hypersensitivity reactions to penicillamine, complement-binding antibodies against penicillamine were detected (349). Patients with Wilson's disease are not known to have an abnormal immune status. The striking variability of penicillamine-induced pathology, including autoimmune reactions such as SLE, is also seen in patients with Wilson's disease, but the proportion of these patients in whom withdrawal is necessary is smaller, about 2–8% (72,79,80,350).

An unusual case report showed that low back pain can be a manifestation of drug hypersensitivity (253).

Anaphylaxis

Although hypersensitivity reactions are frequent, systemic anaphylaxis has only been reported rarely (351).

ANCA-positive vasculitis

Various vasculitic diseases, including Wegener's granulomatosis, microscopic polyangiitis, Churg–Straus syndrome, and crescentic glomerulonephritis, are associated with antineutrophil cytoplasmic antibodies (ANCA) or leukocytoclastic vasculitis. In drug-induced ANCA-positive vasculitis antimyeloperoxidase antibodies are most often found; they produce a perinuclear pattern of staining by indirect immunofluorescence (pANCA), but antiproteinase 3 (anti-PR3) antibodies can also occur (cANCA).

The possible drug causes of ANCA-positive vasculitis with high titers of antimyeloperoxidase antibodies in

30 new patients have been reviewed (124). The findings illustrate that this type of vasculitis is a predominantly drug-induced disorder. Only 12 of the 30 cases were not related to a drug. The most frequently implicated drug was hydralazine (10 cases); the rest involved propylthiouracil (three cases), penicillamine (two cases), allopurinol (two cases), and sulfasalazine.

- A 49-year-old woman with systemic sclerosis, taking penicillamine 750 mg/day, developed a vasculitis, with an orbital pseudotumor and, 2 months later, fatal alveolar hemorrhage. She also had antinuclear antibodies with a homogeneous pattern.
- A 56-year-old woman with systemic sclerosis taking penicillamine 750 mg/day had homogeneous antinuclear antibodies and antibodies to native DNA. Her manifestations of vasculitis were glomerulonephritis with renal insufficiency, pulmonary hemorrhage, and bilateral hemothorax (that is similar to Goodpasture's syndrome).

As the authors pointed out, practically all drugs known to cause ANCA-positive vasculitis (including penicillamine) have also been associated with a lupus-like syndrome, suggesting the possibility of a similar underlying mechanism. However, the presence of discriminating markers (such as anti-elastase and antilactoferrin antibodies) in drug-induced ANCA-positive vasculitis, but not in idiopathic cases, is suggestive of different pathways in these conditions.

In three Japanese patients with penicillamine-associated glomerulonephritis, antimyeloperoxidase ANCA assays were strongly positive (352). These patients had been taking penicillamine for rheumatoid arthritis in daily doses of 100, 200, and 300 mg for 32, 42, and 39 months respectively. All three had proteinuria, hematuria, anemia, and rapidly progressive renal insufficiency. Histological examination showed crescentic glomerulonephritis with granular deposits of IgG, IgM, IgA, C1q, and C3 in the mesangium. Penicillamine was withdrawn and the patients were given steroid pulse therapy, warfarin, and in two cases cyclophosphamide. Renal function gradually improved and the antineutrophil cytoplasmic antibodies disappeared.

- In a 69-year-old man with penicillamine-induced crescentic glomerulonephritis ANCA tests were repeatedly negative (353). He had been taking penicillamine up to 750 mg/day for systemic sclerosis.

Churg–Strauss syndrome
The Churg–Strauss syndrome is a rare disease, with eosinophilia, vasculitis, and granulomas, involving many organ systems (skin, lungs, kidneys, gastrointestinal tract, joints, heart, and central nervous system); rhinitis and asthma are often early manifestations. In one of two patients with the syndrome, penicillamine might have triggered its development (64); however, withdrawing the drug had no effect on the course of the disease and the relation was therefore uncertain.

Dermatomyositis and polymyositis
Penicillamine can cause other serious autoimmune reactions involving the muscles: dermatomyositis, with its characteristic facial rash (354), and polymyositis (56,95,96,321,355–366).

Effects vary from only biochemical abnormalities, through moderate muscular weakness, to severe polymyositis with myolysis and sometimes myocarditis. There can be dysrhythmias, heart block, and Adams–Stokes attacks (362) and deaths have occurred (96). Muscle weakness can cause secondary respiratory failure (56,321). The clinical, pathological, and electromyographic features are similar to those of idiopathic polymyositis.

Antinuclear antibodies are found in about 90% of cases of penicillamine-induced polymyositis, a finding that may be helpful in distinguishing this condition from true polymyositis (357). In one patient anti-Jo-1 antibodies were found, which was thought to be an epiphenomenon and not pathogenic (78). Myositis occurs in about 1% of patients taking penicillamine and appears to be relatively common in Japanese and Indian patients (SEDA-15, 240) (23,355,363). HLA investigations showed that the antigens DR2 and DQw1 are increased in patients with penicillamine-induced myositis, suggesting that myositis occurs in a specific genetic subgroup (363). Of interest is the report of a patient with penicillamine-associated polymyositis who had a relapse after administration of ampicillin (358).

In penicillamine-induced polymyositis, weakness can be the presenting symptom and it may at first be mistaken for myasthenia (56).

The diagnostic pitfalls of penicillamine-induced polymyositis have been reviewed in the light of a report of a patient in whom postural changes were at first mistaken for possible ankylosing spondylitis (367).

IgA deficiency
IgA deficiency is a rare penicillamine-induced immune disorder, which can be accompanied by recurrent upper respiratory tract infections (67,68,368). IgA deficiency is more likely to develop when there is improved rheumatic disease activity, together with other adverse effects (for example rash, thrombocytopenia, proteinuria).

Lupus-like syndrome
Serological features of systemic lupus erythematosus develop in about 7% of patients taking penicillamine (172,227,249–251,369). A clinical lupus-like syndrome is less frequent (about 2%) and is as frequent in rheumatoid arthritis as in Wilson's disease. Characteristic phenomena are polyarthropathy, rash, pleurisy, fever, leukopenia, thrombocytopenia, antinuclear antibodies, and LE cells. The syndrome can be associated with antibodies to native DNA, renal damage, and neurological symptoms. The disorder usually improves in a few weeks or months after stopping penicillamine, but serological tests may remain abnormal for a longer period. Also, type II bullous systemic lupus erythematosus has been attributed to penicillamine (252). Penicillamine is no longer used in juvenile rheumatoid arthritis, in particular because of lack of effect and the possibility of inducing a lupus-like syndrome (370).

- A 6-year-old Taiwanese girl, who had taken penicillamine (dosage not specified) for Wilson's disease for 17 months, developed arthralgia, fever, and oral ulcers (371). She had antinuclear antibodies with a homogeneous pattern at a dilution of 1/5120, and a direct

Coombs' test was positive. On the other hand, anti-DNA antibodies were within the reference range and antibodies against non-histone nuclear antigens (Sm, RNP, SS-A/Ro, SS-B/La, Scl-70) were all negative. She improved with prednisolone, and penicillamine was continued in a lower dosage.

Sjögren's syndrome

There have been two reports of Sjögren's syndrome (keratoconjunctivitis sicca, xerostomia, swelling of the parotids) in suspected association with penicillamine (372,373). In one study, reference was made to a patient with a Henoch–Schönlein-like syndrome as a suspected adverse reaction to penicillamine, but no details were given (374).

Multiple autoimmune reactions

Penicillamine often elicits multiple adverse reactions in the same patient, illustrating its immunomodulatory actions. Examples are listed in Table 4.

In a long-term prospective study of 69 patients taking penicillamine (750 mg/day) for progressive systemic sclerosis, 27 had adverse effects requiring either temporary reduction or complete withdrawal of therapy. Five of these had two, or, in one case, three different reactions (115).

- A 47-year-old woman developed concurrent pemphigus and myasthenia gravis (with ptosis and diplopia), apparently induced by penicillamine (500 mg/day for rheumatoid arthritis) (376).

In another patient, pemphigus, polymyositis, and myasthenia gravis developed simultaneously (111).

- A 67-year-old patient with rheumatoid arthritis had taken penicillamine 600 mg/day for 15 months when a skin eruption developed. Although no intercellular substance or basement membrane antibodies were found, a biopsy showed characteristic intraepidermal blistering. Direct immunofluorescence showed anti-IgG and anti-C3 antibodies, and desmoglein immunolabelling (32–2B) favored drug-induced pemphigus. In addition, acetylcholine receptor antibodies were found. After the withdrawal of penicillamine there was rapid improvement of pemphigus and myasthenia. However, polymyositis was progressive, required high doses of corticosteroids for about 18 months, and improved only slowly.

Table 4 Examples of simultaneous multiple reactions reported with penicillamine

Pulmonary alveolitis, pancytopenia, cholestatic hepatitis, stomatitis, proctitis, skin rash, proteinuria, renal insufficiency (52)
Cholestatic hepatitis with allergic pneumonitis (186)
Pemphigus and nephrosis (minimal change nephropathy) (375)
Pemphigus and myasthenia gravis (376)
Thyroiditis and myasthenia gravis (125)
Polyradiculopathy and nephrosis (70)
Aplastic anemia and cholestatic hepatitis (162)
Gingival hyperplasia, acne, hirsutism, breast gigantism (255)
Agranulocytosis and toxic epidermal necrolysis (167)

Desensitization

The National Taiwan University Hospital has reported successful desensitization with prednisolone in a patient with hypersensitivity to penicillamine (377).

- A 14-year-old boy with Wilson's disease had a rash, fever, and angioedema repeatedly after the administration of penicillamine (600 mg/day). He was given prednisolone 30 mg/day for 2 days and then 20 mg/day. He was given penicillamine in an initial dose of 300 mg/day, which was increased to 600 mg/day in increments of 150 mg over 3 days and subsequently to 900 mg/day. Prednisolone was gradually discontinued over a 4-week interval, and penicillamine was increased to 1.2 g/day without further problems.

Infection risk

In a nested case-control study in Mexican patients with rheumatoid arthritis encompassing 1274 patient years, the risk factors were determined for acquiring infectious diseases (378). In addition to the cumulative doses of methotrexate and the duration of corticosteroids use, the mean daily dose of penicillamine was a risk factor. In one patient the infection was secondary to neutropenia. Tests for a possible immunoglobulin deficiency were not performed.

Long-Term Effects

Mutagenicity

In one experimental study it has been suggested that penicillamine may be mutagenic (379).

Tumorigenicity

There are a few case reports of lymphatic malignancies in patients using penicillamine, but epidemiological data in support of the association are lacking (SEDA-7, 259) (380–382).

Second-Generation Effects

Teratogenicity

Whereas the benefits of penicillamine outweigh the risk in patients with Wilson's disease and probably cysteinuria, there have been a few reports of congenital injury attributed to the use of penicillamine, notably congenital cutis hyperelastica with a fatal course in three infants. Penicillamine should be withdrawn during pregnancy in patients with rheumatoid arthritis (383–385). It should be added, however, that in Wilson's disease it is also worth considering if it is possible to control copper metabolism with less penicillamine or without it altogether.

- A baby with a bilateral cleft lip with total cleft palate was born at 41 weeks to a 22-year-old mother who had taken penicillamine (dosage not specified) throughout an uncomplicated pregnancy for Wilson's disease (386). The child did not have a lax skin.

This case was found as part of a case-control study of 24696 mothers of malformed infants. It was the only case of penicillamine exposure in the entire series.

However, cleft lip has not previously been observed in association with maternal use of penicillamine, and there is little reason for suspecting the drug.

Susceptibility Factors

Genetic factors

Several studies have shown an increased frequency of penicillamine adverse effects in patients with low sulfoxidation activity, especially with regard to proteinuria and probably thrombocytopenia and myasthenia gravis (SED-12, 547) (3,196,387,388). The sulfoxidation capacity is expressed as the sulfoxidation index, calculated as the percentage of administered S-carboxymethyl-L-cysteine (750 mg), excreted as sulfoxides in the urine in 8 hours. A sulfoxidation index above 6% is taken as indicative of relative impairment of sulfoxidation capacity.

Certain adverse reactions to penicillamine are associated with increased or decreased frequencies of HLA antigens (SEDA-8, 235) (SEDA-11, 212) (22,389–396). Most consistently reported are the associations between proteinuria and the antigens B8 and DR3 and between thrombocytopenia and DR4. These associations are not strong enough to include HLA typing into the routine of treatment with penicillamine. The relative risk of toxicity for patients possessing either HLA-DR3 or poor sulfoxidation appeared to be 25 as compared with those possessing neither; if these tests could be simplified, a valuable opportunity would become available for identifying patients at risk (202,387). Racial factors may be involved: proteinuria is less frequent in Japanese people, whereas polymyositis occurs at an increased frequency in India and Japan (202,330).

Age

Although published experience in children is limited, penicillamine has the same pattern of adverse effects as in adults. However, an interesting difference is that taste dysfunction has so far not been reported in children (SED-10, 221) (SEDA-14, 198). In two children with Wilson's disease, penicillamine was thought to have caused persistence of a pre-existing increase in amintransase activity (187).

Other features of the patient

Patients with previous hypersensitivity to penicillin are more likely to experience a rash when taking penicillamine. Cross-allergy to penicillin can occur, but the risk of a severe allergic reaction to penicillamine in penicillin-allergic patients is thought to be low. An important measure to reduce the frequency of adverse reactions of penicillamine is to start with a small dosage (for example 125 mg/day in rheumatoid arthritis), to increase the dosage only slowly, and to maintain treatment with the lowest effective dosage. Nevertheless, serious complications such as nephrosis, pemphigus, alveolitis, and polymyositis have occurred while only 250 mg/day or less was used (SEDA-8, 235) (50,182,355).

The absorption of penicillamine can be significantly altered by alimentary factors. Changing habits, for example taking penicillamine between meals instead of with food, or stopping iron supplements, can precipitate adverse reactions by increased absorption.

Early hypersensitivity reactions are usually transient, and although there is undoubtedly an increased risk, in patients with a history of previous adverse reactions to penicillamine (or gold), re-exposure may not be followed by a relapse (SEDA-10, 218). In the case of serious complications, such as agranulocytosis, profound thrombocytopenia, polymyositis, or Goodpasture's syndrome, the repeated use of penicillamine carries unacceptable risks. Commencing penicillamine in patients with Wilson's disease can aggravate or even precipitate neurological involvement.

Antibodies to the Ro(SSA) cellular antigen (244,397) and circulating cryoglobulins (244) are risk factors for adverse reactions to penicillamine. AntiRo (SSA) antibodies characterize a distinct group of patients with rheumatoid arthritis who are almost exclusively female, express more activated B cell function, have a high prevalence of Sjögren's features, and commonly develop adverse reactions to penicillamine. Rashes and febrile reactions were especially associated with anti-Ro(SSA) antibodies, and renal pathology was more frequent in men (244).

Drug–Drug Interactions

Antacids

Antacids that contain aluminium or magnesium can reduce the absorption of penicillamine by up to 45%, presumably because increased gastric pH favors oxidation to the poorly absorbed disulfide (182,398,399).

Iron compounds

Iron compounds reduce the systemic availability of penicillamine to about 35% and copper excretion to about 28%, probably as a result of catalysis of the oxidation of penicillamine to its disulfide (2,398,400). Even the iron present in certain multivitamin formulations can be sufficient to cause interference, and when a patient who has regularly taken iron stops taking it, increased absorption of penicillamine and adverse effects can ensue (401,402).

Probenecid

When probenecid is co-administered with penicillamine in cystinuria, the efficacy of the penicillamine is significantly reduced (403).

Interference with Diagnostic Tests

Alpha-1 antitrypsin

Penicillamine can cause an artificially abnormal alpha-1 antitrypsin protein pattern, which can result in diagnostic errors (404).

Diagnosis of Adverse Drug Reactions

Reporting adverse reactions

The organization and preliminary results of an intensified voluntary reporting system for rheumatologists in the UK

West Midlands for studying the safety of DMARDs have been described (405).

References

1. Florentine MJ, Sanfilippo DJ 2nd. Elemental mercury poisoning. Clin Pharm 1991;10(3):213–21.

2. Joyce DA. D-penicillamine pharmacokinetics and pharmacodynamics in man. Pharmacol Ther 1989;42(3):405–27.

3. Madhok R, Zoma A, Torley HI, Capell HA, Waring R, Hunter JA. The relationship of sulfoxidation status to efficacy and toxicity of penicillamine in the treatment of rheumatoid arthritis. Arthritis Rheum 1990;33(4):574–7.

4. Moreland LW, Russell AS, Paulus HE. Management of rheumatoid arthritis: the historical context. J Rheumatol 2001;28(6):1431–52.

5. Parkinson S, Alldred A. Drug regimens for rheumatoid arthritis. Hosp Pharm 2002;9:11–15.

6. Sibilia J. Combinaison de traitements de fond dans la polyarthrite rhumatoïde. [Combination therapy for rheumatoid arthritis.] Ann Med Interne (Paris) 2002;153(1):41–52.

7. Capell H, McCarey D, Madhok R, Hampson R. "5D" outcome in 52 patients with rheumatoid arthritis surviving 20 years after initial disease modifying antirheumatic drug therapy. J Rheumatol 2002;29(10):2099–105.

8. Aletaha D, Smolen JS. Laboratory testing in rheumatoid arthritis patients taking disease-modifying antirheumatic drugs: clinical evaluation and cost analysis. Arthritis Rheum 2002;47(2):181–8.

9. Furst DE. The combination of methotrexate, sulfasalazine and hydroxychloroquine is highly effective in rheumatoid arthritis. Clin Exp Rheumatol 1999;17(1):39–40.

10. Blumberg SN, Fox DA. Rheumatoid arthritis: guidelines for emerging therapies. Am J Manag Care 2001;7(6):617–26.

11. Menninger H. Combination therapy for rheumatoid arthritis: update 2001. Aktuel Rheumatol 2001;26:146–58.

12. Russell A, Haraoui B, Keystone E, Klinkhoff A. Current and emerging therapies for rheumatoid arthritis, with a focus on infliximab: clinical impact on joint damage and cost of care in canada. Clin Ther 2001;23(11):1824–38.

13. Lacaille D. Rheumatology: 8. Advanced therapy. CMAJ 2000;163(6):721–8.

14. Madhok R, Kerr H, Capell HA. Recent advances: rheumatology. BMJ 2000;321(7265):882–5.

15. Simon LS. DMARDs in the treatment of rheumatoid arthritis: current agents and future developments. Int J Clin Pract 2000;54(4):243–9.

16. Fries JF. Current treatment paradigms in rheumatoid arthritis. Rheumatology (Oxford) 2000;39(Suppl 1):30–5.

17. Prieur AM, Quartier P. Comparative tolerability of treatments for juvenile idiopathic arthritis. Biodrugs 2000;14:159–83.

18. Cassidy JT. Medical management of children with juvenile rheumatoid arthritis. Drugs 1999;58(5):831–50.

19. Dubois B, D'Hooghe MB, De Lepeleire K, Ketelaer P, Opdenakker G, Carton H. Toxicity in a double-blind, placebo-controlled pilot trial with D-penicillamine and metacycline in secondary progressive multiple sclerosis. Mult Scler 1998;4(2):74–8.

20. Skoumal M, Wottawa A. Long-term observation study of Austrian patients with rheumatoid arthritis. Acta Med Austriaca 2002;29(2):52–6.

21. Pavelka K, Forejtova S, Pavelkova A, Zvarova J, Rovensky J, Tuchynova A. Analysis of the reasons for DMARD therapy discontinuation in patients with rheumatoid arthritis in the Czech and Slovak republics. Clin Rheumatol 2002;21(3):220–6.

22. Moens HJ, Ament BJ, Feltkamp BW, van der Korst JK. Longterm followup of treatment with D-penicillamine for rheumatoid arthritis: effectivity and toxicity in relation to HLA antigens. J Rheumatol 1987;14(6):1115–19.

23. Cooperative Systematic Studies of Rheumatic Disease Group. Toxicity of longterm low dose D-penicillamine therapy in rheumatoid arthritis. J Rheumatol 1987;14(1):67–73.

24. Kutsuna T, Maeda K, Okamoto T. [Long-term results of D-penicillamine treatment in rheumatoid arthritis.] Ryumachi 1986;26(4):270–7.

25. Kashiwazaki S. Current status of D-penicillamine therapy in Japan. Z Rheumatol 1988;47(Suppl 1):38–40.

26. Felson DT, Anderson JJ, Meenan RF. The comparative efficacy and toxicity of second-line drugs in rheumatoid arthritis. Results of two metaanalyses. Arthritis Rheum 1990;33(10):1449–61.

27. De La Mata J, Blanco FJ, Gomez-Reino JJ. Survival analysis of disease modifying antirheumatic drugs in Spanish rheumatoid arthritis patients. Ann Rheum Dis 1995;54(11):881–5.

28. Wolfe F, Hawley DJ, Cathey MA. Termination of slow acting antirheumatic therapy in rheumatoid arthritis: a 14-year prospective evaluation of 1017 consecutive starts. J Rheumatol 1990;17(8):994–1002.

29. Taylor HG, Samanta A. Penicillamine in rheumatoid arthritis. A problem of toxicity. Drug Saf 1992;7(1):46–53.

30. Pincus T, Marcum SB, Callahan LF. Longterm drug therapy for rheumatoid arthritis in seven rheumatology private practices: II. Second line drugs and prednisone. J Rheumatol 1992;19(12):1885–94.

31. Conaghan PG, Brooks P. Disease-modifying antirheumatic drugs, including methotrexate, gold, antimalarials, and D-penicillamine. Curr Opin Rheumatol 1995;7(3):167–73.

32. Huskisson EC. The side effects of penicillamine therapy in rheumatoid arthritis. J Rheumatol Suppl 1981;7:146–8.

33. Raynauld JP, Lee YS, Kornfeld P, Fries JF. Unilateral ptosis as an initial manifestation of D-penicillamine induced myasthenia gravis. J Rheumatol 1993;20(9):1592–3.

34. Jaffe IA. Combination therapy of rheumatoid arthritis—rationale and overview. J Rheumatol Suppl 1990;25:24–7.

35. Bunch TW, O'Duffy JD, Tompkins RB, O'Fallon WM. Controlled trial of hydroxychloroquine and D-penicillamine singly and in combination in the treatment of rheumatoid arthritis. Arthritis Rheum 1984;27(3):267–76.

36. Gibson T, Emery P, Armstrong RD, Crisp AJ, Panayi GS. Combined D-penicillamine and chloroquine treatment of rheumatoid arthritis—a comparative study. Br J Rheumatol 1987;26(4):279–84.

37. Dijkmans BA, de Vries E, de Vreede TM. Synergistic and additive effects of disease modifying anti-rheumatic drugs combined with chloroquine on the mitogen-driven stimulation of mononuclear cells. Clin Exp Rheumatol 1990;8(5):455–9.

38. Horsfall MW, Shaw JP, Highton J, Cranch PJ. Changing patterns in the use of slow acting antirheumatic drugs for the treatment of rheumatoid arthritis. NZ Med J 1998;111(1067):200–3.

39. Jessop JD, O'Sullivan MM, Lewis PA, Williams LA, Camilleri JP, Plant MJ, Coles EC. A long-term five-year randomized controlled trial of hydroxychloroquine, sodium aurothiomalate, auranofin and penicillamine in the treatment of patients with rheumatoid arthritis. Br J Rheumatol 1998;37(9):992–1002.

40. Capell HA, Maiden N, Madhok R, Hampson R, Thomson EA. Intention-to-treat analysis of 200 patients with rheumatoid arthritis 12 years after random allocation to either sulfasalazine or penicillamine. J Rheumatol 1998;25(10):1880–6.

41. Hill J, Bird H, Johnson S. Effect of patient education on adherence to drug treatment for rheumatoid arthritis: a randomised controlled trial. Ann Rheum Dis 2001; 60(9):869–75.

42. Sokka T, Hannonen P. Utility of disease modifying antirheumatic drugs in "sawtooth" strategy. A prospective study of early rheumatoid arthritis patients up to 15 years. Ann Rheum Dis 1999;58(10):618–22.

43. Galindo-Rodriguez G, Avina-Zubieta JA, Russell AS, Suarez-Almazor ME. Disappointing longterm results with disease modifying antirheumatic drugs. A practice based study. J Rheumatol 1999;26(11):2337–43.

44. Grove ML, Hassell AB, Hay EM, Shadforth MF. Adverse reactions to disease-modifying anti-rheumatic drugs in clinical practice. QJM 2001;94(6):309–19.

45. Clements PJ, Furst DE, Wong WK, Mayes M, White B, Wigley F, Weisman MH, Barr W, Moreland LW, Medsger TA Jr, Steen V, Martin RW, Collier D, Weinstein A, Lally E, Varga J, Weiner S, Andrews B, Abeles M, Seibold JR. High-dose versus low-dose D-penicillamine in early diffuse systemic sclerosis: analysis of a two-year, double-blind, randomized, controlled clinical trial. Arthritis Rheum 1999;42(6):1194–203.

46. Pless M, Sandson T. Chronic internuclear ophthalmoplegia. A manifestation of D-penicillamine cerebral vasculitis. J Neuroophthalmol 1997;17(1):44–6.

47. Haerden J, Coolen L, Dequeker J. The effect of D-penicillamine on lung function parameters (diffusion capacity) in rheumatoid arthritis. Clin Exp Rheumatol 1993; 11(5):509–13.

48. Turner-Warwick M. Adverse reactions affecting the lung: possible association with D-penicillamine. J Rheumatol Suppl 1981;7:166–8.

49. Camus P. Manifestations respiratoires associées aux traitements par la D-pénicillamine. [The respiratory complications of D-pénicillamine therapy.] Rev Fr Mal Respir 1982;10(1):7–20.

50. Shettar SP, Chattopadhyay C, Wolstenholme RJ, Swinson DR. Diffuse alveolitis on a small dose of penicillamine. Br J Rheumatol 1984;23(3):220–4.

51. Cannon GW. Antirheumatic drug reactions in the lung. Baillieres Clin Rheumatol 1993;7(1):147–71.

52. Bauer P, Bollaert P, Dopff C, Vignaud JM, Lambert H, Larcan A. Syndrome de détresse respiratoire aiguë d'évolution fatale au cours d'un traitement par D-pénicillamine. [Syndrome of acute respiratory distress with a fatal development in a treatment with D-penicillamine.] Presse Méd 1988;17(19):961–2.

53. Padley SP, Adler BD, Hansell DM, Muller NL. Bronchiolitis obliterans: high resolution CT findings and correlation with pulmonary function tests. Clin Radiol 1993;47(4):236–40.

54. Honda T, Hachiya T, Hayasaka M, Morita M, Nakagawa S, Kusama Y, Kubo K, Sekiguchi M, Kobayashi O. [A case of rheumatoid arthritis with obstructive bronchiolitis appearing after D-penicillamine therapy.] Nihon Kyobu Shikkan Gakkai Zasshi 1993; 31(9):1195–200.

55. Anaya JM, Diethelm L, Ortiz LA, Gutierrez M, Citera G, Welsh RA, Espinoza LR. Pulmonary involvement in rheumatoid arthritis. Semin Arthritis Rheum 1995;24(4):242–54.

56. Jenkins EA, Hull RG, Thomas AL. D-penicillamine and polymyositis: the significance of the anti-Jo-1 antibody. Br J Rheumatol 1993;32(12):1109–10.

57. Drosos AA, Christou L, Galanopoulou V, Tzioufas AG, Tsiakou EK. D-pénicillamine induced myasthenia gravis: clinical, serological and genetic findings. Clin Exp Rheumatol 1993;11(4):387–91.

58. Wang DY. Diagnosis and management of lupus pleuritis. Curr Opin Pulm Med 2002;8(4):312–16.

59. Lauque D, Courtin JP, Fournie B, Oksman F, Pourrat J, Carles P. Syndrome pneumo-rénal induit par la d-penicillamine: syndrome de Goodpasture ou polyartérite microscopique? [Pneumorenal syndrome induced by d-penicillamine: Goodpasture's syndrome or microscopic polyarteritis] Rev Med Interne 1990; 11(2):168–71.

60. Vazquez-Del Mercado M, Mendoza-Topete A, Best-Aguilera CR, Garcia-De La Torre I. Diffuse alveolar hemorrhage in limited cutaneous systemic sclerosis with positive perinuclear antineutrophil cytoplasmic antibodies. J Rheumatol 1996;23(10):1821–3.

61. Storch W. Seltene immunologisch bedingte Asthmaformen. Atemw-Lungenkrkh 1990;16:271–2.

62. Lagier F, Cartier A, Dolovich J, Malo JL. Occupational asthma in a pharmaceutical worker exposed to penicillamine. Thorax 1989;44(2):157–8.

63. Grobbelaar J, Meyers OL. Penicillamine therapy in rheumatoid arthritis. S Afr Med J 1984;65(18):715–17.

64. Stockmann G. Die Stellung des Churg–Strauss-Syndrome zwischen anderen hypereosinophilen, granulomatösen und vaskulitischen Erkrankungen. [The status of Churg–Strauss syndrome among other hypereosinophilic, granulomatous and vasculitic diseases.] Z Rheumatol 1988;47(6):388–96.

65. Presley AP. Penicillamine induced rhinitis. BMJ (Clin Res Ed) 1988;296(6632):1332.

66. Bardach H, Gebhart W, Niebauer G. "Lumpy-bumpy" elastic fibers in the skin and lungs of a patient with a penicillamine-induced elastosis perforans serpiginosa. J Cutan Pathol 1979;6(4):243–52.

67. Stanworth DR. d-Penicillamine-induced immunodeficiency. In: Dawkins RL, Christiansen FT, Zilko PJ, editors. Immunogenetics in Rheumatology: Musculoskeletal Disease and d-Penicillamine. Amsterdam: Excerpta Medica, 1982:358.

68. Negishi M, Kobayashi K, Ide H, et al. A case report of selective IgA deficiency in rheumatoid arthritis treated with d-penicillamine. J Showa Med Assoc 1990;50:205–9.

69. Pool KD, Feit H, Kirkpatrick J. Penicillamine-induced neuropathy in rheumatoid arthritis. Ann Intern Med 1981;95(4):457–8.

70. Pedersen PB, Hogenhaven H. Penicillamin-induced neuropathy in rheumatoid arthritis. Acta Neurol Scand 1990; 81(2):188–90.

71. Mayr N, Graninger W, Wessely P. Polyneuropathie bei chronischer Polyarthritis unter d-Penicillamin: medikamentös induziert? [A chemically induced polyneuropathy in chronic polyarthritis treated with D-penicillamine?] Wien Klin Wochenschr 1983;95(3):86–8.

72. Stremmel W, Meyerrose KW, Niederau C, Hefter H, Kreuzpaintner G, Strohmeyer G. Wilson disease: clinical presentation, treatment, and survival. Ann Intern Med 1991;115(9):720–6.

73. Klingele TG, Burde RM. Optic neuropathy associated with penicillamine therapy in a patient with rheumatoid arthritis. J Clin Neuroophthalmol 1984;4(2):75–8.

74. Knezevic W, Mastaglia FL, Quintner J, Zilko PJ. Guillain–Barré syndrome and pemphigus foliaceus associated with D-penicillamine therapy. Aust NZ J Med 1984;14(1):50–2.

75. Matsubara K, Noda T, Nakano I, Shikano Y, Maeda M, Mori S. A case of progressive systemic sclerosis with acute polyradiculoneuropathy during d-penicillamine therapy. Nishinihon J Dermatol 1990;52:1120–6.

76. Hilz MJ, Druschky KF, Bauer J, Neundorfer B, Schuierer G. Morbus Wilson—kritische Verschlechterung unter hochdosierter parenteraler Penicillamin-Therapie.

[Wilson's disease—critical deterioration under high-dose parenteral penicillamine therapy.] Dtsch Med Wochenschr 1990;115(3):93–7.

77. Pall HS, Williams AC, Blake DR. Deterioration of Wilson's disease following the start of penicillamine therapy. Arch Neurol 1989;46(4):359–61.

78. Veen C, van den Hamer CJ, de Leeuw PW. Zinc sulphate therapy for Wilson's disease after acute deterioration during treatment with low-dose D-penicillamine. J Intern Med 1991;229(6):549–52.

79. Barbosa ER, Scaff M, Canelas HM. Degenera ção hepatolenticular. Avaliação da evolução neurologica em 76 casos tratados. [Hepatolenticular degeneration: evaluation of neurological course in 76 treated cases.] Arq Neuropsiquiatr 1991;49(4):399–404.

80. Tankanow RM. Pathophysiology and treatment of Wilson's disease. Clin Pharm 1991;10(11):839–49.

81. Kher A, Bharucha BA, Kumta NB. Wilson's disease: initial worsening of neurologic syndrome with penicillamine therapy. Indian Pediatr 1992;29(7):927–9.

82. Glass JD, Reich SG, Mahlon R, DeLong MR. Wilson's disease. Development of neurological disease after beginning penicillamine therapy. Arch Neurol 1990;47(5):595–6.

83. Porzio S, Iorio R, Vajro P, Pensati P, Vegnente A. Penicillamine-related neurologic syndrome in a child affected by Wilson disease with hepatic presentation. Arch Neurol 1997;54(9):1166–8.

84. George J, Spokes EG. Myasthenic pseudo-internuclear ophthalmoplegia due to penicillamine. J Neurol Neurosurg Psychiatry 1984;47(9):1044.

85. Reeback J, Benton S, Swash M, Schwartz MS. Penicillamine-induced neuromyotonia. BMJ 1979;1(6176):1464–5.

86. Pinals RS. Diffuse fasciculations induced by D-penicillamine. J Rheumatol 1983;10(5):809–10.

87. Liu GT, Bienfang DC. Penicillamine-induced ocular myasthenia gravis in rheumatoid arthritis. J Clin Neuroophthalmol 1990;10(3):201–5.

88. Katz LJ, Lesser RL, Merikangas JR, Silverman JP. Ocular myasthenia gravis after D-penicillamine administration. Br J Ophthalmol 1989;73(12):1015–18.

89. Ferbert A. D-Penicillamin-induzierte okuläre Myasthenie bei Psoriasisarthritis. [D-penicillamine-induced ocular myasthenia in psoriatic arthritis.] Nervenarzt 1989;60(9):576–9.

90. Chapat-Jolivet F, Wendling D, Moulin T, et al. Myasthénie induite par la d-pénicillamine au cours du traitement de la polyarthrite rhumatoïde. Rhumatologic 1989;41:181–8.

91. Zakarian H, Viallet F, Acquaviva PC, Khalil R. Syndrome myasthénique induit par la d-pénicillamine au cours de la polyarthrite rhumatoïde. Sem Hop Paris 1989;65:2052–6.

92. Tzartos SJ, Morel E, Efthimiadis A, Bustarret AF, D'Anglejan J, Drosos AA, Moutsopoulos HA. Fine antigenic specificities of antibodies in sera from patients with D-penicillamine-induced myasthenia gravis. Clin Exp Immunol 1988;74(1):80–6.

93. Paladini G, Mazzanti G, Mysco G, et al. La sindrome miastenica indotta da d-penicillamina nell'artrite reumatoide: caratteri clinici e genetici. Reumatismo 1988;40:139–44.

94. Cikes N, Momoi MY, Williams CL, Howard FM Jr, Hoagland HC, Whittingham S, Lennon VA. Striational autoantibodies: quantitative detection by enzyme immunoassay in myasthenia gravis, thymoma, and recipients of D-penicillamine or allogeneic bone marrow. Mayo Clin Proc 1988;63(5):474–81.

95. Derman H, Theron HP. A propos de trois observations de syndrome myasthénique induit par la D-pénicillamine. [3 cases of myasthenic syndrome induced by D-penicillamine.] Bull Soc Ophtalmol Fr 1987;87(11):1235–43.

96. Dubost JJ, Soubrier M, Bouchet F, Kemeny JL, Lhopitaux R, Bussiere JL, Sauvezie B. Complications neuromusculaires de la D-pénicillamine dans la polyarthrite rhumatoide. [Neuromuscular complications of D-penicillamine in rheumatoid arthritis.] Rev Neurol (Paris) 1992;148(3):207–11.

97. Norscini N, Lancman M, Doctorovich D, Poeraniec C, Bauso Toselli L, Granillo R. Miastenia gravis inducida por d-penicilamina. Presentacion de un caso y revision de la literatura. Rev Neurol Argent 1990;15:59–62.

98. Kuriyama S, Hosoya T, Sakai O. [D-penicillamine induced myasthenia gravis in a patient with rheumatoid arthritis.] Ryumachi 1991;31(3):298–302.

99. Voltz R, Hohlfeld R, Fateh-Moghadam A, Witt TN, Wick M, Reimers C, Siegele B, Wekerle H. Myasthenia gravis: measurement of anti-AChR autoantibodies using cell line TE671. Neurology 1991;41(11):1836–8.

100. Hanabusa K, Ohtsuki H, Watanabe S, Okano M, Hasebe S, Tadokoro Y. d-Penicillamine-induced ocular myasthenia gravis in rheumatoid arthritis. Folia Ophthalmol Jpn 1993;44:1306–10.

101. Wittbrodt ET. Drugs and myasthenia gravis. An update. Arch Intern Med 1997;157(4):399–408.

102. Chuah SY, Wong NW, Goh KL. Lethargy in a patient with cirrhosis. Postgrad Med J 1997;73(857):177–9.

103. Kato Y, Naito Y, Narita Y, Kuzuhara S. D-penicillamine-induced myasthenia gravis in a case of eosinophilic fasciitis. J Neurol Sci 1997;146(1):85–6.

104. Komal Kumar RN, Patil SA, Taly AB, Nirmala M, Sinha S, Arunodaya GR. Effect of D-penicillamine on neuromuscular junction in patients with Wilson disease. Neurology 2004;63(5):935–6.

105. Morel E, Feuillet-Fieux MN, Vernet-der Garabedian B, Raimond F, D'Anglejan J, Bataille R, Sany J, Bach JF. Autoantibodies in D-penicillamine-induced myasthenia gravis: a comparison with idiopathic myasthenia and rheumatoid arthritis. Clin Immunol Immunopathol 1991;58(3):318–30.

106. Kolarz G, El-Shohoumi M, Maida EM, Scherak O. Azetylcholin rezeptor-Antikorper unter d-Penicillamin-Therapie. Ther Oesterr 1991;6:735–42.

107. Dominkus M, Chlud K, Maida EM, Grisold W. Monitoring of patients with rheumatoid arthritis in longterm administration of D-penicillamine. J Rheumatol 1992;19(10):1648–50.

108. Dominkus M, Grisold W, Albrecht G. Stimulation single fiber EMG study in patients receiving a long-term D-penicillamine treatment for rheumatoid arthritis. Muscle Nerve 1992;15(11):1300–1.

109. Hill M, Beeson D, Moss P, Jacobson L, Bond A, Corlett L, Newsom-Davis J, Vincent A, Willcox N. Early-onset myasthenia gravis: a recurring T-cell epitope in the adult-specific acetylcholine receptor epsilon subunit presented by the susceptibility allele HLA-DR52a. Ann Neurol 1999;45(2):224–31.

110. Hill M, Moss P, Wordsworth P, Newsom-Davis J, Willcox N. T cell responses to D-penicillamine in drug-induced myasthenia gravis: recognition of modified DR1: peptide complexes. J Neuroimmunol 1999;97(1–2):146–53.

111. Jan V, Callens A, Machet L, Machet MC, Lorette G, Vaillant L. Pemphigus polymyosite et myasthénie induites par la D-pénicillamine. [D-penicillamine-induced pemphigus, polymyositis and myasthenia.] Ann Dermatol Venereol 1999;126(2):153–6.

112. Garlepp MI, Dawkins RL, Christiansen FT. HLA antigens and acetylcholine receptor antibodies in penicillamine induced myasthenia gravis. BMJ (Clin Res Ed) 1983;286(6375):1442–3.

113. Andonopoulos AP, Terzis E, Tsibri E, Papasteriades CA, Papapetropoulos T. D-penicillamine induced myasthenia

gravis in rheumatoid arthritis: an unpredictable common occurrence? Clin Rheumatol 1994;13(4):586–8.

114. Fried MJ, Protheroe DT. D-penicillamine induced myasthenia gravis. Its relevance for the anaesthetist. Br J Anaesth 1986;58(10):1191–3.

115. Jimenez SA, Sigal SH. A 15-year prospective study of treatment of rapidly progressive systemic sclerosis with D-penicillamine. J Rheumatol 1991;18(10):1496–503.

116. Gabutti V. Current therapy for thalassemia in Italy. Ann NY Acad Sci 1990;612:268–74.

117. Nores JM, Biacabe B, Bonfils P. Troubles olfactifs d'origine médicamenteuse: analyse et revue de la littérature. [Olfactory disorders due to medications: analysis and review of the literature.] Rev Med Interne 2000; 21(11):972–7.

118. Knudsen L, Weismann K. Taste dysfunction and changes in zinc and copper metabolism during penicillamine therapy for generalized scleroderma. Acta Med Scand 1978;204(1–2):75–9.

119. Tausch G, Broll H, Eberl R. D-Penicillamin (Artamin) als Basistherapie bei chronischer Polyarthritis. [D-penicillamine (Artamin) as basic therapeutic agent in the treatment of chronic rheumatoid arthritis.] Wien Klin Wochenschr 1973;85(4):59–63.

120. Gutierrez Fuentes JA, Vazquez Gallego MC, Fernandez Remis JE, Arroyo Vicente M, Schuller Perez A. Ageusia como manifestacion secundaria del tratiamento con D-penicillamina. [Ageusia as a secondary manifestation of treatment with D-penicillamine.] Rev Clin Esp 1984;172(3):149–51.

121. Schiffman SS. Taste and smell in disease (first of two parts). N Engl J Med 1983;308(21):1275–9.

122. Prieur AM, Piussan C, Manigne P, Bordigoni P, Griscelli C, Reinert P, de Goujon F, Lefur JM, Garnier JM. Arthrite chronique juvénile. Etude en double insu de l'efficacité et de la tolérance de la D-pénicillamine. [Juvenile chronic arthritis. Double-blind study of the efficacy and tolerance of D-penicillamine.] Arch Fr Pediatr 1985;42(2):91–6.

123. Klepach GL, Wray SH. Bilateral serous retinal detachment with thrombocytopenia during penicillamine therapy. Ann Ophthalmol 1981;13(2):201–3.

124. Choi HK, Merkel PA, Walker AM, Niles JL. Drug-associated antineutrophil cytoplasmic antibody-positive vasculitis: prevalence among patients with high titers of antimyeloperoxidase antibodies. Arthritis Rheum 2000;43(2):405–13.

125. Delrieu F, Menkes CJ, Sainte-Croix A, Babinet P, Chesneau AM, Delbarre F. Myasthénie et thyroidite auto-immune au course du traitements de la polyarthrite rhumatoïde par la D-pénicillamine. Etude anatomo-clinique d'un cas. [Myasthenia gravis and autoimmune thyroiditis during the treatment of rheumatoid polyarthritis with D-penicillamine. Anatomoclinical study of 1 case.] Ann Med Interne (Paris) 1976;127(10):739–43.

126. Bertrand JL, Rousset H, Queneau P, Ollagnier M. Thyroïdite auto-immune, une complication rare du traitement à la D-pénicillamine. [Autoimmune thyroiditis. A rare complication of treatment with D-penicillamine.] Therapie 1981;36(3):333–6.

127. Addyman R, Beyeler C, Astbury C, Bird HA. Urinary glucaric acid excretion in rheumatoid arthritis: influence of disease activity and disease modifying drugs. Ann Rheum Dis 1996;55(7):478–81.

128. Benson EA, Healey LA, Barron EJ. Insulin antibodies in patients receiving penicillamine. Am J Med 1985; 78(5):857–60.

129. Herranz L, Rovira A, Grande C, Suarez A, Martinez-Ara J, Pallardo LF, Gomez-Pan A. Autoimmune insulin

130. Becker RC, Martin RG. Penicillamine-induced insulin antibodies. Ann Intern Med 1986;104(1):127–8.

131. Elling P, Elling H. Penicillamine, captopril, and hypoglycemia. Ann Intern Med 1985;103(4):644–5.

132. Vardi P, Brik R, Barzilai D, Lorber M, Scharf Y. Frequent induction of insulin autoantibodies by D-penicillamine in patients with rheumatoid arthritis. J Rheumatol 1992; 19(10):1527–30.

133. Faguer de Moustier B, Burgard M, Boitard C, Desplanque N, Fanjoux J, Tchobroutsky G. Syndrome hypoglycémique auto-immun induit par le pyritinol. [Auto-immune hypoglycemic syndrome induced by pyritinol.] Diabete Metab 1988;14(4):423–9.

134. Sheikh IA, Kaplan AP. Assessment of kininases in rheumatic diseases and the effect of therapeutic agents. Arthritis Rheum 1987;30(2):138–45.

135. Schulze E, Herrmann K, Haustein UF, Krusche U, Rothenburger I. Einfluss von Penicillin und D-Penicillamin auf die Betagalactosidaseaktivität bei Patienten met progressiver Sklerodermie. [Effect of penicillin and D-penicillamine on beta-galactosidase activity in patients with progressive scleroderma.] Dermatol Monatsschr 1988;174(11):661–6.

136. Doornbos DA, Faber JS. Studies on metal complexes of drugs. D-penicillamine and N-acetyl-D-penicillamine. Pharm Weekbl 1964;99:289–309.

137. Doornbos DA. Stability constants of metal complexes of L-cysteine, D-penicillamine, N-acetyl-D-penicillamine and some biguanides. Determination of stoichiometric stability constants by an accurate method for pH measurement. Pharm Weekbl 1968;103(45):1213–27.

138. Kuchinskas EJ, Rosen Y. Metal chelates of DL-penicillamine. Arch Biochem Biophys 1962;97:370–2.

139. Cutolo M, Accardo S, Cimmino MA, Rovetta G, Bianchi G, Bianchi V. Hypocupremia-related hypochromic anemia during D-penicillamine treatment. Arthritis Rheum 1982;25(1):119–20.

140. Dastych M, Jezek P, Richtrova M. Der Einfluss einer Penicillamintherapie auf die Konzentration von Zink, Kupfer, Eisen, Kalzium und Magnesium in Serum und auf deren Ausscheidung in Urin. [Effect of penicillamine therapy on the concentration of zinc, copper, iron, calcium and magnesium in the serum and their excretion in urine.] Z Gastroenterol 1986;24(3):157–60.

141. Klingberg WG, Prasad AS, Oberleas D. Zinc deficiency following penicillamine therapy. In: Prasad AS, editor. Trace Elements in Human Health and Disease. New York: Academic Press, 197951–4.

142. Hammond WP, Miller JE, Starkebaum G, Zweerink HJ, Rosenthal AS, Dale DC. Suppression of in vitro granulocytopoiesis by captopril and penicillamine. Exp Hematol 1988;16(8):674–80.

143. Hamilton JA, Williams N. In vitro inhibition of myelopoiesis by gold salts and D-penicillamine. J Rheumatol 1985;12(5):892–6.

144. Thomas D, Gallus AS, Brooks PM, Tampi R, Geddes R, Hill W. Thrombokinetics in patients with rheumatoid arthritis treated with D-penicillamine. Ann Rheum Dis 1984;43(3):402–6.

145. Singh G, Fries JF, Williams CA, Zatarain E, Spitz P, Bloch DA. Toxicity profiles of disease modifying antirheumatic drugs in rheumatoid arthritis. J Rheumatol 1991; 18(2):188–94.

146. Kay AG. Myelotoxicity of D-penicillamine. Ann Rheum Dis 1979;38(3):232–6.

147. Netter P, Trechot P, Bannwarth B, Faure G, Royer RJ. Effets secondaires de la D-Pénicillamine et du pyritinol.

Etude Coopérative des centres de pharmacovigilance hospitalière français. [Side effects of D-penicillamine and pyritinol. Cooperative study among French hospital drug surveillance centers.] Therapie 1985;40(6):475–9.

148. Edelman J, Maguire KF, Owen ET. Eosinophilia in rheumatoid patients treated with D-penicillamine. J Rheumatol 1984;11(5):624–5.

149. Pedersen-Bjergaard U, Andersen M, Hansen PB. Drug-induced thrombocytopenia: clinical data on 309 cases and the effect of corticosteroid therapy. Eur J Clin Pharmacol 1997;52(3):183–9.

150. Hill HF. Treatment of rheumatoid arthritis with penicillamine. Semin Arthritis Rheum 1977;6(4):361–88.

151. Sanchez-Albisua I, Garde T, Hierro L, Camarena C, Frauca E, de la Vega A, Diaz MC, Larrauri J, Jara P. A high index of suspicion: the key to an early diagnosis of Wilson's disease in childhood. J Pediatr Gastroenterol Nutr 1999;28(2):186–90.

152. Katayama Y, Kohriyama K, Matsui T. In vitro inhibition of hematopoiesis in a patient with systemic sclerosis treated with D-penicillamine. J Rheumatol 1999;26(11):2493–5.

153. Trice JM, Pinals RS, Plitman GI. Thrombotic thrombocytopenic purpura during penicillamine therapy in rheumatoid arthritis. Arch Intern Med 1983;143(7):1487–8.

154. Holdrinet RS, Namdar Z, Haanen C. Thrombotic thrombocytopenic purpura: clinical course and response to therapy in twelve patients. Neth J Med 1988;33(3–4):113–32.

155. Ahmed F, Sumalnop V, Spain DM, Tobin MS. Thrombohemolytic thrombocytopenic purpura during penicillamine therapy. Arch Intern Med 1978;138(8):1292–3.

156. Speth PA, Boerbooms AM, Holdrinet RS, Van de Putte LB, Meyer JW. Thrombotic thrombocytopenic purpura associated with D-penicillamine treatment in rheumatoid arthritis. J Rheumatol 1982;9(5):812–13.

157. Masson C, Bregeon C, Ifrah N, Berton V, Housseau F, Renier JC. Syndrome d'Evans sous D-pénicillamine au cours d'une polyarthrite rhumatoïde. Intérêt de l'association corticoïdes–danazol. [Evans' syndrome caused by D-penicillamine in rheumatoid arthritis. Value of the corticoids–danazol combination.] Rev Rhum Mal Osteoartic 1991;58(7):519–22.

158. Henzgen M, Hein G. Agranulozytose und andere Nebenwirkungen. Erfahrungen mit der d-Penicillamintherapie bei der Rheumatoidarthritis. Z Klin Med 1985;40:521.

159. Umeki S, Konishi Y, Yasuda T, Morimoto K, Terao A. D-penicillamine and neutrophilic agranulocytosis. Arch Intern Med 1985;145(12):2271–2.

160. Ramselaar AC, Dekker AW, Huber-Bruning O, Bijlsma JW. Acquired sideroblastic anaemia after aplastic anaemia caused by D-penicillamine therapy for rheumatoid arthritis. Ann Rheum Dis 1987;46(2):156–8.

161. Ehrlich JC, Van Paasen HC. Een dodelijke bijwerking van penicillamine. Ned Tijdschr Geneeskd 1984;128:1790.

162. Fishel B, Tishler M, Caspi D, Yaron M. Fatal aplastic anaemia and liver toxicity caused by D-penicillamine treatment of rheumatoid arthritis. Ann Rheum Dis 1989;48(7):609–10.

163. Petrides PE, Gerhartz HH. D-penicillamine-induced agranulocytosis: hematological remission upon treatment with recombinant GM-CSF. Z Rheumatol 1991;50(5):328–9.

164. Lowenthal RM, Cohen ML, Atkinson K, Biggs JC. Apparent cure of rheumatoid arthritis by bone marrow transplantation. J Rheumatol 1993;20(1):137–40.

165. Kaufman DW, Kelly JP, Jurgelon JM, Anderson T, Issaragrisil S, Wiholm BE, Young NS, Leaverton P, Levy M, Shapiro S. Drugs in the aetiology of agranulocytosis and aplastic anaemia. Eur J Haematol Suppl 1996;60:23–30.

166. Mary JY, Guiguet M, Baumelou E. Drug use and aplastic anaemia: the French experience. French Cooperative Group for the Epidemiological Study of Aplastic Anaemia. Eur J Haematol Suppl 1996;60:35–41.

167. Ward K, Weir DG. Life threatening agranulocytosis and toxic epidermal necrolysis during low dose penicillamine therapy. Ir J Med Sci 1981;150(8):252–3.

168. Kandola L, Swannell AJ, Hunter A. Acquired sideroblastic anaemia associated with penicillamine therapy for rheumatoid arthritis. Ann Rheum Dis 1995;54(6):529–30.

169. Williams DM. Copper deficiency in humans. Semin Hematol 1983;20(2):118–28.

170. Frieden E. The copper connection. Semin Hematol 1983;20(2):114–17.

171. LaRusso NF, Wiesner RH, Ludwig J, MacCarty RL, Beaver SJ, Zinsmeister AR. Prospective trial of penicillamine in primary sclerosing cholangitis. Gastroenterology 1988;95(4):1036–42.

172. Demelia L, Vallebona E, Perpignano G, Pitzus F. Positivizzazione di sierologia lupica in corso di morbo di Wilson in trattamento con penicillamina. Reumatismo 1991;43:119–24.

173. Capell HA, Marabani M, Madhok R, Torley H, Hunter JA. Degree and extent of response to sulphasalazine or penicillamine therapy for rheumatoid arthritis: results from a routine clinical environment over a two-year period. Q J Med 1990;75(276):335–44.

174. Carpenter EH, Plant MJ, Hassell AB, Shadforth MF, Fisher J, Clarke S, Hothersall TE, Dawes PT. Management of oral complications of disease-modifying drugs in rheumatoid arthritis. Br J Rheumatol 1997;36(4):473–8.

175. Fenton DA, Young ER, Wilkinson JD. Recurrent aphthous ulceration. BMJ (Clin Res Ed) 1983;286:1062.

176. Wassef M, Galian A, Pepin B, Haguenau M, Vassel P, Hautefeuille P, Brazy J. Unusual digestive lesions in a patient with Wilson's disease treated with long-term penicillamine. N Engl J Med 1985;313(1):49.

177. Greene MW, King RC, Alley RS. Management of an oroantral fistula in a patient with Wilson's disease: case report and review of the literature. Oral Surg Oral Med Oral Pathol 1988;66(3):293–6.

178. Rajendran N, Koteeswaran A, Kala M. Penicillamine-induced cheilosis. Indian J Dermatol Venereol Leprol 1985;51:50.

179. Blasberg B, Dorey JL, Stein HB, Chalmers A, Conklin RJ. Lichenoid lesions of the oral mucosa in rheumatoid arthritis patients treated with penicillamine. J Rheumatol 1984;11(3):348–51.

180. Lyle WH. Letter: Peptic ulceration and D-penicillamine. Lancet 1974;2(7875):285.

181. Ramboer C, Verhamme M. D-penicillamine-induced oesophageal ulcers. Acta Clin Belg 1989;44(3):189–91.

182. Perrett D. The metabolism and pharmacology of D-penicillamine in man. J Rheumatol Suppl 1981;7:41–50.

183. Houghton AD, Nadel S, Stringer MD. Penicillamine-associated total colitis. Hepatogastroenterology 1989;36(4):198.

184. Roux H, Bonnefoy-Cudraz M, Antipoff GM. Les complications hépatiques de la d-pénicillamine. Rhumatologie 1984;36:233.

185. Gefel D, Harats N, Lijovetsky G, Eliakim M. Cholestatic jaundice associated with D-penicillamine therapy. Scand J Rheumatol 1985;14(3):303–6.

186. Kumar A, Bhat A, Gupta DK, Goel A, Malaviya AN. D-penicillamine-induced acute hypersensitivity pneumonitis and cholestatic hepatitis in a patient with rheumatoid arthritis. Clin Exp Rheumatol 1985;3(4):337–9.

187. Menara M, Zancan L, Sturniolo GC. Penicillamine hepatotoxicity in the treatment of Wilson's disease. J Pediatr Gastroenterol Nutr 1992;14(3):353–4.

188. Matsukawa Y, Saito N, Nishinarita S, Horie T, Ryu J. Therapeutic effect of tiopronin following D-penicillamine toxicity in a patient with rheumatoid arthritis. Clin Rheumatol 1998;17(1):73–4.

189. Mok MY, Ng WL, Yuen MF, Wong RW, Lau CS. Safety of disease modifying anti-rheumatic agents in rheumatoid arthritis patients with chronic viral hepatitis. Clin Exp Rheumatol 2000;18(3):363–8.

190. Schilsky ML. The irony of treating Wilson's disease. Am J Gastroenterol 2001;96(11):3055–7.

191. Shiono Y, Wakusawa S, Hayashi H, Takikawa T, Yano M, Okada T, Mabuchi H, Kono S, Miyajima H. Iron accumulation in the liver of male patients with Wilson's disease. Am J Gastroenterol 2001;96(11):3147–51.

192. Luca P, Demelia L, Lecca S, Ambu R, Faa G. Massive hepatic haemosiderosis in Wilson's disease. Histopathology 2000;37(2):187–9.

193. Rook AH, Freundlich B, Jegasothy BV, Perez MI, Barr WG, Jimenez SA, Rietschel RL, Wintroub B, Kahaleh MB, Varga J, Heald PW, Steen V, Massa MC, Murphy GF, Perniciaro C, Istfan M, Ballas SK, Edelson RL. Treatment of systemic sclerosis with extracorporeal photochemotherapy. Results of a multicenter trial. Arch Dermatol 1992;128(3):337–46.

194. Stein HB, Schroeder ML, Dillon AM. Penicillamine-induced proteinuria: risk factors. Semin Arthritis Rheum 1986;15(4):282–7.

195. Hall CL, Jawad S, Harrison PR, MacKenzie JC, Bacon PA, Klouda PT, MacIver AG. Natural course of penicillamine nephropathy: a long term study of 33 patients. BMJ (Clin Res Ed) 1988;296(6629):1083–6.

196. Combe C, Deforges-Lasseur C, Chehab Z, De Precigout, Aparicio M. La lithiase cystinique et son traitement par la d-pénicillamine. Semin Hop 1992;68:746–50.

197. Pedersen LM, Nordin H, Svensson B, Bliddal H. Microalbuminuria in patients with rheumatoid arthritis. Ann Rheum Dis 1995;54(3):189–92.

198. DeSilva RN, Eastmond CJ. Management of proteinuria secondary to penicillamine therapy in rheumatoid arthritis. Clin Rheumatol 1992;11(2):216–19.

199. Stephens AD. Cystinuria and its treatment: 25 years experience at St. Bartholomew's Hospital. J Inherit Metab Dis 1989;12(2):197–209.

200. Hill GS. Drug-associated glomerulopathies. Toxicol Pathol 1986;14(1):37–44.

201. Emery P, Panayi G. Penicillamine nephropathy. BMJ (Clin Res Ed) 1988;296(6635):1538.

202. Speerstra F, van de Putte LB, Rasker JJ, Reekers P, Vandenbroucke JP. The relationship between aurothioglucose- and D-penicillamine-induced proteinuria. Scand J Rheumatol 1984;13(4):363–8.

203. Yoshida A, Morozumi K, Suganuma T, Aoki J, Sugito K, Koyama K, Oikawa T, Fujinimi T, Matsumoto Y. [Clinicopathological study of nephropathy in patients with rheumatoid arthritis.] Ryumachi 1991;31(1):14–21.

204. Bar J, Ehrenfeld M, Rozenman J, Perelman M, Sidi Y, Gur H. Pulmonary-renal syndrome in systemic sclerosis. Semin Arthritis Rheum 2001;30(6):403–10.

205. Koseki Y, Terai C, Moriguchi M, Uesato M, Kamatani N. A prospective study of renal disease in patients with early rheumatoid arthritis. Ann Rheum Dis 2001;60(4):327–31.

206. Niederstadt C, Happ T, Tatsis E, Schnabel A, Steinhoff J. Glomerular and tubular proteinuria as markers of nephropathy in rheumatoid arthritis. Rheumatology (Oxford) 1999;38(1):28–33.

207. Verroust PJ. Kinetics of immune deposits in membranous nephropathy. Kidney Int 1989;35(6):1418–28.

208. Isenring P, de Cotret PR, Delage C, Kingma I, Lebel M. d-Penicillamine induced reversible minimal change nephropathy in rheumatoid arthritis. J Nephrol 1991;4:245–8.

209. Dische FE, Swinson DR, Hamilton EB, Parsons V. Immunopathology of penicillamine-induced glomerular disease. J Rheumatol 1984;11(5):584–5.

210. Druet P, Kleinknecht D. Les néphropathies glomérulaires d'origine toxique. [Toxic glomerulonephritis.] Presse Méd 1989;18(37):1840–5.

211. Malaise MG, Davin JC, Mahieu PR, Franchimont P. Elevated antigalactosyl antibody titers reflect renal injury after gold or D-penicillamine in rheumatoid arthritis. Clin Immunol Immunopathol 1986;40(2):356–64.

212. Rehan A, Johnson K. IgM nephropathy associated with penicillamine. Am J Nephrol 1986;6(1):71–4.

213. Ntoso KA, Tomaszewski JE, Jimenez SA, Neilson EG. Penicillamine-induced rapidly progressive glomerulonephritis in patients with progressive systemic sclerosis: successful treatment of two patients and a review of the literature. Am J Kidney Dis 1986;8(3):159–63.

214. Williams AJ, Fordham JN, Barnes CG, Goodwin FJ. Progressive proliferative glomerulonephritis in a patient with rheumatoid arthritis treated with D-penicillamine. Ann Rheum Dis 1986;45(1):82–4.

215. Suda M, Yoshikawa Y, Suzuki T, Dohi Y, Shibata T. [A case report of rheumatoid arthritis which showed acute renal failure, nephrotic syndrome and drug-related lupus-like syndrome caused by D-penicillamine.] Nippon Jinzo Gakkai Shi 1990;32(11):1235–41.

216. Donnelly S, Levison DA, Doyle DV. Systemic lupus erythematosus-like syndrome with focal proliferative glomerulonephritis during D-penicillamine therapy. Br J Rheumatol 1993;32(3):251–3.

217. Rejchrt S, Hrncir Z, Pinterova E. [Rheumatoid arthritis developing into systemic lupus erythematosus during long-term treatment with penicillamine and sulfasalazine.] Vnitr Lek 1991;37(6):597–603.

218. Almirall J, Alcorta I, Botey A, Revert L. Penicillamine-induced rapidly progressive glomerulonephritis in a patient with rheumatoid arthritis. Am J Nephrol 1993;13(4):286–8.

219. Gaertner HV. Drug-associated nephropathy. In: Grundman E, editor. Drug-induced Pathology. Vol. 69. Current Topics in Pathology. Berlin: Springer-Verlag, 198051–4.

220. Karpinski J, Jothy S, Radoux V, Levy M, Baran D. D-penicillamine-induced crescentic glomerulonephritis and antimyeloperoxidase antibodies in a patient with scleroderma. Case report and review of the literature. Am J Nephrol 1997;17(6):528–32.

221. Sadjadi SA, Seelig MS, Berger AR, Milstoc M. Rapidly progressive glomerulonephritis in a patient with rheumatoid arthritis during treatment with high dosage d-penicillamine. Ann Rheum Dis 1985;45:82.

222. Devogelaer JP, Pirson Y, Vandenbroucke JM, Cosyns JP, Brichard S, Nagant de Deuxchaisnes C. D-penicillamine induced crescentic glomerulonephritis: report and review of the literature. J Rheumatol 1987;14(5):1036–41.

223. Leatherman JW, Davies SF, Hoidal JR. Alveolar hemorrhage syndromes: diffuse microvascular lung hemorrhage in immune and idiopathic disorders. Medicine (Baltimore) 1984;63(6):343–61.

224. Macarron P, Garcia Diaz JE, Azofra JA, Martin de Francisco J, Gonzalez E, Fernandez G, Sampedro J. D-penicillamine therapy associated with rapidly progressive glomerulonephritis. Nephrol Dial Transplant 1992;7(2):161–4.

225. Bindi P, Gilson B, Aymard B, Noel LH, Wieslander J. Antiglomerular basement membrane glomerulonephritis following D-penicillamine-associated nephrotic syndrome. Nephrol Dial Transplant 1997;12(2):325–7.

226. Scherberig JE, Sniehotta KP, Miehlke K, Schoeppe W. Nierenbeteiligung bei rheumatoider Arthritis. Nieren Hochdrukkr 1987;16:69.

227. Boers M, Croonen AM, Dijkmans BA, Breedveld FC, Eulderink F, Cats A, Weening JJ. Renal findings in rheumatoid arthritis: clinical aspects of 132 necropsies. Ann Rheum Dis 1987;46(9):658–63.

228. Cantagrel A, Fournie B, Pourrat J, Conte JJ, Fournie A. Hématurie microscopique d'origine rénale au cours de la polyarthrite rhumatoïde. [Renal microscopic hematuria in rheumatoid polyarthritis.] Rev Med Interne 1991;12(1):31–6.

229. Honkanen E, Tornroth T, Pettersson E, Skrifvars B. Membranous glomerulonephritis in rheumatoid arthritis not related to gold or D-penicillamine therapy: a report of four cases and review of the literature. Clin Nephrol 1987;27(2):87–93.

230. Feehally J, Wheeler DC, Mackay EH, Oldham R, Walls J. Recurrent acute renal failure with interstitial nephritis due to D-penicillamine. Ren Fail 1987;10(1):55–7.

231. Nakano M, Ueno M, Nishi S, Shimada H, Hasegawa H, Watanabe T, Kuroda T, Sato T, Maruyama Y, Arakawa M. Analysis of renal pathology and drug history in 158 Japanese patients with rheumatoid arthritis. Clin Nephrol 1998;50(3):154–60.

232. Siafakas CG, Jonas MM, Alexander S, Herrin J, Furuta GT. Early onset of nephrotic syndrome after treatment with D-penicillamine in a patient with Wilson's disease. Am J Gastroenterol 1998;93(12):2544–6.

233. Marchand-Courville S, Dhib M, Fillastre JP, Godin M. Glomerulonéphrites extracapillaires secondaires à la D-pénicillamine. A propos d'une observation et revue de la littérature. [Extracapillary glomerulonephritis secondary to D-penicillamine. Apropos of 1 case and review of the literature.] Nephrologie 1998;19(1):25–32.

234. Phillips D, Phillips B, Mannino D. A case study and national database report of progressive systemic sclerosis and associated conditions. J Womens Health 1998;7(9):1099–104.

235. Haviv YS, Safadi R. Rapid progression of scleroderma possibly associated with penicillamine therapy. Clin Drug Invest 1998;15:61–3.

236. Kyndt X, Ducq P, Bridoux F, Reumaux D, Makdassi R, Gheerbrant JD, Vanhille P. Glomerulonéphrite extracapillaire avec anticorps anti-myeloperoxydase chez 2 malades ayant une sclérodermie systémique traitée par D-pénicillamine. [Extracapillary glomerulonephritis with anti-myeloperoxidase antibodies in 2 patients with systemic scleroderma treated with penicillamine D.] Presse Méd 1999;28(2):67–70.

237. Marlier S, Gisserot O, Yao N, Hecht M, Paris JF, Carli P, Chagnon A. Glomerulonéphrite extracapillaire lors d'un traitement par D-pénicillamine. [Extra-capillary glomerulonephritis induced by D-penicillamine therapy.] Presse Méd 1999;28(13):689–90.

238. Mazhari R, Kimmel PL. Hematuria: an algorithmic approach to finding the cause. Cleve Clin J Med 2002;69(11):870–6.

239. Shannon M, Graef J, Lovejoy FH Jr. Efficacy and toxicity of D-penicillamine in low-level lead poisoning. J Pediatr 1988;112(5):799–804.

240. Bell CL, Graziano FM. The safety of administration of penicillamine to penicillin-sensitive individuals. Arthritis Rheum 1983;26(6):801–3.

241. Oliver I, Liberman UA, DeVries A. Lupus-like syndrome induced by penicillamine in cystinuria. JAMA 1972;220(4):588.

242. Pachoula-Papasteriades C, Boki K, Varla-Leftherioti M, Kappos-Rigatou I, Fostiropoulos G, Economidou J. HLA-A,-B, and -DR antigens in relation to gold and D-penicillamine toxicity in Greek patients with RA. Dis Markers 1986;4(1–2):35–41.

243. Vlachoyiannopoulos PG, Zerva LV, Skopouli FN, Drosos AA, Moutsopoulos HM. D-penicillamine toxicity in Greek patients with rheumatoid arthritis: anti-Ro(SSA) antibodies and cryoglobulinemia are predictive factors. J Rheumatol 1991;18(1):44–9.

244. Shannon MW, Townsend MK. Adverse effects of reduced-dose d-penicillamine in children with mild-to-moderate lead poisoning. Ann Pharmacother 2000;34(1):15–18.

245. Miyagawa S, Yoshioka A, Hatoko M, Okuchi T, Sakamoto K. Systemic sclerosis-like lesions during long-term penicillamine therapy for Wilson's disease. Br J Dermatol 1987;116(1):95–100.

246. Liddle BJ. Development of morphoea in rheumatoid arthritis treated with penicillamine. Ann Rheum Dis 1989;48(11):963–4.

247. Schachter RK. Localized scleroderma. Curr Opin Rheumatol 1990;2(6):947–55.

248. Enzenauer RJ, West SG, Rubin RL. D-penicillamine-induced lupus erythematosus. Arthritis Rheum 1990;33(10):1582–5.

249. Chin GL, Kong NC, Lee BC, Rose IM. Penicillamine induced lupus-like syndrome in a patient with classical rheumatoid arthritis. J Rheumatol 1991;18(6):947–8.

250. Tsankov NK, Lazarova AZ, Vasileva SG, Obreshkova EV. Lupus erythematosus-like eruption due to D-penicillamine in progressive systemic sclerosis. Int J Dermatol 1990;29(8):571–4.

251. Condon C, Phelan M, Lyons JF. Penicillamine-induced type II bullous systemic lupus erythematosus. Br J Dermatol 1997;136(3):474–5.

252. Bannwarth B, Schaeverbeke T, Dehais J. Low back pain associated with penicillamine. BMJ 1991;303(6801):525.

253. Zvulunov A, Grunwald MH, Avinoach I, Halevy S. Transient acantholytic dermatosis (Grover's disease) in a patient with progressive systemic sclerosis treated with D-penicillamine. Int J Dermatol 1997;36(6):476–7.

254. Rose BI, LeMaire WJ, Jeffers LJ. Macromastia in a woman treated with penicillamine and oral contraceptives. A case report. J Reprod Med 1990;35(1):43–5.

255. Pyo JY, Lee WJ, Koo DW. A case of penicillamine dermatopathy. Korean J Dermatol 2001;39:341–3.

256. Melani L, Caproni M, Cardinali C, Antiga E, Bernacchi E, Schincaglia E, Fabbri P. A case of nodular scleroderma. J Dermatol 2005;32(12):1028–31.

257. Sehgal VN, Srivastava G, Aggarwal AK, Behl PN, Choudhary M, Bajaj P. Localized scleroderma/morphea. Int J Dermatol 2002;41(8):467–75.

258. Rencic A, Goyal S, Mofid M, Wigley F, Nousari HC. Bullous lesions in scleroderma. Int J Dermatol 2002;41(6):335–9.

259. Newbold PC. Contact reaction to penicillamine in vaginal secretions. Lancet 1979;1(8130):1344.

260. Iozumi K, Nakagawa H, Tamaki K. Penicillamine-induced degenerative dermatoses: report of a case and brief review of such dermatoses. J Dermatol 1997;24(7):458–65.

261. Dootson G, Sarkany I. D-penicillamine induced dermopathy in Wilson's disease. Clin Exp Dermatol 1987;12(1):66–8.

262. Pasquali Ronchetti I, Quaglino D Jr, Baccarani Contri M, Hayek J, Galassi G. Dermal alterations in patients with Wilson's disease treated with D-penicillamine. J Submicrosc Cytol Pathol 1989;21(1):131–9.

263. Goldstein JB, McNutt NS, Hambrick GW Jr, Hsu A. Penicillamine dermatopathy with lymphangiectases. A clinical, immunohistologic, and ultrastructural study. Arch Dermatol 1989;125(1):92–7.

264. Light N, Meyrick Thomas RH, Stephens A, Kirby JD, Fryer PR, Avery NC. Collagen and elastin changes in D-penicillamine-induced pseudoxanthoma elasticum-like skin. Br J Dermatol 1986;114(3):381–8.

265. Camus JP, Koeger AC. D-Pénicillamine et collagène. [D-penicillamine and collagen.] Ann Biol Clin (Paris) 1986;44(3):296–9.

266. Nimni ME. Penicillamine and collagen metabolism. Scand J Rheumatol Suppl 1979;(28):71–8.

267. Buckley C, Sankey EA, Harris D, Wright S. Case update—progressive skin laxity secondary to penicillamine treatment. Clin Exp Dermatol 1991;16(4):310–11.

268. Narron GH, Zec N, Neves RI, Manders EK, Sexton FM Jr. Penicillamine-induced pseudoxanthoma elasticum-like skin changes requiring rhytidectomy. Ann Plast Surg 1992;29(4):367–70.

269. Bolognia JL, Braverman I. Pseudoxanthoma-elasticum-like skin changes induced by penicillamine. Dermatology 1992;184(1):12–18.

270. Layton AM, Cunliffe WJ. Electrocautery as a successful treatment for penicillamine-induced elastosis perforans serpiginosa. J Dermatol Treat 1991;2:111–12.

271. Dalziel KL, Burge SM, Frith PA, Ryan TJ, Mowat A. Elastic fibre damage induced by low-dose D-penicillamine. Br J Dermatol 1990;123(3):305–12.

272. Sahn EE, Maize JC, Garen PD, Mullins SC, Silver RM. D-penicillamine-induced elastosis perforans serpiginosa in a child with juvenile rheumatoid arthritis. Report of a case and review of the literature. J Am Acad Dermatol 1989;20(5 Pt 2):979–88.

273. Price RG, Prentice RS. Penicillamine-induced elastosis perforans serpiginosa. Tip of the iceberg? Am J Dermatopathol 1986;8(4):314–20.

274. Matsushita A, Hiruma M, Ogawa H, Watanabe S, Saeki T. A case of D-penicillamine-induced elastosis perforans serpiginosa in a women with systemic sclerosis. Nishinihon J Dermatol 1999;61:451–4.

275. Fraysse T, De Wazieres B. Maladie de Wilson et "vieille peau". Pract Med Ther 2001;15:38–9.

276. Hill VA, Seymour CA, Mortimer PS. Penicillamine-induced elastosis perforans serpiginosa and cutis laxa in Wilson's disease. Br J Dermatol 2000;142(3):560–1.

277. Coatesworth AP, Darnton SJ, Green RM, Cayton RM, Antonakopoulos GN. A case of systemic pseudo-pseudoxanthoma elasticum with diverse symptomatology caused by long-term penicillamine use. J Clin Pathol 1998;51(2):169–71.

278. Zacher J, Spath S, Wessinghage D, Waertel G. Basistherapie der chronisch-entzündlichem Gelenkerkrankungen met D-penicillamin und Wundheilungsstörungen bei rheumaorthopädischen Eingriffen. [Basic therapy of chronic inflammatory joint diseases with D-penicillamine and disorders of wound healing in rheumatoid orthopedic interventions.] Z Rheumatol 1988;47(Suppl 1):41–3.

279. Burry HC. Penicillamine and wound healing—a potential hazard? Postgrad Med J 1974;50(Suppl 2):75–6.

280. Mutasim DF, Pelc NJ, Anhalt GJ. Drug-induced pemphigus. Dermatol Clin 1993;11(3):463–71.

281. Brenner S, Halevy S, Livni E, Schewach-Millet M, Sandbank M, Wolf R. Macrophage migration inhibition test in patients with drug-induced pemphigus. Isr J Med Sci 1993;29(1):44–6.

282. Wolf R, Brenner S. Arzneimittelbedingter Pemphigus-Uebersicht. Z Hautkrankh 1991;66:289–93.

283. Zillikens D, Zentner A, Burger M, Hartmann AA, Burg G. Pemphigus foliaceus durch Penicillamin. [Pemphigus foliaceus caused by penicillamine.] Hautarzt 1993;44(3):167–71.

284. Brenner S, Bialy-Golan A, Anhalt GJ. Recognition of pemphigus antigens in drug-induced pemphigus vulgaris and pemphigus foliaceus. J Am Acad Dermatol 1997;36(6 Pt 1):919–23.

285. Penas PF, Buezo GF, Carvajal I, Dauden E, Lopez A, Diaz LA. D-penicillamine-induced pemphigus foliaceus with autoantibodies to desmoglein-1 in a patient with mixed connective tissue disease. J Am Acad Dermatol 1997;37(1):121–3.

286. McGovern TW, Bennion SD. Diffuse blisters and erosions in a patient with limited scleroderma. Penicillamine-induced pemphigus foliaceus (PIPF). Arch Dermatol 1997;133(4):501.

287. Verret JL, Avene IM, Smulevici A, Esparbes M. Les pemphigus induits par la pénicillamine: á propos de trois cas. J Agregres 1983;16:209.

288. Hashimoto K, Shafran KM, Webber PS, Lazarus GS, Singer KH. Anti-cell surface pemphigus autoantibody stimulates plasminogen activator activity of human epidermal cells. A mechanism for the loss of epidermal cohesion and blister formation. J Exp Med 1983;157(1):259–72.

289. Hashimoto K, Singer K, Lazarus GS. Penicillamine-induced pemphigus. Immunoglobulin from this patient induces plasminogen activator synthesis by human epidermal cells in culture: mechanism for acantholysis in pemphigus. Arch Dermatol 1984;120(6):762–4.

290. Bahmer FA, Bambauer R, Stenger D. Penicillamine-induced pemphigus foliaceus-like dermatosis. A case with unusual features, successfully treated by plasmapheresis. Arch Dermatol 1985;121(5):665–8.

291. Tholen S. Arzneimittelbedingter Pemphigus. [Drug-induced pemphigus.] Z Hautkr 1986;61(10):719–23.

292. Walton S, Keczkes K, Robinson AE. A case of penicillamine-induced pemphigus, successfully treated by plasma exchange. Clin Exp Dermatol 1987;12(4):275–6.

293. Kind P, Goerz G, Gleichmann E, Plewig G. Penicillamin induzierter Pemphigus. [Penicillamine-induced pemphigus.] Hautarzt 1987;38(9):548–52.

294. Buckley C, Barry C, Woods R, Dervan P, O'Loughlin S. Penicillamine induced pemphigus—a report of 2 cases. Ir J Med Sci 1988;157(8):267–8.

295. Civatte J. Durch Medikamente induzierte Pemphigus-Erkrankungen. [Drug-induced pemphigus diseases.] Dermatol Monatsschr 1989;175(1):1–7.

296. Willemsen MJ, De Coninck AL, De Raeve LE, Roseeuw DI. Penicillamine-induced pemphigus erythematosus. Int J Dermatol 1990;29(3):193–7.

297. Rasmussen HB, Jepsen LV, Brandrup F. Penicillamine-induced bullous pemphigoid with pemphigus-like antibodies. J Cutan Pathol 1989;16(3):154–7.

298. Shapiro M, Jimenez S, Werth VP. Pemphigus vulgaris induced by D-penicillamine therapy in a patient with systemic sclerosis. J Am Acad Dermatol 2000;42(2 Pt 1):297–9.

299. Weller R, White MI. Penicillamine in the etiology of bullous pemphigoid. Ann Pharmacother 1998;32(12):1368.

300. Verma KK, Pasricha JS. Pemphigus foliaceous induced by penicillamine. Indian J Dermatol Venereol Leprol 1990;56:234–5.

301. Piette-Brion B, de Bast C, Chamoun E, de Dobbeleer G, Andre J, Huybrechts A, Ledoux M, Achten G. Pemphigus superficial apparu lors du traitement d'une polyarthrite rhumatoïde par D-pénicillamine et piroxicam. [Superficial pemphigus during the treatment of rheumatoid polyarthritis with D-penicillamine and piroxicam (Feldene).] Dermatologica 1985;170(6):297–301.

302. Kohn SR. Fatal penicillamine-induced pemphigus foliaceus-like dermatosis. Arch Dermatol 1986;122(1):17.

303. Toth GG, Jonkman MF. Successful treatment of recalcitrant penicillamine-induced pemphigus foliaceus by low-dose intravenous immunoglobulins. Br J Dermatol 1999;141(3):583–5.

304. Korman NJ, Eyre RW, Zone J, Stanley JR. Drug-induced pemphigus: autoantibodies directed against the pemphigus antigen complexes are present in penicillamine and captopril-induced pemphigus. J Invest Dermatol 1991;96(2):273–6.

305. Bedane C, Bernard P, Dang PM, Amici JM, Catanzano G, Bonnetblanc JM. Étude ultrastructurale des antigènescibles du pemphigus foliacé et du pemphigus vulgaire. A propos de deux observations. [Ultrastructural study of pemphigus foliaceus and pemphigus vulgaris antigens. Apropos of 2 cases.] Ann Dermatol Venereol 1991;118(11):888–90.

306. Ruocco V, de Angelis E, Lombardi ML, Pisani M. In vitro acantholysis by captopril and thiopronine. Dermatologica 1988;176(3):115–23.

307. Yokel BK, Hood AF, Anhalt GJ. Induction of acantholysis in organ explant culture by penicillamine and captopril. Arch Dermatol 1989;125(10):1367–70.

308. Lombardi ML, de Angelis E, Rossano F, Ruocco V. Imbalance between plasminogen activator and its inhibitors in thiol-induced acantholysis. Dermatology 1993;186(2):118–22.

309. Bauer-Vinassac D, Menkes CJ, Muller JY, Escande JP. HLA system and penicillamine induced pemphigus in nine cases of rheumatoid arthritis. Scand J Rheumatol 1992;21(1):17–19.

310. Wilkinson SM, Smith AG, Davis MJ, Hollowood K, Dawes PT. Rheumatoid arthritis: an association with pemphigus foliaceous. Acta Derm Venereol 1992;72(4):289–91.

311. Aydemir EH, Is imen A, Aksoy F. d-Penisilamin'e bagli eritem anuler benzeri pemfigus. Deri Hast Frengi Ars 1988;22:247–50.

312. Shuttleworth D, Graham-Brown RA, Hutchinson PE, Jolliffe DS. Cicatricial pemphigoid in D-penicillamine treated patients with rheumatoid arthritis—a report of three cases. Clin Exp Dermatol 1985;10(4):392–7.

313. Peyri J, Servitje O, Ribera M, Henkes J, Ferrandiz C. Cicatricial pemphigoid in a patient with rheumatoid arthritis treated with D-penicillamine. J Am Acad Dermatol 1986;14(4):681.

314. Marti-Huguet T, Quintana M, Cabiro I. Cicatricial pemphigoid associated with D-penicillamine treatment. Arch Ophthalmol 1989;107(8):1115.

315. Hallauer W, Gartner HV, Kronenberg KH, Manz G. Immunkomplexnephritis mit nephrotischem Syndrom unter Therapie mit D-Penizillamin. [Immune complex nephritis with nephrotic syndrome following D-penicillamine therapy.] Schweiz Med Wochenschr 1974;104(12):434–8.

316. Takatsuka H, Takemoto Y, Yamada S, Mori A, Wada H, Fujimori Y, Okamoto T, Kanamaru A, Kakishita E. Similarity between eruptions induced by sulfhydryl drugs and acute cutaneous graft-versus-host disease after bone marrow transplantation. Hematology 2002;7(1):55–7.

317. Powell FC, Rogers RS, Dickson ER. Lichen planus, primary biliary cirrhosis and penicillamine. Br J Dermatol 1982;107(5):616.

318. Kitamura K, Aihara M, Osawa J, Naito S, Ikezawa Z. Sulfhydryl drug-induced eruption: a clinical and histological study. J Dermatol 1990;17(1):44–51.

319. Kitamura K, Aihara M, Osawa J, Naito S, Ikezawa Z. Clinical histological study of drug eruptions induced by sulfhydryl drugs. Proc Jpn Soc Investig Dermatol 1988;12:136–7.

320. Forgie JC, Highet AS. Psoriasiform eruptions associated with penicillamine. BMJ (Clin Res Ed) 1987;294:1101.

321. Jimenez-Balderas FJ, Rangel J, Mintz G. Penicillamine induced myositis: correlation between urinary zinc excretion and serum creatine. J Rheumatol 1991;18(6):945–7.

322. Garcia-Nieto AV, Fernandez Roldan JC, Martinez-Sanchez F, Gonzalez Gomez J, Moreno Gimenez JC. Yellow nail syndrome by d-penicillamine. Actas Dermo-Sifiliogr 1997;88:191–5.

323. Ilchyshyn A, Vickers CF. Yellow nail syndrome associated with penicillamine therapy. Acta Derm Venereol 1983;63(6):554–5.

324. Dubost JJ, Fraysse P, Ristori JM, Rampon S. Syndrome des ongles jaunes avec dilatation des bronches après traitement d'une polyarthrite rhumatoïde par la d-pénicillamine. Semin Hop Paris 1988;64:1548–51.

325. Ichikawa Y, Shimizu H, Arimori S. "Yellow nail syndrome" and rheumatoid arthritis. Tokai J Exp Clin Med 1991;16(5–6):203–9.

326. Bjellerup M. Nail-changes induced by penicillamine. Acta Derm Venereol 1989;69(4):339–41.

327. Sturrock RD, Brooks PM. Penicillamine and creaking joints. BMJ 1974;3(5930):575.

328. Stein HB, Patterson AC, Offer RC, Atkins CJ, Teufel A, Robinson HS. Adverse effects of D-penicillamine in rheumatoid arthritis. Ann Intern Med 1980;92(1):24–9.

329. Halperin EC, Thier SO, Rosenberg LE. The use of D-penicillamine in cystinuria: efficacy and untoward reactions. Yale J Biol Med 1981;54(6):439–46.

330. Butler D, Tiliakos NA. Penicillamine-induced exacerbation of rheumatoid arthritis. South Med J 1986;79(6):778–9.

331. Narvaez J, Alegre-Sancho JJ, Juanola X, Roig-Escofet D. Arthropathy of Wilson's disease presenting as noninflammatory polyarthritis. J Rheumatol 1997;24(12):2494.

332. Dulcine M, Borges C, Vianna MADAG, Neto EFB. Eosinophilic fasciitis with subclinical myopathy with exacerbated myositis after using the d-penicillamine. Rev Bras Reumatol 1999;39:303–6.

333. Sampaio-Barros PD, De Paiva Magalhaes E, Sachetto Z, Samara AM, Marques Neto JF. Bone mineral density in systemic sclerosis. Rev Bras Reumatol 2000;40:153–8.

334. Kahl LE, Medsger TA Jr, Klein I. Massive breast enlargement in a patient receiving D-penicillamine for systemic sclerosis. J Rheumatol 1985;12(5):990–1.

335. Craig HR. Penicillamine induced mammary hyperplasia: report of a case and review of the literature. J Rheumatol 1988;15(8):1294–7.

336. Spaeth M, Berkl M, Miehle W. Mammahyperplasie und d-Penicillamin. Aktuel Rheumatol 1991;16:214–16.

337. Caballeria J, Caballeria L, Cabre J, Bruguera M, Rodes J. Mammary hyperplasia secondary to treatment with d-penicillamine in a patient with Wilson's disease. Gastroenterol Hepatol 1993;16:607–9.

338. O'Hare PM, Frieden IJ. Virginal breast hypertrophy. Pediatr Dermatol 2000;17(4):277–81.

339. Salliere D, Clerc D, Bisson M, Massias P. Gynécomastie transitoire an course d'un traitement par la D-penicillamine. [Transient gynecomastia during treatment with D-penicillamine.] Presse Méd 1984;13(37):2265.

340. Tchebiner JZ. Breast enlargement induced by D-penicillamine. Ann Pharmacother 2002;36(3):444–5.

341. Upponi SS, Jadav AM, Bobrow L, Purushotham AD. Breast hypertrophy related to D-penicillamine? Breast 2001;10:349–50.

342. Rosada M, Fiocco U, De Silvestro G, Doria A, Cozzi L, Favaretto M, Todesco S. Effect of D-pénicillamine on the T cell phenotype in scleroderma. Comparison between treated and untreated patients. Clin Exp Rheumatol 1993;11(2):143–8.

343. Panayi GS, Mills MM. Second-line drug treatment in rheumatoid arthritis associated with depressed autologous mixed lymphocyte reaction. Rheumatol Int 1986;6(1):25–9.

344. Miyachi Y, Yoshioka A, Imamura S, Niwa Y. Decreased hydroxyl radical generation from polymorphonuclear leucocytes in the presence of D-penicillamine and thiopronine. J Clin Lab Immunol 1987;22(2):81–4.

345. Sim E, Dodds AW, Goldin A. Inhibition of the covalent binding reaction of complement component C4 by penicillamine, an anti-rheumatic agent. Biochem J 1989;259(2):415–19.

346. Price EJ, Venables PJ. Drug-induced lupus. Drug Saf 1995;12(4):283–90.

347. Haberhauer G, Broll H. Drug-induced anticentromere antibody? Z Rheumatol 1989;48(2):99–100.

348. Haberhauer G. D-penicillamine (DPA)-induced anticentromere antibody (ACA). Clin Exp Rheumatol 1989;7(3):332–4.

349. Storch W. Antikörper gegen D-penicillamin bei primär biliärer Zirrhose. [Antibodies against D-penicillamine in primary biliary cirrhosis.] Immun Infekt 1990;18(1):22–3.

350. Yarze JC, Martin P, Munoz SJ, Friedman LS. Wilson's disease: current status. Am J Med 1992;92(6):643–54.

351. Tanphaichitr K. D-penicillamine-induced bronchial spasm. South Med J 1980;73(6):788–90.

352. Nanke Y, Akama H, Terai C, Kamatani N. Rapidly progressive glomerulonephritis with D-penicillamine. Am J Med Sci 2000;320(6):398–402.

353. Garcia-Porrua C, Gonzalez-Gay MA, Bouza P. D-penicillamine-induced crescentic glomerulonephritis in a patient with scleroderma. Nephron 2000;84(1):101–2.

354. Kolsi R, Bahloul Z, Hachicha J, Gouiaa R, Jarraya A. Dermatopolymyosite induite par la D-pénicillamine au cours de la polyarthrite rhumatoïde. A propos d'un cas avec revue de la littérature. [Dermatopolymyositis induced by D-penicillamine in rheumatoid polyarthritis. Apropos of 1 case with review of the literature.] Rev Rhum Mal Osteoartic 1992;59(5):341–4.

355. Takahashi K, Ogita T, Okudaira H, Yoshinoya S, Yoshizawa H, Miyamoto T. D-penicillamine-induced polymyositis in patients with rheumatoid arthritis. Arthritis Rheum 1986;29(4):560–4.

356. Matsumura T, Yuhara T, Yamane K, Kono I, Kabashima T, Kashiwagi H. D-penicillamine-induced polymyositis occurring in patients with rheumatoid arthritis: a report of two cases and demonstration of a positive lymphocyte stimulation test to D-penicillamine. Henry Ford Hosp Med J 1986;34(2):123–6.

357. Masson CJ, Menard HA, Audran M, Renier JC, Lussier A, Myhal DM. Polymyosite induite par la D-pénicillamine lors d'arthrite rhumatoïde: à propos de deux cas avec des anticorps antinucléaire. [Polymyositis induced by D-penicillamine treatment of rheumatoid arthritis: apropos of 2 cases with antinuclear antibodies.] Union Med Can 1986;115(12):855–9.

358. Ostensen M, Husby G, Aarli J. Polymyositis with acute myolysis in a patient with rheumatoid arthritis treated with penicillamine and ampicillin. Arthritis Rheum 1980;23(3):375–7.

359. Car J, Lorette G, Jacob C. Dermatomyosite induite par la d-pénicillamine. Semin Hop 1987;63:399.

360. Leden I, Libelius R. Penicillamine-induced polymyositis. Scand J Rheumatol 1985;14(1):90–3.

361. Carroll GJ, Will RK, Peter JB, Garlepp MJ, Dawkins RL. Penicillamine induced polymyositis and dermatomyositis. J Rheumatol 1987;14(5):995–1001.

362. Christensen PD, Sorensen KE. Penicillamine-induced polymyositis with complete heart block. Eur Heart J 1989;10(11):1041–4.

363. Taneja V, Mehra N, Singh YN, Kumar A, Malaviya A, Singh RR. HLA-D region genes and susceptibility to D-penicillamine-induced myositis. Arthritis Rheum 1990;33(9):1445–7.

364. Santos JC, Velasco JA. Polymyositis due to D-penicillamine in a patient with systemic sclerosis. Clin Exp Dermatol 1991;16(1):76.

365. Fukuda S, Murata Y, Takahashi T, Hatada Y, Tsushima Y, Takemori H, Yoshida Y, Okushima T. d-Penicillamine-induced polymyositis in a patient with rheumatoid arthritis. Saishin-Igaku 1990;45:1854–9.

366. Larbre JP, Perret P, Collet P, Llorca G. Antinuclear antibodies during pyrithioxine treatment. Br J Rheumatol 1990;29(6):496–7.

367. Barrera P, den Broeder AA, van den Hoogen FH, van Engelen BG, van de Putte LB. Postural changes, dysphagia, and systemic sclerosis. Ann Rheum Dis 1998;57(6):331–8.

368. Ibel H, Feist D, Endres W, Belohradsky BH. D-Penicillamin-induzierter IgA-Mangel bei der Therapie der Wilsonschen Erkrankung. [D-penicillamine-induced IgA deficiency in the therapy of Wilson's disease.] Klin Padiatr 1990;202(6):427–9.

369. Chalmers A, Thompson D, Stein HE, Reid G, Patterson AC. Systemic lupus erythematosus during penicillamine therapy for rheumatoid arthritis. Ann Intern Med 1982;97(5):659–63.

370. Chikanza IC. Juvenile rheumatoid arthritis: therapeutic perspectives. Paediatr Drugs 2002;4(5):335–48.

371. Lin HC, Hwang KC, Lee HJ, Tsai MJ, Ni YH, Chiang BL. Penicillamine induced lupus-like syndrome: a case report. J Microbiol Immunol Infect 2000;33(3):202–4.

372. May V, Aristoff H, Lecoq G. Syndrome de Gougerot–sjögren induit par la D-pénicillamine. A propos d'un cas. [Gougerot–Sjögren syndrome induced by D-penicillamine. Apropos of a case.] Rev Rhum Mal Osteoartic 1977;44(7–9):497–501.

373. Pruzanski E, editor. Proceedings. International Symposium on Penicillamine, Miami, 1980. J Rheumatol 1981;8(Suppl 7):181.

374. Dubois RS, Rodgerson DO, Hambidge KM. Treatment of Wilson's disease with triethylene tetramine hydrochloride (Trientine). J Pediatr Gastroenterol Nutr 1990;10(1):77–81.

375. Savill JS, Chia Y, Pusey CD. Minimal change nephropathy and pemphigus vulgaris associated with penicillamine treatment of rheumatoid arthritis. Clin Nephrol 1988;29(5):267–70.

376. Jones E, Sobkowski WW, Murray SJ, Walsh NM. Concurrent pemphigus and myasthenia gravis as manifestations of penicillamine toxicity. J Am Acad Dermatol 1993;28(4):655–6.

377. Hsu HL, Huang FC, Ni YH, Chang MH. Steroids used to desensitize penicillamine allergy in Wilson disease. Acta Paediatr Taiwan 1999;40(6):448–50.

378. Hernandez-Cruz B, Cardiel MH, Villa AR, Alcocer-Varela J. Development, recurrence, and severity of infections in Mexican patients with rheumatoid arthritis. A nested case-control study. J Rheumatol 1998;25(10):1900–7.

379. Speit G, Haupter S. Cytogenetic effects of penicillamine. Mutat Res 1987;190(3):197–203.

380. Gilman PA, Holtzman NA. Acute lymphoblastic leukemia in a patient receiving penicillamine for Wilson's disease. JAMA 1982;248(4):467–8.

381. Sheldon P, Wood JK. Remission of arthritis and radiological improvement after combination therapy for non-Hodgkin's lymphoma in a patient with rheumatoid arthritis undergoing treatment with D-penicillamine. Ann Rheum Dis 1985;44(8):556–8.

382. Anonymous. Neoplasms in rheumatoid arthritis: update on clinical and epidemiologic data. Am J Med 1985; 78(1A):1–83.

383. Miehle W. Aktuelles zu D-Penicillamin and Schwangerschaft. [Current aspects of D-penicillamine and pregnancy.] Z Rheumatol 1988;47(Suppl 1):20–3.

384. Rosa FW. Teratogen update: penicillamine. Teratology 1986;33(1):127–31.

385. Frishman WH. Chelation therapy for coronary artery disease: panacea or quackery? Am J Med 2001;111(9):729–30.

386. Martinez-Frias ML, Rodriguez-Pinilla E, Bermejo E, Blanco M. Prenatal exposure to penicillamine and oral clefts: case report. Am J Med Genet 1998;76(3):274–5.

387. Emery P, Panayi GS, Huston G, Welsh KI, Mitchell SC, Shah RR, Idle JR, Smith RL, Waring RH. D-Penicillamine induced toxicity in rheumatoid arthritis: the role of sulphoxidation status and HLA-DR3. J Rheumatol 1984;11(5):626–32.

388. Seideman P, Ayesh R. Reduced sulphoxidation capacity in D-penicillamine induced myasthenia gravis. Clin Rheumatol 1994;13(3):435–7.

389. Dawkins RL, Christiansen FT, Zilko PJ, editors. Immunogenetics in Rheumatology: Musculoskeletal Disease and d-Penicillamine. Amsterdam: Excerpta Medica, 1982:358.

390. Speerstra F, Reekers P, van de Putte LB, Vandenbroucke JP. HLA associations in aurothioglucose- and D-penicillamine-induced haematotoxic reactions in rheumatoid arthritis. Tissue Antigens 1985;26(1):35–40.

391. Welsh KI, Black CM. The major histocompatibility system and its relevance to rheumatological disorders. In: Carson DW, Moll JMH, editors. Recent Advances in Rheumatology. Edinburgh: Churchill Livingstone, 1983;147.

392. Scherak O, Smolen JS, Mayr WR, Mayrhofer F, Kolarz G, Thumb NJ. HLA antigens and toxicity to gold and penicillamine in rheumatoid arthritis. J Rheumatol 1984;11(5):610–14.

393. Dequeker J, Van Wanghe P, Verdickt W. A systematic survey of HLA-A,B,C and D antigens and drug toxicity in rheumatoid arthritis. J Rheumatol 1984;11(3):282–6.

394. Ford PM. HLA antigens and drug toxicity in rheumatoid arthritis. J Rheumatol 1984;11(3):259–61.

395. Bardin T, Dryll A, Ryckewaert A. Système HLA et accidents du traitement de la polyarthrite rhumatoïde par la D-pénicillamine. [HLA system and complications of the treatment of rheumatoid polyarthritis with D-penicillamine.] Rev Rhum Mal Osteoartic 1986;53(1):27–9.

396. Perrier P, Raffoux C, Thomas P, Tamisier JN, Busson M, Gaucher A, Streiff F. HLA antigens and toxic reactions to sodium aurothiopropanol sulphonate and D-penicillamine in patients with rheumatoid arthritis. Ann Rheum Dis 1985;44(9):621–4.

397. Skopouli FN, Andonopoulos AP, Moutsopoulos HM. Clinical implications of the presence of anti-Ro (SSA) antibodies in patients with rheumatoid arthritis. J Autoimmun 1988;1(4):381–8.

398. Osman MA, Patel RB, Schuna A, Sundstrom WR, Welling PG. Reduction in oral penicillamine absorption by food, antacid, and ferrous sulfate. Clin Pharmacol Ther 1983;33(4):465–70.

399. Ifan A, Welling PG. Pharmacokinetics of oral 500-mg penicillamine: effect of antacids on absorption. Biopharm Drug Dispos 1986;7(4):401–5.

400. Lyle WH, Pearcey DF, Hui M. Inhibition of penicillamine-induced cupruresis by oral iron. Proc R Soc Med 1977;70(Suppl 3):48–9.

401. Harkness JA, Blake DR. Penicillamine nephropathy and iron. Lancet 1982;2(8312):1368–9.

402. Muijsers AO, van de Stadt RJ, Henrichs AM, Ament HJ, van der Korst JK. D-penicillamine in patients with rheumatoid arthritis. Serum levels, pharmacokinetic aspects, and correlation with clinical course and side effects. Arthritis Rheum 1984;27(12):1362–9.

403. Yu TF, Roboz J, Johnson S, Kaung C. Studies on the metabolism of D-penicillamine and its interaction with probenecid in cystinuria and rheumatoid arthritis. J Rheumatol 1984;11(4):467–70.

404. Whitehouse DB, Lovegrove JU, Hopkinson DA. Variation in alpha-1-antitrypsin phenotypes associated with penicillamine therapy. Clin Chim Acta 1989; 179(1):109–15.

405. Jobanputra P, Maggs F, Homer D, Bevan J. Monitoring and assessing the safety of disease-modifying antirheumatic drugs: a West Midlands experience. Drug Saf 2002;25(15):1099–105.

Penicillins

See also Beta-lactam antibiotics

General Information

The basic structure of the penicillins consists of a thiazolidine ring, the beta-lactam ring, and a side chain. The beta-lactam ring is essential for antibacterial activity. The side chain determines in large part the antibacterial spectrum and pharmacological properties of a particular penicillin. The rapid emergence of bacteria, particularly *Staphylococcus aureus*, that produce beta-lactamases (penicillinase) has been partly countered by the development of compounds that resist hydrolysis by beta-lactamases and compounds that are more active than penicillin G against Gram-negative species. This has led to the production of many semisynthetic penicillins, the first of which was meticillin, active against beta-lactamase-producing *S. aureus*; followed by ampicillin, active against selected Gram-negative bacilli; carbenicillin, which has activity against *Pseudomonas aeruginosa*; and subsequently many agents with different pharmacological and antimicrobial properties. Some of the more important penicillins are listed in Table 1. Another method of combating beta-lactamase-producing organisms has been the development of beta-lactamase inhibitors.

Clinical experience with penicillins, especially penicillin G and the aminopenicillins, is extensive. These substances are rarely toxic, even when they are given in an extended range of dosages, making them invaluable for use in pregnant women and children. Their major limitation is their propensity to cause allergic reactions.

Use in non-infective conditions

In spite of the fact that most trials of antibiotics in pregnancy have shown that antibiotic administration prolongs pregnancy, the mechanism is unclear. However, it is well established that several antibiotics can alter intracellular calcium concentrations (1–3) or inhibit some enzymes, including various phospholipases (4). It is also well established that bacterial products, such as phospholipases and

Table 1 Some penicillins (all rINNs except where stated)

Beta-lactamase sensitive penicillins	Broad-spectrum penicillins	Beta-lactamase resistant penicillins	Antipseudomonal penicillins
Benzylpenicillin (penicillin G)	Ampicillin	Flucloxacillin	Piperacillin
Benzylpenicillin benethamine	Amoxicillin	Meticillin (pINN)	Ticarcillin (pINN)
Penicillin G procaine	Azlocillin	Oxacillin	
Phenoxymethylpenicillin	Mezlocillin	Cloxacillin	
(penicillin V)	Piperacillin	Dicloxacillin	

endotoxins, can stimulate prostaglandin biosynthesis and release by the human amnion (5). Therefore, because prostaglandin biosynthesis depends on the action of phospholipase A2, a calcium-dependent enzyme (4), it has been hypothesized that antibiotics that interfere with phospholipase A2 might affect prostaglandin biosynthesis and release by the amnion. This hypothesis has been tested by evaluating the effect of ampicillin on the release of prostaglandin E from human amnion (6). The results were clear: ampicillin dose-dependently inhibited the release of prostaglandin E from human amnion in vitro. Moreover, ampicillin reversibly counteracted the rise in prostaglandin E induced by arachidonic acid or oxytocin. The authors concluded that inhibition of prostaglandin E release from amnion is a mechanism whereby ampicillin might prevent some cases of premature delivery, even in the absence of infection.

General adverse effects

Non-allergic reactions to penicillins occur mainly with high doses or are related to renal insufficiency. They consist of convulsions or electrolyte disturbances, with hyperkalemia or sodium retention. The penicillinase-resistant and broad-spectrum penicillins can cause specific adverse reactions. Leukopenia, agranulocytosis, liver damage, and some cases of nephropathy are considered to be due to toxic rather than to allergic mechanisms. Diarrhea is a common complication, whereas severe antibiotic-associated colitis is rare. Hypersensitivity reactions are of great importance and are dealt with in the monograph on beta-lactam antibiotics. They range from mostly harmless skin reactions to life-threatening immediate reactions, including anaphylactic shock, acute bronchial obstruction, and severe skin reactions. Tumor-inducing effects have not been described.

Organs and Systems

Respiratory

Bronchospasm may be a consequence of penicillin allergy (7–12). Acute severe dyspnea with cyanosis has also been observed without symptoms of bronchial obstruction or pulmonary edema (13). Specific mechanisms for such cases have yet to be identified.

Allergic pneumonitis and transient eosinophilic pulmonary infiltrate (Loeffler's syndrome) are rare. These syndromes have also been observed with penicillin hypersensitivity (14–16). In one case, an alveolar allergic reaction, probably due to ampicillin, showed features of an adult respiratory distress syndrome (17).

Nervous system

High doses of penicillins, in the order of several million units/day of penicillin G, can produce myoclonic jerks, hyper-reflexia, seizures, or coma. Drowsiness and hallucinations can occur occasionally (18–20). Such reactions are due to a direct toxic effect and are more likely with high concentrations, as seen with intravenous administration (21,22) and with cardiopulmonary bypass in open-heart surgery (23,24).

Myasthenia gravis can be aggravated by ampicillin (25), a reaction that is well described with aminoglycosides and some other antibiotics.

Intrathecal instillation of more than 10 000 units of penicillin and the topical application of high concentrations of penicillin to the nervous system, especially the brain, during surgery have produced comparable reactions (26). All penicillin formulations can produce this kind of reaction.

Benign intracranial hypertension is an extremely rare reaction to penicillins, possibly allergic (27).

Metabolism

Lipoatrophy can occur after the injection of some drugs, including penicillin (28).

- A 2-year-old boy developed a non-tender, hypopigmented, atrophic patch measuring about 2 × 6 cm on his right buttock. He had been well until 5 months before, when he had received an injection of penicillin into the right buttock.

The incidence of this adverse effect is unknown, as is the mechanism.

In six healthy subjects, ampicillin caused an increase in urinary uric acid excretion; this effect was attributed to competition for active renal tubular reabsorption of urate (SEDA-13, 212).

Electrolyte balance

Potassium penicillin G can significantly alter potassium balance when given in very high doses; 20 million units of potassium penicillin G contains about 30 mmol of potassium, and in patients with renal insufficiency this amount can decisively aggravate potentially lethal hyperkalemia. Similarly, large doses of sodium penicillin G, carbenicillin, or ticarcillin can cause hypernatremia (29,30).

High doses of sodium penicillin can cause urinary potassium loss, presumably by acting as a non-absorbable anion in the distal tubule (30). Apparently by analogous mechanisms a variety of semisynthetic penicillins, including carbenicillin, cloxacillin, mezlocillin, nafcillin, piperacillin, and ticarcillin, caused hypokalemia, mainly in severely ill patients (30–36).

Urinary loss of potassium and interstitial nephritis are well-recognized adverse effects of piperacillin. Since patients in ICU may have increased risks of renal complications, serum electrolyte concentrations have been measured in 43 patients before and after piperacillin administration and in 40 patients who were given other antibiotics (37). The groups were comparable in regard to age and severity of disease and all had normal serum creatinine concentrations before the study. Serum concentrations of magnesium, potassium, and, to a lesser degree, calcium fell significantly 36 hours after the start of therapy in patients who were given piperacillin, but not in patients who were given other antibiotics. The fall was most pronounced in the subgroup of patients who were also given furosemide. The authors concluded that treatment with piperacillin can cause or aggravate electrolyte disorders and tubular dysfunction in ICU patients, even when serum creatinine is normal and that the mechanism is probably exacerbation of pre-existing tubular dysfunction. Serum concentrations of electrolytes, including magnesium, should be regularly monitored and, if necessary, supplements should be given to patients in ICU who are receiving piperacillin. This may hold true for all patients receiving piperacillin.

Hematologic

Since the days when chloramphenicol was more commonly used, it has been recognized that many antimicrobial drug are associated with severe blood dyscrasias, such as aplastic anemia, neutropenia, agranulocytosis, thrombocytopenia, and hemolytic anemia. Information on this association has come predominantly from case series and hospital surveys (38–40). Some evidence can be extracted from population-based studies that have focused on aplastic anemia and agranulocytosis and their association with many drugs, including antimicrobial drugs (41,42). The incidence rates of blood dyscrasias in the general population have been estimated in a cohort study with a nested case-control analysis, using data from a General Practice Research Database in Spain (43). The study population consisted of 822048 patients aged 5–69 years who received at least one prescription (in all 1 507307 prescriptions) for an antimicrobial drug during January 1994 to September 1998. The main outcome measure was a diagnosis of neutropenia, agranulocytosis, hemolytic anemia, thrombocytopenia, pancytopenia, or aplastic anemia. The incidence was 3.3 per 100000 person-years in the general population. Users of antimicrobial drugs had a relative risk (RR), adjusted for age and sex, of 4.4, and patients who took more than one class of antimicrobial drug had a relative risk of 29. Among individual antimicrobial drugs, the greatest risk was with cephalosporins (RR = 14), followed by the sulfonamides (RR = 7.6) and penicillins (RR = 3.1).

An immunologically induced hemolytic anemia due to penicillin or its congeners occurs but is rare (44–47). It typically occurs during treatment with high doses (over 10 million units/day) of penicillin for more than 2 weeks (44,45,48). The dose- and time-dependence of this reaction appear to be explained by the underlying mechanism.

During penicillin treatment the erythrocytes are normally coated with penicillin, thereby forming a penicilloyl bond on their surface (49). A drug-specific IgG antibody is directed against the complete antigen, that is the penicillin–erythrocyte complex, and can be shown in direct and indirect Coombs' tests. Clinical hemolysis therefore requires both sufficient coating of erythrocytes and high anti-penicilloyl IgG titers.

Besides this "hapten" or "penicillin-type" of drug-induced hemolysis, a second less frequent mechanism, the so-called "innocent bystander" mechanism can occur (46,49,50). Penicillin–antibody complexes are only loosely bound to erythrocytes and activate complement, which can be detected on the erythrocyte surface with the complement antiglobulin test ("complement" or "non-gamma" type). This mechanism plays a part in immune hemolytic anemias due to various drugs other than penicillins. The hemolytic reaction can continue for weeks after withdrawal of penicillin, that is as long as sufficient penicillin-coated erythrocytes and specific antibodies remain in circulation.

That any penicillin derivative can cause hemolytic anemia is emphasized by the following case (51).

- A 34-year-old woman with cystic fibrosis took piperacillin 6 g tds for respiratory distress. She had no known allergies, although she had previously had pruritus while taking ceftazidime and tingling in her hands with azlocillin. She had completed courses of amoxicillin and flucloxacillin without adverse effects. After about 2 weeks she complained of headache and nausea and passed pink urine. A diagnosis of hemolytic anemia was established and piperacillin was withdrawn. She was given a blood transfusion, prednisone, and folic acid, with good effect.

Various antibiotics, including azlocillin, aztreonam, cefuroxime, ceftazidime, chloramphenicol, colistin, flucloxacillin, gentamicin, imipenem, meropenem, piperacillin, tazobactam, temocillin, and ticarcillin, were incubated with this patient's serum. Only piperacillin and piperacillin + tazobactam caused agglutination in an indirect agglutination test. The authors concluded that the hemolytic anemia had been caused by piperacillin.

Penicillin has been rarely suspected to cause hemolytic–uremic syndrome (52).

Agranulocytosis and leukopenia are discussed in the monograph on beta-lactam antibiotics. Over the years, several cases of neutropenia after treatment with piperacillin with or without tazobactam have been described, especially in children (53–55).

- A 77-year-old man with chronic obstructive lung disease and pneumonia received piperacillin 4 g + tazobactam 0.5 g every 6 hours (56). The neutrophil count gradually fell to zero after 24 days. Piperacillin + tazobactam was withdrawn and lenograstim was given. Within 4 days, the number of neutrophils started to increase. Lenograstim was withdrawn, and the number of neutrophils returned to normal within a week. He made a full recovery.

Whether the rate of hematological adverse effects is higher for piperacillin + tazobactam than for other penicillins is unclear, as is the question of whether neutropenia is more frequent in children than in adults or more frequent in patients with cystic fibrosis than in patients with other conditions (51). It would anyway be wise to follow patients treated with piperacillin, either alone or in combination with tazobactam, with particular attention.

Thrombocytopenia with penicillins has very rarely been reported (57–61). In two cases with mezlocillin (62) and piperacillin + azobactam (63) antibodies became attached to the platelets in the presence of the incriminated drug. The second of these cases is of particular interest, since drug-dependent antibodies were found in the presence of piperacillin but not tazobactam.

- A young woman developed microangiopathic hemolysis and thrombocytopenia in temporal relation to three separate courses of penicillin or ampicillin (64).

Bleeding disorders with penicillins are discussed in the monograph on beta-lactam antibiotics.

Disseminated intravascular coagulation has been reported during long-term administration of piperacillin (65).

- A 51-year-old man was given piperacillin 2 g bd for osteomyelitis. After close to 4 weeks he developed acute renal insufficiency and superior mesenteric venous thrombosis. His coagulation profile showed disseminated intravascular coagulation. Withdrawal of piperacillin and anticoagulation therapy resulted in clinical improvement and normalization of the laboratory data.

Gastrointestinal

Antibiotic-induced colitis and diarrhea and non-specific gastrointestinal symptoms are discussed in the monograph on beta-lactam antibiotics.

Liver

Penicillin-induced hepatotoxicity may not be as uncommon as has been thought. There have been three reviews. The first was a comparison of the assessment of drug-induced liver injury obtained by two different methods, the Council for International Organizations of Medical Sciences (CIOMS) scale and the Maria & Victorino (M&V) clinical scale (66). Three independent experts evaluated 215 cases of hepatotoxicity reported using a structured reporting form. There was absolute agreement between the two scales in 18% of cases, but there was no agreement in cases of fulminant hepatitis or death. The authors concluded that the CIOMS instrument is more likely to lead to a conclusion compatible with the specialist's empirical approach.

In the second review some syndromes of drug-induced cholestasis were outlined, with lists of typical examples of which drugs cause what (67). The authors stated that the treatment of drug-induced cholestasis is largely supportive and that the offending drug should be withdrawn immediately.

In the third review the authors' intention was to give new insights into basic mechanism of bile secretion and cholestasis (68). Some drug-induced forms of cholestasis appear to be associated with certain HLA class II haplotypes in patients taking co-amoxiclav (SEDA-24; 276). Whether or not this holds true for hepatotoxicity due to other beta-lactam antibiotics is not known.

Co-amoxiclav

Transient rises in serum transaminases are not uncommon after the use of co-amoxiclav, and hepatic dysfunction with jaundice can also occur. Since this effect is thought to be largely due to the clavulanic acid that co-amoxiclav contains rather than the amoxicillin, it is covered in the monograph on beta-lactamase inhibitors.

Isoxazolyl penicillins

Flucloxacillin is the most important cause of antimicrobial drug-induced hepatotoxicity in various countries (69–71). The risk has been estimated in some countries to be in the range of 1 in 10000 to 1 in 30000 prescriptions (72–74). The hepatic injury is often severe and deaths have occurred (73). The course can be prolonged. Cholestasis is the most frequent and prominent feature and the so-called "vanishing bile duct syndrome" can develop. Female sex, increasing age, and duration of therapy are risk factors (75). High daily doses increase the risk (74).

Chronic hepatitis has been reported in a patient with a history of flucloxacillin-induced hepatitis (76).

- A 55-year-old woman with psoriasis was treated with oral 5-methoxypsoralen and UVA photochemotherapy. After 40 treatments over 5 months she became unwell and complained of headaches, nausea, and abdominal pain. Laboratory tests confirmed a diagnosis of hepatitis. Six years earlier she had had flucloxacillin-induced hepatitis.

Hepatitis after 5-methoxypsoralen is supposedly very rare, and the authors gave only one reference, although there have been several more reports after the use of 8-methoxypsoralen. Without discussing possible mechanisms underlying this difference, it might be wise to remember that a previous history of drug-induced hepatitis should be a reminder of the need to consider hepatotoxic reactions in any patient who develops unexplained symptoms while using another drug.

The other isoxazolyl penicillins, that is cloxacillin, dicloxacillin, and oxacillin, can cause similar hepatotoxicity (77–82). However, it is not known whether the incidence is as high as with flucloxacillin. Nor is it known whether the clearly dose-dependent "oxacillin hepatitis" (83–85) is an identical reaction.

In isolated cases, glucocorticoids (77) and ursodeoxycholic acid (86) apparently improved the outcome of hepatitis related to isoxazolyl penicillins.

Other penicillins

Other penicillins have been only very rarely associated with hepatotoxicity. There are isolated reports involving, among others, penicillin G (87), penicillin V (88), ampicillin and amoxicillin (89,90), carbenicillin (91), and nafcillin (92).

- A 28-year-old woman developed upper abdominal pain, weakness, and dark urine 5 days after a single injection of benzylpenicillin 2 million units for suspected strepto-coccal pharyngitis (93). Liver dysfunction persisted for up to 18 months.

The authors rated the likelihood that benzylpenicillin had caused cholestasis as probable and referred to three previous reports in which penicillin was claimed to cause hepatotoxicity.

- A 20-year-old man with abdominal trauma received a single dose of piperacillin (1 g) followed by nine doses of imipenem + cilastatin (500 mg tds for 3 days) and 2 weeks later developed jaundice, fatigue, and pruritus (94). A liver biopsy showed centrilobular cholestasis, portal infiltration with eosinophils, and cholangitis. Lymphocyte transformation tests for piperacillin and imipenem/cilastatin were positive, suggesting an immunological mechanism. He made a full clinical and biochemical recovery after 3 months.

The authors concluded that short-term therapy with piperacillin, imipenem + cilastatin, or the combination could cause the same type of liver damage as described with co-amoxiclav and antistaphylococcal penicillins.

Pancreas

The list of agents associated with pancreatitis is long and diverse and is growing. Drugs such as glucocorticoids, estrogens, diuretics, and cancer chemotherapeutic agents have all been implicated, as have various antibiotics, including tetracyclines, rifampicin, and isoniazid (95). Cases of pancreatitis have been reported after the administration of ampicillin (96) and a penicillin derivative (97).

- A 7-year-old boy developed epigastric pain, nausea, and vomiting, starting 10 days after a course of oral penicillin (dose and derivative not stated). His serum amylase activity was 1260 U/l and lipase 528 U/l; electrolytes and liver functions tests were within the reference ranges. Ultrasonography showed a normal liver, spleen, and gallbladder, but his pancreas was diffusely enlarged.

Urinary tract

Acute tubulointerstitial nephritis has been reported in relation to various penicillins, including penicillin G, ampicillin, and amoxicillin (98–102), dicloxacillin (103), meticillin (104–109), nafcillin (110,111), oxacillin (107), and piperacillin (112–114). However, meticillin is the prototype that has caused this reaction more often than any other beta-lactam.

Meticillin-induced acute interstitial nephritis follows a similar pattern of dose-dependence and time-dependence to that of neutropenia (104,105). This reaction occurred in 16% of all children treated with high-dose meticillin (115). Nephritis occurred after a mean of 17 days and a mean cumulative dose of 120 g.

Fever and hematuria (macroscopic or microscopic) are the dominating symptoms. Rash, eosinophilia in the blood, possibly eosinophiluria, and signs of non-oliguric renal insufficiency can occur but are not always present (107). Acute anuric/oliguric renal insufficiency is rare.

Hemorrhagic cystitis has been observed in connection with meticillin (116) and carbenicillin (117).

A very high dose of amoxicillin (250 mg/kg/day for *Listeria monocytogenes* meningitis) combined with an aminoglycoside led to crystal-induced acute renal insufficiency after 14 days (118).

Drug-induced nephrolithiasis, often seen during the sulfonamide era, is nowadays rare, especially in patients taking beta-lactams. However, it can still occur with penicillins (119).

- A 48-year-old woman with pneumococcal meningitis developed acute oliguric renal insufficiency after taking high-dose amoxicillin (320 mg/kg/day) for 4 days. Amoxicillin crystallization was documented by infrared spectrometry. The outcome was favorable after dosage reduction, a single hemodialysis, and adequate hydration.

As was true for the sulfonamides, the risk of crystalluria due to penicillins is increased by high doses, a low urinary pH, and low urine output.

Skin

Skin reactions are the commonest adverse effects of therapeutically administered penicillins (120). Penicillin-contaminated milk or meat can cause itching or generalized skin reactions (121) or even anaphylaxis (122,123).

Incidence

The overall annual incidence of severe erythema multiforme (toxic epidermal necrolysis and Stevens–Johnson syndrome) is about one case per million, antibiotics being involved in 30–40% (124,125). The clinical differentiation between these syndromes can be difficult (126). Allergic contact dermatitis is usually caused by topical drugs, but is also seen in connection with ingestion, injection, or inhalation (127–129).

The increased frequency of contact eczema due to cloxacillin and bacampicillin may be because they are intensely irritant and lipophilic (130).

Mechanisms

Mechanisms of non-immediate reactions are unclear; but may be immunological and non-immunological. Delayed reactions of the IgE type are known (131). Aminopenicillins seem to be an important cause of non-immediate reactions (132–134). The morbilliform rash that begins 1–10 days after amoxicillin can be caused by a delayed cell-mediated immune reaction (135) as can fixed drug eruptions (136,137), toxic epidermal necrolysis (138–140), bullous erythroderma (141), and contact eczema (142). Investigation of these disorders should include delayed readings of skin tests (135). In patients with chronic urticaria, penicillin allergy was demonstrated by cutaneous tests.

Presentation

In contrast to other drugs, penicillin-induced skin reactions can occur after more than 1 week of therapy (60). The typical presentation is a maculopapular, erythematous, symmetrically disposed rash on the legs, buttocks, and trunk.

In very rare cases, certain penicillins can cause pemphigus vulgaris (143) or pemphigoid-like reactions (144,145).

Linear IgA disease is an acquired subepidermal bullous disease characterized by linear deposits of IgA at the cutaneous basement membrane zone and by circulating IgA anti-basement membrane antibodies. Although the cause of linear IgA disease is usually unknown, a few cases have been reported to follow ingestion of drugs, especially vancomycin and diclofenac. A patient with penicillin G-induced linear IgA disease who had circulating IgA antibodies showed specificity against type VII collagen (146).

- A previously fit, 76-year-old man developed pneumococcal pneumonia and acute confusion. He was given oxygen, digoxin, furosemide, and penicillin G 9.6 g/day. Because his symptoms of infection continued he was then given higher doses of penicillin, together with intravenous dexamethasone, and his condition slowly improved. After 10 days of treatment with penicillin (cumulative dose 125 g), he developed a maculopapular truncal eruption compatible with a drug rash. Penicillin was withdrawn and the eruption faded over several days, but 1 week later he developed a localized blistering eruption with tense clear bullae and erosions on the penis, scrotum, and inner thighs. This became generalized, affecting most of the body, and he developed large erosions over pressure-bearing sites, oral ulcers, and hemorrhagic nasal crusting. He was given oral prednisolone. His blistering abated within a month, steroid therapy was withdrawn after 3 months, and his disease remained in remission at follow-up 12 months later. Histology of the affected skin showed subepidermal bullae and a mixed inflammatory infiltrate in the dermis. Direct immunofluorescence showed linear IgA deposition along the basement membrane. Anti-basement membrane antibodies were demonstrated by indirect immunofluorescence and were identified by Western blotting to be against a 250 kDa antigen in dermal extracts. Monoclonal antibodies to collagen VII co-migrated to the same spot.

Collagen VII is the major target antigen of epidermolysis bullosa acquisita (147). Consequently, it is open for discussion whether such patients should be classified as having IgA epidermolysis bullosa acquisita or collagen VII linear IgA disease. The authors stated that their patient did not have the clinical phenotype of epidermolysis bullosa acquisita, and the diagnosis of drug-induced collagen VII linear IgA disease seems to have been well validated (95).

Allergic contact urticaria has been attributed to amoxicillin (148).

- A 40-year-old male nurse developed facial angioedema, dyspnea, rhinoconjunctivitis, dysphonia, and dysphagia immediately after opening a sachet containing amoxicillin and clavulanic acid (149). Skin prick tests were positive for both amoxicillin and ampicillin, and an open test with amoxicillin resulted in a severe immediate-type reaction with large localized wheals and erythema at 10 minutes. Six months later, when he was asymptomatic, erythema was observed during open tests with ampicillin 5%.

Consort urticaria has been attributed to penicillins and may occur more often than recognized.

- A 22-year-old woman had labial urticaria with oropharyngeal edema some minutes after kissing her boyfriend, who had taken amoxicillin some minutes before kissing her (150). A few months before, she had had generalized urticaria several minutes after taking amoxicillin. A prick test with amoxicillin was positive and a similar test with penicillin G was negative. Total serum IgE was 90 kU/l and a RAST test for amoxicillin was positive (4.74 kU/l).

- Two episodes of urticarial angioedema occurred in a 45-year-old woman (151). The first episode occurred 1 hour after she had taken a fifth dose of bacampicillin 1200 mg. In the second episode, she had mild itching and edema of the lips and moderate cutaneous itching and swelling about 30 minutes after making love with her husband, who was taking bacampicillin 1200 mg bd and had taken a tablet about 2 hours before. He had used a condom as contraception, and so the only contact between their mucosae was by kissing. Her symptoms disappeared 2 hours after she took cetirizine 10 mg. Some months later, her husband took placebo or bacampicillin 120, 360, or 520 mg on different days, and 2 hours after taking the tablets kissed his wife. She developed mild intraoral itching and itching and wheals on the face and arms 20 minutes after kissing her husband after he had taken bacampicillin 360 mg.

Kissing can cause an allergic reaction if one of the lovers is sensitized to a compound that has just been taken by the other. This holds true for both drugs and food (152,153). Whether a similar reaction can occur if the lovers have intercourse without using a condom has neither been reported nor investigated. However, allergic reactions to penicillin during in vitro fertilization and intrauterine insemination are possible, and the authors recommended that in patients who are penicillin-sensitive, penicillin should not be used during transfer of gamete and embryo for assisted reproductive procedures (154).

Pustular drug eruptions due to penicillin (155), amoxicillin (156), ampicillin (157), bacampicillin (158), or imipenem + cilastin (159) seem to form a distinct clinical entity that has to be differentiated from pustular psoriasis, which can be drug-induced as well (159). A history of drug exposure, rapid disappearance of the eruption after the drug is stopped, and eosinophils in the inflammatory infiltrate argue in favor of pustular drug eruptions.

Pseudoallergic reactions are reactions that mimic immunoallergic reactions, but in which a specific immune-mediated mechanism is not involved. The so-called "ampicillin rash," which also occurs with amoxicillin, another aminopenicillin, is an example of a pseudoallergic reaction, which looks like a typical type III allergic rash, but usually occurs at 7–12 days after the start of administration rather than 3–10 days (160). Some major mediators of pseudoallergic reactions have been reviewed (161). The roles of newer putative mechanisms, involving cytokines, kinins, and other host-derived substances, remain to be ascertained. Most important is the fact that currently there are no standardized and validated animal models for predicting pseudoallergic reactions (162). In patients with infectious mononucleosis, the aminopenicillins evoke rashes in a much higher percentage than usual (163). The incidence of rashes in infectious mononucleosis without antibiotics is 3–15%, compared with 40–100% with ampicillin. The underlying mechanism is speculative.

Although several reports have described fixed rashes due to amoxicillin, palmar exfoliation has rarely been described (164).

- Five patients (one man, four women, aged 30–72 years) developed intense palmar rashes and itching during treatment with amoxicillin (doses not stated). All the episodes began after several days of treatment with amoxicillin, either alone or in combination with clavulanic acid. Three of the patients had repeated episodes, and the interval between treatment and onset was shorter each time (down to 5 hours on the third occasion). In all cases the rash was followed by exfoliation and cleared in 7–10 days without residual lesions. Skin prick tests, intradermal tests, and patch tests were performed with several beta-lactams, including amoxicillin, and all were negative. A challenge test with amoxicillin was performed in one patient, and the erythema recurred in 3–4 hours. All five patients tolerated cefuroxime and ceftazidime. Cefalexin was given to one patient only, and palmar exfoliative erythema developed a few days later.

Diagnosis

A maximum of 20% of subjects with a history of allergy-like reactions after administration of a penicillin antibiotic have positive skin or RAST tests (165–167). Tests using benzylpenicillin derivatives or semisynthetic penicillins can almost double positive test results (168,169). Patients with a positive history but negative skin tests run a 1–3% risk of an IgE-mediated reaction and 60% of test-positive patients had evidence of an immediate reaction, including urticaria and angioedema (165).

Management

Penicillins should be avoided in any patient who gives a history of a skin reaction or anaphylaxis to any penicillin derivative. To prevent mild skin reactions becoming severe when they occur, it is advisable to withdraw the culprit antibiotic not only when a type I reaction is suspected but in all kinds of common rashes, in view of a possible epidermolytic process. A diet free of dairy products was curative in 30 of 70 patients with positive tests (170).

Immunologic

Type I reactions

Anaphylactic shock can occur, even after oral administration of penicillin and skin testing. However, anaphylactic shock is less common after oral than parenteral administration (171). In one study the incidence of anaphylactic shock was 0.04% of all patients treated with penicillin (7). It is also low in patients receiving long-term benzathine penicillin (1.2 million units every 4 weeks). Four episodes of anaphylaxis occurred in 0.012% of injections (1.2 reactions to 10 000 injections) (172). Anaphylactic shock resulting in death occurred in 0.002% of all patients treated with penicillin (7) and in 0.003% of those treated with benzathine penicillin (172).

In nearly half of the cases, the course of anaphylactic shock, especially that induced by penicillin and other small molecular substances, is that of a cardiovascular reaction without any other effects suggestive of an allergic mechanism (173–175). There is an extensive list of articles on anaphylactic shock to penicillins (7–10,173,174,176,177). General anesthesia does not inhibit the development of anaphylactic shock in penicillin allergy (178).

Diagnosis

The two most important elements in the evaluation of an individual for the presence or absence of beta-lactam hypersensitivity are the drug history and skin tests. Other diagnostic tools, such as measurement of drug-specific antibodies and lymphocyte transformation tests, are investigational or restricted to specialized laboratories. Standardized and widely used protocols for skin testing only exist for the penicillins and allow assessment of IgE-mediated hypersensitivity. The most commonly used reagents are penicilloyl-polylysine (PPL, which contains multiple penicilloyl molecules coupled to a polylysine carrier) and fresh penicillin followed by minor determinant mixtures (MDM), containing penicilloate, benzylpenicilloate, and benzylpenilloate (179). A survey conducted among members of the American Academy of Allergy and Immunology reported the use of penicilloyl-polylysine and fresh penicillin by 86% and minor determinant mixtures by 40% of those responding to the questionnaire (180).

Skin tests are first applied as a prick test for safety. In the absence of a local or systemic reaction, an intradermal test is performed and interpreted as described elsewhere (181,182). Experience with skin testing in penicillin allergy has been reviewed (176,183). Properly performed sequential testing is considered a safe procedure, and only an estimated 1% or less of penicillin allergic patients will have systemic symptoms while undergoing skin tests. However, at least three deaths have been reported with both epicutaneous and intradermal testing (184).

In a collaborative study in the National Institute of Allergy and Infectious Diseases (NIAID), hospitalized patients were tested with major and minor skin test reagents in order to assess the predictive value of skin testing. Among 600 history-negative patients, 568 had negative skin tests and none had a reaction to penicillin. Among 726 history-positive patients, 566 had a negative skin test and received penicillin, seven of whom (1.2%) had a possibly IgE-mediated reaction. Nine of the 167 patients with positive skin tests were exposed to penicillin, two of whom had reactions compatible with IgE-mediated reactions. These data suggest that overall, 99% of patients with negative skin tests to penicilloyl-polylysine and minor determinant mixtures can safely receive penicillin. A history of a previous reaction slightly increases the risk of an adverse reaction, to 1.2%. Most positive skin tests were detected with penicilloyl-polylysine with or without minor determinant mixtures, and a further 16% reacted to minor determinant mixtures alone (166).

In another study in an outpatient clinic for sexually transmitted diseases, 5063 consecutive patients were tested with penicilloyl-polylysine with and without minor determinant mixtures (167). The role of the history of a previous penicillin reaction was emphasized in this study: 1.7% of history-negative subjects had a positive skin test; in contrast, 7.1% of history-positive patients had a positive skin test, and a previous history of anaphylaxis or urticaria was associated with positive skin tests in 17% and 12% respectively. Penicillin was safe in more than 99% of patients with a negative history and a negative skin test. Reactions were more common (2.9%) in patients with a positive history and a negative skin test. The reactions were mild and self-limiting. Two patients with a history of severe IgE-mediated reaction had mild anaphylactic reactions.

Relatively safe doses for skin testing, provided that one begins with a prick test, are 25 nmol/ml of penicilloyl-polylysine and purified benzylpenicillin. Positive skin tests of the immediate type with penicilloyl-polylysine are usually obtained 2 weeks to 3 months after the clinical reaction (185).

The safety of such an approach has been challenged in a description of three patients who were negative in skin tests with penicilloyl-polylysine and minor determinant mixtures and who tolerated therapeutic doses of benzylpenicillin, but reacted to amoxicillin (173). In an extension of that study, 177 patients who were allergic to beta-lactams were identified using the clinical history, a skin test panel including penicilloyl-polylysine, and minor determinant mixtures, as well as ampicillin and amoxicillin and drug-specific radio-allergosorbent tests. Fifty-four patients (31%) tolerated penicillin G but reacted to amoxicillin with anaphylaxis, urticaria, or angioedema. Skin tests with penicilloyl-polylysine and minor determinant mixtures failed to detect those patients, but tests with amoxicillin were positive in 63% (168).

Canadian data have partly confirmed these findings (169). Benzylpenicillin derivatives and semisynthetic penicillins were applied to 112 patients with a history of an allergic reaction to penicillins. The tests were positive in 21 patients (19%), of whom 10 reacted against the semisynthetic penicillin reagents only. Reports of subjects allergic to flucloxacillin (186), cloxacillin (187), and cefadroxil (188), but not penicillin, lend further support to the concept of side chain-specific allergic reactions (see the monograph on beta-lactam antibiotics).

Management
Fearing penicillin anaphylaxis, many clinicians overdiagnose penicillin allergy in patients who have not had a true allergic reaction. Consequently, penicillins are withheld from many patients who could safely receive them. This was the background to a study whose objectives were to determine the likelihood of true penicillin allergy, taking into consideration the clinical history, and to evaluate the diagnostic value added by appropriate skin testing (189). The authors searched MEDLINE for relevant English-language articles dated 1966 to October 2000. Bibliographies were searched to identify additional articles. Original articles describing the precision of skin tests in the diagnosis of penicillin allergy were included, and studies that did not use both minor and major determinants were excluded; 14 studies met the inclusion criteria.

At least three authors independently reviewed and abstracted the data from all the articles and reached a consensus about any discrepancies. Some of their conclusions are worth remembering:

- 80–90% of all patients who report penicillin allergy have negative skin tests, suggesting that penicillins are withheld from many patients who could safely receive them;
- patients who develop a rash while taking penicillins should not be automatically labeled as allergic without considering other possibilities, including rashes due to ampicillin distinct from allergic rashes, and rashes caused by the infection being treated or by other drugs;
- for patients with a history of immediate (type I) penicillin allergy who have a compelling need for penicillin, skin testing should be performed;
- at least 98% of patients with positive histories of penicillin allergy and negative skin test results can tolerate penicillin without any sequelae.

Desensitization
Patients with a history of penicillin allergy should undergo skin testing with both penicilloyl-polylysine and minor determinant mixtures. Patients with positive skin tests should be treated with another immunologically unrelated compound or should undergo desensitization. The management of patients with a negative skin test but a history of a severe IgE-mediated reaction has to be individualized; options include the use of an alternative compound, desensitization, or the controlled administration of a test dose.

Acute drug desensitization is commonly described as the process by which a drug-allergic individual is converted from a highly sensitive state to a state in which the drug is tolerated. The procedure involves cautious administration of incremental doses of the drug over a short period of time (hours to a few days). In the past it has mainly been considered to be of value in patients in whom IgE antibodies to a particular drug are known or assumed to exist and no alternative treatment agent is available. In clinical practice, most of the desensitization protocols have involved penicillins (190). However, the principle has been applied successfully to other agents as well (191,192), including other antibiotics, insulin, chemotherapeutic agents, vaccines, heterologous sera, and other proteins.

Mechanism   It has been stated that in patients with penicillin-specific IgE antibodies who underwent successful penicillin desensitization, the data suggest that anti-specific, mast cell desensitization is responsible for the tolerant state and that mediator depletion plays no role (190). Additionally, the clinical observation that wheal-and-flare skin responses to penicillin often become negative with successful desensitization, while IgE responses to other antigens remain unchanged, also supports an involvement of an antigen-specific mechanism. Furthermore, both clinical reactivity and skin-test reactivity return within a few days, unless a tolerant state is maintained by continued drug administration. The author stressed that these findings show that the desensitized state depends on the continuous presence of antigen and that clinical sensitivity returns rapidly in the absence of antigen.

However, the underlying mechanisms responsible for the antigen-specific desensitized state are still unclear. It has been hypothesized that IgE receptor aggregation may generate counter-regulatory forces that, instead of causing cell activation, actually extinguish activating signals (191). The key point is that during desensitization, the drug is introduced very slowly and the drug concentration rises gradually. The slow rate of possible receptor aggregation caused by the gradual increase in drug concentration, along with suppression of cellular activation signals, may lead to antigen-specific desensitization and clinical tolerance. It has also been long thought that during desensitization, univalent drug-hapten protein conjugates are formed and may act by inhibiting the cross-linking of drug-specific IgE molecules on mast cells. It is slightly surprising that this prospect has not come into routine therapy.

Procedure   Beta-lactam desensitization should be done in an intensive care unit and any concomitant risk factors for anaphylaxis, such as use of beta-blockers should be corrected. Protocols based on incremental use of the drug orally or parenterally have been described (190,193). The oral route is preferable and is associated with a lower incidence of adverse events, but mild transient reactions are frequent (171,194,195). Pregnant women with limited antibiotic choices have been treated with immunotherapy (196). Repeated administration will maintain a state of anergy, which is often lost after withdrawal (197). At the conclusion of therapy, patients must be informed that after withdrawal, they may once again become allergic to penicillin, with a new reaction to the first subsequent application (197).

Desensitization is not effective in non-IgE-mediated reactions and should therefore not be attempted, for example in cases of serum sickness-like syndromes or Stevens–Johnson syndrome.

Treatment of acute anaphylaxis
For acute anaphylaxis, immediate treatment is essential, with adrenaline followed by intravenous histamine H_1 receptor antagonists, glucocorticoids, fluids, and electrolytes. In view of the frequency of cardiac dysrhythmias and conduction disturbances in patients with anaphylactic shock, they should immediately be monitored (198,199).

Type III reactions
Serum sickness was first described by von Pirquet and Schick in 1905 and was regarded as a syndrome resulting from the administration of heterologous serum or other foreign proteins. The immunopathology of classic serum sickness results from antigen–antibody complex formation with a foreign protein as the antigen. Characteristic symptoms include fever, cutaneous eruptions, edema, arthralgia, and lymphadenopathy. The incidence of classical serum sickness has fallen secondary to the refinement of foreign proteins. However, a serum sickness-like reaction that is clinically similar to classical serum sickness can result from the administration of a number of

non-protein drugs, such as tetracyclines, penicillins, and cephalosporins (200). The reaction typically occurs within 1 month of the start of therapy and resolves after withdrawal.

Serum sickness has been associated with penicillins (201).

- A 39-year-old woman developed the characteristic symptoms for serum sickness, having completed a 5-day course of amoxicillin for a perilingual infection 1 week before. She was treated with prednisone 60 mg/day and diphenhydramine 25–50 mg tds. Her symptoms gradually resolved and the prednisolone dose was tapered over 2 weeks.
- A 29-year-old woman complained of fever, rash, throat and facial swelling, abdominal pain, and increasing joint pain, leaving her wheelchair-bound. Her symptoms started a week after she had completed a 10-day course of penicillin V for a dental abscess. She was given oral methylprednisolone, 40 mg every 6 hours, and over the next few days her symptoms gradually resolved.
- A 29-year-old woman developed symptoms of serum-sickness 2 weeks after completing a 21-day course of co-amoxiclav for sinusitis. She responded to prednisone 40 mg/day.

The authors suggested that serum sickness may be more common than has previously been described and that the reaction may be under-reported or unrecognized.

Second-Generation Effects

Teratogenicity

Early animal studies suggested that malformations could be caused by penicillins. However, this was not confirmed in later, more extensive evaluations (202). Penicillin G, ampicillin, and probably most other penicillins can be safely used in pregnant women and children. Experience with the newer semisynthetic penicillins is not extensive enough to allow definite conclusions regarding their safety for mother and fetus during pregnancy.

Fetotoxicity

Increased antenatal administration of ampicillin for the prevention of neonatal group B streptococcal disease may be responsible for the higher incidence of more severe neonatal sepsis with ampicillin-resistant non-group B streptococci, without a change in the overall infection rate (203,204).

Lactation

The transfer of penicillins (ampicillin, pivampicillin, phenoxymethylpenicillin) into the breast milk of nursing mothers with puerperal mastitis to the breastfed infant is minimal (205). The risk of adverse drug reactions due to penicillins is therefore negligible, unless the infant has penicillin allergy (SEDA-14, 215).

Susceptibility Factors

Renal disease

Toxic effects of penicillins can occur in patients with renal insufficiency if the dosage is not altered (206).

Other features of the patient

Toxic reactions can occur in patients with pre-existing cerebral damage or during cardiopulmonary bypass. Embolic reactions can have severe consequences in patients with pre-existing cardiac or pulmonary disease.

Drug Administration

Drug formulations

Embolic-toxic reactions to penicillin depot formulations were first described in patients with syphilis (207). The symptoms include fear of death, confusion, acoustic and visual hallucinations, and possibly palpitation, tachycardia, and cyanosis (SEDA-8, 559) (175,207–211). Generalized seizures or twitching of the limbs have been observed in children and adults (210,212–216). As a rule, the symptoms abate and disappear within several minutes to an hour. They rarely persist for up to 24 hours. If a cardiovascular reaction with a fall in blood pressure occurs simultaneously with typical symptoms, a combination with anaphylactic shock must be considered (217,218).

Such reactions have been called "pseudo-anaphylactic reactions" or "acute non-allergic reactions" (174,208–210,219–223), "panic attack syndrome," and "acute psychotic reactions" (212,224). In several countries, the term "Hoigné syndrome" is used.

The frequency of such reactions is about 1–3 reactions per 1000 intramuscular injections of penicillin G procaine, the usual dose being about 0.6–1.2 million units (175,213,225–227). Eight of 920 patients with venereal diseases had a definite toxic-like reaction with a dose of 4.8 million units of penicillin G procaine, corresponding to about one in 120 patients (228). In a series of 7700 intramuscular injections with only 400 000 units of penicillin G procaine, there was not one episode (221).

The mechanism is probably embolic (172,207,219,222,225), as has been shown in one case at autopsy, in which emboli of benzathine penicillin crystals were found in the lungs (219).

Some reports suggest that the procaine component may be especially important (213,222). Plasma procaine esterase activity was low in patients with systemic toxic reactions (213). The same symptoms occurred in three patients after erroneous administration of penicillin G procaine by intravenous infusion (222), but also in two after procaine-free antihistamine penicillin was injected intramuscularly (172,225). However, observations of similar symptoms with a procaine-free antihistamine penicillin argue against a central role of the procaine component (SED-8, 560) (175,217,220,221,225).

Drug administration route

Intramuscular injection of high doses of depot formulations of penicillins can lead to painful swelling, especially

when over 600 000–1 000 000 units are given at a single site (229,230). Such reactions occurred in two of 878 patients (0.2%) with intramuscular penicillin G procaine (231). Arthus phenomenon seems to be rare (127,232).

Nicolau syndrome (embolia cutis medicamentosa) is a very rare complication of intramuscular injections, in which there is extensive necrosis of the injected skin area, perhaps due to accidental intra-arterial and/or para-arterial injection (233). It usually occurs in children: in a review of 102 patients, 80 were under 12 years of age (234). Complications can include everything from an ischemic syndrome with local necrosis of the skin, subcutaneous tissue, and muscle, often combined with vascular and nervous system involvement, intestinal and renal hemorrhage, necrosis of the entire leg, and even paraplegia from spinal cord damage (235–241). Necrosis of the forearm has been described in two patients after inadvertent intra-arterial administration of dicloxacillin (242).

Special emphasis should be put on the precautionary measures to be taken when injecting long-acting penicillins or other drugs in crystalline suspensions intramuscularly.

Repeated intramuscular injections into the thighs of newborns and infants can cause severe and widespread muscular contractures of the quadriceps femoris (SEDA-8, 560). In some cases, penicillin was implicated.

Drug–Drug Interactions

Allopurinol

The risk of rashes caused by aminopenicillins does not seem to be increased by parallel treatment with allopurinol (243), as had been suggested before (244).

Aminoglycosides

High doses of parenteral penicillin can inactivate aminoglycosides (245). In patients receiving low doses of aminoglycosides because of reduced renal function this can be clinically important (246,247). Parenteral administration of these drugs in neonatal dosages does not seem to produce relevant inactivation, and so temporal separation of the infusions is not required (248).

Piperacillin protected against aminoglycoside nephrotoxicity without reducing its blood concentration; this was possibly a protective effect of co-administered mineral salts (249).

Ciclosporin

In a study in lung transplant recipients, ciclosporin nephrotoxicity was potentiated by nafcillin (111).

Methotrexate

Beta-lactams are weak organic acids that compete with the renal tubular secretion of methotrexate and its metabolites and reduce their clearance, leading to methotrexate toxicity (250,251). Consecutive aplastic crises have been described, particularly in patients with impaired renal clearance (250,252,253). In contrast, co-administration of flucloxacillin in another study produced a significant but not clinically important reduction in methotrexate AUC (254).

The more basic interactions between piperacillin and methotrexate and its major metabolite 7-hydroxymethotrexate have been studied in rabbits (255). The interaction was mainly caused by reduced renal clearance of both methotrexate and its metabolite. The authors concluded that renal function in patients taking this combination should be monitored, with adequate fluid intake, especially in elderly patients, because dehydration may accelerate the occurrence of toxicity.

Phenytoin

Competitive albumin binding of drugs with high serum protein affinity can increase pharmacologically active unbound concentrations and enhance the metabolism of low clearance drugs. In vitro data suggest a significant increase in unbound phenytoin concentration by high doses of oxacillin, especially with hypoalbuminemia or uremia (256).

Interference with Diagnostic Tests

Pseudoproteinuria

Patients who take penicillin G or ureidopenicillin derivatives in doses over 5 g/day develop pseudoproteinuria. Proteinuria should be evaluated by a bromphenol blue test (Albustix) or after urine dialysis (SEDA-3, 219).

17-ketosteroids

High-dosage penicillin produces abnormally high concentrations of 17-ketogenic steroids in the blood and high concentrations of 17-ketosteroid in the urine (257).

References

1. Cloutier MM, Guernsey L, Sha'afi RI. Duramycin increases intracellular calcium in airway epithelium. Membr Biochem 1993;10(2):107–18.
2. Burroughs SF, Johnson GJ. Beta-lactam antibiotics inhibit agonist-stimulated platelet calcium influx. Thromb Haemost 1993;69(5):503–8.
3. Bird SD, Walker RJ, Hubbard MJ. Altered free calcium transients in pig kidney cells (LLC-PK1) cultured with penicillin/streptomycin. In Vitro Cell Dev Biol Anim 1994;30A(7):420–4.
4. Verheij HM, Slotboom AJ, de Haas GH. Structure and function of phospholipase A2. Rev Physiol Biochem Pharmacol 1981;91:91–203.
5. Romero R, Mazor M, Wu YK, Sirtori M, Oyarzun E, Mitchell MD, Hobbins JC. Infection in the pathogenesis of preterm labor. Semin Perinatol 1988;12(4):262–79.
6. Vesce F, Buzzi M, Ferretti ME, Pavan B, Bianciotto A, Jorizzo G, Biondi C. Inhibition of amniotic prostaglandin E release by ampicillin. Am J Obstet Gynecol 1998; 178(4):759–64.
7. Idsoe O, Guthe T, Willcox RR, de Weck AL. Art und Ausmass der Penizillinnebenwirkungen unter besonderer Berücksichtigung von 151 Todesfällen nach anaphylaktischem Schock. [Nature and extent of penicillin side effects with special reference to 151 fatal cases after anaphylactic shock.] Schweiz Med Wochenschr 1969;99(33):1190–7 contd.
8. Capaul R, Maibach R, Kunzi UP, et al. Atopy, bronchial asthma and previous adverse drug reactions (ADRs): risk factors for ADRs? Post Marketing Surveillance 1993;7:331.
9. Bertelsen K, Dalgaard JB. Penicillindodsfald. 16 secerede Danske tilfaelde. [Death due to penicillin. 16 Danish cases with autopsies.] Nord Med 1965;73:173–7.
10. Hoffman DR, Hudson P, Carlyle SJ, Massello W 3rd. Three cases of fatal anaphylaxis to antibiotics in patients with prior histories of allergy to the drug. Ann Allergy 1989;62(2):91–3.
11. Davies RJ, Hendrick DJ, Pepys J. Asthma due to inhaled chemical agents: ampicillin, benzyl penicillin, 6 amino penicillanic acid and related substances. Clin Allergy 1974; 4(3):227–47.
12. Hoigné R, Braunschweig S, Zehnder D, et al. Drug-induced bronchial asthma attack: epidemiological aspects (communication of CHDM Berne/St. Gallen, Switzerland). Pharmacoepidemiol Drug Saf 1994;3:S90.
13. Hoigne R, Jaeger MD, Hess T, Wymann R, Muller U, Galeazzi R, Maibach R, Kunzi UP. Akute schwere Dyspnoe als Medikamentennebenwirkung. [Acute severe dyspnea as a side effect of drugs. Report from the CHDM (Comprehensive Hospital Drug Monitoring).] Schweiz Med Wochenschr 1990;120(34):1211–16.
14. Reichlin S, Loveless MH, Kane EG. Loeffler's syndrome following penicillin therapy. Ann Intern Med 1953; 38(1):113–20.
15. Wengrower D, Tzfoni EE, Drenger B, Leitersdorf E. Erythroderma and pneumonitis induced by penicillin? Respiration 1986;50(4):301–3.
16. de Hoyos A, Holness DL, Tarlo SM. Hypersensitivity pneumonitis and airways hyperreactivity induced by occupational exposure to penicillin. Chest 1993;103(1):303–4.
17. Poe RH, Condemi JJ, Weinstein SS, Schuster RJ. Adult respiratory distress syndrome related to ampicillin sensitivity. Chest 1980;77(3):449–51.
18. New PS, Wells CE. Cerebral toxicity associated with massive intravenous penicillin therapy. Neurology 1965; 15(11):1053–8.
19. Nicholls PJ. Neurotoxicity of penicillin. J Antimicrob Chemother 1980;6(2):161–5.
20. Schliamser SE, Bolander H, Kourtopoulos H, Norrby SR. Neurotoxicity of benzylpenicillin: correlation to concentrations in serum, cerebrospinal fluid and brain tissue fluid in rabbits. J Antimicrob Chemother 1988;21(3):365–72.
21. Boston Collaborative Drug Surveillance Program. Drug-induced convulsions. Lancet 1972;2(7779):677–9.
22. Smith H, Lerner PI, Weinstein L. Neurotoxicity and "massive" intravenous therapy with penicillin. A study of possible predisposing factors. Arch Intern Med 1967; 120(1):47–53.
23. Currie TT, Hayward NJ, Westlake G, Williams J. Epilepsy in cardiopulmonary bypass patients receiving large intravenous doses of penicillin. J Thorac Cardiovasc Surg 1971;62(1):1–6.
24. Seamans KB, Gloor P, Dobell RA, Wyant JD. Penicillin-induced seizures during cardiopulmonary bypass. A clinical and electroencephalographic study. N Engl J Med 1968;278(16):861–8.
25. Argov Z, Brenner T, Abramsky O. Ampicillin may aggravate clinical and experimental myasthenia gravis. Arch Neurol 1986;43(3):255–6.
26. Reuling JR, Cramer C. Intrathecal penicillin. JAMA 1947;134:16.
27. Schmitt BD, Krivit W. Benign intracranial hypertension associated with a delayed penicillin reaction. Pediatrics 1969;43(1):50–3.

28. Kuperman-Beade M, Laude TA. Partial lipoatrophy in a child. Pediatr Dermatol 2000;17(4):302–3.

29. Wright AJ, Wilkowske CJ. The penicillins. Mayo Clin Proc 1987;62(9):806–20.

30. Brunner FP, Frick PG. Hypokalaemia, metabolic alkalosis, and hypernatraemia due to "massive" sodium penicillin therapy. BMJ 1968;4(630):550–2.

31. Mohr JA, Clark RM, Waack TC, Whang R. Nafcillin-associated hypokalemia. JAMA 1979;242(6):544.

32. Wade JC, Schimpff SC, Newman KA, Fortner CL, Standiford HC, Wiernik PH. Piperacillin or ticarcillin plus amikacin. A double-blind prospective comparison of empiric antibiotic therapy for febrile granulocytopenic cancer patients. Am J Med 1981;71(6):983–90.

33. Rotstein C, Cimino M, Winkey K, Cesari C, Fenner J. Cefoperazone plus piperacillin versus mezlocillin plus tobramycin as empiric therapy for febrile episodes in neutropenic patients. Am J Med 1988;85(1A):36–43.

34. Kibbler CC, Prentice HG, Sage RJ, Hoffbrand AV, Brenner MK, Mannan P, Warner P, Bhamra A, Noone P. A comparison of double beta-lactam combinations with netilmicin/ureidopenicillin regimens in the empirical therapy of febrile neutropenic patients. J Antimicrob Chemother 1989;23(5):759–71.

35. Arevalo A, Mateos F, Otero MJ, Fuertes A. Hipopotasemia inducida por cloxacilina. [Hypopotassemia induced by cloxacillin.] Rev Clin Esp 1996;196(7):494–5.

36. Garcia Diaz B, Plaza S, Garcia Benayas E, Santos D. Hipopotasemia por cloxacilina: un nuevo caso. [Hypopotassemia caused by cloxacillin: a new case.] Rev Clin Esp 1997;197(11):792–3.

37. Polderman KH, Girbes AR. Piperacillin-induced magnesium and potassium loss in intensive care unit patients. Intensive Care Med 2002;28(4):520–2.

38. George JN, Raskob GE, Shah SR, Rizvi MA, Hamilton SA, Osborne S, Vondracek T. Drug-induced thrombocytopenia: a systematic review of published case reports. Ann Intern Med 1998;129(11):886–90.

39. Wright MS. Drug-induced hemolytic anemias: increasing complications to therapeutic interventions. Clin Lab Sci 1999;12(2):115–18.

40. Arneborn P, Palmblad J. Drug-induced neutropenia—a survey for Stockholm 1973–1978. Acta Med Scand 1982;212(5):289–92.

41. Baumelou E, Guiguet M, Mary JY. Epidemiology of aplastic anemia in France: a case-control study. I. Medical history and medication use. The French Cooperative Group for Epidemiological Study of Aplastic Anemia. Blood 1993;81(6):1471–8.

42. International Agranulocytosis and Aplastic Anemia Study Group. Anti-infective drug use in relation to the risk of agranulocytosis and aplastic anemia. Arch Intern Med 1989;149(5):1036–40.

43. Huerta C, Garcia Rodriguez LA. Risk of clinical blood dyscrasia in a cohort of antibiotic users. Pharmacotherapy 2002;22(5):630–6.

44. Petz LD, Fudenberg HH. Coombs-positive hemolytic anemia caused by penicillin administration. N Engl J Med 1966;274(4):171–8.

45. White JM, Brown DL, Hepner GW, Worlledge SM. Penicillin-induced haemolytic anaemia. BMJ 1968;3(609):26–9.

46. Funicella T, Weinger RS, Moake JL, Spruell M, Rossen RD. Penicillin-induced immunohemolytic anemia associated with circulating immune complexes. Am J Hematol 1977;3:219–23.

47. Tuffs L, Manoharan A. Flucloxacillin-induced haemolytic anaemia. Med J Aust 1986;144(10):559–60.

48. Spath P, Garratty G, Petz LD. Immunhämatologische Reaktionen bei Penizillinbehandlung. [Immunohematologic reactions during treatment with penicillin.] Schweiz Med Wochenschr 1973;103(10):383–8.

49. Kerr RO, Cardamone J, Dalmasso AP, Kaplan ME. Two mechanisms of erythrocyte destruction in penicillin-induced hemolytic anemia. N Engl J Med 1972;287(26):1322–5.

50. Harris JW. Studies on the mechanism of a drug-induced hemolytic anemia. J Lab Clin Med 1956;47(5):760–75.

51. Thickett KM, Wildman MJ, Fegan CD, Stableforth DE. Haemolytic anaemia following treatment with piperacillin in a patient with cystic fibrosis. J Antimicrob Chemother 1999;43(3):435–6.

52. Brandslund I, Petersen PH, Strunge P, Hole P, Worth V. Haemolytic uraemic syndrome and accumulation of haemoglobin–haptoglobin complexes in plasma in serum sickness caused by penicillin drugs. Haemostasis 1980;9(4):193–203.

53. Gerber L, Wing EJ. Life-threatening neutropenia secondary to piperacillin/tazobactam therapy. Clin Infect Dis 1995;21(4):1047–8.

54. Ruiz-Irastorza G, Barreiro G, Aguirre C. Reversible bone marrow depression by high-dose piperacillin/tazobactam. Br J Haematol 1996;95(4):611–12.

55. Reichardt P, Handrick W, Linke A, Schille R, Kiess W. Leukocytopenia, thrombocytopenia and fever related to piperacillin/tazobactam treatment—a retrospective analysis in 38 children with cystic fibrosis. Infection 1999;27(6):355–6.

56. Ortega Garcia MP, Guevara Serrano J, Gil Gomez I, Iglesias Iglesias AA, Fernandez Villalba EM. Neutropenia reversibile secundaria al tratamiento con piperacillina/tazobactam. Atencion Pharmaceutica 2002;4:44–8.

57. Schiffer CA, Weinstein HJ, Wiernik PH. Methicillin-associated thrombocytopenia. Ann Intern Med 1976;85(3):338–9.

58. Lee M, Sharifi R. Severe thrombocytopenia due to apalcillin. Urol Int 1987;42(4):313–5.

59. Brocks AP. Thrombocytopenia during treatment with ampicillin. Lancet 1974;2:273.

60. Hsi YJ, Kuo HY, Ouyang A. Thrombocytopenia following administration of penicillin. Report of a case. Chin Med J 1966;85(4):249–51.

61. Olivera E, Lakhani P, Watanakunakorn C. Isolated severe thrombocytopenia and bleeding caused by piperacillin. Scand J Infect Dis 1992;24(6):815–17.

62. Gharpure V, O'Connell B, Schiffer CA. Mezlocillin-induced thrombocytopenia. Ann Intern Med 1993;119(8):862.

63. Perez-Vazquez A, Pastor JM, Riancho JA. Immune thrombocytopenia caused by piperacillin/tazobactam. Clin Infect Dis 1998;27(3):650–1.

64. Parker JC, Barrett DA 2nd. Microangiopathic hemolysis and thrombocytopenia related to penicillin drugs. Arch Intern Med 1971;127(3):474–7.

65. Miyazaki H, Yanagitani S, Matsumoto T, Yoshida K, Amoh Y, Watanabe T, Kubota Y, Inoue K. Hypercoagulopathy with piperacillin administration in osteomyelitis. Intern Med 2000;39(5):424–7.

66. Lucena MI, Camargo R, Andrade RJ, Perez-Sanchez CJ, Sanchez De La Cuesta F. Comparison of two clinical scales for causality assessment in hepatotoxicity. Hepatology 2001;33(1):123–30.

67. Chitturi S, Farrell GC. Drug-induced cholestasis. Semin Gastrointest Dis 2001;12(2):113–24.

68. Trauner M, Boyer JL. Cholestatic syndromes. Curr Opin Gastroenterol 2001;17:242–56.

69. George DK, Crawford DH. Antibacterial-induced hepatotoxicity. Incidence, prevention and management. Drug Saf 1996;15(1):79–85.

70. Farrell GC. Drug-induced hepatic injury. J Gastroenterol Hepatol 1997;12(9–10):S242–50.

71. Pillans PI. Drug associated hepatic reactions in New Zealand: 21 years experience. NZ Med J 1996;109(1028): 315–19.

72. Derby LE, Jick H, Henry DA, Dean AD. Cholestatic hepatitis associated with flucloxacillin. Med J Aust 1993;158(9):596–600.

73. Devereaux BM, Crawford DH, Purcell P, Powell LW, Roeser HP. Flucloxacillin associated cholestatic hepatitis. An Australian and Swedish epidemic? Eur J Clin Pharmacol 1995;49(1–2):81–5.

74. Olsson R, Wiholm BE, Sand C, Zettergren L, Hultcrantz R, Myrhed M. Liver damage from flucloxacillin, cloxacillin and dicloxacillin. J Hepatol 1992;15(1–2):154–61.

75. Fairley CK, McNeil JJ, Desmond P, Smallwood R, Young H, Forbes A, Purcell P, Boyd I. Risk factors for development of flucloxacillin associated jaundice. BMJ 1993;306(6872):233–5.

76. Stephens RB, Cooper A. Hepatitis from 5-methoxy-psoralen occurring in a patient with previous flucloxacillin hepatitis. Australas J Dermatol 1999;40(4):217–19.

77. Goland S, Malnick SD, Gratz R, Feldberg E, Geltner D, Sthoeger ZM. Severe cholestatic hepatitis following cloxacillin treatment. Postgrad Med J 1998;74(867):59–60.

78. Barrio J, Castiella A, Cosme A, Lopez P, Fernandez J, Arenas JI. Hepatotoxicidad pox cloxacilina. [Hepatotoxicity caused by cloxacillin.] Rev Esp Enferm Dig 1997;89(7):559–60.

79. Konikoff F, Alcalay J, Halevy J. Clocaxcillin-induced cholestatic jaundice. Am J Gastroenterol 1987;482–3.

80. Siegmund JB, Tarshis AM. Prolonged jaundice after dicloxacillin therapy. Am J Gastroenterol 1993;88(8): 1299–300.

81. Tauris P, Jorgensen NF, Petersen CM, Albertsen K. Prolonged severe cholestasis induced by oxacillin derivatives. A report on two cases. Acta Med Scand 1985;217(5):567–9.

82. Kleinman MS, Presberg JE. Cholestatic hepatitis after dicloxacillin-sodium therapy. J Clin Gastroenterol 1986;8(1):77–8.

83. Olans RN, Weiner LB. Reversible oxacillin hepatotoxicity. J Pediatr 1976;89(5):835–8.

84. Michelson PA. Reversible high dose oxacillin-associated liver injury. Can J Hosp Pharm 1981;34:83.

85. Onorato IM, Axelrod JL. Hepatitis from intravenous high-dose oxacillin therapy: findings in an adult inpatient population. Ann Intern Med 1978;89(4):497–500.

86. Piotrowicz A, Polkey M, Wilkinson M. Ursodeoxycholic acid for the treatment of flucloxacillin-associated cholestasis. J Hepatol 1995;22(1):119–20.

87. Bauer TM, Bircher AJ. Drug-induced hepatocellular liver injury due to benzylpenicillin with evidence of lymphocyte sensitization. J Hepatol 1997;26(2):429–32.

88. Onate J, Montejo M, Aguirrebengoa K, Ruiz-Irastorza G, Gonzalez de Zarate P, Aguirre C. Hepatotoxicity associated with penicillin V therapy. Clin Infect Dis 1995;20(2):474–5.

89. Davies MH, Harrison RF, Elias E, Hubscher SG. Antibiotic-associated acute vanishing bile duct syndrome: a pattern associated with severe, prolonged, intrahepatic cholestasis. J Hepatol 1994;20(1):112–16.

90. Anderson CS, Nicholls J, Rowland R, LaBrooy JT. Hepatic granulomas: a 15-year experience in the Royal Adelaide Hospital. Med J Aust 1988;148(2):71–4.

91. Wilson FM, Belamaric J, Lauter CB, Lerner AM. Anicteric carbenicillin hepatitis. Eight episodes in four patients. JAMA 1975;232(8):818–21.

92. Presti ME, Janney CG, Neuschwander-Tetri BA. Nafcillin-associated hepatotoxicity. Report of a case and review of the literature. Dig Dis Sci 1996;41(1):180–4.

93. Andrade RJ, Guilarte J, Salmeron FJ, Lucena MI, Bellot V. Benzylpenicillin-induced prolonged cholestasis. Ann Pharmacother 2001;35(6):783–4.

94. Quattropani C, Schneider M, Helbling A, Zimmermann A, Krahenbuhl S. Cholangiopathy after short-term administration of piperacillin and imipenem/cilastatin. Liver 2001;21(3):213–16.

95. Marshall JB. Acute pancreatitis. A review with an emphasis on new developments. Arch Intern Med 1993;153(10): 1185–98.

96. Hanline MH Jr. Acute pancreatitis caused by ampicillin. South Med J 1987;80(8):1069.

97. Sammett D, Greben C, Sayeed-Shah U. Acute pancreatitis caused by penicillin. Dig Dis Sci 1998;43(8):1778–83.

98. Ruley EJ, Lisi LM. Interstitial nephritis and renal failure due to ampicillin. J Pediatr 1974;84(6):878–82.

99. Tannenberg AM, Wicher KJ, Rose NR. Ampicillin nephropathy. JAMA 1971;218(3):449.

100. Kleinknecht D, Vanhille P, Morel-Maroger L, Kanfer A, Lemaitre V, Mery JP, Laederich J, Callard P. Acute interstitial nephritis due to drug hypersensitivity. An up-to-date review with a report of 19 cases. Adv Nephrol Necker Hosp 1983;12:277–308.

101. Gilbert DN, Gourley R, d'Agostino A, Goodnight SH Jr, Worthen H. Interstitial nephritis due to methicillin, penicillin and ampicillin. Ann Allergy 1970;28(8):378–85.

102. Dharnidharka VR, Rosen S, Somers MJ. Acute interstitial nephritis presenting as presumed minimal change nephrotic syndrome. Pediatr Nephrol 1998;12(7):576–8.

103. Hedstrom SA, Hybbinette CH. Nephrotoxicity in isoxazolylpenicillin prophylaxis in hip surgery. Acta Orthop Scand 1988;59(2):144–7.

104. Ditlove J, Weidmann P, Bernstein M, Massry SG. Methicillin nephritis. Medicine (Baltimore) 1977;56(6): 483–91.

105. Galpin JE, Shinaberger JH, Stanley TM, Blumenkrantz MJ, Bayer AS, Friedman GS, Montgomerie JZ, Guze LB, Coburn JW, Glassock RJ. Acute interstitial nephritis due to methicillin. Am J Med 1978;65(5):756–65.

106. Baldwin DS, Levine BB, McCluskey RT, Gallo GR. Renal failure and interstitial nephritis due to penicillin and methicillin. N Engl J Med 1968;279(23):1245–52.

107. Appel GB. A decade of penicillin related acute interstitial nephritis—more questions than answers. Clin Nephrol 1980;13(4):151–4.

108. Woodroffe AJ, Thomson NM, Meadows R, Lawrence JR. Nephropathy associated with methicillin administration. Aust NZ J Med 1974;4(3):256–61.

109. Hansen ES, Tauris P. Methicillin-induced nephropathy. A case with linear deposition of IgG and C3 on the tubular-basement-membrane. Acta Pathol Microbiol Scand [A] 1976;84(5):440–2.

110. Parry MF, Ball WD, Conte JE Jr, et al. Nafcillin nephritis. JAMA 1973;225:178.

111. Jahansouz F, Kriett JM, Smith CM, Jamieson SW. Potentiation of cyclosporine nephrotoxicity by nafcillin in lung transplant recipients. Transplantation 1993;55(5): 1045–8.

112. Dorner O, Piper C, Dienes HP, et al. Akute interstitielle Nephritis nach Piperacillin. Klin Wochenschr 1988;67:682.

113. Soto J, Bosch JM, Alsar Ortiz MJ, Moreno MJ, Gonzalez JD, Diaz JM. Piperacillin-induced acute interstitial nephritis. Nephron 1993;65(1):154–5.

114. Tanaka H, Waga S, Kakizaki Y, Tateyama T, Koda M, Yokoyama M. Acute tubulointerstitial nephritis associated

with piperacillin therapy in a boy with glomerulonephritis. Acta Paediatr Jpn 1997;39(6):698–700.

115. Sanjad SA, Haddad GG, Nassar VH. Nephropathy, an underestimated complication of methicillin therapy. J Pediatr 1974;84(6):873–7.

116. Bracis R, Sanders CV, Gilbert DN. Methicillin hemorrhagic cystitis. Antimicrob Agents Chemother 1977;12(3):438–9.

117. Moller NE. Carbenicillin-induced haemorrhagic cystitis. Lancet 1978;2(8096):946.

118. Boursas M, Benhassine L, Kempf J, Petit B, Vuillemin F. Insuffisance rénale obstructive par cristallurie à l'amoxicilline. [Obstructive renal insufficiency caused by amoxicillin crystalluria.] Ann Fr Anesth Reanim 1997;16(7):908–10.

119. Boffa JJ, De Preneuf H, Bouadma L, Daudon M, Pallot JL. Insuffisance rénale aiguë par cristallisation d'amoxicilline. [Acute renal failure after amoxicillin crystallization.] Presse Méd 2000;29(13):699–701.

120. De Weck AL. Penicillins and cephalosporins. In: Allergic Reactions to Drugs. Heidelberg: Springer-Verlag, 1983:423.

121. Lindemayr H, Knobler R, Kraft D, Baumgartner W. Challenge of penicillin-allergic volunteers with penicillin-contaminated meat. Allergy 1981;36(7):471–8.

122. Schwartz HJ, Sher TH. Anaphylaxis to penicillin in a frozen dinner. Ann Allergy 1984;52(5):342–3.

123. Tscheuschner I. Anaphylaktische Reaktion auf Penicillin nach Genuss von Schweinefleisch. [Penicillin anaphylaxis following pork consumption.] Z Haut Geschlechtskr 1972;47(14):591–2.

124. Schopf E, Stuhmer A, Rzany B, Victor N, Zentgraf R, Kapp JF. Toxic epidermal necrolysis and Stevens–Johnson syndrome. An epidemiologic study from West Germany. Arch Dermatol 1991;127(6):839–42.

125. Roujeau JC, Guillaume JC, Fabre JP, Penso D, Flechet ML, Girre JP. Toxic epidermal necrolysis (Lyell syndrome). Incidence and drug etiology in France, 1981–1985. Arch Dermatol 1990;126(1):37–42.

126. Bastuji-Garin S, Rzany B, Stern RS, Shear NH, Naldi L, Roujeau JC. Clinical classification of cases of toxic epidermal necrolysis, Stevens–Johnson syndrome, and erythema multiforme. Arch Dermatol 1993;129(1):92–6.

127. Fellner MJ. Adverse reactions to penicillin and related drugs. Clin Dermatol 1986;4(1):133–41.

128. Schulz KH, Schopf E, Wex O. Allergische Berufsekzeme durch Ampicillin. [Allergic occupational eczemas caused by ampicillin.] Berufsdermatosen 1970;18(3):132–43.

129. Calkin JM, Maibach HI. Delayed hypersensitivity drug reactions diagnosed by patch testing. Contact Dermatitis 1993;29(5):223–33.

130. Kristofferson A, Ahlstedt S, Enander I. Contact sensitivity in guinea pigs to different penicillins. Int Arch Allergy Appl Immunol 1982;69(4):316–21.

131. Hoigné R, D'Andrea Jaeger M, Wymann R, et al. Time pattern of allergic reactions to drugs. In: Weber E, Lawson DH, Hoigné R, editors. Risk Factors for Adverse Drug Reactions. Agents Actions 1990; Suppl 29:423.

132. de Haan P, Bruynzeel DP, van Ketel WG. Onset of penicillin rashes: relation between type of penicillin administered and type of immune reactivity. Allergy 1986;41(1):75–8.

133. Dolovich J, Ruhno J, Sauder DN, Ahlstedt S, Hargreave FE. Isolated late cutaneous skin test response to ampicillin: a distinct entity. J Allergy Clin Immunol 1988;82(4):676–9.

134. Vega JM, Blanca M, Carmona MJ, Garcia J, Claros A, Juarez C, Moya MC. Delayed allergic reactions to beta-lactams. Four cases with intolerance to amoxicillin or ampicillin and good tolerance to penicillin G and V. Allergy 1991;46(2):154–7.

135. Barbaud AM, Bene MC, Schmutz JL, Ehlinger A, Weber M, Faure GC. Role of delayed cellular hypersensitivity and adhesion molecules in amoxicillin-induced morbilliform rashes. Arch Dermatol 1997;133(4):481–6.

136. Shiohara T, Nickoloff BJ, Sagawa Y, Gomi T, Nagashima M. Fixed drug eruption. Expression of epidermal keratinocyte intercellular adhesion molecule-1 (ICAM-1). Arch Dermatol 1989;125(10):1371–6.

137. Jimenez I, Anton E, Picans I, Sanchez I, Quinones MD, Jerez J. Fixed drug eruption from amoxycillin. Allergol Immunopathol (Madr) 1997;25(5):247–8.

138. Surbled M, Lejus C, Milpied B, Pannier M, Souron R. Syndrome de Lyell consecutif a l'administration d'amoxicilline chez un enfant de 2 ans. [Lyell syndrome after amoxicillin administration in a 2 year old child.] Ann Fr Anesth Reanim 1996;15(7):1095–8.

139. Miyauchi H, Hosokawa H, Akaeda T, Iba H, Asada Y. T-cell subsets in drug-induced toxic epidermal necrolysis. Possible pathogenic mechanism induced by CD8-positive T cells. Arch Dermatol 1991;127(6):851–5.

140. Correia O, Delgado L, Ramos JP, Resende C, Torrinha JA. Cutaneous T-cell recruitment in toxic epidermal necrolysis. Further evidence of CD8+ lymphocyte involvement. Arch Dermatol 1993;129(4):466–8.

141. Hertl M, Bohlen H, Jugert F, Boecker C, Knaup R, Merk HF. Predominance of epidermal CD8+ T lymphocytes in bullous cutaneous reactions caused by beta-lactam antibiotics. J Invest Dermatol 1993;101(6):794–9.

142. Stejskal VD, Forsbeck M, Olin R. Side-chain-specific lymphocyte responses in workers with occupational allergy induced by penicillins. Int Arch Allergy Appl Immunol 1987;82(3–4):461–4.

143. Fellner MJ, Mark AS. Penicillin- and ampicillin-induced pemphigus vulgaris. Int J Dermatol 1980;19(7):392–3.

144. Miralles J, Barnadas MA, Baselga E, Gelpi C, Rodriguez JL, de Moragas JM. Bullous pemphigoid-like lesions induced by amoxicillin. Int J Dermatol 1997;36(1):42–7.

145. Wakelin SH, Allen J, Wojnarowska F. Drug-induced bullous pemphigoid with dermal fluorescence on salt-split skin. J Eur Acad Dermatol Venereol 1996;7:266.

146. Wakelin SH, Allen J, Zhou S, Wojnarowska F. Drug-induced linear IgA disease with antibodies to collagen VII. Br J Dermatol 1998;138(2):310–14.

147. Woodley DT, Burgeson RE, Lunstrum G, Bruckner-Tuderman L, Reese MJ, Briggaman RA. Epidermolysis bullosa acquisita antigen is the globular carboxyl terminus of type VII procollagen. J Clin Invest 1988;81(3):683–7.

148. Gamboa P, Jauregui I, Urrutia I. Occupational sensitization to aminopenicillins with oral tolerance to penicillin V. Contact Dermatitis 1995;32(1):48–9.

149. Conde-Salazar L, Guimaraens D, Gonzalez MA, Mancebo E. Occupational allergic contact urticaria from amoxicillin. Contact Dermatitis 2001;45(2):109.

150. Petavy-Catala C, Machet L, Vaillant L. Consort contact urticaria due to amoxycillin. Contact Dermatitis 2001;44(4):251.

151. Liccardi G, Gilder J, D'Amato M, D'Amato G. Drug allergy transmitted by passionate kissing. Lancet 2002;359(9318):1700.

152. Wuthrich B. Oral allergy syndrome to apple after a lover's kiss. Allergy 1997;52(2):235–6.

153. Wuthrich B, Dascher M, Borelli S. Kiss-induced allergy to peanut. Allergy 2001;56(9):913.

154. Smith YR, Hurd WW, Menge AC, Sanders GM, Ansbacher R, Randolph JF Jr. Allergic reactions to penicillin during in vitro fertilization and intrauterine insemination. Fertil Steril 1992;58(4):847–9.

155. Katz M, Seidenbaum M, Weinrauch L. Penicillin-induced generalized pustular psoriasis. J Am Acad Dermatol 1987;17(5 Pt 2):918–20.

156. Prieto A, de Barrio M, Lopez-Saez P, Baeza ML, de Benito V, Olalde S. Recurrent localized pustular eruption induced by amoxicillin. Allergy 1997;52(7):777–8.

157. Beylot C, Bioulac P, Doutre MS. Pustuloses exanthématiques aiguës généralisées. A propos de 4 cas. [Acute generalized exanthematic pustuloses (four cases).] Ann Dermatol Venereol 1980;107(1–2):37–48.

158. Isogai Z, Sunohara A, Tsuji T. Pustular drug eruption due to bacampicillin hydrochloride in a patient with psoriasis. J Dermatol 1998;25(9):612–15.

159. Spencer JM, Silvers DN, Grossman ME. Pustular eruption after drug exposure: is it pustular psoriasis or a pustular drug eruption? Br J Dermatol 1994;130(4):514–19.

160. Beckmann H. Exantheme unter der Behandlung mit Ampicillin. [Exanthemas during ampicillin treatment.] Munch Med Wochenschr 1971;113(43):1423–9.

161. Dejarnatt AC, Grant JA. Basic mechanisms of anaphylaxis and anaphylactoid reactions. Immunol Allergy Clin North Am 1992;12:33–46.

162. Choquet-Kastylevsky G, Descotes J. Value of animal models for predicting hypersensitivity reactions to medicinal products. Toxicology 1998;129(1):27–35.

163. McCloskey GL, Massa MC. Cephalexin rash in infectious mononucleosis. Cutis 1997;59(5):251–4.

164. Gastaminza G, Audicana MT, Fernandez E, Anda M, Ansotegui IJ. Palmar exfoliative exanthema to amoxicillin. Allergy 2000;55(5):510–11.

165. Terrados S, Blanca M, Garcia J, Vega J, Torres MJ, Carmona MJ, Miranda A, Moya M, Juarez C, Fernandez J. Nonimmediate reactions to betalactams: prevalence and role of the different penicillins. Allergy 1995;50(7):563–7.

166. Sogn DD, Evans R 3rd, Shepherd GM, Casale TB, Condemi J, Greenberger PA, Kohler PF, Saxon A, Summers RJ, VanArsdel PP Jr, et al. Results of the National Institute of Allergy and Infectious Diseases Collaborative Clinical Trial to test the predictive value of skin testing with major and minor penicillin derivatives in hospitalized adults. Arch Intern Med 1992;152(5):1025–32.

167. Gadde J, Spence M, Wheeler B, Adkinson NF Jr. Clinical experience with penicillin skin testing in a large inner-city STD clinic. JAMA 1993;270(20):2456–63.

168. Vega JM, Blanca M, Garcia JJ, Carmona MJ, Miranda A, Perez-Estrada M, Fernandez S, Acebes JM, Terrados S. Immediate allergic reactions to amoxicillin. Allergy 1994;49(5):317–22.

169. Silviu-Dan F, McPhillips S, Warrington RJ. The frequency of skin test reactions to side-chain penicillin determinants. J Allergy Clin Immunol 1993;91(3):694–701.

170. Boonk WJ, van Ketel WG. Chronische urticaria, penicilline-allergie en melkprodukten in de voeding. [Chronic urticaria, penicillin allergy and dairy products in the diet.] Ned Tijdschr Geneeskd 1980;124(42):1771–3.

171. Bochner BS, Lichtenstein LM. Anaphylaxis. N Engl J Med 1991;324(25):1785–90.

172. Markowitz M, Kaplan E, Cuttica R, et al. Allergic reactions to long-term benzathine penicillin prophylaxis for rheumatic fever. International Rheumatic Fever Study Group. Lancet 1991;337(8753):1308–10.

173. Blanca M, Perez E, Garcia J, Miranda A, Fernandez J, Vega JM, Terrados S, Avila M, Martin A, Suau R. Anaphylaxis to amoxycillin but good tolerance for benzyl penicillin. In vivo and in vitro studies of specific IgE antibodies. Allergy 1988;43(7):508–10.

174. Hunziker I, Kunzi UP, Braunschweig S, Zehnder D, Hoigné R. Comprehensive hospital drug monitoring (CHDM): adverse skin reactions, a 20-year survey. Allergy 1997;52(4):388–93.

175. Hoigne R. Akute Nebenreaktionen auf Penicillinpräparate. [Acute side-reactions to penicillin preparations.] Acta Med Scand 1962;171:201–8.

176. Lin RY. A perspective on penicillin allergy. Arch Intern Med 1992;152(5):930–7.

177. Spark RP. Fatal anaphylaxis due to oral penicillin. Am J Clin Pathol 1971;56(3):407–11.

178. Cullen DJ. Severe anaphylactic reaction to penicillin during halothane anaesthesia. A case report. Br J Anaesth 1971;43(4):410–12.

179. Macy E, Richter PK, Falkoff R, Zeiger R. Skin testing with penicilloate and penilloate prepared by an improved method: amoxicillin oral challenge in patients with negative skin test responses to penicillin reagents. J Allergy Clin Immunol 1997;100(5):586–91.

180. Wickern GM, Nish WA, Bitner AS, Freeman TM. Allergy to beta-lactams: a survey of current practices. J Allergy Clin Immunol 1994;94(4):725–31.

181. Levine BB, Redmond AP, Fellner MJ, Voss HE, Levytska V. Penicillin allergy and the heterogenous immune responses of man to benzylpenicillin. J Clin Invest 1966;45(12):1895–906.

182. VanArsdel PP Jr, Larson EB. Diagnostic tests for patients with suspected allergic disease. Utility and limitations. Ann Intern Med 1989;110(4):304–12.

183. Barbaud A, Reichert-Penetrat S, Trechot P, Jacquin-Petit MA, Ehlinger A, Noirez V, Faure GC, Schmutz JL, Bene MC. The use of skin testing in the investigation of cutaneous adverse drug reactions. Br J Dermatol 1998;139(1):49–58.

184. Ressler C, Mendelson LM. Skin test for diagnosis of penicillin allergy—current status. Ann Allergy 1987;59(3):167–70.

185. Erffmeyer JE. Adverse reactions to penicillin. Ann Allergy 1981;47(4):288–300.

186. Baldo BA, Pham NH, Weiner J. Detection and side-chain specificity of IgE antibodies to flucloxacillin in allergic subjects. J Mol Recognit 1995;8(3):171–7.

187. Torres MJ, Blanca M, Fernandez J, Esteban A, Moreno F, Vega JM, Garcia J. Selective allergic reaction to oral cloxacillin. Clin Exp Allergy 1996;26(1):108–11.

188. Sastre J, Quijano LD, Novalbos A, Hernandez G, Cuesta J, de las Heras M, Lluch M, Fernandez M. Clinical cross-reactivity between amoxicillin and cephadroxil in patients allergic to amoxicillin and with good tolerance of penicillin. Allergy 1996;51(6):383–6.

189. Salkind AR, Cuddy PG, Foxworth JW. The rational clinical examination. Is this patient allergic to penicillin? An evidence-based analysis of the likelihood of penicillin allergy. JAMA 2001;285(19):2498–505.

190. Gruchalla RS. Acute drug desensitization. Clin Exp Allergy 1998;28(Suppl 4):63–4.

191. Sullivan TJ. Drug Allergy. In: Middleton E Jr, editor. Allergy—Principles and Practice. 4th ed.CV Mosby Co, 1993:1726.

192. Tidwell BH, Clearly JD, Lorenz KR. Antimicrobial desensitization: a review of published protocols. Hosp Pharm 1997;32:1362–70.

193. Sullivan TJ. Management of patients allergic to antimicrobial drugs. Allergy Proc 1991;12(6):361–4.

194. Sullivan TJ, Yecies LD, Shatz GS, Parker CW, Wedner HJ. Desensitization of patients allergic to penicillin using orally administered beta-lactam antibiotics. J Allergy Clin Immunol 1982;69(3):275–82.

195. Chisholm CA, Katz VL, McDonald TL, Bowes WA Jr. Penicillin desensitization in the treatment of syphilis during pregnancy. Am J Perinatol 1997;14(9):553–4.

196. Wendel GD Jr, Stark BJ, Jamison RB, Molina RD, Sullivan TJ. Penicillin allergy and desensitization in serious infections during pregnancy. N Engl J Med 1985; 312(19):1229–32.

197. Naclerio R, Mizrahi EA, Adkinson NF Jr. Immunologic observations during desensitization and maintenance of clinical tolerance to penicillin. J Allergy Clin Immunol 1983;71(3):294–301.

198. Booth BH, Patterson R. Electrocardiographic changes during human anaphylaxis. JAMA 1970;211(4):627–31.

199. Petsas AA, Kotler MN. Electrocardiographic changes associated with penicillin anaphylaxis. Chest 1973; 64(1):66–9.

200. Mannik M. Serum sickness and pathophysiology of immune complexes. In: Rich RR, Fleisher TA, Schwartz BD, editors. Clinical Immunology, Principles and Practice. St Louis: Mosby Year Book Inc, 1996:1062–71.

201. Tatum AJ, Ditto AM, Patterson R. Severe serum sickness-like reaction to oral penicillin drugs: three case reports. Ann Allergy Asthma Immunol 2001;86(3):330–4.

202. Heinonen OP, Slone D, Shapiro S. Antimicrobial and antiparasitic agents. In: Birth Defects and Drugs in Pregnancy. 4th ed. Boston: John Wright PSG, 1982:296.

203. Joseph TA, Pyati SP, Jacobs N. Neonatal early-onset Escherichia coli disease. The effect of intrapartum ampicillin. Arch Pediatr Adolesc Med 1998;152(1):35–40.

204. Towers CV, Carr MH, Padilla G, Asrat T. Potential consequences of widespread antepartal use of ampicillin. Am J Obstet Gynecol 1998;179(4):879–83.

205. Matheson I, Samseth M, Sande HA. Ampicillin in breast milk during puerperal infections. Eur J Clin Pharmacol 1988;34(6):657–9.

206. Manian FA, Stone WJ, Alford RH. Adverse antibiotic effects associated with renal insufficiency. Rev Infect Dis 1990;12(2):236–49.

207. Batchelor RC, Horne GO, Rogerson HL. An unusual reaction to procaine penicillin in aqueous suspension. Lancet 1951;2(5):195–8.

208. Hoigné R, Schoch K. Anaphylaktischer Schock und akute nichtallergische Reaktionen nach Procain-Penicillin. [Anaphylactic shock and acute nonallergic reactions following procaine-penicillin.] Schweiz Med Wochenschr 1959;89:1350–6.

209. Dry J, Leynadier F, Damecour C, Pradalier A, Herman D. Réaction pseudo-anaphylactique à la procaine-pénicilline G. Trois cas de syndrome de Hoigné. [Pseudo-anaphylactic reaction to procaine-penicillin G. 3 cases of Hoigné's syndrome.] Nouv Presse Med 1976;5(22):1401–3.

210. Schmied C, Schmied E, Vogel J, Saurat JH. Syndrome de Hoigné ou réaction pseudo-anaphylactique à la procaine pénicilline G: un classique d'actualité. [Hoigné's syndrome or pseudo-anaphylactic reaction to procaine penicillin G: a still current classic.] Schweiz Med Wochenschr 1990; 120(29):1045–9.

211. Lewis GW. Acute immediate reactions to penicillin. BMJ 1957;(5028):1151–2.

212. Silber TJ, D'Angelo L. Psychosis and seizures following the injection of penicillin G procaine. Hoigné's syndrome. Am J Dis Child 1985;139(4):335–7.

213. Downham TF 2nd, Cawley RA, Salley SO, Dal Santo G. Systemic toxic reactions to procaine penicillin G. Sex Transm Dis 1978;5(1):4–9.

214. Silber TJ, D'Angelo LJ. Panic attack following injection of aqueous procaine penicillin G (Hoigné syndrome) J Pediatr 1985;107(2):314–15.

215. Berger H, Juchinka H, Tomczyk D, et al. Pseudo-anaphylactic syndrome after procaine penicillin in children. In: Abstracts, 10th Jubilee Congress. Bialystok: Polish Neurology Society, 1977:82.

216. Menke HE, Pepplinkhuizen L. Acute non-allergic reaction to aqueous procaine penicillin. Lancet 1974;2(7882):723–4.

217. Hoigné R, Krebs A. Kombinierte anaphylaktische und embolisch-toxische Reaktion durch akzidentelle intravaskuläre Injektion von Procain-Penicillin. [Combined anaphylactic and embolic-toxic reaction caused by the accidental intravascular injection of procaine penicillin.] Schweiz Med Wochenschr 1964;94:610–14.

218. Kryst L, Wanyura H. Hoigné's syndrome—its course and symptomatology. J Maxillofac Surg 1979;7(4):320–6.

219. Ernst G, Reuter E. Nicht-allergische tödliche Zwischenfälle nach depot-Penicillin. Beitrag zur Pathogenese und Prophylaxe. [Nonallergic fatal incidents following depot penicillin. Pathogenesis and prevention.] Dtsch Med Wochenschr 1970;95(12):618.

220. Bornemann K, Schulz E, Heinecker R. Akute, nicht-allergische Reaktionen nach i.m. Gabe von Clemizol-Penicillin G und Streptomycin. [Acute, non-allergic reactions following i.m. administration of clemizole-penicillin G and streptomycin.] Munch Med Wochenschr 1966;108(15):834–7.

221. Bredt J. Akute nicht-allergische Reaktionen bei Anwendung von Depot-Penicillin. [Acute non-allergic reactions in the use of depot-penicillin.] Dtsch Med Wochenschr 1965;90:1559–63.

222. Galpin JE, Chow AW, Yoshikawa TT, Guze LB. "Pseudoanaphylactic" reactions from inadvertent infusion of procaine penicillin G. Ann Intern Med 1974;81(3):358–9.

223. Kraus SJ, Green RL. Pseudoanaphylactic reactions with procaine penicillin. Cutis 1976;17(4):765–7.

224. Ilechukwu ST. Acute psychotic reactions and stress response syndromes following intramuscular aqueous procaine penicillin. Br J Psychiatry 1990;156:554–9.

225. Clauberg G. Wiederbelebung bei embolisch-toxischer Komplikation. [Resuscitation in embolic and toxic complication caused by intravascular administration of a depot-penicillin.] Anaesthesist 1966;15(8):284–5.

226. Utley PM, Lucas JB, Billings TE. Acute psychotic reactions to aqueous procaine penicillin. South Med J 1966; 59(11):1271–4.

227. Randazzo SD, DiPrima G. Psicosi allucinatoria acuta da penicillina-procaina in sospensione acquosa. [Acute hallucinatory psychoses caused by procaine penicillin in aqueous suspension.] Minerva Dermatol 1959;34(6):422–8.

228. Green RL, Lewis JE, Kraus SJ, Frederickson EL. Elevated plasma procaine concentrations after administration of procaine penicillin G. N Engl J Med 1974;291(5):223–6.

229. Fishman LS, Hewitt WL. The natural penicillins. Med Clin North Am 1970;54(5):1081–99.

230. Lloyd-Roberts GC, Thomas TG. The etiology of quadriceps contracture in children. J Bone Joint Surg Br 1964;46:498–517.

231. Greenblatt DJ, Allen MD. Intramuscular injection-site complications. JAMA 1978;240(6):542–4.

232. Girard JP, Zawodnik S. Diagnostic procedures in drug allergy. In: De Weck AL, Bundgard H, editors. Handbook Exp Pharmacol. Heidelberg: Springer-Verlag; 1983;63:207.

233. Nicolau S. Dermite livédoïde et gangréneuse de la fesse, consécutive aux injections intra-musculaires, dans la syphilis: à propos d'un cas d'embolie artérielle bismuthique. Ann Mal Vener 1925;20:321.

234. Saputo V, Bruni G. La sindrome di Nicolau da preparati di penicillina: analisi della letteratura alla ricercá di potenziali fattori di rischio. [Nicolau syndrome by penicillin preparations: review of the literature in search for potential risk factors.] Pediatr Med Chir 1998;20(2):105–23.

235. Schanzer H, Gribetz I, Jacobson JH 2nd. Accidental intra-arterial injection of penicillin G. A preventable catastrophe. JAMA 1979;242(12):1289–90.

236. Vivell O, Hennewig J. Infarktähnliche Nekrosen nach intramuskulärer Injektion von Antibiotika. Padiatr Prax 1963;2:415.

237. Friederiszick FK. Embolien während intramuskulärer Penicillinbehandlung. Klin Wochenschr 1949;27:173.

238. Deutsch J. Schwere lokale Reaktion nach Benzathin-Penizillin. Ein Beitrag zum Nicolau-Syndrom (Dermatitis livedoides). [Severe local reaction to benzathine penicillin. A contribution to the Nicolau syndrome (dermatitis livedoides).] Dtsch Gesundheitsw 1966;21(51):2433–7.

239. Gerbeaux J, Couvreur J, Lajouanine P, Canet J, Bonvallet. Sur deux cas d'ischémie étendue transitoire après injection intramusculaire de benzathine-pénicilline chez l'enfant. [On 2 cases of transitory extensive ischemia after intramuscular injection of benzathine penicillin in children.] Presse Méd 1966;74(7):299–302.

240. Muller-Vahl H. Adverse reactions after intramuscular injections. Lancet 1983;1(8332):1050.

241. Shaw EB. Transverse myelitis from injection of penicillin. Am J Dis Child 1966;111:548.

242. Ehringer H, Fischer M, Holzner JH, Imhof H, Kubiena K, Lechner K, Pichler H, Schnack H, Seidl K, Staudacher M. Gangrän nach versehentlicher intraaerterieller Injektion von Dicloxacillin. [Gangrene following erroneous intraarterial injection of dicloxacillin.] Dtsch Med Wochenschr 1971;96(26):1127–30.

243. Hoigné R, Sonntag MR, Zoppi M, Hess T, Maibach R, Fritschy D. Occurrence of exanthema in relation to aminopenicillin preparations and allopurinol. N Engl J Med 1987;316(19):1217.

244. Jick H, Porter JB. Potentiation of ampicillin skin reactions by allopurinol or hyperuricemia. J Clin Pharmacol 1981;21(10):456–8.

245. Henderson JL, Polk RE, Kline BJ. In vitro inactivation of gentamicin, tobramycin, and netilmicin by carbenicillin, azlocillin, or mezlocillin. Am J Hosp Pharm 1981;38(8):1167–70.

246. Thompson MI, Russo ME, Saxon BJ, Atkin-Thor E, Matsen JM. Gentamicin inactivation by piperacillin or carbenicillin in patients with end-stage renal disease. Antimicrob Agents Chemother 1982;21(2):268–73.

247. Halstenson CE, Hirata CA, Heim-Duthoy KL, Abraham PA, Matzke GR. Effect of concomitant administration of piperacillin on the dispositions of netilmicin and tobramycin in patients with end-stage renal disease. Antimicrob Agents Chemother 1990;34(1):128–33.

248. Daly JS, Dodge RA, Glew RH, Keroack MA, Bednarek FJ, Whalen M. Effect of time and temperature on inactivation of aminoglycosides by ampicillin at neonatal dosages. J Perinatol 1997;17(1):42–5.

249. Sabra R, Branch RA. Role of sodium in protection by extended-spectrum penicillins against tobramycin-induced nephrotoxicity. Antimicrob Agents Chemother 1990;34(6):1020–5.

250. Ronchera CL, Hernandez T, Peris JE, Torres F, Granero L, Jimenez NV, Pla JM. Pharmacokinetic interaction between high-dose methotrexate and amoxycillin. Ther Drug Monit 1993;15(5):375–9.

251. Yamamoto K, Sawada Y, Matsushita Y, Moriwaki K, Bessho F, Iga T. Delayed elimination of methotrexate associated with piperacillin administration. Ann Pharmacother 1997;31(10):1261–2.

252. Mayall B, Poggi G, Parkin JD. Neutropenia due to low-dose methotrexate therapy for psoriasis and rheumatoid arthritis may be fatal. Med J Aust 1991;155(7):480–4.

253. Dawson JK, Abernethy VE, Lynch MP. Methotrexate and penicillin interaction. Br J Rheumatol 1998;37(7):807.

254. Herrick AL, Grennan DM, Griffen K, Aarons L, Gifford LA. Lack of interaction between flucloxacillin and methotrexate in patients with rheumatoid arthritis. Br J Clin Pharmacol 1996;41(3):223–7.

255. Najjar TA, Abou-Auda HS, Ghilzai NM. Influence of piperacillin on the pharmacokinetics of methotrexate and 7-hydroxymethotrexate. Cancer Chemother Pharmacol 1998;42(5):423–8.

256. Dasgupta A, Sperelakis A, Mason A, Dean R. Phenytoin–oxacillin interactions in normal and uremic sera. Pharmacotherapy 1997;17(2):375–8.

257. Bower BF, McComb R, Ruderman M. Effect of penicillin on urinary 17-ketogenic and 17-ketosteroid excretion. N Engl J Med 1967;277(10):530–2.

Pentagastrin

General Information

Pentagastrin is a short peptide that stimulates the production of gastric acid from the stomach by a direct action on gastrin receptors and of calcitonin from thyroid C cells (1). It also acts on cholecystokinin receptors centrally and stimulates the release of adrenocorticotropin (ACTH) and hence the production of glucocorticoids (2).

Pentagastrin was originally used to test for suppression of gastric acid in patients who had had a vagotomy, and has been used to study gastric physiology and to test the effects of drugs that inhibit gastric acid secretion. It has also been used in the diagnosis of medullary carcinoma of the thyroid because it stimulates the production of calcitonin.

General adverse effects

Pentagastrin often causes adverse effects, which limit its use. Nausea, abdominal cramps, headache, drowsiness, and giddiness can occur. The effect on the stomach is largely dissociated from these unwanted effects. In one series 38 of 40 patients had a feeling of chest tightness (3). In 50 patients parenteral pentagastrin 6 micrograms/kg caused nausea in 14, tremor in 12, and a hot sensation in 11 (4). These effects occurred immediately after injection and continued for several minutes. In four subjects the test had to be stopped because of collapse.

Organs and Systems

Cardiovascular

Pentagastrin causes small transient increases in blood pressure and pulse (5), autonomic effects that are prevented by inhibiting cholecystokinin receptors (6). Atrial fibrillation has been observed (7).

Psychological, psychiatric

In a double-blind placebo-controlled study intravenous pentagastrin led to panic attacks in nine of 19 patients with social phobia, seven of 11 with panic disorder, and two of 19 healthy controls (8). Anxiety, blood pressure, and pulse increased in all three groups.

In a double-blind, placebo-controlled study in seven patients with obsessive-compulsive disorder and seven healthy controls, intravenous pentagastrin 0.6 microgram/kg produced panic-like reactions in six (86%) of the seven patients and only two (29%) of the controls (9).

The anxiety caused by pentagastrin is prevented by inhibiting cholecystokinin receptors (6).

Hematologic

In one case thrombocytopenia was attributed to pentagastrin (10).

Pancreas

- Acute severe abdominal pain occurred in a 25-year-old patient with recurrent duodenal ulcers after subcutaneous injection of pentagastrin (11). Laparotomy showed acute hemorrhagic pancreatitis. Healing and freedom from complaint occurred rapidly with drug therapy.

The authors postulated the following mechanisms: acute exacerbation of chronic pancreatitis, a direct effect of pentagastrin on the pancreas, increased pancreatic secretion due to stimulation by gastric acid, reflux of duodenal contents or bile, arterial hypotension with local acidosis in the pancreas.

Drug–Drug Interactions

Cimetidine

In 150 subjects some, but not all, of the somatic symptoms caused by pentagastrin were abolished by cimetidine; however, the combination of pentagastrin and cimetidine produced a significant incidence of dizziness (12).

References

1. Escalada J, Teruel JL, Pavon I, Vila T, Navarro J, Varela C. Normal calcitonin response to pentagastrin stimulation in patients with chronic renal failure. Acta Endocrinol (Copenh) 1993;129(1):39–41.
2. Abelson JL, Liberzon I. Dose response of adrenocorticotropin and cortisol to the CCK-B agonist pentagastrin. Neuropsychopharmacology 1999;21(4):485–94.
3. Vitale G, Ciccarelli A, Caraglia M, Galderisi M, Rossi R, Del Prete S, Abbruzzese A, Lupoli G. Comparison of two provocative tests for calcitonin in medullary thyroid carcinoma: omeprazole vs pentagastrin. Clin Chem 2002; 48(9):1505–10.
4. Brunner H, Grabner G. Subjektive Vertraglichkeit des Pentagastrintests. [Subjective tolerance of pentagastrin test.] Leber Magen Darm 1978;8(3):165–9.
5. Ewers HR, Brouwers HP, Merguet P, Hengstebeck W. Nebenwirkungen nach Stimulation der Magensekretion mit Pentagastrin. [Side effects after stimulation of gastric secretion with pentagastrin.] Med Klin 1976;71(1):19–23.
6. Lines C, Challenor J, Traub M. Cholecystokinin and anxiety in normal volunteers: an investigation of the anxiogenic properties of pentagastrin and reversal by the cholecystokinin receptor subtype B antagonist L-365,260. Br J Clin Pharmacol 1995;39(3):235–42.
7. Drucker D. Atrial fibrillation after administration of calcium and pentagastrin. N Engl J Med 1981;304(23):1427–8.
8. McCann UD, Slate SO, Geraci M, Roscow-Terrill D, Uhde TW. A comparison of the effects of intravenous pentagastrin on patients with social phobia, panic disorder and healthy controls. Neuropsychopharmacology 1997;16(3): 229–37.
9. de Leeuw AS, Den Boer JA, Slaap BR, Westenberg HG. Pentagastrin has panic-inducing properties in obsessive compulsive disorder. Psychopharmacology (Berl) 1996; 126(4):339–44.
10. Arnved J, Stahl Skov P, Winter K. Pentagastrin-induced thrombocytopenia. Lancet 1985;2(8463):1068–9.
11. Buttner D, Cartsburg R. Akute pankreatitis nach Magensekretionsanalyse unter Pentagastrinstimulation. [Acute pancreatitis following gastric secretion analysis by pentagastrin stimulation.] MMW Munch Med Wochenschr 1978;120(50): 1679–80.
12. Wade A, Wingate D. Use of pentagastrin test as a combined teaching and research project for medical students. Lancet 1980;2(8193):516–19.

Pentamidine

General Information

Pentamidine, an aromatic diamine, has been known since the late 1930s as a treatment for trypanosomiasis and some forms of leishmaniasis. In recent times it has been extensively used in the treatment of *Pneumocystis jiroveci* pneumonia. Its mechanism of action is probably related to inhibition of dihydrofolate reductase and inhibition of oxidative phosphorylation and nucleic acid synthesis, as well as an effect on aerobic glycolysis.

Pharmacokinetics

The pharmacokinetics of pentamidine are incompletely known. It is not absorbed after oral administration and needs to be given parenterally or by aerosol. After intramuscular injection peak concentrations are seen after about 1 hour, and the serum concentration stays about the same for 24 hours. A study of multiple dosing over 2 weeks showed progressive accumulation in the plasma during that time. After multiple intravenous doses the half-life was 12.5 days. After a course of treatment decreasing amounts of pentamidine can be found in the urine for as long as 8 weeks. It seems that pentamidine is stored or bound in the tissues and excreted slowly in the urine and the amount excreted changes only marginally with repeated doses. The highest tissue concentrations have been found in the kidney, followed by the liver and then other tissues, but pentamidine was not found in the brain. Serum concentrations after aerosol therapy are markedly lower than after intravenous therapy. Uptake via the lungs is limited, which explains the lack of serious systemic toxicity seen with aerosol treatment, but also explains the reported occurrence of extrapulmonary *Pneumocystis* infections.

These pharmacokinetic data merit attention, because they may be helpful in preventing toxicity, which seems to be dictated by tissue accumulation rather than serum concentrations; major toxic reactions usually occur only after the first week of parenteral treatment. The pharma-cokinetics may also explain the varied response to treat-ment with aerosolized pentamidine and the more satisfactory results of prophylaxis with the aerosol after initial parenteral treatment (SEDA-13, 824) (SEDA-16, 312). A retrospective study showed efficacy of intrave-nous pentamidine in AIDS patients with *Pneumocystis jiroveci* pneumonia, the most frequent toxic effects being gastrointestinal, especially nausea (SEDA-21, 299).

Observational studies

In an uncontrolled study in French Guiana, intramuscular pentamidine isethionate (two 4 mg/kg injections 48 hours apart) in 198 patients with cutaneous leishmaniasis pro-duced a cure rate of 87%; 80% of treatment failures responded to an identical second course (1). Compared with published studies, adverse events were relatively mild: pain on injection (54%), gastrointestinal effects (53%), and hypotension (8%). There were no dysrhyth-mias or glucose abnormalities. This may reflect the brief course of pentamidine used.

Pentamidine is the drug of choice for the treatment of cutaneous leishmaniasis in Surinam. Pentamidine mesy-late in 235 patients and pentamidine isethionate in 80 patients have been compared in a retrospective study; the cure rate (healing without relapse) was nearly 90% in both groups (2). Relapses occurred in about 10% of patients in both groups. Minor adverse effects, such as pain at the injection site, bitter taste, and nausea, occurred with both drugs in about 65% of patients. Respiratory tract problems occurred in under 10% of patients who took pentamidine isethionate but were uncommon in those who took pentamidine mesylate.

General adverse effects

Pentamidine in therapeutic doses has a high rate of adverse effects (over 50%). Toxicity seems to occur more often in patients with AIDS. Hypotension subsequent to injection or infusion, hypoglycemia, and nephrotoxicity are the major adverse effects. Hepatotoxicity and neutropenia are not uncommon. Compared with the general population there is a high incidence of pancreatitis in patients with AIDS, particularly during aerosol treatment. Hypoglycemia has also been seen after aerosol treatment. Intermittent prophylactic aerosol use causes few adverse effects, apart from cough and bronchial irritation after inhalation. There is a higher incidence of spontaneous pneumothorax with aerosol prophylaxis. There is also a higher incidence of extrapulmonary infections with *P. jiroveci* in patients treated with aerosolized pentamidine. Another disturbing finding was the higher incidence of other opportunistic infections with pentamidine aerosol versus placebo, while pentamidine aerosol was associated with a markedly lower recurrence rate of *P. jiroveci* pneu-monitis in a placebo-controlled pentamidine aerosol study of prophylaxis after initial treatment (SEDA-13, 824). Intramuscular administration of pentamidine brings its own adverse effects: localized pain, erythema, and sterile abscesses are frequent and troublesome (SEDA-13, 824) (3). The use of the Z-track technique for injection mitigates the local effects. Allergic reactions have been reported. There is no information about tumor-inducing effects.

Organs and Systems

Cardiovascular

Severe hypotension can occur after a single intramuscular injection of pentamidine or with rapid intravenous admin-istration, but has been seen with slow infusion as well. Infusing the drug over 60 minutes or more may reduce this risk. Facial flushing, breathlessness, dizziness, and nausea and vomiting can occur at the same time.

Cardiac dysrhythmias, including ventricular tachycar-dia, have been reported during treatment (SEDA-13, 824) (SEDA-16, 331) (4,5). Prolongation of the QT inter-val, which usually precedes the development of ventricu-lar dysrhythmias with pentamidine, occurs in one-third of patients, usually within 2 weeks of starting therapy. Torsade de pointes has been described. Any dysrhythmia can recur many days after the pentamidine has been dis-continued, which is not surprising, in view of the long half-life and tissue accumulation. Electrolyte abnormalities, including low serum magnesium concentrations, have been noticed at times of dysrhythmias (SEDA-16, 315) (SEDA-17, 331) (4–6).

- Torsade de pointes has been reported in a 48-year-old HIV-positive woman treated with intravenous pentami-dine (7).

Local thrombophlebitis can occur after injection of pentamidine, but problems are more often seen at the injection site after intramuscular injection.

Respiratory

Inhalation of pentamidine can cause intolerable coughing. Bronchospasm can occur, especially in cases of asthma; tolerance of inhaled pentamidine is increased in nearly all patients by pretreatment with inhaled beta$_2$-adrenoceptor agonists (SEDA-16, 313) (SEDA-17, 330) (SEDA-18, 290) (4).

In lung function tests, high-dose aerosolized pentami-dine (600 mg/month) was associated with an increased pulmonary residual volume, reduced flow rates, and increased airway reactivity (SEDA-18, 291).

There is an increased incidence of spontaneous pneu-mothorax after the administration of pentamidine by aerosol, which may be connected with the effect on air-way resistance. There was a particularly high frequency of spontaneous pneumothorax in people with hemophilia; the authors suggested that *P. jiroveci* infection and treat-ment resistance had played a role (SEDA-16, 313).

Acute eosinophilic pneumonia after one dose of inhaled pentamidine of 300 mg has been reported; the reaction subsided within 2 weeks but recurred on rechal-lenge (SEDA-18, 292).

Dissemination of lung infection is a potentially serious matter, especially when using pentamidine by the aerosol route. While high alveolar drug concentrations can be reached in the most accessible parts of the lung, systemic absorption is minimal and the organism can spread through the lung and beyond, despite containment of the initial pulmonary infection; in some cases there has been extensive spread of *P. jiroveci* into major organs and the bone marrow (SEDA-16, 313) (SEDA-17, 332). Patients who have been treated with parenteral pentamidine are at a lower risk of disseminated *P. jiroveci* infection than those given aerosol prophylaxis only (SEDA-16, 313) (SEDA-17, 322).

Nervous system

Mild dizziness can occur with pentamidine, but nervous system adverse effects are uncommon.

Psychological, psychiatric

Confusion and hallucinations have occasionally been reported with pentamidine. Magnesium deficiency may affect mental function; a flat affect, slow speech, and mental withdrawal are some of the typical effects (SEDA-13, 825) (6). The symptoms of hypomagnesemia can be ill defined; unexplained symptoms, despite improvement of the *P. jiroveci* infection, demand measurement of the serum magnesium concentration.

Metabolism

Hypoglycemia can be a serious and life-threatening effect of pentamidine and is seen in 10–30% of cases, mainly with parenteral use, although it can also occur with inhalation. In one 21-day study it was equally common with either form of therapy. Higher doses and longer durations of treatment increase the likelihood, as does prior treatment with pentamidine (SEDA-16, 314); uremia also increases the risk. In one study there was nephrotoxicity in all cases with hypoglycemia. The hypoglycemia is the result of a direct toxic effect on the pancreatic beta cells, resulting in insulin release and transient hypoglycemia, which is followed by beta cell destruction and insulin deficiency, which in turn can eventually lead to an irreversible state of diabetes mellitus (SEDA-13, 825) (SEDA-16, 315) (SEDA-17, 331) (4).

Mineral balance

Hypocalcemia has been attributed to pentamidine but not explained (8).

Hypomagnesemia (related to excess urinary excretion of magnesium due to pentamidine) and clinical signs of magnesium deficiency can have psychiatric consequences. Magnesium deficiency itself can affect mental function; a flat affect, slow speech, and mental withdrawal are some of the typical effects (SEDA-13, 825) (6). In one case (6) hypomagnesemia was still present 2 months after intravenous pentamidine treatment, although aerosolized pentamidine was being continued and could have caused hypomagnesemia. Some patients are particularly sensitive to this effect, and previous renal damage (for example by other drugs) can be a risk factor (SEDA-13, 825).

Hematologic

Anemia, leukopenia, or thrombocytopenia occur in less than 5% of cases (SEDA-13, 825). Thrombocytopenia is more likely to occur during prolonged therapy than initially.

Megaloblastic bone marrow changes can occur with prolonged therapy (SEDA-11, 598). Low blood cell counts have been reported even after aerosolized pentamidine.

- Intravenous pentamidine caused megaloblastic anemia in a 38-year-old woman with *Pneumocystis jiroveci* pneumonia (9).

In one patient with AIDS with severe but reversible thrombocytopenia after intravenous pentamidine, the serum during the acute phase contained antiplatelet antibodies that reacted with glycoprotein IIb/IIIa, similar to the reactions observed with quinine-induced thrombocytopenia (SEDA-18, 292). This suggests that even aerosol treatment or environmental exposure will need to be avoided in such patients.

Gastrointestinal

Gastrointestinal complaints due to pentamidine are usually minor. Nausea and vomiting can occur. Dysgeusia has been reported in a few cases with intravenous therapy, but one study of aerosol administration specifically noted its absence (SEDA-13, 825).

Liver

Occasionally, abnormal liver function tests have been seen in patients receiving pentamidine (10).

Pancreas

Episodes of acute pancreatitis and of hemorrhagic pancreatitis have been reported. This may or may not be combined with evidence of damage to pancreatic beta cells (SEDA-13, 825) (SEDA-16, 315) (SEDA-17, 331) (4). However, pancreatitis has also been seen in patients with AIDS who did not receive pentamidine. The risk of pancreatitis seems to be greater in children with CD4 counts under 100×10^6/l. In a case-control study 12 of 44 patients with AIDS and pancreatitis had used pentamidine (SEDA-20, 264).

Urinary tract

Nephrotoxicity is common with pentamidine. In one study, serum creatinine concentrations increased in nine of 10 patients with *P. jiroveci* infection during 2–3 weeks of treatment. The incidence is 20–35% (SEDA-13, 825), and in AIDS higher still, for example 50–65% (SEDA-17, 331) (4). Renal toxicity is more pronounced in patients with diarrhea and probably more severe with intramuscular use, perhaps because of dehydration, which is more readily corrected if the drug is given by infusion. In one study there was evidence of renal toxicity in all patients with pentamidine-induced hypoglycemia, in contrast to an incidence of 38% in the group who remained euglycemic. Because of the marked accumulation of pentamidine, it is conceivable that after an initial period of daily administration a modified treatment regimen, every other day or even twice a week, may prevent renal and pancreatic permanent damage (SEDA-13, 825).

Skin

Rashes can occur with pentamidine but are not common (11).

Local pain at the injection site, local infiltration, and sterile abscesses have been reported after intramuscular pentamidine (2,3).

There have been reports of a Herxheimer reaction and of skin lesions resembling toxic epidermal necrolysis, both in children (SEDA-13, 825).

Musculoskeletal

- Two patients (aged 31 and 38 years) with cutaneous leishmaniasis given intramuscular pentamidine 600 mg twice in 48 hours developed rhabdomyolysis (12). They recovered with fluid replacement and alkaline diuresis.

Drug Administration

Drug formulations

The administration of nebulized pentamidine has an environmental impact; handling the nebulizer, cleaning and preparing it for use, and assisting the patient exposes health-care workers to pentamidine (13). Adverse reactions, such as ocular and pulmonary irritation and irritation of exposed skin, have been reported in health care workers (14).

Drug–Drug Interactions

Potassium-sparing diuretics

Pentamidine is structurally similar to amiloride and can cause severe hyperkalemia if co-prescribed with potassium-sparing diuretic (15). This is a particularly important interaction in patients with AIDS.

References

1. Nacher M, Carme B, Sainte Marie D, Couppie P, Clyti E, Guibert P, Pradinaud R. Influence of clinical presentation on the efficacy of a short course of pentamidine in the treatment of cutaneous leishmaniasis in French Guiana. Ann Trop Med Parasitol 2001;95(4):331–6.
2. Lai A Fat EJ, Vrede MA, Soetosenojo RM, Lai A Fat RF. Pentamidine, the drug of choice for the treatment of cutaneous leishmaniasis in Surinam. Int J Dermatol 2002;41(11):796–800.
3. Cheung TW, Matta R, Neibart E, Hammer G, Chusid E, Sacks HS, Szabo S, Rose D. Intramuscular pentamidine for the prevention of *Pneumocystis carinii* pneumonia in patients infected with human immunodeficiency virus. Clin Infect Dis 1993;16(1):22–5.
4. Masur H. Prevention and treatment of *Pneumocystis* pneumonia. N Engl J Med 1992;327(26):1853–60.
5. Ryan C, Madalon M, Wortham DW, Graziano FM. Sulfa hypersensitivity in patients with HIV infection: onset, treatment, critical review of the literature. WMJ 1998;97(5):23–7.
6. Gradon JD, Fricchione L, Sepkowitz D. Severe hypomagnesemia associated with pentamidine therapy. Rev Infect Dis 1991;13(3):511–12.
7. Kroll CR, Gettes LS. T wave alternans and torsades de Pointes after the use of intravenous pentamidine. J Cardiovasc Electrophysiol 2002;13(9):936–8.
8. Anonymous. Pentamine isethionate. Drugs Today 1985;21:315.
9. Au WY, Ma ES, Kwong YL. Intravenous pentamidine induced megaloblastic anaemia. Haematologica 2002;87(1):ECR06.
10. Bonacini M. Hepatobiliary complications in patients with human immunodeficiency virus infection. Am J Med 1992;92(4):404–11.
11. Leen CL, Mandal BK. Rash due to nebulised pentamidine. Lancet 1988;2(8622):1250–1.
12. Lieber-Mbomeyo A, Lipsker D, Milea M, Heid E. Rhabdomyolyse induite par l'isethionate de pentamidine (Pentacarinat) lors du traitement d'une leishmaniose cutanée. 2 cas. [Rhabdomyolysis induced by pentamidine (Pentacarinat) during treatment of cutaneous leishmaniasis: 2 cases.] Ann Dermatol Venereol 2002;129(1 Pt 1):50–2.
13. Beach JR, Campbell M, Andrews DJ. Exposure of health care workers to pentamidine isethionate. Occup Med (Lond) 1999;49(4):243–5.
14. McDiarmid MA, Fujikawa J, Schaefer J, Weinmann G, Chaisson RE, Hudson CA. Health effects and exposure assessment of aerosolized pentamidine handlers. Chest 1993;104(2):382–5.
15. Perazella MA. Drug-induced hyperkalemia: old culprits and new offenders. Am J Med 2000;109(4):307–14.

Pentamorphone

See also Opioid analgesics

General Information

Pentamorphone is a potent opiate with a rapid onset and short duration of action, similar to that of fentanyl, which has been reported to produce analgesia with limited depression of ventilation (1).

Subjective symptoms in 23 male volunteers who received pentamorphone were pain on injection, headache, tiredness, euphoria, dizziness, visual disturbances, and nausea (2).

Organs and Systems

Cardiovascular

There was no effect on blood pressure or heart rate with pentamorphone doses of 0.015–0.48 micrograms/kg (2).

References

1. Rudo FG, Wynn RL, Ossipov M, Ford RD, Kutcher BA, Carter A, Spaulding TC. Antinociceptive activity of pentamorphone, a 14-beta-aminomorphinone derivative, compared to fentanyl and morphine. Anesth Analg 1989;69(4):450–6.
2. Glass PS, Camporesi EM, Shafron D, Quill T, Reves JG. Evaluation of pentamorphone in humans: a new potent opiate. Anesth Analg 1989;68(3):302–7.

Pentaquine

General Information

Pentaquine is an 8-aminoquinoline that has been used to treat malaria (1,2) and trypanosomiasis (3,4). It has adverse effects very similar to those of primaquine.

References

1. Hall WH, Latts EM. Pentaquine and quinine in the treatment of Korean vivax malaria; a controlled study in 101 patients. J Lab Clin Med 1955;45(4):573–9.
2. Eldin GN, Morcos F. Pentaquine in the treatment of malaria. J Egypt Med Assoc 1952;35(5):330–4.
3. Rubio M, Pizzi T. Accion de la primaquina, pentaquina y pentaquina-quinina, sobre formas sanguaneas virulentas de *Trypanosoma cruzi*. [Effect of primaquine, pentaquine and pentaquine-quinine on virulent blood forms of Trypanosoma cruzi.] Bol Chil Parasitol 1954;9(3):75–9.
4. Neghme A, Agosin M, Christen R, Jarpa A, Atias AV. Ensayos de quimioterapia de la enfermedad de Chagas experimental. VIII. Accion de la cortisona sola y asociada al fosfato de pentaquina o al compuesto de sulfato de quinina-fosfato de pentaquina; estudio histopatologico. [Attempts at the chemotherapy of experimental Chagas' disease. VIII. Effect of cortisone alone and associated with pentaquine phosphate or with the combination of quinine sulfate and pentaquine phosphate; histopathological study.] Bol Inf Parasit Chil 1951;6(3):36.

Pentazocine

General Information

The adverse effects of pentazocine in effective doses are largely typical of its class (1,2), with some quantitative exceptions.

Pentazocine 30 mg had no effect on motor skills but impaired sensory processing and extraocular muscle imbalance (3). Other effects reported in this study were slight respiratory depression (enhanced by concurrent amitriptyline) and feelings of clumsiness, drowsiness, friendliness, and contentedness, and a muzzy head.

The effects of pentazocine were studied in 16 non-abusing volunteers recruited via posters and local newspaper advertisements and were compared with the effects of morphine (4). Pentazocine had dose-related effects on subjective, psychomotor, and physiological variables, and the clinically relevant dose of 30 mg produced a greater magnitude of dysphoric subjective effects than morphine 10 mg and, unlike morphine, impaired psychomotor performance. With pentazocine, peak ratings from the adjective checklist were significantly increased for "dry mouth," "sweating," and "turning of stomach." Compared with morphine, pentazocine led to higher ratings for "drunk," "feel bad," "having pleasant bodily sensations," and "having unpleasant bodily sensations."

Organs and Systems

Psychological, psychiatric

Perceptual disturbances are generally thought to occur more often with pentazocine than with other opioids. Objective definition of such phenomena is difficult, but in a study of postoperative dreaming after the use of pentazocine and morphine as premedicants there was no statistically significant difference between the two drugs (SED-11, 148) (5).

Hematologic

There have been reports of pentazocine-induced agranulocytosis in the absence of other predisposing factors (SED-11, 148) (6).

Skin

Two distinct types of skin lesions have been described in patients taking pentazocine: scleroderma-like changes, subcutaneous abscesses, cellulitis, ulceration, muscle atrophy and granulomas (all of which are well-recognized consequences of pentazocine abuse), and a generalized erythematous desquamative rash.

Severe renal insufficiency associated with toxic epidermal necrolysis has been reported (7).

Long-Term Effects

Drug abuse

Abusers sometimes adulterate the pentazocine with tripelennamine (T's and blues). Medical and psychiatric complications can include seizures, abscesses, depression, psychosis, dysphoria, confusion, and hallucinations (8,9).

Drug dependence

Pentazocine dependence is associated with a mild opioid–like withdrawal syndrome (8,9).

Drug withdrawal

A neonatal withdrawal syndrome has been described, with verification by the detection of pentazocine and its metabolites in the urine of both mother and baby. Within 4 hours of birth the child was irritable, jittery, and hypertonic, with a high-pitched cry, a voracious appetite, and frequent bowel movements. The symptoms improved over 3 days. The mother had abused parenteral pentazocine (23–46 mg) for the previous 10 years and injected the last dose of 46 mg some 10 hours before delivery (10).

Susceptibility Factors

Renal disease

A fatal nephrotic syndrome occurred in a 33-year-old man with renal glomerular disease dependent on pentazocine (SEDA-17, 88).

Other features of the patient

There is evidence that heavy smoking can increase the elimination of pentazocine; thus heavy smokers may require larger doses than non-smokers.

Drug Administration

Drug administration route

Fibrous myopathy and necrotic ulceration can occur at the injection site after repeated parenteral administration (1). Myocutaneous sclerosis and extensive calcinosis at the injection site have also been reported (SEDA-17, 88).

- A 58-year-old nurse who was given parenteral pentazocine developed large sclerotic and infected areas with multiple depressed atrophic scars at sites of prior ulceration; unsterile injection technique could not be excluded as a cause (11).
- A 47-year old woman with a 4-year history of injections of pentazocine into the legs developed very hard thigh and buttock muscles with hard, shiny, hairless overlying skin (12). Imaging showed fibrosis and calcification of the muscles and biopsy showed fibromyopathy. There were associated clinical and electrophysiological polyradiculopathy and multiple mononeuropathy of the lower extremities.
- A 26-year-old woman presented with progressive thickening and tightening of the skin over both her shoulders and buttocks, with resulting movement restrictions (13). She had a 5-year history of multiple intramuscular pentazocine injections for abdominal pain. The site of skin tightening was initially localized to the injection site. The affected areas increased progressively. There was an ill-defined area of hyperpigmented, indurated, "woody hard" skin bound to underlying structures and over her shoulders and buttocks. The diagnosis was pentazocine-induced widespread cutaneous fibrosis and myofibrosis. There was no evidence of scleroderma or dermatomyositis.
- A 38-year-old man, with a painless progressive restriction of flexion around both knee joints for 4 years, had been injecting pentazocine 1–2 ml intramuscularly for 18–20 years (14). The diagnosis was pentazocine-induced fibromyositis and contracture.

Drug overdose

Pentazocine in overdose can cause generalized tonic-clonic seizures, hypertension, hypotonia, dysphoria, hallucinations, delusions, and agitation, with a poor response to naloxone (15). Others have reported status epilepticus, coma, respiratory depression, acidosis, severe hypotension, and ventricular dysrhythmias.

Drug–Drug Interactions

Alcohol

There is increased toxicity in patients who take pentazocine with alcohol, antihistamines, or CNS depressants; one patient developed opioid pulmonary edema and one died (15).

Rhabdomyolysis and acute renal necrosis occurred in a 26-year-old man after concomitant use of pentazocine and alcohol (16).

Methylphenidate

Intravenous injection of a mixture of methylphenidate and pentazocine intended for oral use resulted in death due to granulomatosis associated with pulmonary hypertension (17).

Monoamine oxidase inhibitors

Opioids interact with monoamine oxidase inhibitors, causing CNS excitation and hypertension (18).

Serotonin re-uptake inhibitors

A serious excitatory interaction between fluoxetine and pentazocine has been reported (SEDA-16, 89). The authors commented on the similarity of this syndrome to the reported dangerous interactions between monoamine oxidase inhibitors and narcotic analgesics, and suggested that increased central 5-HT activity may be the basis of the observed interaction.

References

1. Goldstein G. Pentazocine. Drug Alcohol Depend 1985;14(3-4):313–23.
2. Rudra A. Comparison of buprenorphine, morphine, pethidine, and pentazocine as postoperative analgesic after upper abdominal surgery. Calcutta Med J 1989;86:1.
3. Saarialho-Kere U, Mattila MJ, Seppala T. Parenteral pentazocine: effects on psychomotor skills and respiration, and interactions with amitriptyline. Eur J Clin Pharmacol 1988;35(5):483–9.
4. Zacny JP, Hill JL, Black ML, Sadeghi P. Comparing the subjective, psychomotor and physiological effects of intravenous pentazocine and morphine in normal volunteers. J Pharmacol Exp Ther 1998;286(3):1197–207.
5. Heaney RM, Gotlieb N. Granulocytopenia after intravenous abuse of pentazocine and tripelennamine ("Ts and blues"). South Med J 1983;76(5):654–6.
6. Haibach H, Yesus YW, Doggett JJ. Pentazocine-induced agranulocytosis. Can Med Assoc J 1984;130(9):1165–6.
7. Pedragosa R, Vidal J, Fuentes R, Huguet P. Tricotropism by pentazocine. Arch Dermatol 1987;123(3):297–8.
8. Showalter CV. T's and blues. Abuse of pentazocine and tripelennamine. JAMA 1980;244(11):1224–5.
9. Lahmeyer HW, Steingold RG. Medical and psychiatric complications of pentazocine and tripelennamine abuse. J Clin Psychiatry 1980;41(8):275–8.
10. Wu WH, Teng RJ, Shin HY. Neonatal pentazocine withdrawal syndrome—a case report of conservative treatment. Zhonghua Yi Xue Za Zhi (Taipei) 1988;42(3):229–32.
11. Furner BB. Parenteral pentazocine: cutaneous complications revisited. J Am Acad Dermatol 1990;22(4):694–5.
12. Sinsawaiwong S, Phanthumchinda K. Pentazocine-induced fibrous myopathy and localized neuropathy. J Med Assoc Thai 1998;81(9):717–21.
13. Jain A, Bhattacharya SN, Singal A, Baruah MC, Bhatia A. Pentazocine induced widespread cutaneous and myo-fibrosis. J Dermatol 1999;26(6):368–70.
14. Das CP, Thussu A, Prabhakar S, Banerjee AK. Pentazocine-induced fibromyositis and contracture. Postgrad Med J 1999;75(884):361–2.

15. Challoner KR, McCarron MM, Newton EJ. Pentazocine (Talwin) intoxication: report of 57 cases. J Emerg Med 1990;8(1):67–74.

16. Tsai JC, Lai YH, Shin SJ, Chen JH, Torng JK, Tasi JH. Rhabdomyolysis-induced acute tubular necrosis after the concomitant use of alcohol and pentazocine—a case report. Gaoxiong Yi Xue Ke Xue Za Zhi 1987;3(4):299–305.

17. Lundquest DE, Young WK, Edland JF. Maternal death associated with intravenous methylphenidate (Ritalin) and pentazocine (Talwin) abuse. J Forensic Sci 1987;32(3):798–801.

18. Rossiter A, Souney PF. Interaction between MAOIs and opioids: pharmacologic and clinical considerations. Hosp Formul 1993;28(8):692–8.

Pentetrazol

General Information

Pentetrazol (pentylenetetrazol) is a central and respiratory stimulant, similar to doxapram hydrochloride. It is a $GABA_A$ receptor antagonist and is anxiogenic (1). It has been used in respiratory depression and has also been included in multi-ingredient formulations for respiratory tract disorders, including cough, and for the treatment of hypotension and pruritus. However, the general consensus is that pentetrazol does not have a place in the treatment of respiratory depression (2).

Adverse reactions were mild in a controlled study of the efficacy of pentetrazol, alone and in combination with nicotinic acid, in 30 chronic hospitalized elderly patients. Improvement was better with the combined treatment, and only one subject, a 71-year-old woman, developed restlessness, anorexia, and weight loss (3).

Irritability, altered consciousness, and autonomic reactions, together with improvement in thought content and memory testing were noted in a double-blind, placebo-controlled study of pentetrazol 200 mg/day in 20 elderly patients. Nine of the ten patients lost weight (4).

References

1. Jung ME, Lal H, Gatch MB. The discriminative stimulus effects of pentylenetetrazol as a model of anxiety: recent developments. Neurosci Biobehav Rev 2002;26(4):429–39.

2. Hirsh K, Wang SC. Selective respiratory stimulating action of doxapram compared to pentylenetetrazol. J Pharmacol Exp Ther 1974;189(1):1–11.

3. Ananth JV, Deutsch M, Ban TA. Senilex in the treatment of geriatric patients. Curr Ther Res Clin Exp 1971;13(5):316–21.

4. Leckman J, Ananth JV, Ban TA, Lehmann HE. Pentylenetetrazol in the treatment of geriatric patients with disturbed memory function. J Clin Pharmacol New Drugs 1971;11(4):301–3.

Pentoxifylline

General Information

Pentoxifylline (oxipentifylline) is a methylxanthine that antagonizes the vasoconstrictor effects of catecholamines and increases cyclic AMP concentrations, causing smooth muscle to relax. It has also been claimed to correct impaired microcirculation, by improving various factors that disturb blood rheology, and to reduce the generation of toxic free radicals from leukocytes during ischemic leg exercise in patients with intermittent claudication. Pentoxifylline has been used to suppress overproduction of tumor necrosis factor alfa in conditions such as falciparum malaria and rheumatoid arthritis and in transplant recipients, with varied success.

Comparative studies

In 52 adults with cerebral malaria who were randomized to either quinine dihydrochloride alone ($n = 32$) or a combination of quinine and pentoxifylline ($n = 20$), the addition of pentoxifylline significantly improved coma resolution time from 64 to 22 hours and reduced mortality from 25% to 10% (1). Three days after therapy, serum tumor necrosis factor alfa concentrations fell significantly in those who received pentoxifylline. Pentoxifylline caused no serious adverse effects that necessitated withdrawal.

Placebo-controlled studies

The efficacy of pentoxifylline in treating claudication has been evaluated in double-blind, controlled trials in Europe and the USA. Several of these trials have shown that pentoxifylline 400 mg tds increases the walking distance significantly more than placebo in patients with claudication. However, critics remain skeptical about the real value of pentoxifylline, because of a negative correlation between the trial sample sizes and its effects, reflecting an overestimate of drug effect in highly selected trial populations (2). In a trial in almost 300 patients with acute ischemic stroke, the neurological deficit improved more rapidly with pentoxifylline in the initial phase, but the difference was not significant at the end of 1 week (3).

In a placebo-controlled trial in 114 patients with critical limb ischemia, twice-daily intravenous pentoxifylline 600 mg produced unimpressive results (4).

Unwanted effects of pentoxifylline recognized in the double-blind studies were gastrointestinal symptoms (chiefly nausea, vomiting, and bloating) and dizziness. Although common, they required drug withdrawal in only about 3% of patients.

Organs and Systems

Nervous system

Aseptic meningitis has been reported in a patient taking pentoxifylline (5).

- A 37-year-old woman with mixed connective tissue disease took pentoxifylline 400 mg/day for Raynaud's phenomenon. After 12 days she complained of headache, myalgia, and neck pain and developed a fever. She recovered promptly after withdrawal of the drug. A few weeks later, she took a single tablet of pentoxifylline and within 1 hour developed the same symptoms together with chills, vomiting, and diarrhea. Neurological examination was normal, but the cerebrospinal fluid contained a large number of leukocytes. Bacteriological and virological tests were negative.

A diagnosis of aseptic meningitis was made and pentoxifylline was thought to have played a causative role because of the suggestive symptoms after first exposure, the close temporal relation on rechallenge, and the quick recovery after withdrawal. The authors argued that the underlying disease may have had a predisposing role, since aseptic meningitis secondary to pentoxifylline has never been reported in the thousands of patients who have used it for peripheral arterial disease. On the other hand, aseptic meningitis occurs with NSAIDs in patients with connective tissue diseases.

Psychological, psychiatric

Rare cases of hallucinations in elderly people have been ascribed to a stimulant effect of pentoxifylline on the central nervous system (SEDA-18, 219).

Hematologic

A single case of bleeding duodenal ulcer after a single dose of pentoxifylline was reported as being possibly secondary to disturbed platelet function induced by the drug (6). However, the effects of pentoxifylline on platelet function have not been very consistent, and the use of pentoxifylline may have been purely coincidental.

Immunologic

In an open, randomized, controlled trial in 56 children with cerebral malaria, the 26 children who received pentoxifylline 10 mg/kg/day by continuous infusion had significantly shorter periods of coma than the controls. The pentoxifylline recipients showed a trend toward a lower mortality. Pentoxifylline has an inhibitory effect on the synthesis of tumor necrosis factor alfa. The better outcome in the treated group was associated with a fall in tumor necrosis factor alfa serum concentrations on the third day of treatment in a few subjects; this was not seen in the controls (7).

However, in a later, randomized, placebo-controlled trial pentoxifylline neither reduced tumor necrosis factor alfa serum concentrations nor affected the clinical course in 51 patients who received it as adjunctive treatment to standard antimalarial therapy in a dosage of 20 mg/kg/day over 5 days (8).

References

1. Das BK, Mishra S, Padhi PK, Manish R, Tripathy R, Sahoo PK, Ravindran B. Pentoxifylline adjunct improves prognosis of human cerebral malaria in adults. Trop Med Int Health 2003;8(8):680–4.
2. Cameron HA, Waller PC, Ramsay LE. Drug treatment of intermittent claudication: a critical analysis of the methods and findings of published clinical trials, 1965–1985. Br J Clin Pharmacol 1988;26(5):569–76.
3. Hsu CY, Norris JW, Hogan EL, Bladin P, Dinsdale HB, Yatsu FM, Earnest MP, Scheinberg P, Caplan LR, Karp HR. Pentoxifylline in acute nonhemorrhagic stroke. A randomized, placebo-controlled double-blind trial. Stroke 1988;19(6):716–22.
4. Norwegian Pentoxifylline Multicenter Trial Group. Efficacy and clinical tolerance of parenteral pentoxifylline in the treatment of critical lower limb ischemia. A placebo controlled multicenter study. Int Angiol 1996;15(1):75–80.
5. Mathian A, Amoura Z, Piette JC. Pentoxifylline-induced aseptic meningitis in a patient with mixed connective tissue disease. Neurology 2002;59(9):1468–9.
6. Oren R, Yishar U, Lysy J, Livshitz T, Ligumsky M. Pentoxifylline-induced gastrointestinal bleeding. DICP 1991;25(3):315–16.
7. Di Perri G, Di Perri IG, Monteiro GB, Bonora S, Hennig C, Cassatella M, Micciolo R, Vento S, Dusi S, Bassetti D, et al. Pentoxifylline as a supportive agent in the treatment of cerebral malaria in children. J Infect Dis 1995;171(5):1317–22.
8. Hemmer CJ, Hort G, Chiwakata CB, Seitz R, Egbring R, Gaus W, Hogel J, Hassemer M, Nawroth PP, Kern P, Dietrich M. Supportive pentoxifylline in falciparum malaria: no effect on tumor necrosis factor alpha levels or clinical outcome: a prospective, randomized, placebo-controlled study. Am J Trop Med Hyg 1997;56(4):397–403.

Pergolide

General Information

The adverse effects of pergolide, a dopamine receptor agonist, resemble those of bromocriptine (SEDA-10, 118) (SEDA-13, 113).

It is almost universally accepted that directly acting dopamine receptor agonists have less efficacy than levodopa, although the reasons are not clear. Neurologists from London have sought to question this assumption by using cabergoline ($n = 11$) and pergolide ($n = 7$) at considerably higher doses than recommended (1). The actual mean doses were 8.8 and 9.4 mg/day, compared with recommended maxima of 6 and 5 mg/day respectively. The high doses were tolerated by the patients for 2.3–2.5 years; mild dyskinesias ($n = 7$), ankle edema ($n = 3$), and hallucinations ($n = 1$) were the only reported adverse effects. The authors concluded that the therapeutic window for these drugs is apparently much greater than is generally accepted, and that higher doses can be given safely with potentially enhanced efficacy.

In 41 patients with Parkinson's disease who took pergolide, confusion and hallucinations were the adverse effects that were most likely to result in withdrawal of pergolide (2). Symptoms suggestive of dose-related angina pectoris occurred in four patients in the open phase and two patients in the earlier double-blind phase; these symptoms were easily controlled by dosage reduction or withdrawal of pergolide without sequelae. There was leukopenia in one patient.

Organs and Systems

Cardiovascular

Symptoms suggestive of dose-related angina pectoris were observed in a number of patients, either early or late in treatment, but they were easily controlled by dose reduction without sequelae (2).

Pergolide can cause severe hypotension in patients already receiving antihypertensive agents (3).

Respiratory

Pleuropulmonary disease, especially with a fibrotic component, has been reported with all the ergot alkaloids after long-term use.

- A 65-year-old man, who had been taking pergolide 3.5 mg/day for 3 years to treat restless legs syndrome, presented with progressive weight loss, fatigue, and dyspnea (4). The history was of at least 2 years duration. A chest X-ray showed a loculated right hydropneumothorax, and a bloody pleural exudate was aspirated with no cytological evidence of malignancy. An open biopsy showed inflammatory changes and fibrosis. After withdrawal of pergolide and a short course of corticosteroids he made a full clinical and radiological recovery.
- A 73-year-old man who had taken pergolide 1.5 mg/day for 4 months developed dyspnea, bilateral pleural effusions, and severe edema of the legs up to the scrotum (5). There was no pleural thickening or any evidence of cardiac failure or nephrotic syndrome. These clinical features were resistant to diuretic therapy but resolved completely within a month of withdrawal of pergolide. The mechanism of this type of very rare reaction is totally unknown.

Nervous system

Long-term assessment pointed to confusion and hallucinations as the adverse effects most likely to occur requiring withdrawal of the drug (SEDA-15, 3) (2). Owing to its potency as a dopaminergic drug in patients with Parkinson's disease, dyskinesias can occur.

Sleep disorders can occur with pergolide, as with other dopamine receptor agonists.

- A 57-year-old woman and a 61-year-old man taking pergolide 4.5 mg/day and 5 mg/day respectively both suffered sleep disorders; the woman did not suffer from sleepiness but had abrupt sleep episodes, while the man was sleepy for much of the day (6). These were high doses and a reduction to 3 mg/day led to cessation of sleepiness in both patients.

Hematologic

Dose-related leukopenia developed in one patient (2).

Serosae

Most of the dopamine receptor agonists in current use are ergot derivatives, and these are known to cause serosal fibroinflammatory syndromes.

- Three men aged 61–70 years, who had taken pergolide 1–3.75 mg/day for 18–24 months for Parkinson's disease

developed pericardial, pleural, or retroperitoneal fibrosis (one case of each) (7). Despite drug withdrawal, one patient needed pericardial exploration, one was left with residual evidence of severe ureteric obstruction, and one was left with persistent pleural disease.

- Pergolide 3 mg/day has been associated with retroperitoneal fibrosis in an 83-year-old woman after 18 months (8). She required ureteric stents, which were removed 2 years later, after her renal function had remained stable. Because of deterioration in her Parkinson's disease the non-ergot dopamine receptor agonist ropinirole was started and treatment was uneventful after 12 months.
- A 63-year-old British woman with Parkinson's disease was given pergolide in an attempt to minimize motor fluctuations in response to levodopa (9). After taking 4.5 mg/day for 8 months she developed shortness of breath and ankle swelling. This gradually deteriorated over the next year, despite diuretic therapy, and by that time her serum creatinine was 807 µmol/l and her hemoglobin was 8 g/dl. She had bilateral hydronephrosis on ultrasound scanning and a CT scan confirmed retroperitoneal fibrosis, which was successfully treated with nephrostomy and stenting, with resolution of the hydronephrosis. Pergolide was discontinued.

Dutch authors have described four patients, men aged 63–65 years, who had been treated for Parkinson's disease for 3–5 years with various doses (not all specified) of pergolide (10). In three cases pleural fibrosis was demonstrated on biopsy, while in the fourth there was pleural effusion with no histological evidence. On drug withdrawal there was clinical and radiological improvement in three cases but not in the fourth. On reviewing reports of similar adverse drug reactions the authors noted that the age and male preponderance of their patients was in keeping with previous reports. They observed that the dosage was generally higher in patients with retroperitoneal fibrosis compared with those with pleuropulmonary fibrosis. The duration of drug exposure was also a significant risk factor. Clearly, the fact that changes are often irreversible emphasizes the need for early detection and high levels of awareness of these problems.

- A 67-year-old man developed pericardial fibrosis and thickening while taking pergolide for Parkinson's disease (11). The symptoms and signs of heart failure emerged after 11 months, but the possible causative role of the drugs was not suspected for some months while the pericardial changes progressed, as did cardiac failure.

In this case the changes appeared to be wholly reversible on drug withdrawal.

Hair

Treatment with pergolide has very rarely been associated with reversible alopecia (12).

Sexual function

Czech neurologists have described seven men, aged 35–70 years, in whom sexual behavior was greatly increased and who had frequent spontaneous penile erections (13). All had been taking levodopa, to which pergolide 3 mg/day had been added, and all had advanced fluctuating

Parkinson's disease. In one case the dosage of pergolide was halved and in two others ropinirole or entacapone were used as alternatives, in all cases with reduction of the hypersexual symptoms. The other four patients continued to take pergolide, with persistence of the symptoms, to which they and their partners adjusted.

Second-Generation Effects

Teratogenicity

Parkinson's disease is very rare in pregnancy, but has been described (14).

- A 36-year-old woman with a 4-year history of Parkinson's disease, who had been taking pergolide 3 mg/day and levodopa 200 mg/day continued to take it during pregnancy. The end-of-dose wearing-off effect completely disappeared, and reappeared at their previous intensity after delivery. There were no adverse effects in the mother. The baby was healthy at birth and remained so at the time of the report, at the age of 13 months.

References

1. Navan P, Bain PG. Long term tolerability of high dose ergoline derived dopamine agonist therapy for the treatment of Parkinson's disease. J Neurol Neurosurg Psychiatry 2002;73(5):602–3.
2. Ahlskog JE, Muenter MD. Pergolide: long-term use in Parkinson's disease. Mayo Clin Proc 1988;63(10):979–87.
3. Kando JC, Keck PE Jr, Wood PA. Pergolide-induced hypotension. DICP 1990;24(5):543.
4. Danoff SK, Grasso ME, Terry PB, Flynn JA. Pleuropulmonary disease due to pergolide use for restless legs syndrome. Chest 2001;120(1):313–16.
5. Varsano S, Gershman M, Hamaoui E. Pergolide-induced dyspnea, bilateral pleural effusion and peripheral edema. Respiration 2000;67(5):580–2.
6. Schapira AH. Sleep attacks (sleep episodes) with pergolide. Lancet 2000;355(9212):1332–3.
7. Shaunak S, Wilkins A, Pilling JB, Dick DJ. Pericardial, retroperitoneal, and pleural fibrosis induced by pergolide. J Neurol Neurosurg Psychiatry 1999;66(1):79–81.
8. Lund BC, Neiman RF, Perry PJ. Treatment of Parkinson's disease with ropinirole after pergolide-induced retroperitoneal fibrosis. Pharmacotherapy 1999;19(12):1437–8.
9. Mondal BK, Suri S. Pergolide-induced retroperitoneal fibrosis. Int J Clin Pract 2000;54(6):403.
10. Bleumink GS, van der Molen-Eijgenraam M, Strijbos JH, Sanwikarja S, van Puijenbroek EP, Stricker BH. Pergolide-induced pleuropulmonary fibrosis. Clin Neuropharmacol 2002;25(5):290–3.
11. Balachandran KP, Stewart D, Berg GA, Oldroyd KG. Chronic pericardial constriction linked to the antiparkinsonian dopamine agonist pergolide. Postgrad Med J 2002;78(915):49–50.
12. Tabamo RE, Di Rocco A. Alopecia induced by dopamine agonists. Neurology 2002;58(5):829–30.
13. Kanovsky P, Bares M, Pohanka M, Rektor I. Penile erections and hypersexuality induced by pergolide treatment in advanced, fluctuating Parkinson's disease. J Neurol 2002;249(1):112–14.
14. De Mari M, Zenzola A, Lamberti P. Antiparkinsonian treatment in pregnancy. Mov Disord 2002;17(2):428–9.

Perindopril

See also Angiotensin converting enzyme inhibitors

General Information

Perindopril is a prodrug ester of perindoprilat, an ACE inhibitor that has been used in patients with hypertension and heart failure. An updated review of its use in hypertension has appeared (1).

A large French open postmarketing study in 47351 hypertensive patients treated with perindopril for 12 months did not show unexpected adverse effects. The safety profile was similar to that of ACE inhibitors as a class (2).

Organs and Systems

Respiratory

Two cases of pneumonitis have been reported with perindopril (3). The second case was more convincing, because of the result of involuntary rechallenge, but the two cases had typical features of drug-induced pneumonitis. The authors referred to two previous reports of less typical but very likely cases of pneumonitis with captopril.

Skin

UVA photosensitivity induced by perindopril has been reported (4).

References

1. Hurst M, Jarvis B. Perindopril: an updated review of its use in hypertension. Drugs 2001;61(6):867–96.
2. Speirs C, Wagniart F, Poggi L. Perindopril postmarketing surveillance: a 12 month study in 47,351 hypertensive patients. Br J Clin Pharmacol 1998;46(1):63–70.
3. Benard A, Melloni B, Gosselin B, Bonnaud F, Wallaert B. Perindopril-associated pneumonitis. Eur Respir J 1996;9(6):1314–16.
4. Le Borgne G, Leonard F, Cambie MP, Serpier J, Germain ML, Kalis B. UVA photosensitivity induced by perindopril (Coversyl): first reported case. Nouv Dermatol 1996;15:378–80.

Peroxides

See also Disinfectants and antiseptics

General Information

Solutions of hydrogen peroxide containing 5–7% H_2O_2 are used for cleaning wounds and ulcers. The disinfectant and deodorant actions of hydrogen peroxide occur by oxidation of cell materials during the rapid release of oxygen while hydrogen peroxide is in contact with the tissues. The solution does not penetrate well, but the effervescence provides a mechanical means for detaching necrotic tissue from inaccessible parts of wounds. It should not be used in closed body cavities. The germicidal action of hydrogen peroxide is relatively weak and of short duration.

Residues on insufficiently rinsed equipment disinfected by hydrogen peroxide can provoke local irritation, burns, and general reactions. Non-specific inflammation has been reported, with instantaneous blanching and effervescence on the surfaces of the intestinal mucosa during endoscopy (1).

Organs and Systems

Respiratory

Pneumomediastinum caused by subcutaneous emphysema has been reported in a 30-year-old man after the application of hydrogen peroxide solution to a root canal. The patient had acute pulpitis of the lower right third molar, treated by extirpation followed by irrigation with 3% hydrogen peroxide solution. Soon after irrigation, subcutaneous emphysema developed (2).

Hematologic

Hemolysis was reported after hemodialysis therapy with a dialysis fluid inadvertently contaminated with hydrogen peroxide (3).

References

1. Bilotta JJ, Waye JD. Hydrogen peroxide enteritis: the "snow white" sign. Gastrointest Endosc 1989;35(5):428–30.
2. Nahlieli O, Neder A. Iatrogenic pneumomediastinum after endodontic therapy. Oral Surg Oral Med Oral Pathol 1991;71(5):618–19.
3. Gordon SM, Bland LA, Alexander SR, Newman HF, Arduino MJ, Jarvis WR. Hemolysis associated with hydrogen peroxide at a pediatric dialysis center. Am J Nephrol 1990;10(2):123–7.

Perphenazine

See also Neuroleptic drugs

General Information

Perphenazine is a phenothiazine neuroleptic drug.

Organs and Systems

Hematologic

Aplastic anemia, defined by the presence of pancytopenia and a hypocellular bone marrow in the absence of any abnormal blood cells, is a serious reaction that has been attributed to perphenazine in a single case (1).

- A 23-year-old man with schizophrenia taking perphenazine 4 mg bd, benzatropine mesylate 2 mg/day, lithium carbonate 600 mg each morning and 900 mg at bedtime, and famotidine 40 mg/day developed fatigue, shortness of breath, dizziness, light-headedness, and general debility. He had a pancytopenia, which persisted in spite of blood transfusions. Bone-marrow aspiration showed hypocellularity, absent megakaryocytes, reduced erythropoiesis and myelopoiesis, increased iron storage, and a relative excess of lymphoid cells. All medications were withdrawn and he was given lorazepam 2 mg bd. He recovered after 8 months.

Reference

1. Oyewumi LK. Acquired aplastic anemia secondary to perphenazine. Can J Clin Pharmacol 1999;6(3):169–71.

Pertussis vaccines

See also Vaccines

Note on abbreviations

DTP = Diphtheria + tetanus toxoids + pertussis
DTaP = Diphtheria + tetanus toxoids + acellular pertussis
DTwP = Diphtheria + tetanus toxoids + whole cell pertussis

General Information

Whole-cell and acellular pertussis vaccines have been reviewed, with emphasis on the protectivity of the various virulence factors and antigens (1). The authors summarized their review as follows: although *Bordetella pertussis* has at least five proteins required for virulence and an additional two "toxic" components, only serum neutralizing antibodies to pertussis toxin have been shown to confer immunity to pertussis.

Acellular pertussis vaccine

Quality control of acellular pertussis vaccines presents particular problems related to the various methods used for preparation of the active components, the different compositions of the final formulations, and different amounts of antigen. Researchers in the National Institute for Biological Standards and Control in the UK have presented a strategy capable of addressing the key problem areas likely to be encountered with all existing types of acellular pertussis vaccines and combinations (2). Their proposal could be considered as a starting point for improvement of quality control programs for these vaccines.

An overview of clinical trials with a special diphtheria and tetanus toxoids and acellular pertussis (DTaP) vaccine has been published (3). The vaccine contains as pertussis components purified filamentous hemagglutinin, pertactin, and genetically engineered pertussis toxin. The vaccine induces high and long-lasting immunity and is at least as efficacious as most whole-cell pertussis vaccines and similar in efficacy to the most efficacious acellular pertussis vaccines that contain three pertussis antigens. The vaccine is better tolerated than whole cell vaccines and has a similar reactogenicity profile to other acellular vaccines.

A vaccine containing diphtheria and tetanus toxoids and acellular pertussis with reduced antigen content for diphtheria and pertussis (TdaP) has been compared with a licensed reduced adult-type diphtheria–tetanus (Td) vaccine and with an experimental candidate monovalent acellular pertussis vaccine with reduced antigen content (ap) (4). A total of 299 healthy adults (mean age 30 years) were randomized into three groups to receive one dose of the study vaccines. The antibody responses (anti-diphtheria, anti-tetanus, anti-pertussis toxin, anti-pertactin, anti-filamentous hemagglutinin) were similar in all groups. The most frequently reported local symptom was pain at the injection site (62–94%), but there were no reports of severe pain; redness and swelling with a diameter of 5 cm or more occurred in up to 13%. The incidence of local symptoms was similar after TdaP and Td immunization. The most frequently reported general symptoms were headache and fatigue (20–50%). The incidence of general symptoms was similar in the TdaP and Td groups. There were no reports of fever over 39°C. No serious adverse events were reported.

Japanese studies of acellular vaccines

The first generation of the new acellular vaccines was developed in Japan in the late 1970s (Sato). Since late 1981, acellular vaccines have replaced the whole-cell pertussis vaccines for use in the Japanese immunization program. Two types of acellular pertussis vaccine have been produced by six Japanese manufacturers (5,6) (SEDA-12, 276) (SEDA-13, 283) (SEDA-14, 279). No doubt as a result of these measures the rate of reported serious reactions has decreased in Japan. During the period 1975–81, when whole-cell vaccines were given, the rate was 0.4 per million doses, compared with a rate of 0.25 per million doses during the period 1982–84 (7). In 1988, Kumura and Kuno-Sakai (8) summarized the experience gained in Japan since the introduction in 1981 of the new DTP vaccines containing acellular pertussis components. Acellular vaccines seem to be effective in Japan, since in parallel with their wider use the numbers of reported cases of pertussis and pertussis deaths have declined. Reactogenicity (as expressed by fever or local reactions) was very low. Kimura and Kuno-Sakei cited reports of Quincke's edema-like swelling of the whole arm following the third injection (0.17% of vaccinees) and the booster injection (2.61%), respectively. Data on more severe adverse events have been collected from 1970 to 1986 in the framework of the National Adverse Reaction Compensation System (SED-12, 818). Kimura and Kuno-Sakei considered the vaccines to be safe and effective enough to eliminate pertussis in Japan in the future (8).

European studies of acellular vaccines

The epidemiological circumstances in Sweden and in parts of Germany and Italy, where the immunization programs against pertussis using whole-cell vaccine had been discontinued or reduced because of public concern about rare severe adverse events, offered good opportunities to assess the clinical efficacy and safety of acellular pertussis vaccines. In Germany, both controlled field trials and a household contact study were carried out. Different mono-component and multi-component acellular vaccines from European and US manufacturers were used in European trials. They comprised a mono-component vaccine composed only of detoxified pertussis toxin (toxoid); a two-component vaccine composed of pertussis toxin and filamentous hemagglutinin; a three-component vaccine composed of pertussis toxin, filamentous hemagglutinin, Pertactin; and another five-component vaccine composed of pertussis toxin, filamentous hemagglutinin, Pertactin, and fimbriae antigens 2 and 3. In some instances they were compared directly with whole-cell pertussis vaccines. In general, the acellular vaccines were found to be immunogenic, epidemiologically effective, and less reactogenic than the whole-cell pertussis-component vaccines as assessed in terms of fever, pain, fretfulness, and local reactions at the injection site. Based on the results, acellular pertussis vaccines have since been licensed in many countries of the world both for primary and booster immunization. Details regarding the results and conclusions of the large-scale field trials completed in 1994 and 1995 in Germany, Italy, and Sweden have been reviewed (SEDA-19, 298), as have reports on other clinical trials using acellular pertussis vaccines (SED-12, 818) (SEDA-12, 277) (SEDA-13, 283) (SEDA-14, 279) (SEDA-15, 350) (SEDA-16, 382) (SEDA-17, 370) (SEDA-18, 332) (SEDA-20, 289) (SEDA-21, 230). The optimal composition of acellular vaccines has not yet been determined: the number of antigens still varies from one to five, and antigen amounts are also different. Post-licensing studies will therefore be of the utmost importance in studying the induction of herd immunity and possible rare events.

Local effects of acellular vaccines: effect of number of injections

Data on the use of a single DTaP vaccine for four-dose or five-dose series are limited, but the available data show a substantial increase in the frequency and magnitude of local reactions with successive doses. The accompanying tables show reactions after the fourth dose (Table 1) and fifth dose (Table 2). The original data and references are included in the supplementary recommendations of the Advisory Committee on Immunization Practices (ACIP) on the use of DTaP vaccines in a five-dose series (9). Reports from Alberta and British Columbia provinces, Canada, have suggested that the incidence rates of severe local adverse reactions may increase with each dose (third, fourth, fifth) in preschool children (10).

Limb swelling after booster doses of acellular vaccines

Swelling involving the entire thigh or upper arm has been reported after booster doses of different acellular pertussis vaccines, for example in a German study during April 1993 to November 1994 using a fourth dose of Infanrix. There was an increase in thigh circumference in 1.2–3.2% of children; swelling began within 48 hours of a booster

Table 1 Reactions after the fourth dose of DTaP given at 2 or 3 years of age

Local and systemic reactions	ACEL-IMUNE	Tripedia	Infanrix*	Certiva
Pain		19%	26%	19
Erythema	10% ≥2.4 cm	30% ≥2.54 cm	14% ≥2 cm	6% ≥3 cm
Swelling		29% ≥2.54 cm	11% ≥2 cm	5% ≥3 cm
Induration	9% ≥2.4 cm			
Tenderness				
Fever = 38°C	26%		26%	6.3%
Fever = 38.3°C		5.5%		

*To be compared with reactions after the first dose: pain 2%, erythema 0%, swelling 0%, fever ≥38°C 6.3%

Table 2 Reactions after the fifth dose of DTaP administered at entry to school

Local and systemic reactions	ACEL-IMUNE	Tripedia	Infanrix
Pain		2.1% severe pain	1.6% severe pain
Erythema	20% >2–2.4 cm	31% >5 cm	
Swelling		25% >5 cm	30% >5 cm
Induration	14%		21% >5 cm
Tenderness	38%		

dose and the mean duration was 3.9 (range 1–7) days; the mean increase in circumference was 2.2–5.0 cm; in a few children, the swelling interfered with walking.

Similar swelling and substantial local reactions have been observed in fourth-dose and fifth-dose follow-up studies from the Multicenter Acellular Pertussis Trial, which examined 12 different DTaP vaccines, and in recent studies of the fifth dose of Tripedia and Infanrix in Germany. The pathogenesis of both substantial local reactions and limb swelling is unknown. Associations with pertussis toxoid, diphtheria toxoid, or aluminium in the vaccine have been discussed. Because reports to date have suggested that the reactions are self-limited and resolve without sequelae, and in recognition of the benefits of a fifth dose of DTaP, the ACIP has recommended that a history of extensive swelling after the fourth dose should not be considered to be a contraindication to a fifth dose of DTaP. Parents or caregivers of children who receive fourth and fifth doses of a DTaP series should be informed of the increases in reactogenicity that have been observed (9).

Whole-cell pertussis vaccine

Pertussis whole cell vaccine is an adsorbed suspension of inactivated pertussis bacteria. The vaccine is available in monovalent form or in combination with diphtheria and tetanus toxoids (DTP). DTP vaccine is the preparation of choice in routine immunization practice.

Local reactions are common after DTP immunization (40–70% of the vaccinees) but are usually self-limiting (10). A nodule may be palpable at the injection site of adsorbed products for several weeks. Abscess at the injection site has been reported (6–10 per million vaccinees). Mild to moderate fever (38.0–40.4°C) occurs frequently (about 50% of vaccinated infants), generally within several hours of administration, persisting for 1–2 days. Fever and other systemic symptoms are much less common following immunization with preparations not containing the pertussis component. Arthus-type hypersensitivity reactions occur, particularly after booster doses. Rarely,

severe systemic reactions (urticaria, anaphylaxis) have been reported.

The non-neurological adverse effects of whole-cell immunization have been reviewed (SED-12, 815) (SEDA-16, 379) (SEDA-17, 370) (SEDA-18, 330). The most frequent are mild fever, drowsiness, and reduction in appetite; a very small percentage of vaccinees experience more severe fever, redness, swelling, pain, "fussiness", or vomiting.

A follow-up study has been carried out in 105 children with collapse (a hypotonic-hyporesponsive episode or a shock-like syndrome) after their first immunization with DTwP + IPV vaccine (11). Information about subsequent immunizations, health, and development in 101 of the children was supplied by child health-care units. The parents of one child refused further immunization, 16 children completed their schedule with the combination diphtheria + tetanus + poliomyelitis vaccine (DT-IPV), and the other 84 children received further pertussis vaccine (DTP-IPV), totalling 236 doses; 74 children received the complete series of three additional doses. None of the children had recurrent collapse, and other adverse events were only minor. About half were given paracetamol prophylactically for the first subsequent dose; most of them did not take it for further doses. The authors suggested that it is unnecessary to withhold further doses of pertussis vaccine in a child with collapse after a previous dose. It has been suggested that the threat of natural pertussis in non-immunized children should be taken much more into account than the fear of developing a collapse reaction (12). In another study (13) in the USA, one of the 14 children not completely immunized because of a hypotonic-hyporesponsive episode after a previous dose later developed natural pertussis, which lasted for 3 months and was transmitted to both her parents.

Acellular pertussis vaccine versus whole-cell pertussis vaccine

In a randomized, double-blind trial to determine the efficacy of vaccination against *Bordetella* infection, a multi-component acellular pertussis has been compared with a whole-cell product and diphtheria + tetanus toxoids (DT) in 8532 infants aged 2–4 months, who received four doses of either DTwP or DTaP vaccine at 3, 4.5, 6, and 15–18 months of age, and 1739 controls, who received three doses of DT vaccine at 3, 4.5, 15–18 months of age (14). All the vaccines were generally well tolerated. However, adverse reactions were significantly less common after DTaP compared with DTwP vaccine. Persistent inconsolable crying was four times more common in DTwP recipients than in DTaP recipients. High fever, 40.5°C or over, was three times more common in DTwP vaccinees than in DTaP vaccinees. Only one DTaP recipient had a convulsion in temporal relation to immunization.

The 2000 Childhood Immunization Schedule, proposed by the Advisory Committee of Immunization Practices (ACIP), the American Academy of Pediatrics, and the American Academy of Family Physicians, recommended that acellular pertussis vaccines be exclusively chosen for routine use in the USA (15).

One evaluation of the results of two studies in a total of 182 children primed either with acellular or with whole-cell pertussis vaccines at 2, 4, and 6 months of age and boosted with an acellular vaccine has shown that booster doses of acellular vaccine are safe and immunogenic (16). Local adverse reactions after booster immunization with acellular vaccine were more common in children primed with acellular vaccine than in those primed with whole-cell pertussis vaccine (68 versus 33%). In another and similar study, children primed with acellular or whole cell pertussis combined with DT vaccine have been boosted with a recombinant acellular pertussis vaccine combined with DT vaccine. The vaccine was highly immunogenic and safe (17).

From 1991 to 1993 about 27 million doses of DTP vaccine and 5 million doses of DTaP (that is acellular) vaccine were distributed in the USA. The results of a postmarketing comparison of the safety of acellular pertussis vaccines with whole-cell pertussis vaccines have been published. The rates of reported adverse events per 100 000 immunizations were significantly lower after the administration of DTaP vaccine than after DTP vaccine for the following outcomes: all reports (2.9 versus 9.8); fever (1.9 versus 7.5); seizures (0.5 versus 1.7); and hospitalizations (0.2 versus 0.9) (18).

The safety and immunogenicity of 12 acellular pertussis vaccines and one whole-cell pertussis vaccine given as a fourth dose have been compared in 1293 children aged 15–20 months. In general, DTaP vaccines were associated with fewer adverse events than a US-licensed DTwP vaccine (SEDA-22, 342).

A randomized, controlled comparison of two-component, three-component, and five-component acellular pertussis vaccines and a whole-cell pertussis vaccine has been carried out in 82 892 infants who were immunized either at age 3, 5, and 12 months, or at 2, 4, and 6 months. High fever and seizures occurred more often after whole-cell vaccine than after any of the acellular vaccines. Hypotonic-hyporesponsive episodes also occurred significantly more often in the whole-cell group and were more frequent in the acellular groups than previously reported (SEDA-22, 342).

An informal consultation of invited epidemiologists, infectious disease clinicians, immunologists, representatives of regulatory agencies for biological products, and other scientists and public health officials was held in Geneva on 18–19 May 1998 on the control of pertussis using whole-cell and acellular pertussis vaccines. The consultation was called jointly by the Children's Vaccine Initiative and the World Health Organization Global Program on Vaccines. The report of the meeting including the conclusions at full length has been summarized (SEDA-22, 341). The main conclusions read as follows. Whole-cell vaccines of documented quality have proved to be highly effective tools for preventing pertussis. Acellular pertussis vaccines are valuable alternatives to whole-cell vaccines for immunization in infancy. Because of their safety profiles, acellular vaccines may be preferred alternatives in industrialized countries, in which pertussis vaccination with whole-cell vaccines is not widely accepted. In each country, recommendations for the use of pertussis vaccines will be based on local risk–benefit and cost–benefit analyses. The use of acellular vaccines in many circumstances can be further considered for booster doses (fourth and fifth doses) in improving pertussis control after evaluation by local authorities of the epidemiological, cost, and programmatic issues. Additional data on the potential benefit of booster doses using acellular pertussis vaccines in adolescence or older ages are needed. The current control regulations and recommendations for pertussis vaccines (whole-cell and acellular) needs thorough review in the light of recently available scientific data, and appropriate revisions should be made (19).

Comparisons of DTP and DT

An older study in the USA compared the rates of both minor and more serious reactions in 15 752 children 0–6 years of age to DTP vaccine and in 784 children to DT vaccine. The frequencies of minor reactions associated with DTP and DT are shown in Table 3. The reactions after DT were not only less frequent, but also less severe. Convulsions and hypotonic-hyporesponsive episodes each occurred in one per 1750 immunizations (20).

Data from the Monitoring System for Adverse Events Following Immunization (MSAEFI) (SEDA-13, 274) show that the adverse effects rate for DTP vaccine was twice as high as that for DT vaccine. The most reported adverse effect was fever (59% of all reports) followed by

Table 3 Frequencies of minor reactions associated with DTP and DT

Adverse effect	DTP (%)	DT (%)
Fitfulness	53	23
Pain	51	9.9
Fever	47	9.3
Local swelling	41	7.6
Local redness	37	7.6
Drowsiness	32	15
Anorexia	21	7.0
Vomiting	8.2	2.6
Persistent crying	3.1	0.7
High pitched unusual cry	0.1	0

local reactions (36%) (21). Similar results have been published by Dittmann (13.5 severe adverse effects per million vaccinees after DTP immunization and 4.8 reactions per million vaccinees after DT immunization) (22) and by Miller and colleagues (23).

Tetravalent, pentavalent, and hexavalent immunization

DTaP or DTwP vaccine can be combined with other antigens, such as *Haemophilus influenzae* type b (Hib), inactivated poliovirus (IPV), and hepatitis B vaccine. In children DTaP or DTwP vaccines form the basis for such combinations, while in adults it is mostly Td vaccine. Current safety concerns regarding combination vaccines have been defined and reviewed (24). The author concluded that there is no evidence that adding vaccines to combination products increases the burden on the immune system, which can respond to many millions of antigens. Combining antigens usually does not increase adverse effects, but it can lead to an overall reduction in adverse events. Before licensure, combination vaccines undergo extensive testing to assure that the new products are safe and effective.

The frequency, severity, and types of adverse reactions after DTP-Hib immunization in very pre-term babies have been studied (25). Adverse reactions were noted in 17 of 45 babies: nine had major events (apnea, bradycardia, or desaturation) and eight had minor reactions (increased oxygen requirements, temperature instability, poor handling, and feeding intolerance). Babies who had major adverse reactions were significantly younger at the time of immunization than the babies who did not have major reactions. Of 27 babies immunized at 70 days or less, nine developed major reactions compared with none of those who were immunized at over 70 days.

The Hexavalent Study Group has compared the immunogenicity and safety of a new liquid hexavalent vaccine against diphtheria, tetanus, pertussis, poliomyelitis, hepatitis B, and *Haemophilus influenzae* type b (DTP + IPV + HB + Hib vaccine, manufactured by Aventis Pasteur MSD, Lyon, France) with two reference vaccines, the pentavalent DTP + IPV + Hib vaccine and the monovalent hepatitis B vaccine, administrated separately at the same visit (26). Infants were randomized to receive either the hexavalent vaccine ($n = 423$) or (administered at different local sites) the pentavalent and the HB vaccine ($n = 425$) at 2, 4, and 6 months of age. The hexavalent vaccine was well tolerated (for details, see Table 4 and Table 5). At least one local reaction was reported in 20% of injections with hexavalent vaccine compared with 16% after the receipt of pentavalent vaccine or 3.8% after the receipt of hepatitis B vaccine. These reactions were generally mild and transient. At least one systemic reaction was reported in 46% of injections with hexavalent vaccine, whereas the respective rate for the recipients of pentavalent and HB vaccine was 42%. No vaccine-related serious adverse event occurred during the study. The hexavalent vaccine provided immune responses adequate for protection against the six diseases.

Organs and Systems

Nervous system

The question of nervous system complications and persistent brain damage after whole-cell pertussis vaccination has been argued for a long time. During the 1980s it was debated by physicians as well as by the general public in several countries. Reports, publications, and national evaluations of the matter led some countries to change their national pertussis immunization policy. In the autumn of 1981, Japan replaced the whole-cell vaccine with acellular pertussis vaccine developed by Sato in Japan. Sweden ended its pertussis (whole-cell vaccine) immunization program in 1979. As a result of the prominence accorded

Table 4 Percentage rates of local adverse events within 72 hours of immunization in infants given a hexavalent vaccine (Hexavac) or separate injections of the reference vaccines

Events	Hexavac				Pentavac				Hepatitis B Vax II			
	First dose	Second dose	Third dose	All[a]	First dose	Second dose	Third dose	All[a]	First dose	Second dose	Third dose	All[a]
Number of injections	423	420	418	1261	424	418	417	1259	424	418	417	1259
Any local reaction	23[b]	18	20	20	14[b]	16	18	16	3.3	2.6	5.5	3.8
Skin redness ≥2 cm	10	12	14	12	3.5	7.9	9.1	6.8	0.7	1.0	2.9	1.5
Skin redness ≤5 cm	2.8	1.2	1.0	1.6	0.5	0.7	1.0	0.7	0	0	0	0
Skin induration ≥2 cm	15	14	14	15	11	14	16	14	2.6	2.4	4.8	3.3
Skin induration ≥5 cm	2.6	1.5	0.7	1.6	0.3	1.0	0.7	0.6	0	0	0.3	0.1
Other local reactions[c]	2.8	0.5	1.2	1.5	0.9	0.2	0.7	0.6	0.5	0	0.2	0.2

[a] At least one reaction to any of the three primary doses.
[b] Statistically significant between the groups.
[c] Other local reactions: hematoma, injection site pain, local maculopapular rash, local heat.

Table 5 Percentage rates of systemic adverse events within 72 hours of immunization in infants given a hexavalent vaccine (Hexavac) or separate injections of the reference vaccines

Events	Hexavac				Pentavac and Hepatitis B Vax II			
	First dose	Second dose	Third dose	All[a]	First dose	Second dose	Third dose	All[a]
Any systemic events (%)	52[b]	47	38	46	45[b]	42	40	42
Fever >38°C	6.9	19	18	15	4.7	17	22	15
Fever 38.0–38.9°C	6.4	18	14	13	4.2	17	18	18
Fever 39.0–39.9°C	0.5	1.4	3.6	1.8	0.2	0.2	3.4	1.3
Fever >40°C	0	0	0	0	0.2	0	0.5	0.2
Drowsiness	17	9.5	7.7	11	14	9.3	6.0	9.9
Irritability/unusual crying	33	27	21	27	29	23	20	24
Inconsolable crying >3 hours	0.2	0.2	0.2	0.2	0	0	0	0
Vomiting/diarrhea	7.3	5.7	5.0	6.0	6.8	4.3	6.5	5.9
Insomnia	6.1	5.2	3.1	4.8	4.5	4.1	5.0	4.5
Loss of appetite	13	8.3	6.5	9.3	9.2	9.1	7.4	8.6
Other systemic events[c]	4.3	5.0	7.7	5.6	3.8	4.1	6.2	4.7

[a] At least one reaction to any of the three primary doses.
[b] Statistically significant between the groups.
[c] Minor childhood illnesses (for example respiratory or gastrointestinal disorders).

to the risks involved, the pertussis vaccine coverage rates in the UK fell sharply at the beginning of the 1980s, but were increasing again when some large pertussis epidemics occurred as a result of diminished population immunity. In the 1980s, in the erstwhile Federal Republic of Germany, pertussis immunization was only recommended for children at special risk but from 1991 onwards the approach changed again and use of DTP was advised throughout what was now a united Germany. Severe neurological adverse effects of whole-cell pertussis immunization has been reviewed in detail, including reports on the legal cases brought in the English High Court pertussis vaccine trials (SED-12, 817).

It would now seem that the long debate has been resolved. The first step toward its resolution was taken in a review of all information available worldwide which was presented in a report produced in 1991 by the Institute of Medicine of the National Academy of Sciences, Washington (27) (SED-12, 817). It was concluded that:

- there is evidence indicating a causal relation between DTP vaccine and anaphylaxis, febrile seizures and inconsolable crying;
- there is weaker evidence pointing to a relationship between DTP vaccine and acute encephalopathy and hypotonic-hyporesponsive episodes;
- there is no reason to believe in an association between vaccination and the occurrence of infantile spasms, afebrile seizures, hypsarrhythmia, Reye's syndrome, or sudden infant death syndrome;
- there is insufficient evidence to indicate either the presence or absence of a causal relation between DTP vaccine and chronic neurological damage, epilepsy, aseptic meningitis, erythema multiforme or other rash, Guillain–Barré syndrome, hemolytic anemia, juvenile diabetes, learning disabilities and attention-deficit disorder, peripheral mononeuropathy, or thrombocytopenia.

In 1993, Miller and colleagues (28) and Madge and colleagues (29) presented the results of a 10-year follow-up study of the National Childhood Encephalopathy Study

(NCES) carried out in 1976–79. The findings suggested a small excess risk of severe acute neurological events within 7 days of pertussis immunization, but the risk of permanent damage due to the vaccine, if any, was slight. Follow-up of cases and controls from this study for some years has shown that significantly more children with such illnesses die or suffer subsequent educational, behavioural, or neurological deficits than expected by comparison with controls, but the number of cases associated with pertussis vaccine was small and statistically vulnerable.

The committee responsible for the report of the Institute of Medicine concluded in 1994 that the recent findings from the NCES necessitated a review of the conclusion that the evidence is insufficient to indicate a causal relation between DTP and permanent neurological damage. After having reviewed the new NCES data, the committee declared that the balance of evidence was consistent with a causal relation between DTP vaccine and the forms of chronic nervous system dysfunction described in the NCES in children who have a serious acute neurological illness within 7 days after receiving DTP vaccine. This type of serious acute neurological response to DTP is rare. The estimated excess risk ranged from 0 to 10.5 per million immunizations. The evidence remains insufficient to indicate the presence or absence of a causal relation between DTP vaccine and chronic nervous system dysfunction under any other circumstances (30).

Finally, Gangarosa and colleagues have reviewed in detail the so-called pertussis vaccine encephalopathy. Seven epidemiological studies have been conducted; they show that neurological reactions are exceedingly rare with whole-cell pertussis vaccines (SEDA-21, 329).

Susceptibility factors
The (US) Immunization Practices Advisory Committee (ACIP) has recommended that a personal history of a prior convulsion should be evaluated before initiating or continuing immunization with vaccines containing a

pertussis component. The presence of an evolving neurological disorder contraindicates pertussis immunization. Other contraindications to the receipt of pertussis vaccine are hypersensitivity to vaccine components or a history of a severe reaction following an earlier dose (31). Reviewing the data on the relation between a family history of convulsions and immunization with pertussis-containing vaccines, both the ACIP as well as the US Committee on Infectious Diseases considered that a family history of convulsions in parents and siblings was not a contraindication to pertussis immunization. The ACIP and other authors, believe that the use of an antipyretic (for example paracetamol given at a dose of 15 mg/kg at the time of DTP immunization and again 4 hours later) in conjunction with DTP vaccine may be reasonable in children with personal or family histories of convulsions since it will reduce the incidence of post-immunization fever (32,33).

Skin

Bullous pemphigoid has been attributed to DTP-IPV vaccine (34).

- A previous healthy 3.5-month-old infant developed bullous pemphigoid 3 days after receiving a first dose of DTP-IPV vaccine. *Staphylococcus aureus* was isolated from purulent bullae. The lesions resolved rapidly after treatment with antibiotics and methylprednisolone.

The authors mentioned 12 other cases of bullous pemphigoid, reported during the last 5 years, that had possibly been triggered by vaccines (influenza, tetanus toxoid booster, and DTP-IPV vaccine).

Immunologic

Data from the Third National Health and Nutrition Survey (1988–94) have been used to analyse the possible effects of DTP or tetanus immunization on allergies and allergy-related symptoms among 13 944 infants, children, and adolescents aged 2 months to 16 years in the USA (35). The authors concluded that DTP or tetanus immunization increases the risk of allergies and related respiratory symptoms in children and adolescents. However, the small number of non-immunized individuals and the study design limited their ability to make firm causal inferences about the true magnitude of effect.

It has been suggested that the development of a sterile abscess represents an idiosyncratic reaction of some individuals, perhaps genetically determined, which causes a granulomatous response to antigens, irrespective of the location of the vaccine (36). Others maintain that it is caused by a contaminated needle track or to vaccine material coating the outside of the needle, resulting from the lack of a proper injection technique.

Susceptibility Factors

Age

Details regarding the age-related efficacy of the use of paracetamol and the inefficacy of prophylactic paracetamol given in a single dose have been published (SEDA-14, 277).

Drug Administration

Drug formulations

In a study of local and systemic reactions following 9920 DTP immunizations there were significant differences relating to different manufacturers and different vaccine lots (37).

Drug additives

Eight children developed urticaria within 30 minutes after administration of a diphtheria + tetanus + acellular pertussis (DTaP) vaccine that contained gelatin as a stabilizer (38). None of the children had anti-gelatin IgE, and only two had detectable concentrations of anti-toxoid IgE to diphtheria and pertussis toxoids. No methods to measure anti-thiomersal and anti-alum IgE were available. The authors recommended the development of such methods, which could improve research into the causality of adverse effects of this sort.

Drug administration route

The "two-needle strategy," based on the hypothesis that changing the needle on the syringe after drawing up the DTP vaccine and before injecting reduces local reactions by eliminating deposition of aluminium adjuvant in the subcutaneous track of the needle, has been evaluated (39). When immunizing 223 children using this strategy and 200 others using the "one-needle strategy," there was no significant difference in the occurrence of local or systemic reaction.

References

1. Robbins JB, Schneerson R, Bryla DA, Trollfors B, Taranger J, Lagergard T. Immunity to pertussis. Not all virulence factors are protective antigens. Adv Exp Med Biol 1998;452:207–18.
2. Corbel MJ, Xing DK, Bolgiano B, Hockley DJ. Approaches to the control of acellular pertussis vaccines. Biologicals 1999;27(2):133–41.
3. Matheson AJ, Goa KL. Diphtheria–tetanus–acellular pertussis vaccine adsorbed (Triacelluvax; DTaP3-CB): a review of its use in the prevention of *Bordetella pertussis* infection. Paediatr Drugs 2000;2(2):139–59.
4. Van der Wielen M, Van Damme P. Tetanus–diphtheria booster in non-responding tetanus–diphtheria vaccinees. Vaccine 2000;19(9–10):1005–6.
5. Galazka A. Update on acellular pertussis vaccine. WHO/EPI/GEN/88.4. Geneva: World Health Organization, 1988.
6. Aoyama T, Hagiwara S, Murase Y, Kato T, Iwata T. Adverse reactions and antibody responses to acellular pertussis vaccine. J Pediatr 1986;109(6):925–30.
7. Kimura M, Kuno-Sakai H. Pertussis vaccines in Japan. Acta Paediatr Jpn 1988;30(2):143–53.
8. Kimura M, Kuno-Sakai H. Reports on cases of neurological illnesses occurring after administration of acellular pertussis vaccines in Japan. Tokai J Exp Clin Med 1988;13(Suppl):165–70.
9. Advisory Committee on Immunization Practices (ACIP). Use of diphtheria toxoid–tetanus toxoid–acellular pertussis vaccine as a five-dose series. MMWR Recomm Rep 2000;49(RR-13):1–8.

10. Scheifele DW, Meekison W, Arcand T, Humphrey G. Local adverse reactions to DTP vaccine, adsorbed, in Surrey, BC. CMAJ 1989;141:312.

11. Vermeer-de Bondt PE, Labadie J, Rumke HC. Rate of recurrent collapse after vaccination with whole cell pertussis vaccine: follow up study. BMJ 1998;316(7135):902–3.

12. Miller E. Collapse reactions after whole cell pertussis vaccination. BMJ 1998;316(7135):876.

13. Baraff LJ, Shields WD, Beckwith L, Strome G, Marcy SM, Cherry JD, Manclark CR. Infants and children with convulsions and hypotonic-hyporesponsive episodes following diphtheria–tetanus–pertussis immunization: follow-up evaluation. Pediatrics 1988;81(6):789–94.

14. Stehr K, Cherry JD, Heininger U, Schmitt-Grohe S, uberall M, Laussucq S, Eckhardt T, Meyer M, Engelhardt R, Christenson P, Muller W, Neugebauer A, Sailer K, Keller H, Kircher U, Netzel B, Sachsenhauser-Kratzer H, Thelen M, Buck KE, Nath G, Clapier E, Gelius P, Graf zu Castell B, Hess H-J, Maas-Doyle E, Mayer HPR, Renner K, Seltsam I, Seuwen G. A comparative efficacy trial in Germany in infants who received either the Lederle/Takeda acellular pertussis component DTP (DTaP) vaccine, the Lederle whole-cell component DTP vaccine, or DT vaccine. Pediatrics 1998;101(1 Pt 1):1–11.

15. Recommendations of the Advisory Committee on Immunization Practices (ACIP). The 2000 Immunization Schedule. MMWR Morb Mortal Wkly Rep 2000;49:25.

16. Halperin SA, Mills E, Barreto L, Pim C, Eastwood BJ. Acellular pertussis vaccine as a booster dose for seventeen- to nineteen-month-old children immunized with either whole cell or acellular pertussis vaccine at two, four and six months of age. Pediatr Infect Dis J 1995;14(9):792–7.

17. Podda A, Bona G, Canciani G, Pistilli AM, Contu B, Furlan R, Meloni T, Stramare D, Titone L, Rappuoli R, Granoff DM, Bartalini M, Budroni M, De Luca EC, Cascio A, Cascio G, Cossu M, Orto PD, Di Leo G. Effect of priming with diphtheria and tetanus toxoids combined with whole-cell pertussis vaccine or with acellular pertussis vaccine on the safety and immunogenicity of a booster dose of an acellular pertussis vaccine containing a genetically inactivated pertussis toxin in fifteen- to twenty-one-month-old children. Italian Multicenter Group for the Study of Recombinant Acellular Pertussis Vaccine. J Pediatr 1995;127(2):238–43.

18. Rosenthal S, Chen R, Hadler S. The safety of acellular pertussis vaccine vs whole-cell pertussis vaccine. A postmarketing assessment. Arch Pediatr Adolesc Med 1996;150(5):457–60.

19. Children's Vaccine Initiative (CVI) and Global Programme on Immunization of the World Health Organization (WHO). Informal Consultation on control of pertussis with whole cell and acellular vaccines. Report on a meeting May 18–19, 1998. Geneva: World Health Organization, 1999.

20. Cody CL, Baraff LJ, Cherry JD, Marcy SM, Manclark CR. Nature and rates of adverse reactions associated with DTP and DT immunizations in infants and children. Pediatrics 1981;68(5):650–60.

21. Centers for Disease Control. Adverse Events Following Immunization. Surveillance report No. 2, US Department of Health and Human Services, Public Health Service, CDC, Atlanta, GA, 1986.

22. Dittmann S. Atypische Impfverläufe nach Schutzimpfungen. Leipzig: Barth, 1981.

23. Miller DL, Ross EM, Alderslade R, Bellman MH, Rawson NSB. Pertussis immunisation and serious acute neurological illness in children. BMJ 1981;282:1595–9.

24. Halsey NA. Combination vaccines: defining and addressing current safety concerns. Clin Infect Dis 2001;33(Suppl 4):S312–18.

25. Sen S, Cloete Y, Hassan K, Buss P. Adverse events following vaccination in premature infants. Acta Paediatr 2001;90(8):916–20.

26. Mallet E, Fabre P, Pines E, Salomon H, Staub T, Schodel F, Mendelman P, Hessel L, Chryssomalis G, Vidor E, Hoffenbach A, Abeille A, Amar R, Arsene JP, Aurand JM, Azoulay L, Badescou E, Barrois S, Baudino N, Beal M, Beaude-Chervet V, Berlier P, Billard E, Billet L, Blanc B, Blanc JP, Bohu D, Bonardo C, Bossu C. Hexavalent Vaccine Trial Study Group. Immunogenicity and safety of a new liquid hexavalent combined vaccine compared with separate administration of reference licensed vaccines in infants. Pediatr Infect Dis J 2000;19(12):1119–27.

27. In: Howson CP, Howe CJ, Fineberg HV, editors. Adverse effects of pertussis and rubella vaccines. A report of the Committee to Review the Adverse Consequences of Pertussis and Rubella Vaccines. Washington, DC: National Academy Press, 1991.

28. Miller D, Madge N, Diamond J, Wadsworth J, Ross E. Pertussis immunisation and serious acute neurological illnesses in children. BMJ 1993;307(6913):1171–6.

29. Madge N, Diamond J, Miller D, Ross E, McManus C, Wadsworth J, Yule W, Frost B. The National Childhood Encephalopathy study: a 10-year follow-up. A report on the medical, social, behavioural and educational outcomes after serious, acute, neurological illness in early childhood. Dev Med Child Neurol Suppl 1993;68:1–118.

30. Stratton KR, Howe CJ, Johnston RB Jr, editors. DPT Vaccine and Chronic Nervous System Dysfunction: A New Analysis. Washington, DC: National Academy Press, 1994:51–4.

31. Centers for Disease Control (CDC). Diphtheria, tetanus, and pertussis: guidelines for vaccine prophylaxis and other preventive measures. Immunization Practices Advisory Committee. MMWR Morb Mortal Wkly Rep 1985;34(27):405–14, 419–26.

32. Lewis K, Cherry JD, Sachs MH, Woo DB, Hamilton RC, Tarle JM, Overturf GD. The effect of prophylactic acetaminophen administration on reactions to DTP vaccination. Am J Dis Child 1988;142(1):62–5.

33. Anonymous. Prophylactic paracetamol with childhood immunisation? Drug Ther Bull 1990;28(19):73–4.

34. Baykal C, Okan G, Sarica R. Childhood bullous pemphigoid developed after the first vaccination. J Am Acad Dermatol 2001;44(Suppl 2):348–50.

35. Hurwitz EL, Morgenstern H. Effects of diphtheria–tetanus–pertussis or tetanus vaccination on allergies and allergy-related respiratory symptoms among children and adolescents in the United States. J Manipulative Physiol Ther 2000;23(2):81–90.

36. Vulginity V. Sterile abscesses after diphtheria–tetanus toxoids–pertussis vaccination. Pediatr Infect Dis J 1987;6:497.

37. Baraff LJ, Manclark CR, Cherry JD, Christenson P, Marcy SM. Analyses of adverse reactions to diphtheria and tetanus toxoids and pertussis vaccine by vaccine lot, endotoxin content, pertussis vaccine potency and percentage of mouse weight gain. Pediatr Infect Dis J 1989;8(8):502–7.

38. Sakaguchi M, Nakayama T, Inouye S. Cases of systemic immediate-type urticaria associated with acellular diphtheria–tetanus–pertussis vaccination. Vaccine 1998;16(11–12):1138–40.

39. Salomon ME, Halperin R, Yee J. Evaluation of the two-needle strategy for reducing reactions to DPT vaccination. Am J Dis Child 1987;141(7):796–8.

Pethidine

General Information

Pethidine (meperidine) is about one-tenth as potent as morphine in terms of analgesia. It is metabolized in the liver by hydrolysis and conjugation, either directly or via *N*-demethylation to norpethidine. Norpethidine (normeperidine) is significantly less analgesic, with a longer half-life (15–20 hours).

There has been a systematic review of the postoperative analgesic efficacy and adverse effects of pethidine and ketorolac compared with placebo in published randomized, controlled, double-blind studies (1). The authors reviewed studies of moderate to severe postoperative pain relief and the use of single doses by injection (intravenously or intramuscularly) or orally. Studies of epidural, intrathecal, or intravenous administration using patient-controlled analgesia were excluded. Of the 24 placebo-controlled pethidine studies, only 8 met the inclusion criteria and these generated 10 pethidine versus placebo comparisons and 254 patients given pethidine 50 mg or 100 mg intramuscularly. No studies of oral or intravenous pethidine at any dose met the inclusion criteria. Only the eight comparisons of pethidine 100 mg versus placebo ($n = 203$) had sufficient information available for analysis of adverse effects. The overall conclusion was that opioids carry a small but finite risk of serious adverse effects, such as respiratory depression, and a greater risk of minor adverse effects than single-dose injected or oral NSAIDs like ketorolac. Analgesia from the injected opioid or NSAID was equivalent to that achieved with oral NSAIDs. For those who cannot swallow, the choice is injected opioids like pethidine.

In a double-blind, randomized, placebo-controlled study, 40 patients who were scheduled for elective cesarean section under spinal anesthesia were given intrathecal 0.5% hyperbaric bupivacaine 2 ml together with either 5% pethidine 0.2 ml or isotonic saline (2). The pethidine group had a significantly greater incidence of intraoperative nausea or vomiting, with significantly better immediate postoperative analgesia, which was not sustained 4 hours after surgery.

In a randomized, controlled study in 611 mothers, 310 were randomized to intramuscular pethidine up to 300 mg and 301 to epidural 0.25% bupivacaine 10 ml with an infusion of 0.125–0.25% bupivacaine (3). There were no significant differences in analgesic efficacy, adverse effects, or the incidence of backaches.

Organs and Systems

Cardiovascular

- A 70-year-old patient with a metastatic carcinoid tumor of the liver presented with a hypertensive crisis after being given pethidine 10 mg/hour by continuous intravenous infusion (4). The patient remained hypertensive with a systolic blood pressure of 210 mmHg, even after chemoembolization of the tumor. The blood pressure

fell when pethidine was withdrawn and nitroprusside was given. The serum 5-HT concentration was 15 μmol/l (reference range 0.17–0.26) and the urine 5-hydroxyindoleacetic acid concentration was 1311 mg/g of creatinine (reference range less than 10).

The authors postulated that the hypertensive crisis had occurred from the release of 5-HT from the tumor and blockade by pethidine of 5-HT re-uptake.

When used for sedation in children undergoing esophagogastroduodenoscopy, hypoxia with dysrhythmias was more likely to occur with a combination of pethidine and diazepam than with pethidine and midazolam (SEDA-18, 81).

Nervous system

Cases of severe reversible neurotoxicity and parkinsonism are on record (SED-11, 143) (SEDA-18, 82) (5,6). Severe nervous system syndromes may also result from interactions (see the monograph on Opioid analgesics).

Although seizures are uncommon, several cases have been reported, including when pethidine was used in PCA. The metabolite norpethidine is considered to be of significant importance in provoking seizures. Risk factors are renal insufficiency, sickle-cell anemia, high doses of pethidine, and concurrent administration of phenothiazines or drugs that induce hepatic enzymes (SEDA-16, 85) (SEDA-18, 82) (SEDA-19, 85). Myoclonus can occur (7). Norpethidine is twice as likely as pethidine to cause convulsions. The seizures occur at a norpethidine concentration range of 0.38–9.9 μg/ml, and only few reports have described convulsions within the first 24 hours of pethidine treatment.

- A 35-year-old woman, who was admitted for elective laparotomy and ileostomy formation was given patient-controlled analgesic with pethidine for postoperative analgesia (8). The device was set to deliver 20 mg of pethidine with a 5-minute lock-out period and no hourly limit. At 4 hours postoperatively she did not have pethidine-related neurotoxicity, but at 23 hours she had myoclonic jerks and facial twitching followed by a brief generalized tonic-clonic seizure and postictal sequelae. The pethidine was withdrawn and there was no further seizure activity. She had self administered a total of 2700 mg. The norpethidine concentration was 1.8 μg/ml.

Two of three patients with seizures due to norpethidine toxicity (9–11) had renal disease.

- A 46-year-old woman with previous extensive urological problems, including ureteric stricture and recurrent urinary tract infections, was given pethidine in a total cumulative dose of 1500 mg postoperatively over 12 hours when she presented with a single tonic-clonic seizure that lasted 30 seconds. The pethidine concentration was 1200 ng/ml and the norpethidine concentration 2100 ng/ml.
- A 72-year-old patient with end-stage renal insufficiency undergoing peritoneal dialysis developed myoclonic contractions and a generalized tonic-clonic seizure 48 hours after having been given pethidine in a total cumulative dose of 250 mg intravenously and 600 mg

orally. The neurotoxicity resolved after withdrawal of pethidine and 4 hours of hemodialysis.

- A 2-month-old boy presented with muscle rigidity of the arms and legs, catatonia, and an exaggerated startle reflex after being erroneously given a single dose of pethidine 1 mg/kg. The symptoms subsided without any active intervention.

Two case reports have highlighted the potential danger of injecting pethidine into the lateral thigh region, which can cause injury to the femoral nerve branch to the vastus lateralis, causing muscle atrophy (12).

In a retrospective survey of 355 medical records of patients who received intravenous PCA pethidine between 1988 and 1994 the mean consumption by patients who had used over 600 mg/day of pethidine was 13.3 mg/kg/day in asymptomatic patients and 16.9 mg/kg/day in the 2% of patients who presented with central nervous system excitatory signs and symptoms (muscle twitches, jitteriness, agitation, and hallucinations) (13). The authors recommended a maximum safe dose of pethidine by PCA of 10 mg/kg/day for no more than 3 days.

Gastrointestinal

A study in which it was intended to recruit 90 women in labor for a comparison of intrathecal bupivacaine 2.5 mg, fentanyl 25 μg, pethidine 15 mg, and pethidine 25 mg was stopped prematurely after only 34 had been recruited, because of a significant increase in the incidence of nausea and vomiting in the patients who received the two doses of pethidine (14).

Immunologic

Pethidine causes histamine release (7). Of 16 patients given pethidine (mean dose 4.3 mg/kg), 5 had signs of the effects of histamine (hypotension, tachycardia, erythema) and raised histamine concentrations (7).

- A 42-year-old patient presented with generalized pruritus, erythema, urticaria, facial angioedema, dysphagia, dysphonia, and dizziness 15 minutes after a single intramuscular dose of pethidine 100 mg for severe renal colic (15). Prick tests and intradermal tests with pethidine and other compounds confirmed an allergic reaction to pethidine.

Long-Term Effects

Drug dependence

The interaction between the drug-dependent patient and health professional has been investigated in a retrospective study of the medical records of 20 patients with chronic organic pain and perceived as being dependent on pethidine (16). The fact that the patients were perceived as being addicted may have influenced the adequate management of their chronic intractable pain, precipitated poor staff–patient relationships, created a lower pain threshold or tolerance due to anxiety and depression, and led to overuse of placebo, leading to inadequate analgesia. All of these factors may then have led to craving-like behavior and demands for more analgesics, further fuelling the negative stereotyped

perception of the addicted personality. The authors suggested that people with dependence-related problems should be evaluated for suicidal intent; concurrent psychiatric illnesses should be treated; and precipitating factors that make pain worse should be identified. Medical and other staff should be educated about the use of opiate analgesics and concepts of dependence, in order to reduce negative judgmental attitudes and misconceptions.

Second-Generation Effects

Fetotoxicity

Pethidine is commonly used in some countries as an analgesic in maternal labor. The analgesic and adverse effects of intramuscular pethidine 5 mg plus diamorphine 100 mg in labor have been studied in a randomized, double-blind, controlled study in 64 multiparous and 69 nulliparous women (17). There was a significantly higher incidence of low Apgar scores at 1 minute after pethidine compared with diamorphine. The study also confirmed that for women who requested intramuscular narcotic analgesia, neither diamorphine nor pethidine provided good pain relief, suggesting that there is a need to consider alternatives.

Pethidine 50 mg plus promethazine 25 mg given intravenously to 14 mothers in labor caused a significant change in fetal heart rate indices 40 minutes after administration (18). There were significant changes in fetal heart rate acceleration of at least 10 beats/minute, acceleration of at least 15 beats/minute, time spent in episodes of high variation, and short-term variation.

Susceptibility Factors

Renal disease

Norpethidine (normeperidine) accumulates in cases of renal insufficiency (19), leading to symptoms of overdosage.

Hepatic disease

Patients with cirrhosis and acute viral hepatitis can have a 50% reduction in pethidine clearance (SEDA-19, 85).

Drug Administration

Drug dosage regimens

In a double-blind study of 60 patients undergoing elective carpal tunnel release given pethidine 0, 10, 20, 30, 40, or 50 mg in addition to intravenous regional anesthesia with lidocaine 0.5%, the duration of analgesia increased dose-dependently with 0, 10, 20, and 30 μg (20). In those given pethidine 30, 40, and 50 μg there was a significantly higher incidence of sedation, pruritus, nausea, vomiting, and respiratory depression with no increase in analgesic effect. These results support an optimal dose of pethidine 30 mg when used with 0.5% lidocaine for postoperative analgesia.

In a prospective, randomized, single-blind study in 45 men undergoing lower abdominal surgery using one of three doses of intrathecal pethidine (1.2, 1.5, or 1.8 mg/kg) there was no difference in the incidence of adverse effects among the three groups (21). The authors postulated that increasing the dose of pethidine from 1.2 to 1.5 mg/kg increased the duration of analgesia but not the level of sensory block, without an increase in adverse effects.

In 40 patients undergoing prostatectomy with spinal anesthesia with lidocaine 5% (75 mg) intrathecally, either alone or co-administered with pethidine 0.15 or 0.30 mg/kg, the higher dose of pethidine reduced the requirement for parenteral analgesics with a non-significant incidence of pethidine-related adverse effects (22).

Drug administration route

Epidural versus intravenous

In a double-blind, randomized, controlled study, 17 patients undergoing gastrectomy were given epidural PCA pethidine (10 mg bolus and a 4-hourly maximum dose of 3 mg/kg) and were compared with 20 patients after gastrectomy who were given the same regimen intravenously (23). The mean pethidine consumption in the first 24 hours was 33% less in the epidural group than in the intravenous group. Pain scores, adverse effects profiles, patient satisfaction, and patient outcome were similar. However, the sample size was small, and even though the study was intended to be double-blind, the route of pethidine administration and the patient's perception of an intravenous and epidural injection might have caused bias.

Rectal

Rectal pethidine is not advised in children, owing to enormous variability in systemic availability (SEDA-18, 82).

Drug overdose

Cardiac arrest occurred after pethidine overdose (24).

- A 2-month-old boy had a cardiac arrest when he was given a combination of pethidine, promethazine, and chlorpromazine in 10 times the recommended dose by the wrong route (intravenously rather than intramuscularly). Within seconds he became apneic and stiff. Cardiopulmonary resuscitation was instituted, including two intravenous doses of adrenaline 0.06 mg and naloxone 0.6 mg, with recovery 7 minutes after the incident and complete resolution 24 hours later.

Drug–Drug Interactions

Cimetidine

The hepatic metabolism of pethidine can be inhibited by cimetidine, leading to respiratory depression and sedation (25,26).

Phenytoin

Phenytoin enhances the metabolism of pethidine (27).

Selegiline

A syndrome resembling the serotonin syndrome has been reported in a patient taking pethidine plus selegiline (28).

- A woman with Parkinson's disease, taking selegiline 5 mg bd, pergolide 0.75 mg bd, co-careldopa 440 mg qds, imipramine 175 mg qds, and desipramine 25 mg qds, was given pethidine, 325 mg over 3 days, and hydroxyzine for pain. After 2 days she became restless and irritable, and after 4 days she developed delirium, muscle rigidity, sweating, and fever. The symptoms resolved when selegiline was withdrawn.

The authors did not discuss the role of the tricyclic antidepressants in this presentation.

References

1. Smith LA, Carroll D, Edwards JE, Moore RA, McQuay HJ. Single-dose ketorolac and pethidine in acute postoperative pain: systematic review with meta-analysis. Br J Anaesth 2000;84(1):48–58.
2. Yu SC, Ngan Kee WD, Kwan AS. Addition of meperidine to bupivacaine for spinal anaesthesia for Caesarean section. Br J Anaesth 2002;88(3):379–83.
3. Simopoulos TT, Smith HS, Peeters-Asdourian C, Stevens DS. Use of meperidine in patient-controlled analgesia and the development of a normeperidine toxic reaction. Arch Surg 2002;137(1):84–8.
4. Balestrero LM, Beaver CR, Rigas JR. Hypertensive crisis following meperidine administration and chemoembolization of a carcinoid tumor. Arch Intern Med 2000;160(15):2394–5.
5. Lieberman AN, Goldstein M. Reversible parkinsonism related to meperidine. N Engl J Med 1985;312(8):509.
6. Goetting MG, Thirman MJ. Neurotoxicity of meperidine. Ann Emerg Med 1985;14(10):1007–9.
7. Flacke JW, Flacke WE, Bloor BC, Van Etten AP, Kripke BJ. Histamine release by four narcotics: a double-blind study in humans. Anesth Analg 1987;66(8):723–30.
8. McHugh GJ. Norpethidine accumulation and generalized seizure during pethidine patient-controlled analgesia. Anaesth Intensive Care 1999;27(3):289–91.
9. Knight B, Thomson N, Perry G. Seizures due to norpethidine toxicity. Aust NZ J Med 2000;30(4):513.
10. Hassan H, Bastani B, Gellens M. Successful treatment of normeperidine neurotoxicity by hemodialysis. Am J Kidney Dis 2000;35(1):146–9.
11. Baris S, Karakaya D, Sarihasan B. A dose of 1 mg.kg^{-1} meperidine causes muscle rigidity in infants? Paediatr Anaesth 2000;10(6):684.
12. Haber M, Kovan E, Andary M, Honet J. Postinjection vastus lateralis atrophy: 2 case reports. Arch Phys Med Rehabil 2000;81(9):1229–33.
13. Loughnan BA, Carli F, Romney M, Dore CJ, Gordon H. Epidural analgesia and backache: a randomized controlled comparison with intramuscular meperidine for analgesia during labour. Br J Anaesth 2002;89(3):466–72.
14. Booth JV, Lindsay DR, Olufolabi AJ, El-Moalem HE, Penning DH, Reynolds JD. Subarachnoid meperidine (pethidine) causes significant nausea and vomiting during labor. The Duke Women's Anesthesia Research Group. Anesthesiology 2000;93(2):418–21.
15. Anibarro B, Vila C, Seoane FJ. Urticaria induced by meperidine allergy. Allergy 2000;55(3):305–6.

16. Hung CI, Liu CY, Chen CY, Yang CH, Yeh EK. Meperidine addiction or treatment frustration? Gen Hosp Psychiatry 2001;23(1):31–5.

17. Fairlie FM, Marshall L, Walker JJ, Elbourne D. Intramuscular opioids for maternal pain relief in labour: a randomised controlled trial comparing pethidine with diamorphine. Br J Obstet Gynaecol 1999; 106(11):1181–7.

18. Solt I, Ganadry S, Weiner Z. The effect of meperidine and promethazine on fetal heart rate indices during the active phase of labor. Isr Med Assoc J 2002;4(3):178–80.

19. Kaiko RF, Foley KM, Grabinski PY, Heidrich G, Rogers AG, Inturrisi CE, Reidenberg MM. Central nervous system excitatory effects of meperidine in cancer patients. Ann Neurol 1983;13(2):180–5.

20. Reuben SS, Steinberg RB, Lurie SD, Gibson CS. A dose-response study of intravenous regional anesthesia with meperidine. Anesth Analg 1999;88(4):831–5.

21. Hansen D, Hansen S. The effects of three graded doses of meperidine for spinal anesthesia in African men. Anesth Analg 1999;88(4):827–30.

22. Murto K, Lui AC, Cicutti N. Adding low dose meperidine to spinal lidocaine prolongs postoperative analgesia. Can J Anaesth 1999;46(4):327–34.

23. Chen PP, Cheam EW, Ma M, Lam KK, Ngan Kee WD, Gin T. Patient-controlled pethidine after major upper abdominal surgery: comparison of the epidural and intravenous routes. Anaesthesia 2001;56(11):1106–12.

24. Brown ET, Corbett SW, Green SM. Iatrogenic cardiopulmonary arrest during pediatric sedation with meperidine, promethazine, and chlorpromazine. Pediatr Emerg Care 2001;17(5):351–3.

25. Knodell RG, Holtzman JL, Crankshaw DL, Steele NM, Stanley LN. Drug metabolism by rat and human hepatic microsomes in response to interaction with H$_2$-receptor antagonists. Gastroenterology 1982;82(1):84–8.

26. Lee HR, et al Effect of histamine H$_2$-receptors on fentanyl metabolism. Pharmacology 1982;24:145.

27. Pond SM, Kretschzmar KM. Effect of phenytoin on meperidine clearance and normeperidine formation. Clin Pharmacol Ther 1981;30(5):680–6.

28. Zornberg GL, Bodkin JA, Cohen BM. Severe adverse interaction between pethidine and selegiline. Lancet 1991;337(8735):246.

Phenazone

General Information

Phenazone, commonly known as antipyrine, is still used therapeutically in some countries, although it is now used mainly as a marker of hepatic enzyme drug metabolizing activity. It is an old compound with little recent investigation, usually taken in combination with other analgesics, and an exact analysis of its adverse effects is impossible. Phenazone seems to have a low toxicity index, in correspondence with its weak anti-inflammatory effect. Allergic reactions are very rare (SEDA-6, 92) (SEDA-14, 92) (SEDA-16, 108), but subjects undergoing the phenazone test should be informed of the potential risk.

Organs and Systems

Hematologic

Hemolysis can occur in patients with glucose-6-phosphate dehydrogenase deficiency. An immediate reaction after a single test dose, in the form of latent leukopenia, has also been reported (1), with previous sensitization to pyrazolone derivatives as the most probable explanation. Agranulocytosis has been observed in six women after the use of a phenazone-containing cream (SEDA-18, 101).

Gastrointestinal

Only chronic abuse of phenazone, probably together with other more aggressive antipyretics, can cause gastric symptoms (2).

Urinary tract

Phenazone nephrotoxicity is well-established, but information is limited. Experimental papillary necrosis can easily be provoked; analgesic nephropathy is probably a real danger with antipyrine, especially when it is combined with a stronger inhibitor of prostaglandin synthesis. The effect is probably toxic, since inhibition of prostaglandins is not a marked characteristic of phenazone. Two reports have suggested a causal link between phenazone and renal carcinoma, as is well-known for phenacetin (3,4), but this has not been confirmed.

Skin

Urticarial rashes and erythema are the most common adverse effects of phenazone, followed by maculopapular eruptions, erythema multiforme, erythema nodosum, or even angioedema (5).

References

1. Kadar D, Kalow W. Acute and latent leukopenic reaction to antipyrine. Clin Pharmacol Ther 1980;28(6):820–2.

2. Drtil J, Sandz Z. Veranderungen der Magenschleimhaut nach Gebrauch einiger Antiasthmatika und Analgetika Antipyretika. [Changes in the gastric mucosa following the use of various antiasthmatics and analgesics-antipyretics.] Z Gesamte Inn Med 1968;23(8):236–40.

3. Johansson S, Angervall L, Bengtsson U, Wahlqvist L. Uroepithelial tumors of the renal pelvis associated with abuse of phenacetin-containing analgesics. Cancer 1974;33(3):743–53.

4. Shabert P, Nagel R, Leistenschneider W. Zur Frage der Koinzidenz von Tumoren der oberen Harnwege mit chronischer Einnahme analgetischer Substanzen. In: Haschek H, editor. Internationales Symposium uber Probleme des Phenacetin Abusus. Vienna: Facta Publication, Verlag H, Egerman, 1973:257.

5. Zurcher K, Krebs A. Nebenwirkungen interner Arzneimittel auf die Haut unter besonderer Berudcksichtigung neuerer Medikamente. [Cutaneous side effects of systemic drugs with special reference to recently introduced medicaments. I.] Dermatologica 1970;141(2):119–29.

Phenazopyridine

General Information

Phenazopyridine, an azo dye, is used as a urinary tract analgesic. However, because of toxicity, the standard use of phenazopyridine as part of a fixed-dose combination no longer seems justified.

Organs and Systems

Nervous system

Aseptic meningitis was diagnosed in a patient who had three distinct episodes of fever and confusion after taking phenazopyridine (SEDA-13, 84).

Hematologic

Hematological adverse effects of phenazopyridine include methemoglobinemia and hemolytic anemia, particularly after overdosage (1,2).

Liver

Liver toxicity has been reported with phenazopyridine (3).

Urinary tract

Because of nephrotoxicity (oliguria, cylindruria, and reduced creatinine clearance, with crystal deposits in renal tubules and interstitial tissue) (4) phenazopyridine should not be used in patients with suspected renal disease and insufficiency, or in patients with glucose-6-phosphate dehydrogenase deficiency. Bladder stones have also been described (5).

Skin

Yellow discoloration of the nails has been attributed to long-term therapy with phenazopyridine (6).

References

1. Jeffery WH, Zelicoff AP, Hardy WR. Acquired methemoglobinemia and hemolytic anemia after usual doses of phenazopyridine. Drug Intell Clin Pharm 1982;16(2):157–9.
2. Green ED, Zimmerman RC, Ghurabi WH, Colohan DP. Phenazopyridine hydrochloride toxicity: a cause of drug-induced methemoglobinemia. JACEP 1979;8(10):426–31.
3. Goldfinger SE, Marx S. Hypersensitivity hepatitis due to phenazopyridine hydrochloride. N Engl J Med 1972;286(20):1090–1.
4. Alano FA Jr, Webster GD Jr. Acute renal failure and pigmentation due to phenazopyridine (Pyridium). Ann Intern Med 1970;72(1):89–91.
5. Mulvaney WP, Beck CW, Brown RR. Urinary phenazopyridine stones. A complication of therapy. JAMA 1972;221(13):1511–12.
6. Amit G, Halkin A. Lemon-yellow nails and long-term phenazopyridine use. Ann Intern Med 1997;127(12):1137.

Phencyclidine

General Information

Phencyclidine or 1-(1-phenylcyclohexy-1) piperidine (known as PCP or "angel dust") was originally developed as an anesthetic, but was abused as an illicit drug from the late 1960s onwards. It is an antagonist at the N-methyl-d-aspartate (NMDA) subtype of glutamate receptors and a dopamine receptor agonist. It has anticholinergic properties through blockade of ion channels in acetylcholine receptors. It is still used in some countries as an anti-parkinsonian agent (SED-11, 86) (1–3).

The psychoactive effects of phencyclidine are stimulant and similar to the effects of hallucinogens. Hallucinations are often bizarre, frightening, and challenging. Aggressive behavior, usually with amnesia, is common. Self-destructive actions are also seen. Overdosage is associated with paresthesia, slurred speech, ataxia, and later catatonia, dilated pupils, and coma, with tachycardia, hypertension, and dysrhythmias. Seizures and deaths have occurred (SED-11, 86) (4).

References

1. Balster RL, Wessinger WD. Central nervous system depressant effects of phencyclidine. In: Kameka JM, Domino EF, Geneste P, editors. Phencyclidine and Related Amylcyclohexylamines. Preset and Future Applications. Ann Arbor, MI: NPP Books, 1983:291–309.
2. McCarron MM, Schulze BW, Thompson GA, Conder MC, Goetz WA. Acute phencyclidine intoxication: incidence of clinical findings in 1,000 cases. Ann Emerg Med 1981;10(5):237–42.
3. Peterson RC, Stillman RC. Phencyclidine. A review. Rockville, MD: National Institute on Drug Abuse, 1978.
4. Garey RE. PCP (Phencyclidine): an update. J Psychedelic Drugs 1979;11(14):265–75.

Phenelzine

See also Monoamine oxidase inhibitors

General Information

Phenelzine is a non-selective monoamine oxidase (MAO) inhibitor.

Organs and Systems

Nervous system

A potential risk of using a non-selective inhibitor in patients with Parkinson's disease is illustrated by separate reports of the appearance of parkinsonism in patients taking phenelzine (1,2).

- Speech blockage, so called, has been reported in a 34-year-old woman who had taken phenelzine 45 mg/day for 2 months (3). The adverse effect disappeared on withdrawal and did not recur when her depression was successfully treated with maprotiline 175 mg/day.

Psychological, psychiatric

In a carefully controlled 3-week comparison of phenelzine (up to 90 mg/day, mean 77 mg) and imipramine (up to 150 mg/day, mean 139 mg), four patients developed antisocial behavior, three overt paranoid psychosis, and one a hypertensive crisis, despite all precautions to avoid interacting foods and drugs (4).

There has also been a report of delusional parasitosis with phenelzine (SEDA-17, 14).

Dose-related visual hallucinations have been reported in a patient with macular degeneration taking phenelzine (the Charles Bonnet syndrome); the authors discussed the possibility that deprivation-induced visual phenomena had been intensified by increased central monoamine concentrations (5).

Nutrition

Authors who reported a case of carpal tunnel syndrome due to pyridoxine deficiency in a patient taking tranylcypromine (SEDA-9, 21) later collected data (6) on six patients taking phenelzine (up to 75 mg/day for up to 4 months). All developed low concentrations of pyridoxine and a variety of symptoms, including numbness, paresthesia, and edema of the hands, as well as an "electric shock" sensation in the head, neck, and arms. The symptoms resolved completely after the addition of pyridoxine 150–300 mg/day to the treatment regimen.

Hematologic

Leukopenia and agranulocytosis are well-recognized complications of treatment with tricyclic antidepressants and have been reported with some second-generation compounds. In a report of leukopenia in a patient taking phenelzine, attention was drawn to five other unpublished cases and to previous published reports involving isocarboxazid, tranylcypromine, and tryptamine (7).

Long-Term Effects

Drug withdrawal

In a study of the use of phenelzine in continuation therapy after recovery from an acute episode of depression, relapse rates were higher in patients subjected to tapered withdrawal than in those who continued taking the therapeutic dose (8).

In a study of the effects of sudden drug withdrawal in 34 patients taking phenelzine and 17 taking tricyclic antidepressants who had been treated for a mean duration of over 9 months, depressed patients taking phenelzine had significantly more symptoms than depressed patients taking tricyclic antidepressants, and a third of them relapsed, compared with a quarter taking the tricyclic (9). At 3 months follow-up 47% of the patients taking phenelzine had resumed treatment compared with 23% taking the tricyclic. An attempt to distinguish between withdrawal symptoms and relapse on the basis of the rapidity and severity of symptoms was unsuccessful, but about a third

of the patients in both groups developed new symptoms of adrenergic hyperactivity, including anxiety and perceptual disturbances.

Acute psychotic symptoms have been reported in two young women shortly after withdrawal of long-term phenelzine 90 mg/day (10).

Tumorigenicity

A single case of angiosarcoma in the liver has been reported in a patient taking phenelzine (11); similar tumors have occurred in mice treated with phenelzine.

Drug–Drug Interactions

Amantadine

A possible hypertensive interaction of phenelzine with amantadine in Parkinson's disease has been reported (SEDA-10, 17).

Clonazepam

A flushing reaction has been associated with an interaction of phenelzine with clonazepam (SEDA-17, 17).

Venlafaxine

There have been reports of serotonin toxicity when venlafaxine was combined with therapeutic doses of conventional MAO inhibitors (SEDA-20, 21). The serotonin syndrome has been reported in four patients who were switched from the MAO inhibitor phenelzine to venlafaxine (12). In two of them, the 14-day washout period recommended when switching from phenelzine to other antidepressant drugs had elapsed.

- A 25-year-old woman, who had taken phenelzine (45 mg/day) for refractory migraine and tension headache, suffered intolerable adverse effects (weight gain, edema, and insomnia). Phenelzine was withdrawn and 15 days elapsed before she took a single dose of 37.5 mg of venlafaxine. Within 1 hour she developed agitation, twitching, shakiness, sweating, and generalized erythema with hyperthermia (38°C). Her symptoms resolved within 3 hours with no sequelae.

This suggests that even after the recommended 2-week washout from MAO inhibitors, venlafaxine can provoke serotonin toxicity in some patients.

References

1. Teusink JP, Alexopoulos GS, Shamoian CA. Parkinsonian side effects induced by a monoamine oxidase inhibitor. Am J Psychiatry 1984;141(1):118–19.
2. Gillman MA, Sandyk R. Parkinsonism induced by a monoamine oxidase inhibitor. Postgrad Med J 1986;62(725):235–6.
3. Goldstein DM, Goldberg RL. Monoamine oxidase inhibitor-induced speech blockage. J Clin Psychiatry 1986;47(12):604.
4. Evans DL, Davidson J, Raft D. Early and late side effects of phenelzine. J Clin Psychopharmacol 1982;2(3):208–10.
5. Galynker I, Kampf R, Rosenthal R. Dose-related visual hallucinations in macular degeneration patients receiving phenelzine. Am J Psychiatry 1994;151(3):450.

6. Stewart JW, Harrison W, Quitkin F, Liebowitz MR. Phenelzine-induced pyridoxine deficiency. J Clin Psychopharmacol 1984;4(4):225–6.
7. Tipermas A, Gilman HE, Russakoff LM. A case report of leukopenia associated with phenelzine. Am J Psychiatry 1984;141(6):806–7.
8. Davidson J, Raft D. Use of phenelzine in continuation therapy. Neuropsychobiology 1984;11(3):191–4.
9. Tyrer P. Clinical effects of abrupt withdrawal from tricyclic antidepressants and monoamine oxidase inhibitors after long-term treatment. J Affect Disord 1984;6(1):1–7.
10. Liskin B, Roose SP, Walsh BT, Jackson WK. Acute psychosis following phenelzine discontinuation. J Clin Psychopharmacol 1985;5(1):46–7.
11. Daneshmend TK, Scott GL, Bradfield JW. Angiosarcoma of liver associated with phenelzine. BMJ 1979;1(6179):1679.
12. Diamond S, Pepper BJ, Diamond ML, Freitag FG, Urban GJ, Erdemoglu AK. Serotonin syndrome induced by transitioning from phenelzine to venlafaxine: four patient reports. Neurology 1998;51(1):274–6.

Phenindamine

See also Antihistamines

General Information

Phenindamine is an antihistamine that is reputed to cause stimulation rather than sedation in some patients. However, in one small study the central nervous system effects of phenindamine were intermediate between those of terfenadine and diphenhydramine (1).

Reference

1. Witek TJ Jr, Canestrari DA, Miller RD, Yang JY, Riker DK. The effects of phenindamine tartrate on sleepiness and psychomotor performance. J Allergy Clin Immunol 1992;90(6 Pt 1):953–61.

Pheniramine

See also Antihistamines

General Information

Pheniramine is a first-generation antihistamine.

Organs and Systems

Skin

Skin reactions with parenteral pheniramine maleate are uncommon. Relapsing generalized multiple evanescent pruritic erythematous weals after antihistamine and steroid injections have been reported in a 29-year-old woman (1).

Cutaneous reactions have also been reported with pheniramine in eye-drops (2).

- A 30-year old woman who used pheniramine eye-drops for allergic oculorhinitis developed eyelid dermatitis (2). Patch testing showed positive reactions on days 2 and 3.

References

1. Yeon Jin Kim, Jin Hyouk Choi, Jang Seok Bang, Moo Kyu Suh, Jeong Woo Lee, Tae Hoon Kim. A case of pheniramine maleate-aggravated chronic urticaria. Korean J Dermatol 2000;38:1414–16.
2. Parente G, Pazzaglia M, Vincenzi C, Tosti A. Contact dermatitis from pheniramine maleate in eyedrops. Contact Dermatitis 1999;40(6):338.

Phenmetrazine and phendimetrazine

See also Anorectic drugs

General Information

Phenmetrazine and phendimetrazine are central stimulants and indirect sympathomimetics related to dexamfetamine. Phendimetrazine is about 30% rapidly metabolized to phenmetrazine (1). Their reported adverse effects include glossitis, stomatitis, dry mouth, nausea, abdominal pain, cramps, constipation, difficulty in micturition, and headache.

Organs and Systems

Cardiovascular

A dilated cardiomyopathy has been associated with chronic consumption of phendimetrazine (2).

Nervous system

The main adverse effects of phenmetrazine reflect central nervous system stimulation and resemble those of other stimulants. There have been reports of encephalopathy as a result of phenmetrazine toxicity. There were also two cases of damage to the central nervous system after long-term treatment with phenmetrazine; in one, there were disseminated lesions, and in the other, hemiparesis and sensory motor aphasia (3).

Urinary tract

Phendimetrazine has reportedly caused acute interstitial nephritis (4).

Long-Term Effects

Drug abuse

There are many reports of abuse of phenmetrazine. Nervousness, hyperexcitability, euphoria, and insomnia, although less frequent than with amphetamines, have been observed with average doses. Dizziness, headache, nausea, dryness of the mouth, and urticaria have also been recorded. With large doses these adverse reactions were more pronounced. Paranoid psychosis was produced in addicts, and with chronic ingestion psychotic manifestations were evident as with amphetamine.

In Sweden, phenmetrazine has been extensively abused and misused, sometimes with intravenous use. Addicts who had previously been taking morphine stated that phenmetrazine gave them a sense of well-being and overconfidence. There was a high incidence of criminal activity in phenmetrazine users whose primary objective was obtaining money for the drug. Their average doses were 3060 tablets at a time, repeated 4–5 times a day (SED-9, 15).

Second-Generation Effects

Teratogenicity

Very rarely, congenital defects in the newborn have been associated with phenmetrazine consumption by the expectant mother.

References

1 Hager W, Thiede D, Wink K. Primär vaskuläre pulmonale Hypertonie und Appetitzügler. [Primary vascular pulmonary hypertension and appetite suppressants.] Med Klin 1971;66(11):386–90.
2 Rostagno C, Caciolli S, Felici M, Gori F, Neri Serneri GG. Dilated cardiomyopathy associated with chronic consumption of phendimetrazine. Am Heart J 1996;131(2):407–9.
3 Czarnecka E, Mazurkiewicz H. Encefalopatie toksyczne po diugotrwalym przyjmowaniu fenmetrazyny. Wiad Lek 1972;25:1977.
4 Markowitz GS, Tartini A, D'Agati VD. Acute interstitial nephritis following treatment with anorectic agents phentermine and phendimetrazine. Clin Nephrol 1998;50(4):252–4.

Phenobarbital

See also Antiepileptic drugs

General Information

Because it is cheap and of unquestioned efficacy, phenobarbital is still widely prescribed around the world, although in developed countries its use has fallen since the introduction of drugs that are better tolerated. Its most common adverse effects are sedation (to which partial tolerance develops), cognitive dysfunction, and in children hyperkinesia and other behavioral disturbances.

In a randomized trial in newly diagnosed patients, adverse effects leading to withdrawal were more common with phenobarbital (22%, mostly drowsiness and lethargy) than with all other drugs combined (carbamazepine 11%, phenytoin 3%, valproate 5%) (1).

Pretreating patients with phenobarbital can reduce the impact of adverse events when primidone is introduced.

Of 30 patients with intractable partial epilepsy pretreated with phenobarbital before starting primidone (500 mg/day increasing by 125–250 mg/day every 3 weeks until adverse events or a seizure-free state was reached), 26 tolerated the introduction of primidone with minimal or no adverse events (2). Only one patient had to discontinue primidone during the initial 4 weeks because of severe dizziness. Three other patients had dizziness severe enough to interfere with their activities and this disappeared in two patients after the dose was lowered.

Organs and Systems

Nervous system

Unusual manifestations of neurological toxicity of phenobarbital include regression of developmental milestones mimicking a neurodegenerative disorder in young children (SEDA-19, 72) and unilateral choreiform hyperkinesia as a possible withdrawal symptom (SEDA-22, 82).

In a 12-month trial in 109 epileptic children randomized to monotherapy with phenobarbital (maintenance dosage 3.0 mg/kg/day) or phenytoin (5.0 mg/kg/day) in rural India there were no significant differences in either efficacy or toxicity (3). In particular, behavioral adverse effects were not more common with phenobarbital. The findings suggest that phenobarbital is an acceptable first-line agent for childhood epilepsy in rural settings in developing countries.

In 114 patients, of whom 72% took phenobarbital, one had ataxia due to phenobarbital toxicity (4).

Psychological, psychiatric

Phenobarbital-induced behavioral disturbances, especially hyperkinesia, are especially common in children, with an incidence of 20–50%; drug withdrawal is required in 20–30% of cases. It is unclear whether and to what extent adults are affected in this way.

Skin

Rare effects of phenobarbital include erythroderma and an atypical lymphocytosis that mimics cutaneous T cell lymphoma (SEDA-18, 67).

Toxic epidermal necrolysis has been reported in a 62-year-old woman and a 72-year-old man who had taken phenobarbital 100 and 150 mg/day respectively (5).

Musculoskeletal

The incidence of barbiturate-induced Dupuytren's contracture, frozen shoulder, Ledderhose syndrome, Peyronie's disease, fibromas, and joint pains may be up to 10% (6). Most affected patients develop connective tissue changes in the first year, although these become disabling at a later stage. These complications should be recognized early, since they are often reversible (SED-12, 137) (7).

Immunologic

Giant cell myocarditis has been reported in a patient taking phenytoin, phenobarbital, and mephobarbital and in one taking primidone (8).

Death

The efficacy of a single intramuscular dose of phenobarbital (20 mg/kg) in preventing seizures in childhood cerebral malaria has been the subject of a randomized, placebo-controlled study in 340 children in Kenya (9). Seizure frequency was significantly lower with phenobarbital than placebo: 18 versus 46 children had three or more seizures of any duration (OR = 0.32; 95% CI = 0.18, 0.58). However, mortality was doubled (30 versus 14 deaths; OR = 2.39; CI = 1.28, 4.64). The frequency of respiratory arrest was higher with phenobarbital than with placebo, and mortality was greatly increased in children who received phenobarbital plus three or more doses of diazepam (OR = 32; CI = 1.2, 814). The authors felt that although phenobarbital was effective, the risks were too high to recommend using it.

Second-Generation Effects

Teratogenicity

There is an association of phenobarbital with oral clefts and cardiac malformations (10). This is also the case for methylphenobarbital (10).

Fetotoxicity

After prenatal exposure to anticonvulsants, small head size has been observed in neonates and cognitive impairment in infancy. However, it is currently unknown whether these effects are permanent or disappear later in life. Head size and cognition have been studied in adults who had been exposed in utero to phenobarbital plus phenytoin and who as neonates had a significantly smaller occipitofrontal circumference than neonates who had been exposed to phenobarbital alone or controls (mean difference 0.7 cm) (11). There was no difference in cognitive functioning between the exposed and the control groups, and most of the exposed subjects had normal intellectual capacity. However, 12% of the exposed subjects versus 1% of the controls had persistent learning problems. In addition, more of the exposed subjects were mentally retarded. The authors concluded that the combination of phenobarbital plus phenytoin reduced neonatal head size, which was not associated with reduced cognitive functioning in adulthood, but was associated with learning problems and mental retardation.

Susceptibility Factors

Patients with brain metastases treated with radiotherapy seem to have increased susceptibility to phenobarbital-induced toxic epidermal necrolysis (SEDA-19, 72). In a 53-year-old man taking phenobarbital, eruptions were limited to the sites of radiation, which were multiple (12).

Drug–Drug Interactions

Clozapine

Compared with 15 patients taking clozapine alone, seven patients taking similar dosages in combination with phenobarbital had significantly lower plasma clozapine concentrations (232 versus 356 ng/ml) (13). Plasma norclozapine concentrations did not differ between the two groups, whereas clozapine N-oxide concentrations were significantly higher in the phenobarbital group. These findings suggest that phenobarbital stimulates the metabolism of clozapine, probably by inducing its N-oxidation and demethylation. Although the clinical implications remain to be defined, an increase in clozapine dosage requirements may be considered in patients co-medicated with phenobarbital.

References

1. Heller AJ, Chesterman P, Elwes RD, Crawford P, Chadwick D, Johnson AL, Reynolds EH. Phenobarbitone, phenytoin, carbamazepine, or sodium valproate for newly diagnosed adult epilepsy: a randomised comparative monotherapy trial. J Neurol Neurosurg Psychiatry 1995;58(1):44–50.
2. Kanner AM, Parra J, Frey M. The "forgotten" cross-tolerance between phenobarbital and primidone: it can prevent acute primidone-related toxicity. Epilepsia 2000;41(10):1310–14.
3. Pal DK, Das T, Chaudhury G, Johnson AL, Neville BG. Randomised controlled trial to assess acceptability of phenobarbital for childhood epilepsy in rural India. Lancet 1998;351(9095):19–23.
4. Adamolekun B, Mielke J, Ball D, Mundanda T. An evaluation of the management of epilepsy by primary health care nurses in Chitungwiza, Zimbabwe. Epilepsy Res 2000;39(3):177–81.
5. Devidal R, Guy C, Perrot JL, Cathebras P, Ferron C, Ollagnier M. Syndrome de Lyell et phénobarbital: à propos de deux cas. [Lyell's syndrome and phenobarbital: two cases.] Thérapie 2000;55(1):225–7.
6. Falasca GF, Toly TM, Reginato AJ, Schraeder PL, O'Connor CR. Reflex sympathetic dystrophy associated with antiepileptic drugs. Epilepsia 1994;35(2):394–9.
7. Schmidt D. Connective tissue disorders induced by antiepileptic drugs. In: Oxley J, Janz D, Meinardi H, editors. Chronic Toxicity of Antiepileptic Drugs. New York: Raven Press, 1983:115.
8. Daniels PR, Berry GJ, Tazelaar HD, Cooper LT. Giant cell myocarditis as a manifestation of drug hypersensitivity. Cardiovasc Pathol 2000;9(5):287–91.
9. Crawley J, Waruiru C, Mithwani S, Mwangi I, Watkins W, Ouma D, Winstanley P, Peto T, Marsh K. Effect of phenobarbital on seizure frequency and mortality in childhood cerebral malaria: a randomised, controlled intervention study. Lancet 2000;355(9205):701–6.
10. Arpino C, Brescianini S, Robert E, Castilla EE, Cocchi G, Cornel MC, de Vigan C, Lancaster PA, Merlob P, Sumiyoshi Y, Zampino G, Renzi C, Rosano A, Mastroiacovo P. Teratogenic effects of antiepileptic drugs: use of an International Database on Malformations and Drug Exposure (MADRE). Epilepsia 2000;41(11):1436–43.
11. Dessens AB, Cohen-Kettenis PT, Mellenbergh GJ, Koppe JG, van De Poll NE, Boer K. Association of prenatal phenobarbital and phenytoin exposure with small head size at birth and with learning problems. Acta Paediatr 2000;89(5):533–41.
12. Duncan KO, Tigelaar RE, Bolognia JL. Stevens–Johnson syndrome limited to multiple sites of radiation therapy in a patient receiving phenobarbital. J Am Acad Dermatol 1999;40(3):493–6.
13. Facciola G, Avenoso A, Spina E, Perucca E. Inducing effect of phenobarbital on clozapine metabolism in patients with chronic schizophrenia. Ther Drug Monit 1998;20(6):628–30.

Phenols

See also Disinfectants and antiseptics

General Information

Phenol is a benzyl alcohol and a major oxidized metabolite of benzene that was introduced into medicine as an antiseptic (1). Although it can be prepared in an aqueous solution or in glycerine, it appears to be more effective when mixed in aqueous compounds. At a concentration of 0.2% it is bacteriostatic and at over 1% bactericidal (2). In addition to its uses as an antiseptic and disinfectant, phenol is also used as a sclerosant, as a local anesthetic on the skin, and as an analgesic, by injection into nerves or spinally, but its use was limited by severe adverse effects. Current medical uses include cosmetic face peeling, nerve injections, and topical anesthesia. It is also an ingredient of various topical formulations, and is used as an environmental disinfectant.

Systemic adverse effects can occur through absorption from intact skin or wounds, by ingestion, or by absorption of vapor through the skin or via the lungs. They include central nervous stimulation followed by depression, seizures, coma, tachycardia, hypotension, dysrhythmias, pulmonary edema, metabolic acidosis, and hepatic and renal injury. Serious adverse reactions due to percutaneous absorption can occur and death has been described several times. The signs and symptoms of phenol toxicity have been reviewed (3–7) and are listed in Table 1.

Nonoxynols are ethoxylated alkyl phenols that are synthesized from alkylbenzene nonoxynol by reacting it with ethylene oxide to produce ethylene oxide polymers of various lengths. Each nonoxynol is followed by a number that indicates the approximate number of ethylene oxide groups it contains. In cosmetic products, nonoxynols are used as emulsifying, wetting, foaming, and solubilizing agents. They are used in hair and skin products, and in bath, shaving, and fragrance formulations (8). The non-ionic surfactant properties of nonoxynols allow them to be used in a wide variety of industrial, household, agricultural, and pharmaceutical products. Nonoxynol-9 and nonoxynol-10 are surface-active agents used in antiseptic formulations, such as Hibitane solution, Betadine solution, Hexomedine transcutanée, and Hexomedine ointment. They are the most commonly used spermicidal contraceptives and have been recommended in the prevention of sexually transmitted diseases and in human immunodeficiency virus prophylaxis (9).

Pentachlorphenol is a disinfectant that is used in commercial laundries. In 1967 a hospital laundry accidentally used a product containing sodium pentachlorphenolate for a final rinse in the laundering of diapers and infants' bed linen. Twenty newborn infants developed sweating, tachycardia, tachypnea, hepatomegaly, and metabolic acidosis. Six children with severe reactions were subjected to exchange blood transfusion and in each instance there was a dramatic improvement. Two babies died before exchange transfusion could be carried out; postmortem examination showed fatty change in the liver and hydropic and fatty degeneration in the renal tubules and myocardium. There were toxic concentrations of pentachlorphenol in the serum of one patient and autopsy tissue of another.

The phenol derivatives paratertiary butylphenol and amylphenol are used in proprietary germicides.

The permeability of the human epidermis to many phenolic compounds correlates with their lipophilic pattern. However, phenolic compounds appear to produce denaturation in the skin, and an additional increase in permeability is attributed to the resulting damage to the epidermis. Complications of topical phenol, notably cardiac dysrhythmias, including death, can be caused by phenol face peels (10).

Phenol is so rapidly absorbed through the skin that severe systemic effects and even death can result within minutes to hours.

- A 90% solution of phenol spilled over the left sole and shoe of a 47-year-old tanker driver (11). He neither removed his soaked shoe nor attempted to decontaminate himself. He continued driving for 4.5 hours, after which he had vertigo and faintness. Fire fighters removed him from the vehicle, took off his shoes and clothes, and thoroughly washed his leg with copious amount of water. On admission to hospital he was alert but confused, his heart rate was 146/minute, his blood pressure 160/100 mmHg, and there was tense swelling and blue-black discoloration of his left foot, ankle, and distal part of the leg (3% total body surface area), with hypalgesia and hypesthesia over the affected area. His leg was irrigated with large amounts of water, longitudinal incisions of his left foot were performed, and he was transferred to the intensive care unit. Shortly afterwards, he developed rapid atrial fibrillation, ventricular extra beats, reduced blood pressure (90/60 mmHg), and fever of 38.3°C. He was treated with intravenous crystalloids, verapamil, dopamine, and phenylephrine. All the systemic symptoms resolved in 24 hours. Blood and urine cultures were negative. Over the next 3 weeks he was treated with 0.25% troclosene dressings and 1% micronized silver sulfadiazine, until the swelling resolved and the wound had healed. On discharge from hospital and at a 4-month follow up, only blue-black discoloration was noted.

Phenol can be applied percutaneously by the use of a monopolar needle electrode or by open injection when the nerve is exposed surgically. In addition, main nerve trunks or motor branches can be injected, depending on the clinical indication.

Table 1 The signs and symptoms of phenol toxicity

System	Symptoms
Cardiovascular	Cyanosis, cardiac dysrhythmias, electrocardiographic abnormalities, circulatory failure, collapse
Respiratory	Respiratory failure
Nervous system	Dizziness, coma
Sensory systems	Darkening of the cornea
Hematologic	Methemoglobinemia
Gastrointestinal	Abdominal pain
Urinary tract	Hemoglobinuria
Skin	Darkening of the face and hands

Organs and Systems

Cardiovascular

Phenol is cardiotoxic, and various cardiac dysrhythmias have been noted after application to the skin, or less commonly when it has been used for neurolysis. Ventricular extra beats occurred during topical application of phenol and croton oil in hexachlorophene soap and water for chemical peeling of a giant hairy nevus (12). Three of sixteen children treated with motor point blocks for cerebral palsy with a phenolic solution under halothane anesthesia developed cardiac dysrhythmias (13). Severe cardiac dysrhythmias followed by circulatory arrest occurred in an elderly patient with pancreatic cancer, injected with a phenolic solution to produce splanchnic neurolysis (14). The authors recommended that ethanol should replace phenol for this purpose.

In New Zealand, a patient died with brain damage after a cardiac arrest after being exposed to a chemical face peeling solution containing 64% phenol, Exoderm (15). The New Zealand Ministry of Health issued a public statement concerning the safety of phenol solutions.

Respiratory

Acute life-threatening epiglottitis developed in one patient after the use of a throat spray containing the equivalent of 1.4% phenol. The reaction may have been anaphylactic or a direct toxic effect (16).

Nervous system

Early reports suggested that phenol caused selective damage only to small sensory nerve fibers (17). However, later studies showed that in concentrations of 1–7% it caused indiscriminate damage to efferent and afferent nerve fibers (18). At concentrations under 1%, phenol appears to have a local anesthetic affect, which is fully reversible (19). However, at higher concentrations it causes both Wallerian degeneration and axonal demyelination, leading to muscle denervation. After injection of 2% aqueous phenol there can be damage to the microcirculation around nerves, leading to occlusion of small blood vessels and fibrosis in the injected area (20).

The most common adverse effect of phenol injection is pain during injection, often described as a burning or stinging sensation. It can be associated with edema several hours after injection. The application of ice and the use of non-steroidal anti-inflammatory drugs often help to minimize the discomfort. In some studies, lidocaine mixed with phenol has been used to help diminish the local pain response associated with injection (21).

The most worrying adverse effect related to phenol injection is dysesthesia, caused by involvement of sensory nerve axons when perineural injection is attempted. Dysesthesia has been reported from a few days to about 2 weeks after injection; most patients describe a neuropathic component, including a burning pain with light tactile stimulation and involvement of only a small portion of the sensory distribution of the nerve that was blocked (22).

Sensory loss or loss of voluntary motor strength are not uncommon in the first few days after chemical neurolysis

with phenol (23), but permanent loss, other than motor changes associated with the reduction in hypertonia, is less frequent (24,25). A muscle that is already weak is more susceptible to further weakening with chemical neurolysis (26).

- Loss of all sensation and strength after chemical neurolysis occurred in the distribution of the posterior tibial nerve after mixed sensorimotor block of this nerve, in this case after five blocks of the nerve or its motor branches over several years. Some strength and partial sensation returned after surgical lysis of excessive fibrous tissue at the site where the injection had been performed (27).

Chemoneurectomy with aqueous phenol injection in 116 selected patients with spastic cerebral palsy, in whom 246 peripheral nerves were blocked, caused complications in 11 patients (28). Five patients, in whom the posterior tibial nerve was blocked, developed paresthesia: one had complete loss of sensation, which recovered spontaneously after a couple of days; and three had pain at the site of injection or in the distribution of the injected nerve, lasting for a few days to a month. In another study there was a 3% complication rate in 98 blocks (29), while adverse effects occurred in nine of 150 blocks, with muscle weakness in eight cases and painful paresthesia in one (30).

Liver

Neonatal jaundice has been associated with the use of phenolic disinfectants in nurseries, not only when used in excessive concentrations, but also when applied in the recommended dilution (SEDA-5, 258) (SEDA-8, 246) (SEDA-11, 484).

Chronic liver disease has been attributed to long-term household poisoning with pentachlorphenol (31).

Skin

Phenol-related contact pemphigus has been described (22).

- A 32-year-old otherwise healthy woman developed oral erosive lesions of 6 weeks duration and a bullous eruption on her legs, back, and chest of 2 weeks duration. She had bullae and erosions on the left thigh and bullae on the legs, back, abdomen, and chest. There was no family history of pemphigus. Pemphigus vulgaris was diagnosed, and she was given prednisone 100 mg/day. She went home for weekends during hospitalization, and returned to hospital each time with worse lesions. She reported working with a cleaning agent that she had begun using before the onset of the disease. The cleaning agent contained nonyl phenol, and she challenged herself at her next visit home by putting the same agent on her hands for a full day. As a result, new bullae appeared in the mouth. She was advised to stop using the product and was discharged a few days later taking prednisone 80 mg/day, which was tapered as the disease subsided. No new lesions appeared after 1 year of follow-up.

Depigmentation has been attributed to germicides (O-Syl® and Ves-Phene®), containing a mixture of the phenol derivatives paratertiary butylphenol and amylphenol, in five hospital workers and seven other patients who had used them as household disinfectants. Patch tests with the phenolic components of the disinfectants on the patients and controls showed that virtually any moderately irritating phenolic compound can depigment the skin, but of those tested, paratertiary butylphenol and amylphenol most often depigmented the skin without producing toxic inflammation. Initial signs of depigmentation appeared 6 months after using the phenolic mixtures. Within 1 year, two of five patients noted a spontaneous return of pigment; another continued to use the product and there was no evidence of repigmentation (SEDA-11, 485) (32).

Musculoskeletal

Intramuscular injection of phenol can cause pain and swelling in the muscle (33,34). Sometimes, a firm nodular swelling develops in the calf 1–3 weeks after intramuscular neurolysis (35), particularly when larger quantities of phenol are injected into the intramuscular branches of the tibial nerve. This can usually be avoided by limiting the quantity of phenol injected to the minimum necessary and by applying cold packs to the injected area after the procedure.

Muscle necrosis and round cell infiltrates have been seen in histological studies of animal muscle recently injected with phenol, but not after a few months have passed (36).

Immunologic

Contact dermatitis in patients exposed to nonoxynols was initially considered to result from irritation, but allergic reactions have also been reported (37). Nonoxynol contact allergy has been described in two patients who developed contact photosensitivity to nonoxynol-l0 in the antiseptic product Hexomedine transcutanée (38). Among 32 control subjects, 13 had positive photopatch tests to Hexomedine transcutanée and four had positive photopatch tests to nonoxynol-10. Surprisingly, the authors observed that only undiluted nonoxynol was phototoxic. In another study, nonoxynol-9 was found to be rarely sensitizing and compatible with latex and silicone lubricants used in condoms (39).

There is evidence of immunosuppressive effects due to interference by dibenzo-p-dioxin and/or dibenzofuran with the chemical properties of pentachlorphenol (SEDA-11, 485) (40).

Death

Phenol can be fatal in the newborn.

- A 1-day-old child died 11 hours after 2% phenol had been applied to the umbilicus. The postmortem blood concentration of phenol was 125 µg/ml (SEDA-11, 485)(7).
- A 6-day-old child developed cerebral symptoms, circulatory failure, and methemoglobinemia after application of a phenol camphor solution (30% phenol, 60% camphor) to a skin ulcer. The child recovered after exchange transfusion (SEDA-11, 485)(7).

Drug Administration

Drug administration route

A phenol solution of 89% was mistakenly sprayed into the nostrils of a 79-year-old man (41). Immediately, blanching and local erythema developed. It was expected that the patient would develop a significant local burn and possibly systemic toxicity, but neither developed. This may have been due to the amount sprayed or the relatively small body surface area covered by the phenol.

References

1. Glenn MB, Elovic E. Chemical denervation for the treatment of hypertonia and related motor disordrers: phenol and botulinum toxin. J Head Trauma Rehabil 1997;12:40–62.
2. Felsenthal G. Pharmacology of phenol in peripheral nerve blocks: a review. Arch Phys Med Rehabil 1974;55(1):13–16.
3. Truppman ES, Ellenby JD. Major electrocardiographic changes during chemical face peeling. Plast Reconstr Surg 1979;63(1):44–8.
4. Del Pizzo A, Tanski A. Chemical face peeling—malignant therapy for benign disease? Plast Reconstr Surg 1980;66(1):121–3.
5. Ruedemann R, Deichmann WB. Blood phenol level after topical application of phenol-containing preparations. JAMA 1953;152(6):506–9.
6. Deichmann WB. Local and systemic effects following skin contact with phenol—a review of the literature. J Ind 1949;31:146.
7. Hinkel GK, Kintzel HW. Phenolvergiftungen bei Neugeborenen durch kutane Resorption. [Phenol poisoning of a newborn through skin resorption.] Dtsch Gesundheitsw 1968;23(51):2420–2.
8. Christian MS. Cosmetic ingredient review: final report on the safety assessment of nonoxynols 2, 4, 8, 9, 10, 12, 14, 15, 30, 40 and 50. J Am Coll Toxicol 1983;2:35–60.
9. Bird KD. The use of spermicide containing nonoxynol-9 in the prevention of HIV infection. AIDS 1991;5(7):791–6.
10. Botta SA, Straith RE, Goodwin HH. Cardiac arrhythmias in phenol face peeling: a suggested protocol for prevention. Aesthetic Plast Surg 1988;12(2):115–17.
11. Bentur Y, Shoshani O, Tabak A, Bin-Nun A, Ramon Y, Ulman Y, Berger Y, Nachlieli T, Peled YJ. Prolonged elimination half-life of phenol after dermal exposure. J Toxicol Clin Toxicol 1998;36(7):707–11.
12. Warner MA, Harper JV. Cardiac dysrhythmias associated with chemical peeling with phenol. Anesthesiology 1985;62(3):366–7.
13. Morrison JE Jr, Matthews D, Washington R, Fennessey PV, Harrison LM. Phenol motor point blocks in children: plasma concentrations and cardiac dysrhythmias. Anesthesiology 1991;75(2):359–62.
14. Gaudy JH, Tricot C, Sezeur A. Troubles du rythme cardiaque graves après phénolisation splanchnique peropératoire. [Serious heart rate disorders following perioperative splanchnic nerve phenol nerve block.] Can J Anaesth 1993;40(4):357–9.
15. Anonymous. Failure to provide the necessaries of life. NZ Med J 2003;116(1168):1.
16. Ho SL, Hollinrake K. Acute epiglottitis and Chloraseptic. BMJ 1989;298(6687):1584.
17. Moller JE, Helweg-Larsen J, Jacobsen E. Histopathological lesions in the sciatic nerve of the rat following perineural application of phenol and alcohol solutions. Dan Med Bull 1969;16(4):116–19.
18. Bodine-Fowler SC, Allsing S, Botte MJ. Time course of muscle atrophy and recovery following a phenol-induced nerve block. Muscle Nerve 1996;19(4):497–504.

19. Burkel WE, McPhee M. Effect of phenol injection into peripheral nerve of rat: electron microscope studies. Arch Phys Med Rehabil 1970;51(7):391–7.

20. Glenn MB. Nerve blocks. In: Glenn M, Whyte J, editors. The Practical Management of Spasticity in Children and Adults. Philadelphia: Lea & Febiger, 1990:227–58.

21. Petrillo CR, Knoploch S. Phenol block of the tibial nerve for spasticity: a long-term follow-up study. Int Disabil Stud 1988;10(3):97–100.

22. Goldberg I, Sasson O, Brenner S. A case of phenol-related contact pemphigus. Dermatology 2001;203(4):355–6.

23. Khalili AA, Betts HB. Peripheral nerve block with phenol in the management of spasticity. Indications and complications. JAMA 1967;200(13):1155–7.

24. Tardieu G, Tardieu C, Hariga J, Gagnard L. Treatment of spasticity in injection of dilute alcohol at the motor point or by epidural route. Clinical extension of an experiment on the decerebrate cat. Dev Med Child Neurol 1968;10(5):555–68.

25. Copp EP, Harris R, Keenan J. Peripheral nerve block and motor point block with phenol in the management of spasticity. Proc R Soc Med 1970;63(9):937–8.

26. Khalili AA, Benton JG. A physiologic approach to the evaluation and the management of spasticity with procaine and phenol nerve block: including a review of the physiology of the stretch reflex. Clin Orthop Relat Res 1966;47:97–104.

27. Glenn MB. Nerve blocks for the treatment of spasticity. Phys Med Rehabil State of the Art Rev 1994;3:481–505.

28. Yadav SL, Singh U, Dureja GP, Singh KK, Chaturvedi S. Phenol block in the management of spastic cerebral palsy. Indian J Pediatr 1994;61(3):249–55.

29. Copp EP, Keenan J. Phenol nerve and motor point block in spasticity. Rheumatol Phys Med 1972;11(6):287–92.

30. Helweg-Larsen J, Jacobsen E. Treatment of spasticity in cerebral palsy by means of phenol nerve block of peripheral nerves. Dan Med Bull 1969;16(1):20–5.

31. Brandt M, Schmidt E, Schmidt FW. Chronische Lebererkrankung durch laugjahrige Intoxikation in Haushalt mit Pentachlorphenol. [Chronic liver disease caused by long term household poisoning with pentachlorophenol.] Verh Dtsch Ges Inn Med 1977;83:1609–11.

32. Kahn G. Depigmentation caused by phenolic detergent germicides. Arch Dermatol 1970;102(2):177–87.

33. Halpern D, Meelhuysen FE. Phenol motor point block in the management of muscular hypertonia. Arch Phys Med Rehabil 1966;47(10):659–64.

34. Garland DE, Lilling M, Keenan MA. Percutaneous phenol blocks to motor points of spastic forearm muscles in head-injured adults. Arch Phys Med Rehabil 1984;65(5):243–5.

35. Mullins RJ, Richards C, Walker T. Allergic reactions to oral, surgical and topical bovine collagen. Anaphylactic risk for surgeons. Aust NZ J Ophthalmol 1996;24(3):257–60.

36. Halpern D, Meelhuysen FE. Duration of relaxation after intramuscular neurolysis with phenol. JAMA 1967;200(13):1152–4.

37. Dooms-Goossens A, Deveylder H, de Alam AG, Lachapelle JM, Tennstedt D, Degreef H. Contact sensitivity to nonoxynols as a cause of intolerance to antiseptic preparations. J Am Acad Dermatol 1989;21(4 Pt 1):723–7.

38. Michel M, Dompmartin A, Moreau A, Leroy D. Contact photosensitivity to nonoxynol used in antiseptic preparations. Photodermatol Photoimmunol Photomed 1994;10(5):198–201.

39. Fisher AA. Allergic contact dermatitis to nonoxynol-9 in a condom. Cutis 1994;53(3):110–1.

40. Dickson D. PCP dioxins found to pose health risks. Nature 1980;283(5746):418.

41. Durback-Morris LF, Scharman EJ. Accidental intranasal administration of phenol. Vet Hum Toxicol 1999;41(3):157.

Phenoperidine

General Information

Phenoperidine is a potent opioid analgesic often used in neuroleptanalgesia and as a respiratory depressant in ventilated patients.

Organs and Systems

Cardiovascular

Intracranial hypertension occurred within 1 minute in a patient with a severe head injury who received phenoperidine 1 mg intravenously. It was associated with a reduction in arterial blood pressure. A similar reaction occurred when a second 1 mg bolus was given 8 hours later (SED-11, 146) (1).

Reference

1. Grummitt RM, Goat VA. Intracranial pressure after phenoperidine. Anaesthesia 1984;39(6):565–7.

Phenoxybenzamine

General Information

Phenoxybenzamine is a non-selective irreversible alpha-adrenoceptor antagonist. It is given orally in total daily doses up to 60 mg in pheochromocytoma, and lower doses have been used to relieve bladder obstruction before surgery. The maximum effect may be delayed because of irregular absorption, and even after intravenous use it may not be attained for 1 hour. Some of the most severe effects, that is hypotension and syncope with tachycardia, can therefore occur unexpectedly. In a review of published reports from 1966 to 2002 phenoxybenzamine improved bladder function in adult men with retention due to inguinal hernioplasty, in women with retention caused by vaginal repair, and in children with myelomeningocele, in whom there was also a reduced incidence of urinary tract infections (1). The most common adverse events were dizziness, impotence and ejaculatory dysfunction, and nasal stuffiness. No drug-related tumors were reported. Phenoxybenzamine can also cause miosis, lassitude, and gastrointestinal upsets.

Organs and Systems

Cardiovascular

In patients with myocardial infarction, in whom phenoxybenzamine has been used to improve circulation, it can cause or aggravate pulmonary edema; this could be explained by severe hyponatremia during treatment with phenoxybenzamine (SEDA-13, 113).

Psychological, psychiatric

Panic attacks have been described in one case, a week after withdrawal of the drug; the causal association was not certain (SEDA-17, 163).

Susceptibility Factors

Renal disease

Because a large proportion is renally excreted, dosages should be reduced in renal disease.

Other features of the patient

In view of the nature of its effects, phenoxybenzamine should be used sparingly in cardiovascular disease.

Drug Administration

Drug administration route

When phenoxybenzamine is injected intradermally or when it is extravasated during intravenous administration, it can cause both extremely severe necrotic reactions and an allergic response.

Reference

1. Te AE. A modern rationale for the use of phenoxybenzamine in urinary tract disorders and other conditions. Clin Ther 2002;24(6):851–61.

Phentermine

See also Anorectic drugs

General Information

Despite the withdrawal of the fenfluramines, the appetite suppressants phendimetrazine and phentermine have remained in widespread use for the treatment of obesity.

With phentermine, adverse effects due to stimulation of the central nervous system are less than with dexamfetamine, although in one study withdrawal because of adverse effects was as high as 16 of 177 patients (9%); 2 of 13 healthy young volunteers withdrew because of unacceptable stimulation (1).

Organs and Systems

Cardiovascular

In a systematic review of 1279 patients taking fenfluramine, dexfenfluramine, or phentermine, evaluated in seven uncontrolled cohort studies, 236 (18%) and 60 (5%) had aortic and mitral regurgitation respectively (2). Pooled data from six controlled cohort studies yielded, for aortic regurgitation, a relative risk ratio of 2.32 (95% CI = 1.79, 3.01) and an attributable rate of 4.9% and, for mitral regurgitation, a relative risk ratio of 1.55 (95% CI = 1.06, 2.25) with an attributable rate of 1.0%. Only one case of valvular heart disease was detected in 57 randomized controlled trials, but this was judged unrelated to drug therapy. The authors concluded that the risk of valvular heart disease is significantly increased by the appetite suppressants. Nevertheless, valvulopathy is much less common than suggested by previous less methodologically rigorous studies.

Spontaneous rupture of a retroperitoneal aneurysm occurred in a 70-year-old woman who had been taking phentermine hydrochloride, 30 mg/day, for about 1 month (3). Other long-term medications included fluoxetine and amitriptyline, and she had no history of coronary artery disease, hypertension, diabetes, or complications of pregnancy. Although it is plausible that phentermine could have contributed to the ruptured aneurysm, other possibilities should be considered, particularly rupture of an anomalous retroperitoneal blood vessel.

Fatal pulmonary hypertension occurred in a 32-year-old man who had been taking phentermine in unknown doses for 4 months (SED-9, 16).

Nervous system

Insomnia is one of the most common adverse effects of phentermine. In a survey in Edinburgh, 20% of the subjects taking phentermine reported insomnia compared with 6% of those taking placebo (SED-9, 13).

Urinary tract

Phentermine can cause allergic interstitial nephritis (4).

- A 47-year-old mildly obese woman began a weight reduction program that included anorectic therapy with phentermine and phendimetrazine. She had normal renal function at the start of therapy. After 3 weeks of treatment she fell ill and discontinued treatment. She was subsequently found to have leukocyturia, a rash on her face and chest, and a rise in serum creatinine from 67 to 175 μmol/l (0.8–2.1 mg/dl). Renal biopsy confirmed the diagnosis of acute interstitial nephritis. She was treated with corticosteroids, and her renal function returned to normal.

Long-Term Effects

Drug abuse

Some cases of toxic psychosis have been reported with abuse doses of phentermine (5).

Drug–Drug Interactions

Fluoxetine

Following the withdrawal of the fenfluramines, alternative combinations have been explored as appetite suppressants. In an open study of a combination of phentermine + fluoxetine in 16 obese patients with binge-eating disorder, in the setting of cognitive behavioral therapy, there were significant reductions in weight, binge frequency, and psychological distress by the end of treatment; however, the patients regained most of the weight within 1 year (6). At follow-up at 18 months there was still a reduction in binge eating in patients who continued maintenance treatment. The results did not support the long-term value of adding phentermine + fluoxetine to cognitive behavioral therapy for binge-eating disorder. It is worth emphasizing that it is not known whether phentermine + fluoxetine is also associated with cardiac valvulopathy. Moreover, the recognition that phentermine is a monoamine oxidase inhibitor (7) raises further concerns about its safety.

References

1. Malcolm AD, Mace PM, Outar KP, Pawan GL. Experimental evaluation of anorexigenic agents in man: a pilot study. Proc Nutr Soc 1972;31(1):12A–14A.
2. Loke YK, Derry S, Pritchard-Copley A. Appetite suppressants and valvular heart disease—a systematic review. BMC Clin Pharmacol 2002;2(1):6.
3. Sobel RM. Ruptured retroperitoneal aneurysm in a patient taking phentermine hydrochloride. Am J Emerg Med 1999;17(1):102–3.
4. Markowitz GS, Tartini A, D'Agati VD. Acute interstitial nephritis following treatment with anorectic agents phentermine and phendimetrazine. Clin Nephrol 1998; 50(4):252–4.
5. Munro JF. Clinical aspects of the treatment of obesity by drugs: a review. Int J Obes 1979;3(2):171–80.
6. Devlin MJ, Goldfein JA, Carino JS, Wolk SL. Open treatment of overweight binge eaters with phentermine and fluoxetine as an adjunct to cognitive-behavioral therapy. Int J Eat Disord 2000;28(3):325–32.
7. Maher TJ, Ulus IH, Wurtman RJ. Phentermine and other monoamine-oxidase inhibitors may increase plasma serotonin when given with fenfluramines. Lancet 1999; 353(9146):38.

Phentolamine

General Information

Phentolamine is a non-selective alpha-adrenoceptor antagonist. It is used to treat hypertensive crises attributable to the effects of noradrenaline, as in pheochromocytoma and during the interaction of monoamine oxidase inhibitors with amine-containing medicaments and foods (1). Its adverse effects are similar to those of phenoxybenzamine.

Reference

1. Tuncel M, Ram VC. Hypertensive emergencies: etiology and management. Am J Cardiovasc Drugs 2003;3(1):21–31.

Phenylbutazone

See also Non-steroidal anti-inflammatory drugs

General Information

Phenylbutazone was originally a solubilizing agent for aminopyrine and was first used to treat rheumatoid arthritis and allied disorders in 1949. Phenylbutazone and its related compounds were used worldwide until the early 1980s when, following growing concern about their safety, Ciba-Geigy published its own international assessment on phenylbutazone (Butazolidine) and oxyphenbutazone (Tanderil), which summarized reports on 1182 deaths associated with them from their initial use until 1982 (SEDA-9, 85). The report showed that the percentage of serious unwanted effects was high for both drugs, and in both cases the most frequent problems were dermatological and hematological, closely followed by gastrointestinal disorders.

Since 1983 phenylbutazone and oxyphenbutazone have been removed from the market in many countries or have been limited to specific indications. In 1985, Ciba-Geigy decided to stop sales of systemic dosage forms of oxyphenbutazone worldwide and to reduce the indications for phenylbutazone (SEDA-9, 85) (SEDA-10, 78). Nevertheless, phenylbutazone is still to be found in many places. Phenylbutazone and its congeners are now used only for ankylosing spondylitis and sometimes for acute gout, psoriatic arthritis, and active rheumatoid arthritis in patients who have not responded to other therapy, including other NSAIDs. For other indications, less toxic alternatives suffice (1,2).

All combinations of butazone derivatives and a corticosteroid have been removed from the market, even in Germany, one of the most lenient countries in the regulation of phenylbutazone use.

Significant adverse effects can affect up to 40% of patients (3).

Pyrazinobutazone is pyrazine phenylbutazone, which is metabolized to phenylbutazone (4).

General adverse effects

Most of the adverse effects of phenylbutazone are on the gastrointestinal system; they include symptoms ranging from gastric irritation to ulcer perforation and bleeding. Salt and water retention leads to edema, which is undesirable in older patients, and even to congestive heart failure. Hematological adverse effects include blood dyscrasias, lymphadenopathy, and agranulocytosis. Hepatotoxicity and nephrotoxicity occur (5). Headache is common, but other nervous system effects are mild. Acute poisoning can be successfully treated by hemoperfusion (6). Hypersensitivity reactions can be very severe (7); asthma and systemic lupus erythematosus have been reported. Tumor-inducing effects have not been reported.

Organs and Systems

Cardiovascular

Salt and water retention (see the section on Fluid balance in this monograph) are particularly dangerous for patients with impaired cardiac function. Hypertension due to increased plasma volume readily occurs.

Respiratory

Left ventricular failure can result in pleural effusions. Asthma can be provoked. Cross-reactivity with aspirin has been noted (8). A picture resembling allergic alveolitis has been described (9).

Nervous system

Therapeutic doses of phenylbutazone can be followed by headache, dizziness, and vertigo (10). Overdose can cause coma and convulsions (11).

Sensory systems

Phenylbutazone can damage the eyes. Conjunctivitis, damage to the cornea with vascularization and scarring, adhesion of the lids to the eyeballs, amblyopia, retinal hemorrhage, and even blindness have been reported (12).

Psychological, psychiatric

Psychomotor reactions to phenylbutazone when driving have been reported (13).

Endocrine

Because of interference with iodine uptake, hypothyroidism and goiter can result (14). The condition is reversible, but an obstructive syndrome due to thyroid enlargement has been observed (14).

Fluid balance

As many as 10% of patients show signs of salt and fluid retention and edema (7). Increased intravascular fluid volume is responsible for dilution anemia and increasing cardiac load (SED-8, 216). There is still no explanation for the water-retaining effect, but it might reflect increased production of antidiuretic hormone.

Hematologic

Phenylbutazone causes blood dyscrasias (SED-8, 213) (SEDA-2, 92) (7,15). The most serious adverse effect is aplastic anemia which, according to Swedish and British sources, ends fatally in almost 50% of cases (15,16,17). More than 1100 deaths are on record with the principal manufacturer (SEDA-8, Essay).

Specific anti-platelet antibodies can cause thrombocytopenic purpura (18), which can be fatal. The increased risk of leukemia after phenylbutazone could be secondary to bone marrow depression (SED-9, 143) (19).

Agranulocytosis and liver injury have been described in a patient with Reiter's syndrome who took pyrazinobutazone for 6 weeks (20). Other causes of agranulocytosis and hepatic damage were excluded and a lymphocyte transformation test showed significant lymphocyte proliferation in response to pyrazinobutazone.

Gastrointestinal

A potent gastric and intestinal irritant, phenylbutazone can cause ulcers and bleeding. In one study in 1975, when the drug was widely used, 19% of 241 cases had acute

gastrointestinal bleeding due to phenylbutazone (21). According to the UK's Committee on Safety of Medicines, 120 of 1967 adverse reactions attributed to phenylbutazone and its metabolite oxyphenbutazone involved gastrointestinal bleeding, and 32 ended fatally (22). The risk of developing a peptic ulcer during phenylbutazone therapy is estimated at 1–3% (SED-8, 214). Perforation has also been repeatedly observed (21,23). Other adverse effects are nausea, vomiting, abdominal pain, heartburn, diarrhea, and abdominal discomfort.

Even rectal and enteric-coated formulations can cause adverse reactions in the upper gastrointestinal tract. In one double-blind, crossover trial, plain naproxen caused fewer gastrointestinal adverse effects than enteric-coated phenylbutazone (Butacote) (24).

Phenylbutazone suppositories can cause rectal irritation, with mucosal defects, severe hemorrhagic proctitis (25), perforation of the large bowel, and necrotizing colitis (26).

Gastrointestinal toxicity has been reported in a patient treated short-term with pyrazinobutazone (27).

Liver

Hepatotoxicity has been clearly documented (28). Phenylbutazone causes three types of liver damage through three separate pathogenic mechanisms:

1. acute hepatic necrosis after overdosage, related to the hepatotoxicity of phenylbutazone and/or its metabolites;
2. mild hepatocellular damage (with or without cholestasis) and granulomas (sometimes also found at extrahepatic sites, with varying degrees of steatosis); these changes are the result of hypersusceptibility and possibly a certain degree of toxicity;
3. more pronounced hepatocellular damage with cholestasis but without granulomas; toxicity plays a more important role than hypersusceptibility.

Concomitant treatment with other hepatotoxic agents can predispose to phenylbutazone-induced liver toxicity.

Urinary tract

Although adverse renal effects can occur with any NSAID, phenylbutazone-induced nephrotoxicity has mainly been reported when the drug was taken in association with other anti-inflammatory agents (SED-8, 215) or when taken alone in a high dose (29).

Skin

Skin eruptions, Quincke's edema, and even epidermal necrolysis (SEDA-5, 100) (30,31) can develop during or after phenylbutazone therapy.

Considerable local irritation and pain at the site of injection are sometimes followed by necrosis. Sterile abscess formation has also been reported (32).

Long-Term Effects

Mutagenicity

Phenylbutazone infusion for 10 days induced chromosomal abnormalities in patients with rheumatoid arthritis (33), although the significance of this finding is not clear.

Second-Generation Effects

Lactation

If phenylbutazone is taken during lactation, only small amounts are found in the milk (34).

Susceptibility Factors

Age

The risk of adverse reactions to phenylbutazone increases with age (SED-8, 213) (17).

Other features of the patient

The specific risks of salt and water retention in cardiac and renal disease have already been mentioned. The potential for ulcerogenic activity should be kept in mind if phenylbutazone is given to a patient with a history of peptic ulceration. Patients who are hypersensitive to other drugs (especially aspirin) should be carefully monitored when taking phenylbutazone.

Drug Administration

Drug overdose

Acute intoxication with phenylbutazone is dominated by metabolic acidosis, which can progress to coma, seizures, hypotension, shock, and oliguria. Kidney and liver reactions, acute bone marrow depression, and acute perforation of peptic ulcer have all been described (5,11,35).

Drug–Drug Interactions

Antihypertensive agents

Inhibition of the effect of antihypertensive agents by phenylbutazone can probably be explained by salt and water retention (36).

Aspirin

Phenylbutazone interferes with the tubular excretion of aspirin (3).

Coumarin anticoagulants

Phenylbutazone displaces warfarin from binding sites on serum albumin, temporarily increasing its effects before the clearance of warfarin increases because of an increase in the unbound fraction (37). If that were the only mechanism, this interaction would not be important. However, phenylbutazone also inhibits the metabolism of S-warfarin and induces the metabolism of R-warfarin (38); the half-life of racemic warfarin is unchanged, but because the S isomer is more potent than the R isomer, the action of warfarin is potentiated (SED-9, 144) (36,39).

Oral hypoglycemic drugs

Phenylbutazone can potentiate the hypoglycemic effects of the sulfonylureas acetohexamide (40), chlorpropamide (41), tolbutamide (42), and glibenclamide (43). One

mechanism of this interaction is interference with tubular excretion (3).

Penicillins

Phenylbutazone interferes with the tubular excretion of penicillins (3).

Phenytoin

Phenylbutazone can reduce the clearance of phenytoin by inhibiting CYP2C9 (44).

Sulfonamides

Phenylbutazone can displace sulfonamides from protein-binding sites (SED-9, 144) (45).

Interference with Diagnostic Tests

Thyroid function tests

Phenylbutazone inhibits thyroid uptake of iodine and/or competes for protein-binding sites with thyroxine (SED-9, 145) (46,47), and can thus interfere with the use of thyroid function tests.

References

1. Anonymous. BGA "loose" Butazone Coombs warning. Scrip 1985;974:8.
2. Anonymous. Mofebuzone restriction explained. Scrip 1985;965:1.
3. Martindale: The Extra Pharmacopoeia. 28th ed. London: The Pharmaceutical Press, 1983:273.
4. von Bruchhausen V, Lohmann H, O'svath J. The pharmacokinetic profile of pyrazinobutazone in man. Arzneimittelforschung 1978;28(12):2337–43.
5. Prescott LF, Critchley JA, Balali-Mood M. Phenylbutazone overdosage: abnormal metabolism associated with hepatic and renal damage. BMJ 1980;281(6248):1106–7.
6. Berlinger WG, Spector R, Flanigan MJ, Johnson GF, Groh MR. Hemoperfusion for phenylbutazone poisoning. Ann Intern Med 1982;96(3):334–5.
7. Adverse Drug Reactions Advisory Committee. Phenylbutazone. Med J Aust 1979;2:553.
8. Szczeklik A, Gryglewski RJ, Czerniawska-Mysik G. Relationship of inhibition of prostaglandin biosynthesis by analgesics to asthma attacks in aspirin-sensitive patients. BMJ 1975;1(5949):67–9.
9. Thurston JG, Marks P, Trapnell D. Lung changes associated with phenylbutazone treatment. BMJ 1976;2(6049):1422–3.
10. Rechenberg HK. Phenylbutazone. London: Edward Arnold Ltd, 1962:113–20, 125–5, 131.
11. Anvik T. Akutt forgittning med fenylbutazon. [Acute poisoning with phenylbutazone.] Tidsskr Nor Laegeforen 1970;90(2):95–7.
12. Willetts GS. Ocular side-effects of drugs. Br J Ophthalmol 1969;53(4):252–62.
13. Linnoila M, Seppala M, Mattila MJ. Acute effect of antipyretic analgesics alone or in combination with alcohol on human psychomotor skills related to driving. Br J Clin Pharmacol 1974;1:477.
14. Schwarzmann E, Quast M. Kasuistische Betrachtungen zur Phenylbutazon-Struma. Dtsch Gesundheitsw 1973;28:1417.
15. Bottiger LE, Westerholm B. Drug-induced blood dyscrasias in Sweden. BMJ 1973;3(5875):339–43.

16. Bottiger LE. Phenylbutazone, oxyphenbutazone and aplastic anaemia. BMJ 1977;2(6081):265.

17. Inman WH. Study of fatal bone marrow depression with special reference to phenylbutazone and oxyphenbutazone. BMJ 1977;1(6075):1500–5.

18. Davidson C, Manohitharajah SM. Drug-induced antiplatelet antibodies. BMJ 1973;3(5879):545.

19. Hartwich G, Lutz H. Leukämieentstehung nach benzol und phenylbutazon. [Leukemia origin after benzene and phenylbutazone.] Verh Dtsch Ges Inn Med 1973;79:394–6.

20. Maria VA, da Silva JA, Victorino RM. Agranulocytosis and liver damage associated with pyrazinobutazone with evidence for an immunological mechanism. J Rheumatol 1989;16(11):1484–5.

21. Schwenke W, Schwenke G, Willgeroth C. Die grosse obere Gastrointestinalblutung unter besonderer Berucksichtigung der akuten Magenschleimhäutlasionen durch Medikamente. Z Gesamte Inn Med Ihre Grenzgeb 1975;30:198.

22. Cuthbert MF. Adverse reactions to non-steroidal antirheumatic drugs. Curr Med Res Opin 1974;2(9):600–10.

23. Schwabe H. Magenperforation und Blutung nach langeren Gaben von Antirheumatika. 2. [Stomach perforation and hemorrhage after long-term administration of antirheumatic agents.] Z Allgemeinmed 1975;51(25):1097–8.

24. Ansell BM, Major G, Liyanage SP, Gumpel JM, Seifert MH, Mathews JA, Engler C. A comparative study of Butacote and Naprosyn in ankylosing spondylitis. Ann Rheum Dis 1978;37(5):436–9.

25. Cheli R, Ciancamerla G. Proctiti emorragiche da medicamenti locali. [Hemorrhagic proctitis due to local drugs.] Minerva Gastroenterol 1974;20(2):56.

26. Liaras H, Neidhardt JH, Tairraz JP, Lesbros F, Guelpa G. Les entérites et colites aiguës nécrosantes: essai nosologique et pathogenique—étude clinique: à propos de 8 cas. [Acute necrosing colitis and enteritis. Nosologic and pathogenic attempt. Clinical study (apropos of 8 cases).] J Chir (Paris) 1968;96(6):501–18.

27. Ritschard T, Filippini L. Nebenwirkungen nichtsteroidaler Antirheumatika auf den unteren Intestinaltrakt. [Side effects of non-steroidal antirheumatic agents on the lower intestinal tract.] Dtsch Med Wochenschr 1986;111(41):1561–4.

28. Benjamin SB, Ishak KG, Zimmerman HJ, Grushka A. Phenylbutazone liver injury: a clinical-pathologic survey of 23 cases and review of the literature. Hepatology 1981;1(3):255–63.

29. Wigley RA. The New Zealand experience. Aust NZ J Med 1976;6(Suppl 1):37–44.

30. Eischbeck R, Huhle G, Stiller D, Zucker G. Durch immunologische in vitro Untersuchungen gesicherte hochgradige Phenylbutazon Uberempfindlichkeit bei einem Fall von Morbus Lyell. Dtsch Gesundheitsw 1975;30:2331.

31. Zurcher K, Krebs A. Nebenwirkungen interner Arzneimittel auf die Haut unter besonderer Berudcksichtigung neuerer Medikamente. [Cutaneous side effects of systemic drugs with special reference to recently introduced medicaments. I.] Dermatologica 1970;141(2):119–29.

32. Hadida A, Groulier P. Nécrose de la fesse après une injection de phénylbutazone. Marseille Chir 1968;20:270.

33. Vormittag W, Kolarz G. Chromosomenuntersuchungen vor und nach Infusionstherapie mit Phenylbutazon. [Chromosome studies before and after phenylbutazone infusion therapy.] Arzneimittelforschung 1979;29(8):1163–8.

34. Strobel E, Herrmann B. [On the problem of the passage of oxyphenbutazone into the fetal circulation and maternal milk.] Arzneimittelforschung 1962;12:302–5.

35. Farber D, Liel E. Phenylbutazon-Vergiftung in Kindesalter. Tadgl Prax 1968;9:231.

36. Polak F. Die hemmende Wirkung von Phenylbutazon auf die durch einige Antihypertonika hervorgerufene Blutdrucksenkung bei Hypertonikern. [The inhibitory effect of phenylbutazone on lowered blood pressure produced by antihypertensives in hypertensive patients.] Z Gesamte Inn Med 1967;22(12):375–6.

37. Lewis RJ, Trager WF, Chan KK, Breckenridge A, Orme M, Roland M, Schary W. Warfarin. Stereochemical aspects of its metabolism and the interaction with phenylbutazone. J Clin Invest 1974;53(6):1607–17.

38. O'Reilly RA, Goulart DA. Comparative interaction of sulfinpyrazone and phenylbutazone with racemic warfarin: alteration in vivo of free fraction of plasma warfarin. J Pharmacol Exp Ther 1981;219(3):691–4.

39. Aggeler PM, O'Reilly RA, Leong L, Kowitz PE. Potentiation of anticoagulant effect of warfarin by phenylbutazone. N Engl J Med 1967;276(9):496–501.

40. Field JB, Ohta M, Boyle C, Remer A. Potentiation of acetohexamide hypoglycemia by phenylbutazone. N Engl J Med 1967;277(17):889–94.

41. Shah SJ, Bhandarkar SD, Satoskar RS. Drug interaction between chlorpropamide and non-steroidal anti-inflammatory drugs, ibuprofen and phenylbutazone. Int J Clin Pharmacol Ther Toxicol 1984;22(9):470–2.

42. Szita M, Gachalyi B, Tornyossy M, Kaldor A. Interaction of phenylbutazone and tolbutamide in man. Int J Clin Pharmacol Ther Toxicol 1980;18(9):378–80.

43. Schulz E, Koch K, Schmidt FH. [Potentiation of the hypoglycemic effect of sulfonylurea derivatives by drugs. II. Pharmacokinetics and metabolism of glibenclamide (HB 419) in presence of phenylbutazone.] Eur J Clin Pharmacol 1971;4(1):32–7.

44. Levy RH. Cytochrome P450 isozymes and antiepileptic drug interactions. Epilepsia 1995;36(Suppl 5):S8–13.

45. Wardell WM. Drug displacement from protein binding: source of the sulphadoxine liberated by phenylbutazone. Br J Pharmacol 1971;43(2):325–34.

46. Aly FW, Hadam W, Kallee E, Kloss G. Veränderungen des freien Thyroxins unter kurzfristiger Phenylbutazon-Behandlung. Nucl -Med (Stuttg) 1970;(Suppl):195–8.

47. Bartha KG. Iodine kinetics of the organism under the influence of phenylbutazone. Acta Med Acad Sci Hung 1971;28(3):271–7.

Phenylephrine

General Information

Phenylephrine is seldom given systemically but is still commonly used as a mydriatic for both diagnostic and therapeutic purposes. Ocular application of phenylephrine 10% in pledget form is used to produce hemostasis in laser-assisted in-situ keratomileusis (LASIK) surgery and other ophthalmic surgical procedures. Phenylephrine is in some countries available in a non-prescription concentration of 0.12% for use as an ocular decongestant. Phenylephrine (up to 10 mg intramuscularly) has similar properties and uses to other alpha-adrenoceptor agonists.

The incidence of adverse effects is high with 10% phenylephrine, but less with lower concentrations. Systemic reactions also increase with increased frequency of use and when phenylephrine is applied in a pledget. The package inserts for 10% phenylephrine in the USA and Australia require that the drug should not be used more often than once an hour. A large number of severe systemic reactions, including death, have been reported in more than 20 articles in peer-reviewed ophthalmic journals. For this reason 10% phenylephrine eye-drops should be used with caution in patients with cardiac disease, significant hypertension, or advanced arteriosclerosis, and in frail elderly people.

It can never be emphasized enough that the eyes are a potential route for systemic drug administration. This has been illustrated by a British case of pulmonary edema in a child, apparently attributable to systemic absorption of phenylephrine eye-drops (1).

- An 8-year-old boy was admitted for unilateral retinal detachment surgery. Phenylephrine 2.5% and cyclopentolate 1% as premedication were prescribed but not given. In theatre the assistant surgeon administered 2–5 drops of 10% phenylephrine to the right eye. During the operation the boy developed bradycardia and was given glycopyrrolate, but shortly afterwards the systolic arterial pressure rose to 211 mmHg and the pulse rate to 160 beats/minute, with multifocal atrial and ventricular ectopic beats. Labetalol was given and the pulse and blood pressure fell to normal, but he then developed clinical and radiological signs of pulmonary edema, which resolved spontaneously.

The management of this case was subsequently criticized by correspondents in the same journal (2). They suggested that a lower ocular dose of phenylephrine should be used routinely, that oxymetazoline might in any case be safer, and that labetalol might have been hazardous, owing to its beta-blocking properties. In their reply the authors pointed out that they used the lowest concentration of phenylephrine available for ocular use, that oxymetazoline is not licensed for use as a mydriatic agent, and that the patient had tachycardia and ventricular extra beats, which made the beta-blocking properties of labetalol clinically desirable.

It is always wise to advocate nasolacrimal occlusion by digital compression of the lacrimal drainage system when using phenylephrine eye-drops in patients at risk or in patients in whom higher concentrations are necessary (3).

Organs and Systems

Cardiovascular

The FDA and the National Registry of Drug-induced Ocular Side Effects (Casey Eye Institute, Portland, Oregon) have received 11 reports of adverse systemic reactions to a single dose of topical ocular phenylephrine 10% applied in pledget form (4). There were eight men and three women, aged 1–76 years. Most of the patients noted systemic effects within minutes of applying phenylephrine, and the adverse systemic reactions included severe hypertension, pulmonary edema, cardiac dysrhythmias, cardiac arrest, and subarachnoid hemorrhage. Ophthalmologists should be warned not to apply phenylephrine in this way, which is believed to be contraindicated in ophthalmic surgery, especially when other medications may be used (SED-14, 1643).

A 10% solution of phenylephrine has sometimes caused extremely severe cardiovascular complications, including myocardial infarction.

In newborn infants the benefit of accurate assessment of gestational age by examination of the anterior vascular capsule of the lens and the value of funduscopic examination in ill premature babies must be weighed against the possible risks of the associated increase in blood pressure produced by the pupillary dilators. Since there is no increase in mydriatic effect with repeated instillation or increasing concentration, and their small body mass places premature neonates at increased risk of phenylephrine overdose, it is prudent to use the lowest possible concentration, as well as the most effective combination of mydriatics for indirect ophthalmoscopy in premature infants when such examination is absolutely necessary. The hypertensive effect is likely to be maximal at some time within the first 20 minutes, and whenever possible (or when risk factors are present) the blood pressure should be monitored.

- A child developed cardiac dysrhythmias, severe hypertension, and pulmonary edema after the intraoperative administration of ocular phenylephrine (1).
- A 2-month-old child given perioperative phenylephrine drops during cataract extraction developed ventricular extra beats, very severe hypertension, and pulmonary edema requiring intensive therapy (5). Extubation was possible within 3 hours, and she recovered with no untoward consequences.

The authors commented that changes in arterial blood pressure are well described with phenylephrine eye-drops, especially in infants. Clearly precise dosage is difficult in these very young patients and they suggested that microdrops might be a safer mode of administration.

Ear, nose, throat

When used as a nasal decongestant, phenylephrine can cause local nasal irritation and even perforation of the anterior nasal septum.

- A 69-year-old woman developed perforation of the nasal septum after overuse of a common over-the-counter nasal spray containing phenylephrine (6).

The authors attributed this effect to both vasoconstriction and physical irritation.

Nervous system

It has been suggested that sodium bisulfite, a preservative in phenylephrine solutions for injection, may have been responsible for transient neurological symptoms that have been observed in some patients (7). However, the original authors rejected this, since the dose of bisulfite was small and since there is uncertain evidence whether the compound is neurotoxic in any case. Another correspondent commented that tetracaine itself may be more toxic than other local anesthetics: the authors did not address this point in their reply (8).

Sensory systems

With phenylephrine, several cases of allergic blepharoconjunctivitis have been seen, even at low concentrations; the reaction begins 3–4 hours after drug application, persists for 12 hours, and regresses gradually within 72 hours

(9). Biopsy of the conjunctiva reveals marked infiltration with cells of various types; there is some evidence that a sensitization mechanism is involved.

However, blepharoconjunctivitis can occur (SEDA-17, 162), as can other complications.

- Acute periorbital dermatitis and conjunctivitis occurred in a 69-year-old man given phenylephrine 5% eye-drops for ophthalmological examination (10). Subsequent patch-testing was strongly positive for phenylephrine eye-drops.

There have been responses to last year's report of occurring after the addition of phenylephrine to tetracaine spinal anesthesia. It has been suggested that sodium bisulfite, a preservative in phenylephrine solutions for injection, may have been responsible for transient neurological symptoms that have been observed in some patients (7). However, the original authors rejected this, since the dose of bisulfite was small and since there is uncertain evidence whether the compound is neurotoxic in any case. Another correspondent commented that tetracaine itself may be more toxic than other local anesthetics: the authors did not address this point in their reply (8).

Skin

There have been a few reports of allergic contact dermatitis caused by phenylephrine, and little is known about cross-reactivity between the phenylephrine, adrenaline, and ephedrine.

- A 62-year-old man developed contact dermatitis after using phenylephrine eye-drops (Neosynerphin POS) (11). The inflammation affected both eyelids symmetrically and resolved rapidly on withdrawal of the eye-drops and application of topical glucocorticoids. Skin-testing confirmed hypersensitivity to phenylephrine but no cross-sensitization to ephedrine or adrenaline.

Immunologic

Phenylephrine was the drug that most often caused sensitization in patients with contact allergy after the application of mydriatic eye-drops. Since several eye-drops are often used in the same patient, it is always important to find out which drug or preservative is the allergen (10–13).

Long-Term Effects

Drug abuse

Abuse of alpha-adrenoceptor agonist nose-drops can cause a chronic rhinitis (14) and psychoses (15).

Susceptibility Factors

Phenylephrine should be used cautiously in elderly people and in patients with hypertension, coronary heart disease, aneurysms, and diabetic autonomic neuropathy (SEDA-21, 487).

Drug–Drug Interactions

Monoamine oxidase inhibitors

Patients taking monoamine oxidase inhibitors, anticholinergic drugs (such as tricyclic antidepressants), propranolol, reserpine, guanethidine, and methyldopa should be monitored closely if phenylephrine is used (SEDA-16, 542) (16).

Tetracaine

When phenylephrine was used together with tetracaine in spinal anesthesia, 10 of 80 patients developed transient dysesthesia (SEDA-22, 155). Provocation of myocardial ischemia (17), acute edema of the lung (18), and ischemic colitis (SEDA-22, 155) were not so clear-cut.

References

1. Baldwin FJ, Morley AP. Intraoperative pulmonary oedema in a child following systemic absorption of phenylephrine eyedrops. Br J Anaesth 2002;88(3):440–2.
2. Krovvidi H, Kulkarni PR. Management of intraoperative pulmonary oedema in a child following systemic absorption of phenylephrine eyedrops. Br J Anaesth 2002;89(2):343–4.
3. Hempel S, Senn P, Pakdaman F, Schmid MK, Suppiger M, Schipper I. Einfluss der Pupillenerweiterung mit Phenylephrin 5% auf das perioperative Kreislaufverhalten. [Perioperative circulatory side effects of topical 5% phenylephrine for mydriasis.] Klin Monatsbl Augenheilkd 1999;215(5):298–304.
4. Fraunfelder FW, Fraunfelder FT, Jensvold B. Adverse systemic effects from pledgets of topical ocular phenylephrine 10%. Am J Ophthalmol 2002;134(4):624–5.
5. Greher M, Hartmann T, Winkler M, Zimpfer M, Crabnor CM. Hypertension and pulmonary edema associated with subconjunctival phenylephrine in a 2-month-old child during cataract extraction. Anesthesiology 1998;88(5):1394–6.
6. Vilensky W. Illicit and licit drugs causing perforation of the nasal septum. J Forensic Sci 1982;27(4):958–62.
7. Tanaka M, Nishikawa T. Is phenylephrine of sodium bisulfite neurotoxic? Anesthesiology 1998;89(1):272–3.
8. Lambert DH. Transient neurologic symptoms when phenylephrine is added to tetracaine spinal anesthesia—an alternative. Anesthesiology 1998;89(1):273.
9. Mehelas TJ, Kollarits CR, Martin WG. Cystoid macular edema presumably induced by dipivefrin hydrochloride (Propine). Am J Ophthalmol 1982;94(5):682.
10. Wigger-Alberti W, Elsner P, Wuthrich B. Allergic contact dermatitis to phenylephrine. Allergy 1998;53(2):217–18.
11. Erdmann SM, Sachs B, Merk HF. Allergic contact dermatitis from phenylephrine in eyedrops. Am J Contact Dermat 2002;13(1):37–8.
12. Villarreal O. Reliability of diagnostic tests for contact allergy to mydriatic eyedrops. Contact Dermatitis 1998;38(3):150–4.
13. Rafael M, Pereira F, Faria MA. Allergic contact blepharoconjunctivitis caused by phenylephrine, associated with persistent patch test reaction. Contact Dermatitis 1998;39(3):143–4.
14. Bogacka E. Leki naczyniokurczace w leczeniu obturacji nosa. [Decongestants in treatment of nasal obstruction.] Otolaryngol Pol 1999;53(3):347–52.
15. Snow SS, Logan TP, Hollender MH. Nasal spray "addiction" and psychosis: a case report. Br J Psychiatry 1980;136:297–9.

16. Fraunfelder FT. Pupil dilation using phenylephrine alone or in combination with tropicamide. Ophthalmology 1999;106(1):4.

17. Hecker RB, Hays JV, Champ JD, Rubal BJ. Myocardial ischemia and stunning induced by topical intranasal phenylephrine pledgets. Mil Med 1997;162(12):832–5.

18. Benatar-Haserfaty J, Mariscal-Ortega A, Candela-Toha AM, Puig-Flores JA. Fenilefrina por via conjuntival y edema agudo de pulmon. [Conjunctival phenylephrine and acute edema of the lung.] Rev Esp Anestesiol Reanim 1997;44(7):287–9..

Phenylpropanolamine (norephedrine)

General Information

In the past, phenylpropanolamine was marketed extensively in over-the-counter products for a variety of indications, and dietary supplements were marketed with no premarket safety evaluation, at least by the Food and Drug Administration (FDA), since for dietary supplements that include an ingredient marketed in the USA before 15 October 1994 no FDA review is required. Because many of these products were promoted as foodstuffs, consumers may have assumed that they are safe (SEDA-21, 5). It has been used as an anorectic agent in doses of 3–25 mg/day.

However, adverse effects from therapeutic and toxic doses of phenylpropanolamine have often been reported (SEDA-9, 2) (SEDA-10, 3) (SEDA-11, 1), and recently it has been implicated as a cause of stroke and other neurological events. In November 2000, the US FDA asked all manufacturers to recall the product voluntarily.

Organs and Systems

Cardiovascular

Much of the concern over the free sale of phenylpropanolamine relates to its cardiovascular effects. Although the commonly recommended 75 mg dose has no significant effect on blood pressure in healthy volunteers, 150 mg causes significant albeit transient hypertension lasting several hours (1). Hypertensive crises have been reported, for example after a 600 mg overdose (SEDA-18, 158). However, field experience suggests that, because of individual variations in sensitivity, the risks to some patients are greater than these findings suggest. In single doses of 50 mg, phenylpropanolamine increased diastolic blood pressure to over 100 mmHg in 12% of adults.

Phenylpropanolamine can also, on occasion, cause cardiac dysrhythmias in mild overdosage.

A transient cardiomyopathy without hypertension occurred in a girl of 14 who had taken only a small overdose (2) and another in an adult woman (SEDA-17, 163).

A warning was issued by the Swiss Pharmaceutical Association that phenylpropanolamine can cause severe sympathomimetic adverse effects, including hypertensive crises, dysrhythmias, and tachycardia (3) (SEDA-5, 11) (SEDA-7, 12).

Nervous system

Although it has been thought to have relatively little stimulant effect on the central nervous system, phenylpropanolamine can produce restlessness, anxiety, insomnia, and tremor; its central stimulant effects are in practice often masked by manufacturers' practice of combining it with an antihistamine.

In a consecutive stroke registry since 1988, 22 patients (10 men and 12 women) had strokes associated with over-the-counter sympathomimetic drugs (4). There was intracerebral hemorrhage in 17, subarachnoid hemorrhage in 4, and ischemic stroke in 1. Stroke was associated with the use of phenylpropanolamine (75–675 mg) in 16 patients.

- Stroke occurred in an 8-year-old boy on chronic peritoneal dialysis after he took phenylpropanolamine (5). He developed occipital infarcts and was found to have extremely high concentrations of phenylpropanolamine in his blood and dialysis fluid. Although the voluntary recall was in effect, the family already had a bottle of phenylpropanolamine at home.

In a case-control study, 2078 men and women (702 patients and 1376 controls), age range 18–49 years, were recruited from 43 US hospitals if they had had a subarachnoid or intracerebral hemorrhage within 30 days before enrolment and no previously diagnosed brain lesion (6). For women, the adjusted odds ratio was 17 (95% CI = 1.5, 182) for the association between the use of appetite suppressants containing phenylpropanolamine and the risk of a hemorrhagic stroke. For men and women combined, the adjusted odds ratio was 16 (1.4, 184). The authors suggested that phenylpropanolamine in appetite suppressants is an independent risk factor for hemorrhagic stroke in women. There was a trend toward an increased risk of stroke with cough and cold remedies in women (OR = 3.1; CI = 0.9, 11).

- A 37-year-old woman took an over-the-counter formulation containing phenylpropanolamine 100 mg (7). About 90 minutes later she developed very severe bilateral headache resistant to analgesics. Her blood pressure was 180/100 mmHg but fell rapidly to 110/70 mmHg. A CT scan showed multiple small frontal and parietal hemorrhages, and angiography showed extensive segmental vasospasm. She was treated with nimodipine and prednisolone, followed by verapamil. She made an uneventful recovery, and there was angiographic resolution of the vascular lesions.

The authors reviewed a number of other case reports of phenylpropanolamine-induced cerebral vasospasm associated with hemorrhages and drew a parallel with similar effects of amfetamines.

Psychological, psychiatric

Psychosis has been attributed to phenylpropanolamine (8,9). Risk factors include symptoms or a history of mood spectrum disorder, a history of psychosis, female sex, and a family history of psychiatric disorder.

Although irritability and insomnia are frequent in adults, behavioral disturbances (restlessness, irritability, aggressiveness, and sleep disturbances), seizures, and delirium with hallucinations have been most often observed in children (SEDA-11, 1) (10).

Immunologic

Phenylpropanolamine can give rise to severe allergic reactions with dyspnea, urticaria, and facial swelling (11).

Long-Term Effects

Drug abuse

As with several other sympathomimetics, phenylpropanolamine is often sold illegally in special packages as a look-alike for more euphoriant/alerting stimulants. Both the absolute increase in use and the changes in the type of user have been associated with many reports of overdose consequences, including hypertension, cardiac dysrhythmias (SEDA-9, 10, 11), cerebral hemorrhage (SEDA-11, 2) (12,13), neuropsychiatric symptoms, including agitation and acute psychosis, and seizures (SEDA-9, 4) (14).

Susceptibility Factors

Age

Children appear to be sensitive to therapeutic doses of pseudoephedrine in the development of hallucinosis as well as irritability and insomnia syndromes (15,16).

Drug–Drug Interactions

Caffeine

Pharmacokinetic and pharmacodynamic interactions between caffeine 250 mg and phenylpropanolamine 25 mg have been investigated in six healthy subjects in a double-blind, placebo-controlled study. Coadministration of caffeine and phenylpropanolamine produced an additive increase in blood pressure, not attributable to a pharmacokinetic interaction and despite the fact that phenylpropanolamine attenuated the responses of adrenaline and renin to caffeine (17).

However, in another study in 16 healthy subjects who took caffeine 400 mg plus phenylpropanolamine 75 mg, the peak plasma–caffeine concentration was significantly higher than after caffeine alone. There were greater increases in both systolic and diastolic blood pressures, and adverse effects were more frequent after the combination than after either drug alone or after placebo (18).

Indinavir

A hypertensive crisis has been reported in a patient receiving triple therapy for HIV prophylaxis, including indinavir (19).

- A 28-year-old female medical resident was given zidovudine, lamivudine, and indinavir after a needle-stick injury involving an HIV-positive patient. She had a long history of sinus complaints and was taking a phenylpropanolamine-containing formulation intermittently. Ten days after starting prophylactic therapy she took phenylpropanolamine, although the dose was not stated, and 6 hours later developed right-sided headache, weakness of the left arm, and a blood pressure of 220/120 mmHg. CT and MRI scans of the brain were normal. Her blood pressure and neurological signs resolved during treatment with nimodipine and aspirin, though the weakness returned briefly.

It seems very likely that the protease inhibitor indinavir inhibited the metabolism of phenylpropanolamine by cytochrome P450 (predominantly CYP3A4), increasing circulating concentrations, and causing systemic and cerebral vasoconstriction.

Indometacin

Severe systemic hypertension developed in a patient who took indometacin shortly after taking an appetite suppressant (Trimolets) containing phenylpropanolamine (20). The hypertension was attributed to inhibition of prostaglandin synthesis by indometacin, which exacerbated the sympathomimetic effects of phenylpropanolamine. However, in 14 young, healthy, normotensive women who were randomized double-blind to modified-release phenylpropanolamine 75 mg/day or placebo for 4 days, modified-release indometacin 75 mg bd had no significant effect on mean systolic or diastolic blood pressures (21).

Neuroleptic drugs

Neuroleptic malignant-like syndrome has been reported when phenylpropanolamine was combined with neuroleptic drugs (22).

References

1. Lake CR, Zaloga G, Clymer R, Quirk RM, Chernow B. A double dose of phenylpropanolamine causes transient hypertension. Am J Med 1988;85(3):339–43.
2. Chin C, Choy M. Cardiomyopathy induced by phenylpropanolamine. J Pediatr 1993;123(5):825–7.
3. Anonymous. Norephedrin (Phenylpropanolamin) statt Nord-pseudoephedrin als Appetitzügler? Schweiz Apoth Ztg 1977;115:430.
4. Cantu C, Arauz A, Murillo-Bonilla LM, Lopez M, Barinagarrementeria F. Stroke associated with sympathomimetics contained in over-the-counter cough and cold drugs. Stroke 2003;34(7):1667–72.
5. Delorio NM. Cerebral infarcts in a pediatric patient secondary to phenylpropanolamine, a recalled medication. J Emerg Med 2004;26(3):305–7.
6. Kernan WN, Viscoli CM, Brass LM, Broderick JP, Brott T, Feldmann E, Morgenstern LB, Wilterdink JL, Horwitz RI. Phenylpropanolamine and the risk of hemorrhagic stroke. N Engl J Med 2000;343(25):1826–32.
7. Veyrac G, Huguenin H, Guillon B, Chiffoleau A, Thajte N, Bourin M, Jolliet P. Hémorragie cérébroméningée et angiopathie cérébrale aiguë associées à la prise de phénylopropanolamine: un nouveau cas. [Cerebral meningeal hemorrhage and acute cerebral angiopathy associated with the taking of phenylpropanolamine: a new case.] Therapie 2001;56(3):323–7.

8. Cornelius JR, Soloff PH, Reynolds CF 3rd. Paranoia, homicidal behavior, and seizures associated with phenylpropanolamine. Am J Psychiatry 1984;141(1):120–1.

9. Marshall RD, Douglas CJ. Phenylpropanolamine-induced psychosis: Potential predisposing factors. Gen Hosp Psychiatry 1994;16(5):358–60.

10. Dupuis L, Spielberg S. Oral decongestants: facts and fiction. On Contin Pract 1985;12:22.

11. Speer F, Carrasco LC, Kimura CC. Allergy to phenylpropanolamine. Ann Allergy 1978;40(1):32–4.

12. McDowell JR, LeBlanc HJ. Phenylpropanolamine and cerebral hemorrhage. West J Med 1985;142(5):688–91.

13. Kikta DG, Devereaux MW, Chandar K. Intracranial hemorrhages due to phenylpropanolamine. Stroke 1985;16(3):510–12.

14. Lake CR, Gallant S, Masson E, Miller P. Adverse drug effects attributed to phenylpropanolamine: a review of 142 case reports. AM J Med 1990;89(2):195–208.

15. Sankey RJ, Nunn AJ, Sills JA. Visual hallucinations in children receiving decongestants. Br Med J (Clin Res Ed) 1984;288(6427):1369.

16. Bain J. Visual hallucinations in children receiving decongestants. Br Med J 1984;288:1688.

17. Brown NJ, Ryder D, Branch RA. A pharmacodynamic interaction between caffeine and phenylpropanolamine. Clin Pharmacol Ther 1991;50(4):363–71.

18. Lake CR, Rosenberg DB, Gallant S, Zaloga G, Chernow B. Phenylpropanolamine increases plasma caffeine levels. Clin Pharmacol Ther 1990;47(6):675–85.

19. Khurana V, de la Fuente M, Bradley TP. Hypertensive crisis secondary to phenylpropanolamine interacting with triple-drug therapy for HIV prophylaxis. Am J Med 1999;106(1):118–19.

20. Lee KY, Beilin LJ, Vandongen R. Severe hypertension after ingestion of an appetite suppressant (phenylpropanolamine) with indomethacin. Lancet 1979;1(8126):1110–11.

21. McKenney JM, Wright JT Jr, Katz GM, Goodman RP. The effect of phenylpropanolamine on 24-hour blood pressure in normotensive subjects administered indomethacin. DICP 1991;25(3):234–9.

22. Castellani S. Catatonia associated with phenylpropanolamine overdose and fluphenazine treatment: case report. J Clin Psychiatry 1985;46(7):288–9.

Phenytoin and fosphenytoin

See also Antiepileptic drugs

General Information

Phenytoin is the only widely used hydantoin and, unless otherwise specified, effects discussed here refer to phenytoin. Other hydantoin derivatives include ethotoin (rINN), mephenytoin (rINN), and albutoin (rINN) (all of which are obsolete), and fosphenytoin (rINN). The latter is a water-soluble prodrug that is rapidly hydrolysed to phenytoin after intravenous or intramuscular injection. It causes fewer adverse reactions near the injection site (pain, phlebitis, tissue necrosis, purple hand syndrome) than phenytoin.

The effects of phenytoin have been studied in 39 patients with acute mania (1). One patient dropped out because of tachycardia and one required a dosage reduction because of nystagmus.

Comparative studies

Intravenous phenytoin and intravenous fosphenytoin have been compared in an open, randomized study in 256 emergency department patients who were given 279 doses (2). The mean phenytoin-equivalent dose was similar in the two groups. Adverse events occurred with similar frequencies, but slightly more often with fosphenytoin (phenytoin 9.1%, fosphenytoin 16%). The most common events were pruritus, pain on infusion, and paresthesia. Only one patient developed hypotension, with fosphenytoin. Thus, this study has not demonstrated obvious advantages of fosphenytoin.

General adverse reactions

Phenytoin can cause vestibulocerebellar, oculomotor, and cognitive dysfunction. It can also cause gingival hyperplasia, hirsutism, and acromegaly-like facial features. Movement disorders, symptoms of peripheral neuropathy, and endocrine changes are uncommon. Interstitial nephritis, interstitial pneumonia, and hepatotoxicity are rare. High intravenous doses are cardiotoxic.

Hypersusceptibility reactions

Hypersusceptibility reactions range from relatively common mild rashes to life-threatening Stevens–Johnson syndrome and toxic epidermal necrolysis. Hepatic, cardiac, muscular, pulmonary, hematological, reticuloendothelial, and renal reactions and systemic lupus erythematosus are uncommon.

Tumorigenesis

Pseudolymphoma and a condition resembling malignant lymphoma are very rare.

Organs and Systems

Cardiovascular

Intravenous phenytoin can cause cardiac dysrhythmias, hypotension, and potentially fatal cardiovascular collapse, especially if the highest recommended infusion rate (50 mg/minute or 1 mg/kg/minute in children) is exceeded. One case of hypersensitivity myocarditis was probably initiated by phenytoin, although carbamazepine may have contributed (SED-13, 142) (3).

After intravenous use, the most common vascular complication is the so-called purple-glove or purple-limb syndrome, defined as the progressive development of edema, discoloration, and pain in the limb; sequelae include soft-tissue necrosis and limb ischemia. Retrospective analysis of data from 152 patients treated with intravenous phenytoin identified nine (6%) who developed this syndrome: they had received a greater mean initial dose of phenytoin (500 versus 300 mg) and a larger dose over 24 hours (800 versus 500 mg), and they tended to be older (72 versus 49 years) than those without the complication (4). In one case surgical therapy was required; the others resolved conservatively within 1 month. Extravasation of intravenously injected phenytoin has caused tissue necrosis requiring amputation (SEDA-18, 67). Purple glove syndrome has generally been reported after intravenous phenytoin.

- In a 49-year-old otherwise healthy woman undergoing craniotomy for aneurysm clipping, inadvertent overdose with phenytoin (1500 mg) by rapid infusion caused intraoperative sinus arrest, which was managed successfully with standard resuscitative measures (5).

This report highlights the cardiovascular risk of intravenous phenytoin, particularly when high infusion rates are used.

However, the purple-glove syndrome can also occasionally occur after oral administration.

- A 10-year-old boy took phenytoin 100 mg/day and his seizures were well controlled (6). However, a pharmacist gave him about 1000 mg of phenytoin instead of the prescribed dose, and several hours later he became drowsy and his hands and feet turned dark purple with marked swelling. Phenytoin was withdrawn after 4 days and the swelling and discoloration of his hands and feet improved gradually and disappeared 11 days later.

The incidence of purple-glove syndrome associated with intravenous phenytoin has been assessed in a prospective review of 179 consecutive exposures (7). There were only three mild cases (1.7%).

However, the purple-limb syndrome was recorded in 20 of 67 patients who received intravenous phenytoin over a 5-month period (8). Affected cases tended to be older (median age 70 years versus 57 years in non-affected cases), and all resolved spontaneously within 3 weeks. These data suggest that the incidence of the syndrome may have been underestimated in the past, possibly owing to its delayed onset, frequent occurrence in patients with impaired communication abilities, and its usually mild self-limiting course.

In 775 patients who received intravenous phenytoin, valproate, or placebo, intravenous site reactions occurred in 25% of patients who received phenytoin (9). Most of the events (70%) occurred in the first intravenous site, and all occurred in peripheral administration sites. When patients who received the drug by central line were excluded, the estimated incidence was 30%. There were fewer adverse events when phenytoin was given alone than when it was given together with valproate.

Fosphenytoin-induced QT interval prolongation has been reported (10).

- A 23-year-old man was given intravenous fosphenytoin (equivalent to phenytoin 1500 mg or 20.5 mg/kg) over 85 minutes. He was normocalcemic before the infusion. During the infusion he had prolongation of the QT interval and reductions in the concentrations of total and ionized serum calcium. Plasma phenytoin concentrations were within the target range during the electrocardiographic changes, and the blood pressure was stable.

Fosphenytoin is metabolized by phosphatases to yield phenytoin plus inorganic phosphate. Binding of calcium by phosphate could have lowered the serum concentration of ionized calcium.

Respiratory

Interstitial pneumonitis is extremely rare with phenytoin (11). The clinical features are fever, dyspnea, hypoxemia, and bilateral radiographic infiltrates. It responds to

withdrawal and corticosteroids. Bronchiolitis obliterans organizing pneumonia in the context of a severe hypersensitivity syndrome also improved rapidly with high-dose steroids (SEDA-22, 90).

Nervous system

Ataxia, dysarthria, fatigue, dizziness, tremor, and nystagmus are relatively common in patients with phenytoin intoxication. Sedation occurs only at high serum drug concentrations; however, toxic effects at relatively low serum concentrations can occur when drug binding to plasma proteins is impaired (SEDA-18, 67). Uncommon effects include seizure exacerbation (12), reversible monoplegia or hemiplegia (13), reversible spastic rigidity, hyper-reflexia and clonus, hyperkinetic disorders, choreoathetosis (14), hemiballismus (15), hemichoreiform movements, local dystonia in the foot, myoclonus (16), and reversible parkinsonism (SED-13, 143).

- A 13-year-old girl developed left partial motor status epilepticus with severe postictal hemiparesis (15). An MRI scan showed a right frontoparietal hyperintense T2-weighted signal. Treatment with phenytoin, carbamazepine, and phenobarbital caused the seizures to abate but left choreic-like flinging movements, consistent with hemiballismus, 2 days later. On phenytoin withdrawal, the symptoms gradually abated, with mild residual dystonia at 14 months.

The authors speculated that the lesion might have rendered the cortex more susceptible to phenytoin, causing unilateral toxicity.

Three patients with severe myoclonic epilepsy in infancy developed choreoathetosis after an increase in phenytoin dosage; it resolved when the phenytoin dosage was reduced (17). In one, an ictal SPECT showed reduced perfusion in the basal ganglia contralateral to the unilateral choreoathetosis. Polypharmacy, including carbamazepine and zonisamide, may have facilitated the onset of choreoathetosis.

Phenytoin can aggravate symptoms and worsen outcome in patients with Baltic myoclonic epilepsy (SED-13, 140) (18) and susceptibility to neurological complications can be increased in patients with organic brain disorders.

Long-term phenytoin can cause cerebellar degeneration, but this is probably rare (SED-13, 143) (19), (SEDA-19, 73); irreversible cerebellar atrophy after acute intoxication is extremely rare (SEDA-21, 73).

- Distal lower extremity paresthesia in stocking distribution and motor weakness with loss of the Achilles tendon reflex, associated with reduced sensory conduction velocity, occurred in an 18-year-old girl a few hours after the administration of phenytoin (7.5 mg/kg) (20). The condition regressed after phenytoin withdrawal.

Peripheral neuropathy is a known adverse effect of phenytoin, but this is the first report of an acute neuropathy within less than 1 week of treatment.

Cerebellar atrophy has been reported in association with phenytoin intoxication (21).

Pre-existing myasthenia gravis can be aggravated by phenytoin (SEDA-7, 78).

Sensory systems

Taste

- Ageusia occurred in a 52-year-old man within a few hours of an intravenous infusion of phenytoin 750 mg for the control of seizures (22). The condition persisted for 2 weeks during oral phenytoin treatment and cleared in about 1 week when phenobarbital was substituted.

The time course in this case strongly suggested that phenytoin was responsible.

Psychological, psychiatric

Phenytoin has been implicated in psychiatric adverse effects with or without other signs of toxicity, and at serum concentrations above or below the upper limit of the target range, but the actual incidence of these reactions is unknown (23).

- A 9-year-old boy with seizures developed intermittent complex visual hallucinations during therapy with fosphenytoin and, on a separate occasion, carbamazepine (24).

Five patients with Down's syndrome and dementia, aged 44–67 years, taking phenytoin had progressive cognitive decline (25). This resolved once the drug was withdrawn. Cognitive decline was not related to high serum concentrations. Older patients with Down's syndrome might be especially sensitive to the effects of phenytoin.

Endocrine

Phenytoin can cause a rise in growth hormone concentration (26).

Phenytoin can cause acromegaly-like facial features, possibly related to its osteogenic actions (SEDA-20, 65).

Hematologic

Megaloblastic anemia and pancytopenia have been rarely attributed to phenytoin (27,28), whereas aplastic anemia has been observed with mephenytoin (29).

Single cases of a hemophilia-like disorder (SED-13, 144) (30), hemolytic anemia associated with renal insufficiency (31), and pure red cell aplasia (SED-12, 129) (32), have been reported.

Mouth and teeth

Gingival hyperplasia is a well-known adverse effect of phenytoin. It occurs in at least one-third of patients, although it can be prevented by careful dental hygiene (SED-13, 144) (33), and does not occur in edentulous mouths. In one case generalized palatal hyperplasia occurred in a patient in whom retained roots and teeth were suspected of having perpetuated a pre-extraction lesion; a subsequently placed complete denture initiated a midpalatal hyperplasia (34).

In 114 patients, of whom 20% took phenytoin, 5 taking phenytoin had gingival hyperplasia (35), which can on occasion be extensive.

- A 17-year-old boy took phenytoin 300 mg/day unsupervised for 2 years and developed coarsening of the facial features, extensive gingival hyperplasia, and cerebellar ataxia (36). The gingival hyperplasia resolved within 3 months of withdrawal but the ataxia persisted.

Gastrointestinal

Phenytoin was implicated in a case of reversible hypertrophy of the submandibular salivary gland, but cause and effect were speculative (SEDA-18, 67).

Liver

Chronic hepatitis is rarely caused by phenytoin (SEDA-18, 67). When it occurs, the signs of hepatotoxicity usually appear after 1–8 weeks in acute cases, and after 4 months to several years in chronic cases (37). Among 16 acute cases, there was fever in 75%, rash in 63%, jaundice in 44%, hepatomegaly in 13%, and lymphadenopathy and splenomegaly in 60% (37). Less common symptoms included sore throat, malaise, chills, myalgia, and pruritus. The condition can be fatal.

- A 51-year-old woman developed hepatitis while taking phenytoin 300 mg/day (38).

The authors did not discuss the possible role of paracetamol, which was co-administered in a dosage of 4 g/day (see Paracetamol section under Drug–Drug Interactions in this monograph).

Urinary tract

There has been one report of autoimmune interstitial nephritis associated with tubular deposits of phenytoin and circulating antitubular basement-membrane antibodies (SED-13, 144) (39).

Skin

Acne and hirsutism are not uncommon in patients taking phenytoin. Of 61 women who had taken phenytoin 100–300 mg/day for 1–5 years, more than half had coarse facial features from a combination of several degrees of acne, hirsutism, and gingival hyperplasia (40).

Skin rashes occur in about 10% of patients. They are generally mild and their incidence varies seasonally (SED-13, 144) (41).

Diffuse fasciitis with eosinophilia (a variant of scleroderma) (42), reversible nodular cutaneous pseudolymphoma, acromelanosis (43), hypertrophic retroauricular folds, and severe forms of erythema multiforme (Stevens–Johnson syndrome and toxic epidermal necrolysis) (44,45) are all rare (SED-13, 144) (SEDA-22, 90) (33).

- Toxic epidermal necrolysis has been reported in a 28-year-old woman who had taken phenytoin for 20 days (46). Phenytoin was cytotoxic in vitro to the patient's lymphocytes.
- A 49-year-old man with post-traumatic epilepsy taking phenytoin developed severe rhinophyma; he also had gingival hyperplasia (47).

Nothing in the history of this case pointed definitively to a cause and effect association.

Subacute cutaneous lupus erythematosus has been reported in a patient taking phenytoin (48).

- A 73-year-old woman who had taken phenytoin for 5 years developed erythematous, macular, annular lesions over her upper chest, back, and arms. She was also taking propafenone and nifedipine. Routine hematology and biochemistry were normal, except for leukopenia and a raised gamma-glutamyltranspeptidase. There were no antinuclear antibodies, but antibodies against Ro, La, and histone proteins were detectable. A skin biopsy was consistent with subacute cutaneous lupus erythematosus. She was given topical steroids, and all medications, apart from phenytoin, were withdrawn. However, as her eruption persisted, the phenytoin was tapered and withdrawn. Her rash cleared within 6 months. Over the next year there was no photosensitivity or recurrence, but Ro and La antibodies remained positive.

Interpretation of this report is confounded by the presence of concomitant treatments and the lack of quick resolution of the symptoms on phenytoin withdrawal. Furthermore, the autoantibodies did not normalize at 6 months.

Reproductive system

- An 18-year-old man with heterozygous point mutation in the defective allele of CYP2C9 and CYP2C19 (two enzymes involved in phenytoin metabolism) developed gynecomastia about 1 month after phenytoin dosage was increased from 175 to 190 mg/day, resulting in a serum phenytoin concentration of 68 µmol/l (49).

Phenytoin has been rarely implicated in gynecomastia, and whether the cytochrome P450 genotype played a contributory role was unclear. The patient was also taking zonisamide, which has also rarely been associated with gynecomastia.

Immunologic

The phenytoin hypersensitivity syndrome ranges from a simple rash to a fulminant fatal illness with exfoliative dermatitis, vasculitis, and disseminated intravascular coagulation. Features include variable combinations of fever, eosinophilia, lymphadenopathy, hepatosplenomegaly, atypical lymphocytes, blood dyscrasias, serum sickness, hepatitis, and renal insufficiency.

Angioimmunoblastic lymphadenopathy, systemic lupus erythematosus, polymyositis, and serum sickness have been noted in individual cases (SED-13, 144) (50,51).

IgA depression is seen in about 10% of patients (52). There has been one report of deficiency of IgG2 and IgG4 (SEDA-17, 73) and one of panhypogammaglobulinemia (SEDA-16, 73).

- A 32-year-old man developed acute lung injury and renal insufficiency after 4 days of starting to take phenytoin (53). The symptoms mimicked a renopulmonary syndrome, and resolved completely after withdrawal of phenytoin and the addition of steroids.

Giant cell myocarditis has been reported in a patient taking phenytoin, phenobarbital, and mephobarbital and in one taking primidone (54).

Lupus-like syndrome has been attributed to phenytoin (55).

- A 67-year-old white man who had taken phenytoin 300 mg/day for about 15 years developed fever, pericarditis, severe abdominal pain, malaise, and weight loss. He had a positive antinuclear antibody in a titer of 1:80 in a homogeneous pattern, a strongly positive antihistone antibody test, a raised erythrocyte sedimentation rate (115 mm/hour), and a neutrophilia (21×10^9/l). All these abnormalities resolved within a few weeks of withdrawal. Rechallenge was not performed.

The long delay between the start of therapy in this case and the clinical presentation makes it highly likely that phenytoin was not implicated and that recovery was spontaneous.

There has been a report of hypersensitivity to phenytoin (which had been previously well tolerated) after a hypersensitivity reaction to carbamazepine (56).

- A 19-year-old man with partial epilepsy took phenytoin 300 mg/day for over 6 months. Carbamazepine was introduced and after about 6 weeks (while taking phenytoin 300 mg/day and carbamazepine 600 mg/day) he developed fever, anorexia, a sore throat, bloody diarrhea, a diffuse, erythematous, maculopapular rash and palatal petechiae, tender cervical lymphadenopathy, and mild splenomegaly. His liver enzymes were raised and he had a leukocytosis with eosinophilia. Phenytoin and carbamazepine were withdrawn, and he was given prednisone and sodium valproate 1000 mg/day. The rash resolved, as did other manifestations of what was thought to be a hypersensitivity reaction. About a year later, phenytoin was reintroduced starting at 100 mg/day. He developed a sore throat after taking the first dose and a widespread rash after the second dose. There was no evidence of hepatic or hematological dysfunction. Phenytoin was withdrawn and the rash resolved in 1 week.

Cross-sensitivity among aromatic antiepileptic drugs occurs in about 50% of patients with a hypersensitivity reaction. It has previously been described on first exposure to each of the offending drugs (57). However, this patient developed an allergic rash on his second exposure to phenytoin, having previously tolerated it for 6 months. This suggests that carbamazepine may have altered his response to phenytoin.

Long-Term Effects

Mutagenicity

Neuroblastoma has been rarely reported in association with the fetal hydantoin syndrome. Phenytoin can cause pseudolymphoma and rarely a condition resembling malignant lymphoma (SED-13, 142). Pseudolymphoma is usually characterized by lymphadenopathy, fever, and a diffuse erythematous macular skin eruption, although a presentation without fever and rash has been described (SEDA-20, 65).

Tumorigenicity

Pseudolymphomatous reactions, pseudomalignant histiocytosis, a reaction resembling mycosis fungoides, and malignant lymphoma have been noted in individual cases (SED-13, 144) (58,59).

Susceptibility Factors

Genetic factors

- A 40-year-old man who developed toxic signs and a high serum phenytoin concentration (130 μmol/l) on a low dosage (187.5 mg/day) was found to be heterozygous for the Leu359 allele of CYP2C9 and for the *3 allele of CYP2C19 (60).

Phenytoin is metabolized by both cytochromes and the mutations probably explained the adverse reaction.

Other features of the patient

Patients receiving cranial irradiation and patients with malignant gliomas may be at particular risk of severe skin reactions to phenytoin (SEDA-18, 68) (SEDA-20, 58). Neurological adverse effects can be enhanced in patients with a recent history of severe traumatic brain injury.

Several reports have suggested that patients with brain tumors who undergo radiation therapy while taking phenytoin may be at increased risk of developing Stevens–Johnson syndrome. A 47-year-old black man (61) and four other patients, including one who died (62), were seen in a 24-month period in one department. A review of 20 similar reported cases showed no relation to the dosage of phenytoin or radiation therapy, or to the histological type of the tumor.

Drug Administration

Drug contamination

Phenytoin poisoning has been reported in a patient who took Chinese proprietary medicines containing phenytoin, carbamazepine, and valproate (63). The manufacturer's information leaflet did not mention any of these prescription drugs.

Drug administration route

Intravenous phenytoin has been associated with fatal hemodynamic complications and serious reactions at the injection site, including skin necrosis and amputation of extremities. Fosphenytoin, a phenytoin prodrug, has the same pharmacological properties but none of the injection site and cardiac rhythm complications after intravenous administration (64).

The extent of absorption and tolerability of intramuscular fosphenytoin has been assessed in a double-blind study in which patients received 10 mg/kg dose of intramuscular fosphenytoin in one gluteus muscle and intramuscular saline in the other (65). More than half the patients had serum concentrations in the target range at 30 minutes. There was no pain at either the fosphenytoin or saline injection sites in 46% of patients and no difference in pain at 60 minutes and thereafter.

Drug overdose

The saturable kinetics of phenytoin results in an increased half-life in overdose and a protracted clinical course, which can last a week or more (66). The most common initial finding in mild toxicity is nystagmus. As concentrations increase, ataxia, decreased coordination, hyperreflexia, slurred speech, and diplopia can occur. Progressive increases result in confusion, lethargy, and coma. Various attempts to increase elimination, including dialysis, hemoperfusion, diuresis, and plasmapheresis, have been ineffective and are not without risk. Meticulous supportive care, including ventilation if necessary, should provide a good clinical outcome. Multiple-dose activated charcoal may be helpful in shortening the duration of symptoms.

Severe poisoning in a hypoalbuminemic neonate responded unusually to peritoneal dialysis, possibly because of reduced phenytoin binding to plasma proteins (SEDA-16, 73).

Serum phenytoin concentrations in overdose have been studied in nine patients aged 20–66 years (67). The serum phenytoin concentrations were initially 136–230 μmol/l and fell linearly (that is with zero-order kinetics); the elimination rate varied from 19 to 41 μmol/l/day. In those with the highest serum concentrations at presentation there was a delay before the fall in concentrations began.

- The apparent effectiveness of charcoal hemoperfusion has been reported in a 19-year-old woman who took about 5 g of phenytoin (68). The plasma concentrations of total and unbound phenytoin fell rapidly, from 160 and 14 μmol/l to 65 and 6 μmol/l respectively, after 3 hours of hemoperfusion. The total phenytoin half-life was 3.9 hours. The protein-bound fraction was constant (91%) throughout.

Drug–Drug Interactions

Atorvastatin

In a 50-year-old woman with familial hypercholesterolemia and epilepsy, the addition of phenytoin caused a marked reduction in the lipid response to atorvastatin, an effect that was reversible after withdrawal of the anticonvulsant (69). It is likely that phenytoin reduced the efficacy of atorvastatin by inducing its metabolism.

Cimetidine

The combined use of cimetidine and phenytoin led to severe thrombocytopenia in four of 1512 neurosurgical patients (70).

Cyclophosphamide

In three patients treated with cyclophosphamide, phenytoin co-medication increased the formation of the S-enantiomer (but not the R-enantiomer) of the dechloroethylated cyclophosphamide metabolite (71). The findings also suggested that phenytoin increased the clearance of both R- and S-cyclophosphamide to 4-hydroxycyclophosphamide (the activation pathway). The clinical relevance of these findings is unclear.

Isradipine

Isradipine, an inhibitor of CYP450, provoked phenytoin intoxication in one patient (72).

Lamotrigine

Choreoathetosis is a rare adverse effect of some anticonvulsants, but has especially been associated with phenytoin. In a retrospective survey, three of 39 adults and one of 38 children developed choreoathetosis acutely when lamotrigine was added to phenytoin or vice versa (73). The effect was reversible by withdrawing one of the drugs. It was calculated that the risk of choreoathetosis is increased more than 50-fold when these drugs are combined, possibly owing to a pharmacodynamic interaction.

Losartan

The interaction of losartan with phenytoin has been studied in a randomized, crossover study in 16 healthy volunteers (74). Losartan, a CYP2C9 substrate, had no effect on the pharmacokinetics of phenytoin. However, phenytoin inhibited the CYP2C9-mediated conversion of losartan to its active metabolite, thus potentially reducing its efficacy.

Nelfinavir

In a 30-year-old man stabilized on phenytoin, the addition of nelfinavir was associated with a fall in serum phenytoin concentration and seizure recurrence (75). However, other drugs were also added or withdrawn during the observation period and the role of nelfinavir in this possible interaction is speculative.

Paracetamol

It has been proposed that phenytoin can exacerbate the hepatotoxic effects of paracetamol (76).

- A 55-year-old woman with a community-acquired pneumonia had unexplained moderate rises in hepatic enzyme activities while taking paracetamol 1300–6200 mg/day and phenytoin 350 mg/day. Paracetamol was withdrawn, and her chemistry normalized within 2 weeks.

The authors suggested that induction of CYP3A4 by phenytoin had encouraged the formation of a hepatotoxic metabolite of paracetamol.

Simvastatin

- In a 50-year-old woman with familial hypercholesterolemia and epilepsy, the addition of phenytoin caused a marked reduction in the lipid response to simvastatin, an effect that was reversible after withdrawal of the anticonvulsant (69).

It is likely that phenytoin reduced the efficacy of simvastatin by inducing its metabolism.

Ticlopidine

A careful study in six patients showed that ticlopidine 250 mg bd caused a two-fold increase in the Michaelis–Menten constant of phenytoin, indicating inhibition of phenytoin metabolism (77). These results are consistent with the known inhibitory activity of ticlopidine on CYP2C19, and suggest that phenytoin dosage requirements can be reduced by ticlopidine.

Valproate

The pharmacokinetic interaction of phenytoin with valproate is complicated (78–80). Initially, the total serum phenytoin concentration falls, because valproate displaces phenytoin from protein binding sites and so the unbound fraction increases, with a consequent increase in clearance. Because of the change in unbound fraction the total plasma concentration effect curve is shifted to the left, and a lower total concentration is as effective as the total phenytoin concentration was in the absence of valproate. However, valproate also inhibits the metabolism of phenytoin and so the serum phenytoin concentration then starts to rise and there is a risk of toxicity.

Phenytoin reduces serum valproate concentrations by inducing its metabolism (81). This may cause the formation of a hepatotoxic metabolite of valproate (82).

In 775 patients who received intravenous phenytoin, valproate, or placebo, intravenous site reactions occurred in 25% of patients who received phenytoin (9). Most of the events (70%) occurred in the first intravenous site, and all occurred in peripheral administration sites. When patients who received the drug by central line were excluded, the estimated incidence was 30%. There were more adverse events when phenytoin was given together with valproate than when it was given alone.

Food–Drug Interactions

The interaction of oral phenytoin with enteral feeding formulations has been reviewed (83). Four prospective, randomized, controlled trials in healthy volunteers showed no interaction. However, numerous anecdotal reports and studies have shown dramatic reductions in serum phenytoin concentrations in patients receiving enteral feeding formulations. The authors therefore concluded that this interaction occurs in patients but not in healthy volunteers.

Diagnosis of Adverse Drug Reactions

The usual target range for plasma concentrations is 40–80 µmol/l (10–20 µg/ml).

References

1. Mishory A, Yaroslavsky Y, Bersudsky Y, Belmaker RH. Phenytoin as an antimanic anticonvulsant: a controlled study. Am J Psychiatry 2000;157(3):463–5.
2. Coplin WM, Rhoney DH, Rebuck JA, Clements EA, Cochran MS, O'Neil BJ. Randomized evaluation of adverse events and length-of-stay with routine emergency department use of phenytoin or fosphenytoin. Neurol Res 2002;24(8):842–8.
3. Taliercio CP, Olney BA, Lie JT. Myocarditis related to drug hypersensitivity. Mayo Clin Proc 1985;60(7):463–8.

4. O'Brien TJ, Cascino GD, So EL, Hanna DR. Incidence and clinical consequence of the purple glove syndrome in patients receiving intravenous phenytoin. Neurology 1998; 51(4):1034–9.

5. Berry JM, Kowalski A, Fletcher SA. Sudden asystole during craniotomy: unrecognized phenytoin toxicity. J Neurosurg Anesthesiol 1999;11(1):42–5.

6. Yoshikawa H, Abe T, Oda Y. Purple glove syndrome caused by oral administration of phenytoin. J Child Neurol 2000;15(11):762.

7. Burneo JG, Anandan JV, Barkley GL. A prospective study of the incidence of the purple glove syndrome. Epilepsia 2001;42(9):1156–9.

8. Meara FM, O'Brien TJ, Cook MJ, Vajda FJ. Prospective study of the incidence of local cutaneous reactions (the purple limb syndrome) in patients receiving i.v. phenytoin. Epilepsia 1999;40(Suppl 7):145.

9. Anderson GD, Lin Y, Temkin NR, Fischer JH, Winn HR. Incidence of intravenous site reactions in neurotrauma patients receiving valproate or phenytoin. Ann Pharmacother 2000;34(6):697–702.

10. Keegan MT, Bondy LR, Blackshear JL, Lanier WL. Hypocalcemia-like electrocardiographic changes after administration of intravenous fosphenytoin. Mayo Clin Proc 2002;77(6):584–6.

11. Michael JR, Rudin ML. Acute pulmonary disease caused by phenytoin. Ann Intern Med 1981;95(4):452–4.

12. Osorio I, Burnstine TH, Remler B, Manon-Espaillat R, Reed RC. Phenytoin-induced seizures: a paradoxical effect at toxic concentrations in epileptic patients. Epilepsia 1989;30(2):230–4.

13. Abdulhadi MH, Notman DD, Cardon GC, Johnston PM. Phenytoin toxicity: a cause of reversible monoplegia. Cleve Clin J Med 1987;54(5):438–9.

14. Haider Y, Abbott RJ. Phenytoin-induced choreoathetosis. Postgrad Med J 1990;66(782):1089.

15. Micheli F, Lehkuniec E, Gatto M, Pelli M, Asconape J. Hemiballism in a patient with partial motor status epilepticus treated with phenytoin. Funct Neurol 1993;8(2):103–7.

16. Duarte J, Sempere AP, Cabezas MC, Marcos J, Claveria LE. Postural myoclonus induced by phenytoin. Clin Neuropharmacol 1996;19(6):536–8.

17. Saito Y, Oguni H, Awaya Y, Hayashi K, Osawa M. Phenytoin-induced choreoathetosis in patients with severe myoclonic epilepsy in infancy. Neuropediatrics 2001; 32(5):231–5.

18. Eldridge R, Iivanainen M, Stern R, Koerber T, Wilder BJ. "Baltic" myoclonus epilepsy: hereditary disorder of childhood made worse by phenytoin. Lancet 1983;2(8354):838–42.

19. Koller WC, Glatt SL, Fox JH. Phenytoin-induced cerebellar degeneration. Ann Neurol 1980;8(2):203–4.

20. Yoshikawa H, Abe T, Oda Y. Extremely acute phenytoin-induced peripheral neuropathy. Epilepsia 1999; 40(4):528–9.

21. Hironishi M. [Cerebellar atrophy associated with phenytoin intoxication.] No To Shinkei 2000;52(3):264–5.

22. Zeller JA, Machetanz J, Kessler C. Ageusia as an adverse effect of phenytoin treatment. Lancet 1998; 351(9109):1101.

23. Wong I, Tavernor S, Tavernor R. Psychiatric adverse effects of anticonvulsant drugs: incidence and therapeutic implications. CNS Drugs 1997;8:492–509.

24. Nousiainen I, Kalviainen R, Mantyjarvi M. Color vision in epilepsy patients treated with vigabatrin or carbamazepine monotherapy. Ophthalmology 2000;107(5):884–8.

25. Tsiouris JA, Patti PJ, Tipu O, Raguthu S. Adverse effects of phenytoin given for late-onset seizures in adults with Down syndrome. Neurology 2002;59(5):779–80.

26. Franceschi M, Perego L, Cavagnini F, Cattaneo AG, Invitti C, Caviezel F, Strambi LF, Smirne S. Effects of long–term antiepileptic therapy on the hypothalamic–pituitary axis in man. Epilepsia 1984;25(1):46–52.

27. Hawkins CF, Meynell MJ. Megaloblastic anaemia due to phenytoin sodium. Lancet 1954;267(6841):737–8.

28. Iivanainen M, Savolainen H. Side effects of phenobarbital and phenytoin during long-term treatment of epilepsy. Acta Neurol Scand Suppl 1983;97:49–67.

29. Troupin AS, Ojemann LM, Dodrill CB. Mephenytoin: a reappraisal. Epilepsia 1976;17(4):403–14.

30. O'Reilly RA, Hamilton RD. Acquired hemophilia, meningioma, and diphenylhydantoin therapy. J Neurosurg 1980;53(5):600–5.

31. Yoshida K, Takeda K, Asano Y, Hosoda S. Diphenylhydantoin induced hemolytic anemia and acute renal failure. Jpn J Med 1980;19:202.

32. Kaku K, Kawakatsu S, Matsumoto N, Miwa S. Pure red cell aplasia and diphenylhydantoin. Bull Yamaguchi Med Sch 1980;27:33.

33. Schmidt D. Adverse Effects of Antiepileptic Drugs. New York: Raven Press, 1982.

34. Dreyer WP, Thomas CJ. Diphenylhydantoinate-induced hyperplasia of the masticatory mucosa in an edentulous epileptic patient. Oral Surg Oral Med Oral Pathol 1978;45(5):701–6.

35. Adamolekun B, Mielke J, Ball D, Mundanda T. An evaluation of the management of epilepsy by primary health care nurses in Chitungwiza, Zimbabwe. Epilepsy Res 2000;39(3):177–81.

36. Sharma S, Dasroy SK. Images in clinical medicine. Gingival hyperplasia induced by phenytoin. N Engl J Med 2000;342(5):325.

37. Mullick FG, Ishak KG. Hepatic injury associated with diphenylhydantoin therapy. A clinicopathologic study of 20 cases. Am J Clin Pathol 1980;74(4):442–52.

38. Colombo-Arnet E. Phenytoin-induzierte Hypersensitivitätsreaktion mit Leberversagen. [Phenytoin-induced hypersensitivity reaction with liver failure.] Schweiz Rundsch Med Prax 2000;89(16):675–7.

39. Hyman LR, Ballow M, Knieser MR. Diphenylhydantoin interstitial nephritis. Roles of cellular and humoral immunologic injury. J Pediatr 1978;92(6):915–20.

40. Trevisol-Bittencourt PC, da Silva VR, Molinari MA, Troiano AR. Phenytoin as the first option in female epileptic patients? Arq Neuropsiquiatr 1999;57(3B):784–6.

41. Leppik IE, Lapora J, Loewenson R. Seasonal incidence of phenytoin allergy unrelated to plasma levels. Arch Neurol 1985;42(2):120–2.

42. Buchanan RR, Gordon DA, Muckle TJ, McKenna F, Kraag G. The eosinophilic fasciitis syndrome after phenytoin (Dilantin) therapy. J Rheumatol 1980;7(5):733–6.

43. Kanwar AJ, Jaswal R, Thami GP, Bedi GK. Acquired acromelanosis due to phenytoin. Dermatology 1997; 194(4):373–4.

44. Janinis J, Panagos G, Panousaki A, Skarlos D, Athanasiou E, Karpasitis N, Pirounaki M. Stevens–Johnson syndrome and epidermal necrolysis after administration of sodium phenytoin with cranial irradiation. Eur J Cancer 1993;29A(3):478–9.

45. Schmidt D, Kluge W. Fatal toxic epidermal necrolysis following reexposure to phenytoin: a case report. Epilepsia 1983;24(4):440–3.

46. Eisen ER, Fish J, Shear NH. Management of drug-induced toxic epidermal necrolysis. J Cutan Med Surg 2000;4(2):96–102.

47. Jaramillo MJ, Stewart KJ, Kolhe PS. Phenytoin induced rhinophyma treated by excision and full thickness skin grafting. Br J Plast Surg 2000;53(6):521–3.

48. Ross S, Ormerod AD, Roberts C, Dwyer C, Herriot R. Subacute cutaneous lupus erythematosus associated with phenytoin. Clin Exp Dermatol 2002;27(6):474–6.

49. Ikeda A, Hattori H, Odani A, Kimura J, Shibasaki H. Gynaecomastia in association with phenytoin and zonisamide in a patient having a CYP2C subfamily mutation. J Neurol Neurosurg Psychiatry 1998;65(5):803–4.

50. Rodriguez-Garcia JL, Sanchez-Corral J, Martinez J, Bellas C, Aguado M, Serrano M. Phenytoin-induced benign lymphadenopathy with solid spleen lesions mimicking a malignant lymphoma. Ann Oncol 1991;2(6):443–5.

51. Tsund SH, Lin TI. Angioimmunoblastic lymphoadenopathy in a patient taking diphenylhydantoin. Ann Clin Lab Med 1981;11:542.

52. Ruff ME, Pincus LG, Sampson HA. Phenytoin-induced IgA depression. Am J Dis Child 1987;141(8):858–61.

53. Polman AJ, van der Werf TS, Tiebosch AT, Zijlstra JG. Early-onset phenytoin toxicity mimicking a renopulmonary syndrome. Eur Respir J 1998;11(2):501–3.

54. Daniels PR, Berry GJ, Tazelaar HD, Cooper LT. Giant cell myocarditis as a manifestation of drug hypersensitivity. Cardiovasc Pathol 2000;9(5):287–91.

55. Siragusa RJ, Ramos-Caro FA, Edwards NL, Flowers FP. Drug-induced lupus due to phenytoin. J Pharm Technol 2000;16:5–7.

56. Klassen BD, Sadler RM. Induction of hypersensitivity to a previously tolerated antiepileptic drug by a second antiepileptic drug. Epilepsia 2001;42(3):433–5.

57. Arroyo S, de la Morena A. Life-threatening adverse events of antiepileptic drugs. Epilepsy Res 2001;47(1–2):155–74.

58. Gutierrez-Rave Pecero VM, Luque Marquez R, Ayerza Lerchundi MA, Fernandez Jurado A. Phenytoin-induced hemocytophagic histiocytosis indistinguishable from malignant histiocytosis. South Med J 1991; 84(5):649–50.

59. Jeng YM, Tien HF, Su IJ. Phenytoin-induced pseudolymphoma: reevaluation using modern molecular biology techniques. Epilepsia 1996;37(1):104–7.

60. Ninomiya H, Mamiya K, Matsuo S, Ieiri I, Higuchi S, Tashiro N. Genetic polymorphism of the CYP2C subfamily and excessive serum phenytoin concentration with central nervous system intoxication. Ther Drug Monit 2000; 22(2):230–2.

61. Micali G, Linthicum K, Han N, West DP. Increased risk of erythema multiforme major with combination anticonvulsant and radiation therapies. Pharmacotherapy 1999; 19(2):223–7.

62. Khafaga YM, Jamshed A, Allam AA, Mourad WA, Ezzat A, Al Eisa A, Gray AJ, Schultz H. Stevens–Johnson syndrome in patients on phenytoin and cranial radiotherapy. Acta Oncol 1999;38(1):111–16.

63. Lau KK, Lai CK, Chan AW. Phenytoin poisoning after using Chinese proprietary medicines. Hum Exp Toxicol 2000;19(7):385–6.

64. DeToledo JC, Ramsay RE. Fosphenytoin and phenytoin in patients with status epilepticus: improved tolerability versus increased costs. Drug Saf 2000;22(6):459–66.

65. Pryor FM, Gidal B, Ramsay RE, DeToledo J, Morgan RO. Fosphenytoin: pharmacokinetics and tolerance of intramuscular loading doses. Epilepsia 2001;42(2):245–50.

66. Larsen JR, Larsen LS. Clinical features and management of poisoning due to phenytoin. Med Toxicol Adverse Drug Exp 1989;4(4):229–45.

67. Chua HC, Venketasubramanian N, Tjia H, Chan SP. Elimination of phenytoin in toxic overdose. Clin Neurol Neurosurg 2000;102(1):6–8.

68. Kawasaki C, Nishi R, Uekihara S, Hayano S, Otagiri M. Charcoal hemoperfusion in the treatment of phenytoin overdose. Am J Kidney Dis 2000;35(2):323–6.

69. Murphy MJ, Dominiczak MH. Efficacy of statin therapy: possible effect of phenytoin. Postgrad Med J 1999; 75(884):359–60.

70. Yue CP, Mann KS, Chan KH. Severe thrombocytopenia due to combined cimetidine and phenytoin therapy. Neurosurgery 1987;20(6):963–5.

71. Williams ML, Wainer IW, Embree L, Barnett M, Granvil CL, Ducharme MP. Enantioselective induction of cyclophosphamide metabolism by phenytoin. Chirality 1999;11(7):569–74.

72. Cachat F, Tufro A. Phenytoin/isradipine interaction causing severe neurologic toxicity. Ann Pharmacother 2002; 36(9):1399–402.

73. Beach RL, Zaatreh M, Tennison M, D'Cruz ON. Apparent pharmacodynamic interaction between lamotrigine and phenytoin causing chorea. Epilepsia 1999;40(Suppl 7):145.

74. Fischer TL, Pieper JA, Graff DW, Rodgers JE, Fischer JD, Parnell KJ, Goldstein JA, Greenwood R, Patterson JH. Evaluation of potential losartan–phenytoin drug interactions in healthy volunteers. Clin Pharmacol Ther 2002; 72(3):238–46.

75. Honda M, Yasuoka A, Aoki M, Oka S. A generalized seizure following initiation of nelfinavir in a patient with human immunodeficiency virus type 1 infection, suspected due to interaction between nelfinavir and phenytoin. Intern Med 1999;38(3):302–3.

76. Brackett CC, Bloch JD. Phenytoin as a possible cause of acetaminophen hepatotoxicity: case report and review of the literature. Pharmacotherapy 2000;20(2):229–33.

77. Donahue S, Flockhart DA, Abernethy DR. Ticlopidine inhibits phenytoin clearance. Clin Pharmacol Ther 1999; 66(6):563–8.

78. Perucca E, Hebdige S, Frigo GM, Gatti G, Lecchini S, Crema A. Interaction between phenytoin and valproic acid: plasma protein binding and metabolic effects. Clin Pharmacol Ther 1980;28(6):779–89.

79. Bruni J, Gallo JM, Lee CS, Perchalski RJ, Wilder BJ. Interactions of valproic acid with phenytoin. Neurology 1980;30(11):1233–6.

80. Friel PN, Leal KW, Wilensky AJ. Valproic acid–phenytoin interaction. Ther Drug Monit 1979;1(2):243–8.

81. May T, Rambeck B. Serum concentrations of valproic acid: influence of dose and comedication. Ther Drug Monit 1985;7(4):387–90.

82. Levy RH, Rettenmeier AW, Anderson GD, Wilensky AJ, Friel PN, Baillie TA, Acheampong A, Tor J, Guyot M, Loiseau P. Effects of polytherapy with phenytoin, carbamazepine, and stiripentol on formation of 4-ene-valproate, a hepatotoxic metabolite of valproic acid. Clin Pharmacol Ther 1990;48(3):225–35.

83. Au Yeung SC, Ensom MH. Phenytoin and enteral feedings: does evidence support an interaction? Ann Pharmacother 2000;34(7–8):896–905.

Phosphates

General Information

Sodium phosphates are considered to be dangerous (1), particularly because of their effects on electrolyte balance. An oral solution of sodium phosphates (dibasic sodium phosphate + monobasic sodium phosphate) is used as a laxative for the relief of occasional constipation and is used as part of a bowel-cleansing regimen in preparing patients for surgery or colonoscopy.

The FDA has limited the container size for oral solutions of sodium phosphates to not more than 90 ml in over-the-counter laxatives, because of reports of deaths associated with overdosage of oral solutions of sodium phosphates when the product was packaged in a larger container and a larger than intended dose was taken inadvertently. The agency has also required warning and direction statements to inform consumers that exceeding the recommended dose of oral and rectal sodium phosphates products in a 24-hour period can be harmful.

In 194 patients randomized to receive either sodium picosulfate or fleet phosphate soda before barium enema, there was no difference in the quality of bowel preparation, but picosulfate was easier to take and better tasting and it provoked less nausea and vomiting (2).

Organs and Systems

Endocrine

A 39-year-old woman with oncogenic osteomalacia caused by an osteosarcoma of the right scapula developed tertiary hyperparathyroidism after taking oral phosphate and vitamin D (3). The uniqueness of this case was the co-existence of hyperparathyroidism and oncogenic osteomalacia. All patients previously reported as having developed tertiary hyperparathyroidism with phosphate supplements had taken them for 10–14 years before diagnosis, but this patient had taken it for only 2 years. The proposed mechanism is that exogenous phosphate stimulates parathyroid activity through sequestration of calcium.

Electrolyte balance

From 1987 to October 31, 2001 the Canadian Adverse Drug Reaction Monitoring Program received 10 reports of serious electrolyte disturbances (hypocalcemia, hyperphosphatemia, hypernatremia, and hypokalemia), acidosis, dehydration, renal insufficiency, and tetany in patients who had taken more than 45 ml of the solution, in patients at risk of these complications, and/or in patients using multiple purgatives for bowel preparation (4). In view of these reports, Johnson & Johnson, Merck Consumer Pharmaceuticals, and Pharmascience Inc, in consultation with Health Canada, each issued a letter to all health professionals, giving information related to the safe use of sodium phosphates oral solution. The identification, characterization, and management of drug-related adverse events depend on the active participation of health care professionals in adverse drug reaction reporting programs. Health care professionals are asked to report any suspected adverse reactions in patients who have taken sodium phosphates oral solution.

The Austrian Adverse Drug Reactions Advisory Committee received three reports of severe electrolyte disturbances associated with an oral bowel-cleansing solution containing sodium phosphate solution (Fleet Phospho-Soda Buffered Saline Laxative Mixture), used as a bowel preparation for colonoscopy (5). Prescribers are advised to be aware of complications of the use of phosphate enemas, particularly in infants, elderly or debilitated patients, patients with congestive heart failure, and patients with impaired renal function.

Gastrointestinal

Four cases have suggested an association between oral sodium phosphate and microscopic focal cryptitis (6). The three men and one woman, aged 31–56 years, all had symptoms suggestive of irritable bowel syndrome and had not taken any antibiotics, NSAIDs, or immunosuppressive drugs before the onset symptoms. Colonoscopy was normal. There was no microbiological evidence of an infective cause, and routine biochemistry and hematology laboratory tests were normal. Histology was distinct from infective, ischemic, or inflammatory bowel disease. However, rebiopsy after withdrawal of the drug was not performed in any patient.

Rectal necrosis has been described in a child after phosphate enemas (7).

Susceptibility Factors

Age

Children

Although phosphate enemas are used in preparing children's bowels for colonoscopy and have been described as being safe and ideal for this purpose (8), in children under 5 years they carry risks of significant morbidity due to hyperphosphatemia, hypocalcemia, hypokalemia and dehydration (9). Phosphate toxicity associated with enteral sodium phosphate has been reported in more than 20 children (10,11). Two died, and one had severe neurological sequelae; these three children had either gastrointestinal or renal abnormalities, and one was very premature. Fatal phosphate toxicity has been reported in a 17-month-old child who had no apparent renal or gastrointestinal abnormality after a relatively small dose of hypertonic phosphate enema (12). Hypocalcemic tetany developed in children after the administration of phosphate enemas (10,11). The authors advised against the use of phosphate enemas in children under 2 years, and they recommend use only with extreme caution in children aged 2–5 years, especially when there is underlying bowel disease or renal dysfunction.

Elderly people

In elderly patients, phosphate enemas (Fleet Enema) have caused serious adverse effects.

- A 77-year-old patient with diverticular disease, who received phosphate enemas in preparation for a barium enema, developed hyperphosphatemia and hypocalcemic coma (13).

This case suggests that caution is required in administering phosphate enemas to patients with abnormal colonic mucosa.

- A Fleet Enema was given to a 91-year-old patient who lapsed into coma and died a few hours afterwards, despite treatment with phosphate binders and calcium (14).

Another similar case has been described (15).

Renal disease

Adults with normal excretory functions should not be at risk, but those with renal failure are likely to experience complications (SEDA-17, 425) (SEDA-18, 374).

Drug Administration

Drug overdose

A 46-year-old woman, with hepatic encephalopathy complicating cirrhosis due to hepatitis B and C infection, developed fatal hypernatremia, hyperphosphatemia, and hypocalcemia following the erroneous administration of a total of six sodium phosphate enemas (133 ml each) over 36 hours (16).

References

1. Anonymous. Laxatives containing sodium phosphates—package size limitations and warnings. WHO Pharm Newslett 1998;112:2.
2. Macleod AJ, Duncan KA, Pearson RH, Bleakney RR. A comparison of Fleet Phospho-soda with Picolax in the preparation of the colon for double contrast barium enema. Clin Radiol 1998;53(8):612–14.
3. Huang QL, Feig DS, Blackstein ME. Development of tertiary hyperparathyroidism after phosphate supplementation in oncogenic osteomalacia. J Endocrinol Invest 2000;23(4):263–7.
4. Anonymous. Sodium phosphates oral solution. Risk of electrolyte shift if maximum dose is exceeded. WHO Pharmaceuticals Newslett 2002;2:4.
5. Anonymous. Oral phosphate bowel preparations—electrolyte disturbances. Pharm Newslett 1997;5,6:9.
6. Wong NA, Penman ID, Campbell S, Lessells AM. Microscopic focal cryptitis associated with sodium phosphate bowel preparation. Histopathology 2000;36(5):476–8.
7. Goldman M. Phosphate enemas in childhood. BMJ 1991;302(6787):1273–4.
8. Abubakar K, Goggin N, Gormally S, Durnin M, Drumm B. Preparing the bowel for colonoscopy. Arch Dis Child 1995;73(5):459–61.
9. Hunter MF, Ashton MR, Griffiths DM, Ilangovan P, Roberts JP, Walker V. Hyperphosphataemia after enemas in childhood: prevention and treatment. Arch Dis Child 1993;68(2):233–4.
10. Craig JC, Hodson EM, Martin HC. Phosphate enema poisoning in children. Med J Aust 1994;160(6):347–51.
11. Helikson MA, Parham WA, Tobias JD. Hypocalcemia and hyperphosphatemia after phosphate enema use in a child. J Pediatr Surg 1997;32(8):1244–6.
12. Ismail EA, Al-Mutairi G, Al-Anzy H. A fatal small dose of phosphate enema in a young child with no renal or gastrointestinal abnormality. J Pediatr Gastroenterol Nutr 2000;30(2):220–1.
13. Rohack JJ, Mehta BR, Subramanyam K. Hyperphosphatemia and hypocalcemic coma associated with phosphate enema. South Med J 1985;78(10):1241–2.
14. Spinrad S, Sztern M, Grosskopf Y, Graff E, Blum I. Treating constipation with phosphate enema: an unnecessary risk. Isr J Med Sci 1989;25(4):237–8.
15. Pitcher DE, Ford RS, Nelson MT, Dickinson WE. Fatal hypocalcemic, hyperphosphatemic, metabolic acidosis following sequential sodium phosphate-based enema administration. Gastrointest Endosc 1997; 46(3):266–8.
16. Egesel T, Sivri B, Asik M, Altun B, Bayraktar Y. A fatal complication of sodium-phosphate enema. Turk J Gastroenterol 2000;11:338–40.

Phosphodiesterase type III, selective inhibitors of

See also Individual drugs

General Information

There is a range of bipyridines that are selective inhibitors of a specific isoenzyme of phosphodiesterase, F-III. These include amrinone, enoximone (fenoximone), milrinone, pimobendan, sulmazole, and vesnarinone. Their clinical pharmacology has been reviewed (1).

The pharmacology, clinical pharmacology, uses, therapeutic value, and adverse effects of positive inotropic drugs other than digitalis have been reviewed (2–6), as has the suggestion that their long-term use may be deleterious (6). Apart from the selective inhibitors of phosphodiesterase type III, these drugs include some beta-adrenoceptor agonists and partial agonists, such as dobutamine, dopamine, ibopamine, pirbuterol, prenalterol, and xamoterol, and calcium sensitizers.

The under-reporting of the results of clinical trials in patients with heart failure has been reviewed (7). Some trials that have been unpublished or published only in abstract or preliminary form have involved drugs with positive inotropic effects, such as the phosphodiesterase inhibitor vesnarinone (SEDA-23, 195), the beta-adrenoceptor partial agonist xamoterol, and the dopamine receptor agonist ibopamine.

Although the phosphodiesterase inhibitors are effective in the treatment of acute cardiac failure in various settings, overall mortality during long-term treatment of heart failure is increased, and these drugs should not be used for that purpose (8).

References

1. Frielingsdorf J, Kiowski W. Pharmacology and clinical use of newer inotropic agents. Anaesth Pharmacol Rev 1994; 2:332–41.
2. Colucci WS, Wright RF, Braunwald E. New positive inotropic agents in the treatment of congestive heart failure. Mechanisms of action and recent clinical developments. N Engl J Med 1986;314(5):290–9;1986;314(6):349–58.
3. Webster MW, Sharpe DN. Adverse effects associated with the newer inotropic agents. Med Toxicol 1986;1(5):335–42.
4. Rocci ML Jr, Wilson H. The pharmacokinetics and pharmacodynamics of newer inotropic agents. Clin Pharmacokinet 1987;13(2):91–109.
5. Leier CV. Current status of non-digitalis positive inotropic drugs. Am J Cardiol 1992;69(18):G120–8.
6. Sasayama S. What do the newer inotropic drugs have to offer? Cardiovasc Drugs Ther 1992;6(1):15–18.
7. van Veldhuisen DJ, Poole-Wilson PA. The underreporting of results and possible mechanisms of "negative" drug trials in patients with chronic heart failure. Int J Cardiol 2001; 80(1):19–27.
8. Nony P, Boissel JP, Lievre M, Leizorovicz A, Haugh MC, Fareh S, de Breyne B. Evaluation of the effect of phosphodiesterase inhibitors on mortality in chronic heart failure patients. A meta-analysis. Eur J Clin Pharmacol 1994;46(3):191–6.

Photochemotherapy (PUVA)

General Information

Photochemotherapy, which consists of oral (and sometimes topical) administration of psoralens (the furocoumarins 5-methoxypsoralen, 8-methoxypsoralen, and trioxysalen) plus long-wave ultraviolet radiation, known as PUVA, is a well-established effective treatment for psoriasis, which has also been used for vitiligo (1), mycosis fungoides, alopecia areata, dyshidrotic eczema, atopic dermatitis, and certain other skin diseases. Guidelines for treatment have been recommended (2,3).

Bathwater delivery of psoralens ("Bath PUVA") is an attractive alternative to oral administration, since it virtually lacks systemic adverse effects and the rapid decline of photosensitivity after bath PUVA enables the patient to pursue daily activities without restrictions (4). Trioxysalen bath PUVA does not have carcinogenic effects (5).

Guidelines for topical PUVA therapy, including bath and local immersion PUVA therapy, have been published by the British Photodermatology Group (6).

Short-term reactions are not uncommon. They include erythema, burns, nausea, pruritus, headache, and dizziness. Hypersensitivity reactions, which are uncommon, include drug fever, skin rashes, and bronchial asthma. Long-term treatment increases the risk of non-melanoma skin cancers and possibly of cutaneous melanoma.

Organs and Systems

Cardiovascular

A rise in ambient temperature can have cardiovascular effects. In high-risk conditions, cardiovascular monitoring during treatment has been advised (SEDA-6, 148), although patients with cardiovascular disease and hypertension are also reported to tolerate PUVA therapy without evidence of cardiovascular stress (7).

Edema of the legs has been noted occasionally.

Respiratory

Bronchial asthma and coughing attacks have been attributed to methoxsalen allergy (8).

Nervous system

Dizziness, headache, and itching are well-known immediate adverse effects (SEDA-3, 132). Persistent skin pain can be serious (9).

Sensory systems

Although several cases of cataracts presumably or probably induced by PUVA have been reported (10,11), the risk appears to be small when recommendations to prevent ocular complications (12) are strictly adhered to (13). Other ocular symptoms after PUVA include photophobia, conjunctivitis, keratitis, and dry eyes (SEDA-7, 166). Adequately protecting the eyes from the sun reduces the risk of acute toxic effects on the cornea and conjunctivae (14).

Visual field defects have been described in some patients (15).

Metabolism

Severe hyperlipidemia possibly related to PUVA has been observed once (SEDA-19, 155).

Hematologic

There have been reports of acute leukemia (SEDA-10, 125) and neutropenia (SEDA-5, 151) during PUVA and one dubious report of preleukemia (SEDA-4, 105). Transformation of stable chronic myelomonocytic leukemia to acute myeloid leukemia has been attributed to PUVA (SEDA-14, 124). These events may all have been purely coincidental and not causally related, as PUVA does not appear to increase the risk of non-cutaneous malignancies (16).

Gastrointestinal

Nausea and diarrhea sometimes occur (17).

Liver

Slight transient rises in liver enzymes have been reported during PUVA treatment, but they were usually attributable to pre-existing liver disease or the use of alcohol or other drugs. However, there have been two reports of liver damage clearly attributable to PUVA (18,19). It is rare for liver enzymes to rise after topical 8-methoxypsoralen (20).

Urinary tract

In 12 of 106 patients treated with PUVA an increase in serum creatinine to abnormal values was noted. In one patient a renal biopsy showed uncharacteristic glomerulonephritis (SEDA-5, 151).

Nephrotic syndrome has been reported in a patient treated with PUVA for polymorphic light eruption (SEDA-9, 132).

Skin

Phototoxicity with erythema, burns, localized edema, and blistering can occur in up to 11% of patients treated with PUVA (SEDA-22, 165) (21). Other cutaneous adverse effects that are related or possibly related to PUVA are listed in Table 1.

PUVA can cause pemphigus vulgaris, bullous pemphigoid, and pemphigus foliaceus. In one case intermittent flares continued for 2 years after the withdrawal of PUVA (22).

Immunologic

Concerns that PUVA therapy can cause systemic lupus erythematosus (SLE) and other connective tissue diseases, such as giant cell arteritis (SEDA-6, 147), have been raised by several reports (SED-12, 336) (30), (SEDA-15, 139) (SEDA-17, 183). There have been several studies of the incidence of serum antinuclear antibodies in patients who have received PUVA, with both

Table 1 Adverse effects of PUVA on the skin, hair, and nails

Acne (SEDA-3, 132)
Actinic lichenoid dermatitis (SEDA-12, 130)
Allergic contact dermatitis to methoxsalen (8-methoxypsoralen)
Allergic cutaneous vasculitis (SEDA-6, 146)
Bacterial infections, such as folliculitis and erysipelas
Bowen's disease and Bowenoid lesions
Bullous eruptions, including phototoxic bullae, acrobullous
   eruptions, and (rarely) bullous pemphigoid (SEDA-21, 160) (23)
Dermatomyositis (SEDA-19, 155)
Disseminated epidermolytic acanthoma (SEDA-12, 130)
Disseminated superficial actinic porokeratosis (SEDA-6, 147)
   (SEDA-11, 136)
Epidermal dystrophy
Exacerbation of polymorphic light eruption
Generalized exanthematous pustulosis (SEDA-20, 153)
Granuloma annulare (SEDA-4, 105)
Herpes simplex infection
Herpes zoster infection
Hirsutism (SEDA-6, 146)
Hypertrichosis
Kaposi's varicelliform eruption
Keratoacanthoma (SEDA-9, 131)
Lichen planus (SEDA-6, 147)
Lupus erythematosus (SEDA-15, 140) (SEDA-17, 183)
Lymphomatoid papulosis (SEDA-16, 151)
Mycosis fungoides, inflammatory flare-up (SEDA-20, 153)
Nail pigmentation (SEDA-8, 152)
Neurofibroma (SEDA-15, 142)
Papular phototoxic reaction
Pemphigus vulgaris (24)
Photoallergic dermatitis (SEDA-15, 141)
Photo-oncolysis (SEDA-3, 152) (SEDA-4, 105)
Pigment alterations, notably PUVA lentigines (SEDA-9,130);
   absence of PUVA lentigines may be an indicator of a lower risk
   of PUVA malignancy (25)
Psoriasis of the nails
Pustular psoriasis
PUVA keratoses (26)
Rosacea
Scleroderma-like changes
Seborrheic dermatitis of the face
Senile elastosis
Subungual bleeding
Suppression of induction and expression of delayed cutaneous
   hypersensitivity (27)
Urticaria (28)
Verruciform xanthoma (SEDA-20, 153)
Vitiligo (SEDA-22, 165) (29)

positive and negative results. Current evidence suggests that frequent evaluation of antinuclear antibodies during treatment of patients with uncomplicated psoriasis with an initially negative antinuclear antibody test and with no symptoms of connective tissue diseases is unnecessary (31).

Hypersensitivity reactions occur infrequently and have included drug fever, skin rashes, and bronchial asthma. Anaphylaxis to 5-methoxypsoralen has been reported (32).

- A 36-year-old woman had been treated for a polymorphic light eruption with two annual courses of PUVA, three times weekly for 6 weeks, plus oral 5-methoxypsoralen 60 mg, without any adverse effects. However, during the fourth course, 30 minutes after

taking 5-methoxypsoralen 60 mg, she developed intense pruritus of the palms, spreading to the body. This was followed by erythema of the palms and symmetrical erythematous patches and urticarial lesions on the trunk. She had dizziness and slight difficulty in breathing. Her symptoms cleared within an hour after intravenous administration of an antihistamine and cortisone. Two months later skin prick tests with 5-methoxypsoralen were negative, but placebo-controlled oral provocation with 5-methoxypsoralen 20 mg resulted in symptoms similar to those she had experienced during PUVA.

Body temperature

Influenza-like symptoms have been attributed to psoralens (33).

- A 54-year-old man treated with photochemotherapy for disabling hand eczema developed flu-like symptoms, which lasted for 48 hours and occurred repeatedly within 2 hours after oral methoxsalen 50 mg. In addition to a fever up to 39°C, he had headache, nausea and vomiting, fatigue, dyspepsia, and muscle aches.

Although no attempt was made to isolate any viruses, the multiple positive rechallenges, in combination with a time-course compatible with methoxsalen pharmacokinetics, suggested a drug-related event.

Long-Term Effects

Tumorigenicity

Cutaneous carcinogenicity
In a review of the English language literature on the risk of non-melanoma skin cancer from photochemotherapy in the treatment of psoriasis (34) the following were the conclusions:

(a) PUVA is an independent dose-related carcinogen in humans and can initiate and promote the formation of squamous cell carcinoma (35). The relation of basal cell carcinoma to PUVA alone is not well established.

(b) The carcinogenic risk of PUVA is not simply dose-related and skin type; geographic location and other well-established co-carcinogenic risk factors must be taken into account.

(c) Three factors are important co-carcinogens with PUVA: a history of arsenic exposure, ionizing radiation therapy, and skin cancer. Other factors believed to be related to increased risk include skin types I and II.

(d) Factors that appear to be associated with little or no risk of PUVA-related carcinogenesis include methotrexate (although a study from Sweden (36) has suggested otherwise), topical tar, and ultraviolet B (UVB). Exceptions to this include simultaneous use of methotrexate and PUVA, and high exposure of the genital skin to UVB/tar. Retinoids may prove to be negatively correlated with skin cancer.

(e) The dose-related increased risk of cutaneous squamous cell carcinoma from PUVA is independent of skin type (I–IV), although the absolute risk is much higher in skin types I and II.

(f) Men treated with PUVA without genital protection are at high risk of developing dose-related invasive squamous cell carcinoma of the penis and the scrotum (SEDA-15, 141).

(g) PUVA-induced squamous cell carcinoma is not biologically aggressive. Nevertheless, metastases have been observed in some patients, emphasizing the need for continued monitoring (37).

(h) There is no definitive degree of cumulative PUVA exposure above which carcinogenicity can be predicted. However, the risk of squamous cell carcinoma is less in patients with skin types II, III, and IV, no risk factors, and a cumulative exposure below 1000 J/cm². Of patients treated with over 2000 J/cm², even those without risk factors, at least 20% will develop squamous cell carcinomas and 50% atypical squamous keratoses (35). Patients with skin type I should be monitored more rigorously than others.

The following recommendations were made

(a) Whenever possible, exclude patients with a history of ionizing radiation therapy, skin cancer, or arsenic exposure.

(b) Shield the male genital skin at all times during PUVA treatment.

(c) Use the European dosage protocol (lower doses and less frequent irradiations than the US protocol) whenever possible.

(d) Reduce PUVA dosage by combining or cycling with other treatments. Avoid maintenance therapy if possible.

(e) Use PUVA in younger patients only when necessary.

(f) Monitor patients with skin type I closely.

(g) Monitor patients prospectively and at least annually for keratoses and cutaneous carcinoma, particularly after cumulative exposure of more than 1000 J/cm².

Risk of melanoma
The PUVA Follow up Study was a prospective evaluation of 1380 patients who started using PUVA for psoriasis in 1975 and 1976. There was a modest but significantly increased risk of malignant melanoma in PUVA-treated patients ($n = 822$), beginning 15 years after first exposure (SEDA-22, 166) (38,39). Incidence rates during 1996–1999 were 10-fold higher than those expected from incidence data in the general population (data available only for 1992–1996). There was a non-significant trend toward a higher incidence of melanoma in patients who had received more courses of PUVA (over 200). High degrees of exposure to PUVA, a period of at least 15 years from the time of the first exposure, or both are required before the risk of melanoma increases substantially. Despite the fact that melanoma is lethal if left untreated, this observation does not necessitate abandonment of PUVA (40). This risk should be weighed against the substantial efficacy of PUVA therapy in severe psoriasis. However, it does suggest that the guidelines for treating psoriasis with PUVA should be rigidly observed (41). Patients receiving long-term treatment should be carefully followed

throughout their lives and those who are at increased risk of melanoma should not be given this treatment.

Non-cutaneous cancers
Long-term PUVA does not increase the risk of non-cutaneous cancer, including lymphomas or leukemia (16).

Second-Generation Effects

Pregnancy

Although PUVA therapy should not be begun during pregnancy or lactation, the theoretical mutagenic and teratogenic effect of PUVA does not carry any significant risk of abnormal delivery (42,43).

Susceptibility Factors

Relative contraindications to PUVA therapy include a history of arsenic intake, previous ionizing radiation, long-term use of cytostatic drugs, skin cancer, cataracts, and severe cardiovascular disease. In patients with photosensitive dermatoses and in patients who are using systemic photosensitizing drugs, PUVA should be administered with caution. The possible long-term adverse effects should be taken into consideration, especially when young patients are candidates for photochemotherapy. Uncontrolled use of psoralens may lead to life-threatening burns (27).

Drug–Drug Interactions

Emollients

The use of emollients before PUVA can significantly interfere with UV light transmission during photochemotherapy (44).

Phenytoin

Phenytoin can reduce the serum concentrations of methoxsalen, probably by inducing its metabolism (45).

References

1. Grimes PE. Psoralen photochemotherapy for vitiligo. Clin Dermatol 1997;15(6):921–6.
2. Lowe NJ, Chizhevsky V, Gabriel H. Photo(chemo)therapy: general principles. Clin Dermatol 1997;15(5):745–52.
3. Lauharanta J. Photochemotherapy. Clin Dermatol 1997;15(5):769–80.
4. Degitz K, Plewig G, Rocken M. Rapid decline in photosensitivity after 8-methoxypsoralen bathwater delivery. Arch Dermatol 1996;132(11):1394–5.
5. Hannuksela A, Pukkala E, Hannuksela M, Karvonen J. Cancer incidence among Finnish patients with psoriasis treated with trioxsalen bath PUVA. J Am Acad Dermatol 1996;35(5 Pt 1):685–9.
6. Halpern SM, Anstey AV, Dawe RS, Diffey BL, Farr PM, Ferguson J, Hawk JL, Ibbotson S, McGregor JM, Murphy GM, Thomas SE, Rhodes LE. Guidelines for topical PUVA: a report of a workshop of the British photodermatology group. Br J Dermatol 2000;142(1):22–31.

7. Chappe SG, Roenigk HH Jr, Miller AJ, Beeaff DE, Tyrpin L. The effect of photochemotherapy on the cardiovascular system. J Am Acad Dermatol 1981;4(5):561–6.

8. Ramsay B, Marks JM. Bronchoconstriction due to 8-methoxypsoralen. Br J Dermatol 1988;119(1):83–6.

9. Burrows NP, Norris PG. Treatment of PUVA-induced skin pain with capsaicin. Br J Dermatol 1994;131(4):584–5.

10. Lerman S, Megaw J, Gardner K. Psoralen—long-wave ultraviolet therapy and human cataractogenesis. Invest Ophthalmol Vis Sci 1982;23(6):801–4.

11. Woo TY, Wong RC, Wong JM, Anderson TF, Lerman S. Lenticular psoralen photoproducts and cataracts of a PUVA-treated psoriatic patient. Arch Dermatol 1985;121(10):1307–8.

12. Lerman S, Megaw J, Willis I. Potential ocular complications from PUVA therapy and their prevention. J Invest Dermatol 1980;74(4):197–9.

13. Stern RS. Ocular lens findings in patients treated with PUVA. Photochemotherapy Follow-Up-Study. J Invest Dermatol 1994;103(4):534–8.

14. Calzavara-Pinton PG, Carlino A, Manfredi E, Semeraro F, Zane C, De Panfilis G. Ocular side effects of PUVA-treated patients refusing eye sun protection. Acta Dermatol Venereol Suppl (Stockh) 1994;186:164–5.

15. Fenton DA, Wilkinson JD. Dose-related visual-field defects in patients receiving PUVA therapy. Lancet 1983;1(8333):1106.

16. Stern RS, Vakeva LH. Noncutaneous malignant tumors in the PUVA follow-up study: 1975–1996. J Invest Dermatol 1997;108(6):897–900.

17. Agren-Jonsson S, Tegner E. PUVA therapy for palmoplantar pustulosis. Acta Derm Venereol 1985;65(6):531–5.

18. Bjellerup M, Bruze M, Hansson A, Krook G, Ljunggren B. Liver injury following administration of 8-methoxypsoralen during PUVA therapy. Acta Dermatol Venereol 1979;59(4):371–2.

19. Pariser DM, Wyles RJ. Toxic hepatitis from oral methoxsalen photochemotherapy (PUVA). J Am Acad Dermatol 1980;3(3):248–50.

20. Park YM, Kim TY, Kim HO, Kim CW. Reproducible elevation of liver transaminases by topical 8-methoxypsoralen. Photodermatol Photoimmunol Photomed 1994;10(6):261–3.

21. Morison WL, Marwaha S, Beck L. PUVA-induced phototoxicity: incidence and causes. J Am Acad Dermatol 1997;36(2 Pt 1):183–5.

22. Aghassi D, Dover JS. Pemphigus foliaceus induced by psoralen-UV-A. Arch Dermatol 1998;134(10):1300–1.

23. Grabbe S, Schutte B, Bruckner-Tuderman L, Schwarz T. PUVA-induzierte akrobullöse Dermatose. [PUVA-induced acro-bullous dermatosis.] Hautarzt 1996;47(6):465–8.

24. Fryer EJ, Lebwohl M. Pemphigus vulgaris after initiation of psoralen and UVA therapy for psoriasis. J Am Acad Dermatol 1994;30(4):651–3.

25. Ophaswongse S, Maibach H. Topical nonsteroidal antiinflammatory drugs: allergic and photoallergic contact dermatitis and phototoxicity. Contact Dermatitis 1993;29(2):57–64.

26. Payne CM, Bladin C, Colchester AC, Bland J, Lapworth R, Lane D. Argyria from excessive use of topical silver sulphadiazine. Lancet 1992;340(8811):126.

27. Nettelblad H, Vahlqvist C, Krysander L, Sjoberg F. Psoralens used for cosmetic sun tanning: an unusual cause of extensive burn injury. Burns 1996;22(8):633–5.

28. Bech-Thomsen N, Wulf HC. 8-Methoxypsoralen urticaria. J Am Acad Dermatol 1994;31(6):1063–4.

29. White SI, Friedmann PS, Moss C, Simpson JM. Recovery of cutaneous immune responsiveness after PUVA therapy. Br J Dermatol 1988;118(3):403–7.

30. Bruze M, Krook G, Ljunggren B. Fatal connective tissue disease with antinuclear antibodies following PUVA therapy. Acta Dermatol Venereol 1984;64(2):157–60.

31. Calzavara-Pinton P, Franceschini F, Rastrelli M, Manera C, Zane C, Cattaneo R, De Panfilis G. Antinuclear antibodies are not induced by PUVA treatment in patients with uncomplicated psoriasis. J Am Acad Dermatol 1994;30(6):955–8.

32. Legat FJ, Wolf P, Kranke B. Anaphylaxis to 5-methoxypsoralen during photochemotherapy. Br J Dermatol 2001;145(5):821–2.

33. Van Coevorden AM, Coenraads PJ. Severe influenzalike symptoms associated with methoxsalen photochemotherapy. Arch Dermatol 2002;138(6):840–1.

34. Studniberg HM, Weller P. PUVA, UVB, psoriasis, and nonmelanoma skin cancer. J Am Acad Dermatol 1993;29(6):1013–22.

35. Lever LR, Farr PM. Skin cancers or premalignant lesions occur in half of high-dose PUVA patients. Br J Dermatol 1994;131(2):215–19.

36. Lindelof B, Sigurgeirsson B. PUVA and cancer: a case-control study. Br J Dermatol 1993;129(1):39–41.

37. Stern R. Metastatic squamous cell cancer after psoralen photochemotherapy. Lancet 1994;344(8937):1644–5.

38. Stern RS; Nichols KT, Vakeva LH. Malignant melanoma in patients treated for psoriasis with methoxsalen (psoralen) and ultraviolet A radiation (PUVA). The PUVA Follow-Up Study. N Engl J Med 1997;336(15):1041–5.

39. Stern RS; PUVA Follow up Study. The risk of melanoma in association with long-term exposure to PUVA. J Am Acad Dermatol 2001;44(5):755–61.

40. Wolff K. Should PUVA be abandoned? N Engl J Med 1997;336(15):1090–1.

41. Morison WL, Baughman RD, Day RM, Forbes PD, Hoenigsmann H, Krueger GG, Lebwohl M, Lew R, Naldi L, Parrish JA, Piepkorn M, Stern RS, Weinstein GD, Whitmore SE. Consensus workshop on the toxic effects of long-term PUVA therapy. Arch Dermatol 1998;134(5):595–8.

42. Gunnarskog JG, Kallen AJ, Lindelof BG, Sigurgeirsson B. Psoralen photochemotherapy (PUVA) and pregnancy. Arch Dermatol 1993;129(3):320–3.

43. Garbis H, Elefant E, Bertolotti E, Robert E, Serafini MA, Prapas N. Pregnancy outcome after periconceptional and first-trimester exposure to methoxsalen photochemotherapy. Arch Dermatol 1995;131(4):492–3.

44. Gabard B, Treffel P, Bieli E, Schwab S. Emollients and photo(chemo)therapy: a call for caution. Dermatology 1996;192(3):242–5.

45. Staberg B, Hueg B. Interaction between 8-methoxypsoralen and phenytoin. Consequence for PUVA therapy. Acta Dermatol Venereol 1985;65(6):553–5.

Physical contraceptives— intrauterine devices

General Information

Intrauterine contraceptive devices (IUCDs) have been reviewed (1,2). Most are composed of bland synthetic materials or contain in addition a small amount of metallic copper. Others are designed to release either progesterone or a synthetic progestogen (for example levonorgestrel) (3,4). IUCDs that release levonorgestrel are somewhat more effective than copper-containing devices, while those that release progesterone are less effective (5).

Copper-containing IUCDs (6,7) became popular because local inflammatory reactions in the endometrium are more marked and the contraceptive effect is thus more pronounced (SEDA-21, 234) (8). In addition, copper ions released from IUCDs reach concentrations in the luminal fluids of the genital tract that are toxic to spermatozoa and embryos. The ability of copper to induce the generation of free radicals and the formation of malonaldehyde may be involved in its contraceptive effect.

Migration of IUCDs

Migration of IUCDs is relatively rare, although they have been found in the omentum, rectosigmoid, peritoneum, bladder, appendix, small bowel, adnexa, and iliac vein. Most authors have recommended removal of copper-containing devices, because of the potential for inflammatory reactions, which can cause bowel obstruction and perforation (9). Two cases of migration of IUCDs to the bowel have been reported.

- A 29-year-old woman who had had a Copper 7 IUCD inserted 3 years before developed amenorrhea (10). The intrauterine contraceptive was not in the uterine cavity and X-ray showed that it was positioned over the sacrum just to the right of the midline and outside the uterus. It later moved to the cecum and became completely embedded in the muscular layer after penetrating the serosal surface.
- A Copper-T IUCD migrated to the rectal lumen in a 36-year-old woman with menorrhagia for 3 month and a history of Copper-T insertion 6 years before (11).
- A 28-year-old pregnant woman developed an ileal perforation 4 weeks after the insertion of a Multiload-Cu 375 IUCD (12).

The last report documents the shortest interval between insertion and proven bowel injury by an IUCD.

Organs and Systems

Skin

Perimenstrual dermatitis has been attributed to a copper-containing IUCD (13).

- A 41-year-old woman had a 2-year history of a recurrent, self-healing skin rash associated with abdominal pain. She had had cholinergic urticaria since 1995 and had had a copper-containing IUCD inserted 12 years before. The eruption followed a cyclical pattern, invariably appearing 3–7 days before the menses and tending to improve spontaneously with the onset of bleeding. This non-itchy rash was associated with abdominal distension and cramps that followed a similar course. She had multiple non-itchy symmetrical erythematous papules on the upper trunk, neck, and arms. Patch-testing was positive for copper sulfate. The IUCD was removed and the abdominal symptoms subsided at the following cycle. Progressive resolution of the dermatitis was observed. No cutaneous eruption was observed after 8 months and no new lesions developed after a further 5 months.

Reproductive system

Although the effect of a progestogen in an IUCD is primarily local, the amounts released are sufficient to have some systemic effects. In particular, there are partial and variable effects on ovulation, which seem to cause a greater risk of functional ovarian cysts (14,15).

Menstrual disturbances

The authors of a balanced review of hormone-releasing intrauterine systems concluded that while with large-size devices that release high doses (for example 20 micrograms/day) pregnancy rates and the incidence of ectopic pregnancy are extremely low, users are more likely to have amenorrhea and device expulsion (16). Compared with users of a subdermal hormonal implant (Norplant-2), women who used LNG-20 were more likely to have oligomenorrhea but less likely to have prolonged bleeding and spotting.

The fibrinolytic activity of menstrual blood in wearers of Lippes loops exceeds that of patients with menorrhagia, while the values in users of the Cu-T (200) are in the same range as in normally menstruating and untreated women. In users of Lippes loops no fibrin was found in the endometrial stroma. This may explain the increased blood loss associated with the use of the Lippes loop, which can be severe enough to cause anemia (17).

Oligomenorrhea is a common adverse effect of IUCDs; during the first year after insertion; some 16% of users experience 90 days or more of amenorrhea, which is substantially more common than with a bland IUCD.

Early experience in 22 women who used a device releasing both copper and norgestrel ("Gynefix-Norgestrel") suggested that it was well tolerated and that the amount of menstrual bleeding was less than with the conventional copper-only "Gynefix" product (18).

In women who used a variant that released levonorgestrel 20 micrograms/day from a polymer cylinder covered with a membrane that controlled the rate of release, both the volume of menstrual blood loss and the number of bleeding days were reduced, and during the first year of use 20% of women developed amenorrhea (19). There was an initial increase in the mean number of bleeding and spotting days, but in 3–6 months the number of bleeding and spotting days was the same as observed in users of copper IUCDs. The variation between individuals was wide and unpredictable, but the method was claimed to be well accepted by users, with typical annual continuation rates above 80% in various studies. However, premature removal of the system was often required because of unwanted effects; in a nationwide study in Finland, the continuation rates at 1, 2, 3, 4, and 5 years were 93, 87, 81, 75, and 65% respectively (20). The symptoms most strongly associated with premature removal were excessive bleeding and spotting, infections, and pain. The risk of premature removal was markedly lower among women who had occasional or total absence of menstruation. Premature removal was less likely in the oldest age group. British experience showed a clear need to counsel women in advance about the possibility of early disruption of the bleeding pattern, including the chance of oligomenorrhea or amenorrhea, if they are not to become discouraged and abandon the treatment entirely (21).

The FibroPlant is a levonorgestrel-releasing device derived from the earlier GyneFix principle. Experience with two forms of this frameless "fibrous delivery system," which releases smaller doses (10 or 14 micrograms/day), suggested that it was as effective and well tolerated as other types of device (22). However, the irregular bleeding that can occur with devices of this type can complicate and delay the recognition of endometrial cancer (23).

Ectopic pregnancy

It is not known whether the risk of ectopic pregnancy is increased in women using an IUCD (24,25). The proportion of such pregnancies has been reported as 6–8%, or higher. Primary ovarian pregnancies also develop in IUCD users, suggesting that ovarian implantation is not fully prevented (26).

The proportion of pregnancies that are ectopic is higher with devices that release either levonorgestrel or progesterone than with copper IUCDs, although the rates vary inversely with the hormonal content; at the most common dosages, the ectopic pregnancy rate for progesterone-containing devices (releasing 65 mg/day) was three times that with IUCDs containing levonorgestrel (releasing 20 mg/day).

Use of a variant that released levonorgestrel 20 micrograms/day from a polymer cylinder covered with a membrane that controlled the rate of release resulted in extrauterine pregnancies in one per 5000 users per year (19).

Chronic inflammatory and degenerative changes

There is a positive correlation between high copper loss from an IUCD and the development of menorrhagia or pathological lesions, such as cervical dysplasia and endometrial cytopathology (27). Evidence of endometrial carcinoma was not found in endometrial aspirates from 189 women who had used Copper-T-200 devices for 1–10 years, but five cases of endometrial hyperplasia (2.67%) were encountered in women in the series, all of whom had worn copper devices for 6 years or more. Inflammatory changes in the endometrial cells were found in 12 cases (6.2%), 11 of 12 having worn the device for over 3 years. It is possible that constant exposure to copper may be responsible for persistence of chronic inflammatory changes in endometrial cells, which could be the precursors of hyperplastic changes. It is not clear whether the dissolved copper is also responsible for the temporarily increased predisposition to bacterial contamination and the somewhat increased risk of pelvic inflammatory disease, seen especially in young nulliparous women using this type of contraceptive method.

In endometrial specimens in which copper-containing IUCDs had been embedded there was evidence of severe, degenerative changes in abnormal cells on the surface of the device and also in the endometrium and occasionally also in the muscle layer of the uterus (28,29). These were characterized by pyknosis of the endometrial cells and altered intracellular components. There were relatively few microtubuli in the endometrial cells. Copper ions escaping to the surface of the device may have been responsible for local endometrial damage.

Uterine and extrauterine infections

Progesterone-releasing devices have to be replaced annually, and since there is always a risk of microbacterial contamination of the endometrium on IUCD insertion this brings with it some risk of pelvic inflammatory disease. The risk is less with an IUCD that releases levonorgestrel 20 mg/day, which remains effective for several years. There is even some evidence of an actual protective effect against pelvic inflammatory disease (30); in a comparative study, the 36-month rate of pelvic inflammatory disease was significantly lower for a levonorgestrel device (0.5 per 100 woman-years) than for a copper-releasing IUCD (2.0 per 100). The pregnancy rate in this study was also very significantly lower (0.3 for the progestogen device compared with 3.7 for the copper device), as was the rate of ectopic pregnancies (0.03 compared with 0.25). The rate of expulsion was similar, while the rates of removal because of amenorrhea and the hormonally related adverse effects were significantly higher with the levonorgestrel-releasing device than the copper IUCD.

If copper-containing fragments of IUCDs perforate the uterine wall and enter the peritoneal cavity, acute inflammatory reactions and peritoneal adhesions can occur. Laparoscopic removal is then not only as a rule impossible but may also be dangerous because of the marked peritoneal reaction surrounding the copper part of the device. Laparotomy has therefore been suggested as the primary measure in such cases. Whether copper devices result more commonly in perforation than non-copper devices is not entirely clear, nor is the question answered whether copper increases the risk of extrauterine pregnancies, although older evidence suggested this as a risk (SED-9, 371).

Immunologic

Immunological and hypersensitivity reactions beyond the uterus are uncommon, but they can occur. Rashes, including generalized urticaria and eczematoid eruptions, have occurred as a result of allergy to the copper released from IUCDs, although they are extremely rare (SEDA-11, 204) (SEDA-12, 186) (SEDA-21, 235). One woman who had worn a copper-containing device for 12 months developed widespread urticaria and angioedema of the eyelids and the labia majora and minora for about 6 months (31). She also had persistent symptoms of premenstrual and postmenstrual spotting and leukorrhea for about 6 months. A patch test was positive with 1% copper sulfate, as was an in vitro lymphocyte-stimulating test with copper. An endometrial biopsy showed vulvovaginitis, with hyperplasia of the cervical canal and T cell and eosinophilic granulocyte infiltration. Removal of the device caused complete remission.

The incidence of salpingitis and other pelvic inflammation is believed to be higher in users of IUCDs. A study of cervical smears in women using IUCD contraception compared with others using other methods of contraception showed that the incidence of cervical inflammation was higher in the former (32).

Genital tract actinomycosis has come increasingly to the fore (33,34). In one study in Britain, the pelvic smears of nearly one-third of women using plastic devices were positive for *Actinomyces*-like organisms, compared with two of 165 women using copper-loaded IUCDs and none in a series of oral contraceptive users. There was a highly significant correlation between the presence of these organisms on smear and pain or other symptoms of pelvic inflammatory disease.

Current users of IUCDs suffer more often from acute rather than chronic pelvic inflammatory disease (1.51 compared with 0.54 times per 1000 woman-years). In ex-users the situation was reversed, chronic pelvic inflammatory disease being more common (0.95 compared with 0.48 times per 1000 woman-years) (35).

Second-Generation Effects

Fetotoxicity

Although copper-containing IUCDs are very effective, pregnancies do occur and the question of possible second-generation effects has to be considered. In one case the neonate showed significantly increased copper and ceruloplasmin concentrations, whereas maternal concentrations were within the reference range. Whether such exposure to copper can cause harm is not clear; because of the pharmacological effects of copper, it has been suspected of having mutagenic and carcinogenic potential. Until now, there is no clear evidence that harm is actually done. Five published cases scattered throughout the literature in which incomplete closure of the neural tube was found (36) could have been coincidental, bearing in mind the large number of pregnancies in which exposure to copper must occur in this way. In various species of animals which have been studied (rat, rabbit, hamster, sheep) no teratogenicity of intrauterine copper was detected (SED-11, 442).

Drug–Drug Interactions

Immunosuppressants

Two pregnancies (with normal outcomes) have been described in renal transplant patients using an IUCD. It seems that an intact immune system is needed for effective contraception by IUCD, and that immunosuppressive therapy can render an IUCD ineffective. Immunosuppressed patients should be advised to use another means of contraception (37).

References

1. Rehan N, Inayatullah A, Chaudhary I. Norplant: reasons for discontinuation and side-effects. Eur J Contraceptive Reprod Health Care 2000;5(2):113–18.
2. Riphagen FE. Intrauterine application of progestins in hormone replacement therapy: a review. Climacteric 2000;3(3):199–211.
3. Odlind V. Review: new methods for fertility regulation in women. Clin Reprod Fertil 1987;3:221.
4. Andersson K, Tybo G. Levonova: intrauterine release of 20 micrograms of levonorgestrel/24 hours. In: Anonymous. Workshop on Contraceptive Methods. Uppsala. Swedish Medical Products Agency, 1994:2.
5. Sivin I. Dose- and age-dependent ectopic pregnancy risks with intrauterine contraception. Obstet Gynecol 1991;78(2):291–8.
6. Fortney JA, Feldblum PJ, Raymond EG. Intrauterine devices. The optimal long-term contraceptive method? J Reprod Med 1999;44(3):269–74.
7. Thonneau P, Goulard H, Goyaux N. Risk factors for intrauterine device failure: a review. Contraception 2001;64(1):33–7.
8. Ortiz ME, Croxatto HB, Bardin CW. Mechanisms of action of intrauterine devices. Obstet Gynecol Surv 1996;51(Suppl 12):S42–51.
9. Kassab B, Audra P. Le sterilet migrateur. A propos d'un cas et revue de la littérature. [The migrating intrauterine device. Case report and review of the literature.] Contracept Fertil Sex 1999;27(10):696–700.
10. Sarkar P. Translocation of a copper 7 intra-uterine contraceptive device with subsequent penetration of the caecum: case report and review. Br J Fam Plann 2000;26(3):161.
11. Banerjee N, Kriplani A, Roy KK, Bal S, Takkar D. Retrieval of lost Copper-T from the rectum. Eur J Obstet Gynecol Reprod Biol 1998;79(2):211–12.
12. Chen CP, Hsu TC, Wang W. Ileal penetration by a Multiload-Cu 375 intrauterine contraceptive device. A case report with review of the literature. Contraception 1998;58(5):295–304.
13. Pujol RM, Randazzo L, Miralles J, Alomar A. Perimenstrual dermatitis secondary to a copper-containing intrauterine contraceptive device. Contact Dermatitis 1998;38(5):288.
14. Robinson GE, Bounds W, Kubba AA, Adams J, Guilleband J. Functional ovarian cysts associated with the levonorgestrel releasing intrauterine device. J Fam Plan 1989;14:131–2.
15. Barbosa I, Bakos O, Olsson SE, Odlind V, Johansson ED. Ovarian function during use of a levonorgestrel-releasing IUD. Contraception 1990;42(1):51–66.
16. French RS, Cowan FM, Mansour D, Higgins JP, Robinson A, Procter T, Morris S, Guillebaud J. Levonorgestrel-releasing (20 microgram/day) intrauterine systems (Mirena) compared with other methods of reversible contraceptives. BJOG 2000;107(10):1218–25.
17. Hefnawi F, Saleh A, Kandil O, El-Sheikha Z, Hassanein M, Askalani H. Fibrinolytic activity of menstrual blood in normal and menorrhagic women and in women wearing the Lippes Loop and the Cu-T (200). Int J Gynaecol Obstet 1979;16(5):400–7.
18. Wildemeersch D, Dhont M, Temmerman M, Delbarge W, Schacht E, Thiery M. GyneFix-LNG: preliminary clinical experience with a copper and levonorgestrel-releasing intrauterine system. Eur J Contracept Reprod Health Care 1999;4(1):15–19.
19. Lahteenmaki P, Rauramo I, Backman T. The levonorgestrel intrauterine system in contraception. Steroids 2000;65(10–11):693–7.
20. Backman T, Huhtala S, Blom T, Luoto R, Rauramo I, Koskenvuo M. Length of use and symptoms associated with premature removal of the levonorgestrel intrauterine system: a nation-wide study of 17,360 users. BJOG 2000;107(3):335–9.
21. Cox M, Blacksell S. Clinical performance of the levonorgestrel intra-uterine system in routine use by the UK Family Planning and Reproductive Health Research Network: 12-month report. Br J Fam Plann 2000;26(3):143–7.
22. Wildemeersch D, Schacht E. Endometrial suppression with a new 'frameless' levonorgestrel releasing intrauterine system in perimenopausal and postmenopausal women: a pilot study. Maturitas 2000;36(1):63–8.
23. Wong CY. Irregular bleeding with levonorgestrel IUS may delay cancer diagnosis. Br J Fam Plann 2000;26:61.
24. Anonymous. Unanswered questions on ectopic pregnancy. BMJ 1980;280(6223):1127–8.

25. Vessey MP, Yeates D, Flavel R. Risk of ectopic pregnancy and duration of use of an intrauterine device. Lancet 1979;2(8141):501–2.

26. Shamai A, Peretz BA, Kerner H, Paldi E. Four cases of primary ovarian pregnancy and two of them associated with an intrauterine device. Infertility 1979;2:233.

27. Engineer AD, Misra JS, Tandon P. Copper loss & cyto-pathological changes associated with copper IUD use. Indian J Med Res 1983;78:42–8.

28. Patai K, Balogh I. Clinicopathological problems of tissue effects caused by IUDs containing copper. Mag Noorv Lapja 1988;51:240.

29. Patai K, Balogh I, Szarvas Z. Clinicopathological problems of the local tissue effect of copper-containing IUDs. II. Electron-microscopic study of the endometrial scraping. Acta Chir Hung 1989;30(2):133–8.

30. Toivonen J, Luukkainen T, Allonen H. Protective effect of intrauterine release of levonorgestrel on pelvic infection: three years' comparative experience of levonorgestrel- and copper-releasing intrauterine devices. Obstet Gynecol 1991;77(2):261–4.

31. Purello D'Ambrosio F, Ricciardi L, Isola S, Gangemi S, Cilia M, Levanti C, Marcazzo A. Systemic contact dermatitis to copper-containing IUD. Allergy 1996;51(9):658–9.

32. Bulgaresi P, Confortini M, Galanti L, Gargano D. Inflammatory changes and cervical intraepithelial neoplasia in IUD users. Cervix Low Female Genital Tract 1989;7(3):207–12.

33. Duguid HL, Parratt D, Traynor R. *Actinomyces*-like organisms in cervical smears from women using intrauterine contraceptive devices. BMJ 1980;281(6239):534–7.

34. Leeton J. Female genital actinomycosis and the intrauterine device. Med J Aust 1980;1(11):518.

35. Vessey MP, Yeates D, Flavel R, McPherson K. Pelvic inflammatory disease and the intrauterine device: findings in a large cohort study. BMJ (Clin Res Ed) 1981;282(6267):855–7.

36. Graham D, Enkin M, deSa D. Neural tube defects in association with copper intrauterine devices. Int J Gynaecol Obstet 1980;18(6):404–5.

37. Zerner J, Doil LK, Drewry J, Leeber D. Intrauterine contraceptive device failures in renal transplant patients. J Reprod Med 1981;26:99.

Physical contraceptives— spermicides

General Information

Modern spermicides are produced in a variety of formulations, including gels, foams, creams, suppositories, pessaries, capsules, foaming tablets, and melting films. Spermicides are also used in conjunction with other methods, such as diaphragms, condoms, and sponges, but also with intrauterine contraceptive devices and methods based on fertility awareness (1).

Contraceptive sponges are controversial: do they act by delivering spermicides or as barriers? However, it has been shown conclusively that the newest forms of sponges, which provide not one but a combination of three active spermicides, act much more like spermicides than as simple vaginal barriers.

Spermicides are relatively inexpensive and widely available over the counter in most countries. All currently used formulations contain the non-ionic detergent nonoxinol-9, usually in a dose of 70–230 mg, but the newest formulations may contain octoxynol or benzalkonium chloride (2). All chemical agents used in spermicides disrupt the sperm cell membrane and finally rupture the cell.

Spermicides, especially in certain communities, have important advantages over the more modern methods of contraception: they are immediately reversible, are available over the counter without prescription, can be used by breastfeeding women, and are under direct female control.

However, spermicides also have adverse effects. They can cause local irritation in the woman or her partner, especially if they are used several times a day and can very rarely cause local allergic reactions in the woman or her partner.

Nonoxinols

Nonoxinols (ethoxylated alkyl phenols) are synthesized from alkylbenzene nonoxinol by reacting it with ethylene oxide to produce ethylene oxide polymers of various lengths. Each nonoxinol is followed by a number that indicates the approximate number of ethylene oxide groups it contains. In cosmetic products, nonoxinols are used as emulsifying, wetting, foaming, and solubilizing agents. They are used in hair and skin products, and in bath, shaving, and fragrance formulations (3). The non-ionic surfactant properties of nonoxinols allow them to be used in a wide variety of industrial, household, agricultural, and pharmaceutical products. Nonoxinol-9 and -10 are surface-active agents used in antiseptic formulations, such as Hibitane (chlorhexidine), Betadine (povidone-iodine), and Hexomedine (hexamidine). They are the most commonly used spermicidal contraceptives and have been recommended in the prevention of sexually transmitted diseases and in human immunodeficiency virus prophylaxis (4).

Carbomers

Carbomers are acrylic acid polymers that are used for a variety of purposes. They are used in pharmaceutical processes as suspending agents, gel bases, emulsifiers, and binding agents. They are also used as artificial tears. Carbomer 974P is a carbomer that is the major non-aqueous component (5% polymer, 94% water) of a proprietary formulation called BufferGel, which also contains dibasic potassium phosphate, magnesium sulfate, dibasic sodium phosphate, sorbic acid, monobasic sodium phosphate, and disodium EDTA. It is a buffering agent, a microbicide, and a spermicide. It is formulated in an aqueous gel at pH 3.9, which acidifies twice its volume of semen to a pH of 5 and maintains the protective acidity of the vagina. It is used vaginally as a spermicide that also protects against HIV infection and possibly other sexually transmitted diseases.

The safety of BufferGel has been evaluated in a high-dose tolerance trial in 98 women, of whom 91 (26 sexually abstinent and 65 sexually active) completed the study (5). Reasons for withdrawal included: an inability to adhere to the protocol ($n = 1$); breakthrough menstrual bleeding ($n = 2$); the presence of yeast on day 7 (two asymptomatic cases and one symptomatic case); and refusal to continue ($n = 1$). The percentage of women with at least one sign or symptom judged by a clinician as potentially related to the product was 29% in India, 33% in Thailand, 35% in Malawi, and 33% in Zimbabwe. There were no differences in the proportions of sexually abstinent and sexually active women with at least one potentially product-related sign or symptom at each study site. In all, there were 45 potentially product-related signs and symptoms. Two were judged to be definitely related to the product (vaginal itching after product insertion) and 43 as possibly or probably related. All were categorized as mild (84%) or moderate (16%). Excluding participants who withdrew by day 7, 71% of the signs and symptoms resolved during the trial and 24% within 3 days of product withdrawal at the end of the trial; 5% persisted at the end of the trial (one woman was given treatment for a yeast infection and one was not re-evaluated for itching). Minor self-reported symptoms of irritation of limited duration accounted for 64% of reported signs and symptoms and were approximately equally distributed across study sites. They included vulvar and vaginal itching or burning, burning when urinating, and genital rash. The overall rate of symptoms of irritation for all sites combined was 0.58 events per woman-week of observation (95% CI = 0.3, 0.88). Other signs and symptoms included lower abdominal pain or backache, symptomatic yeast infection, and vaginal discharge.

Organs and Systems

Urinary tract

Urinary tract infections are quite common, although not very serious adverse effects of spermicides. For several years, the rate of urinary tract infections in young, sexually active women caused by the use of spermicides has been uncertain and has not been thoroughly evaluated. Since this phenomenon was observed, special surveys have been carried out and several have confirmed a higher risk of urinary tract infection among women who use a diaphragm with spermicides, compared with sexually active women who use other types of contraception (6). Finally, women who use spermicides are at higher risk of urinary tract infection than women who use other methods of contraception. Users of diaphragms and other barrier methods (including spermicide-coated male condoms) in conjunction with spermicides have increased degrees of introital and periurethral colonization with coliform organisms and *Staphylococcus saprophyticus*, leading to urinary tract infection (7).

In a large case control study in the USA, 96 sexually active young women with acute urinary tract infections caused by *S. saprophyticus* and 629 control patients without urinary tract infections were interviewed (7). Exposure to spermicide-coated condoms during the previous month was associated with a higher risk of urinary tract infections. Younger age, intercourse frequency, prior urinary tract infections and frequency of exposure to spermicide-coated condoms were independent predictors. Among women exposed to spermicide-coated condoms, 74% of urinary tract infections caused by *S. saprophyticus* were attributable to this exposure. The

authors concluded that spermicide-coated condoms were associated with an increased risk of urinary tract infections caused by *S. saprophyticus*.

Skin

Contact dermatitis in patients exposed to nonoxinols was initially considered to result from irritation, but allergic reactions have also been reported (8). Nonoxinol contact allergy has been described in two patients who developed contact photosensitivity to nonoxinol-l0 in the antiseptic product Hexomedine transcutanée (hexamidine) (9). Among 32 control subjects, 13 had positive photopatch tests to Hexomedine transcutanée and four had positive photopatch tests to nonoxinol-10. Surprisingly, the authors observed that only undiluted nonoxinol was phototoxic, and in another study, nonoxinol-9 was found to be rarely sensitizing and compatible with latex and silicone lubricants used in condoms (10).

Second-Generation Effects

Teratogenicity

Use of spermicides in the year before pregnancy or during pregnancy has been associated with adverse reproductive outcomes, including spontaneous abortion and Down syndrome. In a preliminary analysis, an association was found between spermicide use at conception and tetraploid and hypertriploid conceptions (11). An association between the use of vaginal spermicides and birth defects has been suggested (12).

Spermicide use for more than a year at any time before conception was more common in cases aborting a trisomic conception than in controls. The association varied with maternal age, and was confined to women aged 30 years or older (13). However, it has since been concluded that there is no convincing evidence of an increased risk of fetal abnormalities in women who become pregnant while using spermicides, or in women who have used them before realizing that they were pregnant (14).

References

1. Lech MM. Spermicides 2002: an overview. Eur J Contracept Reprod Health Care 2002;7(3):173–7.
2. Aubeny E, Colau JC, Nandeuil A. Local spermicidal contraception: a comparative study of the acceptability and safety of a new pharmaceutical formulation of benzalkonium chloride, the vaginal capsule, with a reference formulation, the pessary. Eur J Contracept Reprod Health Care 2000;5(1):61–7.
3. Christian MS. Cosmetic ingredient review: final report on the safety assessment of nonoxynols 2, 4, 8, 9, 10, 12, 14, 15, 30, 40 and 50. J Am Coll Toxicol 1983;2:35–60.
4. Bird KD. The use of spermicide containing nonoxynol-9 in the prevention of HIV infection. AIDS 1991;5(7):791–6.
5. van De Wijgert J, Fullem A, Kelly C, Mehendale S, Rugpao S, Kumwenda N, Chirenje Z, Joshi S, Taha T, Padian N, Bollinger R, Nelson K. Phase 1 trial of the topical microbicide BufferGel: safety results from four international sites. J Acquir Immune Defic Syndr 2001;26(1):21–7.
6. Strom BL, Collins M, West SL, Kreisberg J, Weller S. Sexual activity, contraceptive use, and other risk factors

for symptomatic and asymptomatic bacteriuria. A case-control study. Ann Intern Med 1987;107(6):816–23.

7. Fihn SD, Boyko EJ, Chen CL, Normand EH, Yarbro P, Scholes D. Use of spermicide-coated condoms and other risk factors for urinary tract infection caused by *Staphylococcus saprophyticus*. Arch Intern Med 1998; 158(3):281–7.

8. Dooms-Goossens A, Deveylder H, de Alam AG, Lachapelle JM, Tennstedt D, Degreef H. Contact sensitivity to nonoxynols as a cause of intolerance to antiseptic preparations. J Am Acad Dermatol 1989;21(4 Pt 1):723–7.

9. Michel M, Dompmartin A, Moreau A, Leroy D. Contact photosensitivity to nonoxynol used in antiseptic preparations. Photodermatol Photoimmunol Photomed 1994; 10(5):198–201.

10. Fisher AA. Allergic contact dermatitis to nonoxynol-9 in a condom. Cutis 1994;53(3):110–11.

11. Strobino B, Kline J, Stein Z, Susser M, Warburton D. Exposure to contraceptive creams, jellies and douches and their effect on the zygote. Am J Epidemiol 1980; 223:434.

12. Manjuck JE. Relationship of vaginal spermicides to birth defects. J Fla Med Assoc 1989;76(3):316–21.

13. Strobino B, Kline J, Lai A, Stein Z, Susser M, Warburton D. Vaginal spermicides and spontaneous abortion of known karyotype. Am J Epidemiol 1986; 123(3):431–43.

14. Simpson JL, Phillips OP. Spermicides, hormonal contraception and congenital malformations. Adv Contracept 1990;6(3):141–67.

Phytolaccaceae

See also Herbal medicines

General Information

The genera in the family of Phytolaccaceae (Table 1) include pokeweed.

Phytolacca americana

Phytolacca americana (pokeweed) contains powerful mitogens (pokeweed mitogen), including phytolacain, used to study cell function.

Adverse effects
Severe emesis and diarrhea, accompanied by tachycardia, have been observed after ingestion of raw leaves and after drinking tea prepared from the powdered root of *P. americana* (pokeweed).

Table 1 The genera of Phytolaccaceae

Agdestis (agdestis)
Gisekia (gisekia)
Petiveria (petiveria)
Phytolacca (pokeweed)
Rivina (rivina)
Stegnosperma (stegnosperma)
Trichostigma (alpine clubrush)

In one case Mobitz type I heart block was associated with vomiting due to pokeweed, which resolved after intravenous promethazine (1). The authors suggested that the heart block had been due to increased vagal tone associated with severe gastrointestinal colic.

Reference

1. Hamilton RJ, Shih RD, Hoffman RS. Mobitz type I heart block after pokeweed ingestion. Vet Hum Toxicol 1995; 37(1):66–7.

Picenadol

General Information

Picenadol is a racemic mixture of an *N*-methyl-4-phenyl-piperidine derivative. It has mixed agonist–antagonist properties, because the dextrorotatory isomer is a potent opioid agonist and the levorotatory isomer is an opioid antagonist. Picenadol also has anticholinergic activity. Its adverse effects include drowsiness, dizziness, and light-headedness (SEDA-16, 90). In a double-blind comparison of the analgesic potency and adverse effects profiles of a single oral dose of picenadol 25 mg with codeine 60 mg and placebo, few adverse effects were reported. Drowsiness was the most frequent, with an incidence of 16% (1).

Picenadol 75 mg was reportedly distinguishable from morphine by sedation, dysphoria, and hallucinatory activity, probably due to anticholinergic activity; at lower doses it was morphine-like (SEDA-16, 90).

Reference

1. Brunelle RL, George RE, Sunshine A, Hammonds WD. Analgesic effect of picenadol, codeine, and placebo in patients with postoperative pain. Clin Pharmacol Ther 1988;43(6):663–7.

Picibanil

General Information

Picibanil (OK 432) is derived from *Streptococcus pyogenes* and has been used in the treatment of cancers, lymphangiomas, and viral infections. Low-grade fever, nausea and vomiting, and an inflammatory reaction at the injection site were commonly reported, whereas joint pain and mild liver dysfunction were seldom described.

Organs and Systems

Fluid balance

Hyponatremia due to the syndrome of inappropriate secretion of antidiuretic hormone (SIADH) has been attributed to picibanil (1).

- A 59-year-old woman with a previous history of squamous cell carcinoma of the esophagus developed a metastatic lung tumor 4 years later. A right lower lobectomy was performed, and intrapleural picibanil was instilled on postoperative days 4, 5, and 9 for pulmonary fistula with prolonged air leakage. On day 13 she had fatigue, nausea, and drowsiness. Her serum sodium concentration was 106 mmol/l and there was a 2.5-fold increase in serum antidiuretic hormone concentration. She recovered completely after fluid restriction and sodium supplementation.

The author thought that SIADH had resulted from severe pleurisy secondary to intrapleural administration of picibanil rather than to direct stimulation of antidiuretic hormone release.

Hematologic

Hemolytic anemia, presumably of immune origin, has been reported in a patient taking picibanil (2).

References

1. Hanagiri T, Muranaka H, Hashimoto M, Nagashima A. A syndrome of inappropriate secretion of antidiuretic hormone associated with pleuritis caused by OK-432. Respiration 1998;65(4):310–12.
2. Nomura S, Kanoh T. Immune hemolytic anemia associated with streptococcal preparation OK-432. Cancer 1987;59(8): 1409–11.

Picrotoxin

General Information

Picrotoxin is a non-nitrogenous plant derivative that is a powerful stimulant of all parts of the central nervous system, acting on the chloride ionophore–aminobutyric acid complex in a manner opposite to that of barbiturates (1). Its adverse effects resemble those of nikethamide; picrotoxin 20 mg can cause severe poisoning.

Reference

1 Obata K. The inhibitory action of aminobutyric acid, a probable synaptic transmitter. Int Rev Neurobiol 1972; 15:167–87.

Piketoprofen

See also Non-steroidal anti-inflammatory drugs

General Information

Piketoprofen is an NSAID that has been used topically as the hydrochloride salt.

Organs and Systems

Skin

A photoallergic contact dermatitis followed topical administration of piketoprofen in a 46-year-old man after 3 days; photopatch testing for piketoprofen was positive (1).

Reference

1. Bujan JJ, Morante JM, Guemes MG, Del Pozo Losada J, Capdevila EF. Photoallergic contact dermatitis from piketoprofen. Contact Dermatitis 2000;43(5):315.

Pilocarpine

General Information

Pilocarpine is an antagonist at acetylcholine receptors (1). While it is mainly used in the eye in the treatment of glaucoma, pilocarpine is still occasionally used for other purposes, for example for treating salivary gland hypofunction and xerostomia. When used in this way, cardiovascular tolerance was good but there was a high incidence of sweating, flushing, increased frequency of micturition, increased nasal secretion, and lacrimation (SEDA-18, 174).

Reference

1. Wiseman LR, Faulds D. Oral pilocarpine: a review of its pharmacological properties and clinical potential in xerostomia. Drugs 1995;49(1):143–55.

Pimecrolimus

General Information

Pimecrolimus is a non-steroidal ascomycin derivative with topical anti-inflammatory activity. In a 1% cream it is effective and safe in atopic dermatitis in infants, children, and adults (1–3), although its efficacy has been questioned (4).

Organs and Systems

Skin

The main adverse effect of pimecrolimus is local skin irritation, with a stinging or burning sensation, which occurs in 30% of patients. Typically, children have less skin irritation than adults. Adverse effects such as local immunosuppression and an increased risk of local bacterial and viral infections (notably eczema herpeticum) are less common than with topical glucocorticoids (5). In addition, there is a lack of skin atrophy (6,7). However, topical corticosteroids have the advantage of better skin penetration than pimecrolimus and will therefore continue to be used for more heavily keratinized skin such as in psoriasis (8).

Tinea incognito has been attributed to pimecrolimus (9).

- A 6-year-old boy developed a small, erythematous, slightly scaly, pruritic plaque near his right eye, which was treated with twice-daily pimecrolimus cream. After 2–3 days, the itching and erythema completely resolved, but a rough scaly plaque persisted. After 1–2 weeks, the itching gradually returned and the lesion began to increase in size. Multiple similar lesions appeared several centimeters from the initially affected area. Pimecrolimus was withdrawn and topical nystatin + triamcinolone ointment was prescribed. The eruption continued to spread, with multiple annular scaly papules and plaques with central clearing. There was excoriation and mild inflammation around all affected areas. A potassium hydroxide examination of the lesions showed numerous hyphae. The nystatin + triamcinolone was withdrawn and oral griseofulvin was prescribed. The eruption improved dramatically after 3 weeks and eventually cleared completely after 5 weeks of treatment. Topical 2% ketoconazole cream was applied twice a day during the final 2 weeks of treatment.

References

1. Van Leent EJ, Graber M, Thurston M, Wagenaar A, Spuls PI, Bos JD. Effectiveness of the ascomycin macrolactam SDZ ASM 981 in the topical treatment of atopic dermatitis. Arch Dermatol 1998;134(7):805–9.
2. Eichenfield LF, Lucky AW, Boguniewicz M, Langley RG, Cherill R, Marshall K, Bush C, Graeber M. Safety and efficacy of pimecrolimus (ASM 981) cream 1% in the treatment of mild and moderate atopic dermatitis in children and adolescents. J Am Acad Dermatol 2002;46(4):495–504.
3. Weinberg JM. Formulary review of therapeutic alternatives for atopic dermatitis: focus on pimecrolimus. J Manag Care Pharm 2005;11(1):56–64.
4. Anonymous. Pimecrolimus: new preparation. Me-too: too many risks, not beneficial enough in atopic dermatitis. Prescrire Int 2004;13(74):209–12.
5. Lubbe J, Pournaras CC, Saurat JH. Eczema herpeticum during treatment of atopic dermatitis with 0.1% tacrolimus ointment. Dermatology 2000;201(3):249–51.
6. Soter NA, Fleischer AB Jr, Webster GF, Monroe E, Lawrence I. Tacrolimus ointment for the treatment of atopic dermatitis in adult patients: part II, safety. J Am Acad Dermatol 2001;44(Suppl 1):S39–46.
7. Reitamo S, Wollenberg A, Schopf E, Perrot JL, Marks R, Ruzicka T, Christophers E, Kapp A, Lahfa M, Rubins A, Jablonska S, Rustin M. Safety and efficacy of 1 year of tacrolimus ointment monotherapy in adults with atopic dermatitis. The European Tacrolimus Ointment Study Group. Arch Dermatol 2000;136(8):999–1006.
8. Nghiem P. "Topical immunomodulators?" Introducing old friends and a new ally, tacrolimus. J Am Acad Dermatol 2001;44(1):111–13.
9. Crawford KM, Bostrom P, Russ B, Boyd J. Pimecrolimus-induced tinea incognito. Skinmed 2004;3(6):352–3.

Pimobendan

See also Phosphodiesterase type III, selective inhibitors of

General Information

Pimobendan is an inhibitor of phosphodiesterase type III with calcium sensitizing properties in the myocardium. It has been associated with a worrisome albeit non-significant increase in mortality in patients with chronic congestive heart failure (1).

Reference

1. Lubsen J, Just H, Hjalmarsson AC, La Framboise D, Remme WJ, Heinrich-Nols J, Dumont JM, Seed P. Effect of pimobendan on exercise capacity in patients with heart failure: main results from the Pimobendan in Congestive Heart Failure (PICO) trial. Heart 1996;76(3):223–31.

Pimozide

See also Neuroleptic drugs

General Information

Pimozide is a diphenylbutylpiperidine neuroleptic drug, structurally similar to the butyrophenones.

Organs and Systems

Cardiovascular

Pimozide can cause QT interval prolongation and torsade de pointes; a total of 40 reports (16 deaths) of serious cardiac reactions, mainly dysrhythmias, were reported to the Committee on Safety of Medicines in the UK from 1971 to 1995 (1).

Drug Administration

Drug overdose

In a study of overdosages of different neuroleptic drugs, pimozide had the lowest fatality index (the number of deaths divided by the number of prescriptions) (2).

Drug–Drug Interactions

Clarithromycin

In 12 healthy volunteers given oral pimozide 6 mg after 5 days of treatment with clarithromycin (500 mg bd) or placebo, pimozide significantly prolonged the QT_c interval in the first 20 hours in both groups (maximum changes in QT_c 16 and 13 ms respectively) (3).

References

1. Committee on Safety of Medicines—Medicines Control Agency. Cardiac arrhythmias with pimozide (Orap). Curr Probl Pharmacovigilance 1995;21:1.
2. Buckley N, McManus P. Fatal toxicity of drugs used in the treatment of psychotic illnesses. Br J Psychiatry 1998; 172:461–4.
3. Desta Z, Kerbusch T, Flockhart DA. Effect of clarithromycin on the pharmacokinetics and pharmacodynamics of pimozide in healthy poor and extensive metabolizers of cytochrome P450 2D6 (CYP2D6). Clin Pharmacol Ther 1999;65(1):10–20.

Pinaverium bromide

General Information

Pinaverium bromide is an anticholinergic drug (1). Like emepronium bromide, it can cause inflammation and ulceration in the mouth and esophagus (SEDA-6, 143).

Reference

1. Guslandi M. Profilo farmacologico-clinico del pinaverio bromuro. [The clinical pharmacological profile of pinaverium bromide.] Minerva Med 1994;85(4):179–85.

Pindolol

See also Beta-adrenoceptor antagonists

General Information

Pindolol is a beta-adrenoceptor antagonist with beta$_2$-adrenoceptor agonist action and some membrane-stabilizing activity (1).

Organs and Systems

Nervous system

Pindolol can cause resting tremor in some patients (2).

References

1. Aellig WH, Clark BJ. Is the ISA of pindolol beta$_2$-adrenoceptor selective? Br J Clin Pharmacol 1987; 24(Suppl 1):S21–8.
2. Hod H, Har-Zahav J, Kaplinsky N, Frankl O. Pindolol-induced tremor. Postgrad Med J 1980;56(655):346–7.

Pipebuzone

See also Non-steroidal anti-inflammatory drugs

General Information

Pipebuzone is a combination of phenylbutazone with piperazine, produced in an unsuccessful attempt to improve the tolerance of phenylbutazone. Typical phenylbutazone reactions (abdominal, hematological, renal, allergic, and rectal irritation from suppositories) were common (SED-9, 145) (1–3).

References

1. Poulain D. Bilan de l'utilisation de l'élarzone dausse en chirurgie gynécologique et obstétricale. A propos de 228 cas. Arch Med Ouest 1976;8:117.
2. Chovelon R, Hovasse BM. Expérimentation de l'élarzone-dausse, nouvel antiinflammatoire, dans les affectations des voies respiratoires chez les personnes âgées. Med Int Pol 1975;10:179.
3. Pelissier P, Colas IJ, Beaulieux J. Expérimentation de l'élarzone dausse dans un service de chirurgie vasculaire. J Méd Lyon 1974;55:709.

Pipecuronium bromide

See also Neuromuscular blocking drugs

General Information

Pipecuronium bromide is a bisquaternary steroid analogue of pancuronium. In vitro pipecuronium reversibly inhibits both human red cell acetylcholinesterase and human plasma cholinesterase to an extent that might have clinical implications (1). Its potency is similar to that of pancuronium and its onset and duration are also approximately the same. Accumulation can occur (2), and maintenance doses should be one-quarter to one-sixth of the initial dose to achieve a similar effect, depending on the anesthetic technique used.

From animal investigations hepatic uptake appears to be a factor in the drug's total plasma clearance, but renal excretion seems to be the main route of elimination. Ligation of renal pedicles in dogs (3) resulted in reduced elimination of pipecuronium, with a four-fold increase in mean residence time and a four-fold increase in hepato-biliary elimination, which did not compensate for the loss of urinary excretion. In humans, about 40% of pipecuronium is excreted unchanged in the urine together with another 15% as 3-hydroxypipecuronium in 24 hours (4). The half-life is around 135–160 minutes.

Organs and Systems

Cardiovascular

No histamine release has been reported with pipecuronium, and vagolytic or sympathomimetic effects are not seen in the usual dose range. Rarely, significant hypotension has been reported (2), but this was transient and occurred during an unstable phase of anesthesia. Bradycardia has also been seen (2) but is usually mild (5), and probably due to the vagotonic effects of co-administered drugs, as is seen with vecuronium and atracurium (that is a minor disadvantage of the relaxant's lack of vagolytic or sympathomimetic effects). Usually, no significant changes in heart rate or blood pressure are seen (6–8), even with doses up to three times the ED_{95} (9,10). Cardiovascular stability has also been reported in cardiac patients (11), including patients in ASA classes II and III about to undergo coronary artery bypass grafting who received doses up to 0.15 mg/kg (12) and those who received high-dose fentanyl anesthesia (13). The absence of tachycardia in these high-risk cardiac patients, in whom any increase in myocardial oxygen demand is unwanted, was considered an advantage of pipecuronium.

Susceptibility Factors

Renal disease

As expected, renal dysfunction is associated with an increase in volume of distribution, a decrease in plasma clearance (1.6 versus 2.4 ml/kg/minute), and an increase in half-life (263 versus 137 minutes) compared with patients with normal renal function (14). In the latter study there was no statistically significant prolongation of the mean duration of action of pipecuronium, but there was a much greater variation in those with renal insufficiency, with 25% recovery times (after 0.07 mg/kg) of 30–267 minutes (controls 55–198 minutes). These patients were also undergoing renal transplantation and most of the replacement kidneys would be expected to have some function and some glomerular excretion of pipecuronium. Prolongation of pipecuronium blockade should be expected in patients with renal insufficiency.

Drug–Drug Interactions

Barbiturates

Thiobutobarbital prolongs the duration of action of pipecuronium in dogs (15), but no interaction with barbiturates has been reported in man.

General anesthetics

In patients who have been exposed to volatile anesthetic agents for 30 minutes or so there is an increase in potency of pipecuronium to such an extent that doses can be reduced by about one-third with isoflurane (16) or

enflurane (10) compared with those required for balanced anesthesia. Halothane appears to be associated with relatively minor changes in potency (16). When the same doses of pipecuronium are given, the duration of blockade is significantly longer during isoflurane anesthesia than during neuroleptanesthesia (17); halothane is also associated with a prolonged action but to a lesser extent.

References

1. Simon G, Biro K, Karpati E, Tuba Z. The effect of the steroid muscle relaxant pipecurium bromide on the acetylcholinesterase activity of red blood cells in vitro. Arzneimittelforschung 1980;30(2a):360–3.
2. Wittek L, Gecsenyi M, Barna B, Hargitay Z, Adorjan K. Report on clinical test of pipecurium bromide. Arzneimittelforschung 1980;30(2a):379–83.
3. Khuenl-Brady KS, Sharma M, Chung K, Miller RD, Agoston S, Caldwell JE. Pharmacokinetics and disposition of pipecuronium bromide in dogs with and without ligated renal pedicles. Anesthesiology 1989;71(6):919–22.
4. Wierda JM, Karliczek GF, Vandenbrom RH, Pinto I, Kersten-Kleef UW, Meijer DK, Agoston S. Pharmacokinetics and cardiovascular dynamics of pipecuronium bromide during coronary artery surgery. Can J Anaesth 1990;37(2):183–91.
5. Boros M, Szenohradszky J, Marosi G, Toth I. Comparative clinical study of pipecurium bromide and pancuronium bromide. Arzneimittelforschung 1980;30(2a):389–93.
6. Alant O, Darvas K, Pulay I, Weltner J, Bihari I. First clinical experience with a new neuromuscular blocker pipecurium bromide. Arzneimittelforschung 1980;30(2a):374–9.
7. Bunjatjan AA, Miheev VI. Clinical experience with a new steroid muscle relaxant: pipecurium bromide. Arzneimittelforschung 1980;30(2a):383–5.
8. Newton DE, Richardson FJ, Agoston S. Preliminary studies in man with pipecurium bromide (Arduan), a new steroid neuromuscular blocking agent. Br J Anaesth 1982;54:P789.
9. Larijani GE, Bartkowski RR, Azad SS, Seltzer JL, Weinberger MJ, Beach CA, Goldberg ME. Clinical pharmacology of pipecuronium bromide. Anesth Analg 1989;68(6):734–9.
10. Foldes FF, Nagashima H, Nguyen HD, Duncalf D, Goldiner PL. Neuromuscular and cardiovascular effects of pipecuronium. Can J Anaesth 1990;37(5):549–55.
11. Barankay A. Circulatory effects of pipecurium bromide during anaesthesia of patients with severe valvular and ischaemic heart diseases. Arzneimittelforschung 1980;30(2a):386–9.
12. Tassonyi E, Neidhart P, Pittet JF, Morel DR, Gemperle M. Cardiovascular effects of pipecuronium and pancuronium in patients undergoing coronary artery bypass grafting. Anesthesiology 1988;69(5):793–6.
13. Stanley JC, Carson IW, Gibson FM, McMurray TJ, Elliott P, Lyons SM, Mirakhur RK. Comparison of the haemodynamic effects of pipecuronium and pancuronium during fentanyl anaesthesia. Acta Anaesthesiol Scand 1991;35(3):262–6.
14. Caldwell JE, Canfell PC, Castagnoli KP, Lynam DP, Fahey MR, Fisher DM, Miller RD. The influence of renal failure on the pharmacokinetics and duration of action of pipecuronium bromide in patients anesthetized with halothane and nitrous oxide. Anesthesiology 1989;70(1):7–12.
15. Pulay I, Alant O, Darvas K, Weltner J, Zeteny Z. Respiration paralysing and circulatory effects of a new

non-depolarizing relaxant, pipecurium bromide, in anaesthetized dogs. Arzneimittelforschung 1980;30(2a):358–60.

16. Pittet JF, Tassonyi E, Morel DR, Gemperle G, Richter M, Rouge JC. Pipecuronium-induced neuromuscular blockade during nitrous oxide–fentanyl, isoflurane, and halothane anesthesia in adults and children. Anesthesiology 1989; 71(2):210–13.

17. Wierda JM, Richardson FJ, Agoston S. Dose-response relation and time course of action of pipecuronium bromide in humans anesthetized with nitrous oxide and isoflurane, halothane, or droperidol and fentanyl. Anesth Analg 1989; 68(3):208–13.

Piperaceae

See also Herbal medicines

General Information

The family of Piperaceae contains three genera:

1. *Lepianthes* (lepianthes)
2. *Peperomia* (peperomia)
3. *Piper* (pepper).

Piper methysticum

The rhizome of *Piper methysticum* (kava kava) has been used for hundreds of years in the South Pacific islands as a recreational drug, the main constituents of which are non-alkaloidal pyrone derivatives. These compounds cause sedation and centrally induced muscle relaxation. Kava has also been marketed in the West as a herbal pharmaceutical for use in the treatment of anxiety, for which it seems to be effective (1). However, the formulation used indigenously is an aqueous extract, while the pharmaceutical formulation is prepared from a lipid extract. Thus, the formulation that has been used in the West may contain compounds that are not present in the drink that is commonly prepared in the South Pacific and may therefore have different adverse effects (2). This may explain the risk of liver damage that has been seen in the West, not having previously been reported.

Kava contains the pyridine alkaloid pipermethystine, the chalcone flavokavain, the norsesquiterpenoid dihydrokavain, and the pyran tetrahydroyangonin.

Adverse effects

The acute and chronic effects of kava were first described by the 19th-century German toxicologist Louis Lewin (3) in his book *Phantastica* (1924).

A carefully prepared kava beverage taken in small quantity occasioned only slight and agreeable modifications of sensibility. In this form it is a stimulating beverage after the imbibition whereof hardships can be endured more easily. It refreshes the fatigued body and brightens and sharpens the intellectual faculties. Appetite is augmented, especially if it is taken half an hour before meals . . . After doses that are not too strong a state of happy carelessness, content, and well-being appears without any physical or mental excitation. It is a

real euphoric state which is accompanied by an increased muscular efficiency. At the beginning speech is fluent and lively and the hearing becomes more sensible to subtle impressions. Kava has a soothing effect. Those who drink it are never choleric, angry, aggressive and noisy, as in the case of alcohol. Both natives and whites look upon it as a sedative in case of accidents. Reason and consciousness remain unaffected. After the consumption of greater quantities, however, the limbs become weary, the muscles seem out of control of the will, the gait is slow and unsteady, and the subject appears half drunk. An urgent desire to lie down manifests itself. The eye sees objects before it but is unable to identify them with exactness. In the same way the ears hear everything, but the individual is unable to account for what he hears. Everything becomes more and more diffuse. The drinker succumbs to fatigue, and experiences a desire to sleep which is stronger than all other impressions. He becomes somnolent and finally falls asleep. Many Europeans have themselves experienced this action of kava which paralyses the senses like magic and finally leads to deep sleep. Frequently a state of somnolent torpor accompanied by incoherent dreams and occasionally erotic visions remains without sleep supervening.

The sleep is similar to that produced by alcohol, out of which the individual can be awakened only with difficulty. If moderate quantities have been consumed it occurs twenty to thirty minutes later, and lasts from two to eight hours according to the degree of habituation of the subject. If the beverage is concentrated, that is contains a large amount of the resinous components of kava, intoxication comes on much more rapidly. The drinkers are found lying in the very places where they have been drinking. Occasionally a short state of nervous trembling occurs before they fall asleep. No excitation precedes these symptoms.

The kava drinker is incessantly tormented with the craving for his favourite beverage, which he cannot prepare for himself. It is a repugnant spectacle to see old and white-haired people, degenerate through prolonged abuse of the drug, going from house to house in order to beg for freshly prepared kava and often meeting with a refusal. Mental weakness has also been stated to follow from kavaism. It is said that old kava habitues have red, inflamed, bloodshot eyes, dull, bleary, and diminished in their functions. They become extremely emaciated, their hands tremble, and finally they cannot bring the drinking vessel to their mouths. Numerous cutaneous diseases of the natives of the South Seas, especially a kind of scaly eruption which results in a parchment-like state of the skin, have been attributed to the abuse of kava.

Nervous system

In a pilot study, 24 patients with stress-induced insomnia were treated for 6 weeks with kava 120 mg/day, followed by a 2-week washout period and then treatment with valerian 600 mg/day for another 6 weeks (4). Stress was measured in three areas, including social, personal, and life events, and insomnia was assessed by evaluating the time taken to fall asleep, the number of hours slept, and waking mood. Total stress severity and insomnia were significantly improved by both compounds, with no significant differences. The most commonly reported adverse events were vivid dreams with valerian (16%) and dizziness with kava (12%).

In 24 patients treated with kava for generalized anxiety disorder for 4 weeks in an open, crossover, randomized trial, two dosage schedules were compared: 120 mg od and 45 mg tds (5). There were significant reductions in mean Hamilton Anxiety Rating Scale scores, irrespective of dose schedule, treatment order, or sex. The impact of adverse effects was relatively low, and only one patient had to withdraw from the study (tds schedule) because of nausea. There was daytime drowsiness in 33% of patients taking the thrice-daily regimen compared with 9% in those taking a once-daily dose.

Parkinsonism has been attributed to kava (6).

- A 45-year-old woman with a family history of essential tremor developed severe and persistent parkinsonism after taking kava extract for anxiety for 10 days. Her symptoms improved with anticholinergic drugs.

The authors concluded that kava derivatives can produce severe parkinsonism in individuals with a genetic susceptibility.

Liver

There have been reports of liver damage with lipid kava extracts (1), and it has therefore been banned in several countries.

- A 39-year-old woman had been treated for toxic hepatitis of unknown cause (7). When she represented with hepatitis-like symptoms and high liver enzymes, toxic hepatitis was diagnosed. Other causes for the liver pathology were excluded and it was noted that before both exacerbations, she had self-prescribed kava. When the kava was withdrawn, the liver pathology normalized and she made an uneventful recovery.
- A 60-year-old patient, who had taken no medications other than kava extract, developed liver and kidney failure and progressive encephalopathy (8). Viral, metabolic, and autoimmune causes were excluded. Liver biopsy was consistent with toxic liver damage. The patient eventually received an orthotopic liver transplant and made a good recovery.
- A 50-year-old man developed jaundice. He had noticed fatigue for a month, a "tanned" skin, and dark urine (9). The medical history was unremarkable, apart from slight anxiety, for which he had been taking three or four capsules of kava extract daily for 2 months. He took no other drugs and did not consume alcohol. Liver function tests showed very large increases in transaminases. He subsequently developed stage IV encephalopathy but made a good recovery after liver transplantation.
- A 34-year-old woman developed toxic hepatitis after taking kava-kava (10). Ultrasound showed an enlarged echogenic liver, and histology showed centrilobular necrosis and periportal inflammation. After withdrawal of the kava the changes resolved completely. This case illustrates the high hepatotoxic potential of kava-kava.
- A 33-year-old woman took a kava extract equivalent to 210 mg of kavalactones daily for 3 weeks (11). She

developed malaise, loss of appetite, and jaundice. Her liver enzymes were raised 3-fold to 60-fold. Viral hepatitis was excluded and liver biopsy confirmed toxic hepatitis. Kava was withdrawn, and within 8 weeks the liver enzymes returned to normal. A lymphocyte transformation test showed strong concentration-dependent T cell reactivity to kava. Phenotyping of CYP2D6 activity showed that she was a poor metabolizer.

The authors of the last report concluded that the liver damage in this case was due to an immune-mediated reaction, possibly mediated by a reactive metabolite of kava, even though she was a poor metabolizer.

Kava has been associated with toxic liver damage in six cases reported from Switzerland (12). In one patient, the liver damage was so extensive that liver transplantation became necessary. Histological data from four patients were consistent with an allergic mechanism. In several cases, other medications with hepatotoxic potential had been taken concurrently. Symptoms generally occurred at between 3 weeks and 4 months and involved daily doses that contained kavapyrones 60–210 mg. Most instances involved acetone extracts. The leading kava extract, Laitan, was subsequently withdrawn from the Swiss market.

Australia's Therapeutic Goods Administration initiated a voluntary recall of all complementary medicines containing kava after the death of a woman who used a medicine containing kava (13). Sponsors and retailers were asked to remove all products containing kava from the market immediately. Consumers were advised to discard kava-containing products in their possession.

The Federal Institute of Germany has withdrawn all products that contain kava and kavaine from the German market because of the risk of hepatotoxicity and insufficiently proven efficacy. The regulation included homeopathic products with dilutions up to D4. The German regulation applies to all kava-containing pharmaceutical formulations. Moreover, following a provisional opinion from the UK Committee on Safety of Medicines (CSM), the Medicines and Healthcare products Regulatory Agency (MHRA) has consulted on a proposal to prohibit the sale, supply, or importation of unlicensed medicinal products containing kava in the UK. The CSM reviewed the issue of kava-associated liver toxicity following the emergence of safety concerns in Europe. At that time, stocks of kava were voluntarily withdrawn by the herbal sector while the safety concerns were under investigation. Currently the MHRA is aware of 68 cases worldwide of suspected kava-associated liver problems, including 6 cases of liver failure that resulted in transplant, and 3 deaths. In the UK there have been three reports of kava-associated liver toxicity. The CSM has advised consumers to stop taking medicinal products containing kava, and to seek medical advice if they feel unwell or have concerns about possible liver problems.

Finally, the FDA has advised consumers of the potential for liver injury by kava-containing dietary supplements. People who have liver disease or liver problems or who are taking medicines that can affect the liver have been advised to consult a physician before using kava-containing supplements (14). Consumers who use kava-containing dietary supplements and who have signs of illness associated with liver disease should also consult a physician. The FDA has issued a letter to healthcare professionals informing them of the consumer advice and has urged consumers and healthcare professionals to report injuries that may be related to the use of kava.

The incidence of liver damage with kava seems to be less than one case per million daily doses (15). The mechanism of the effect is currently unclear. It has been suggested that supervised, monitored, short-term medication with kava would still do more good than harm (16). However, the FDA will continue to investigate the relation, if any, between the use of dietary supplements containing kava and liver damage.

Skin
Allergic skin reactions (17) and other adverse effects, including dermatological problems and neurological symptoms, have been described in individuals using such formulations. Heavy chronic consumption of kava-kava can lead to a pellagroid dermopathy that appears to be unrelated to niacin deficiency (18).

- A 36-year-old woman developed a generalized rash, severe itching with erythema, and papules 4 days after discontinuing a kava formulation (Antares), which she had taken in a dosage of 120 mg/day for 3 weeks (19). The condition improved with glucocorticoids and antihistamines, but the itching lasted several weeks. Patch tests with the kava extract were positive.

Musculoskeletal
Rhabdomyolysis has been attributed to kava (20).

- A 29-year-old man developed severe diffuse muscle pain and passed dark urine a few hours after taking a herbal combination product containing guaraná 500 mg, Ginkgo biloba 200 mg, and kava 100 mg. His blood creatine kinase activity and myoglobin concentration were raised and there were no signs of an underlying metabolic myopathy. His condition improved within 6 weeks.

The authors suggested that the methylxanthine-like effects of guaraná and the antidopaminergic and neuromuscular blocking properties of kava had caused the rhabdomyolysis in this patient.

Drug overdose

- A 34-year-old Tongan man complained of sore eyes, headache, generalized muscle weakness, and abdominal pain (21). He was disoriented and hallucinating. His family reported that he had been drinking large quantities of kava daily for about 14 years. Chronic kava intoxication was treated with intravenous Plasmalyte (a crystalloid solution) and he recovered within a day.

References

1. Stevinson C, Huntley A, Ernst E. A systematic review of the safety of kava extract in the treatment of anxiety. Drug Saf 2002;25(4):251–61.
2. Jamieson DD, Duffield PH, Cheng D, Duffield AM. Comparison of the central nervous system activity of the aqueous and lipid extract of kava (*Piper methysticum*). Arch Int Pharmacodyn Ther 1989;301:66–80.
3. Aronson JK. Louis Lewin—Meyler's predecessor. In: Aronson JK, editor. Side Effects of Drugs Annual. Amsterdam: Elsevier, 2004;27:xxv–xxix.
4. Wheatley D. Kava and valerian in the treatment of stress-induced insomnia. Phytother Res 2001;15(6):549–51.
5. Wheatley D. Kava-kava (LI 150) in the treatment of generalized anxiety disorder. Prim Care Psychiatry 2001;7:97–100.
6. Meseguer E, Taboada R, Sanchez V, Mena MA, Campos V, Garcia De Yebenes J. Life-threatening parkinsonism induced by kava-kava. Mov Disord 2002;17(1):195–6.
7. Strahl S, Ehret V, Dahm HH, Maier KP. Nedrotisierende Hepatitis nach Einnahme pflanzlicher Heilmittel. [Necrotizing hepatitis after taking herbal remedies.] Dtsch Med Wochenschr 1998;123(47):1410–14.
8. Kraft M, Spahn TW, Menzel J, Senninger N, Dietl KH, Herbst H, Domschke W, Lerch MM. Fulminantes Leberversagen nach Einnahme des planzlichen Antidepressivums Kava-Kava. [Fulminant liver failure after administration of the herbal antidepressant Kava-Kava.] Dtsch Med Wochenschr 2001;126(36):970–2.
9. Escher M, Desmeules J, Giostra E, Mentha G. Hepatitis associated with kava, a herbal remedy for anxiety. BMJ 2001;322(7279):139.
10. Weise B, Wiese M, Plotner A, Ruf BR. Toxic hepatitis after intake of kava-kava. Vergauungskrankheiten 2002;20:166–9.
11. Russmann S, Lauterburg BH, Helbling A. Kava hepatotoxicity. Ann Intern Med 2001;135(1):68–9.
12. Stoller A. Leberschädigungen unter Kava-Extrakten. Schweiz Arztez 2000;24:1335–6.
13. Anonymous. Kava-kava. More withdrawals due to hepatotoxic risks. WHO Pharmaceuticals Newslett 2002;3:4–5.
14. Anonymous. Kava-kava. Further investigations into *Piper methysticum* and liver injury. WHO Pharmaceuticals Newslett 2002;2:2–3.
15. Ernst E. Safety concerns about kava. Lancet 2002;359(9320):1865.
16. Teschke R. Hepatotoxizität durch Kava–Kava. Deutsch Arzteblatt 2002;99:A3411–18.
17. Suss R, Lehmann P. Haematogenes Kontaktekzem durch pflanzliche Medikamente am Beispiel des Kavawurzelextraktes. [Hematogenous contact eczema cause by phytogenic drugs exemplified by kava root extract.] Hautarzt 1996;47(6):459–61.
18. Ruze P. Kava-induced dermopathy: a niacin deficiency? Lancet 1990;335(8703):1442–5.
19. Schmidt P, Boehncke WH. Delayed-type hypersensitivity reaction to kava-kava extract. Contact Dermatitis 2000;42(6):363–4.
20. Donadio V, Bonsi P, Zele I, Monari L, Liguori R, Vetrugno R, Albani F, Montagna P. Myoglobinuria after ingestion of extracts of guaraná, *Ginkgo biloba* and kava. Neurol Sci 2000;21(2):124.
21. Chanwai LG. Kava toxicity. Emerg Med 2000;12:142–5.

Piperaquine

General Information

Piperaquine is a synthetic 4-aminoquinoline with high blood schizonticidal activity, similar to that of chloroquine (SEDA-13, 810). There is some evidence that piperaquine is active against chloroquine-resistant *Plasmodium falciparum*, but laboratory studies suggest a degree of cross-resistance. Piperaquine 600 mg/month was well tolerated. Its reported adverse effects included headache, dizziness, vomiting, and diarrhea.

Organs and Systems

Gastrointestinal

The novel combination (Artekin™) of dihydroartemisinin and piperaquine has been assessed in 106 patients (76 children and 30 adults) with uncomplicated *P. falciparum* malaria in Cambodia (1). The respective doses of dihydroartemisinin and piperaquine, which were given at 0, 8, 24, and 32 hours, were 9.1 and 74 mg/kg in children and 6.6 and 53 mg/kg in adults. All the patients became aparasitemic within 72 hours. Excluding the results in one child who died on day 4, there was a 97% 28-day cure rate (99% in children and 92% in adults). Patients who had recrudescent infections used low doses of Artekin. Adverse effects, most commonly gastrointestinal complaints, were reported by 22 patients (21%) but did not necessitate premature withdrawal.

Reference

1. Denis MB, Davis TM, Hewitt S, Incardona S, Nimol K, Fandeur T, Poravuth Y, Lim C, Socheat D. Efficacy and safety of dihydroartemisinin-piperaquine (Artekin) in Cambodian children and adults with uncomplicated falciparum malaria. Clin Infect Dis 2002;35(12):1469–76.

Piperazine

General Information

Piperazine is an antihelminthic drug that selectively blocks the neuromuscular cholinergic receptors of worms. It is readily absorbed, but has a highly variable half-life. The adult oral dose of 4 g of piperazine hydrate has been used extensively in the treatment of ascariasis. A very old drug, it is still considered sufficiently safe for use, although in most developed countries it has been abandoned, primarily because of concerns about possible carcinogenicity and electroencephalographic changes (SEDA-12, 267).

General adverse effects

In most patients, piperazine is free of adverse reactions. Mild gastrointestinal disturbances may occur; neurotoxicity is rare. Eczematous skin reactions, lacrimation, rhinorrhea, joint pains, productive cough, and bronchospasm can develop after sensitization, especially with occupational exposure. Urticaria has also been reported. When hypersensitivity reactions occur it should be withdrawn and not used again in the same patient. Mononitrosylation of piperazine can occur in the stomach, releasing the potential carcinogen *N*-mononitrosopiperazine, but there is no direct proof of risk in human subjects.

Organs and Systems

Cardiovascular

Cardiac conduction defects have been described in patients taking piperazine (1).

Respiratory

Allergic respiratory reactions can occur in patients taking piperazine, resulting in cough and bronchospasm (2).

Nervous system

Headache, dizziness, and somnolence occur in a small proportion of individuals who take piperazine (3). More serious neurological reactions occur rarely, but tend to be reported in young children, in people with neurological or renal disease, or after overdosage. Symptoms in such cases include ataxia, paresthesia, undue clumsiness, myoclonus, and nystagmus. Choreiform movements and an electroencephalogram with prominent slow waves have been reported as well as an exacerbation of petit mal (4) and absence seizures (5). In a child, horizontal nystagmus and hypotonia have been reported after a normal dose (6).

- A previously well 23-month-old girl was given piperazine 65 mg/kg/day for 7 days for a suspected worm infestation and developed cerebellar ataxia after 8 days (7). Over the next 48 hours her symptoms gradually settled. She made a complete recovery 5 days later.

Sensory systems

Piperazine can cause a range of visual effects, including dry eyes, bulging eyes, difficulty in focusing, and double vision (8).

Reports of cataract after piperazine have not been authenticated (9).

Hematologic

One suspected case of hemolysis after piperazine treatment was published but it appeared as long ago as 1971 and the patient had G6PD deficiency (10).

A case of temporary thrombocytopenia has been described (11), probably due to prior sensitization by ethylenediamine (a stabilizer in some creams), with which piperazine cross-reacts.

Gastrointestinal

Nausea, vomiting, abdominal pain, and diarrhea can occur occasionally with piperazine (12).

Liver

A single incident resembling viral hepatitis after piperazine and recurring after further dosage has been reported (13).

Skin

Erythema and rarely allergic reactions can occur in patients taking piperazine (12).

Second-Generation Effects

Teratogenicity

There is no evidence that piperazine has any second-generation effects; it has been used extensively in pregnancy without untoward incidents, but as a precaution WHO advises against administration in the first trimester.

Drug–Drug Interactions

Chlorpromazine

High doses of piperazine can enhance the adverse effects of chlorpromazine and other phenothiazines (14,15).

Pyrantel

Piperazine can antagonize the antihelminthic efficacy of pyrantel and vice versa (16).

References

1. Gouffault J, Van den Driessche J, Pony JC, Courgeon P, Thomas R. Les troubles de conduction induits par la pipérazine: étude clinique et expérimentale. [Conduction disorders induced by piperazine; clinical and experimental study.] Arch Mal Coeur Vaiss 1973;66(10):1289–95.
2. McCullagh SF. Allergenicity of piperazine: a study in environmental aetiology. Br J Ind Med 1968;25(4):319–25.
3. Onuaguluchi G, Mezue WC. Some effects of piperazine citrate on skeletal muscle and central nervous system. Arch Int Pharmacodyn Ther 1987;290(1):104–16.
4. Vallat JN, Vallat JM, Texier J, Leger J. Les signes neurologiques d'intoxication par la pipérazine (à propos de deux observations recentes). [Neurologic manifestations of piperazine poisoning (apropos of 2 cases).] Bord Med 1972;5(4):391–400.
5. Yohai D, Barnett SH. Absence and atonic seizures induced by piperazine. Pediatr Neurol 1989;5(6):393–4.
6. Bomb BS, Bedi HK. Neurotoxic side-effects of piperazine. Trans R Soc Trop Med Hyg 1976;70(4):358.
7. Shroff R, Houston B. Unusual cerebellar ataxia: "worm wobble" revisited. Arch Dis Child 2002;87(4):333–4.
8. Frauenfelder FT, editor. Drug-Induced Ocular Side Effects and Drug Interactions. 3rd ed. Philadelphia: Lea & Febiger, 1989:494–580.
9. Radnot M, Varga M. Structure histologique de la cataracte causée par le pipérazine. [Histologic structure of cataracts caused by piperazine.] Ann Ocul (Paris) 1969;202(4):325–9.
10. Buchanan N, Cassel R, Jenkins T. G-6-PD deficieny and piperazine. BMJ 1971;2(753):110.
11. Cork MJ, Cooke NJ, Mellor E. Pruritus ani, piperazine, and thrombocytopenia. BMJ 1990;301(6765):1398.
12. Point G. Incidents neurologiques lors de l'utilisation de la pipérazine comme vermifuge. [Neurologic complications during the use of piperazine as a vermifuge.] Pediatrie 1965;20(5):600–4.
13. Hamlyn AN, Morris JS, Sarkany I, Sherlock S. Piperazine hepatitis. Gastroenterology 1976;70(6):1144–7.
14. Sturman G. Interaction between piperazine and chlorpromazine. Br J Pharmacol 1974;50(1):153–5.
15. Boulos BM, Davis LE. Hazard of simultaneous administration of phenothiazine and piperazine. N Engl J Med 1969;280(22):1245–6.
16. Aubry ML, Cowell P, Davey MJ, Shevde S. Aspects of the pharmacology of a new anthelmintic: pyrantel. Br J Pharmacol 1970;38(2):332–44.

Piperidolate

General Information

Piperidolate is an anticholinergic drug that has been used to treat premature labor and digestive disorders (1). Doses of 50 mg are usual for treating pyloric spasm. The effects and adverse effects at this dose are both small.

Reference

1. Plancherel P. Klinischer Vergleich zwischen Dactil und Dactilase bei Verdauungsstorungen. [Clinical comparison of Dactil and Dactilase in digestive disorders.] Praxis 1969;58(40):1275–8.

Piracetam

General Information

Piracetam is a so-called "nootropic" drug, one of a class of drugs that affect mental function (1). In healthy volunteers it improves the higher functions of the brain involved in cognitive processes, such as learning and memory. Its mechanisms of action are not known but may include increased cholinergic neurotransmission.

A meta-analysis of 19 double-blind, placebo-controlled trials in elderly patients with dementia or cognitive impairment showed significant improvement with piracetam (2).

Piracetam has also been used to treat fetal distress during labor, but there is insufficient evidence to assess its efficacy (3).

Organs and Systems

Nervous system

Piracetam 80–100 mg/day for 4 months has been evaluated in a randomized, double-blind, placebo-controlled, crossover study in 25 children with Down syndrome (4). Piracetam did not enhance cognition or behavior but was associated with adverse events: 18 children completed the study, 4 withdrew, and 3 were excluded at baseline. The adverse events were related to the nervous system and included aggression ($n = 4$), agitation/irritability ($n = 2$), sexual arousal ($n = 2$), poor sleep ($n = 1$), and reduced appetite ($n = 1$).

References

1 Vernon MW, Sorkin EM. Piracetam. An overview of its pharmacological properties and a review of its therapeutic use in senile cognitive disorders. Drugs Aging 1991;1(1):17–35.
2 Waegemans T, Wilsher CR, Danniau A, Ferris SH, Kurz A, Winblad B. Clinical efficacy of piracetam in cognitive impairment: a meta-analysis. Dement Geriatr Cogn Disord 2002;13(4):217–24.

3   Hofmeyr GJ, Kulier R. Piracetam for fetal distress in labour. Cochrane Database Syst Rev 2002;(1):CD001064.

4   Lobaugh NJ, Karaskov V, Rombough V, Rovet J, Bryson S, Greenbaum R, Haslam RH, Koren G. Piracetam therapy does not enhance cognitive functioning in children with Down syndrome. Arch Pediatr Adolesc Med 2001;155(4):442–8.

Pirazolac

See also Non-steroidal anti-inflammatory drugs

General Information

Pirazolac, a pyrazoloacetic acid derivative, caused heartburn, upper abdominal pain, cutaneous adverse effects (rashes, exacerbation of pre-existing eczema), and eosinophilia in early clinical studies (1). In two comparative studies it was withdrawn in 15–20% of patients, that is more often than the comparator NSAIDs (indometacin, sulindac) (SEDA-16, 111).

Reference

1   Symmons D, Clark B, Panayi G, Geddawi M. Differential dosing study of pirazolac, a new non-steroidal anti-inflammatory agent, in patients with rheumatoid arthritis. Curr Med Res Opin 1985;9(8):542–7.

Pirenzepine

General Information

Pirenzepine is an anticholinergic drug with selective effects on muscarinic M_1 receptors. It therefore inhibits gastric acid secretion in the stomach. When it was introduced it was claimed that in the doses necessary to affect gastric acid secretion it would be almost entirely free of other muscarinic (atropine-like) effects. However, although muscarinic adverse effects, such as dry mouth and difficulty in accommodation, are less common with pirenzepine than with atropine, they can still occur in about half the patients who take the drug (1). Cardiac conduction effects resulting in sinus tachycardia, atrial fibrillation, and nodal tachycardia can also occur.

Granulocytopenia and thrombocytopenia are on record (SED-12, 944) (2).

References

1   Londong W, Londong V, Federle C, Tanswell P, Voderholzer U. Pharmacokinetic and pharmacodynamic studies in man simulating acute and chronic treatment with oral pirenzepine. Eur J Clin Pharmacol 1989;36(4):369–74.

2   Stricker BH, Meyboom RH, Bleeker PA, van Wieringen K. Blood disorders associated with pirenzepine. BMJ (Clin Res Ed) 1986;293(6554):1074.

Piretanide

See also Diuretics

General Information

Piretanide is a close relative of furosemide, with diuretic and kinetic properties very similar to those of furosemide and bumetanide (1,2). Its potency lies somewhere between the two. As with some other diuretics, attempts have been made to show specific advantages for piretanide, for example that it is a "potassium-stable" diuretic. However, there is no good evidence that it has such advantages (SEDA-10, 188) (SEDA-15, 213).

References

1   Clissold SP, Brogden RN. Piretanide. A preliminary review of its pharmacodynamic and pharmacokinetic properties, and therapeutic efficacy. Drugs 1985;29(6):489–530.

2   Knauf H, Mutschler E. Das Wirkprofil von Diuretika. Piretanid im Vergleich zu Thiaziden und Autikaliure tika. Internist (Berl) 1992;33(suppl 1):S16–22.

Piribedil

General Information

Piribedil is a piperazine derivative, a dopamine receptor agonist, which has been mainly used for the treatment of depression and Parkinson's disease. It has also been recommended for the treatment of patients with intermittent claudication, without convincing evidence.

Somnolence is a common adverse effect and can occur at low doses (SED-10, 346) (SEDA-10, 119). Among 50 patients with Parkinson's disease who had recently taken piribedil, 3 satisfied the clinical description of sleep attacks (1).

At higher doses gastrointestinal effects (anorexia and nausea) occur in 13% of patients taking a gradually increasing dose up to 120 mg/day (2). At very high doses (240 mg/day), changes in liver function tests occasionally occur. After intravenous administration (1.5–3.0 mg/hour for 6 hours) drowsiness, cold extremities, and spontaneous erections are common (SED-9, 317) (SEDA-2, 185) (SEDA-5, 207).

In 49 Filipino patients with Parkinson's disease and motor fluctuations the most common adverse effects of piribedil in a dosage of up to 150 mg/day were hallucinations (20%), dyskinesias (20%), dizziness (8%), and sleepiness (6%) (3).

References

1   Tan EK. Piribedil-induced sleep attacks in Parkinson's disease. Fundam Clin Pharmacol 2003;17(1):117–19.

2   Velho-Gronberg P, Paal G, Grossmann W. Parkinson tremor: clinical and electrophysiological assessments

of the response to piribedil. Psychol Med (Paris) 1979; 11:235.

3. Evidente VG, Esteban RP, Domingo FM, Carbajal LO, Parazo MA. Piribedil as an adjunct to levodopa in advanced Parkinson's disease: the Asian experience. Parkinsonism Relat Disord 2003;10(2):117–21.

Piridoxilate

General Information

Piridoxilate, an equimolar mixture of glyoxylic acid and pyridoxine, is marketed in a few countries (for example France) for peripheral arterial occlusive disease and functional venous disorders.

Organs and Systems

Urinary tract

A few reports have dealt with the occurrence of calcium oxalate renal calculi associated with long-term administration of piridoxilate.

- A 23-year-old man developed acute renal insufficiency due to hyperoxaluria and intratubular deposits of oxalate crystals after attempting suicide with an overdose of piridoxilate (SEDA-11, 180).
- An old woman developed end-stage chronic renal insufficiency and histological evidence of renal oxalosis ascribed to 10 years of piridoxilate treatment; renal function did not improve after withdrawal of the drug, and chronic hemodialysis was required (1).

Reference

1. Mousson C, Justrabo E, Rifle G, Sgro C, Chalopin JM, Gerard C. Piridoxilate-induced oxalate nephropathy can lead to end-stage renal failure. Nephron 1993;63(1):104–6.

Piritrexim

General Information

Piritrexim is a lipid-soluble analogue of methotrexate that has been used to treat methotrexate-resistant tumors (1). It is given with leucovorin (folinic acid) to minimize hematological toxicity. Myelosuppression is the major dose-limiting adverse effect. In 35 patients with urothelial carcinomas there was WHO grade 3/4 thrombocytopenia in four, granulocytopenia in one, and anemia in three; grade 3 non-hematological toxicity consisted of neuropathy in five patients, hepatotoxicity in two, nausea in two, and pulmonary toxicity and rash in one each (2). Piritrexim also causes facial flushing, periorbital edema, and pruritus, and anaphylactic shock has been reported (SEDA-18, 289).

References

1. Liu G, Bailey HH, Arzoomanian RZ, Alberti D, Binger K, Volkman J, Feierabend C, Marnocha R, Wilding G, Thomas JP. Gemcitabine, Paclitaxel, and Piritrexim: a phase I study. Am J Clin Oncol 2003;26(3):280–4.
2. Roth BJ, Manola J, Dreicer R, Graham D, Wilding G; Eastern Cooperative Oncology Group. Piritrexim in advanced, refractory carcinoma of the urothelium (E3896): a phase II trial of the Eastern Cooperative Oncology Group. Invest New Drugs 2002;20(4):425–9.

Piroxicam

See also Non-steroidal anti-inflammatory drugs

General Information

Piroxicam was the first of the oxicam compounds, and is by far the most widely used. It is an inhibitor of prostaglandin synthesis and platelet aggregation. Its long half-life (36–48 hours) allows it to be given in a single daily dose. Adverse effects data from 46 trials in 3827 patients, 2716 on short-term treatment (less than 12 weeks), have been reviewed (SEDA-6, 1) (1). In 20 controlled trials in 816 patients, adverse effects occurred in 27%, causing withdrawal in 2.2%. However, an uncontrolled study registered adverse effects in only 16% of patients. Allowing for all analyses and reviews, the overall adverse effects profile of piroxicam seems to be qualitatively the same as that of other NSAIDs, with gastrointestinal complaints at the top of the list.

Reactions involving the gastrointestinal system occur in up to 40% of patients. The approximately 1% incidence of peptic ulcer appears to be dose-related, as it rises to 7% in patients who take dosages higher than 20 mg/day for several weeks (2). Nervous system reactions are the second most frequent types of adverse effect. Changes in laboratory findings (creatinine, aspartate transaminase, alanine transaminase) are frequent, but they have little clinical relevance. Hypersensitivity reactions do not seem to be a problem with piroxicam treatment, although skin or mucosal reactions have been reported. Shock has been described. Tumor-inducing effects have not been reported.

Cinnoxicam is the cinnamate ester of piroxicam; its adverse effects are similar. Gastrointestinal effects (81%), nervous system effects (4%), and cutaneous effects (4%) were most common in a multicenter post-marketing surveillance study of 2969 patients; 12% had adverse effects (SEDA-16, 113). Cinnoxicam cream can cause itchy erythema, edema, vesicles, and exudation (SEDA-20, 94).

Organs and Systems

Respiratory

In two cases piroxicam caused pulmonary infiltrates and eosinophilia (SEDA-19, 99).

Nervous system

Adverse effects in about 11% of patients include head-ache, dizziness, drowsiness, fatigue, and sweating (3).

Sensory systems

Eyes
Blurred vision and burning eyes have been described with piroxicam (SEDA-5, 107).

Ears
Permanent sensorineural hearing loss and tinnitus have been described with piroxicam (4).

Electrolyte balance

Severe hyponatremia, characterized by increasing confusion and disorientation, has been reported (SEDA-13, 83).

Hyperkalemia has often been linked to prolonged use of piroxicam, especially in the elderly (SEDA-8, 110) (SEDA-10, 87).

Hematologic

Piroxicam can cause thrombocytopenia, including a case of thrombocytopenic purpura due to an immunological mechanism (SEDA-13, 83). As an inhibitor of prostaglandin synthesis, piroxicam also inhibits platelet aggregation and prolongs bleeding time.

Leukopenia has been reported; the leukocyte count returned to normal after withdrawal (5). Agranulocytosis in a woman who took piroxicam for 3 days disappeared rapidly after withdrawal (SEDA-14, 95).

Aplastic anemia, which resolved fully after withdrawal, has been described (SEDA-17, 114).

Gastrointestinal

Gastrointestinal effects are the most frequent adverse effects of piroxicam. Although epigastric distress, nausea, abdominal pain, constipation, flatulence, and diarrhea have all been reported, they rarely interfere with treatment.

Esophageal lesions have been recorded in young healthy volunteers taking piroxicam (6).

An unusual case of gastrocolic fistula occurred in an old man who had taken piroxicam for 2 months (7).

Peptic ulceration and gastrointestinal bleeding were recorded in 1–1.4% of patients taking piroxicam 20 mg/day, and the incidence of ulceration increased to 6.9% at a dosage of 40 mg/day. A comparative study of gastrointestinal blood loss after aspirin 972 mg qds for 4 days versus different doses of piroxicam (20 mg od, 5 mg qds, and 10 mg qds) showed that piroxicam did not increase fecal blood loss, whereas aspirin did. Gastroscopic evidence of irritation was also greater with aspirin (8). The debate on the ulcerogenicity and relative safety of piroxicam continues, as new reports are published (SEDA-10, 85) (SEDA-11, 97) (SEDA-12, 91). As the perfect epidemiological study has yet not been carried out, the only thing that can be said is that piroxicam's ulcerogenicity increases with dosage and that 20 mg/day constitutes high-dose therapy, especially in elderly women.

Piroxicam can cause diaphragm-like strictures of the intestinal tract (9).

- A 65 year-old woman who had taken piroxicam for the previous 3 years presented with frequent episodes of abdominal bloating and cramping, sometimes associated with nausea and vomiting, and loss of weight. Small bowel examination showed several mid-ileal strictures associated with proximal dilated bowel.

Liver

Transient rises in aspartate transaminase and alanine transaminase can occur (10). Biopsy-proven hepatitis was noted in one patient who was also taking other medications (SEDA-5, 107). Cases of acute hepatitis have been described. Two elderly women developed acute hepatocellular injury, which progressed to fatal subacute hepatic necrosis (SEDA-12, 93) (11,12).

Urinary tract

Piroxicam reduces renal blood flow by inhibition of renal prostaglandins. It can cause transient and probably insignificant rises in urea or blood urea nitrogen, without increases in serum creatinine concentrations. Renal function should be monitored during long-term therapy and piroxicam should be avoided in renal insufficiency. An occasional patient develops edema and dysuria.

Hematuria with purpuric rash and Henoch–Schönlein purpura have been described (13).

Fatal acute renal insufficiency due to diffuse interstitial nephritis has been described in a young man (SEDA-14, 95).

Skin

Minor, often transient, skin rashes are relatively common, as with other NSAIDs. Light-induced skin eruptions have been reported to national ADR monitoring centers in several countries and generally occur only 1–6 days after the start of therapy. They are characterized by pruritic, papulovesicular, or bullous eruptions, usually restricted to exposed areas. Clinical, histological, and provocation studies are not conclusive in distinguishing the eruptions as photoallergic or phototoxic (SEDA-13, 76) (SEDA-15, 103) (14). Cross-reactivity between thiosalicylic acid and piroxicam supports the hypothesis that piroxicam-induced photosensitive reactions have a photoallergic mechanism and occur soon after starting therapy when patients have previously been sensitized to thiosalicylate (SEDA-16, 113) (15). The wide range of adverse skin effects include several types of rashes, urticaria, vasculitis, and life-threatening reactions (toxic epidermal necrolysis, erythema multiforme, and pemphigus) (SEDA-8, 110) (SEDA-11, 192) (SEDA-13, 77). Fixed drug eruptions have also been described (SEDA-16, 113).

- After piroxicam intake and sun exposure a patient with Sjögren's syndrome developed the typical cutaneous lesions and serological markers of systemic lupus erythematosus, despite drug withdrawal (16).

Susceptibility Factors

Renal disease

Reduced piroxicam excretion increases the risk of gastro-intestinal adverse effects. Most reports of these effects refer to elderly women, since impaired renal function in the elderly can lower excretion of the drug by 33%. Dosages should be as low as possible, and certainly not above 20 mg/day in these patients.

Drug Administration

Drug formulations

The adverse effects profile of suppositories, soluble tablet formulations, and standard capsules are similar (SEDA-13, 83). A parenteral formulation of piroxicam caused somnolence more often than diclofenac in a double-blind study, but diclofenac provoked more gastric discomfort and nausea than piroxicam. Local adverse effects of both drugs were pain, burning, and induration at the site of injection (SEDA-15, 103).

In an attempt to reduce gastric toxicity, piroxicam has been complexed with cyclodextrins. In healthy volunteers piroxicam beta-cyclodextrin is less toxic than either piroxicam or indometacin; gastrointestinal adverse effects were the most frequent (SEDA-16, 113).

A fast-dissolving form of piroxicam that can be taken under the tongue infrequently causes local adverse effects, including stomatitis, mucosal erythema, and dysesthesia (SEDA-20, 95).

Drug–Drug Interactions

Furosemide

Furosemide natriuresis and kaliuresis can be reduced by short-term treatment with piroxicam in hypertensive patients with impaired renal function (SEDA-16, 113).

Lithium

Piroxicam can increase the risk of lithium toxicity (17).

Phenazone

The half-life of phenazone (antipyrine) was prolonged and its metabolic clearance significantly reduced in proportion to the dose of piroxicam administered to healthy young volunteers (SEDA-16, 113).

References

1. Pitts NE. Ubersicht udber die mit Piroxicam in klinischen Untersuchungen gewonnenen Erfahrungen. Aktuel Rheumatol 1980;5:53.
2. Pisko EJ, Rahaman MA, Turner RA, et al. Long term efficacy and safety of piroxicam in the treatment of rheumatoid arthritis. Curr Ther Res 1980;27:852.
3. Dessain P, Estabrooks TF, Gordon AJ. Piroxicam in the treatment of osteoarthrosis: a multicentre study in general practice involving 1218 patients. J Int Med Res 1979; 7(5):335–43.
4. Vernick DM, Kelly JH. Sudden hearing loss associated with piroxicam. Am J Otol 1986;7(2):97–8.
5. Box J, Box P, Turner R, Pisko E. Piroxicam and rheumatoid arthritis: a double blind 16-week study comparing piroxicam and phenylbutazone. In: Piroxicam, International Congress and Symposium Series No. 1, Royal Soceity of Medicine. 1978:40.
6. Santucci L, Patoia L, Fiorucci S, Farroni F, Favero D, Morelli A. Oesophageal lesions during treatment with piroxicam. BMJ 1990;300(6730):1018.
7. Carver N, Wedgwood KR, Ralphs DN. Iatrogenic gastro-colic fistula associated with non-steroidal anti-inflammatory drug administration. Br J Clin Pract 1990;44(12):759–61.
8. Bianchine JR, Procter RR, Thomas FB. Piroxicam, aspirin, and gastrointestinal blood loss. Clin Pharmacol Ther 1982;32(2):247–52.
9. Abrahamian GA, Polhamus CD, Muskat P, Karulf RE. Diaphragm-like strictures of the ileum associated with NSAID use: a rare complication. South Med J 1998; 91(4):395–7.
10. Blackburn WD Jr, Prupas HM, Silverfield JC, Poiley JE, Caldwell JR, Collins RL, Miller MJ, Sikes DH, Kaplan H, Fleischmann R, et al. Tenidap in rheumatoid arthritis. A 24-week double-blind comparison with hydroxychloroquine-plus-piroxicam, and piroxicam alone. Arthritis Rheum 1995;38(10):1447–56.
11. Planas R, De Leon R, Quer JC, Barranco C, Bruguera M, Gassull MA. Fatal submassive necrosis of the liver associated with piroxicam. Am J Gastroenterol 1990;85(4):468–70.
12. Honein K, Attali P, Pelletier G, Ink O. Hépatite aiguë due au piroxicam: un nouveau cas. [Acute hepatitis due to piroxicam: a new case.] Gastroenterol Clin Biol 1988;12(1):79.
13. Goebel KM, Mueller-Brodmann W. Reversible overt nephropathy with Henoch–Schönlein purpura due to piroxicam. BMJ (Clin Res Ed) 1982;284(6312):311–12.
14. Ljunggren B. The piroxicam enigma. Photodermatol 1989;6(4):151–3.
15. Mammen L, Schmidt CP. Photosensitivity reactions: a case report involving NSAIDs. Am Fam Physician 1995; 52(2):575–9.
16. Roura M, Lopez-Gil F, Umbert P. Systemic lupus erythematosus exacerbated by piroxicam. Dermatologica 1991; 182(1):56–8.
17. Kerry RJ, Owen G, Michaelson S. Possible toxic interaction between lithium and piroxicam. Lancet 1983;1(8321): 418–19.

Pirprofen

See also Non-steroidal anti-inflammatory drugs

General Information

In an open, non-comparative trial in 1506 patients, the adverse effects of pirprofen were mainly gastrointestinal, and consisted mostly of epigastric pain. There were single cases of an attack of asthma, iron deficiency anemia, leukopenia, and an increase in serum transaminases to more than 10 times normal (1). In a long-term trial, 9.7% of over 3000 patients stopped treatment because of poor tolerability. The manufacturers decided to discontinue marketing it worldwide, saying that this was a commercial decision (SEDA-16, 111).

Organs and Systems

Liver

Laboratory signs of hepatic damage were documented in 37 patients, including three cases of hepatitis (2); pirprofen can definitely be considered hepatotoxic.

References

1. Daubresse AJ. Pirprofen for the treatment of rheumatic disorders and post-traumatic lesions. Acta Ther 1984;10:97.
2. Salliere D, Alcalay M. Rangasil en traitement prolongé. Rheumatologie 1986;38:131.

Pizotifen

See also Antihistamines

General Information

Pizotifen is a 5-HT receptor antagonist chemically related to the tricyclic antidepressants, with a five-membered third ring containing a sulfur atom. It has been suggested that pizotifen has effects and adverse effects resembling those of amitriptyline (1). However, it is pharmacologically similar to the antihistamine cyproheptadine and shares its adverse effects, including drowsiness and increased appetite. When used in migraine it causes increased weight; conversely, when it is used to improve appetite, sleepiness and dizziness are common.

Organs and Systems

Metabolism

In 47 patients with severe migraine unresponsive to clonidine, pizotifen 1.5 mg for 6 months more than halved the incidence of attacks in 30 patients and 12 became headache-free. Weight gain was a problem in some subjects (2). In an open, multicenter study of the use of pizotifen 1.5 mg at night to prevent migraine in 834 patients, the most frequent adverse effects were drowsiness, although in one-third of the affected patients this was transient, and weight gain, with an average increase of 0.7 kg over 2 months (3).

Long-Term Effects

Drug withdrawal

Severe weight loss has been reported after withdrawal of chronic pizotifen (4).

Drug Administration

Drug overdose

An acute overdose of 30 mg pizotifen caused pyrexia and anticholinergic effects, with resolution after 10 hours (5).

References

1. Olgiati S, Calobrisi A. Clinical results with pizotyline in depression. Dis Nerv Syst 1974;35:35.
2. Peet KM. Use of pizotifen in severe migraine: a long-term study. Curr Med Res Opin 1977;5(2):192–9.
3. Crowder D, Maclay WP. Pizotifen once daily in the prophylaxis of migraine: results of a multi-centre general practice study. Curr Med Res Opin 1984;9(4):280–5.
4. Jowett NI. Severe weight loss after withdrawal of chronic pizotifen treatment. J Neurol Neurosurg Psychiatry 1998;65(1):137.
5. Griffiths AP, Penn ND, Tindall H. A report of acute overdosage of the anti-serotonergic drug pizotifen. Postgrad Med J 1987;63(735):59–60.

Placebo

General Information

Since the first paper in 1945 (1), thousands of papers have been published on placebos. However, little attention has been paid to data on placebos in clinical pharmacology studies. The conditioning model of placebo has been elegantly illustrated in a crossover study in hypertensive patients (2). The use of placebos has been reviewed (3).

The impact of experimental conditions on the results of 109 double-blind, placebo-controlled clinical pharmacology studies conducted in 1228 healthy volunteers has been reported (4). The subjects were young (aged 18–40 years) or old (65–80 years). The treatment was oral placebo (capsules, tablets, or suspension) and the adverse effects were spontaneously reported and/or observed by the investigators. The overall incidence of adverse effects was 19%, with an increased number of complaints in the elderly subjects. After single dosing of placebo, the most common events were headache, drowsiness, and weakness. After repeated dosing, there was an increased incidence of weakness, reaching 7% (compared with 2.5% after a single dose), while the incidences of the other major symptoms were unchanged. A lower overall incidence (7%) of adverse events has been reported after free interviews (5), while in another study there was a higher frequency (6).

Experimental conditions in phase I trials have been described as being potentially responsible for changes in serum transaminase activities (7,8), perhaps ascribable to dietary factors and rest.

Bed-rest experiments have previously shown changes in homeostasis (for example, glucose-induced insulin release) but no change in plasma catecholamine concentrations.

References

1. Pepper OHP. A note on placebo. Ann J Pharm 1945;117:409–12.
2. Suchman AL, Ader R. Classic conditioning and placebo effects in crossover studies. Clin Pharmacol Ther 1992;52(4):372–7.

3. Evans D. Placebo. The Belief Effect. London: Harper Collins, 2003.
4. Rosenzweig P, Brohier S, Zipfel A. The placebo effect in healthy volunteers: influence of experimental conditions on the adverse events profile during phase I studies. Clin Pharmacol Ther 1993;54(5):578–83.
5. Sibille M, Deigat N, Olagnier V, Durand DV, Levrat R. Adverse events in phase one studies: a study in 430 healthy volunteers. Eur J Clin Pharmacol 1992;42(4):389–93.
6. Dhume VG, Agshikar NV, Diniz RS. Placebo-induced side effects in healthy volunteers. Clinician 1975;39:289–90.
7. Kanamary M, Nagashima S, Uematsu T, Nakashima M. Influence of 7-day hospitalisation for phase I study on the biochemical laboratory tests of healthy volunteers. Jpn J Clin Pharmacol Ther 1989;20:493–4.
8. Mikines KJ, Dela F, Tronier B, Galbo H. Effect of 7 days of bed rest on dose-response relation between plasma glucose and insulin secretion. Am J Physiol 1989;257(1 Pt 1):E43–8.

Plague vaccine

See also Vaccines

General Information

Plague vaccine is a suspension of the formaldehyde-killed encapsulated form of *Yersinia pestis*. Primary immunization involves three doses given intramuscularly.

The Working Group on Civilian Biodefense has developed consensus-based recommendations for measures to be taken by medical and public health professionals following the use of plague as a biological weapon against a civilian population (1). They concluded that an aerosolized plague weapon could cause fever, cough, chest pain, and hemoptysis, with signs consistent with severe pneumonia 1–6 days after exposure. Rapid evolution of disease would occur in the 2–4 days after the onset of symptoms and would lead to septic shock with a high mortality if early treatment was not instituted. They advised early treatment and prophylaxis with streptomycin or gentamicin or one of the tetracycline or fluoroquinolone classes of antimicrobials.

General adverse effects

General malaise, headache, fever, mild lymphadenopathy, or erythema and induration at the injection site have been reported following the administration of plague vaccine (10% of vaccinees); these effects are more common with repeated injections. Sterile abscesses and hypersensitivity reactions (urticaria, asthma) occur rarely (2).

Organs and Systems

Immunologic

Known allergy to any of the plague vaccine constituents (beef protein, soya, casein, phenol) contraindicates immunization. Severe local or systemic reactions following previous doses contraindicate revaccination (2).

References

1. Inglesby TV, Dennis DT, Henderson DA, Bartlett JG, Ascher MS, Eitzen E, Fine AD, Friedlander AM, Hauer J, Koerner JF, Layton M, McDade J, Osterholm MT, O'Toole T, Parker G, Perl TM, Russell PK, Schoch-Spana M, Tonat K. Plague as a biological weapon: medical and public health management. Working Group on Civilian Biodefense. JAMA 2000;283(17):2281–90.
2. Committee on Immunization. Guide for Adult Immunization. Philadelphia: American College of Physicians, 1985:65.

Plantaginaceae

See also Herbal medicines

General Information

The family of Plantaginaceae contains two genera:

1. *Littorella* (littorella)
2. *Plantago* (plantain).

Plantago species

Plantago species have traditionally been used for many purposes in folk medicine (1,2). Plantain seeds are widely used as bulk laxatives under the names of "psyllium" (from *Plantago psyllium* or *Plantago indica*) and "ispaghula" (from *Plantago ovata*). They are covered in the monograph on laxatives.

References

1. Grigorescu E, Stanescu U, Basceanu V, Aur MM. Controlul fitochimic si microbiologic al unor specii utilizate in medicina populara. II. *Plantago lanceolata* L., *Plantago media* L., *Plantago major*. [Phytochemical and microbiological control of some plant species used in folk medicine. II. *Plantago lanceolata* L., *Plantago media* L., *Plantago major* L.] Rev Med Chir Soc Med Nat Ias; 1973;77(4):835–41.
2. Samuelsen AB. The traditional uses, chemical constituents and biological activities of *Plantago major* L. A review. J Ethnopharmacol 2000;71(1–2):1–21.

Plasma products

General Information

Plasma products are used to substitute plasma proteins and in plasma exchange. Fresh frozen plasma is used as a source of coagulation factors in deficiency, if no purified factors are available.

Intensive plasma exchange has been studied in the treatment of numerous diseases, above all in Waldenström's macroglobulinemia, hypercholesterolemia, hyperviscosity syndrome, thrombotic thrombocytopenic purpura, systemic lupus erythematosus, myasthenia gravis, hemolytic-uremic syndrome, Goodpasture's syndrome, Guillain–Barré syndrome, and several other autoimmune diseases. Its potential benefit is attributable to the removal of a variety of harmful substances from plasma, such as antibodies, antigens, immune complexes, toxins, or abnormal plasma components. If the circulating substance is a cause of the disease, the plasma exchange can be effective. However, its therapeutic potential in many diseases has not yet been precisely defined.

The performance of intensive plasma exchange (removal from an adult of 2–3 liters of plasma with substitution of fresh plasma to maintain the patient's blood volume) requires separation of plasma from cells, so that the patient's own cells can be returned. There are two methods of plasma separation: centrifugal flow separation and flow filtration (1,2).

Intensive plasma exchange is relatively safe. It is generally well tolerated, and only a few serious complications have been reported. The potential complications (3–5) include transient hypotension, nausea, urticaria, abdominal discomfort, fever, hypothermia, air or microaggregate embolism, hypocalcemia (citrate effect) with paresthesia, tetany, and cardiac depression, thrombocytopenia (often observed), coagulation factor depletion and depletion of various intravascular proteins, visual scotomata, hepatitis, vasovagal reactions, and reactions associated with phlebotomy (phlebitis, hematoma).

The fluid volume and protein removed by plasmapheresis must be replaced. Among the solutions available for replacement therapy are fresh frozen plasma and human albumin solutions.

Fresh frozen plasma

Fresh frozen plasma is defined as the fluid portion of 1 unit of human blood that has been centrifuged and separated and then frozen at $-18°C$ (or below) within 6 hours of collection. It is used to reverse the effects of oral anticoagulants (for example during surgery or bleeding episodes) (6). Its use has increased considerably in most countries within the past 20–25 years (7), in spite of mounting evidence of its potential risks, such as the transmission of viral infections. Allo-immunization occurs infrequently, with the formation of Rh antibodies in response to contaminating stroma of red blood cells, and as with any intravenous administered fluid, hypervolemia and cardiac failure can occur (8). Anti-A and anti-B in the plasma can hemolyse the recipient's red cells if ABO-compatible fresh frozen plasma is not used (9). Other disadvantages of fresh frozen plasma are the large volume that needs to be given, the risk of viral transmission, and the variable quantities of clotting factors it contains. Quarantine fresh frozen plasma, when the unit is used after the next consecutive donation of the same donor has been found to be negative in virus screening assays, is a safe alternative.

Organs and Systems

Cardiovascular

Hypotension is a sometimes severe adverse effect of the administration of plasma proteins. It may be associated with the presence of a potent prekallikrein activator, the Hageman factor degradation product, which is thought to initiate the production of kinin from fibrinogen in the recipient's blood. The kinin then produces systemic hypotension.

In five of eight patients treated with fresh frozen plasma to achieve rapid correction of anticoagulation after warfarin-related intracranial hemorrhage, there were complications of fluid overload (10). In two of these patients congestive heart failure developed, resulting in myocardial infarction and renal insufficiency respectively. Two patients had supraventricular tachydysrhythmias and one developed pulmonary edema.

Respiratory

The incidence of transfusion-related acute lung injury is 0.16–0.24% per transfusion of blood products and is the cause of 15% of all fatal complications of blood transfusion (11). Specific antigen–antibody reactions involving donor antibodies specific for leukocyte antigens of the recipients cause activation of neutrophils and aggregation in small pulmonary vessels (11). The complement and cytokine cascade is activated, leading to capillary leakage.

- In a 58-year-old man transfusion of a unit fresh frozen plasma resulted in acute lung injury, caused by antibodies of the donor specific for the neutrophil antigen NB1 (11).

NB1 has a phenotype frequency of 97%.

Immunologic

Immunological adverse effects of the administration of plasma range from mild urticaria and flushing to fatal anaphylaxis. Such reactions can occur either during the infusion or some minutes after. Mild reactions often start locally and have a tendency to spread. In more severe cases dyspnea, arthralgia, and fever occur. Stabilizers or other additives in plasma protein preparations may be of significance in provoking these reactions. In addition, protein aggregates in the preparations may participate in anaphylactoid reactions, including acute pulmonary injury. Severe reactions have occasionally been encountered.

Development of an antibody response

The development of an antibody response against a deficient or genetically different protein can cause post-transfusion complications. The main problems are antibodies against antihemophilia factors, for example directed against factor VIII or factor IX, which may be produced in hemophiliacs after repeated transfusions and inhibit the therapeutic effect. Another problem arises when antibody formation occurs in IgA-deficient subjects who receive IgA-containing products and produce anti-IgA antibodies. Inhibitors of coagulation proteins and antibodies to IgA are described in the monographs on coagulation proteins and immunoglobulins.

Body temperature

Fever can occur 10–15 minutes after the start of an infusion of plasma. It is often accompanied by headache, nausea, and shivering. These symptoms often disappear when the infusion is discontinued.

References

1. Heal JM, Bailey G, Helphingstine C, Thiem PA, Leddy JP, Buchholz DH, Nusbacher J. Non-centrifugal plasma collection using cross-flow membrane plasmapheresis. Vox Sang 1983;44(3):156–66.
2. Wiltbank TB, Castino F, Grapka BH, Daniels JR, Solomon BA, Friedman LI. Filtration plasmapheresis in vivo. Transfusion 1981;21(5):502–10.
3. Barton JC. Nonhemolytic, noninfectious transfusion reactions. Semin Hematol 1981;18(2):95–121.
4. Braunstein AH, Oberman HA. Transfusion of plasma components. Transfusion 1984;24(4):281–6.
5. Patten E, Reddi CR, Riglin H, Edwards J. Delayed hemolytic transfusion reaction caused by a primary immune response. Transfusion 1982;22(3):248–50.
6. Cartmill M, Dolan G, Byrne JL, Byrne PO. Prothrombin complex concentrate for oral anticoagulant reversal in neurosurgical emergencies. Br J Neurosurg 2000;14(5):458–61.
7. Ring J, Messmer K. Incidence and severity of anaphylactoid reactions to colloid volume substitutes. Lancet 1977;1(8009):466–9.
8. National Institutes of Health Consensus Conference. Fresh frozen plasma: indications and risks. Transfus Med Rev 1987;1(3):201–4.
9. Jones J. Abuse of fresh frozen plasma. BMJ (Clin Res Ed) 1987;295(6593):287.
10. Boulis NM, Bobek MP, Schmaier A, Hoff JT. Use of factor IX complex in warfarin-related intracranial hemorrhage. Neurosurgery 1999;45(5):1113–19.
11. Leger R, Palm S, Wulf H, Vosberg A, Neppert J. Transfusion-related lung injury with leukopenic reaction caused by fresh frozen plasma containing anti-NB1. Anesthesiology 1999;91(5):1529–32.

Platelet glycoprotein IIb/IIIa antagonists

General Information

Platelet membrane glycoprotein IIb/IIIa receptor inhibitors have been approved in various countries for the treatment of patients scheduled for percutaneous transluminal coronary angioplasty or coronary atherectomy to prevent ischemic complications (1). They are antagonists at an adhesion receptor on the platelet membrane, the glycoprotein IIb/IIIa, which binds some ligands implicated in platelet aggregation, fibrinogen, and von Willebrand factor, and is involved in the common final pathway whereby various stimuli cause platelet activation. They therefore reduce platelet aggregation regardless of the mechanism by which the platelet is activated, and are currently the most powerful inhibitors of platelet aggregation available.

The first drug to be developed in this family was the monoclonal antibody abciximab, which is covered in a separate monograph. Other GP IIb/IIIa blockers include peptides (eptifibatide) or small molecules such as

tirofiban and lamifiban. Other small molecules that are orally active are in development (2).

For the drugs so far used in major clinical trials (eptifibatide, tirofiban, lamifilan, roxifiban, and sibrafiban) the available data suggest that the commonest adverse events are episodes of bleeding, mostly minor and essentially at the vascular access site, without an excess of intracranial hemorrhage. There is also a low incidence of thrombocytopenia with these non-antibody drugs; two cases were reported in a study of the use of roxifiban in 98 patients with chronic stable angina pectoris (3).

References

1. Ferguson JJ, Kereiakes DJ, Adgey AA, Fox KA, Hillegass WB Jr, Pfisterer M, Vassanelli C. Safe use of platelet GP IIb/IIIa inhibitors. Am Heart J 1998;135(4):S77–89.
2. Topol EJ, Byzova TV, Plow EF. Platelet GPIIb-IIIa blockers. Lancet 1999;353(9148):227–31.
3. Murphy J, Wright RS, Gussak I, Williams B, Daly RN, Cain VA, Pieniaszek HJ, Sy SK, Ebling W, Simonson K, Wilcox RA, Kopecky SL. The use of Roxifiban (DMP754), a novel oral platelet glycoprotein IIb/IIIa receptor inhibitor, in patients with stable coronary artery disease. Am J Cardiovasc Drugs 2003;3(2):101–12.

Platinum-containing cytostatic drugs

See also Cytostatic and immunosuppressant drugs

General Information

Although the main platinum-containing cytotoxic drugs, cisplatin (rINN), carboplatin (rINN), and oxaliplatin (rINN), share some structural similarities, there are marked differences between them in therapeutic uses, pharmacokinetics, and adverse effects profiles (1–4). Compared with cisplatin, carboplatin has inferior efficacy in germ-cell tumors, head and neck cancers, and bladder and esophageal carcinomas, whereas the two drugs appear to have comparable efficacy in ovarian cancer, extensive small-cell lung cancers, and advanced non-small-cell lung cancers (5–7).

Oxaliplatin belongs to the group of diaminocyclohexane (DACH) platinum compounds. It is the first platinum-based drug that has marked efficacy in colorectal cancer when given in combination with 5-fluorouracil and folinic acid (8,9).

Nedaplatin has been registered in Japan, whereas other derivatives, like satraplatin (JM216, which is the only orally available platinum derivative), ZD0473, BBR3464, and SPI-77 (a liposomal formulation of cisplatin), are still under investigation (10–13).

Other platinum-containing compounds under investigation include dexormaplatin, enloplatin, eptaplatin, iproplatin, lobaplatin, miboplatin, miriplatin, ormaplatin, picoplatin, sebriplatin, spiroplatin, and zeniplatin.

The adverse effects of platinum compounds have been reviewed (14).

Mechanism of action

Although the precise mechanism of the cytotoxic action of the platinum-containing compounds has not been fully elucidated, they are thought to act by causing interstrand and intrastrand cross-links in DNA, particularly including two adjacent guanine or two adjacent guanine-adenine bases (15–18). In comparison with cisplatin- or carboplatin-induced DNA lesions, diaminocyclohexane (DACH) platinum DNA adduct formation has been associated with greater cytotoxicity and inhibition of DNA synthesis. In addition, there appears to be a complete lack of cross-resistance between oxaliplatin and cisplatin, which may be related to the bulky DACH carrier ligand of oxaliplatin, hindering DNA repair mechanisms within tumor cells (8,9).

Pharmacokinetics

There are significant pharmacokinetic differences among cisplatin, carboplatin, and oxaliplatin. Cisplatin is the most highly protein-bound (>90%), followed by oxaliplatin (85%) and carboplatin (24–50%).

The negligible nephrotoxicity of oxaliplatin and carboplatin compared with cisplatin may be related to their slower rates of conversion to reactive species. As a result, intensive hydration is not warranted during carboplatin or oxaliplatin infusion, in contrast to cisplatin (1,8–10). In the case of macromolecular platinum-protein complex formation, decomposition proceeds rather slowly, which may explain why the urinary excretion of total platinum is increased for a long time after treatment, particularly in patients who have been given cisplatin (19,20).

In contrast to cisplatin, carboplatin is primarily eliminated (about 75%) by glomerular filtration, whereas tubular secretion appears to be of minor importance (2–4). It has therefore been recommended that the dose of carboplatin be adjusted according to the individual glomerular filtration rate, in order to avoid high plasma drug concentrations when the dose is calculated according to body surface area (21–23). Individualized carboplatin therapy helps to avoid abnormally high drug concentrations in patients with renal dysfunction and subtherapeutic concentrations in patients with an unexpectedly high glomerular filtration rate (24,25).

Pharmacokinetic-pharmacodynamic correlations between AUC, response rates, and the extent of myelosuppression have been examined retrospectively in patients with advanced ovarian carcinoma (21,24). AUC values below 4 minutes/mg/ml and exceeding 7 minutes/mg/ml cannot be recommended; the former is associated with low response rates and the latter is associated with more pronounced neutropenia and thrombocytopenia without higher response rates. Doses of carboplatin are generally calculated by the Calvert formula (26):

$$\text{Carboplatin dose} = \text{AUC (minutes.mg/ml)} \times (\text{GFR} + 25)$$

However, it is still debatable which method most accurately predicts individual values of glomerular filtration rate or creatinine clearance. Whereas the Cr-EDTA method is the most accurate method of estimating glomerular filtration rate, most clinicians do not use it routinely, and prefer to collect urine for estimation of creatinine clearance. Alternatively, the use of special formulae has been proposed, for example Wright's formula and the formulae of Cockcroft & Gault or Jelliffe (27–29). However, calculation of the glomerular filtration rate or creatinine clearance using such formulae has been associated with some bias in different ranges, regardless of which formula has been used.

After intravenous administration of oxaliplatin, about 33% and 40% of the dose is bound to erythrocytes and plasma proteins. The half-life averages 26 days, which is in accordance with the normal life expectancy of erythrocytes (12–50 days). Oxaliplatin undergoes rapid non-enzymatic biotransformation to form a variety of reactive platinum intermediates, which bind rapidly and extensively to plasma proteins and erythrocytes. The antineoplastic and toxic properties appear to reside in the non-protein bound fraction, whereas platinum bound to plasma proteins or erythrocytes is considered to be pharmacologically inactive. Biotransformation produces DACH-platinum dichloride, 1,2-DACH-platinum dicysteinate, 1,2-DACH-platinum diglutathionate, 1,2-DACH-platinum monoglutathionate, and 1,2-DACH-platinum methionine. The erythrocyte contains only thiol derivatives, whereas all derivatives can be recovered from the plasma.

The platinum-containing metabolites of oxaliplatin are predominantly excreted in the urine (about 50% of the dose within 3 days), whereas drug excretion via the feces is of minor importance (about 5% of the dose after 11 days). The mean total platinum half-life averages 9 days after oxaliplatin administration (130 mg/m^2 intravenously) (8,9). There is a strong negative correlation between the mean plasma concentration of unbound oxaliplatin and renal function; however, moderate renal impairment does not increase the risk of acute toxicity associated with oxaliplatin (30).

General adverse effects

The comparative toxicity and mutagenic effects of platinum anticancer drugs have been reviewed (31).

Of the clinically established platinum compounds, cisplatin has the most toxic effects on organs like the nervous system, the organ of Corti, and the kidneys in a dose-dependent fashion. The dose per cycle has therefore usually been limited to 100–120 mg/m^2 intravenously, in order to avoid drug-induced irreversible organ dysfunction (12,13). The complete spectrum of late or long-term adverse effects of cisplatin in survivors of testicular cancer has been reviewed (32).

In contrast to cisplatin, myelotoxicity represents the most prominent adverse effect of carboplatin. Based on its lower organ toxicity and its better predictable pharmacokinetic behavior, carboplatin has extensively replaced cisplatin in combination chemotherapy for the treatment of ovarian cancer and extensive small cell and non-small cell lung cancer. For other indications, one has to weigh the possibly inferior efficacy of carboplatin against the more pronounced undesirable adverse effects of cisplatin, which may limit its long-term use. Based on its marked organ toxicity, high-dose cisplatin-containing regimens are not feasible, in contrast to carboplatin, which is part of several dose-intensified combination chemotherapy regimens (12,13).

Like carboplatin, oxaliplatin does not usually cause nephrotoxicity. In addition, both drugs are only moderately emetogenic, in contrast to cisplatin. The most important dose-limiting adverse effect of oxaliplatin is a sensory peripheral neuropathy, which has two different forms:

1. a unique acute peripheral sensory (and motor) toxicity that often occurs during or within hours after drug infusion and which is rapidly reversible and aggravated by cold;
2. a peripheral sensory neuropathy related to the cumulative dose, which is generally moderate and slowly reversible, in contrast to the forms that have been described after cisplatin administration.

BBR3464

BBR3464 is the first congener of a novel group of platinum compounds, the so-called cationic trinuclear platins. It binds to DNA more rapidly than cisplatin, which results in long-range interstrand and intrastrand cross-links. It is more potent than cisplatin, and very low dosages were effective in phase I trials. With a 1-hour intravenous infusion of 1.1 mg/m^2 every 28 days, diarrhea (preceded by abdominal cramps), nausea/vomiting, and neutropenia were the most prominent drug-related adverse effects. There were no signs of drug-related nephrotoxicity, neurotoxicity, or lung dysfunction (12,13,33).

Heptaplatin

Heptaplatin (cis-malonate[(4R,5R)-4,5-bis(aminomethyl)-2-isopropyl-1,3-dioxolane]platinum(II), SKI-2053R, Sunpla) has high antitumor activity against various cancer cell lines, including cisplatin-resistant tumor cells. Preliminary results suggested that it is less nephrotoxic than cisplatin. However, a comparative trial showed that intravenous heptaplatin 400 mg/m^2 was more nephrotoxic than intravenous cisplatin 60 mg/m^2 in terms of uremia and proteinuria, which occurred despite the use of hyperosmolar mannitol and appropriate concomitant hydration (fluid intake at least 3500 ml/day) (34,35).

Nedaplatin

Nedaplatin (cis-diammineglycolatoplatinum, CDGP, 254-S) has some structural similarities to cisplatin and carboplatin. Since 1995 it has been available for therapeutic use in Japan. In phase II trials, it had promising antineoplastic activity in patients with head and neck cancers, non-small cell lung cancers, esophageal cancer, testicular tumors, and cervical cancer. A distinct number of patients with ovarian cancer have responded to nedaplatin (for example 100 mg/m^2 intravenously) even after relapsing following treatment with cisplatin/carboplatin and cyclophosphamide. Its pharmacokinetic behavior is similar to that of carboplatin. It causes less nephrotoxicity than cisplatin, but hematological toxicity is dose-limiting. Other adverse effects include nausea/vomiting and mild peripheral neuropathy (12,13,36). Although nedaplatin is less nephrotoxic than cisplatin, incidental cases of severe nephrotoxicity have occurred. In addition, ototoxicity, similar to that observed after cisplatin, has been documented. Nedaplatin is excreted primarily unchanged by glomerular filtration, and there is a formula for predicting the clearance of unbound platinum after its administration (37).

Satraplatin

Satraplatin (bis-acetato-ammine-dichloro-cyclohexylamine-platinum, JM 216, BMS-182751) is the first oral platinum compound among the third-generation platinum complexes with activity in platinum-sensitive and some platinum-resistant preclinical models. Adverse effects were generally modest (grades I and II), including nausea, fatigue, anorexia, diarrhea, and altered taste. In addition, myelosuppression and rare cases of grades II and III increases in serum creatinine were reported. During phase II trials satraplatin was given in a dose of 120 mg/m^2/day for 5 consecutive days every 3 weeks in untreated patients with lung cancer or 30 mg/m^2/day for 14 consecutive days every 5 weeks in patients with metastatic squamous cell carcinoma. There was no nephrotoxicity or neurotoxicity (38–40). Pharmacokinetic studies showed that very little intact parent compound reached the systemic circulation after oral administration, perhaps because of extensive metabolic biotransformation or rapid reaction of platinum(II) species with DNA or other compounds. One of the intermediate compounds released during biotransformation is JM118, which has a longer half-life than the parent compound. Its particular role in the overall activity of satraplatin is still being investigated (41).

SPI-77

SPI-77 is a stealth liposomal dosage form of cisplatin. One of the main features of stealth liposomes is that they are pegylated on the liposomal surface. Compared with conventional liposomes (for example DaunoXome or Myocet) the half-life of the liposome and its embedded drug in plasma is significantly increased by this modification, because degradation by cells of the mononuclear phagocytic system is impaired; the cells are thereby, as it were, tricked. Liposomal encapsulation of cisplatin has been suggested to reduce systemic drug exposure and may help to increase drug delivery into tumor tissue. Pharmacokinetic studies have shown a slow rate of release of cisplatin from the liposomes, resulting in low systemic exposure to unbound drug. In contrast to conventional cisplatin, the incidence of gastrointestinal toxicity after SPI-77 was low, and so prophylactic antiemetics could be avoided. In addition, renal toxicity has not been observed, which also makes hydration before or after chemotherapy unnecessary. Extensive neurological measurements did not show any adverse effects. In conclusion, the toxicity profile of SPI-77 is encouraging compared with conventional cisplatin. However, despite its favorable pharmacokinetic behavior, enhanced platinum accumulation in tumor tissue has not yet been detected (42–44).

Tetraplatin

The further development of the third-generation platinum derivative tetraplatin (ormaplatin, *trans*-D, L-1,2-diaminocyclohexane tetrachloroplatinum) has been abandoned, because drug-induced severe motor and sensory peripheral neuropathy occurred even at low cumulative doses. The high neurotoxic potential of tetraplatin may be associated with its pharmacokinetics: it is rapidly metabolized to 1,2-DACH-platinum dichloride, which was 3.8 times more neurotoxic than oxaliplatin in a neurite outgrowth assay (45).

ZD0473

ZD0473 (formerly AMD473, JM473) was developed in order to overcome acquired or intrinsic (de novo) resistance to cisplatin. Based on the steric bulk of its methyl-substituted pyridine moiety, thiol substitution and drug inactivation is hindered compared with cisplatin. In several in-vitro studies, ZD0473 was active even in cisplatin-refractory tumor cells, whose key mechanism of resistance was based on thiol substitution. In addition, ZD0473 is also active in cisplatin-resistant tumor cells, in which resistance is based on altered drug transport mechanisms or enhanced DNA repair.

Based on encouraging preclinical results, ZD0473 entered clinical phase I/II trials in several solid tumors, including non-small cell lung cancers, mesothelioma, head and neck cancers, and ovarian carcinoma. Its most prominent adverse effects included myelosuppression and nausea/vomiting. Thrombocytopenia and neutropenia were the dose-limiting adverse effects at intravenous doses of 130–150 mg/m^2. In contrast to cisplatin, neurotoxicity, ototoxicity, and renal toxicity have not yet been reported during or after treatment with ZD0473 (12,13,33,36).

Organs and Systems

Cardiovascular

Asymptomatic sinus bradycardia (for example 30–40/minute) is observed within 30 minutes to 2 hours after the start of cisplatin infusion. When cisplatin is withdrawn normal rhythm is restored. Because patients who receive platins are not routinely monitored, drug-induced sinus bradycardia may not be detected in practice. However, several case reports have included heavily pretreated patients, which makes a direct relation between cisplatin administration and the onset of cardiotoxic symptoms much more difficult to assess. In conclusion, no dosage adjustment appears to be warranted in patients with cisplatin-induced sinus bradycardia; however, attention should be paid to patients with resting bradycardia or those using medications known to slow the heart rate (46,47).

- A 60-year-old woman with a squamous cell lung carcinoma developed a paroxysmal supraventricular tachycardia during administration of cisplatin 20 mg/m^2 and etoposide 75 mg/m^2. The dysrhythmia appeared to be related to cisplatin since normal rhythm was restored after cisplatin was withdrawn (48).

Orthostatic hypotension was reported in "several" of 126 patients given cisplatin 50 mg/m^2 on days 1, 8, 29, and 36 as part of treatment for lung cancer in combination with etoposide and chest radiotherapy (49).

There have been 21 reports of life-threatening disease affecting large arteries in patients treated with cisplatin, bleomycin, and vinblastine in combination for germ cell tumors (50,51). Five patients died during or after therapy, three from acute myocardial infarction, one from rectal infarction, and one from cerebral infarction. Other patients who developed major vascular disease, including coronary artery and cerebrovascular disease, have been reported. Symptoms occurred acutely in some (within 48 hours of starting therapy), and after months or years had elapsed in others.

Reduced peripheral circulation, Raynaud's phenomenon, and polyneuropathy have been described after the combined use of cisplatin, bleomycin, and vinblastine for testicular tumors. Of eight cases with polyneuropathy that were investigated, it was not possible to confirm a causative association between Raynaud's phenomenon and the chemotherapy (52).

Platinum compounds have rarely been described to cause phlebitis after intravenous administration (53).

Respiratory

Seven patients died from irreversible respiratory failure after receiving combined cisplatin plus bleomycin chemotherapy; five had raised serum creatinine and all received cisplatin before the bleomycin (54). The authors recommended extreme caution with this combination, and suggested that bleomycin should precede the cisplatin infusion.

Ear, nose, throat

- A 67-year-old white woman with a small cell lung cancer was given six courses of cisplatin and etoposide once every 4 weeks and after the last course developed acute shortness of breath, hoarseness, and stridor, due to bilateral vocal cord paralysis (55).

Nervous system

The neurotoxicity of platinum-containing compounds has been reviewed (56,57), as has the prevention of cisplatin-associated neurotoxicity (58). In experimental measurements of sensory nerve conduction velocity: oxaliplatin caused the most impairment, followed by cisplatin, carboplatin, and satraplatin (JM216) (59). The cumulative incidence of grade 2 peripheral sensory neuropathy with oxaliplatin was 19% (60).

Conventional dosages of carboplatin have been associated with the lowest risk of peripheral neuropathy (for example mild paresthesia) among the approved platinum compounds. It has been estimated that about 4–6% of patients who receive carboplatin develop a peripheral neuropathy. Patients over 65 years of age or patients pretreated with other neurotoxic agents may be at a slightly higher risk (61).

A 47% incidence of peripheral neuropathy of all grades has been reported with cisplatin (62), and a 31% off-therapy deterioration of peripheral neuropathy presenting as muscle cramps and demyelination syndromes has been described (63). Cisplatin causes a well-recognized reversible sensory peripheral neuropathy, starting with depressed deep tendon reflexes and loss of vibration sense, progressing to a sensory ataxia (64). This may be age-related, as the use of high-dose cisplatin in children with neuroblastoma has not been associated with peripheral neuropathy (65). Motor nerves are spared (66). There have also been case reports of cerebral herniation and coma, severe encephalopathy, tonic-clonic seizures with concomitant visual disturbances and changed mental state, insomnia, anxiety, and parkinsonian symptoms. The symptoms generally resolved within several weeks (67–71). In some studies, the nervous system effects were the consequence of cisplatin-induced electrolyte disturbances (for example hyponatremia, hypocalcemia, or hypomagnesemia), rather than a direct action of the platinum derivative in the nervous system (72–74). For example, mental status improved in one patient who was given 3% sodium chloride in order to increase the serum sodium from 118 to 128 mmol/l, whereas diazepam, phenytoin, phenobarbital, and dexamethasone were ineffective (75).

Presentation

In about 90% of patients, oxaliplatin is associated with acute neurosensory toxicity, including dysesthesia and paresthesia. Neurosensory toxicity affects the fingers, toes, perioral and oral regions, and the pharyngolaryngeal tract (in about 1–2% of cases), which is generally induced or aggravated by coldness. As a result, patients should be instructed to avoid exposure to cold. Such symptoms can occur during or shortly after the first course of oxaliplatin. The symptoms are commonly mild and disappear within a few hours or days. Some patients also develop muscle cramps or spasms. The risk of acute neuropathy appears to be lower if oxaliplatin is given in a dosage of 85 mg/m^2 every 2 weeks rather than 130 mg/m^2 every 3 weeks. A further strategy to reduce the risk of acute recurrent pseudolaryngospasm is to increase the infusion duration from 2 to 6 hours during subsequent cycles (76,77). The prophylactic use of infusions containing calcium and magnesium sulfate before and after oxaliplatin can prevent acute neurotoxic symptoms (78).

- A woman developed bilateral blindness and lumbosacral myelopathy within 1 month of having received an autologous bone marrow transplant, cisplatin 55 mg/m^2, carmustine 600 mg/m^2, and cyclophosphamide 1875 mg/m^2 (79).

In addition to the acute neurotoxic symptoms caused by oxaliplatin, about 10–15% of patients develop a moderate neuropathy, particularly after cumulative intravenous doses of 700–800 mg/m^2. The symptoms of cumulative neuropathy include non-cold-related dysesthesia, paresthesia, superficial and deep sensory loss, and eventually sensory ataxia and functional impairment, which persists between treatment cycles. Most of these symptoms usually resolve a few weeks or months after oxaliplatin withdrawal. Lower cumulative doses (for example 510–765 mg/m^2) and higher cumulative doses exceeding 1020 mg/m^2 have been associated with incidences of cumulative grade 3 neurotoxicity of 3.2% and 50% respectively (8,9,76,77). In addition, higher cumulative doses, exceeding 1000 mg/m^2, have been associated with severe, atypical neurotoxic symptoms, such as micturition

disturbances and Lhermitte's sign, mimicking cord disease. However, these signs have been observed in only a few patients so far (3.3% in phase 3 trials). Both symptoms appear to be reversible after oxaliplatin withdrawal (80). In some patients oxaliplatin treatment is feasible for as long as 18 months (for example cumulative oxaliplatin dose over 3000 mg/m^2) with no signs of dysesthesia or paresthesia causing functional impairment, indicating high interindividual variability with respect to sensitivity to oxaliplatin-induced cumulative neuropathy (76,77). Whether cumulative sensory neuropathy can occur as a result of accumulation of dichloro-DACH-platinum, a biotransformation product of DACH-platinum, in the axonal and dorsal root ganglia neurons, needs further investigation (45).

Persistent Lhermitte's sign (an electric-like sensation induced by flexion of the neck) suggestive of irreversible spinal cord toxicity has been reported in a patient taking cisplatin and etoposide (81). Of four patients with oxaliplatin neurotoxicity, two presented with Lhermitte's sign, one had urinary retention, and one had both (82). All had received cumulative doses of 1248–2040 mg/m^2, which is more than the generally accepted neurotoxic threshold for oxaliplatin (1000 mg/m^2).

Peripheral paresthesia has been reported 5 years after adjuvant cisplatin-based treatment for stages I and II testicular cancer (83).

Four of eight children developed acute neurological toxicity. Three had seizures and one had transient blindness after high-dose cisplatin (200 mg/m^2) given by continuous infusion over 5 days, followed 10 days later by a further 2 days with 40 mg/m^2/day. These children had the greatest deterioration in renal function, and they may have had impaired clearance of and increased exposure to cisplatin (84).

Peripheral neuropathy with clinical signs and/or symptoms was found in 80% of patients who had received a cumulative dose of 576 mg/m^2 of cisplatin. There was a dose-related reduction in sensory action potential amplitudes (85). The clinical and neurophysiological time progression of the severity of cisplatin polyneuropathy during and after treatment with cisplatin up to a cumulative dose of 600 mg/m^2 has been described (86).

The paraneoplastic neuropathy experienced by women with epithelial ovarian cancer receiving cisplatin has been attributed in certain cases to the drug (87).

- A woman with cancer of the ovary and a man with oat cell carcinoma both developed paresthesia of all four limbs, reduced control of fine movements, and unstable gait after receiving a cumulative dose of 500 mg/m^2 of cisplatin (88). There was distal hypesthesia, with conservation of temperature and pain sensation, areflexia, and sensory ataxia. The woman also had continuous pseudoathetosis. Neurophysiological studies showed absence of peripheral and central sensory potentials and of H-reflexes, normal electromyography, normal motor conduction, and normal mixed silent period.

The target organ in cisplatin neurotoxicity is the dorsal root ganglion. This patient had a syndrome that clinically and neurophysiologically suggested diffuse neuropathic involvement of the dorsal ganglion, in which absence of sensory and H-reflex potentials showed that the small myelinic cells were not altered, consistent with the preservation of pain and temperature sensation.

- A woman developed bilateral blindness and lumbosacral myelopathy within 1 month of having received an autologous bone marrow transplant, cisplatin 55 mg/m^2, carmustine 600 mg/m^2, and cyclophosphamide 1875 mg/m^2 (79).

Encephalopathy has also been reported.

- A 50-year-old woman with carcinoma of the cervix was treated with radiotherapy and six courses of cisplatin (75 mg/m^2 every 3 weeks; total dose 810 mg) (89). The therapy was completed with no obvious acute complications, but 12 weeks after the last course, she developed sudden blindness associated with occipital headache. She had mild global cognitive deficits and intermittent myoclonic jerking of both arms. Her visual acuity was limited to light perception in both eyes; her pupils were symmetrical with no afferent pupillary deficit. Anterior segment examination and dilated fundoscopy were normal; no ocular movements were elicited when a large plain mirror was held in front of her. The rest of the neurological examination was normal. Serum magnesium was reduced to 0.1 mmol/l (reference range 0.7–1.2 mmol/l). Electroencephalography showed diffuse slowing confirming an encephalopathy.
- An 84-year-old woman with adenocarcinoma of the ovary had two fully reversible episodes of non-convulsive encephalopathy, each following a course of cisplatin-based chemotherapy, confirming a causal relation (90). She developed acute confusion, a partial left homonymous hemianopia and a left extinction hemiparesthesia 7 and 10 days after treatment. Brain MRI showed long-standing cerebral microvascular changes and an electroencephalogram showed right-sided parieto-occipital periodic lateralized epileptiform discharges over a generalized background slowing of activity.

In view of the similarity to posterior leukoencephalopathy, the second case suggests regional endovascular injury rather than direct cerebral toxicity as the initial event in the evolution of encephalopathy.

Strokes have been reported in patients receiving cisplatin.

- A 21-year-old woman with a mixed germ cell tumor of the left ovary was given intravenous chemotherapy including etoposide 100 mg/m^2 on days 1–5, cisplatin 20 mg/m^2 on days 1–5, and bleomycin 30 units on days 2, 8, and 15, all of which she tolerated very well (91). Three weeks later she received a second cycle, which was complicated by an episode of dizziness on day 8. The following day she had an episode of transient dysphasia for 10 minutes. Her third course was uneventful until day 7, when she collapsed with a severe right-sided hemiparesis and dysphasia. Left-sided total anterior circulation infarction was confirmed on MRI scan.
- A 31-year-old man with a seminoma had an orchidectomy, followed by chemotherapy with cisplatin, etoposide, and bleomycin (92). A day after the end of the second course of chemotherapy he became comatose with a heart rate of 150/minute and a systolic blood

pressure of 80 mmHg. Cranial angiography showed a thrombosis of the basilar artery and a cranial CT scan showed cerebellar infarction but no brain metastases.

However, the use of other drugs in these patients makes it difficult to assign causality to cisplatin.

Infusions of cisplatin into the axillary artery have led to a bronchial plexopathy rather than the more commonly described lumbosacral nerve plexus lesion (93).

In five patients cerebral herniation followed cisplatin therapy (94). However, all had evidence of an intracerebral tumor with mass effect and the herniation of the brain was thought to be multifactorial rather than directly attributable to cisplatin.

Auditory brainstem responses have been used to detect ototoxicity from cisplatin and carboplatin when used in combination therapy (95).

Mechanism and susceptibility factors

The mechanism of cisplatin-induced neurotoxicity has not been fully explained. Cisplatin appears to affect neurons in the dorsal root ganglia. It has also been suggested that it can act as a calcium channel blocker, altering intracellular calcium homeostasis and leading to apoptosis of exposed neurons, such as those of the dorsal root ganglia. Cisplatin-induced sensory neuropathy is predominantly characterized by symptoms such as numbness and tingling, paresthesia of the upper and lower extremities, reduced deep-tendon reflexes, and leg weakness with gait disturbance. The first symptoms are often observed after a cumulative dose of 300–600 mg/m^2. Risk factors include diabetes mellitus, alcohol consumption, or inherited neuropathies. Advanced age has not been identified as an independent risk factor when there is no co-morbidity (67–70).

The acute neurotoxic effects of oxaliplatin may result from drug-related inhibition of voltage-gated sodium currents (96). It has been suggested that oxalate ions, which are released during oxaliplatin metabolism, might be responsible for the inhibitory effects on the voltage-gated sodium channels, because of their calcium-chelating activity. Whether there are calcium-sensitive, voltage-gated sodium channels that can be affected by oxalate-induced calcium depletion or whether an indirect effect through changes in intracellular calcium-dependent regulatory mechanisms contributes to oxaliplatin-induced sensory neuropathy needs further investigation (97).

The risk of oxaliplatin-induced neurosensory toxicity may be increased after surgery. Of 12 patients with metastatic colorectal cancer, seven reported immediate postoperative aggravation of pre-existing neurotoxicity. Before surgery, they had only acral paresthesia without any functional impairment, whereas after surgery they complained of major worsening of symptoms, including loss of hand grip strength, leading to dependence in dressing, eating, and use of the toilet, or loss of sensitivity, interfering with walking, which could persist for several months (98). The authors speculated that perioperative hemolysis had caused an increase in unconjugated bilirubin and the release of ultrafilterable oxaliplatin, which had previously been confined to the intraerythrocytic compartment. In addition, diffusion of ultrafilterable oxaliplatin out of erythrocytes into the plasma during hemodilution can contribute to the undesirable perioperative increase in unbound oxaliplatin in the plasma.

There is a correlation between the total dose of cisplatin and the vibratory perception threshold of the hand (99).

Dose-relatedness

When three different schedules of cisplatin were evaluated with regard to the drug's neurotoxicity, using the same dose of 450 mg/m^2 for each of the schedules, it was found that cisplatin-induced peripheral neuropathy depended on both total-dose and single-dose intensity (100).

Neurotoxicity in 22 adolescents was related to the prior cumulative dose of cisplatin that had been received; the relative risk increased 3.2-fold up to a dose of 600 mg/m^2, and 4.1-fold up to a dose of 1340 mg/m^2 (101).

By comparing 50 mg/m^2 weekly with 75 mg/m^2 3 times weekly, using detailed neurological and neurophysiological examination, it has been concluded that cisplatin neuropathy is either of sensory or axonal type, and that both are related to total and single doses (102). However, others have suggested that cisplatin-induced peripheral neurotoxicity is related to dose intensity rather than to the total dose received (103).

A 4-year follow-up of comparison of a combination of cyclophosphamide with cisplatin either 50 mg/m^2 or 100 mg/m^2 in ovarian cancer has been reported (104). Peripheral neuropathy was dose-limiting and persistent. Ten of 31 patients had significant toxicity in the high-dose group compared with one of 24 in the low-dose group.

High-dose cisplatin therapy

The use of aggressive hydration using hypertonic saline and sodium thiosulfate, with dose-scheduling, reduces the risks of dose-limiting nephrotoxicity of cisplatin, and this has made possible the use of high-dose cisplatin (over 200 mg/m^2/course). However, such doses can cause severe chronic peripheral neuropathy, ototoxicity, and myelosuppression, although these effects can be reduced by lengthening the infusion time of cisplatin (65). Peripheral neuropathy is the commonest manifestation of cisplatin neurotoxicity; with high-dose administration the incidence and severity increase with the total dose, and it appears to be age-related. It was not seen in 47 children treated with high-dose cisplatin (40 mg/m^2/day for 5 days) for neuroblastoma (105). Autonomic neuropathy, motor neuropathy, and denervation changes in muscles occur occasionally.

In a clinical and electrophysiological study of eight patients treated with high-dose cisplatin (800–1400 mg) plus etoposide and bleomycin, all developed a peripheral sensory neuropathy (106). A reduction in vibratory sensation was the earliest manifestation of the neuropathy and the findings were compatible with primary damage to the dorsal root ganglia with a central-distal axonopathy. No motor nerve abnormalities were detected, apart from one patient with carpal tunnel syndrome, but two patients had prolonged brain-stem auditory-evoked potentials, indicating a central transmission defect. In another clinical and electrophysiological study of seven patients treated with

cisplatin, the sensory neuropathy was also axonal, with considerable involvement of proprioception (107). Postmortem study in one case showed degeneration of the posterior columns of the spinal cord and evidence of neuronal loss in the lumbar spinal ganglion.

Eleven patients referred for neurological evaluation after cisplatin infusion into the internal or external iliac arteries for pelvic or lower limb tumors all developed symptoms within 48 hours of nerve or plexus dysfunction within the territory supplied by the cannulated artery (108). The lumbosacral plexus was affected in nine patients, the femoral nerve in one, and the peroneal nerve in one. The doses of cisplatin ranged from 50 to 160 mg/m^2 and they did not correlate with the severity or course of the neuropathy. Small-vessel injury and infarction or a direct toxic effect are likely explanations.

Time-course

In a study of the time-course and prognosis of cisplatin-induced neurotoxicity (for example sural nerve sensory action, conduction velocity, and vibration threshold in the left big toe) in 29 patients with metastatic germ cell tumors, the onset of paresthesia was delayed (109). After completion of chemotherapy (3–4 cycles) only 11% of the patients had neurotoxic symptoms, whereas 3 months later the proportion was 65%. Cisplatin-induced neurological disorders should therefore be evaluated at 1–4 months after the end of weekly cisplatin administration, because during this time the most severe form of cisplatin neurotoxicity is to be expected. There was resolution of symptoms in most of the patients over the next 12 months, suggesting that in some individuals a long period of regeneration is required to restore axonal sensory function. In patients with mild signs of cisplatin-related neuropathy, retreatment is generally feasible after several months (110,111).

Management

Among several thiol compounds, glutathione may provide neuroprotection in patients treated with cisplatin without altering its antineoplastic activity. This protective role may be based on blockade of the accumulation of p53 protein in response to platinum in dorsal root ganglia, thereby hindering platinum-based apoptosis (57,112).

The melanocortin Org 2766, an ACTH analogue, which is not yet available for clinical use, alleviates neurotoxicity due to vinca alkaloids and cisplatin, perhaps by enhancing neural repair. However, whereas preliminary results suggested some neuroprotection in women with ovarian cancer treated with cisplatin, these results were not confirmed in a randomized, multicenter, double-blind, placebo-controlled dose-finding study, even with higher doses of Org 2766 (113).

There is evidence that amifostine can reduce the frequency of cisplatin-induced peripheral neuropathy, allowing higher mean cumulative doses to be used. However, some of the results should be interpreted with caution, because the studies included patients who differed in respect to treatment regimen, disease states, and pretreatment status. The underlying protective effect of amifostine may be based on its capacity to scavenge free radicals and prevent cisplatin DNA adduct formation in several organs, including the dorsal root ganglia (57).

In a pilot study in 15 patients, subcutaneous amifostine was given 20 minutes before oxaliplatin, in order to counteract oxaliplatin-induced peripheral neurosensory toxicity. In 10 patients, this regimen reduced the severity of cumulative neuropathy without compromising anti-tumor efficacy; the amifostine was well tolerated (114).

There is increasing evidence that acute oxaliplatin-induced neurotoxicity can be improved by intravenous infusion of calcium gluconate 1000 mg and magnesium sulfate heptahydrate 1000 mg before and after oxaliplatin. It has recently been shown that this strategy could reduce the incidence of acute neurotoxic symptoms, including laryngopharyngeal dysesthesia. Of 101 patients with advanced colorectal cancers who received folinic acid (leucovorin), 5-fluorouracil, and oxaliplatin ($85 \text{ mg/m}^2/2$ weeks, 20 patients; $100 \text{ mg/m}^2/2$ weeks, 22 patients; $130 \text{ mg/m}^2 /3$ weeks, 59 patients), 63 received infusions of calcium and magnesium (1 g each) before and after oxaliplatin administration (treatment group); 38 patients (control group) did not receive infusions of calcium + magnesium. The median cumulative dose of oxaliplatin was 910 (range 255–2340) mg/m^2 in the calcium/magnesium group and 650 (range 255–1450) mg/m^2 in the control group. At the end of treatment, 27% had neuropathy (any grade) compared with 75% in the control group; 1.6% and 26% had pharyngolaryngeal dysesthesia; and 5% and 24% had grade 3 neuropathy. However, further studies are warranted before this regimen can be generally recommended for reducing the risk of acute neurosensory symptoms associated with oxaliplatin infusion (77,115).

Carbamazepine is a potent sodium channel blocker and has therefore been studied in the prevention of oxaliplatin-induced neuropathy (116). The doses of carbamazepine were adjusted to produce serum concentrations in the range 30–60 µg/ml. None of the patients who took carbamazepine reported symptoms of peripheral neurotoxicity; however, two patients (one who forgot to take carbamazepine and one who stopped taking it because he felt tired) developed grade-1 peripheral sensory neurotoxicity. These symptoms were abolished when carbamazepine was restarted. One can therefore speculate that the concomitant use of carbamazepine may allow the use of a higher cumulative dose of oxaliplatin without the occurrence of grade-4 neuropathy. However, a multicenter trial is warranted to confirm these encouraging preliminary results (117).

In 15 patients with metastatic colorectal cancer who were given gabapentin (100 mg bd or tds) if neuropathic symptoms developed with oxaliplatin, the symptoms disappeared in all patients, even in those who received up to 14 courses of oxaliplatin. Withdrawal of gabapentin resulted in recurrence. However, a controlled trial is required to verify these encouraging preliminary results.

It has been suggested that chronomodulated delivery of oxaliplatin might reduce the incidence of platinum-induced neurotoxicity (118,119). In a randomized, multicenter trial in patients with previously untreated metastases from colorectal cancer, 93 patients were assigned chronotherapy and 93 were assigned constant-rate infusion (120). Chronotherapy reduced the rate of severe mucositis

five-fold and halved the rate of functional impairment from peripheral sensitive neuropathy. Median and 3-year survival times were similar in the two groups.

Preliminary results have suggested that glutathione may be neuroprotective in patients receiving oxaliplatin (121).

Sensory systems

Eyes

Ocular effects, including optic neuritis, papilledema, and retrobulbar neuritis, are uncommon adverse effects of cisplatin-containing cancer chemotherapy. The risk of retinal toxicity is restricted to high-dose cisplatin therapy (for example 200 mg/m^2 over 5 days) and can result in blurred vision and altered color perception, which can persist for several months. In contrast to cisplatin, carboplatin is seldom involved in drug-induced visual disturbances. In two cases there was a relation between the administration of carboplatin ($800–1200 \text{ mg/m}^2$) and the occurrence of clinical cortical blindness (122). However, both patients had impaired renal function before the start of therapy with carboplatin.

- Ocular toxicity of cisplatin has been reported in a 47-year-old woman who experienced rapid uncontrollable eye movements associated with hypomagnesemia and hypocalcemia in the presence of renal tubular damage (123).

Ears

Cisplatin is ototoxic (95).

Frequency

In serial audiometric testing in 66 patients receiving cisplatin 100 mg/m^2 per course, of 39 evaluable patients, 54% had no or mild hearing loss, 36% developed early hearing loss and 10% had late loss. If early hearing loss occurred and treatment was nevertheless continued, the speech frequencies were eventually affected in 71% of patients (124).

Dose-relatedness

Tinnitus and bilateral high-frequency hearing loss (threshold 3000 Hz) have been observed in up to 31% of patients treated with initial intravenous doses of cisplatin of 50 mg/m^2. There is considerable individual variation in susceptibility to cisplatin-induced ototoxicity, and both peak plasma concentrations and cumulative dose are important. Transient reversible tinnitus occurs commonly, even after low doses, but hearing impairment is more dose-dependent and affected by age, renal function, pre-existing inner ear damage and concomitant loop diuretic and/or aminoglycoside treatment. In in-vitro studies, selective damage to hair cells in the cochlea and in the supporting cells in the cochlear and vestibular parts of the labyrinth has been shown, with arrest of morphogenesis and cytodifferentiation. Morphological changes in the stria vascularis have been noted (125).

An attempt has been made to quantify the ototoxic effects of cisplatin in children by cumulative platinum dose and decibel hearing loss at certain predetermined frequencies. The findings provide useful insight into this toxicity (126). In a study of cisplatin ototoxicity in children it was concluded that 77% experienced ototoxicity with a median cumulative dose of 360 mg/m^2 (127). However, when cisplatin was given by continuous infusion rather than bolus administration in 39 children with germ cell tumors, only one, who had received a total cumulative dose of 500 mg/m^2, had evidence of significant ototoxicity over 6 years after diagnosis (128).

In a series of 154 audiograms, ototoxicity increased with cumulative dosage of cisplatin and low-dose or monthly regimens caused the lowest toxicity (129). Patients who were given high doses over short periods of time, or who developed tinnitus and hearing loss in the speech frequencies, were at the highest risk. In a small series of patients it was confirmed that pretreatment hearing loss does not increase the risk of cisplatin ototoxicity (130). It has been postulated that cisplatin ototoxicity is inversely related to the patient's age (131). A 600 mg/m^2 plateau dose of cisplatin, beyond which hearing loss shows no apparent further deterioration in children and adolescents, has been described (132).

Presentation
Progressive hearing loss develops as a result of repeated administration of cisplatin, until a threshold plateau is reached at 3000–8000 Hz (133). Hearing loss greater than 20 dB with frequency as 5% at 1000 Hz, 31% at 2000 Hz, 59% at 4000 Hz, and 95% at 8000 Hz is described (132). This is the result of damage to the organ of Corti. The ototoxicity is bilateral, symmetrical, progressive, and irreversible. Following one course of cisplatin (150–225 mg/m^2) the mean hearing loss recorded was 27 dB at 8000 Hz, 21 dB at 6000 Hz, and 11 dB at 4000 Hz. Development of hearing loss is independent of pretreatment hearing function (134). Sudden bilateral deafness without tinnitus has been described after a single course of cisplatin at a dose of 120 mg/m^2; the patients showed only slight improvement after 4 weeks (135).

Of 186 women receiving cisplatin 50 mg/m^2 4-weekly for gynecological cancers, 40 developed significant hearing loss of at least 15 dB, but there was no significant loss in the speech frequency range (125). Prior hearing acuity did not influence the incidence or extent of the deterioration.

Susceptibility factors
Susceptibility factors include young age, previous cranial irradiation, pre-existing renal dysfunction or inner ear damage, and the concomitant use of other potentially ototoxic agents, such as aminoglycosides, loop diuretics, or tirapazamine (129,136–142). Previous use of an aminoglycoside increases the risk of ototoxicity. Younger patients and patients who had undergone prior cranial irradiation are more particularly susceptible to audiological changes, which progress in severity with increasing dose (143).

Mechanisms
The mechanisms of cisplatin-induced damage to the outer hairy cells of the cochlea may include the formation of highly reactive oxygen radicals and depletion of glutathione (144). The role of amifostine and glutathione

in preventing cisplatin-induced ototoxicity has therefore been studied (145,146). The data are not sufficient to support the use of glutathione in this indication. In contrast, there is some evidence that amifostine may provide protection (147). No ototoxicity developed in 18 patients who received amifostine over 15 minutes, 15–20 minutes before the intravenous administration of cisplatin 50–120 mg/m^2 over 20 minutes. There was transient hearing loss and mild persistent audiometric abnormalities in only 30% of the patients who received cisplatin 150 mg/m^2.

Animal experiments show that cisplatin is only weakly vestibulotoxic (148), and clinical vestibular toxicity is found less often than hearing loss. Of 10 patients who received 80–550 mg cisplatin, clinical features of vestibulotoxicity were analysed in addition to hearing, and patients underwent audiometry, body sway, caloric, and optokinetic and pendular rotation testing (149). Four patients sustained significant hearing loss, five had tinnitus, and three complained of dizziness, giddiness, and/or unsteadiness rather than vertigo. These symptoms were transient, and they occurred usually after several weeks of administration; they were not consistently dose-related. Spontaneous nystagmus was observed in seven and positional nystagmus in six. Caloric and body sway tests were abnormal in the early stages in several patients. The findings were suggestive of a cumulative toxic effect.

In an in-vitro study of the adverse effect of cisplatin on hair cells and other inner ear structures, aimed at determining whether selective damage occurs in inner ear hair cells and whether morphogenesis and cytodifferentiation are influenced by low cisplatin concentrations, even at low cisplatin concentrations (0.1 µg/ml) there was selective damage to hair cells. Incubation at a cisplatin concentration of 1 µg/ml caused morphological damage in the supporting cochlear and vestibular cells, and 10 µg/ml caused total collapse of the membranous labyrinth. Drug exposure arrested morphogenesis as well as cytodifferentiation (150).

Auditory brainstem responses have been used to detect ototoxicity from cisplatin and carboplatin when used in combination therapy (95). The method can detect early high frequency damage due to these drugs up to two or three cycles earlier than conventional audiometry.

The ototoxicity of cisplatin has been studied using distortion-product otoacoustic emissions (DPOAEs) and conventional pure-tone audiometry (151). Cisplatin ototoxicity was detected on average one cycle earlier with DPOAEs than with pure-tone audiometry. The authors suggested that this was because DPOAEs are more sensitive to outer hair cell damage.

Carboplatin and oxaliplatin
In one study only 1.1% of evaluable patients taking carboplatin had ototoxic symptoms, such as tinnitus, or subclinical audiographic changes (152). However, in a series of closely monitored patients there was an incidence of 27% (129). It has also been estimated that 19% of patients receiving carboplatin have significant hearing loss greater than 30 dB; the hearing loss is cumulative and maximum at 8000 Hz; the authors reported two of these patients with hearing loss greater than 10 dB at

1000 Hz. The overall conclusion is that with low-dose, short-schedule, carboplatin therapy, routine audiometry is not justified (152).

After otoacoustic emission testing in 19 children who received cisplatin the authors suggested that this is better at detecting the early cochlear damage associated with cisplatin ototoxicity than traditional pure-tone audiometry, particularly in children, in whom early detection is of the utmost importance (153). In patients who receive high-dose carboplatin, preliminary results suggest that there may be a correlation between the risk of ototoxicity and carboplatin serum concentrations (AUC) during the first course. Patients with high-grade ototoxicity had higher median carboplatin AUCs than patients without any symptoms (122,154).

In another study, carboplatin-induced ototoxicity was reported in 32% of exposed patients. This was similar to cisplatin ototoxicity, although at a lower frequency (4000–8000 Hz) than the often-quoted 6000–8000 Hz for cisplatin. The extent of otic damage was proportional to the dose of carboplatin (155).

Audiological testing has been recommended for patients receiving high-dose carboplatin therapy, following hearing problems in a series of 10 patients with ovarian cancer (156).

There is no evidence that oxaliplatin causes ototoxicity (157).

Smell

About 30% of patients treated with cisplatin have been reported to have some degree of anosmia, which in 1% is severe or complete; the sense of smell returns to normal within 3–4 months of completing cisplatin therapy (158).

Endocrine

The endocrine effects of cisplatin-based chemotherapy were studied in 22 men 9–24 or more months after completion of treatment for germ cell tumors (159). Mean basal FSH and stimulated LH and FSH concentrations were increased but serum testosterone concentrations were similar to untreated controls. Younger patients (under 25 years old) appeared more resistant to these effects of chemotherapy, and the hormonal abnormalities recovered with time.

The long-term effects on Leydig cell function of chemotherapy in 244 patients with germ cell tumors have been studied by measuring concentrations of sex hormone-binding globulin, luteinizing hormone, and follicle-stimulating hormone at least 74 months after chemotherapy (160). The population was divided into groups by cumulative cisplatin exposure (above and below 400 mg/m^2). Low-dose cisplatin exposure had no effect on Leydig cell function, but cumulative high-dose chemotherapy caused persistent impairment.

Metabolism

- Hyperosmolar non-ketotic hyperglycemia occurred in a 61-year-old patient 6 days after a first cycle of cisplatin therapy (161). The patient recovered with conventional conservative management.

Electrolyte balance

Hyponatremia is rare, and persistent hyponatremia very rare in patients taking cisplatin (162). In a detailed description of the biochemical abnormalities that can result from renal tubular dysfunction after cisplatin therapy, it was noted that hypocalciuria is more common than hypomagnesemia, and that there tends to be a state of reduced serum bicarbonate. The most severe renal tubular damage caused by cisplatin is characterized by hypocalciuria, total body magnesium deficiency, and hypokalemic metabolic alkalosis (163).

Other electrolyte disturbances induced by cisplatin include hypocalcemia, hypophosphatemia, hyponatremia, and hypokalemia (164,165). However, these changes are rarely associated with symptoms (166,167).

Metal metabolism

Magnesium

About 75% of patients treated with cisplatin develop hypomagnesemia (serum concentrations below 1.5 mmol/l), which appears to be associated with drug-induced renal tubular damage (168–171). The symptoms include tetany, muscular weakness, tremulousness, dizziness, personality changes, and perioral and peripheral paresthesia (172). Magnesium supplementation is generally recommended during treatment courses with cisplatin (168,170). Sometimes, hypomagnesemia resolves rather slowly and can last several weeks. A significant reduction in serum magnesium and other effects associated with progressive renal dysfunction appear to correlate with high cumulative doses of carboplatin (for example a median cumulative dose of 2590 mg/m^2 in children or in adults undergoing high-dose chemotherapy with peripheral blood stem cell support).

Renal magnesium wasting is the main mechanism responsible for the hypomagnesemia associated with cisplatin (172), and it can be associated with enhanced tubular reabsorption of calcium and consequent hypocalciuria (173). This dissociation in the renal handling of calcium and magnesium is similar to what is found in Bartter's syndrome. The site of the renal tubular defect in these conditions is not known, but there is evidence that active renal tubular transport systems are disrupted.

In a prospective study of 28 patients who received a total of 82 doses of cisplatin, hypomagnesemia occurred in all patients and was associated with significant and prolonged dose-related magnesium wasting. Serum magnesium was 1.8 mg/dl after the fourth dose. Examination of the urine sediment 2–4 days after each dose of cisplatin showed renal tubular epithelial cells, suggesting that cisplatin directly injures the tubules, leading to reduced tubular reabsorption of magnesium, renal magnesium wasting, and hypomagnesemia (174). In another study, patients receiving cisplatin and concomitant magnesium supplementation developed significantly less renal tubular damage, as assessed by urine N-acetyl-β-D-glucosaminidase (175). No patient developed clinical signs of hypomagnesemia when intravenous or oral supplementation of magnesium was given as soon as the serum magnesium fell to or below 0.45 mmol/l. In patients receiving intracavitary cisplatin in high doses (100–200 mg/m^2), together with intravenous thiosulfate, there was a lower incidence of hypomagnesemia as a result of the thiosulfate; thiosulfate probably inactivated cisplatin before it reached the kidney, by complex formation (176).

Hypomagnesemia secondary to cisplatin administration can be severe enough to present as generalized seizures (172). It more commonly presents with muscular weakness, tremulousness, peripheral paresthesia, tetany, and personality changes. It is dose-related and schedule-related. Loss of magnesium can be prevented by prophylactic magnesium infusion before and during cisplatin administration (177), but this is not universally recommended because of the risk of acute uremia (178).

Zinc

Hyperzincuria and hypozincemia can occur concurrently in patients treated with cisplatin, due to variable excretion of zinc in these cases (179).

Hematologic

Compared with cisplatin and oxaliplatin, carboplatin has the highest myelotoxic potential. Carboplatin-induced myelosuppression is dose-related and results in thrombocytopenia and neutropenia. At conventional doses (AUC 4–7 minutes/μg/ml) about 20–40% of patients develop thrombocytopenia (platelet counts below $50 \times 10^9/l$). In contrast, severe neutropenia is less pronounced with conventional doses; about 16–21% of patients develop neutrophil counts less than $1 \times 10^9/l$. The lowest leukocyte and platelet counts usually occur at 14–28 days after drug administration. The hemoglobin concentration was below 11 g/dl in 71–91% of patients and below 8 g/dl in 8–21% (155). The severity of drug-induced thrombocytopenia is inversely correlated with the endogenous formation and release of thrombopoietin, which is an important cytokine for de novo platelet formation in the bone marrow. In contrast to conventional dosages, high-dose chemotherapy containing carboplatin is generally associated with severe and life-threatening forms of hematological toxicity, requiring the prophylactic use of recombinant hemopoietic growth factors, such as G-CSF, and peripheral blood stem cell support (180).

Underlying risk factors, which predispose patients to more severe forms of myelosuppression, include lower initial blood cell counts, renal impairment, poor performance status, extensive prior chemotherapy, and advanced age. There is a strong correlation between carboplatin pharmacokinetics and the severity of myelosuppressive adverse effects; an AUC-adapted dosage of carboplatin is therefore highly recommended during conventional dose chemotherapy (22,23,155).

Cisplatin belongs to the most important causative agents for the induction of treatment-related anemia requiring the prophylactic use of erythropoietin or intermittent transfusion of erythrocytes, whereas drug-induced leukopenia and thrombocytopenia are generally mild and transient (180,181). In a pharmacokinetic study, non-protein-bound platinum concentrations in patients with significant falls in hemoglobin (3 g/dl or more) were significantly higher (mean 53 ng/ml) than in patients who did not have significant falls in hemoglobin. The authors suggested that early and simple platinum pharmacokinetic control on the day after first drug administration might be useful in targeting patients who are likely to develop more severe forms of cisplatin-related anemia (182).

Myelosuppression caused by oxaliplatin is generally mild. Grade 3/4 anemia, neutropenia, and thrombocytopenia are observed in only 2–3% of patients. In combination with fluorouracil/folinic acid, the frequency is slightly higher, depending on the dose of fluorouracil (8,9).

Cisplatin causes an increase in erythropoietin, but anemias associated with platinum therapy are independent of this mechanism (183).

Forty patients with lung cancer, treated with a combination of cisplatin, mitomycin, vinblastine, doxorubicin, cyclosphosphamide, and methotrexate, had a significant post-treatment increase in fibrinopeptide A and a fall in fibrinolytic activity, reflected by a fall in functional tissue activator; this appeared to be cumulative, depending on the extent of drug exposure (184).

Gastrointestinal

Of the approved platinum compounds, cisplatin has the greatest emetogenic potential (185). Whereas about 65–94% of patients who receive conventional dosages of carboplatin complain of mild to moderate nausea or vomiting, more than 90% of those who receive cisplatin can have more than 10 vomiting episodes within the first day of administration in the absence of effective antiemetic therapy. An emetogenic episode occurring within 24 hours after drug administration is usually classified as acute emesis; nausea and vomiting that occur thereafter are classified as delayed emesis and may persist over several days. There appears to be a correlation between the time of cisplatin administration and the severity of drug-induced vomiting (186). When cisplatin was given in the morning (0500 hours) vomiting was greater than when it was given in the evening (1700 hours). However, the prophylactic use of a 5-HT$_3$ receptor antagonist reduced the time-of-day dependency. 5-HT$_3$ receptor antagonists, such as dolasetron, granisetron, ondansetron, palonosetron, or tropisetron, particularly in combination with dexamethasone, reduce the severity of acute emesis occurring within the first 24 hours after cisplatin. In contrast, the satisfactory prevention of delayed emesis remains a challenge. There is increasing evidence that the introduction of a novel class of antiemetic agents, the neurokinin-1-receptor antagonists, such as MK869 (aprepitant), may be associated with additional benefit in combination with a 5-HT$_3$ receptor antagonist in reducing cisplatin-induced nausea and vomiting, both acute and delayed (187).

Nausea, vomiting, and diarrhea are common adverse effects of oxaliplatin and carboplatin, but they are generally mild to moderate, and both are less emetogenic than cisplatin. However, patients who have previously received cisplatin may be at greater risk of vomiting with carboplatin or oxaliplatin (1,8,9).

In an endoscopic study of the acute gastroduodenal toxicity of intravenous cisplatin 10 mg/m^2 and etoposide 107 mg/m^2 (mean dose) given for three doses, a significant number of patients developed gastroduodenal lesions, several of which progressed (188).

Liver

Mild reversible increases in liver function tests can occur in patients who have received platinum compounds (189). However, the platinum compounds are generally not classified as hepatotoxic drugs.

Urinary tract

Cisplatin

Of the approved platinum compounds, cisplatin has the greatest nephrotoxic potential, and the nephrotoxicity is often dose-limiting (190). If dosages exceed 100 mg/m^2 per course or per day, nephrotoxicity is the most severe drug-related adverse effect. It is mainly due to proximal tubular dysfunction (191), with hydropic degeneration, necrosis, and occasional tubular atrophy. Fragments of distal tubular cells have been demonstrated in the urine of patients receiving chemotherapy that included cisplatin (192). The risk is reduced by adequate hydration, which lowers drug concentrations in the renal tubules. Impaired renal function can persist for at least 6 months after treatment has been withdrawn. Indicators of cisplatin-related renal tubular toxicity include changes in creatinine clearance or in urinary alanine aminopeptidase and N-acetyl-β-D-glucosaminidase activities. Blood urea nitrogen and serum creatinine are poor indicators of early renal damage. The nephrotoxicity of cisplatin is primarily tubular, although changes in renal blood flow and glomerular filtration also occur, and hypomagnesemia is common (SEDA-12) (193,194).

The mechanisms of cisplatin-induced nephrotoxicity have not been fully elucidated. Like several nephrotoxic heavy metals (for example mercury), cisplatin can accumulate in the kidney, where it can interact with sulfhydryl compounds, resulting in increased membrane fragility and depletion of intracellular glutathione. There is some evidence that cisplatin can induce apoptosis and necrosis of kidney cells dose-dependently. In vitro studies have suggested that the constitutive expression of antiapoptotic proteins (for example bcl-X) might be inversely correlated with the sensitivity of renal tubular cells (146,195–197).

Cisplatin-induced nephrotoxicity can be detected by a rise in blood urea or by a fall in creatinine clearance. Tubular dysfunction can cause hyponatremia (72), hypokalemia, hypomagnesemia (173), and hypophosphatemia. Inappropriate ADH secretion may be partly responsible for hyponatremia (191).

In experiments in mice, the trace element selenium, which interacts with heavy metals, reduces the renal, intestinal, hepatic, and hematological toxicity of cisplatin without affecting its antitumor activity (198).

Regarding prolongation of infusion, it has been suggested that there is a correlation between higher plasma platinum concentrations and the risk of cisplatin-induced nephrotoxicity. If platinum concentrations exceed 6 µg/ml, more patients develop nephrotoxicity. These drug concentrations were measured shortly after the end of infusion (for example 5 minutes after intravenous infusions of 100–120 mg/m^2), suggesting that high blood concentrations rather than trough concentrations may be predictively important. As a result, prolongation of cisplatin infusion (for example 6 hours)

has been proposed to reduce the risk of cisplatin-induced renal insufficiency (147,199). However, in practice, a 1-hour infusion remains the common standard.

In 35 children who had taken cisplatin for a maximum of 2 years, nephrotoxicity was not related to total dose but was less severe in children who received cisplatin in doses below 40 mg/m^2/day (200). During follow-up for 2 years there was partial but significant recovery of renal function.

The effect of age on nephrotoxicity after treatment with ifosfamide or cisplatin has been studied (201). Children aged 5 years or less had more severe proximal tubular toxicity associated with ifosfamide than older patients. They also had significantly lower plasma phosphate concentrations and a higher fractional excretion of glucose. There was no evidence of glomerular or distal renal tubular damage after ifosfamide and there was no difference between the older and younger children in any other aspect of renal function. In general, age predicts independently the likelihood and severity of genitourinary toxicity caused by cisplatin in combination chemotherapy (202).

Several supportive measures have been proposed in order to circumvent cisplatin-induced nephrotoxicity. These include:

- adequate hydration before and during cisplatin administration and afterwards, in combination with an osmotic diuretic such as mannitol (the current standard method);
- prolongation of the infusion time (for example 6 hours instead of 2 hours);
- fractionation over several days;
- the use of a chronomodulated schedule;
- the use of nephroprotective agents, such as organic thiosulfate compounds.

Sodium thiosulfate protects against cisplatin-induced nephrotoxicity by reacting covalently with cisplatin in the renal tubules. Other protectors include probenecid, orgotein, fosfomycin (203), amifostine (2-[3-aminopropyl)amino]ethylphosphorothioic acid, WR-2721, ethyofos), and anthiol. Experimental study drugs that may be useful in renal protection include BNP7787 (dimesna), selenium, and silibinin (146,204–212). The beneficial role of furosemide is uncertain.

Amifostine is an organic thiophosphate. It is a prodrug, because dephosphorylation by tissue-bound alkaline phosphatase is necessary to form its active metabolite, WR-1065. It protects normal tissues against the toxic effects of radiation, cisplatin, and alkylating agents in animals, perhaps through free radical scavenging, hydrogen ion donation, and the prevention or removal of DNA platinum adducts (213). Amifostine has been used in the pretreatment of patients with metastatic melanoma before administration of cisplatin 60–150 mg/m^2 in an uncontrolled trial of 36 patients (214). There was a response rate of 53% and a low incidence of nephrotoxicity; transient nephrotoxicity occurred in 4% of 82 courses of amifostine given with cisplatin 120 mg/m^2.

In a randomized study, 242 patients with advanced ovarian cancer received intravenous cisplatin 100 mg/m^2 and cyclophosphamide 1000 mg/m^2 once every 3 weeks with or without amifostine 910 mg/m^2. Besides a significant reduction in chemotherapy-induced neutropenia and thrombocytopenia, amifostine produced significant protection against cisplatin-induced nephrotoxicity. Creatinine clearance fell by more than 40% in 60% of the control group compared with 12% of those in the treated group. In addition, the incidence of cisplatin-related hypomagnesemia was less pronounced in the patients who received amifostine.

Dose fractionation over several days has been associated with less kidney damage. The glomerular filtration rate was maintained in patients who received cisplatin 20 mg/m^2/day over 5 consecutive days (215,216). However, patients still had a significant increase in sensitive urinary markers, such as low molecular weight proteins, N-acetyl-β-D-glucosaminidase (NAG), and α–1-microglobulin, showing that conventional approaches can reduce but not completely prevent nephrotoxicity (146,195).

Chronomodulated administration of cisplatin can also reduce drug-induced organ toxicity, for example nephrotoxicity (217,218). Administration of cisplatin in the evening caused markedly less nephrotoxicity and neurotoxicity than morning administration. There is also increasing evidence that all platinum-based anticancer drugs are better tolerated if they are given in the late afternoon or early evening, with less frequent and severe nephrotoxicity, thrombocytopenia, and cumulative peripheral neuropathy after cisplatin, carboplatin, and oxaliplatin. As chronomodulated scheduling appears to affect the adverse effects of all platinum compounds, the mechanism may be based on circadian variation in renal tubular excretion and plasma filtration of platinum compounds, increased plasma protein binding, and reduced tissue susceptibility at about 1600 hours (217–219).

In several studies, intravenous amifostine (910 mg/m^2) preserved glomerular filtration rate when it was co-administered with cisplatin-containing regimens (213). Even after two cycles containing intravenous cisplatin 50 mg/m^2 plus intravenous ifosfamide and etoposide or paclitaxel, glomerular filtration rate can fall by more than 30%, but concomitant use of amifostine prevented this. Even lower dosages of intravenous amifostine (for example 740 mg/m^2) may be effective (220,221).

Because preclinical results suggested that intracellular glutathione may be involved in the modulation of cisplatin-induced toxicity, several trials (two uncontrolled and two randomized) have been conducted to evaluate the efficacy and tolerability of standard doses of cisplatin with concomitant glutathione. In some studies, glutathione reduced cisplatin-related toxicity without impairing its antineoplastic activity (113). However, a cisplatin dose-escalation study with concomitant administration of glutathione had to be terminated prematurely because of unacceptable ototoxicity. Glutathione has not yet received FDA approval for chemoprotection.

Carboplatin

When carboplatin is used in doses that cause similar hematological toxicity to cisplatin, it has negligible renal, neurological, and auditory toxicity (222,223). In combination with other cytotoxic agents, the maximum tolerated dose is less than normal because of the risk of myelosuppression (224). However, if the dose is increased, as in acute non-lymphocytic leukemia, high-tone hearing loss and renal impairment can occur (225). In this study, all but one patient who developed these adverse effects had also received aminoglycoside antibiotics.

Concomitant intravenous hydration and monitoring is not needed when carboplatin is given in conventional dosages. However, during dose-intensified treatment with carboplatin, the risk of impaired renal function increases. In addition, other nephrotoxic drugs, such as ifosfamide, are often part of those high-dose combination regimens. During a study of the use of high-dose carboplatin (1500 mg/m^2/day or more) on 3 consecutive days, the nephrotoxic profile was comparable to a standard single dose of cisplatin (216).

Ultra-high-dose carboplatin can be safely administered as long as clinicians individualize and adjust the therapy to renal function using ^{51}Cr-EDTA glomerular filtration rate; there was only one death attributed to carboplatin in 31 patients who died of acute renal insufficiency (226).

Mild to moderate reduction in creatinine clearance with rises in serum urea and creatinine were reported in 14% of patients receiving carboplatin in a dose of 400 mg/m^2 for gynecological malignancies. Of the patients who received carboplatin 400 mg/m^2 with vincristine but without hydration for lung cancer, 19% developed renal changes.

During a 2-year follow-up of 23 children receiving carboplatin there were falls in both glomerular filtration rate to 22 ml/minute and serum magnesium concentration to 0.17 mmol/l (166). The authors thought that the fall in glomerular filtration rate, although statistically significant, was not clinically significant, but they were unsure about the long-term clinical effects of the low magnesium.

Intensified carboplatin-containing regimens can predispose patients to drug-induced renal dysfunction when cisplatin has previously been used or when renal function is already impaired (167,227).

In a randomized study of the prophylactic use of amifostine during dose-intensified chemotherapy including carboplatin and ifosfamide, patients in the control arm had a median loss of glomerular filtration rate of 37% compared with baseline after one cycle, and 35% of these patients had glomerular filtration rates below 60 ml/minute on day 10 after treatment. In patients who received amifostine during dose-intensified chemotherapy, the glomerular filtration rate fell only by a median of 10% and no patient developed a glomerular filtration rate below 60 ml/minute by day 10 (228).

Oxaliplatin

Oxaliplatin, when given alone or in combination with fluorouracil, is considered not to be nephrotoxic (166,167,227). There has been a single case of acute tubular necrosis probably caused by oxaliplatin and not related to dehydration or pre-renal insufficiency (229).

Skin

Even in cases of accidental extravasation, the risk of skin ulceration is low. Severe cisplatin-related extravasation injury appears to be primarily restricted to the use of high concentrations (for example 0.75 mg/ml) and infusion over a short time. In such circumstances it is advisable to give a local injection of isotonic thiosulfate solution (0.16 mol/l). Since carboplatin is more slowly activated than cisplatin to active DNA binding moieties and is more water-soluble, there have been no reports of severe carboplatin extravasation and no antidote is necessary (230,231).

- Accidental subcutaneous administration of oxaliplatin resulted in a red-brown painful swelling and sclerosis of the skin within 8 days (232). The symptoms were worst 1 week after extravasation and lasted for about 5 weeks, but the patient, a 52-year-old woman, recovered fully. Acute intervention included local fluid instillation to dilute the extravasation, removal of the cannula, cold packs, and a gel containing aescin and diethylamine salicylate.

Two other cases of oxaliplatin extravasation have been reported (233). Both occurred when the intraport needle disconnected. The initial symptoms were swelling and tenderness at the port site. The patients developed severe inflammation after 3 days. Treatment included local cool packs, diclofenac ointment, and oral indometacin, morphine, or dexamethasone. The authors avoided saline instillation because sodium chloride and oxaliplatin may be incompatible in combination (119). Both patients recovered without any sign of local necrosis and long-term sequelae (233)

Sexual function

Sexual function in men can be compromised by cisplatin + vinblastine + bleomycin chemotherapy. Of 54 patients, 29 had disorders of sexual function 2 years after completion of treatment (234). Ejaculatory dysfunction was tentatively linked to chemotherapy in 30% of those affected. There was reduced libido, usually reversible, in 40 at the time of chemotherapy.

Reproductive system

A cumulative dose–response toxic effect of cisplatin affects gonadal function when the drug is used in children around puberty; this damage is reversible in girls, but not in boys (235).

Immunologic

Cisplatin can cause anaphylactic shock, asthma, or urticaria (236). Hypersensitivity reactions, probably of type I, have also been reported after the administration of cisplatin, carboplatin, and oxaliplatin (237–243). Life-threatening allergy to cisplatin has also been reported after 16 doses of cisplatin 20 mg/m^2/week (244). These allergic reactions can include respiratory dysfunction (for example wheezing, dyspnea), gastro-intestinal discomfort (for example abdominal cramps, diarrhea), and rashes (for example pruritus, urticaria, facial erythema, and swelling). The risk of exfoliative dermatitis is very low. In most patients, the first signs of hypersensitivity reactions usually occurred after the administration of multiple intravenous courses containing platinum compounds. Whether patients who are hypersensitive to one platinum compound also react to another cannot be excluded, since some case reports have suggested possible cross-reactions among platinum compounds (245). Sometimes, successful retreatment may be feasible through premedication with glucocorticoids and antihistamines (240).

The frequency of carboplatin-induced hypersensitivity reactions is 2–9%. Of more than 200 patients 16 had allergic reactions to carboplatin (246). According to one retrospective analysis, mild carboplatin-related hypersensitivity reactions, with itching and mild erythema, occurred in 20 of 194 patients, whereas 12 patients developed severe forms of reactions, including diffuse erythroderma, rigor, facial swelling, throat and chest tightness, tachycardia, bronchospasm, and hypertension or hypotension (243). The most important interventive measures in patients with severe forms of hypersensitivity reactions include intravenous adrenaline, glucocorticoids, and antihistamines.

Severe anaphylaxis has been reported in five patients who had already received several cycles (5–12) containing oxaliplatin 100 mg/m^2 every 2 weeks (241). The predominant symptoms included reduced systolic blood pressure, flushing, sweating, headache, tachycardia, and respiratory distress. If retreatment with the causative platinum compound is required in such cases, premedication with a glucocorticoid and antihistamine may prevent recurrence. However, symptoms can occur despite premedication, making drug withdrawal necessary.

There was a 12% incidence rate of hypersensitivity reactions in 205 women who received carboplatin as part of their treatment for gynecological malignancies (247). In trying to characterize these reactions, the authors noted that in about half of the patients, the reaction developed after more than half of their carboplatin had been infused, with a median number of exposures to carboplatin of eight cycles before the reaction.

An effective carboplatin desensitization protocol has been reported in a child with hypersensitivity, allowing additional months of carboplatin treatment (248). After premedication with diphenhydramine, ranitidine, and methylprednisolone, eight dilutions of carboplatin (0.01–50.0 mg) were given intravenously at 15-minute intervals at a rate of 1 mg/minute. Subsequently, carboplatin 600 mg was given as a continuous infusion over 3 hours without adverse effects. Whether desensitization is generally suitable for overcoming allergic adverse events should be tested prospectively (249).

The term "oxaliplatin-induced hypersensitivity reaction" can refer to:

1. acuteneurosensory symptoms;
2. a cytokine release syndrome related to increased plasma concentrations of interleukin-6 and tumor necrosis factor alfa;
3. an immunological reaction involving antibody formation and histamine release (238).

In order to prove an underlying allergic disorder, an intradermal skin test with commercial formulations of the platinum compound in different concentrations (for example 0.003–1 mg/ml) can be done (250).

Body temperature

Oxaliplatin is generally well tolerated. Some patients develop fever, which appears to be related to a transient increase in cytokines, particularly interleukin-6 and tumor necrosis factor alfa. In one study the oxaliplatin-induced increase in body temperature correlated with a marked increase in interleukin-6 serum concentrations (peak 133 pg/ml) (251). Interleukin-6 is a proinflammatory cytokine, which stimulates acute phase proteins and B lymphocytes. Premedication with metamizol, dexamethasone, and clarithromycin, which interferes with interleukin-6, did not prevent the fever. The roles of interleukin-6 and tumor necrosis factor alfa in the development of fever is strengthened by the observation that their serum concentrations fell during resolution of the fever (252).

Death

- Fatal acute tumor lysis syndrome has been reported in a 74-year-old woman who received cisplatin (50 mg/m^2 on day 1) and fluorouracil (1000 mg/m^2 by continuous infusion for 5 days) for vulvar carcinoma (253).

Whilst this is a well known complication of chemotherapy, particularly with hematological tumors, it is extremely rare as a complication of neoadjuvant chemotherapy for gynecological tumors.

Long-Term Effects

Tumorigenicity

There is some evidence that platinum compounds are mutagenic in bacteria and can cause chromosomal aberrations in animal cells in tissue culture (254). The risk of secondary leukemia in 28 971 patients with ovarian cancers receiving platinum-based chemotherapy has been evaluated; 96 developed a secondary leukemia (255). The authors concluded that the risk of developing a secondary leukemia while receiving a platinum-based protocol may be increased four-fold. The relative risks for carboplatin and cisplatin were estimated at 6.5 and 3.3 respectively. The relative risks of leukemia after cumulative doses of platinum of less than 500, 500–749, 750–999, and 1000 mg were 1.9, 2.1, 4.1, and 7.6 respectively. The delay between the start of platinum-containing chemotherapy and the occurrence of secondary malignancies was 2.8–7.7 years. In children who received an average cumulative dose of cisplatin of 600 mg/m^2, the estimated incidence of chemotherapy-induced leukemia was 1.5% (256). Concomitant radiation therapy or administration of other carcinogenic agents increases the risk.

Second-Generation Effects

Fertility

There is experimental evidence that several anticancer drugs can cause abnormalities of sperm chromosomes. Preliminary data have suggested that after platinum-containing chemotherapy for testicular cancer, penetration of oocytes can be severely impaired. Cytogenetic study of the spermatozoa has shown that many of the abnormalities correspond to structural aberrations that may not have a pathogenic effect in the production of abortions or children with chromosome abnormalities (257).

In men receiving chemotherapy, the sperm count will return to normal within 2 years of discontinuing chemotherapy in 78% of cases; however, intensive treatment, such as with doses of cisplatin in excess of 500 mg/m^2, reduces the probability of full recovery of normal spermatogenesis (258).

A Danish study group has reported a fertility problem of 53% in patients with unilateral germ cell tumors, but there was no significant difference between orchidectomy and cisplatin-based chemotherapy or subdiaphragmatic irradiation (259). Eight patients remained infertile despite evident recovery of spermatogenesis, and all 22 children conceived post-treatment were born normal and without malformations.

Gonadal function was evaluated in 59 men and 31 women after successful treatment of germ-cell tumors with the POMB/ACE regimen (cisplatin, vincristine, methotrexate, and bleomycin + dactinomycin, cyclophosphamide, and etoposide) (260). Most of the patients recovered fertility; 81% of the men who did not receive para-aortic radiotherapy, whose original tumor bulk was less than 5 cm in diameter, and whose duration of chemotherapy was less than 6 months recovered, compared with 32% who had larger tumors or who received longer courses of chemotherapy, or both. Fertility and pregnancies were undisturbed in 24 women with invasive trophoblastic tumors treated with methotrexate alone, with methotrexate and dactinomycin in combination, or with other combination chemotherapy (261). There were nine subsequent pregnancies, with the birth of eight healthy babies, and one woman requested a termination of pregnancy.

The long-term prognosis for sperm counts after chemotherapy with and without radiation in 71 males treated for non-Hodgkin's lymphoma on the CHOP-Bleomycin combination has been studied (262). Pelvic radiotherapy and cumulative cyclophosphamide dosages of greater than 9.5 g/m^2 are associated independently and in combination with a greater risk of permanent sterility.

Teratogenicity

Cisplatin and related compounds cross the placenta and can therefore cause fetal damage. Cisplatin is teratogenic in mice and embryotoxic in mice and rats. The platins should only be used during pregnancy in life-threatening situations. The patient should be informed of the potential hazard to the fetus (263).

Drug Administration

Drug administration route

There have been several reports of local neurotoxicity after intra-arterial cisplatin. In 63 patients pretreated with low-dose cisplatin given by arterial infusion for head and neck cancer (up to 25 mg/day for 1–10 days), before definitive local treatment, cranial nerve palsies developed on the same side as the cannulated artery in four cases (264). There was ipsilateral involvement of the 9th, 10th, 11th, and 12th cranial nerves in two patients, and the 7th and 12th nerves alone were affected in the other two patients. The palsies appeared at the end of treatment or up to 10 days later and only the 12th nerve palsy in one of the patients with multiple cranial nerve involvement recovered completely. In each patient, no other cause for paresis was found and CT scans showed that the nerves were not infiltrated by tumor. The cumulative dose of cisplatin administered to these four patients was less than that received by the unaffected 59 patients (median 200 mg, range 160–250; compared with 250 mg, range 160–400).

Drug overdose

Irreversible renal insufficiency has been described after accidental overdosage with cisplatin.

- In a 68-year-old woman who received an accidental overdose of cisplatin (480 mg), there was severe vomiting and myelosuppression, irreversible renal insufficiency, and deafness; other effects included seizures, hallucinations, loss of vision, and hepatotoxicity (265).

Drug–Drug Interactions

Antiepileptic drugs

Plasma concentrations of antiepileptic drugs (for example carbamazepine, valproic acid, phenytoin) should be measured more frequently during cisplatin-containing cancer chemotherapy (266,267).

- Cisplatin caused subtherapeutic carbamazepine and valproic acid concentrations in a 38-year-old woman with epilepsy undergoing cytotoxic cancer chemotherapy with doxorubicin and cisplatin, resulting in tonic-clonic seizures; the mechanism was not clear (266).

Etoposide

- A 52-year-old patient with glioblastoma developed severe ocular and orbital toxicity after receiving intracarotid etoposide phosphate and carboplatin (268). Acutely non-pupillary block angle-closure glaucoma developed secondary to uveal effusion in the ipsilateral eye. Four days later, severe orbital inflammation resulted in reduced visual acuity, proptosis, optic neuropathy, and total external ophthalmoplegia.

Fluorouracil

The combination of cisplatin 100 mg/m^2 with 5-fluorouracil 1000 mg/m^2 for 7 days caused angina and ischemic electrocardiographic changes, suggesting synergistic cardiotoxicity (269). There have also been cases of arterial occlusive events (270) and myocardial infarction (271,272), in some cases with evidence of coronary vascular spasm (273,274).

In 39 patients given low-dose continuous fluorouracil and cisplatin 20 mg/m^2/week for 8 weeks, there was a very low incidence of renal toxicity, although electrolyte abnormalities, particularly hyponatremia and hypomagnesemia, were as expected (244).

Irinotecan

The concomitant use of irinotecan as a 1-hour infusion immediately following a 2-hour infusion of oxaliplatin resulted in more severe hypersalivation and abdominal pain than irinotecan monotherapy (275). Acute intervention with atropine alleviated these adverse effects. When the drugs were separated by 1 day, the cholinergic symptoms were not exacerbated. The authors postulated that oxaliplatin might have some acetylcholinesterase inhibitory activity.

Lithium

Some data have suggested that cisplatin-containing chemotherapy can alter lithium clearance through impaired renal function, and lithium therapy should be closely monitored during treatment with cisplatin-containing regimens (276).

Mesna

Platinum agents are combined with ifosfamide in the treatment of cancer. The possibility that mesna may interfere with the anticancer effects of platinum agents has been investigated using cultured malignant glioma cells (277). Mesna protected tumor cell lines from the cytotoxic effect of the platinum agents. This in-vitro study emphasizes the importance of specifying in detail the infusion schedules of mesna and platinum agents.

Methotrexate

A patient with no other risk factors developed irreversible nephrotoxicity after four cycles of carboplatin 300 mg/m^2 and methotrexate 50 mg/m^2 (278). This appears to have been an additive effect of drugs that are not individually nephrotoxic until much higher doses.

Nephrotoxic drugs

Based on its considerable nephrotoxic potential, cisplatin should be given after, rather than before, other anticancer drugs and other drugs with a low therapeutic index (for example aminoglycoside antibiotics or bleomycin) that are primarily excreted in the urine in unchanged form. Concomitant use of potentially nephrotoxic agents (for example conventional amphotericin, tacrolimus) with cisplatin should be avoided (279,280).

Neurotoxic drugs

The concomitant or previous use of potentially neurotoxic drugs (for example paclitaxel, vinca alkaloids, or hexamethylmelamine) can increase the risk of peripheral neuropathy due to platinum compounds (68,69).

Paclitaxel

There is some evidence that there is a clinically significant pharmacokinetic interaction of paclitaxel with cisplatin. When cisplatin was given before paclitaxel, the clearance rate of paclitaxel was 25% less than when the two drugs were given in the opposite sequence. In consequence, neutropenia was more profound with the former schedule (281). In addition, in experimental studies, cytotoxicity increased when human ovarian carcinoma cells were exposed to paclitaxel before cisplatin, whereas the interaction was antagonistic when a 1-hour exposure to cisplatin was followed by a 20-hour exposure to taxol, or when the cells were exposed to cisplatin and taxol for 1 hour concurrently (282). The biochemical basis of this interaction has not been elucidated. The pharmacodynamic interaction may be related to cisplatin-induced alterations in cell-specific and non-specific binding sites for paclitaxel (283). In view of these results, paclitaxel should be given before cisplatin (284). There does not appear to be a similar interaction of paclitaxel with carboplatin (285).

Both cisplatin and paclitaxel are neurotoxic, the toxicity being dose-limiting and cumulative; neurotoxicity due to the combination has been suggested to be synergistic; after five cycles of chemotherapy, 96% of 44 patients had grade 1 toxicity and 52% grade 2 toxicity; 18% with grade 2 or 4 toxicity were withdrawn (286).

Vincristine

In 86 patients treated with cisplatin-based chemotherapy for testicular cancer, cumulative exposure (over 400 mg/m^2) and a previous history of noise exposure were significant susceptibility factors for irreversible ototoxicity; high doses of vincristine (greater than 6 mg/m^2) significantly increased the risk of reversible ototoxicity (287).

References

1. Go RS, Adjei AA. Review of the comparative pharmacology and clinical activity of cisplatin and carboplatin. J Clin Oncol 1999;17(1):409–22.

2. Lipp HP, Bokemeyer C. Clinical pharmacokinetics of cytostatic drugs: efficacy and toxicity (2.2. platinum compounds as anticancer drugs). In: Lipp HP, editor. Anticancer drug toxicity; prevention, management and clinical pharmacokinetics. New York-Basel: Marcel Dekker Inc, 1999:61–81.

3. Woloschuk DM, Pruemer JM, Cluxton RJ Jr. Carboplatin: a new cisplatin analogue. Drug Intell Clin Pharm 1988; 22(11):843–9.

4. Calvert AH, Harland SJ, Newell DR, Siddik ZH, Jones AC, McElwain TJ, Raju S, Wiltshaw E, Smith IE, Baker JM, Peckham MJ, Harrap KR. Early clinical studies with cis-diammine-1,1-cyclobutane dicarboxylate platinum II. Cancer Chemother Pharmacol 1982;9(3):140–7.

5. Lokich J, Anderson N. Carboplatin versus cisplatin in solid tumors: an analysis of the literature. Ann Oncol 1998; 9(1):13–21.

6. Vermorken JB, ten Bokkel Huinink WW, Eisenhauer EA, Favalli G, Belpomme D, Conte PF, Kaye SB. Advanced ovarian cancer. Carboplatin versus cisplatin. Ann Oncol 1993;4(Suppl 4):41–8.

7. Markman M. Carboplatin and cisplatin: are they equivalent in efficacy in "optimal residual" advanced ovarian cancer? J Cancer Res Clin Oncol 1996;122(8):443–4.

8. Wiseman LR, Adkins JC, Plosker GL, Goa KL. Oxaliplatin: a review of its use in the management of metastatic colorectal cancer. Drugs Aging 1999;14(6):459–75.

9. Culy CR, Clemett D, Wiseman LR. Oxaliplatin. A review of its pharmacological properties and clinical efficacy in metastatic colorectal cancer and its potential in other malignancies. Drugs 2000;60(4):895–924.

10. van Hennik MB, van der Vijgh WJ, Klein I, Elferink F, Vermorken JB, Winograd B, Pinedo HM. Comparative pharmacokinetics of cisplatin and three analogues in mice and humans. Cancer Res 1987;47(23):6297–301.

11. O'Dwyer PJ, Stevenson JP, Johnson SW. Clinical pharmacokinetics and administration of established platinum drugs. Drugs 2000;59(Suppl 4):19–27.

12. Judson I, Kelland LR. New developments and approaches in the platinum arena. Drugs 2000;59(Suppl 4):29–36.

13. Clark DL, Andrews PA, Smith DD, DeGeorge JJ, Justice RL, Beitz JG. Predictive value of preclinical toxicology studies for platinum anticancer drugs. Clin Cancer Res 1999;5(5):1161–7.

14. Zanotti KM, Markman M. Prevention and management of antineoplastic-induced hypersensitivity reactions. Drug Saf 2001;24(10):767–79.

15. Reed E, Yuspa SH, Zwelling LA, Ozols RF, Poirier MC. Quantitation of cis-diamminedichloroplatinum II (cisplatin)-DNA-intrastrand adducts in testicular and ovarian cancer patients receiving cisplatin chemotherapy J Clin Invest 1986;77(2):545–50.

16. Poirier MC, Reed E, Litterst CL, Katz D, Gupta-Burt S. Persistence of platinum-ammine-DNA adducts in gonads and kidneys of rats and multiple tissues from cancer patients. Cancer Res 1992;52(1):149–53.

17. Poirier MC, Reed E, Zwelling LA, Ozols RF, Litterst CL, Yuspa SH. Polyclonal antibodies to quantitate cis-diamminedichloroplatinum(II)—DNA adducts in cancer patients and animal models. Environ Health Perspect 1985;62:89–94.

18. Knox RJ, Friedlos F, Lydall DA, Roberts JJ. Mechanism of cytotoxicity of anticancer platinum drugs: evidence that cis-diamminedichloroplatinum (II) differ only in the kinetics of their interaction with DNA. Cancer 1986;11:643–5.

19. Gietema JA, Meinardi MT, Messerschmidt J, Gelevert T, Alt F, Uges DR, Sleijfer DT. Circulating plasma platinum more than 10 years after cisplatin treatment for testicular cancer. Lancet 2000;355(9209):1075–6.

20. Schierl R, Rohrer B, Hohnloser J. Long-term platinum excretion in patients treated with cisplatin. Cancer Chemother Pharmacol 1995;36(1):75–8.

21. Jodrell DI, Egorin MJ, Canetta RM, Langenberg P, Goldbloom EP, Burroughs JN, Goodlow JL, Tan S, Wiltshaw E. Relationships between carboplatin exposure and tumor response and toxicity in patients with ovarian cancer. J Clin Oncol 1992;10(4):520–8.

22. Bokemeyer C, Lipp HP. Is there a need for pharmacokinetically guided carboplatin dose schedules? Onkologie 1997;20:343–5.

23. Bergh J. Is pharmacokinetically guided chemotherapy dosage a better way forward? Ann Oncol 2002;13(3):343–4.

24. Jodrell DI. Formula-based dosing for carboplatin. Eur J Cancer 1999;35(9):1299–301.

25. Millward MJ, Webster LK, Toner GC, Bishop JF, Rischin D, Stokes KH, Johnston VK, Hicks R. Carboplatin dosing based on measurement of renal function—experience at the Peter MacCallum Cancer Institute. Aust NZ J Med 1996;26(3):372–9.

26. Calvert AH, Newell DR, Gumbrell LA, O'Reilly S, Burnell M, Boxall FE, Siddik ZH, Judson IR, Gore ME, Wiltshaw E. Carboplatin dosage: prospective evaluation of a simple formula based on renal function. J Clin Oncol 1989;7(11):1748–56.

27. Dooley MJ, Poole SG, Rischin D, Webster LK. Carboplatin dosing: gender bias and inaccurate estimates of glomerular filtration rate. Eur J Cancer 2002;38(1):44–51.

28. Wright JG, Boddy AV, Highley M, Fenwick J, McGill A, Calvert AH. Estimation of glomerular filtration rate in cancer patients. Br J Cancer 2001;84(4):452–9.

29. Wright JG, Calvert AH, Highley MS, Roberts JT, MacGill A, Fenwick J, Boddy AV. Accurate prediction

of renal function for carboplatin. Proc Am Assoc Cancer Res 1999;40:Abstract 2542.

30. Massari C, Brienza S, Rotarski M, Gastiaburu J, Misset JL, Cupissol D, Alafaci E, Dutertre-Catella H, Bastian G. Pharmacokinetics of oxaliplatin in patients with normal versus impaired renal function. Cancer Chemother Pharmacol 2000;45(2):157–64.

31. Yarema KJ. Comparative toxicities and mutagenics of platinum anticancer drugs. Drug Inf J 1995;29:s1633–44.

32. Vaughn DJ, Gignac GA, Meadows AT. Long-term medical care of testicular cancer survivors. Ann Intern Med 2002;136(6):463–70.

33. Piccart MJ, Lamb H, Vermorken JB. Current and future potential roles of the platinum drugs in the treatment of ovarian cancer. Ann Oncol 2001;12(9):1195–203.

34. Kim NK, Im SA, Kim DW, Lee MH, Jung CW, Cho EK, Lee JT, Ahn JS, Heo DS, Bang YJ. Phase II clinical trial of SKI-2053R, a new platinum analogue, in the treatment of patients with advanced gastric adenocarcinoma. Cancer 1999;86(7):1109–15.

35. Ahn JH, Kang YK, Kim TW, Bahng H, Chang HM, Kang WC, Kim WK, Lee JS, Park JS. Nephrotoxicity of heptaplatin: a randomized comparison with cisplatin in advanced gastric cancer. Cancer Chemother Pharmacol 2002;50(2):104–10.

36. Christian MC. The current status of new platinum analogues. Semin Oncol 1992;19(6):720–33.

37. Ishibashi T, Yano Y, Oguma T. A formula for predicting optimal dosage of nedaplatin based on renal function in adult cancer patients. Cancer Chemother Pharmacol 2002;50(3):230–6.

38. Fokkema E, Groen HJ, Bauer J, Uges DR, Weil C, Smith IE. Phase II study of oral platinum drug JM216 as first-line treatment in patients with small-cell lung cancer. J Clin Oncol 1999;17(12):3822–7.

39. Trudeau M, Stuart G, Hirte H, Drouin P, Plante M, Bessette P, Dulude H, Lebwohl D, Fisher B, Seymour L. A phase II trial of JM-216 in cervical cancer: an NCIC CTG study. Gynecol Oncol 2002;84(2):327–31.

40. Fokkema E, de Vries EG, Meijer S, Groen HJ. Lack of nephrotoxicity of new oral platinum drug JM216 in lung cancer patients. Cancer Chemother Pharmacol 2000; 45(1):89–92.

41. Carr JL, Tingle MD, McKeage MJ. Rapid biotransformation of satraplatin by human red blood cells in vitro. Cancer Chemother Pharmacol 2002;50(1):9–15.

42. Meerum Terwogt JM, Groenewegen G, Pluim D, Maliepaard M, Tibben MM, Huisman A, ten Bokkel Huinink WW, Schot M, Welbank H, Voest EE, Beijnen JH, Schellens JM. Phase I and pharmacokinetic study of SPI-77, a liposomal encapsulated dosage form of cisplatin. Cancer Chemother Pharmacol 2002; 49(3):201–10.

43. Vail DM, Kurzman ID, Glawe PC, O'Brien MG, Chun R, Garrett LD, Obradovich JE, Fred RM 3rd, Khanna C, Colbern GT, Working PK. STEALTH liposome-encapsulated cisplatin (SPI-77) versus carboplatin as adjuvant therapy for spontaneously arising osteosarcoma (OSA) in the dog: a randomized multicenter clinical trial. Cancer Chemother Pharmacol 2002;50(2):131–6.

44. Schiller JH. Small cell lung cancer: defining a role for emerging platinum drugs. Oncology 2002;63(2):105–14.

45. Luo FR, Wyrick SD, Chaney SG. Comparative neurotoxicity of oxaliplatin, ormaplatin, and their biotransformation products utilizing a rat dorsal root ganglia in vitro explant culture model. Cancer Chemother Pharmacol 1999; 44(1):29–38.

46. Tassinari D, Sartori S, Drudi G, Panzini I, Gianni L, Pasquini E, Abbasciano V, Ravaioli A, Iorio D. Cardiac arrhythmias after cisplatin infusion: three case reports and a review of the literature. Ann Oncol 1997;8(12):1263–7.

47. Altundag O, Celik I, Kars A. Recurrent asymptomatic bradycardia episodes after cisplatin infusion. Ann Pharmacother 2001;35(5):641–2.

48. Fassio T, Canobbio L, Gasparini G, Villani F. Paroxysmal supraventricular tachycardia during treatment with cisplatin and etoposide combination. Oncology 1986;43(4):219–20.

49. Albain KS, Rusch VW, Crowley JJ, Rice TW, Turrisi AT 3rd, Weick JK, Lonchyna VA, Presant CA, McKenna RJ, Gandara DR, et al. Concurrent cisplatin/etoposide plus chest radiotherapy followed by surgery for stages IIIA (N2) and IIIB non-small-cell lung cancer: mature results of Southwest Oncology Group phase II study 8805. J Clin Oncol 1995;13(8):1880–92.

50. Samuels BL, Vogelzang NJ, Kennedy BJ. Vascular toxicity following vinblastine, bleomycin, and cisplatin therapy for germ cell tumours. Int J Androl 1987;10(1):363–9.

51. Samuels BL, Vogelzang NJ, Kennedy BJ. Severe vascular toxicity associated with vinblastine, bleomycin, and cisplatin chemotherapy. Cancer Chemother Pharmacol 1987;19(3):253–6.

52. Heier MS, Nilsen T, Graver V, Aass N, Fossa SD. Raynaud's phenomenon after combination chemotherapy of testicular cancer, measured by laser Doppler flowmetry. A pilot study. Br J Cancer 1991;63(4):550–2.

53. Dorr RT. Managing extravasations of vesicant chemotherapy drugs. In: Lipp HP, editor. Anticancer Drug Toxicity; Prevention, Management and Clinical Pharmacokinetics. New York-Basel: Marcel Dekker Inc, 1999:279–318.

54. Rabinowits M, Souhami L, Gil RA, Andrade CA, Paiva HC. Increased pulmonary toxicity with bleomycin and cisplatin chemotherapy combinations. Am J Clin Oncol 1990;13(2):132–8.

55. Taha H, Irfan S, Krishnamurthy M. Cisplatin induced reversible bilateral vocal cord paralysis: an undescribed complication of cisplatin. Head Neck 1999;21(1):78–9.

56. Windebank AJ. Chemotherapeutic neuropathy. Curr Opin Neurol 1999;12(5):565–71.

57. Screnci D, McKeage MJ. Platinum neurotoxicity: clinical profiles, experimental models and neuroprotective approaches. J Inorg Biochem 1999;77(1–2):105–10.

58. Alberts DS, Noel JK. Cisplatin-associated neurotoxicity: can it be prevented? Anticancer Drugs 1995;6(3):369–83.

59. Wilson RH, Lehky T, Thomas RR, Quinn MG, Floeter MK, Grem JL. Acute oxaliplatin-induced peripheral nerve hyperexcitability. J Clin Oncol 2002;20(7):1767–74.

60. Levi F, Zidani R, Brienza S, Dogliotti L, Perpoint B, Rotarski M, Letourneau Y, Llory JF, Chollet P, Le Rol A, Focan C. A multicenter evaluation of intensified, ambulatory, chronomodulated chemotherapy with oxaliplatin, 5-fluorouracil, and leucovorin as initial treatment of patients with metastatic colorectal carcinoma. International Organization for Cancer Chronotherapy. Cancer 1999;85(12):2532–40.

61. Heinzlef O, Lotz JP, Roullet E. Severe neuropathy after high dose carboplatin in three patients receiving multidrug chemotherapy. J Neurol Neurosurg Psychiatry 1998; 64(5):667–9.

62. van der Hoop RG, van der Burg ME, ten Bokkel Huinink WW, van Houwelingen C, Neijt JP. Incidence of neuropathy in 395 patients with ovarian cancer treated with or without cisplatin. Cancer 1990;66(8):1697–702.

63. Siegal T, Haim N. Cisplatin-induced peripheral neuropathy. Frequent off-therapy deterioration, demyelinating syndromes, and muscle cramps. Cancer 1990;66(6):1117–23.

64. Gessini L, Jandolo B, Pollera C, et al. Neuropatia da cisplatino: un nuovo tipo di polineuropatia assonale ascendente progressiva. Riv Neurobiol 1987;33:75.

65. Holleran WM, DeGregorio MW. Evolution of high-dose cisplatin. Invest New Drugs 1988;6(2):135–42.

66. Riggs JE, Ashraf M, Snyder RD, Gutmann L. Prospective nerve conduction studies in cisplatin therapy. Ann Neurol 1988;23(1):92–4.

67. Mollman JE. Cisplatin neurotoxicity. N Engl J Med 1990;322(2):126–7.

68. Cersosimo RJ. Cisplatin neurotoxicity. Cancer Treat Rev 1989;16(4):195–211.

69. Tuxen MK, Hansen SW. Neurotoxicity secondary to antineoplastic drugs. Cancer Treat Rev 1994;20(2):191–214.

70. Higa GM, Wise TC, Crowell EB. Severe, disabling neurologic toxicity following cisplatin retreatment. Ann Pharmacother 1995;29(2):134–7.

71. Dewar J, Lunt H, Abernethy DA, Dady P, Haas LF. Cisplatin neuropathy with Lhermitte's sign. J Neurol Neurosurg Psychiatry 1986;49(1):96–9.

72. Mariette X, Paule B, Bennet P, Clerc D, Bisson M, Massias P. Cisplatin and hyponatremia. Ann Intern Med 1988;108(5):770–1.

73. Mune T, Yasuda K, Ishii M, Matsunaga T, Miura K. Tetany due to hypomagnesemia induced by cisplatin and doxorubicin treatment for synovial sarcoma. Intern Med 1993;32(5):434–7.

74. Gonzalez C, Villasanta U. Life-threatening hypocalcemia and hypomagnesemia associated with cisplatin chemotherapy. Obstet Gynecol 1982;59(6):732–4.

75. Ritch PS. Cis-dichlorodiammineplatinum II-induced syndrome of inappropriate secretion of antidiuretic hormone. Cancer 1988;61(3):448–50.

76. Cassidy J, Misset JL. Oxaliplatin-related side effects: characteristics and management. Semin Oncol 2002;29(5 Suppl 15):11–20.

77. Gamelin E, Gamelin L, Bossi L, Quasthoff S. Clinical aspects and molecular basis of oxaliplatin neurotoxicity: current management and development of preventive measures. Semin Oncol 2002;29(5 Suppl 15):21–33.

78. Cersosimo RJ. Oxaliplatin-associated neuropathy: a review. Ann Pharmacother 2005;39(1):128–35.

79. Wang MY, Arnold AC, Vinters HV, Glasgow BJ. Bilateral blindness and lumbosacral myelopathy associated with high-dose carmustine and cisplatin therapy. Am J Ophthalmol 2000;130(3):367–8.

80. Taieb S, Trillet-Lenoir V, Rambaud L, Descos L, Freyer G. L'hermite sign and urinary retention: atypical presentation of oxaliplatin neurotoxicity in four patients. Cancer 2002;94(9):2434–40.

81. List AF, Kummet TD. Spinal cord toxicity complicating treatment with cisplatin and etoposide. Am J Clin Oncol 1990;13(3):256–8.

82. Taieb S, Trillet-Lenoir V, Rambaud L, Descos L, Freyer G. L'hermite sign and urinary retention: atypical presentation of oxaliplatin neurotoxicity in four patients. Cancer 2002;94(9):2434–40.

83. Nichols CR, Roth BJ, Williams SD, Gill I, Muggia FM, Stablein DM, Weiss RB, Einhorn LH. No evidence of acute cardiovascular complications of chemotherapy for testicular cancer: an analysis of the Testicular Cancer Intergroup Study. J Clin Oncol 1992;10(5):760–5.

84. Highley M, Meller ST, Pinkerton CR. Seizures and cortical dysfunction following high-dose cisplatin administration in children. Med Pediatr Oncol 1992;20(2):143–8.

85. Sghirlanzoni A, Silvani A, Scaioli V, Pareyson D, Marchesan R, Boiardi A. Cisplatin neuropathy in brain tumor chemotherapy. Ital J Neurol Sci 1992;13(4):311–15.

86. LoMonaco M, Milone M, Batocchi AP, Padua L, Restuccia D, Tonali P. Cisplatin neuropathy: clinical course and neurophysiological findings. J Neurol 1992; 239(4):199–204.

87. Cavaletti G, Bogliun G, Marzorati L, Marzola M, Pittelli MR, Tredici G. The incidence and course of paraneoplastic neuropathy in women with epithelial ovarian cancer. J Neurol 1991;238(7):371–4.

88. Cano JR, Catalan B, Jara C. Neuronopatia por cisplatino. [Neuronopathy due to cisplatin.] Rev Neurol 1998; 27(158):606–10.

89. Al-Tweigeri T, Magliocco AM, DeCoteau JF. Cortical blindness as a manifestation of hypomagnesemia secondary to cisplatin therapy: case report and review of literature. Gynecol Oncol 1999;72(1):120–2.

90. Lyass O, Lossos A, Hubert A, Gips M, Peretz T. Cisplatin-induced non-convulsive encephalopathy. Anticancer Drugs 1998;9(1):100–4.

91. Gamble GE, Tyrrell P. Acute stroke following cisplatin therapy. Clin Oncol (R Coll Radiol) 1998;10(4):274–5.

92. Doehn C, Buttner H, Fornara P, Jocham D. Fatal basilar artery thrombosis after chemotherapy for testicular cancer. Urol Int 2000;65(1):43–5.

93. Kahn CE Jr, Messersmith RN, Samuels BL. Brachial plexopathy as a complication of intraarterial cisplatin chemotherapy. Cardiovasc Intervent Radiol 1989;12(1):47–9.

94. Walker RW, Cairncross JG, Posner JB. Cerebral herniation in patients receiving cisplatin. J Neurooncol 1988;6(1):61–5.

95. De Lauretis A, De Capua B, Barbieri MT, Bellussi L, Passali D. ABR evaluation of ototoxicity in cancer patients receiving cisplatin or carboplatin. Scand Audiol 1999;28(3):139–43.

96. Grolleau F, Gamelin L, Boisdron-Celle M, Lapied B, Pelhate M, Gamelin E. A possible explanation for a neurotoxic effect of the anticancer agent oxaliplatin on neuronal voltage-gated sodium channels. J Neurophysiol 2001; 85(5):2293–7.

97. Adelsberger H, Quasthoff S, Grosskreutz J, Lepier A, Eckel F, Lersch C. The chemotherapeutic oxaliplatin alters voltage-gated Na(+) channel kinetics on rat sensory neurons. Eur J Pharmacol 2000;406(1):25–32.

98. Gornet JM, Savier E, Lokiec F, Cvitkovic E, Misset JL, Goldwasser F. Exacerbation of oxaliplatin neurosensory toxicity following surgery. Ann Oncol 2002;13(8):1315–18.

99. Oshita F, Saijo N, Shinkai T, Eguchi K, Sasaki Y, et al. Correlation between total dose of cisplatin and vibratory perception threshold in chemotherapy-induced peripheral neuropathy of cancer patients. Cancer J 1992;5:165–9.

100. Cavaletti G, Marzorati L, Bogliun G, Colombo N, Marzola M, Pittelli MR, Tredici G. Cisplatin-induced peripheral neurotoxicity is dependent on total-dose intensity and single-dose intensity. Cancer 1992;69(1):203–7.

101. Pratt CB, Goren MP, Meyer WH, Singh B, Dodge RK. Ifosfamide neurotoxicity is related to previous cisplatin treatment for pediatric solid tumors. J Clin Oncol 1990;8(8):1399–401.

102. Marzorati L, Bogluin G, Cavaletti G, Tredici G, Pittelli MR. Neurotoxicity of two different cisplatin treatments. Rev Neurobiol 1990;26:459–64.

103. Pollera CF, Pietrangeli A, Giannarelli D. Cisplatin-induced peripheral neurotoxicity: relationship to dose intensity. Ann Oncol 1991;2(3):212.

104. Kaye SB, Paul J, Cassidy J, Lewis CR, Duncan ID, Gordon HK, Kitchener HC, Cruickshank DJ, Atkinson RJ, Soukop M, Rankin EM, Davis JA, Reed NS, Crawford SM, MacLean A, Parkin D, Sarkar TK, Kennedy J, Symonds RP. Mature results of a randomized trial of two doses of cisplatin for the treatment of ovarian cancer. Scottish Gynecology Cancer Trials Group. J Clin Oncol 1996;14(7):2113–19.

105. Philip T, Ghalie R, Pinkerton R, Zucker JM, Bernard JL, Leverger G, Hartmann O. A phase II study of high-dose

cisplatin and VP-16 in neuroblastoma: a report from the Société Française d'Oncologie Pédiatrique. J Clin Oncol 1987;5(6):941–50.

106. Daugaard GK, Petrera J, Trojaborg W. Electrophysiological study of the peripheral and central neurotoxic effect of cisplatin. Acta Neurol Scand 1987;76(2):86–93.

107. Amiel H, Gherardi R, Giroux C, et al. Neuropathie au cisplatine. Ann Med Interne 1987;138:101.

108. Castellanos AM, Glass JP, Yung WK. Regional nerve injury after intra-arterial chemotherapy. Neurology 1987; 37(5):834–7.

109. von Schlippe M, Fowler CJ, Harland SJ. Cisplatin neurotoxicity in the treatment of metastatic germ cell tumour: time course and prognosis. Br J Cancer 2001;85(6):823–6.

110. Quasthoff S, Hartung HP. Chemotherapy-induced peripheral neuropathy. J Neurol 2002;249(1):9–17.

111. van den Bent MJ, van Putten WL, Hilkens PH, de Wit R, van der Burg ME. Retreatment with dose-dense weekly cisplatin after previous cisplatin chemotherapy is not complicated by significant neuro-toxicity. Eur J Cancer 2002;38(3):387–91.

112. Gill JS, Windebank AJ. Cisplatin-induced apoptosis in rat dorsal root ganglion neurons is associated with attempted entry into the cell cycle. J Clin Invest 1998;101(12):2842–50.

113. Cavaletti G, Zanna C. Current status and future prospects for the treatment of chemotherapy-induced peripheral neurotoxicity. Eur J Cancer 2002;38(14):1832–7.

114. Penz M, Kornek GV, Raderer M, Ulrich-Pur H, Fiebiger W, Scheithauer W. Subcutaneous administration of amifostine: a promising therapeutic option in patients with oxaliplatin-related peripheral sensitive neuropathy. Ann Oncol 2001;12(3):421–2.

115. Gamelin E, Gamelin L, Delva R, Guerin-Meyer V, Morel A, Boisdron-Celle M. Prevention of oxaliplatin peripheral sensory neuropathy by Ca+ gluconate/Mg+ chloride infusions: a retrospective study. Proc Am Soc Clin Oncol 2002;21:A624.

116. McLean MJ, Macdonald RL. Carbamazepine and 10,11-epoxycarbamazepine produce use- and voltage-dependent limitation of rapidly firing action potentials of mouse central neurons in cell culture. J Pharmacol Exp Ther 1986;238(2):727–38.

117. Eckel F, Schmelz R, Adelsberger H, Erdmann J, Quasthoff S, Lersch C. Prophylaxe der Oxaliplatin-induzierten Neuropathie mit Carbamazepin. Eine Pilotstudie. [Prevention of oxaliplatin-induced neuropathy by carbamazepine. A pilot study.] Dtsch Med Wochenschr 2002;127(3):78–82.

118. Levi FA, Zidani R, Vannetzel JM, Perpoint B, Focan C, Faggiuolo R, Chollet P, Garufi C, Itzhaki M, Dogliotti L, et al. Chronomodulated versus fixed-infusion-rate delivery of ambulatory chemotherapy with oxaliplatin, fluorouracil, and folinic acid (leucovorin) in patients with colorectal cancer metastases: a randomized multi-institutional trial. J Natl Cancer Inst 1994;86(21):1608–17.

119. Levi F, Metzger G, Massari C, Milano G. Oxaliplatin: pharmacokinetics and chronopharmacological aspects. Clin Pharmacokinet 2000;38(1):1–21.

120. Levi F, Zidani R, Misset JL. Randomised multicentre trial of chronotherapy with oxaliplatin, fluorouracil, and folinic acid in metastatic colorectal cancer. International Organization for Cancer Chronotherapy. Lancet 1997;350(9079):681–6.

121. Cascinu S, Catalano V, Cordella L, Labianca R, Giordani P, Baldelli AM, Beretta GD, Ubiali E, Catalano G. Neuroprotective effect of reduced glutathione on oxaliplatin-based chemotherapy in advanced colorectal cancer: a randomized, double-blind, placebo-controlled trial. J Clin Oncol 2002;20(16):3478–83.

122. McKeage MJ. Comparative adverse effect profiles of platinum drugs. Drug Saf 1995;13(4):228–44.

123. Bachmeyer C, Decroix Y, Medioni J, Dhote R, Benfiguig K, Houillier P, Grateau G. Coma, crise convulsive et troubles de l'oculomotricité hypomagnésémiques et hypocalcémiques après chimiothérapie par sels de platine. [Hypomagnesemic and hypocalcemic coma, convulsions and ocular motility disorders after chemotherapy with platinum compounds.] Rev Med Interne 1996;17(6):467–9.

124. Blakley BW, Myers SF. Patterns of hearing loss resulting from cis-platinum therapy. Otolaryngol Head Neck Surg 1993;109(3 Pt 1):385–91.

125. Laurell G, Engstrom B, Hirsch A, Bagger-Sjoback D. Ototoxicity of cisplatin. Int J Androl 1987;10(1):359–62.

126. Cohen BH, Zweidler P, Goldwein JW, Molloy J, Packer RJ. Ototoxic effect of cisplatin in children with brain tumors. Pediatr Neurosurg 1990–91;16(6):292–6.

127. Pasic TR, Dobie RA. Cis-platinum ototoxicity in children. Laryngoscope 1991;101(9):985–91.

128. Gupta AA, Capra M, Papaioannou V, Hall G, Maze R, Dix D, Weitzman S. Low incidence of ototoxicity with continuous infusion of cisplatin in the treatment of pediatric germ cell tumors. J Pediatr Hematol Oncol 2006;28(2):91–4.

129. Waters GS, Ahmad M, Katsarkas A, Stanimir G, McKay J. Ototoxicity due to cis-diamminedichloroplatinum in the treatment of ovarian cancer: influence of dosage and schedule of administration. Ear Hear 1991;12(2):91–102.

130. Durrant JD, Rodgers G, Myers EN, Johnson JT. Hearing loss—risk factor for cisplatin ototoxicity? Observations. Am J Otol 1990;11(5):375–7.

131. Vantrappen G, Rector E, Debruyne F. Cisplatinum ototoxiciteit: Klinische studie. [The ototoxicity of cisplatin: a clinical study.] Acta Otorhinolaryngol Belg 1990;44(4):415–21.

132. Skinner R, Pearson AD, Amineddine HA, Mathias DB, Craft AW. Ototoxicity of cisplatinum in children and adolescents. Br J Cancer 1990;61(6):927–31.

133. Kopelman J, Budnick AS, Sessions RB, Kramer MB, Wong GY. Ototoxicity of high-dose cisplatin by bolus administration in patients with advanced cancers and normal hearing. Laryngoscope 1988;98(8 Pt 1):858–64.

134. Laurell G, Borg E. Ototoxicity of cisplatin in gynaecological cancer patients. Scand Audiol 1988;17(4):241–7.

135. Domenech J, Santabarbara P, Carulla M, Traserra J. Sudden hearing loss in an adolescent following a single dose of cisplatin. ORL J Otorhinolaryngol Relat Spec 1988;50(6):405–8.

136. Aguilar-Markulis NV, Beckley S, Priore R, Mettlin C. Auditory toxicity effects of long-term cis-dichlorodiammineplatinum II therapy in genitourinary cancer patients. J Surg Oncol 1981;16(2):111–23.

137. Berg AL, Spitzer JB, Garvin JH Jr. Ototoxic impact of cisplatin in pediatric oncology patients. Laryngoscope 1999;109(11):1806–14.

138. Melamed LB, Selim MA, Schuchman D. Cisplatin ototoxicity in gynecologic cancer patients. A preliminary report. Cancer 1985;55(1):41–3.

139. Hallmark RJ, Snyder JM, Jusenius K, Tamimi HK. Factors influencing ototoxicity in ovarian cancer patients treated with cis-platinum based chemotherapy. Eur J Gynaecol Oncol 1992;13(1):35–44.

140. Chapman P. Rapid onset hearing loss after cisplatinum therapy: case reports and literature review. J Laryngol Otol 1982;96(2):159–62.

141. Cvitkovic E. Cumulative toxicities from cisplatin therapy and current cytoprotective measures. Cancer Treat Rev 1998;24(4):265–81.

142. Laurell G, Beskow C, Frankendal B, Borg E. Cisplatin administration to gynecologic cancer patients. Long-term effects on hearing. Cancer 1996;78(8):1798–804.

143. Weatherly RA, Owens JJ, Catlin FI, Mahoney DH. Cis-platinum ototoxicity in children. Laryngoscope 1991;101(9):917–24.

144. Moroso MJ, Blair RL. A review of cis-platinum ototoxicity. J Otolaryngol 1983;12(6):365–9.

145. Peters U, Preisler-Adams S, Hebeisen A, Hahn M, Seifert E, Lanvers C, Heinecke A, Horst J, Jurgens H, Lamprecht-Dinnesen A. Glutathione S-transferase genetic polymorphisms and individual sensitivity to the ototoxic effect of cisplatin. Anticancer Drugs 2000;11(8):639–43.

146. Kelsen DP, Alcock N, Young CW. Cisplatin nephrotoxicity. Correlation with plasma platinum concentrations. Am J Clin Oncol 1985;8(1):77–80.

147. Foster-Nora JA, Siden R. Amifostine for protection from antineoplastic drug toxicity. Am J Health Syst Pharm 1997;54(7):787–800.

148. Caston J, Doinel L. Comparative vestibular toxicity of dibekacin, habekacin and cisplatin. Acta Otolaryngol 1987;104(3–4):315–21.

149. Kobayashi H, Ohashi N, Watanabe Y, Mizukoshi K. Clinical features of cisplatin vestibulotoxicity and hearing loss. ORL J Otorhinolaryngol Relat Spec 1987;49(2):67–72.

150. Anniko M, Sobin A. Cisplatin: evaluation of its ototoxic potential. Am J Otolaryngol 1986;7(4):276–93.

151. Ozturan O, Jerger J, Lew H, Lynch GR. Monitoring of cisplatin ototoxicity by distortion-product otoacoustic emissions. Auris Nasus Larynx 1996;23:147–51.

152. Kennedy IC, Fitzharris BM, Colls BM, Atkinson CH. Carboplatin is ototoxic. Cancer Chemother Pharmacol 1990;26(3):232–4.

153. Stavroulaki P, Apostolopoulos N, Segas J, Tsakanikos M, Adamopoulos G. Evoked otoacoustic emissions—an approach for monitoring cisplatin induced ototoxicity in children. Int J Pediatr Otorhinolaryngol 2001;59(1):47–57.

154. de Lemos ML. Application of the area under the curve of carboplatin in predicting toxicity and efficacy. Cancer Treat Rev 1998;24(6):407–14.

155. Bauer FP, Westhofen M, Kehrl W. Zur Ototoxizität des Zytostatikums Carboplatin loei Patienten mit Kopf-Hals-Tumoren. [The ototoxicity of the cytostatic drug carboplatin in patients with head-neck tumors.] Laryngorhinootologie 1992;71(8):412–15.

156. Cavaletti G, Bogliun G, Zincone A, Marzorati L, Melzi P, Frattola L, Marzola M, Bonazzi C, Cantu MG, Chiari S, Galli A, Bregni M, Gianni MA. Neuro- and ototoxicity of high-dose carboplatin treatment in poor prognosis ovarian cancer patients. Anticancer Res 1998;18(5B):3797–802.

157. Cavaletti G, Tredici G, Petruccioli MG, Donde E, Tredici P, Marmiroli P, Minoia C, Ronchi A, Bayssas M, Etienne GG. Effects of different schedules of oxaliplatin treatment on the peripheral nervous system of the rat. Eur J Cancer 2001;37(18):2457–63.

158. Soni N, Bajaj B. Toxic effects of cisplatin on olfaction. Pak J Otolaryngol 1991;7:23–5.

159. Bosl GJ, Bajorunas D. Pituitary and testicular hormonal function after treatment for germ cell tumours. Int J Androl 1987;10(1):381–4.

160. Gerl A, Muhlbayer D, Hansmann G, Mraz W, Hiddemann W. The impact of chemotherapy on Leydig cell function in long term survivors of germ cell tumors. Cancer 2001;91(7):1297–303.

161. Sakakura C, Hagiwara A, Kin S, Yamamoto K, Okamoto K, Yamaguchi T, Sawai K, Yamagishi H. A case of hyperosmolar nonketotic coma occurring during chemotherapy using cisplatin for gallbladder cancer. Hepatogastroenterology 1999;46(29):2801–3.

162. Orbo A, Simonsen E. Cisplatin-induced sodium and magnesium wastage. Eur J Cancer 1992;28A(6–7):1294.

163. Bianchetti MG, Kanaka C, Ridolfi-Luthy A, Hirt A, Wagner HP, Oetliker OH. Persisting renotubular sequelae after cisplatin in children and adolescents. Am J Nephrol 1991;11(2):127–30.

164. Blachley JD, Hill JB. Renal and electrolyte disturbances associated with cisplatin. Ann Intern Med 1981;95(5): 628–32.

165. Hutchison FN, Perez EA, Gandara DR, Lawrence HJ, Kaysen GA. Renal salt wasting in patients treated with cisplatin. Ann Intern Med 1988;108(1):21–5.

166. English MW, Skinner R, Pearson AD, Price L, Wyllie R, Craft AW. Dose-related nephrotoxicity of carboplatin in children. Br J Cancer 1999;81(2):336–41.

167. Mulder PO, Sleijfer DT, de Vries EG, Uges DR, Mulder NH. Renal dysfunction following high-dose carboplatin treatment. J Cancer Res Clin Oncol 1988; 114(2):212–14.

168. Lajer H, Daugaard G. Cisplatin and hypomagnesemia. Cancer Treat Rev 1999;25(1):47–58.

169. Schilsky RL, Barlock A, Ozols RF. Persistent hypomagnesemia following cisplatin chemotherapy for testicular cancer. Cancer Treat Rep 1982;66(9):1767–9.

170. Macaulay VM, Begent RH, Phillips ME, Newlands ES. Prophylaxis against hypomagnesaemia induced by cis-platinum combination chemotherapy. Cancer Chemother Pharmacol 1982;9(3):179–81.

171. Vogelzang NJ, Torkelson JL, Kennedy BJ. Hypomagnesemia, renal dysfunction, and Raynaud's phenomenon in patients treated with cisplatin, vinblastine, and bleomycin. Cancer 1985;56(12):2765–70.

172. Bellin SL, Selim M. Cisplatin-induced hypomagnesemia with seizures: a case report and review of the literature. Gynecol Oncol 1988;30(1):104–13.

173. Mavichak V, Coppin CM, Wong NL, Dirks JH, Walker V, Sutton RA. Renal magnesium wasting and hypocalciuria in chronic cis-platinum nephropathy in man. Clin Sci (Lond) 1988;75(2):203–7.

174. Lam M, Adelstein DJ. Hypomagnesemia and renal magnesium wasting in patients treated with cisplatin. Am J Kidney Dis 1986;8(3):164–9.

175. Willox JC, McAllister EJ, Sangster G, Kaye SB. Effects of magnesium supplementation in testicular cancer patients receiving cis-platin: a randomised trial. Br J Cancer 1986;54(1):19–23.

176. Markman M, Cleary S, Howell SB. Hypomagnesemia following high-dose intracavitary cisplatin with systemically administered sodium thiosulfate. Am J Clin Oncol 1986;9(5):440–3.

177. Kibirige MS, Morris-Jones PH, Addison GM. Prevention of cisplatin-induced hypomagnesemia. Pediatr Hematol Oncol 1988;5(1):1–6.

178. Bauer FP, Westhofen M. Vestibulotoxische Effekte des zytostatikums Carboplatin bei Patienten mit Kopf-Hals-Tumoren. [Vestibulotoxic effects of the cytostatic drug carboplatin in patients with head and neck tumors.] HNO 1992;40(1):19–24.

179. Sweeney JD, Ziegler P, Pruet C, Spaulding MB. Hyperzincuria and hypozincemia in patients treated with cisplatin. Cancer 1989;63(11):2093–5.

180. Kuzur ME, Greco FA. Cisplatin-induced anemia. N Engl J Med 1980;303(2):110–11.

181. Kunikane H, Watanabe K, Fukuoka M, Saijo N, Furuse K, Ikegami H, Ariyoshi Y, Kishimoto S. Double-blind randomized control trial of the effect of recombinant human erythropoietin on chemotherapy-induced anemia in patients with non-small cell lung cancer. Int J Clin Oncol 2001;6(6):296–301.

182. Pivot X, Guardiola E, Etienne M, Thyss A, Foa C, Otto J, Schneider M, Magne N, Bensadoun RJ, Renee N, Milano G. An analysis of potential factors allowing an individual prediction of cisplatin-induced anaemia. Eur J Cancer 2000;36(7):852–7.

183. Hasegawa I, Tanaka K. Serum erythropoietin levels in gynecologic cancer patients during cisplatin combination chemotherapy. Gynecol Oncol 1992;46(1):65–8.

184. Ruiz MA, Marugan I, Estelles A, Navarro I, Espana F, Alberola V, San Juan L, Aznar J, Garcia-Conde J. The influence of chemotherapy on plasma coagulation and fibrinolytic systems in lung cancer patients. Cancer 1989;63(4):643–8.

185. Louvet C, Lorange A, Letendre F, Beaulieu R, Pretty HM, Courchesne Y, Neemeh JA, Monte M, Latreille J. Acute and delayed emesis after cisplatin-based regimen: description and prevention. Oncology 1991;48(5):392–6.

186. Kobayashi M, To H, Tokue A, Fujimura A, Kobayashi E. Cisplatin-induced vomiting depends on circadian timing. Chronobiol Int 2001;18(5):851–63.

187. Campos D, Pereira JR, Reinhardt RR, Carracedo C, Poli S, Vogel C, Martinez-Cedillo J, Erazo A, Wittreich J, Eriksson LO, Carides AD, Gertz BJ. Prevention of cisplatin-induced emesis by the oral neurokinin-1 antagonist, MK-869, in combination with granisetron and dexamethasone or with dexamethasone alone. J Clin Oncol 2001;19(6):1759–67.

188. Sartori S, Nielsen I, Maestri A, Beltrami D, Trevisani L, Pazzi P. Acute gastroduodenal mucosal injury after cisplatin plus etoposide chemotherapy. Clinical and endoscopic study. Oncology 1991;48(5):356–61.

189. Cavalli F, Tschopp L, Sonntag RW, Zimmermann A. A case of liver toxicity following cis-dichlorodiammineplatinum(II) treatment. Cancer Treat Rep 1978;62(12):2125–6.

190. Bergevin P. Nephrotoxicity of cisplatin (cis-diamminedichloroplatinum (II)). Drug Today 1988;24:403.

191. Daugaard G, Abildgaard U, Holstein-Rathlou NH, Bruunshuus I, Bucher D, Leyssac PP. Renal tubular function in patients treated with high-dose cisplatin. Clin Pharmacol Ther 1988;44(2):164–72.

192. Falkenberg FW, Mondorf U, Pierard D, Gauhl C, Mondorf AW, Mai U, Kantwerk G, Meier U, Rindhage A, Rohracker M. Identification of fragments of proximal and distal tubular cells in the urine of patients under cytostatic treatment by immunoelectron microscopy with monoclonal antibodies. Am J Kidney Dis 1987;9(2):129–37.

193. Safirstein R, Wiston J. Cisplatin nephrotoxicity. J UOEH 1987;9(Suppl):216–22.

194. Safirstein R, Winston J, Moel D, Dikman S, Guttenplan J. Cisplatin nephrotoxicity: insights into mechanism. Int J Androl 1987;10(1):325–46.

195. Anand AJ, Bashey B. Newer insights into cisplatin nephrotoxicity. Ann Pharmacother 1993;27(12):1519–25.

196. Tay LK, Bregman CL, Masters BA, Williams PD. Effects of cis-diamminedichloroplatinum(II) on rabbit kidney in vivo and on rabbit renal proximal tubule cells in culture. Cancer Res 1988;48(9):2538–43.

197. Blochl-Daum B, Pehamberger H, Kurz C, Kyrle PA, Wagner O, Muller M, Monitzer B, Eichler HG. Effects of cisplatin on urinary thromboxane B2 excretion. Clin Pharmacol Ther 1995;58(4):418–24.

198. Imura N, Naganuma A, Satoh M, Koyama Y. Depression of toxic effects of anticancer agents by selenium or pretreatment with metallothionein inducers. J UOEH 1987;9(Suppl):223–9.

199. Stewart DJ, Dulberg CS, Mikhael NZ, Redmond MD, Montpetit VA, Goel R. Association of cisplatin nephrotoxicity with patient characteristics and cisplatin administration methods. Cancer Chemother Pharmacol 1997;40(4):293–308.

200. Skinner R, Pearson AD, English MW, Price L, Wyllie RA, Coulthard MG, Craft AW. Cisplatin dose rate as a risk factor for nephrotoxicity in children. Br J Cancer 1998;77(10):1677–82.

201. Skinner R, Pearson AD, Price L, Coulthard MG, Craft AW. The influence of age on nephrotoxicity following chemotherapy in children. Br J Cancer Suppl 1992;18:S30–5.

202. Hargis JB, Anderson JR, Propert KJ, Green MR, Van Echo DA, Weiss RB. Predicting genitourinary toxicity in patients receiving cisplatin-based combination chemotherapy: a Cancer and Leukemia Group B study. Cancer Chemother Pharmacol 1992;30(4):291–6.

203. Saito M, Masaki T, Kato H, Numasaka K. [A clinical evaluation of the protective effect of fosfomycin (FOM) against the cis-diamminedichloroplatinum (CDDP)-induced nephrotoxicity.] Hinyokika Kiyo 1988;34(5):782–9.

204. Pinzani V, Bressolle F, Haug IJ, Galtier M, Blayac JP, Balmes P. Cisplatin-induced renal toxicity and toxicity-modulating strategies: a review. Cancer Chemother Pharmacol 1994;35(1):1–9.

205. Hausheer FH, Kanter P, Cao S, Haridas K, Seetharamulu P, Reddy D, Petluru P, Zhao M, Murali D, Saxe JD, Yao S, Martinez N, Zukowski A, Rustum YM. Modulation of platinum-induced toxicities and therapeutic index: mechanistic insights and first- and second-generation protecting agents. Semin Oncol 1998;25(5):584–99.

206. Bokemeyer C, Fels LM, Dunn T, Voigt W, Gaedeke J, Schmoll HJ, Stolte H, Lentzen H. Silibinin protects against cisplatin-induced nephrotoxicity without compromising cisplatin or ifosfamide anti-tumour activity. Br J Cancer 1996;74(12):2036–41.

207. Markman M, Cleary S, Howell SB. Nephrotoxicity of high-dose intracavitary cisplatin with intravenous thiosulfate protection. Eur J Cancer Clin Oncol 1985;21(9):1015–18.

208. Hayes DM, Cvitkovic E, Golbey RB, Scheiner E, Helson L, Krakoff IH. High dose cis-platinum diamine dichloride: amelioration of renal toxicity by mannitol diuresis. Cancer 1977;39(4):1372–81.

209. Howell SB, Pfeifle CL, Wung WE, Olshen RA, Lucas WE, Yon JL, Green M. Intraperitoneal cisplatin with systemic thiosulfate protection. Ann Intern Med 1982;97(6):845–51.

210. Abe R, Akiyoshi T, Baba T. "Two-route chemotherapy" using cisplatin and its neutralizing agent, sodium thiosulfate, for intraperitoneal cancer. Oncology 1990;47(5):422–6.

211. Leeuwenkamp OR, van der Vijgh WJ, Neijt JP, Pinedo HM. Reaction kinetics of cisplatin and its mono-aquated species with the (potential) renal protecting agents (di)mesna and thiosulfate. Estimation of the effect of protecting agents on the plasma and peritoneal AUCs of CDDP. Cancer Chemother Pharmacol 1990;27(2):111–14.

212. Daugaard G, Holstein-Rathlou NH, Leyssac PP. Effect of cisplatin on proximal convoluted and straight segments of the rat kidney. J Pharmacol Exp Ther 1988;244(3):1081–5.

213. Koukourakis MI. Amifostine in clinical oncology: current use and future applications. Anticancer Drugs 2002; 13(3):181–209.

214. Glover D, Glick JH, Weiler C, Fox K, Guerry D. WR-2721 and high-dose cisplatin: an active combination in the treatment of metastatic melanoma. J Clin Oncol 1987;5(4):574–8.

215. Hartmann JT, Kollmannsberger C, Kanz L, Bokemeyer C. Platinum organ toxicity and possible prevention in patients with testicular cancer. Int J Cancer 1999;83(6):866–9.

216. Hartmann JT, Fels LM, Franzke A, Knop S, Renn M, Maess B, Panagiotou P, Lampe H, Kanz L, Stolte H, Bokemeyer C. Comparative study of the acute nephrotoxicity from standard dose cisplatin +/– ifosfamide and high-

dose chemotherapy with carboplatin and ifosfamide. Anticancer Res 2000;20(5C):3767–73.

217. Hrushesky WJ. Circadian timing of cancer chemotherapy. Science 1985;228(4695):73–5.

218. Hrushesky WJ, Borch R, Levi F. Circadian time dependence of cisplatin urinary kinetics. Clin Pharmacol Ther 1982;32(3):330–9.

219. Levi F, Benavides M, Chevelle C, Le Saunier F, Bailleul F, Misset JL, Regensberg C, Vannetzel JM, Reinberg A, Mathe G. Chemotherapy of advanced ovarian cancer with 4'-O-tetrahydropyranyl doxorubicin and cisplatin: a randomized phase II trial with an evaluation of circadian timing and dose-intensity. J Clin Oncol 1990;8(4):705–14.

220. Hartmann JT, Fels LM, Knop S, Stolt H, Kanz L, Bokemeyer C. A randomized trial comparing the nephrotoxicity of cisplatin/ifosfamide-based combination chemotherapy with or without amifostine in patients with solid tumors. Invest New Drugs 2000;18(3):281–9.

221. Hartmann JT, Knop S, Fels LM, van Vangerow A, Stolte H, Kanz L, Bokemeyer C. The use of reduced doses of amifostine to ameliorate nephrotoxicity of cisplatin/ifosfamide-based chemotherapy in patients with solid tumors. Anticancer Drugs 2000;11(1):1–6.

222. ten Bokkel Huinink WW, van der Burg ME, van Oosterom AT, Neijt JP, George M, Guastalla JP, Veenhof CH, Rotmensz N, Dalesio O, Vermorken JB. Carboplatin in combination therapy for ovarian cancer. Cancer Treat Rev 1988;15(Suppl B):9–15.

223. Anderson H, Wagstaff J, Crowther D, Swindell R, Lind MJ, McGregor J, Timms MS, Brown D, Palmer P. Comparative toxicity of cisplatin, carboplatin (CBDCA) and iproplatin (CHIP) in combination with cyclophosphamide in patients with advanced epithelial ovarian cancer. Eur J Cancer Clin Oncol 1988;24(9):1471–9.

224. Calvert AH, Horwich A, Newlands ES, Begent R, Rustin GJ, Kaye SB, Harris AL, Williams CJ, Slevin ML. Carboplatin or cisplatin? Lancet 1988;2(8610):577–8.

225. Lee EJ, Egorin MJ, Van Echo DA, Cohen AE, Tait N, Schiffer CA. Phase I and pharmacokinetic trial of carboplatin in refractory adult leukemia. J Natl Cancer Inst 1988;80(2):131–5.

226. Lyttelton MP, Newlands ES, Giles C, Bower M, Guimaraes A, O'Reilly S, Rustin GJ, Samson D, Kanfer EJ. High-dose therapy including carboplatin adjusted for renal function in patients with relapsed or refractory germ cell tumour: outcome and prognostic factors. Br J Cancer 1998;77(10):1672–6.

227. Hardy JR, Tan S, Fryatt I, Wiltshaw E. How nephrotoxic is carboplatin? Br J Cancer 1990;61(4):644.

228. Hartmann JT, von Vangerow A, Fels LM, Knop S, Stolte H, Kanz L, Bokemeyer C. A randomized trial of amifostine in patients with high-dose VIC chemotherapy plus autologous blood stem cell transplantation. Br J Cancer 2001;84(3):313–20.

229. Pinotti G, Martinelli B. A case of acute tubular necrosis due to oxaliplatin. Ann Oncol 2002;13(12):1951–2.

230. Marnocha RS, Hutson PR. Intradermal carboplatin and ifosfamide extravasation in the mouse. Cancer 1992; 70(4):850–3.

231. Al-Lamki Z, Pearson P, Jaffe N. Localized cisplatin hyperpigmentation induced by pressure. A case report. Cancer 1996;77(8):1578–81.

232. Baur M, Kienzer HR, Rath T, Dittrich C. Extravasation of oxaliplatin (Eloxatin®) – clinical course. Onkologie 2000;23(5):468–71.

233. Kretzschmar A, Thuss-Patience PC, Pink D, Benter T, Jost D, Scholz C, Reichardt P. Extravasations of oxaliplatin. Proc Am Soc Clin Oncol 2002;21:A2900.

234. Nijman JM, Schraffordt Koops H, Oldhoff J, Kremer J, Sleijfer DT. Sexual function after surgery and combination chemotherapy in men with disseminated nonseminomatous testicular cancer. J Surg Oncol 1988;38(3):182–6.

235. Wallace WH, Shalet SM, Crowne EC, Morris-Jones PH, Gattamaneni HR, Price DA. Gonadal dysfunction due to cis-platinum. Med Pediatr Oncol 1989;17(5):409–13.

236. Khan A, Hill JM, Grater W, Loeb E, MacLellan A, Hill N. Atopic hypersensitivity to cis-dichlorodiammineplatinum(II) and other platinum complexes. Cancer Res 1975; 35(10):2766–70.

237. Saunders MP, Denton CP, O'Brien ME, Blake P, Gore M, Wiltshaw E. Hypersensitivity reactions to cisplatin and carboplatin—a report on six cases. Ann Oncol 1992;3(7):574–6.

238. Goldberg A, Altaras MM, Mekori YA, Beyth Y, Confino-Cohen R. Anaphylaxis to cisplatin: diagnosis and value of pretreatment in prevention of recurrent allergic reactions. Ann Allergy 1994;73(3):271–2.

239. Rose PG, Fusco N, Fluellen L, Rodriguez M. Carboplatin hypersensitivity reactions in patients with ovarian and peritoneal carcinoma. Int J Gynecol Obstet 1998;8:365–8.

240. Schiavetti A, Varrasso G, Maurizi P, Castello MA. Hypersensitivity to carboplatin in children. Med Pediatr Oncol 1999;32(3):183–5.

241. Tournigand C, Maindrault-Goebel F, Louvet C, de Gramont A, Krulik M. Severe anaphylactic reactions to oxaliplatin. Eur J Cancer 1998;34(8):1297–8.

242. Weidmann B, Mulleneisen N, Bojko P, Niederle N. Hypersensitivity reactions to carboplatin. Report of two patients, review of the literature, and discussion of diagnostic procedures and management. Cancer 1994; 73(8):2218–22.

243. Polyzos A, Tsavaris N, Kosmas C, Arnaouti T, Kalahanis N, Tsigris C, Giannopoulos A, Karatzas G, Giannikos L, Sfikakis PP. Hypersensitivity reactions to carboplatin administration are common but not always severe: a 10-year experience. Oncology 2001;61(2):129–33.

244. Williamson SK, Tangen CM, Maddox AM, Spiridonidis CH, Macdonald JS. Phase II evaluation of low-dose continuous 5-fluorouracil and weekly cisplatin in advanced adenocarcinoma of the stomach. A Southwest Oncology Group study. Am J Clin Oncol 1995;18(6):484–7.

245. Dold F, Hoey D, Carberry M, Musket A, Friedberg V, Mitchell E. Hypersensitivity in patients with metastatic colorectal carcinoma undergoing chemotherapy with oxaliplatin. Proc Am Soc Clin Oncol 2002;21:A1478.

246. Hendrick AM, Simmons D, Cantwell BM. Allergic reactions to carboplatin. Ann Oncol 1992;3(3):239–40.

247. Markman M, Kennedy A, Webster K, Elson P, Peterson G, Kulp B, Belinson J. Clinical features of hypersensitivity reactions to carboplatin. J Clin Oncol 1999;17(4):1141.

248. Sims-McCallum RP. Outpatient carboplatin desensitization in a pediatric patient with bilateral optic glioma. Ann Pharmacother 2000;34(4):477–8.

249. Goldberg A, Confino-Cohen R, Fishman A, Beyth Y, Altaras M. A modified, prolonged desensitization protocol in carboplatin allergy. J Allergy Clin Immunol 1996; 98(4):841–3.

250. Meyer L, Zuberbier T, Worm M, Oettle H, Riess H. Hypersensitivity reactions to oxaliplatin: cross-reactivity to carboplatin and the introduction of a desensitization schedule. J Clin Oncol 2002;20(4):1146–7.

251. Ulrich-Pur H, Penz M, Fiebiger WC, Schull B, Kornek GV, Scheithauer W, Raderer M. Oxaliplatin-induced fever and release of IL-6. Oncology 2000;59(3):187–9.

252. Chiche D, Pico JL, Bernaudin JF, Chouaib S, Wollman E, Arnoux A, Denizot Y, Nitenberg G. Pulmonary edema and shock after high-dose aracytine-C for lymphoma;

possible role of TNF-alpha and PAF. Eur Cytokine Netw 1993;4(2):147–51.

253. Khalil A, Chammas M, Shamseddine A, Seoud M. Fatal acute tumor lysis syndrome following treatment of vulvar carcinoma: case report. Eur J Gynaecol Oncol 1998;19(4):415–16.

254. Beck DJ, Brubaker RR. Mutagenic properties of cis-plantinum(II)diammino-dichloride in *Escherichia coli*. Mutat Res 1975;27(2):181–9.

255. Travis LB, Holowaty EJ, Bergfeldt K, Lynch CF, Kohler BA, Wiklund T, Curtis RE, Hall P, Andersson M, Pukkala E, Sturgeon J, Stovall M. Risk of leukemia after platinum-based chemotherapy for ovarian cancer. N Engl J Med 1999;340(5):351–7.

256. Duffner PK, Krischer JP, Horowitz ME, Cohen ME, Burger PC, Friedman HS, Kun LE. Second malignancies in young children with primary brain tumors following treatment with prolonged postoperative chemotherapy and delayed irradiation: a Pediatric Oncology Group study. Ann Neurol 1998;44(3):313–16.

257. Pont J, Albrecht W. Fertility after chemotherapy for testicular germ cell cancer. Fertil Steril 1997;68(1):1–5.

258. Meistrich ML, Chawla SP, Da Cunha MF, Johnson SL, Plager C, Papadopoulos NE, Lipshultz LI, Benjamin RS. Recovery of sperm production after chemotherapy for osteosarcoma. Cancer 1989;63(11):2115–23.

259. Hansen PV, Glavind K, Panduro J, Pedersen M. Paternity in patients with testicular germ cell cancer: pretreatment and post-treatment findings. Eur J Cancer 1991; 27(11):1385–9.

260. Rustin GJ, Pektasides D, Bagshawe KD, Newlands ES, Begent RH. Fertility after chemotherapy for male and female germ cell tumours. Int J Androl 1987;10(1):389–92.

261. Richter P, Buchholz K, Lotze W. Schwangerschaftsverlauf und Geburt nach zytostatischer Behandlung von Throphoblasttumoren. [Course of pregnancy and labor following cytostatic treatment of trophoblastic tumors.] Zentralbl Gynakol 1987;109(9):586–9.

262. Pryzant RM, Meistrich ML, Wilson G, Brown B, McLaughlin P. Long-term reduction in sperm count after chemotherapy with and without radiation therapy for non-Hodgkin's lymphomas. J Clin Oncol 1993;11(2):239–47.

263. Lamont EB, Schilsky RL. Gonadal toxicity and teratogenicity after cytotoxic chemotherapy. In: Lipp HP, editor. Anticancer Drug Toxicity; Prevention, Management and Clinical Pharmacokinetics. New York-Basel: Marcel Dekker Inc, 1999:491–523.

264. Frustaci S, Barzan L, Comoretto R, Tumolo S, Lo Re G, Monfardini S. Local neurotoxicity after intra-arterial cisplatin in head and neck cancer. Cancer Treat Rep 1987;71(3):257–9.

265. Chu G, Mantin R, Shen YM, Baskett G, Sussman H. Massive cisplatin overdose by accidental substitution for carboplatin. Toxicity and management. Cancer 1993;72(12):3707–14.

266. Neef C, de Voogd-van der Straaten I. An interaction between cytostatic and anticonvulsant drugs. Clin Pharmacol Ther 1988;43(4):372–5.

267. Dofferhoff AS, Berendsen HH, vd Naalt J, Haaxma-Reiche H, Smit EF, Postmus PE. Decreased phenytoin level after carboplatin treatment. Am J Med 1990; 89(2):247–8.

268. Lauer AK, Wobig JL, Shults WT, Neuwelt EA, Wilson MW. Severe ocular and orbital toxicity after intra-carotid etoposide phosphate and carboplatin therapy. Am J Ophthalmol 1999;127(2):230–3.

269. Coninx P, Nasca S, Lebrun D, Panis X, Lucas P, Garbe E, Legros M. Sequential trial of initial chemotherapy for advanced cancer of the head and neck. DDP versus DDP + 5-fluorouracil. Cancer 1988;62(9):1888–92.

270. Stefenelli T, Kuzmits R, Ulrich W, Glogar D. Acute vascular toxicity after combination chemotherapy with cisplatin, vinblastine, and bleomycin for testicular cancer. Eur Heart J 1988;9(5):552–6.

271. Sasaki M, Suzuki A, Ishihara T. [A case of acute myocardial infarction after treatment with cisplatin.] Gan To Kagaku Ryoho 1989;16(6):2289–91.

272. Tsutsumi I, Ozawa Y, Kawakami A, Fujii H, Asamoto H. [Acute myocardial infarction induced by lung cancer chemotherapy with cisplatin and eto poside.] Gan To Kagaku Ryoho 1990;17(3 Pt 1):413–7.

273. Murin J, Kasper J, Danko J, Cerna M, Bulas J, Uhliar R. Vznik infarktu myokardu u chorebo liecenebo 5-fluorouracilom. [The development of myocardial infarct in a patient treated with 5-fluorouracil.] Vnitr Lek 1989; 35(10):1020–4.

274. Mazoyer G, Assouline D, Fourchard V, Kalb JC. Cardiotoxicité du 5 fluoro-uracile. A propos d'une observation. [Cardiotoxicity of 5 fluoro-uracil. Apropos of a case.] Rev Mal Respir 1989;6(6):551–3.

275. Dodds HM, Bishop JF, Rivory LP. More about: irinotecan-related cholinergic syndrome induced by coadministration of oxaliplatin. J Natl Cancer Inst 1999;91(1):91–2.

276. Beijnen JH, Vlasveld LT, Wanders J, ten Bokkel Huinink WW, Rodenhuis S. Effect of cisplatin-containing chemotherapy on lithium serum concentrations. Ann Pharmacother 1992;26(4):488–90.

277. Jäger AH, Bogdahn U, Apfel R, Pfeufer B, Dekant A. In vitro studies on interaction of 4-hydroperoxyifosfamide and 2-mercaptoethanesulphonate in malignant gliomas. J Cancer Res Clin Oncol 1993;119(12):721–6.

278. Dogliotti L, Bertetto O, Berruti A, Clerico M, Fanchini L, Sicora W, Faggiuolo R. Combination chemotherapy with carboplatin and methotrexate in the treatment of advanced urothelial carcinoma. A phase II study. Am J Clin Oncol 1995;18(1):78–82.

279. Haas A, Anderson L, Lad T. The influence of aminoglycosides on the nephrotoxicity of cis-diamminedichloroplatinum in cancer patients J Infect Dis 1983;147(2):363.

280. Sleijfer S, van der Mark TW, Schraffordt Koops H, Mulder NH. Enhanced effects of bleomycin on pulmonary function disturbances in patients with decreased renal function due to cisplatin. Eur J Cancer 1996;32A(3):550–2.

281. Rowinsky EK, Gilbert MR, McGuire WP, Noe DA, Grochow LB, Forastiere AA, Ettinger DS, Lubejko BG, Clark B, Sartorius SE, et al. Sequences of taxol and cisplatin: a phase I and pharmacologic study. J Clin Oncol 1991;9(9):1692–703.

282. Jekunen AP, Christen RD, Shalinsky DR, Howell SB. Synergistic interaction between cisplatin and taxol in human ovarian carcinoma cells in vitro. Br J Cancer 1994;69(2):299–306.

283. Vanhoefer U, Harstrick A, Wilke H, Schleucher N, Walles H, Schroder J, Seeber S. Schedule-dependent antagonism of paclitaxel and cisplatin in human gastric and ovarian carcinoma cell lines in vitro. Eur J Cancer 1995;31A(1):92–7.

284. Sonnichsen DS, Relling MV. Clinical pharmacokinetics of paclitaxel. Clin Pharmacokinet 1994;27(4):256–69.

285. Baker AF, Dorr RT. Drug interactions with the taxanes: clinical implications. Cancer Treat Rev 2001;27(4):221–33.

286. Wasserheit C, Frazein A, Oratz R, Sorich J, Downey A, Hochster H, Chachoua A, Wernz J, Zeleniuch-Jacquotte A, Blum R, Speyer J. Phase II trial of paclitaxel and cisplatin in women with advanced breast cancer: an active regimen with limiting neurotoxicity. J Clin Oncol 1996;14(7):1993–9. Erratum in: J Clin Oncol 1996;14(12):3175.

287. Bokemeyer C, Berger CC, Hartmann JT, Kollmannsberger C, Schmoll HJ, Kuczyk MA, Kanz L. Analysis of risk factors for cisplatin-induced ototoxicity in patients with testicular cancer. Br J Cancer 1998; 77(8):1355–62.

Pneumocandins

General Information

The pneumocandins are a class of anti-*Pneumocystis* agents, thought to act by inhibiting the synthesis of beta-1,3-glucan, a component of the *Pneumocystis jiroveci* cyst wall. Chemical modification of the poorly water-soluble pneumocandins resulted in L-693,989, which can be given by aerosol. In rats, this compound prevents *P. jiroveci* pneumonia after daily or weekly administration, without evidence of toxicity. Since there is no counterpart for beta-1,3-glucan synthesis in humans, there are no obvious reasons to suspect mechanism-based toxicity with this class of compounds. More effective compounds are being studied (1).

Reference

1. Powles MA, McFadden DC, Liberator PA, Anderson JW, Vadas EB, Meisner D, Schmatz DM. Aerosolized L-693,989 for *Pneumocystis carinii* prophylaxis in rats. Antimicrob Agents Chemother 1994;38(6):1397–401.

Pneumococcal vaccine

See also Vaccines

General Information

Two types of pneumococcal vaccine are available, polysaccharide vaccine and conjugated polysaccharide vaccine.

Pneumococcal vaccine is composed of a saline solution containing the purified capsular polysaccharides of 23 types of *Streptococcus pneumoniae*. The improved 23-valent vaccine, which replaced a 14-valent vaccine at the beginning of the 1980s, contains antigens to pneumococcal types that are responsible for about 85% of bacteremic pneumococcal pneumonia.

Pneumococcal vaccines produced by different manufacturers are currently available, for example "Pneumovax 23" produced by Merck Sharp & Dohme and "Pnu-Imune 23" produced by Lederle Laboratories. Each vaccine dose (0.5 ml) contains 25 µg of each polysaccharide antigen. Immunization is recommended for people who are at increased risk of developing pneumococcal disease because of underlying chronic health conditions and for older people. About 50% of vaccinees develop mild adverse effects, such as erythema and pain at the injection site. Fever, myalgia, and severe local reactions have been reported in under 1% of vaccinees. Severe systemic reactions, such as anaphylaxis have been rarely reported.

Incidental case reports relate to small vessel vasculitis after combined pneumococcal-influenza immunization (1), severe febrile reactions with leukocytosis (2), Sweet's syndrome (3), thrombocytopenia (4,5), and keratoacanthoma at the injection site (6).

Patients with AIDS have an impaired antibody response to pneumococcal vaccine. Adverse effects in symptomatic and asymptomatic HIV-infected vaccinees were not different from those in HIV-negative persons (7).

Note on abbreviations

DtaP = Diphtheria + tetanus toxoids + acellular pertussis
DTwP = Diphtheria + tetanus toxoids + whole cell pertussis
Hib = *Haemophilus influenzae* type b
OPV = oral poliovirus vaccine
PPV = pneumococcal polysaccharide vaccine

Pneumococcal polysaccharide vaccine

The question of whether revaccination with 23-valent pneumococcal polysaccharide vaccine (PPV) at least 5 years after the first vaccination is associated with more frequent or more serious adverse events than those after the first vaccination has been studied in patients aged 50–74 years who had never been vaccinated with PPV ($n = 901$) or who had been vaccinated once at least 5 years before enrolment ($n = 513$) (8). After one dose of PPV, local injection site reactions and prevaccination concentrations of type-specific antibodies were measured. Those who were re-vaccinated were more likely than those who received their first vaccinations to report a local injection site reaction of at least 10.2 cm (4 in.) in diameter within 2 days of vaccination (55/513 versus 29/901, or 11 versus 3%). The reactions resolved by a median of 3 days after vaccination. The highest rate was among revaccinated patients who were immune competent and did not have chronic illnesses: 15% (33/228) compared with 3% (10/337) among comparable patients receiving their first vaccinations. The risk of these local reactions correlated significantly with prevaccination geometric mean antibody concentrations. The authors concluded that physicians and patients should be aware that self-limited local injection site reactions occur more often after revaccination compared with a first vaccination; however, this risk does not represent a contraindication to revaccination with PPV in recommended patients.

Pneumococcal conjugated polysaccharide vaccines

Pneumococcal polysaccharides are not immunogenic in infants, but improved immunogenicity of polysaccharide-protein conjugates has been demonstrated. One of the major problems in developing a successful vaccine against *S. pneumoniae* is the large number of different serotypes involved. More than 83 serotypes of the bacterium are known to cause disease, although about 10 of these account for up to 70% of disease in young children. The frequency of the serotypes can vary from year to year, from one age group to another, and on a geographical basis. Various conjugated vaccines that include different serotype variations are already licensed (the heptavalent conjugated vaccine Prevnar/Prevenar), under development or undergoing clinical trial (9- and 11-valent conjugated vaccines). If the vaccines prove to be successful, it is estimated that their use could reduce child deaths from pneumococcal pneumonia by up to 25%, saving over 250 000 lives a year worldwide. The development of conjugate pneumococcal vaccines has also been driven by the high incidence of inner ear infections and the severity of meningitis due to *S. pneumoniae* in industrialized countries. The results of some clinical trials with different vaccines of this type have been reviewed (SEDA-22, 344).

The immunogenicity of 7-valent pneumococcal-conjugate vaccine plus 23-valent pneumococcal vaccine in 11 children has been compared with the immunogenicity of 23-valent vaccine alone in 12 children up to 2 years of age with sickle cell disease (9). IgG pneumococcal antibody concentrations were higher with combined administration, with no increase in adverse effects after immunization with 23-valent vaccine.

In 2000, the first heptavalent conjugated pneumococcal vaccine, Prevnar, which contains polysaccharides of pneumococcal serotypes 4, 6B, 9V, 14, 19F, and 23F, and oligosaccharide of serotype 18C, conjugated to the protein carrier CRM 197 (non-toxic variant of diphtheria toxin), was licensed in the USA (covering 90% of pneumococcal serotypes found in young children in the USA) and in all EU member states, as well as in selected other countries in 2001. In a randomized, double-blind study, 302 healthy infants in the Northern California Kaiser Permanente Health Plan received either the pneumococcal vaccine or meningococcal group C conjugate vaccine as a control at 2, 4, and 6 months of age and a booster at 12–15 months of age (10). The immunogenicity and safety of simultaneous administration of vaccines used in the routine immunization program of children (DTwP or DTaP, Hib and OPV or hepatitis B vaccine) were also evaluated. Local reactions after pneumococcal, DTwP-Hib, and DTaP plus Hib vaccine were statistically less severe at the

pneumococcal vaccine site than at the DTwP-Hib sites (Table 1). There were 12 emergency room visits and 8 hospitalizations that occurred soon after immunization (otitis, febrile illness, urinary tract infection, burns), but none was thought to be related to the vaccine. One hypotensive-hyporesponsive episode 15 minutes after pneumococcal vaccine, DTwP-Hib/HB, and OPV, with complete recovery within 1 hour, was considered to have been vaccine-related. After the booster dose of pneumococcal vaccine, the geometric mean titers of all seven serotypes increased significantly (compared with the values after dose 3 and before dose 4) to antibodies considered as protective. When vaccine was administered at the same time as the booster dose of DTaP and Hib vaccines, there were lower antibody titers for some of the antigens than the antibody response when the pneumococcal vaccine was given separately. Because the geometric mean titers of the booster responses were all generally high and all subjects achieved similar percentages above predefined antibody titers, these differences were considered to be probably not clinically significant. Summarizing their results the authors concluded that the pneumococcal vaccine was safe and immunogenic.

A comprehensive technical overview on the epidemiology and prevention of pneumococcal disease, including the use of polysaccharide and conjugate vaccines has been provided (11).

Further results of field trials on the efficacy, safety, and immunogenicity of heptavalent conjugated pneumococcal vaccine have appeared. Between October 1995 and August 1998, 37 868 infants were included in a double-blind trial (12). At 2, 4, 6, and 12–15 months of age they were randomly assigned to receive either the pneumococcal conjugate vaccine or meningococcal conjugate vaccine. More than 95% of pneumococcal vaccine recipients developed = 0.15 µg/ml antibodies against all serotypes included in the vaccine. As of April 1999, a vaccine efficacy of 97% (prevention of invasive pneumococcal disease caused by vaccine serotypes) was calculated; in addition, there was a significant impact on otitis media. Data on reactogenicity of the conjugate pneumococcal and meningococcal vaccines are provided in Table 2 and Table 3. Local reactions were analysed separately for children who had received DTaP and DTwP vaccine simultaneously. Local and systemic reactions were generally relatively mild with either vaccine, and more severe local and systemic reactions were uncommon and self-limiting. There were significant differences in outpatient clinic visits for seizures (11 pneumococcal vaccine recipients versus 23 controls), but none of the subcategories of seizure (febrile seizures, epilepsy, afebrile seizures) was significantly different. There were four cases of sudden infant death syndrome (SIDS) (0.2/1000) in the pneumococcal vaccine group and eight in the controls (0.4/1000). This rate is similar to the rate of 0.5/1000 children observed in the general infant population of California.

Recent advances in conjugated pneumococcal vaccines selected from current literature have been reviewed, including studies with experimental tetravalent and pentavalent conjugated vaccines and vaccines conjugated to various proteins (13).

Table 1 Local reactions within 48 hours of injection in infants given conjugated pneumococcal, DTwP-Hib, and DtaP + Hib vaccines

Reaction	Number of children	Infants		Toddlers
		Pneumococcal vaccine (%)	DTwP-Hib (%)	DtaP + Hib (%)
Redness				
Dose 1	183	17	18	
Dose 2	159	18	29	
Dose 3	160	16	22	
Dose 4	110	9.1		6.1
Swelling				
Dose 1	183	10	19	
Dose 2	159	11	20	
Dose 3	160	9.0	21	
Dose 4	110	6.4		3.7
Tenderness				
Dose 1	183	24	27	
Dose 2	159	21	26	
Dose 3	160	23	28	
Dose 4	110	16		9.8

Table 2 Local reactions comparing pneumococcal conjugate (PNCRM7) and meningococcal conjugate (MnCC) as well as each of these with DtaP

Reaction	PNCRM7 (%)	DTaP (%)	P value	MnCC (%)	DtaP (%)	P value	PNCRM7 versus MnCC (P value)
Redness							
Dose 1	10	6.7	<0.001	6.5	5.6	0.345	0.124
Dose 2	12	11	0.512	7.6	11	0.011	0.003
Dose 3	14	11	0.143	9.3	8.2	0.557	0.011
Dose 4	11	3	0.004	4.5	4.0	0.999	0.226
Redness >3 cm							
Dose 1	0.3	0.0	0.500	0.1	0.3		0.999
Dose 2	0.0	0.2	0.999	0.2	0.4	0.999	0.481
Dose 3	0.2	0.2		1.3	0.8	0.999	0.105
Dose 4	0.6	0.6	0.999	0.0	0.0	0.625	0.255
Swelling							
Dose 1	9.8	6.6	0.002	4.2	4.3	0.999	0.013
Dose 2	12	11	0.312	5.1	7.4	0.080	0.001
Dose 3	10	10	0.999	6.9	8.3	0.473	0.001
Dose 4	12	5.5	0.013	4.5	3.4	0.688	0.247
Swelling >3 cm							
Dose 1	0.1	0.1		0.0	0.0		0.999
Dose 2	0.4	0.6	0.999	0.2	0.0	0.999	0.999
Dose 3	0.5	1.0	0.500	0.3	0.5	0.999	0.999
Dose 4	0.6	0.6	0.999	0.0	0.0		0.224
Tenderness							
Dose 1	18	16	0.053	18	19	0.265	0.970
Dose 2	19	17	0.080	15	16	0.677	0.069
Dose 3	15	13	0.265	12	12	0.999	0.280
Dose 4	23	18	0.096	15	15	0.999	0.052

Table 3 Fever within 48 hours of vaccination among infants receiving PNCRM7 or MnCC vaccine[*]

Reaction	PNCRM7		MnCC		P value
	%	Number	%	Number	
Fever ≥38°C					
Dose 1	15	709	9.4	710	0.001
Dose 2	24	556	11	507	0.001
Dose 3	19	461	12	414	0.003
Dose 4	21	224	17	230	0.274
Fever >39°C					
Dose 1	0.9	709	0.3	710	0.178
Dose 2	2.5	556	0.8	507	0.029
Dose 3	1.7	461	0.7	414	0.180
Dose 4	1.3	224	1.7	230	0.999

[*]Concomitantly with DTaP and other recommended vaccines; MnCC, meningococcal conjugate.

23-valent pneumococcal polysaccharide vaccine

The efficacy of polysaccharide vaccine in preventing invasive pneumococcal disease, pneumonia, and death has been assessed in a double-blind, randomized, placebo-controlled trial in 1392 HIV1-infected adults in Uganda (14). The vaccine was well tolerated. However, it was ineffective and is not recommended for use in HIV1-infected individuals. Reassessment of recommendations for polysaccharide vaccine immunization may be necessary in some countries. The authors suggested that the vaccine causes destruction of polysaccharide-responsive B cell clones.

In another clinical trial the immunogenicity and safety of polysaccharide vaccine has been assessed in 21 renal transplant recipients (15). Protective antibody titers were reached at 6 and 12 weeks after immunization in all recipients, bar one. No local or systemic adverse effects were observed.

Organs and Systems

Immunologic

Arthus reactions and systemic reactions have commonly been reported after booster doses of polysaccharide vaccine and are thought to result from antigen–antibody reactions involving antibodies induced by the previous immunization (16). Data on revaccination of children are not yet sufficient to provide a basis for recommendation.

An allergic reaction has been described to 23-valent polysaccharide pneumococcal vaccine (17).

- A 2-year-old child developed bronchospasm and cutaneous and laryngeal edema immediately after the injection of a 23-valent polysaccharide pneumococcal vaccine. The symptoms resolved within 1 hour of treatment with antihistamines, glucocorticoids, and aerosols. Skin tests and specific IgE tests showed that the pneumococcal antigens were responsible for the anaphylaxis.

Susceptibility Factors

Age

In an evaluation of simultaneous immunization in 85 elderly subjects, pre-immunization pneumococcal antibodies were associated with more reactions, both local and systemic, after vaccination (18). A rise in temperature (9% of vaccinees), and pain at the injection site (5% of vaccinees) were significantly associated with raised preimmunization pneumococcal polysaccharide antibody concentrations.

Other features of the patient

The immunogenicity and safety of pneumococcal polysaccharide vaccine have been studied in renal allograft recipients, dialysis patients (19), children and adolescents with sickle-cell anemia (SED-11, 682) (SEDA-12, 277), people with diabetes mellitus (SED-11, 682), and children with nephrotic syndrome (20). When comparing the results with healthy persons there were no significant differences.

The problems connected with pneumococcal disease and its prevention in HIV-infected individuals have been reviewed (21). Pneumococcal disease occurs significantly more often in HIV-infected individuals, with pneumococcal pneumonia rates 5.5–17.5 times greater than population-based estimates in the USA, and the increasing rate of penicillin-resistant strains of S. pneumoniae highlight the need for improved prevention strategies. Studies of pneumococcal disease in HIV infection have repeatedly shown that over 85% of the isolates from bacteremic patients, in both the USA and Africa, are of serotypes included in the 23-valent vaccine. However, the proportion of HIV-positive individuals who respond to 23-valent pneumococcal polysaccharide vaccine has been shown in some but not all studies to be slightly reduced compared with age-matched controls but comparable to other high-risk groups, such as elderly people, in whom clinical efficacy has been established. Some studies have suggested a trend toward a lower response rate as the CD4 cell count falls. The reason for concern about the safety of pneumococcal immunization in HIV-infected individuals is the reported association between immunization and increasing HIV virus load.

Much of this concern arises from extrapolation from published data on influenza immunization. However, there are some data on pneumococcal immunization alone. In 32 HIV-positive patients with a median CD4 cell count of $242 \times 10^6/l$, who received Pneumovax and tetanus toxoid there was no change in plasma HIV-1 RNA at 20–56 days after immunization (22). In contrast there were marked increases in plasma viral RNA (1.6–586 times) reported in 12 asymptomatic HIV-positive individuals (mean CD4 cell count $374 \times 10^6/l$). More recently, a study of patients with more advanced disease found that HIV-1 RNA and DNA were unaffected by either conjugate or polysaccharide pneumococcal vaccine up to 309 days after immunization (23). In summary, the authors of the review (21) recommended that HIV-infected individuals be immunized with pneumococcal vaccine and that immunization should be carried out as early as possible in the course of HIV infection.

Drug–Drug Interactions

Influenza vaccine

In a study of the interaction between 23-valent pneumococcal polysaccharide vaccine and influenza vaccine, 152 adults with chronic respiratory disease were randomized to receive both vaccines either simultaneously or at an interval of 1 month (24). There were no significant differences in serological responses between the groups. The incidence and severity of both local and systemic adverse effects were also similar: there were mild local reactions in 38 and 36% and systemic reactions in five and three of the vaccinees respectively.

References

1. Houston TP. Small-vessel vasculitis following simultaneous influenza and pneumococcal vaccination. NY State J Med 1983;83(11–12):1182–3.
2. Gabor EP, Seeman M. Acute febrile systemic reaction to polyvalent pneumococcal vaccine. JAMA 1979;242(20):2208–9.
3. Maddox PR, Motley RJ. Sweet's syndrome: a severe complication of pneumococcal vaccination following emergency splenectomy. Br J Surg 1990;77(7):809–10.
4. Citron ML, Moss BM. Pneumococcal-vaccine-induced thrombocytopenia. JAMA 1982;248(10):1178.
5. Kelton JG. Vaccination-Associated relapse of immune thrombocytopenia. JAMA 1981;245(4):369–70.
6. Bart RS, Lagin S. Keratoacanthoma following pneumococcal vaccination: a case report. J Dermatol Surg Oncol 1983;9(5):381–2.
7. Centers for Disease Control (CDC). Pneumococcal polysaccharide vaccine. MMWR Morb Mortal Wkly Rep 1989;38(5):64–8, 73–6.
8. Jackson LA, Benson P, Sneller VP, Butler JC, Thompson RS, Chen RT, Lewis LS, Carlone G, DeStefano F, Holder P, Lezhava T, Williams WW. Safety of revaccination with pneumococcal polysaccharide vaccine. JAMA 1999;281(3):243–8.
9. Vernacchio L, Neufeld EJ, MacDonald K, Kurth S, Murakami S, Hohne C, King M, Molrine D. Combined schedule of 7-valent pneumococcal conjugate vaccine followed by 23-valent pneumococcal vaccine in children and young adults with sickle cell disease. J Pediatr 1998;133(2):275–8.
10. Shinefield HR, Black S, Ray P, Chang I, Lewis N, Fireman B, Hackell J, Paradiso PR, Siber G, Kohberger R, Madore DV, Malinowski FJ, Kimura A, Le C, Landaw I, Aguilar J, Hansen J. Safety and immunogenicity of heptavalent pneumococcal CRM197 conjugate vaccine in infants and toddlers. Pediatr Infect Dis J 1999;18(9):757–63.
11. Overturf GD, Peter G, Pickering LK, MacDonald NE, Chilton L, Jacobs RF, Delage G, Dowell SF, Orenstein WA, Patriarca PA, Myers MG, Ledbetter EO, Kim J. American Academy of Pediatrics. Committee on Infectious Diseases. Technical report: prevention of pneumococcal infections, including the use of pneumococcal conjugate and polysaccharide vaccines and antibiotic prophylaxis. Pediatrics 2000;106(2 Pt 1):367–76.
12. Black S, Shinefield H, Fireman B, Lewis E, Ray P, Hansen JR, Elvin L, Ensor KM, Hackell J, Siber G, Malinoski F, Madore D, Chang I, Kohberger R, Watson W, Austrian R, Edwards K, Aguilar J, Bartlett M, Bergeb R, Burman M, Dorfman S, Easter W, Finkel A, Froehlich H, Glauber J, Herz A, Honeychurch D, Kleinrock R. Efficacy, safety and immunogenicity of heptavalent pneumococcal conjugate vaccine in children. Northern California Kaiser Permanente Vaccine Study Center Group. Pediatr Infect Dis J 2000;19(3):187–95.
13. Dabelstein D, Cromer B. Selections from current literature. Recent advances in conjugated pneumococcal vaccination. Fam Pract 2000;17(5):435–41.

14. French N, Nakiyingi J, Carpenter LM, Lugada E, Watera C, Moi K, Moore M, Antvelink D, Mulder D, Janoff EN, Whitworth J, Gilks CF. 23-valent pneumococcal polysaccharide vaccine in HIV-1-infected Ugandan adults: double-blind, randomised and placebo controlled trial. Lancet 2000;355(9221):2106–11.

15. Kazancioglu R, Sever MS, Yuksel-Onel D, Eraksoy H, Yildiz A, Celik AV, Kayacan SM, Badur S. Immunization of renal transplant recipients with pneumococcal polysaccharide vaccine. Clin Transplant 2000;14(1):61–5.

16. Centers for Disease Control (CDC). Update: pneumococcal polysaccharide vaccine usage—United States. MMWR Morb Mortal Wkly Rep 1984;33(20):273–6, 281.

17. Ponvert C, Ardelean-Jaby D, Colin-Gorski AM, Soufflet B, Hamberger C, de Blic J, Scheinmann P. Anaphylaxis to the 23-valent pneumococcal vaccine in child: a case-control study based on immediate responses in skin tests and specific IgE determination. Vaccine 2001;19(32):4588–91.

18. Sankilampi U, Honkanen PO, Pyhala R, Leinonen M. Associations of prevaccination antibody levels with adverse reactions to pneumococcal and influenza vaccines administered simultaneously in the elderly. Vaccine 1997;15(10):1133–7.

19. Rytel MW, Dailey MP, Schiffman G, Hoffmann RG, Piering WF. Pneumococcal vaccine immunization of patients with renal impairment. Proc Soc Exp Biol Med 1986;182(4):468–73.

20. Halsey NA, Spika JS, Lum GM, Schiffman GS, Lauer BA. Adverse reactions to pneumococcal polysaccharide vaccine in children. Pediatr Infect Dis 1982;1(1):34–6.

21. Moore D, Nelson M, Henderson D. Pneumococcal vaccination and HIV infection. Int J STD AIDS 1998;9(1):1–7.

22. Katzenstein TL, Gerstoft J, Nielsen H. Assessments of plasma HIV RNA and CD4 cell counts after combined Pneumovax and tetanus toxoid vaccination: no detectable increase in HIV replication 6 weeks after immunization. Scand J Infect Dis 1996;28(3):239–41.

23. Kroon FP, Van Furth R, Bruisten SM. The effects of immunization in human immunodeficiency virus type 1 infection. N Engl J Med 1996;335(11):817–8.

24. Fletcher TJ, Tunnicliffe WS, Hammond K, Roberts K, Ayres JG. Simultaneous immunisation with influenza vaccine and pneumococcal polysaccharide vaccine in patients with chronic respiratory disease. BMJ 1997;314(7095):1663–5.

Poaceae

See also Herbal medicines

General Information

The genera in the family of Poaceae (Table 1) include bamboo, barley, cane, fescue, lawn grass, oats, pappus, and rice.

Anthoxanthum odoratum

Anthoxanthum odoratum (sweet vernal grass) contains anticoagulant coumarins, which cause bleeding in cattle that consume the grass.

Adverse effects
In 125 Turkish patients with rhinitis and/or symptoms of asthma reactivity to *Dermatophagoides* as an indoor

Table 1 The genera of Poaceae

Achnatherum (needle grass)
Achnella (rice grass)
Acrachne (goose grass)
Aegilops (goat grass)
Aegopogon (relax grass)
Agropyron (wheat grass)
Agropogon (agropogon)
Agrostis (bent grass)
Aira (hair grass)
Allolepis (Texas salt)
Alloteropsis (summer grass)
Alopecurus (foxtail)
Ammophila (beach grass)
Ampelodesmos (Mauritanian grass)
Amphicarpum (maidencane)
Amphibromus (wallaby grass)
Andropogon (blue stem)
Anthaenantia (silky scale)
Anthephora (oldfield grass)
Anthoxanthum (vernal grass)
Apera (silkybent)
Apluda (Mauritian grass)
Arctagrostis (polar grass)
Arctophila (pendant grass)
Aristida (three awn)
Arrhenatherum (oat grass)
Arthraxon (carp grass)
Arthrostylidium (climbing bamboo)
Arundinaria (cane)
Arundinella (rabo de gato)
Arundo (giant reed)
Avena (oat)
Axonopus (carpet grass)

Bambusa (bamboo)
Beckmannia (slough grass)
Blepharidachne (desert grass)
Blepharoneuron (drop seed)
Bothriochloa (beard grass)
Bouteloua (grama)
Brachiaria (signal grass)
Brachyelytrum (short husk)
Brachypodium (false brome)
Briza (quaking grass)
Bromus (brome)
Buchloe (buffalo grass)

Calamagrostis (reed grass)
Calamovilfa (sand reed)
Calammophila (calammophila)
Catabrosa (whorl grass)
Cathestecum (false grama)
Cenchrus (sandbur)
Chasmanthium (wood oats)
Chloris (windmill grass)
Chrysopogon (false beard grass)
Chusquea (chusquea bamboo)
Cinna (wood reed)
Cladoraphis (bristly love grass)
Coelorachis (joint tail grass)
Coix (Job's tears)
Coleanthus (moss grass)
Cortaderia (pampas grass)
Corynephorus (club awn grass)
Cottea (cotta grass)
Crypsis (prickle grass)
Ctenium (toothache grass)

Continued

Table 1 Continued

Cutandia (Memphis grass)
Cymbopogon (lemon grass)
Cynodon (Bermuda grass)
Cynosurus (dogstail grass)

Dactylis (orchard grass)
Dactyloctenium (crowfoot grass)
Danthonia (oat grass)
Dasyochloa (woolly grass)
Dasypyrum (mosquito grass)
Deschampsia (hair grass)
Desmazeria (fern grass)
Diarrhena (beak grain)
Dichanthelium (rosette grass)
Dichanthium (blue stem)
Dichelachne (plume grass)
Diectomis (folded leaf grass)
Digitaria (crab grass)
Dinebra (viper grass)
Dissanthelium (Catalina grass)
Dissochondrus (false brittle grass)
Distichlis (salt grass)
Dupontia (tundra grass)

Echinochloa (cockspur grass)
Ehrharta (veldt grass)
Eleusine (goose grass)
Elionurus (balsam scale grass)
Elyhordeum (barley)
Elyleymus (wild rye)
Elymus (wild rye)
Enneapogon (feather pappus grass)
Enteropogon (umbrella grass)
Entolasia (entolasia)
Eragrostis (love grass)
Eremochloa (centipede grass)
Eremopyrum (false wheat grass)
Eriochloa (cup grass)
Eriochrysis (moco de pavo)
Erioneuron (woolly grass)
Euclasta (mock bluestem)
Eustachys (finger grass)

Festuca (fescue)
Fingerhuthia (Zulu fescue)

Garnotia (lawn grass)
Gastridium (nit grass)
Gaudinia (fragile oat)
Glyceria (manna grass)
Gymnopogon (skeleton grass)
Gynerium (wild cane)

Hackelochloa (pitscale grass)
Hainardia (barb grass)
Helictotrichon (alpine oat grass)
Hemarthria (joint grass)
Hesperostipa (needle and thread)
Heteropogon (tanglehead)
Hierochloe (sweet grass)
Hilaria (curly mesquite)
Holcus (velvet grass)
Hordeum (barley)
Hymenachne (marsh grass)
Hyparrhenia (thatching grass)
Hypogynium (West Indian bluestem)

Ichnanthus (bed grass)
Imperata (satin tail)
Isachne (blood grass)

Ischaemum (muraina grass)
Ixophorus (Central America grass)

Jarava (rice grass)

Karroochloa (South African oat grass)
Koeleria (June grass)

Lagurus (hare's tail grass)
Lamarckia (goldentop grass)
Lasiacis (small cane)
Leersia (cut grass)
Leptochloa (sprangle top)
Leptochloopsis (limestone grass)
Leptocoryphium (lanilla)
Lepturus (thin tail)
Leucopoa (spike fescue)
Leymus (wild rye)
Limnodea (Ozark grass)
Lithachne (diente de perro)
Lolium (rye grass)
Luziola (water grass)
Lycurus (wolf's tail)

Melica (melic grass)
Melinis (stink grass)
Mibora (sand grass)
Microchloa (small grass)
Microstegium (brown top)
Milium (millet grass)
Miscanthus (silver grass)
Molinia (moor grass)
Monanthochloe (shore grass)
Monroa (false buffalo grass)
Muhlenbergia (muhly)

Nardus (mat grass)
Nassella (tussock grass)
Neeragrostis (creeping love grass)
Neostapfia (Colusa grass)
Neyraudia (neyraudia)

Olyra (carrycillo)
Opizia (opizia)
Oplismenus (basket grass)
Orcuttia (Orcutt grass)
Oryza (rice)
Oryzopsis (rice grass)

Panicum (panic grass)
Pappophorum (pappus grass)
Parapholis (sickle grass)
Pascopyrum (wheat grass)
Paspalidium (watercrown grass)
Paspalum (crown grass)
Pennisetum (fountain grass)
Phalaris (canary grass)
Phanopyrum (savannah panic grass)
Pharus (stalk grass)
Phippsia (ice grass)
Phleum (timothy)
Phragmites (reed)
Phyllostachys (bamboo)
Piptatherum (rice grass)
Piptochaetium (spear grass)
Pleuraphis (galleta grass)
Pleuropogon (semaphore grass)
Poa (blue grass)
Polypogon (rabbit's foot grass)
Polytrias (Java grass)
Psathyrostachys (wild rye)
Pseudoroegneria (wheat grass)

Pseudelymus
   (foxtail wheat grass)
Pseudosasa (arrow bamboo)
Ptilagrostis (false needle grass)
Puccinellia (alkali grass)

Redfieldia (blowout grass)
Reimarochloa (reimar grass)
Rostraria (hair grass)
Rottboellia (itch grass)
Rytidosperma (wallaby grass)

Saccharum (sugar cane)
Sacciolepis (cupscale grass)
Sasa (broad leaf bamboo)
Schedonnardus (tumble grass)
Schismus (Mediterranean grass)
Schizachne (false melic)
Schizachyrium (little bluestem)
Schizostachyum
   (Polynesian 'ohe)
Sclerochloa (hard grass)
Scleropogon (burro grass)
Scolochloa (river grass)
Scribneria (Scribner's grass)
Secale (rye)
Setaria (bristle grass)
Sinocalamus (wide leaf bamboo)
Sorghastrum (Indian grass)
Sorghum (sorghum)
Spartina (cord grass)
Sphenopholis (wedge scale)
Sporobolus (drop seed)
Steinchisma (gaping grass)
Stenotaphrum (St. Augustine grass)
Swallenia (dune grass)

Taeniatherum (Medusa head)
Themeda (kangaroo grass)
Thinopyrum (wheat grass)
Thuarea (Kuroiwa grass)
Torreyochloa
   (false manna grass)
Trachypogon (crinkle awn grass)
Tragus (burr grass)
Trichoneura (Silveus' grass)
Tridens (tridens)
Triplasis (sand grass)
Tripogon (five minute grass)
Tripsacum (gama grass)
Trisetum (oat grass)
Triticum (wheat)
Tuctoria (spiral grass)

Uniola (sea oats)
Urochloa (signal grass)

Vahlodea (hair grass)
Vaseyochloa (Texas grass)
Ventenata (North Africa grass)
Vetiveria (vetiver grass)
Vulpia (fescue)

Willkommia (willkommia)

Zea (corn)
Zizania (wild rice)
Zizaniopsis (cut grass)
Zoysia (lawn grass)

allergen was 50% ($n = 63$); in pollen allergic patients ($n = 100$) sensitivity to Poaceae was the most common (69%), and among them positivity to *A. odoratum* was 45% (1). Sensitivity to grass pollen was the same in patients from urban and rural areas (72 versus 71%).

Reference

1. Harmanci E, Metintas E. The type of sensitization to pollens in allergic patients in Eskisehir (Anatolia), Turkey. Allergol Immunopathol (Madr) 2000;28(2):63–6.

Podophyllum derivatives

General Information

Podophyllum is a powerful skin irritant and antimitotic agent, widely used in the topical treatment of condylomata acuminata. The anticancer topoisomerase inhibitors, tenoposide and etoposide, are podophyllotoxins.

The signs and symptoms of systemic toxicity (1,2) (SED-9, 240) include:

- cyanosis, tachycardia, electrocardiographic changes;
- stertorous respiration;
- polyneuritis, ataxia, coma, agitation, delirium, confusion, lethargy, muscular weakness, paresthesia;
- leukopenia, leukocytosis, thrombocytopenia, anemia;
- nausea, vomiting, abdominal pain, paralytic ileus;
- raised liver enzymes;
- oliguria, anuria, hematuria;
- urticaria;
- fever.

Intrauterine death and teratogenicity have not been demonstrated convincingly.

Podophyllum emodi (Indian podophyllum)

Proresid (mitopodozide), a mixture of more than 20 derivatives of *Podophyllum emodi*, has been used for many years in some countries as a disease-modifying agent in rheumatoid arthritis. A microtubulin antagonist, it is comparable with colchicine and griseofulvin. Its use has been limited because treatment is often complicated by severe diarrhea, abdominal pain, nausea, and vomiting. Leukopenia and thrombocytopenia have been reported (3,4).

Etoposide and teniposide are semisynthetic derivatives of podophyllin, which was originally isolated from the root of the Indian podophyllum plant. They inhibit topoisomerase II and are dealt with in a separate monograph.

Podophyllum peltatum (American mandrake)

The resin prepared from the dried rhizome and roots of *Podophyllum peltatum* contains podophyllotoxin, α-peltatin, and β-peltatin. When applied topically, it is a strong irritant to the skin and mucous membranes and can lead to poisoning because of systemic absorption. When taken by mouth, it has a drastic laxative action and produces violent peristalsis. Ingestion of large doses can result in severe neuropathic toxicity (SEDA-11, 426). The oral and local use of the resin should be avoided during pregnancy, as this has been associated with teratogenicity and fetal death.

- A 31-year-old man took an unknown amount of *Podophyllum peltatum*, thinking it to be *Mandragora officinarum*; he developed severe nausea and vomiting and recovered uneventfully (5).

Dysosma pleianthum (bajiaolian)

Dysosma pleianthum (bajiaolian), a species of mayapple, has been widely used for thousands of years in China as a general remedy and for the treatment of snake bite, weakness, condyloma acuminata, lymphadenopathy, and tumors. Podophyllotoxin is one of its main ingredients. Five people who drank infusions of bajiaolian developed nausea, vomiting, diarrhea, abdominal pain, thrombocytopenia, leukopenia, abnormal liver function tests, sensory ataxia, altered consciousness, and persistent peripheral tingling or numbness (6).

Long-Term Effects

Tumorigenicity

Etoposide and teniposide are prominent causes of secondary malignancies, particularly secondary myeloid and lymphoid leukemias. The risk appears to be related to both the schedule and the cumulative dose, and it may be aggravated by addition of alkylating agents and/or radiotherapy (7,8). There are differences between the chromosomal abnormalities and the subsequent acute myeloid leukemia associated with the alkylating agents and those following topoisomerase inhibition by epipodophyllotoxins (9). The alkylating agents cause abnormalities of chromosomes five and seven, singly or together, and the epipodophyllotoxins damage the 11q23 chromosome locus (10).

Second-Generation Effects

Teratogenicity

Podophyllum is likely to be teratogenic (11,12) because of its effects on topoisomerase.

- A woman who applied podophyllum resin five times for a duration of 4 hours from the 23rd to the 29th week of pregnancy gave birth to a child with a simian crease on the left hand and a preauricular skin tag (11).

Drug Administration

Drug overdose

Fatal podophyllum toxicity has been reported.

- When a 59-year-old man took 10 g of podophyllum in a fatal suicide attempt he did not develop symptoms until 10 hours later, with loss of reflexes, coma, and marked lactic acidosis; there were nuclear and cytoplasmic changes in circulating leukocytes (1). Despite hemoperfusion, he died after 39 hours.

References

1. Cassidy DE, Drewry J, Fanning JP. Podophyllum toxicity: a report of a fatal case and a review of the literature. J Toxicol Clin Toxicol 1982;19(1):35–44.
2. Miller RA. Podophyllin. Int J Dermatol 1985;24(8):491–8.
3. Lysholm J, Weitoft T. Proresid in the long-term treatment of rheumatoid arthritis. Scand J Rheumatol 1988;17(6):465–8.
4. Weitoft T, Lysholm J. Side effects of Proresid in the treatment of chronic arthritis. Scand J Rheumatol 1988;17(1):63–6.
5. Frasca T, Brett AS, Yoo SD. Mandrake toxicity. A case of mistaken identity. Arch Intern Med 1997;157(17):2007–9.
6. Kao WF, Hung DZ, Tsai WJ, Lin KP, Deng JF. Podophyllotoxin intoxication: toxic effect of bajiaolian in herbal therapeutics. Hum Exp Toxicol 1992;11(6):480–7.
7. Pui CH, Ribeiro RC, Hancock ML, Rivera GK, Evans WE, Raimondi SC, Head DR, Behm FG, Mahmoud MH, Sandlund JT. Acute myeloid leukemia in children treated with epipodophyllotoxins for acute lymphoblastic leukemia. N Engl J Med 1991;325(24):1682–7.
8. Hawkins MM, Wilson LM, Stovall MA, Marsden HB, Potok MH, Kingston JE, Chessells JM. Epipodophyllotoxins, alkylating agents, and radiation and risk of secondary leukaemia after childhood cancer. BMJ 1992;304(6832):951–8.
9. Pedersen-Bjergaard J, Philip P. Two different classes of therapy-related and de-novo acute myeloid leukemia? Cancer Genet Cytogenet 1991;55(1):119–24.
10. Rubin CM, Arthur DC, Woods WG, Lange BJ, Nowell PC, Rowley JD, Nachman J, Bostrom B, Baum ES, Suarez CR. Therapy-related myelodysplastic syndrome and acute myeloid leukemia in children: correlation between chromosomal abnormalities and prior therapy. Blood 1991;78(11):2982–8.
11. Karol MD, Conner CS, Watanabe AS, Murphrey KJ. Podophyllum: suspected teratogenicity from topical application. Clin Toxicol 1980;16(3):283–6.
12. Chamberlain MJ, Reynolds AL, Yeoman WB. Medical memoranda. Toxic effect of podophyllum application in pregnancy. BMJ 1972;3(823):391–2.

Poldine methylsulfate

General Information

Poldine methylsulfate is an anticholinergic drug that has been used to reduce gastric acid secretion in patients with peptic ulceration (1) and has been administered by iontophoresis in the treatment of palmar and plantar hyperhidrosis (2). Its adverse effects are those expected of an anticholinergic drug.

References

1. Bieberdorf FA, Walsh JH, Fordtran JS. Effect of optimum therapeutic dose of poldine on acid secretion, gastric acidity, gastric emptying, and serum gastrin concentration after a protein meal. Gastroenterology 1975;68(1):50–7.
2. Hill BH. Poldine iontophoresis in the treatment of palmar and plantar hyperhidrosis. Australas J Dermatol 1976;17(3):92–3.

Poliomyelitis vaccine

See also Vaccines

Note on abbreviations

DTP = Diphtheria + tetanus toxoids + pertussis
DtaP = Diphtheria + tetanus toxoids + acellular pertussis
Hib = *Haemophilus influenzae* type b
IPV = inactivated poliomyelitis vaccine
OPV = oral poliovirus vaccine
PRP-T-Hib = conjugated Hib vaccine (tetanus toxoid linked to Hib capsular polysaccharide)

General Information

There are two types of poliomyelitis vaccines available. One is prepared from polioviruses that as a rule have been inactivated by formaldehyde. Inactivated poliomyelitis vaccine (IPV) is given parenterally. The second group of polio vaccines comprises attenuated strains of live polioviruses (oral poliomyelitis vaccine, OPV), which are given orally; these live vaccines are the most widely used.

Inactivated poliomyelitis vaccine

Inactivated poliomyelitis vaccine produced by improvements in manufacturing technology (potency-enhanced IPV-eIPV was licensed in 1987) is used for routine immunization in an increasing number of countries (for example in Finland, France, Germany, Iceland, the Netherlands, Norway, Sweden, and certain provinces of Canada) and is recommended in other countries for certain specific purposes, for example for persons with underlying immunological disorders or non-immunized adults exposed to high risk. A few countries (for example Denmark, Hungary, Italy, Lithuania, and Israel) use a mixed schedule, starting primary immunization with IPV followed by OPV.

The US 2000 childhood immunization schedule, proposed by the Advisory Committee of Immunization Practices (ACIP), the American Academy of Pediatrics, and the American Academy of Family Physicians, recommended an all-IPV schedule for routine use in the USA, aimed at the elimination of the rare vaccine-associated paralytic poliomyelitis (1). Since 1 January 2000, all children have received four doses of IPV at ages 2 months, 4 months, 6–18 months, and 4–6 years.

Some other industrialized countries that use OPV in their routine immunization programs, and which had no wild poliomyelitis cases for many years but some vaccine-associated poliomyelitis, are reassessing their immunization strategy. They are considering new concepts of shifting from OPV to IPV or from OPV to mixed schedules. This change could help to prevent vaccine-associated poliomyelitis mostly occurring after the first dose of OPV immunization.

Serious adverse effects after IPV immunization have not been documented (2). Because IPV contains streptomycin and neomycin, there is a possibility of allergic reactions in those who are sensitive to these antibiotics. Although it has been postulated that IPV, like some viral infections, might trigger Guillain–Barré syndrome, there is inadequate evidence to accept or reject such an association (3); in this respect it may differ from the oral vaccine.

Oral polio vaccine

In contrast to IPV, OPV causes important problems, including vaccine-associated polio and prolonged polio virus excretion.

Combination vaccines

The safety, immunogenicity, and lot consistency of five-component pertussis combination vaccine (DtaP + IPV + PRP-T-Hib) in infants have been compared to those of a whole-cell pertussis combination vaccine (DTwP + IPV + PRP-T-Hib), as have separate and combined injections of DTP + IPV and Hib. The combination vaccine DtaP + IPV + Hib were comparable or superior regarding safety and immunogenicity to the combination vaccine containing the whole cell pertussis component. There was no interaction between acellular pertussis and PRP-T-Hib, a feature that distinguishes this combination vaccine from some others, which depress anti-PRP responses. The combination vaccine DtaP + IPV + Hib produced significantly lower rates of local and systemic reactions than did the combination vaccine containing the whole-cell pertussis component. Local reactions, such as redness, swelling, and tenderness occurred two to three times more often after combination vaccine containing whole cell pertussis than after combination vaccines with acellular pertussis components. Fever was three times more common after whole cell combination vaccine. Fever over 40°C was rare in all vaccinees, because of the use of paracetamol prophylaxis. Systemic reactions, such as fussiness, crying, reduced activity, and anorexia, were about twice as frequent with whole cell vaccine as with acellular pertussis vaccine. Both local and systemic reactions persisted longer after whole cell vaccine than after acellular pertussis vaccine. There were no significant differences between reaction rates among infants given DtaP + IPV vaccine combined with PRP-T-Hib vaccine in the same syringe compared with those given separate injections, except for local redness after the first dose (4).

Hexavalent immunization

The Hexavalent Study Group has compared the immunogenicity and safety of a new liquid hexavalent vaccine against diphtheria, tetanus, pertussis, poliomyelitis, hepatitis B and *Haemophilus influenzae* type b (DTP + IPV + HB + Hib vaccine, manufactured by Aventis Pasteur MSD, Lyon, France) with two reference vaccines, the pentavalent DTP + IPV + Hib vaccine and the monovalent hepatitis B vaccine, administrated separately at the same visit (5). Infants were randomized to receive either the hexavalent vaccine (*n* = 423) or (administered at different local sites) the pentavalent and the HB vaccine (*n* = 425) at 2, 4, and 6 months of age. The hexavalent vaccine was well tolerated (for details see the monograph on Pertussis vaccines). At least one local reaction was reported in 20% of injections with hexavalent vaccine compared with 16% after the receipt of pentavalent vaccine or 3.8% after the receipt of hepatitis B vaccine. These reactions were generally mild and transient. At least one systemic reaction was reported in 46% of injections with hexavalent vaccine, whereas the respective rate for the recipients of pentavalent and HB vaccine was 42%. No vaccine-related serious adverse event occurred during the study. The hexavalent vaccine provided immune responses adequate for protection against the six diseases.

Polio vaccines as a possible cause of AIDS

There is a hypothesis that the HIV virus might have jumped the species barrier from monkey to people via a contaminated polio vaccine because the vaccine was manufactured in primary monkey kidney tissue known to be sometimes contaminated with monkey viruses. The existing evidence, including tests of poliovirus seed stocks, more than 20 vaccine lots, and serum samples from vaccine recipients makes this hypothesis highly improbable (6,7).

Contamination of polio vaccines with simian papovavirus 40 (SV40)

The problem of early polio vaccines produced in the 1950s and early 1960s, and, in some instances, contaminated with the monkey virus SV40 (simian virus 40) has been discussed (8). From 1954 to 1962, millions of people were immunized with polio vaccines, which during that period contained SV40 as an unrecognized contaminant. Some studies sought to investigate possible causation between the receipt of the vaccine and the development of tumors. The results were not convincing (SEDA-15, 355) (SED-12,821). At a workshop in 1997 some of the scientific questions concerned were again considered (9). The presentations by polio vaccine manufacturers and the UK National Institute for Biological Standards and Control provided convincing evidence that currently used polio vaccine was free of SV40.

Critical assessment of virological and epidemiological data suggests a probable causative role for SV40 in certain human cancers, but that additional studies are necessary to prove etiology (8). To help answer these issues, the World Health Organization has provided the following statement (10): "Investigations from several medical research institutions have detected the presence of simian virus 40 (SV40) genome in certain rare human tumors, notably mesotheliomas, osteosarcomas, and brain tumors. SV40, which is known to induce tumors in laboratory rodents, is a polyomavirus identified in 1960 as a contaminant of some batches of primary rhesus monkey kidney cells used to produce polio vaccine in the 1950s. Soon after its discovery, measures to exclude the virus from polio and other vaccines were rapidly introduced into WHO Requirements for the Manufacture and Quality Control of Polio Vaccines, and these have been rigorously applied by vaccine manufacturers. For over 30 years now, polio vaccines made in primary monkey kidney cells have been shown to be free of live SV40."

The use of new and highly sensitive polymerase chain reaction (PCR) techniques for the detection of the SV40 genome in batches of oral polio vaccines from several manufacturers has confirmed that the measures taken have been effective in excluding SV40 from vaccines.

There is no doubt that the early batches of polio vaccine that were used between 1955 and 1963 contained SV40. Epidemiological studies between 1960 and 1974 failed to show an association between exposure to SV40-contaminated vaccines and human tumors. More recent epidemiological data from tumor registers, involving more than 60 million person years of observation, have likewise found no differences in tumor incidence that could be attributable to SV40-contaminated polio vaccines. The latest data published in the Journal of the National Cancer Institute, USA, suggest that SV40 may be present in humans more commonly than had previously been thought, and raises the possibility of transmission of the virus among humans. Whether the antibodies that have been detected are due to exposure to SV40 or to cross-reacting human polyomaviruses is not known. Neither is it certain that SV40 strains now present in the human population originated from the use of the early polio vaccines. Despite almost 40 years of observation, there is still no evidence that SV40 contamination of some early batches of polio vaccine has had any adverse effect on human health.

"The River" by Edward Hooper

The hypothesis that oral polio vaccine played a key role in the current AIDS epidemic was raised again by Edward Hooper, who has worked many years for the BBC and the UN in Africa and some years ago wrote a book called "Slim," in which he described the AIDS epidemic in East Africa. His book "The River. A journey to the source of HIV and AIDS," published in 1999 (11), raised great public attention and was discussed in BBC Press Releases and in the New York Times. Leading experts in virology and AIDS research published comments in Science and other scientific journals. "The River" is a thoroughly researched, well-written book and deserves to be taken seriously. Hooper carefully collected data and events describing the first phases of HIV infection and AIDS, as well as the early development and implementation of polio vaccines. His book reflects some hundreds of interviews, including the leading researchers in the related fields, and he has documented more than 4000 references.

The hypothesis is based on the following facts and assumptions. In 1957 and 1958, Koprowski, from the Wistar Institute in Philadelphia, was administering oral polio vaccine in Africa (pre-licensure field trials in Burundi, Rwanda, and the North-East Congo) near Stanleyville (now Kisangani) in Congo. Not far from the base, chimpanzees for use in medical research were housed in Camp Lindi and might have carried a primate immunodeficiency virus (PIV). Chimpanzee kidneys for hepatitis research were shipped from Camp Lindi to the Virological Department of the Children Hospital in Philadelphia in 1958 and 1959. Hooper suggests that "it could be that [kidneys from these chimpanzees] ended up at the Wistar", the laboratory in Philadelphia where polio vaccines were manufactured, where they contaminated vaccines with PIV. The polio vaccine that was supposed to be contaminated with PIV was then used in the Congo, transmitting the virus that evolved into HIV-1, the starting point of the worldwide HIV-1 epidemic. Over the next 20 years, infected humans progressed to AIDS, and the disease became visible in central Africa in the mid-to-late 1970s.

Does Hooper prove his hypothesis beyond a shadow of doubt? No, but he makes a powerful case for soberly and squarely addressing the issue.

There are also strong arguments against the hypothesis. Polio vaccines were first propagated in kidney cultures of rhesus and cynomolgus macaques, and later in African green monkeys. Plotkin and Koprowski categorically stated in a letter to the editor of the New York Times (7 December 1999) that no chimpanzee tissues were used in the Wistar Institute for polio vaccine production. They added that two independent analyses of the probable timing of the crossover of HIV from chimpanzees into humans give dates earlier than 1957–59, the years in which the Wistar polio vaccine was used in the Congo (12). It should also be mentioned that the vaccine manufactured in Wistar at that time was not only used in Africa but also in Sweden, Poland, and the US. One vial of Wistar's oral polio vaccine stored in Stockholm has already tested negative. Garrett and colleagues in England experimentally examined the survival of human and simian immunodeficiency viruses in oral polio vaccine formulations; no live retrovirus came through the procedure. Wistar declared that they would release lab specimens from a polio vaccine project carried out at the end of the 1950s in Africa for examination in two independent laboratories, in order to dispel claims that Wistar scientists inadvertently caused the AIDS epidemic.

It should be mentioned that the majority of scientists believe that the AIDS epidemic began after the simian immunodeficiency virus was transmitted from chimpanzees to humans during the slaughter of chimpanzees as early as the 1930s (13–16).

Finally, it is worth repeating the statement of the US Centers for Disease Control and Prevention, issued in 1992 but still valid (17): "The suggestion that HIV, the AIDS virus, originated as a result of inadvertent inoculation of an HIV-like virus present in monkey kidney cell cultures used to prepare polio vaccine is one of a number of unsubstantiated hypotheses. The weight of scientific evidence does not support this idea and there is no more reason to believe this hypothesis than many other which have been considered and rejected on scientific grounds."

Nevertheless, there are important lessons to be learned from Hooper's book. For many years, virologists and regulatory authorities have been worried that using permanent cell lines for vaccine virus propagation may somehow transfer cancer-causing properties and animal viruses. African green monkey kidneys are still used as the main cell substrate for oral polio vaccine. Millions of doses have been made from simian immunodeficiency virus (SIV)-positive monkeys before screening was introduced. Now there are well-tested non-oncogenic cell substrates, and it is time to reopen the debate on the use of primary cells versus cell lines for live attenuated virus vaccines. There is also a need to strengthen research on the sources of AIDS. However, the main focus of AIDS research should be prevention and treatment.

Global eradication of poliomyelitis and immunization

Using oral vaccine, the global campaign to eradicate polio achieved a more than 90% reduction in the number of polio cases worldwide in the 11 years since it was launched, and is on track to eradicate polio (18). It is to be expected that in a few years both poliomyelitis and polio vaccines will be confined to history books and science museums. Polio immunization will stop for good. When the final goal of global eradication is achieved, a decision on when and how to stop polio immunization will be necessary. Such a decision has not yet been prepared. Different scenarios are under discussion: continuation of universal immunization programs, sequential removal of one or two of the Sabin strains of OPV, change to an all-IPV program, and discontinuation of OPV immunization simultaneously worldwide or selectively country by country (19). The Technical Consultative Group for the World Health Organization on the Global Eradication of Poliomyelitis has the task of elaborating a proposal for final approval by the World Health Assembly (20).

Organs and Systems

Cardiovascular

Myopericarditis has been attributed to Td-IPV vaccine (21).

- A 31-year-old man developed arthralgia and chest pain 2 days after Td-IPV immunization and had an acute myopericarditis. He recovered within a few days with high-dose aspirin.

The authors discussed two possible causal mechanisms, natural infection or an immune complex-mediated mechanism. Infection was excluded by negative bacterial and viral serology and a favorable outcome resulted within a few days without antimicrobial drug treatment.

Nervous system

Vaccine-associated poliomyelitis
There is no doubt that OPV can cause poliomyelitis in a minority of recipients and their contacts. The risk is very low, but the seriousness of such a complication is evident. Various case reports and national surveys of vaccine-associated poliomyelitis, as well as studies quantifying this risk for OPV, have been published (SED-12, 820) (SEDA-16, 390) (SEDA-18, 336). The main conclusions from the field study that WHO conducted over a period of 15 years in 13 countries were as follows:

- The type 1 strain is almost never implicated in vaccine-associated poliomyelitis cases.
- The type 2 strain is an occasional cause of paralysis, commoner in contacts of the vaccine than in recipients.
- Most of the very small number of cases that do occur are due to type 3, both in vaccine recipients and in contacts.

In general, the risk of vaccine-associated poliomyelitis is less than one per million children immunized. The type 1 strain has been confirmed to be as safe and effective as any biological substance can be. The type 2 strain is safe for recipients of the vaccine but on rare occasions can cause paralysis in contacts, so that any contact whose immunization status is doubtful should be immunized at the same time as the original vaccinee. The type 3 strain is much less stable genetically than the two strains and requires constant monitoring in the laboratory and in the field (22).

Frequency

The risk of vaccine-associated poliomyelitis has remained exceedingly low but stable since the mid-1960s. In all, 260 cases of vaccine-associated poliomyelitis were reported in the USA between 1961 and 1989. Cases of vaccine-associated poliomyelitis appeared to occur randomly in time and space. One potential cluster of vaccine-associated poliomyelitis consisting of six cases occurring over an 18-month period in Indiana was investigated during the period 1980–89. These cases were not shown to be epidemiologically related.

Using the total number of 80 vaccine-associated poliomyelitis cases in the USA from 1980 to 1989 as a numerator, the overall risk of vaccine-associated poliomyelitis was one case per 2.5 million doses of trivalent OPV distributed. The overall risk of vaccine-associated poliomyelitis was 9.7 times greater after the first dose of OPV than after all subsequent doses. The overall risk of recipient vaccine-associated poliomyelitis was one case per 6.8 million doses. The risk among OPV recipients was 29.0 times higher after the first dose than after subsequent doses. Comparing the first dose of OPV to subsequent doses, the lowest relative risk was found in immunologically abnormal persons. Whereas the average annual rate of vaccine-associated poliomyelitis for the period 1980–89 was 0.34 cases per million population, the annual incidence of vaccine-associated poliomyelitis among immunologically competent infants, who were used as the reference group, was 7.6 cases per 10 million population. Children under 1 year of age with a primary immunodeficiency were at highest risk of vaccine-associated poliomyelitis (annual rate of 16 216 cases per 10 million population, or 0.16%), which is more than 2000 times higher than the rate in the reference group. Among household contacts of children below 6 years of age, the annual rate of contact vaccine-associated poliomyelitis was 0.45 cases per 10 million population. For the remaining US population, the annual rate of vaccine-associated poliomyelitis was 0.14 cases per 10 million population. Summarizing their experience (23), the authors of the 1980–89 study distinguish three groups at risk of vaccine-associated poliomyelitis:

- recipients of OPV, especially infants receiving their first dose of OPV;
- persons in contact with OPV recipients, mostly unimmunized or inadequately immunized adults;
- immunologically abnormal individuals.

There has been a retrospective cohort study of cases of acute flaccid paralysis reported to the Ministry of Health in Brazil between 1989 and 1995 (24,25). For the first dose of OPV the estimated risk was one case of vaccine-associated paralytic poliomyelitis per 2.39 million doses; for total doses of OVP the risk was one case in 13.03 million doses. Most of the cases of vaccine-associated

paralytic poliomyelitis were in children with a mean age of 1 year. Paralysis of the lower limbs caused by poliovirus type 2 was dominant.

Poliomyelitis caused by vaccine-derived polioviruses Between 12 July and 18 November 2000, a total of 19 people (aged between 9 months and 21 years) with acute flaccid paralysis were identified in the Dominican Republic; one case occurred in Haiti (August 2000) (26). The case in Haiti and three of the cases in the Dominican Republic were laboratory-confirmed with poliovirus type 1 isolates. All cases were either unimmunized or incompletely immunized. The outbreak was unusual, because the virus is derived from oral polio vaccine virus, with 97% genetic similarity to the parental OPV strain. Normally, vaccine-derived isolates are more than 99.5% similar to the parent strain. In contrast, wild polioviruses normally have less than 82% genetic similarity to OPV. The differences in nucleotide sequences suggest that the virus causing the outbreak has been circulating for about 2 years in the area in which immunization coverage is very low, and that the virus had accumulated genetic changes that restored the essential properties of wild poliovirus. A mass immunization with OPV brought the outbreak under control.

Causative strains

In an outbreak in Egypt during 1988–93, 32 cases of polio were associated with vaccine-derived poliovirus type 2 (27). Nucleotide sequence analysis performed during 1999 showed that all isolates were related (93–96% similarity) to the OPV 2 vaccine strain. The isolates were not related (less than 81% similarity) to the wild poliovirus type 2 that had been indigenous in Egypt. OPV was probably low in the affected communities.

Between 15 March and 26 July 2001, three cases of acute flaccid paralysis associated with vaccine-derived polioviruses type 1 were reported in the Philippines (28). There was a 3% genetic sequence difference between OPV type 1 virus and the vaccine-derived isolates.

Mechanism

The molecular biological findings connected with the occurrence of vaccine-associated poliomyelitis have been summarized (29). There is convincing evidence that the Sabin 2 and 3 viruses themselves can revert to a neurovirulent phenotype on passage in man. The authors report that a point mutation in the 5'-non-coding region of the genome of the poliovirus type 3 vaccine consistently reverts to the wild type in viruses isolated from cases of vaccine-associated poliomyelitis.

Prolonged poliovirus excretion

Molecular studies of poliovirus isolates have suggested that viral replication of vaccine-related polioviruses may have persisted for as long as 7 years in a patient with vaccine-associated paralytic poliomyelitis, in whom common variable immunodeficiency syndrome had previously been diagnosed (SEDA-21, 336).

DTP injections

The risk of DTP injection in provoking paralytic poliomyelitis during a large poliomyelitis outbreak in Oman has been evaluated (30). Health center immunization records for 70 children aged 5–24 months with confirmed poliomyelitis and 692 control children were reviewed. A significantly higher proportion of case-patients received a DTP injection within 30 days before onset of paralysis compared with controls (43 versus 28%). All the patients for whom this information was available had paralysis of the injected limb. This study, which provided the first quantitative estimate in this respect, confirmed that injections are an important cause of provocative poliomyelitis and stressed the recommendation to avoid unnecessary injections during poliomyelitis outbreaks.

Multiple injections

Studies in 1994–95 in Romania produced evidence that multiple (unnecessary) injections may actually increase the risk of vaccine-associated poliomyelitis (SEDA-19, 302).

Between 1976 and 1985, seven cases of neurological disease were reported to have occurred in Germany among young children after simultaneous administration of oral poliovirus vaccine and diphtheria–tetanus toxoids or diphtheria–tetanus–pertussis vaccine (31). However, the virological data were incomplete; only one case was confirmed by the isolation of a vaccine-like polio virus, and in three cases the clinical symptoms did not correspond to poliomyelitis. The author concluded that in some cases the simultaneous administration of injectable vaccines cannot be excluded as a cause for paralysis.

Acute disseminated encephalomyelitis

Acute disseminated encephalomyelitis associated with polio vaccine has been reported (32).

- A 6-year-old girl developed acute disseminated encephalomyelitis, and polio vaccine virus type 2 was isolated from her cerebrospinal fluid and pharynx. The virus was sequenced throughout the 5′ non-coding region of the genome by polymerase chain reaction and was determined to have undergone various mutations at nucleotides 481, 500, 795, and 1195. The clinical signs of disease had completely disappeared 2 months later.

Guillain–Barré syndrome

Coincident with the mass nationwide campaign of OPV immunization that interrupted the transmission of wild poliovirus in Finland in 1985, with 4.5 million doses of OPV being administered, there was an unexpected rise in the occurrence of Guillain–Barré syndrome. In 10 cases of Guillain–Barré syndrome with onset of symptoms within 10 weeks after OPV immunization, no specific agents were found (33). The authors concluded that live attenuated polioviruses might trigger Guillain–Barré syndrome.

The authors of a report of the Institute of Medicine concluded that the evidence favored a causal relation between OPV and Guillain–Barré syndrome, but considered the evidence inadequate to accept or to reject a causal relation between OPV and transverse myelitis (SEDA-18, 325) (3).

The available reports on a possible association between polio vaccine and Guillain–Barré syndrome have been reviewed (34). The conclusion of a 1994 US Institute of

Medicine committee that the evidence favored acceptance of a causal relation was mainly based on two reports from Finland (35,36). An earlier study of Guillain–Barré syndrome and oral polio vaccine has been extended to include hospital reports from the whole of Finland for 1981–6, during which time an oral polio vaccine campaign was carried out to control an outbreak of poliomyelitis (37). The rise in the numbers of cases of Guillain–Barré syndrome started before the immunization campaign. Because there had also been an influenza epidemic during that time, the researchers acknowledged that the increase in the incidence of Guillain–Barré syndrome could also have been associated with influenza. Data from the Americas are also not supporting an association between oral polio immunization campaigns and Guillain–Barré syndrome (38).

Sensory systems

Optic neuritis has been attributed to Td-IPV vaccine (39).

- Ten days after receiving Td-IPV vaccine a 56-year-old woman developed acute unilateral optic neuritis. Complete remission occurred within 6 weeks of prednisolone treatment. No other causes were found.

Gastrointestinal

Intussusception probably causally related to rotavirus vaccine (SEDA-23, 354) prompted studies to answer the question of whether polio vaccine could also cause intussusception. A workshop held in Atlanta on 15–16 June 2000 brought together experts from various fields with the primary investigators of the studies. The participants concluded that the available evidence favored rejection of a causal relation between OPV and intussusception (40).

Skin

Bullous pemphigoid has been attributed to DTP-IPV vaccine (41).

- A previously healthy 3.5-month-old infant developed bullous pemphigoid 3 days after receiving a first dose of DTP-IPV vaccine. *Staphylococcus aureus* was isolated from purulent bullae. The lesions resolved rapidly after treatment with antibiotics and methylprednisolone.

The authors mentioned 12 other cases of bullous pemphigoid, reported during the last 5 years, that had possibly been triggered by vaccines (influenza, tetanus toxoid booster, and DTP-IPV vaccine).

Second-Generation Effects

Pregnancy

Pregnancy is not a contraindication to the use of IPV. Although there is no convincing evidence documenting adverse effects of OPV on the developing fetus, and some evidence points to safety, it is widely considered prudent to avoid immunizing pregnant women, especially during the first 4 months of pregnancy. However, if immediate protection against poliomyelitis is needed, poliomyelitis immunization is recommended (42,43).

In order to interrupt poliovirus transmission during an outbreak of wild poliomyelitis in Israel in 1988, some 90% of the population, including pregnant women, were immunized with trivalent OPV. In a study of the abortions that occurred within 4 months of immunization compared with figures from a similar period in the previous year, the number of spontaneous abortions did not differ between women immunized during the first trimester of pregnancy and the controls (44). The authors concluded that OPV administered during early pregnancy has no adverse effect on the embryo or placenta that would cause increased fetal deaths or spontaneous abortions, nor does it seem to cause a higher rate of congenital anomalies.

An analysis of the OPV mass campaign in Finland suggested that OPV during early pregnancy had no harmful effects on fetal development (45). There were no significant deviations from the baseline prevalence for all malformations. However, when the vaccine is administered later in pregnancy the prospects may be different.

- Irreparable damage to the anterior horn cells of the cervical and thoracic cord occurred in a 20-week-old fetus whose mother was immune to poliomyelitis before conceiving but who was inadvertently given OPV at 18 weeks gestation (46).

Susceptibility Factors

There are no known contraindications to the use of IPV. OPV should not be given to persons who are immunocompromised due to immunodeficiency diseases, leukemia, lymphoma or generalized malignancy or who are immunosuppressed due to therapy with glucocorticoids, alkylating drugs, antimetabolites, or radiation. If poliomyelitis immunization is indicated in such persons, IPV should be used. OPV should also be avoided when immunizing household contacts of immunocompromised patients.

In the view of the WHO, live vaccines should in general not be given to immunocompromised individuals, but in developing countries, the risk of poliomyelitis in nonimmunized infants is high and the risk from these vaccines, even in the presence of symptomatic HIV infection, appears to be lower (47).

The Immunization Advisory Committees of many developed countries recommend that OPV should not be given to children and young adults who are immunocompromised due to AIDS or other clinical manifestations of HIV infection. OPV can be given to asymptomatic infected persons. However, because family members may be immunocompromised due to AIDS or HIV infection, it seems prudent to use IPV (48).

References

1. Recommendations of the Advisory Committee (ACIP). The 2000 Immunization Schedule. MMWR Morb Mortal Wkly Rep 2000;49:25.
2. Centers for Disease Control. Adverse Events Following Immunization. Surveillance Report No. 2, US Department of Health and Human Services. Atlanta, GA: Public Health Service, CDC, 1986.
3. Stratton KR, Howe CJ, Johnson Jr. RB Jr, editors. Adverse Events Associated with Childhood Vaccines. Washington, DC: National Academy of Sciences, 1994.
4. Mills E, Gold R, Thipphawong J, Barreto L, Guasparini R, Meekison W, Cunning L, Russell M, Harrison D, Boyd M, Xie F. Safety and immunogenicity of a combined five-component pertussis-diphtheria-tetanus-inactivated poliomyelitis-Haemophilus B conjugate vaccine administered to infants at two, four and six months of age. Vaccine 1998;16(6):576–85.
5. Mallet E, Fabre P, Pines E, Salomon H, Staub T, Schodel F, Mendelman P, Hessel L, Chryssomalis G, Vidor E, Hoffenbach A, Abeille A, Amar R, Arsene JP, Aurand JM, Azoulay L, Badescou E, Barrois S, Baudino N, Beal M, Beaude-Chervet V, Berlier P, Billard E, Billet L, Blanc B, Blanc JP, Bohu D, Bonardo C, Bossu C. Hexavalent Vaccine Trial Study Group. Immunogenicity and safety of a new liquid hexavalent combined vaccine compared with separate administration of reference licensed vaccines in infants. Pediatr Infect Dis J 2000;19(12):1119–27.
6. Anonymous. Wkly Epidemiol Rec 1985;35:269.
7. Curtis T. Possible origins of AIDS. Science 1992;256(5061):1260–1.
8. Butel JS, Lednicky JA. Cell and molecular biology of simian virus 40: implications for human infections and disease. J Natl Cancer Inst 1999;91(2):119–34.
9. Griffiths E. Personal communication, 1997.
10. World Health Organization. Hot topics: statement on simian virus (SV40) and polio vaccine. http://www.who.int/vaccines-diseases/safety/hottop/sv40.htm, 14/09/2000.
11. Hooper E. The River: a journey to the source of HIV and AIDS. Boston, New York, London: Little, Brown and Company, 1999.
12. Plotkin SA, Koprowski H. New York Times, 7 December 1999.
13. Wakefield AJ, Pittilo RM, Sim R, Cosby SL, Stephenson JR, Dhillon AP, Pounder RE. Evidence of persistent measles virus infection in Crohn's disease. J Med Virol 1993;39(4):345–53.
14. van der Meijden AP. Practical approaches to the prevention and treatment of adverse reactions to BCG. Eur Urol 1995;27(Suppl 1):23–8.
15. Vegt PD, van der Meijden AP, Sylvester R, Brausi M, Holtl W, de Balincourt C, Andriole GL. Does isoniazid reduce side effects of intravesical bacillus Calmette–Guérin therapy in superficial bladder cancer? Interim results of European Organization for Research and Treatment of Cancer Protocol 30911. J Urol 1997;157(4):1246–9.
16. Tuncer S, Tekin MI, Ozen H, Bilen C, Unal S, Remzi D, Lamm DL. Detection of Bacillus Calmette–Guérin in the blood by the polymerase chain reaction method of treated bladder cancer patients. J Urol 1997;158(6):2109–12.
17. US Department of Health and Human Services, Public Health Service, Centers for Disease Control. Origin of HIV. Press release, 6 March 1992.
18. World Health Organization. Bovine spongiform encephalitis and oral polio vaccine. Position statement. October 2000. http://www.who.int/vaccines-diseases/safety/hottop/bse.htm, 11/10/2000.
19. Wood DJ, Sutter RW, Dowdle WR. Stopping poliovirus vaccination after eradication: issues and challenges. Bull World Health Organ 2000;78(3):347–57.
20. Technical Consultative Group to the World Health Organization on the Global Eradication of Poliomyelitis. "Endgame" issues for the global polio eradication initiative. Clin Infect Dis 2002;34(1):72–7.
21. Boccara F, Benhaiem-Sigaux N, Cohen A. Acute myopericarditis after diphtheria, tetanus, and polio vaccination. Chest 2001;120(2):671–2.

22. Cockburn WC. The work of the WHO Consultative Group on Poliomyelitis Vaccines. Bull World Health Organ 1988;66(2):143–54.

23. Strebel PM, Sutter RW, Cochi SL, Biellik RJ, Brink EW, Kew OM, Pallansch MA, Orenstein WA, Hinman AR. Epidemiology of poliomyelitis in the United States one decade after the last reported case of indigenous wild virus-associated disease. Clin Infect Dis 1992;14(2):568–79.

24. de Oliveira LH, Struchiner CJ. Vaccine-associated paralytic poliomyelitis in Brazil, 1989–1995. Rev Panam Salud Publica 2000;7(4):219–24.

25. de Oliveira LH, Struchiner CJ. Vaccine-associated paralytic poliomyelitis: a retrospective cohort study of acute flaccid paralyses in Brazil. Int J Epidemiol 2000;29(4):757–63.

26. Anonymous. Poliomyelitis, Dominican Republic and Haiti. Wkly Epidemiol Rec 2000;75(49):397–9.

27. Anonymous. Acute flaccid paralysis associated with circulating vaccine-derived poliovirus, Philippines, 2001. Wkly Epidemiol Rec 2001;76(41):319–20.

28. Centers for Disease Control and Prevention (CDC). Circulation of a type 2 vaccine-derived poliovirus—Egypt, 1982–1993. MMWR Morb Mortal Wkly Rep 2001;50(3): 41–2, 51.

29. Evans DM, Dunn G, Minor PD, Schild GC, Cann AJ, Stanway G, Almond JW, Currey K, Maizel JV Jr. Increased neurovirulence associated with a single nucleotide change in a noncoding region of the Sabin type 3 poliovaccine genome. Nature 1985;314(6011):548–50.

30. Sutter RW, Patriarca PA, Suleiman AJ, Brogan S, Malankar PG, Cochi SL, Al-Ghassani AA, el-Bualy MS. Attributable risk of DTP (diphtheria and tetanus toxoids and pertussis vaccine) injection in provoking paralytic poliomyelitis during a large outbreak in Oman. J Infect Dis 1992;165(3):444–9.

31. Ehrengut W. Role of provocation poliomyelitis in vaccine-associated poliomyelitis. Acta Paediatr Jpn 1997;39(6): 658–62.

32. Ozawa H, Noma S, Yoshida Y, Sekine H, Hashimoto T. Acute disseminated encephalomyelitis associated with poliomyelitis vaccine. Pediatr Neurol 2000;23(2):177–9.

33. Kinnunen E, Farkkila M, Hovi T, Juntunen J, Weckstrom P. Incidence of Guillain-Barré syndrome during a nationwide oral poliovirus vaccine campaign. Neurology 1989;39(8):1034–6.

34. Salisbury DM. Association between oral poliovaccine and Guillain-Barré syndrome? Lancet 1998;351(9096):79–80.

35. Uhari M, Rantala H, Niemela M. Cluster of childhood Guillain-Barré cases after an oral poliovaccine campaign. Lancet 1989;2(8660):440–1.

36. Uhari M, Rantala H, Niemela M. Cluster of childhood Guillain–Barré cases after an oral poliovaccine campaign. Lancet 1989;2(8660):440–1.

37. Kinnunen E, Junttila O, Haukka J, Hovi T. Nationwide oral poliovirus vaccination campaign and the incidence of Guillain–Barré syndrome. Am J Epidemiol 1998; 147(1):69–73.

38. Olive JM, Castillo C, Castro RG, de Quadros CA. Epidemiologic study of Guillain–Barré syndrome in children <15 years of age in Latin America. J Infect Dis 1997;175(Suppl 1):S160–4.

39. Burkhard C, Choi M, Wilhelm H. Optikusneuritis als Komplikaton einer Tetanus–Diphtherie–Poliomyelitis–Schutzimpfung: ein Fallbericht. [Optic neuritis as a complication in preventive tetanus-diphtheria-poliomyelitis vaccination: a case report.] Klin Monatsbl Augenheilkd 2001;218(1):51–4.

40. Anonymous. Oral poliovirus vaccine (OPV) and intussusception. Wkly Epidemiol Rec 2000;75(43):345–7.

41. Baykal C, Okan G, Sarica R. Childhood bullous pemphigoid developed after the first vaccination. J Am Acad Dermatol 2001;44(Suppl 2):348–50.

42. Centers for Disease Control (CDC). Poliomyelitis prevention. MMWR Morb Mortal Wkly Rep 1982;31(3): 22–6, 31–4.

43. Department of Health and Social Security. Immunization against infectious disease. London: Her Majesty's Stationery Office, 1992.

44. Ornoy A, Arnon J, Feingold M, Ben Ishai P. Spontaneous abortions following oral poliovirus vaccination in first trimester. Lancet 1990;335(8692):800.

45. Harjulehto T, Aro T, Hovi T, Saxen L. Congenital malformations and oral poliovirus vaccination during pregnancy. Lancet 1989;1(8641):771–2.

46. Burton AE, Robinson ET, Harper WF, Bell EJ, Boyd JF. Fetal damage after accidental polio vaccination of an immune mother. J R Coll Gen Pract 1984; 34(264):390–4.

47. Global Advisory Group of the Expanded Programme on Immunization (EPI). Report on the meeting 13–17 October, 1986, New Delhi. WHO/EPI/Geneva/87/1, 1986.

48. Centers for Disease Control (CDC). Immunization of children infected with human T-lymphotropic virus type III/lymphadenopathy-associated virus. MMWR Morb Mortal Wkly Rep 1986;35(38):595–8, 603–6.

Polyacrylonitrile

General Information

Polyacrylonitrile is a constituent of dialysis membranes (1).

Organs and Systems

Immunologic

Non-IgE-mediated anaphylactic reactions to polyacrylonitrile membranes have been reported (2,3). The effects are enhacing in those using ACE inhibitors (4,5), perhaps because of an effect of bradykinin (6), which is released by the membranes (2,8,9) and whose metabolism is inhibited by ACE inhibitors. The effects also occur to a lesser extent in those taking angiotensin receptor antagonists (7) and in those with C1 esterase inhibitor deficiency (10). Treating the membranes with polyethyleneimine prevents bradykinin release (11).

The FDA has issued a safety alert about life-threatening anaphylactoid reactions associated with the concurrent use of angiotensin converting enzyme (ACE) inhibitors and polyacrylonitrile dialyzers (12). The warning was followed by increased reports in the literature and to the FDA of severe, sudden and sometimes fatal reactions. Symptoms include nausea, abdominal cramps, burning, angioedema, and shortness of breath, leading rapidly to severe hypotension. When these symptoms are recognized, dialysis should be stopped immediately and aggressive treatment for anaphylactoid reactions begun. Antihistamines do not relieve the symptoms. The mechanism of this interaction has not been established, and the incidence and scope of the problem are unknown.

References

1. Ebo DG, Bosmans JL, Couttenye MM, Stevens WJ. Haemodialysis-associated anaphylactic and anaphylactoid reactions. Allergy 2006;61(2):211–20.

2. Tielemans C, Madhoun P, Lenaers M, Schandene L, Goldman M, Vanherweghem JL. Anaphylactoid reactions during hemodialysis on AN69 membranes in patients receiving ACE inhibitors. Kidney Int 1990;38:982–4.

3. Parnes EL, Shapiro WB. Anaphylactoid reactions in hemodialysis patients treated with the AN69 dialyzer. Kidney Int 1991;40:1148–52.

4. Brunet P, Jaber K, Berland Y, Baz M. Anaphylactoid reactions during hemodialysis and hemofiltration: role of associating AN69 membrane and angiotensin I-converting enzyme inhibitors. Am J Kidney Dis 1992;19:444–7.

5. Rousaud BF, Garcia JM, Camps EM, Cubells TD, Comamala MR. ACE inhibitors and anaphylactoid reactions to high-flux membrane dialysis (AN69): clinical aspects. Nephron 1992;60:487.

6. Schaefer RM, Fink E, Schaefer L, Barkhausen R, Kulzer P, Heidland A. Role of bradykinin in anaphylactoid reactions during hemodialysis with AN69 dialyzers. Am J Nephrol 1993;13:473–7.

7. John B, Anijeet HK, Ahmad R. Anaphylactic reaction during haemodialysis on AN69 membrane in a patient receiving angiotensin II receptor antagonist. Nephrol Dial Transplant 2001;16:1955–6.

8. Schulman G, Hakim R, Arias R, Silverberg M, Kaplan AP, Arbeit L. Bradykinin generation by dialysis membranes: possible role in anaphylactic reaction. J Am Soc Nephrol 1993;3:1563–9.

9. Fink E, Lemke HD, Verresen L, Shimamoto K. Kinin generation by hemodialysis membranes as a possible cause of anaphylactoid reactions. Braz J Med Biol Res 1994;27:1975–83.

10. Ebo DG, Stevens WJ, Bosmans JL. An adverse reaction to angiotensin-converting enzyme inhibitors in a patient with neglected C1 esterase inhibitor deficiency. J Allergy Clin Immunol 1997;99:425–6.

11. Thomas M, Valette P, Mausset AL, Dejardin P. High molecular weight kininogen adsorption on hemodialysis membranes: influence of pH and relationship with contact phase activation of blood plasma. influence of pretreatment with poly(ethyleneimine). Int J Artif Organs 2000;23:20–6.

12. Anonymous. Severe allergic reactions associated with dialysis and ACE inhibitors. FDA Med Bull 1992;22(1):4.

Polygeline

General Information

Polygeline is a plasma volume expander used as a 3.5% solution with electrolytes in the management of hypovolemic shock. It is also used in extracorporeal perfusion fluids, as a perfusion fluid for isolated organs, as fluid replacement in plasma exchange, and as a carrier solution for insulin.

Organs and Systems

Urinary tract

The effects of two modified gelatin preparations (Plasmion and Haemaccel) on renal function have been studied in 15 patients (1). In both groups proteinuria appeared as soon as perfusion began, with a peak as high as 6 g/l at the third hour. At the same time, low-molecular weight proteinuria (<30 kDa) was observed. Beta$_2$-microglobulinuria was significantly increased. The authors suggested that proteinuria was due either to inhibited tubular reabsorption of filtered protein, caused by gelatin, or to the amino acids, arginine and lysine, which are released as a result of gelatin hydrolysis. The pathological significance of this finding is unexplained.

Immunologic

Anaphylactic reactions associated with parenteral gelatin products are relatively common. The number of reports to the UK licensing authority now approaches 300, involving 127 patients, with 7 deaths. Most of these reactions are associated with multiconstituent gelatin-containing products, such as Gelofusine. An anaphylactic reaction due solely to the use of Gelofusine in a patient with non-hemorrhagic hypovolemia has been reported (2).

- A 57-year-old man presented with a 3-day history of lower abdominal pain and vomiting. He was hemodynamically stable but febrile, with tenderness and guarding in the lower abdomen. He was given intravenous fluids and antibiotics and mini-laparotomy was performed. Although 6 liters of crystalloids were given, his urine output was minimal, so 500 ml of Gelofusine was prescribed. Within 10 minutes he developed an urticarial rash, with wheals on his face and chest and difficulty in breathing. The infusion was stopped and replaced with crystalloids via a new administration set. Intravenous chlorphenamine and hydrocortisone improved his condition and the operation was completed without further complications.

Anaphylactic reactions to gelatins occur in about 0.1% of patients. Such reactions are more common in atopic patients and men and often occur within 10 minutes of starting the infusion. The authors recommended the use of allergy identification jewellery in such individuals, to reduce the possibility of life-threatening reactions.

The allergic reactions that have been described in association with polygeline are thought to be caused by direct histamine release as a result of allergenic stimulation of mast cells. These cases raise the questions of whether polygeline is appropriate for bronchoreactive patients and whether such patients should be protected by histamine receptor blockade.

- A 46-year-old man with diabetes mellitus and a history of allergy to penicillin, seafood, and soap had spinal anesthesia, and his systolic blood pressure fell to 90 mmHg (3). He was given 500 ml of gelafundin. Within minutes, he complained of pruritus along the drip site. There was no rash or urticaria, but the infusion was stopped immediately. He became restless, had copious oral secretions, complained of dyspnea, quickly lost consciousness, and was bradycardic and hypotensive, with a systolic blood pressure of 65 mmHg. He was given Hartman's solution, Haesteril 6%, adrenaline, and atropine. He had a markedly raised IgE concentration (16 000 IU/ml). He eventually recovered.

The authors suggested that the sequence of events strongly suggested an anaphylactic reaction to gelafundin, and they concluded that while polygelines are useful volume substitutes they should be used carefully in atopic individuals or those with previous drug allergies. Etherified starch is considered a safer alternative in such patients.

- Suspected polygeline-induced anaphylaxis occurred in an 83-year-old woman within 1 minute of receiving an infusion of about 10 ml (exact dose not stated) of polygeline after induction of anesthesia for left thoracotomy (4). Her arterial blood pressure fell to 30 mmHg and there were no palpable pulses and no detectable cardiac output, but she was successfully resuscitated. About 1 month later she showed a strongly positive reaction to polygeline on skin testing. It is believed that modification of the manufacturing process of polygeline has reduced the incidence of associated adverse reactions, although there have been no large-scale studies to estimate the current incidence.

Three cases of acute anaphylactoid reactions to polygeline have been described from Australia. The reactions were serious and the explanation for them was unclear. All three patients were either normovolemic or mildly hypovolemic at the time of the event (5).

In a comparison of 4% human albumin solution, gelatin, and dextran 40, given as replacement fluids during plasma exchange, the gelatin solution induced two immediate allergic reactions and one delayed reaction (among 37 patients exposed). There was no cross-reactive allergy between the two colloids. Dextran 1000 injections were well tolerated. Gelatin infusions were associated with 10 times more episodes of hypovolemia (5.6 compared with 0.62%). This difference is probably explained by the faster elimination of gelatin from the vascular compartment, and it suggests that a larger volume of gelatin is required compared with dextran 40 for the same volume of plasma exchanged (6).

An IgE-mediated anaphylactic reaction to polygeline (Haemaccel, Hoechst Marion Roussel) has been reported (7).

- A 33-year-old woman with supraventricular tachycardia and a history of cadaveric renal transplantation for end-stage renal insufficiency, who was taking an immunosuppressant, enalapril, and simvastatin, was given intravenous adenosine and polygeline 500 ml. After 30 minutes she developed generalized urticaria. Promethazine and hydrocortisone did not ameliorate her symptoms and an hour later she developed angioedema of the lips and tongue, but no airway obstruction, bronchospasm, or hypotension. The reaction resolved with subcutaneous adrenaline. Skin prick tests 2 weeks later showed hypersensitivity to polygeline but not to latex (a possible contaminant).

The authors suggested that the positive skin prick reaction showed that the cause was an IgE-mediated anaphylactic reaction, rather than an anaphylactoid reaction, although this was not confirmed by independent tests.

Susceptibility Factors

Patients with underlying bronchial asthma and pheochromocytoma are thought to be particularly at risk of acute histamine release due to polygeline.

- A 45-year-old woman, who had used salbutamol and budesonide inhalers and oral theophylline for asthma and who had developed bronchospasm during induction of general anesthesia 6 weeks before, was readmitted for surgery under spinal anesthesia (8). During the procedure she developed two episodes of hypotension, which was corrected with fluids and intravenous mephentermine 6 mg. When blood loss reached 750 ml she was given an infusion of polygeline 3.5%, and 10 minutes later complained of respiratory difficulty and developed severe respiratory distress. Polygeline was withdrawn and she was given 100% oxygen with halothane by face mask. The oxygen saturation fell by more than 80% and she developed severe bradycardia and ventricular fibrillation. She was resuscitated.

The authors concluded that the severe reaction in this case had been due to polygeline, despite careful preparation of the patient with glucocorticoids and antihistamines. They recommended that polygeline should be avoided in any patient with reactive airway disease. Preoperative antihistamines and glucocorticoids may not prevent reactions induced by polygeline administration in such patients.

Drug Administration

Drug formulations

Using a computer-aided model for the prediction of pseudoallergic reactions from prospective data collected from 581 patients in a controlled clinical trial with an outdated formulation of polygeline, accurate prediction of 86% of the patients who had a systemic reaction was possible (9). The data were handled by multivariate analysis using the independence Bayes model. The predictive accuracy of other reactions was poor. A history of allergy was recorded in 26% of the patients who had systemic reactions and in 12 and 13% of the patients with no systemic or skin reactions. However, these differences were not statistically significant.

References

1. Lazard T, Deswartes-Pipien I, Tenenhaus D, Voitot H, Drupt F, Desveaux N, Cousin MT. Protéinurie après perfusion de gélatine. [Proteinuria after infusion of gelatin. Comparison of Plasmion and Haemaccel.] Therapie 1989;44(4):269–74.
2. Jenkins SC, Clifton MA. Gelofusine allergy—the need for identification jewellery. Ann R Coll Surg Engl 2002; 84(3):206–7.
3. Ong EL. A case of hypersensitivity to gelafundin. Singapore Med J 2001;42(4):176–7.
4. Duffy BL, Harding JN, Fuller WR, Peake SL. Cardiac arrest following Haemaccel. Anaesth Intensive Care 1994;22(1):90–2.

5. Prevedoros HP, Bradburn NT, Harrison GA. Three cases of anaphylactoid reaction to Haemaccel. Anaesth Intensive Care 1990;18(3):409–12.

6. Bombail-Girard D, Boulechfar H, Tangre M, Landillon N, Bussel A. Etude comparative de l'efficacité et de la tolérance de deux substituts de plasma utilisés comme solution de remplissage au cours des échanges plasmatiques. [Comparative study of the efficacy and tolerability of 2 plasma substitutes used as vascular-loading solutions during plasma exchange.] Ann Med Interne (Paris) 1990;141(7):611–14.

7. Chew GY, Phan TG, Quin JW. Anaphylactic or anaphylactoid reaction to Haemaccel? Med J Aust 1999;171(7):387–8.

8. Kathirvel S, Podder S, Batra YK, Malhotra N, Mahajan R. Severe life threatening reaction to Haemaccel in a patient with bronchial asthma. Eur J Anaesthesiol 2001;18(2):122–3.

9. Ennis M, Ohmann C, Lorenz W, Zaczyk R, Schoning B. Prediction of risk for pseudoallergic reactions and histamine release in patients undergoing anaesthesia and surgery: a computer-aided model using independence-Bayes. Agents Actions 1988;23(3–4):366–9.

Polygonaceae

See also Herbal medicines

General Information

The genera in the family of Polygonaceae (Table 1) include buckwheat and rhubarb.

Table 1 The genera of Polygonaceae

Antenoron (antenoron)
Antigonon (antigonon)
Aristocapsa (spiny cape)
Brunnichia (buckwheat vine)
Centrostegia (centrostegia)
Chorizanthe (spineflower)
Coccoloba (coccoloba)
Dedeckera (July gold)
Dodecahema (spineflower)
Emex (three-corner jack)
Eriogonum (buckwheat)
Fagopyrum (buckwheat)
Gilmania (golden carpet)
Goodmania (spine cape)
Hollisteria (hollisteria)
Homalocladium (homalocladium)
Koenigia (koenigia)
Lastarriaea (lastarriaea)
Mucronea (spine flower)
Muehlenbeckia (maidenhair vine)
Nemacaulis (cottonheads)
Oxyria (mountain sorrel)
Oxytheca (oxytheca)
Polygonella (jointweed)
Polygonum (knotweed)
Pterostegia (pterostegia)
Rheum (rhubarb)
Rumex (dock)
Stenogonum (buckwheat)
Systenotheca (spineflower)

Polygonum species

Some species of *Polygonum* (knotweed) contain stilbene phytoestrogens, including resveratrol. *Polygonum tinctorium* contains indirubin, an isomer of indigo, which inhibits interferon-gamma production by human myelomonocytic HBL-38 cells and interferon-gamma and interleukin-6 production by murine splenocytes with no effect on the proliferation of either cells (1). *Polygonum multiflorum* contains compounds that inhibit calmodulin-depleted erythrocyte calcium-dependent ATPase (2). *Polygonum pennsylvanicum* contains vanicosides, glycosides that inhibit protein kinase C (3).

Adverse effects

Hepatitis has been attributed to *P. multiflorum* (4).

- *Polygonum multiflorum* (Shou wu Pian) was prescribed by a Chinese herbalist for a 46-year-old woman with graying hair (5). After taking it for 2 weeks she developed signs and symptoms of hepatitis. The history revealed no plausible cause for hepatitis and viral infection was ruled out. After withdrawal of the *P. multiflorum* her liver enzymes normalized and she recovered fully.
- A 31-year-old pregnant Chinese woman developed hepatitis after consuming Shou wu Pian; tests for viral hepatitis were negative and there was no evidence of other systemic disease (6).

Rheum palmatum

Rheum palmatum (rhubarb) contains the anthranoids sennosides and rhein. In a study of patients taking regular doses of rhubarb-containing Kampo medicines (extracts or decoctions) and patients taking excess doses there was tolerance to initial stimulant pain in the abdomen during excess use (7). The authors proposed that the absence of tenderness on pressure over the umbilical region could predict increasing or excess use of rhubarb.

In 14 616 patients who used various Kampo medicines, some of which contained rhubarb, there was no association between the use of rhubarb and the development of gastric carcinoma (8).

References

1. Kunikata T, Tatefuji T, Aga H, Iwaki K, Ikeda M, Kurimoto M. Indirubin inhibits inflammatory reactions in delayed-type hypersensitivity. Eur J Pharmacol 2000;410(1):93–100.

2. Grech JN, Li Q, Roufogalis BD, Duck CC. Novel Ca(2+)-ATPase inhibitors from the dried root tubers of *Polygonum multiflorum*. J Nat Prod 1994;57(12):1682–7.

3. Zimmermann ML, Sneden AT. Vanicosides A and B, protein kinase C inhibitors from *Polygonum pensylvanicum*. J Nat Prod 1994;57(2):236–42.

4. Mazzanti G, Battinelli L, Daniele C, Mastroianni CM, Lichtner M, Coletta S, Costantini S. New case of acute hepatitis following the consumption of Shou Wu Pian, a Chinese herbal product derived from *Polygonum multiflorum*. Ann Intern Med 2004;140(7):W30.

5. Park GJ, Mann SP, Ngu MC. Acute hepatitis induced by Shou-Wu-Pian, a herbal product derived from *Polygonum multiflorum* J Gastroenterol Hepatol 2001;16(1):115–17.

6. But PP, Tomlinson B, Lee KL. Hepatitis related to the Chinese medicine Shou-wu-pian manufactured from *Polygonum multiflorum*. Vet Hum Toxicol 1996;38(4):280–2.
7. Mantani N, Kogure T, Sakai S, Kainuma M, Kasahara Y, Niizawa A, Shimada Y, Terasawa K. A comparative study between excess-dose users and regular-dose users of rhubarb contained in Kampo medicines. Phytomedicine 2002; 9(5):373–6.
8. Mantani N, Sekiya N, Sakai S, Kogure T, Shimada Y, Terasawa K. Rhubarb use in patients treated with Kampo medicines—a risk for gastric cancer? Yakugaku Zasshi 2002;122(6):403–5.

Polyhexanide

See also Disinfectants and antiseptics

General Information

Polyhexanide is a polymerized form of chlorhexidine, used as a disinfectant (1).

Organs and Systems

Immunologic

Severe anaphylaxis occurred in an 18-year-old woman and a 15-year-old man when polyhexanide was used to clean surgical wounds (2). Immediate-type hypersensitivity to polyhexanide was suggested by positive skin prick tests. Both patients had previously been exposed to chlorhexidine, but skin tests with chlorhexidine were negative.

References

1. Kramer A, Behrens-Baumann W. Prophylactic use of topical anti-infectives in ophthalmology. Ophthalmologica 1997;211(Suppl 1):68–76.
2. Olivieri J, Eigenmann PA, Hauser C. Severe anaphylaxis to a new disinfectant: polyhexanide, a chlorhexidine polymer. Schweiz Med Wochenschr 1998;128(40):1508–11.

Polymyxins

General Information

The polymyxins are antibacterial agents that are produced from different strains of *Bacillus polymyxa*. Because of their poor tissue distribution and their substantial nephrotoxicity and neurotoxicity, they are mainly restricted to topical use. However, they can be considered for serious systemic infections caused by multidrug-resistant Gram-negative bacteria (1–4).

The polymyxins that are used clinically are polymyxin B (rINN) and colistin (pINN, formerly known as polymyxin E). Colistimethate sodium (rINN, also called colistin methanesulfonate and colistin sulfomethate sodium) is prepared from colistin.

The polymyxins are cationic, basic, and amphipathic polypeptides that interact with lipopolysaccharides in the outer membrane of bacilli. They potently neutralize endotoxin, reduce blood endotoxin concentrations in patients with septic shock during direct hemoperfusion over immobilized polymyxin B fibers, and are bactericidal for many Gram-negative rods, even in resting bacteria. Alteration of the cell wall is also thought to be the mechanism of damage to renal epithelia and to the nervous system.

The polymyxins are effective against Gram-negative bacteria, with the exception of *Proteus* and *Neisseria* (*Branhamella*). They have in the past been used particularly to treat infections due to *Pseudomonas*, including inhalation therapy in patients with cystic fibrosis (5). They are prescribed in mg or units; 1 mg of polymyxin B corresponds to 10 000 units and 1 mg of colistin corresponds to 20 000–30 000 units.

After intravenous colistimethate (5 mg/kg/day) the CSF concentration was 25% of the serum concentration in a patient with meningitis (6). For life-threatening meningitis due to such organisms, polymyxins can also be given intrathecally as adjunctive therapy (7). Polymyxins are also used in regimens of selective decontamination of the digestive tract (8).

Observational studies

In a randomized study of the effects of a triple antibiotic ointment (polymyxin B + bacitracin + neomycin) and simple gauze-type dressings on scarring of dermabrasion wounds, the ointment was superior to the simple dressing in minimizing scarring; the beneficial effect on pigmentary changes was especially pronounced (9).

General adverse effects

Even in patients with normal renal function, adverse reactions have occurred in up to 25%, contributing to death in 5% (10). At therapeutically equivalent doses, suggestions of differences in nephrotoxicity or neurotoxicity between polymyxin B and colistin are not convincing. In view of their potential for adverse effects, the polymyxins have now been largely replaced by other antibacterial drugs.

Organs and Systems

Respiratory

The polymyxins are bronchial irritants, probably by histamine release (11). This reaction can be very rapid and resistant to bronchodilators.

In 58 children with bronchoconstriction in response to nebulized colistin, FEV_1 was significantly reduced for 15 minutes (12). In 20 children the reduction was greater than 10% from baseline FEV_1 and was still at that level in five children after 30 minutes. Subjective assessment, baseline FEV_1, and serum IgE did not distinguish susceptible children.

In 62 children with cystic fibrosis there was increased dyspnea in seven and pharyngitis in three in response to nebulized colistimethate (80 mg dissolved in 3 ml of preservative-free isotonic saline, by inhalation twice daily for 4 weeks) (13).

Nervous system

During treatment with any of the polymyxins, neurotoxicity can occur in up to 7% of patients with normal renal function. Circumoral paresthesia, vasomotor instability, ataxia, dizziness, convulsions of varying severity, and apnea have been reported. Of 31 patients with cystic fibrosis 21 had one or more adverse effects attributed to colistin (14). The most common reactions involved reversible neurological effects, including oral and perioral paresthesia ($n = 16$), headache ($n = 5$), and lower limb weakness ($n = 5$). All of these effects, although bothersome, were benign and reversible. There was no relation between the occurrence of any colistin-associated adverse effect and plasma colistin concentration or colistin pharmacokinetics.

Meningeal irritation rarely occurs in daily doses of 50 000 units (5 mg) given intrathecally, but higher doses can cause a stiff neck with CSF pleocytosis (15).

In animals the polymyxins can cause neuromuscular blockade similar to that observed with the aminoglycosides, aggravated by curare, ether, and suxamethonium, and antagonized by calcium. This can be noted first as fatiguability 1–26 hours after dosing, and can progress to severe muscular weakness, including respiratory paralysis (11). This complication has been reported both in neurologically normal subjects exposed to high plasma concentrations of the polymyxins, and also in some individuals with concentrations that were considered to be in the target range. Particularly at risk are patients with myasthenia gravis, who may require increased doses of neostigmine.

In patients with chronic pulmonary disease, polymyxin-induced neuromuscular block can result in fatal apnea. Finally, after anesthesia involving muscle relaxants the polymyxins can cause relapse of muscle weakness and inadequate ventilation (16).

Effective treatment of polymyxin-induced neuromuscular blockade requires awareness of the complication, with appropriate supervision and immediate ventilatory support, if required. Calcium gluconate and neostigmine are not of proven efficacy and should not be relied on (11).

Sensory systems

The polymyxins are occasionally ototoxic (17).

Electrolyte balance

Hyponatremia, hypokalemia, and hypocalcemia, with corresponding clinical manifestations, have occurred in patients treated for 3 weeks with doses of polymyxin B over 2 g/m^2 body surface (18,19). These abnormalities were interpreted as consequences of polymyxin-induced nephrotoxicity. Hyperchloremia and a negative anion gap seem to result from the polycationic properties of polymyxin B (20).

Urinary tract

Adverse reactions involving the kidneys occur in about 20% of patients receiving polymyxins (10). The potential for kidney damage seems to be related to age. Whereas in neonates and young infants colistimethate 20 mg/kg may be well tolerated, children over 2 years should not receive more than 10 mg/kg/day and adults even less.

Nephrotoxicity occurs more often in patients with pre-existing impairment of renal function. Doses must be adjusted in patients with renal insufficiency, because colistin is excreted principally by the kidneys, and raised blood concentrations can further impair renal function (21).

Intermittent proteinuria was observed on urinalysis in 14 of 31 patients with cystic fibrosis, and one patient developed reversible, colistin-induced nephrotoxicity (14). There was no relation between the occurrence of any colistin-associated adverse effect and plasma colistin concentration or colistin pharmacokinetics.

Skin

Topical polymyxin B was the predominant allergen in patients who underwent patch-testing for evaluation of eczema of the external ear canal (22).

Immunologic

Compared with their toxic effects, allergic reactions to the polymyxins are relatively unimportant. Nevertheless, drug fever and maculopapular eruptions and other skin lesions have been observed in few patients (23,24).

In 145 patients with eczema of the external ear canal, allergic contact dermatitis was diagnosed in one-third; topical therapeutic agents, especially neomycin sulfate and probably polymyxin B, were the dominating allergens (22).

Long-Term Effects

Drug resistance

The Gram-negative organism *Burkholderia pseudomallei* is the pathogen that causes melioidosis. This bacterium is intrinsically resistant to the killing action of cationic antimicrobial peptides, including polymyxins. An in vitro study has now identified genetic loci that are associated with resistance to polymyxins in a virulent clinical isolate (25). In patients with cystic fibrosis *Pseudomonas aeruginosa* synthesized specific lipid A structures containing palmitate and aminoarabinose, which were associated with resistance to cationic antibiotics and increased inflammatory responses (1).

A two-component regulatory system has been characterized that is involved in the resistance of *P. aeruginosa* in response to external magnesium concentrations (26). Similarly, the PmrA/PmrB two-component system of *Salmonella enterica* that mediates modifications in the lipopolysaccharide, resulting in resistance to polymyxins, has been characterized in more detail (27). The pqaB locus affected polymyxin B resistance in *Salmonella typhi* (28).

All hemolytic and cytotoxic *Aeromonas* species that have been isolated from water samples from various sources were resistant to polymyxin B (29). Resistance to polymyxin B was also found in *Vibrio vulnificus* (30).

Resistance to colistin has been analysed in 44 adults with cystic fibrosis treated with inhaled colistin. Five developed polymyxin resistance (31). After therapy *P. aeruginosa* became sensitive to polymyxins within a few months, enabling the reintroduction of colistin for antibacterial treatment.

Second-Generation Effects

Teratogenicity

Colistin, and probably also polymyxin B, crosses the placenta (32). Although there is no evidence that the polymyxins are teratogenic, they should be avoided in pregnancy.

Drug Administration

Drug formulations

A food additive (flavored BMI-60) may help to mask the bitter taste of polymyxin B sulfate tablets (33).

Drug administration route

Bolus intravenous colistin (160 mg in 10 ml of saline tds) has been studied in a phase I open study during acute respiratory exacerbations in adults with cystic fibrosis and chronic *P. aeruginosa* infection; patients without total indwelling venous access systems had mild to moderate injection-like pain (34).

Intramuscular injection of the sulfates of polymyxin or colistin often causes pain at the site of injection; with sodium colistimethate this adverse reaction is largely absent (35).

In a study of the intrathecal administration of colistin adverse events were not reported (36). This may be an effective alternative treatment of bacterial meningitis caused by multidrug-resistant Gram-negative rods.

During sepsis, toxins (for example released from bacteria) can cause shock, disseminated intravascular coagulation, multiorgan dysfunction, and death. Apheresis may be a way of reducing the amounts of toxins and other harmful compounds in the circulation, and polymyxin B may serve as an adsorber. In three patients with septic shock, direct hemoperfusion using a polymyxin B-immobilized fiber column was carried out after antibacterial and antishock therapy. As a result, cardiovascular instabilities improved without increasing the supply of catecholamines (37). Furthermore, in seven patients with endotoxic shock after laparotomy undergoing hemoperfusion with the polymyxin B-immobilized fiber, there was an early increase in urine volume, attributable to increased glomerular filtration independent of systemic hemodynamic factors (38).

Drug overdose

If patients have high plasma concentrations of polymixins, neither hemodialysis nor peritoneal dialysis is effective in eliminating them (39). Exchange transfusion has been proposed (40,41).

Drug–Drug Interactions

Neuromuscular blocking drugs

There may be difficulty in reversing neuromuscular blockade if polymyxin is given in combination with neuromuscular blocking drugs (42).

References

1. Ernst RK, Yi EC, Guo L, Lim KB, Burns JL, Hackett M, Miller SI. Specific lipopolysaccharide found in cystic fibrosis airway *Pseudomonas aeruginosa*. Science 1999;286(5444):1561–5.
2. Asanuma Y, Furuya T, Tanaka J, Sato T, Shibata S, Koyama K. The application of immobilized polymyxin B fiber in the treatment of septic shock associated with severe acute pancreatitis: report of two cases. Surg Today 1999;29(11):1177–82.
3. Nakamura T, Ebihara I, Shoji H, Ushiyama C, Suzuki S, Koide H. Treatment with polymyxin B-immobilized fiber reduces platelet activation in septic shock patients: decrease in plasma levels of soluble P-selectin, platelet factor 4 and beta-thromboglobulin. Inflamm Res 1999; 48(4):171–5.
4. Hellman J, Warren HS. Antiendotoxin strategies. Infect Dis Clin North Am 1999;13(2):371–86, ix.
5. Mordasini C, Aebischer CC, Schoch OD. Zur inhalativen Antibiotika-Therapie bei Patienten mit zystischer Fibrose und *Pseudomonas*-Befall. [Inhalational antibiotic therapy in patients with cystic fibrosis and *Pseudomonas* infection.] Schweiz Med Wochenschr 1997;127(21):905–10.
6. Jimenez-Mejias ME, Pichardo-Guerrero C, Marquez-Rivas FJ, Martin-Lozano D, Prados T, Pachon J. Cerebrospinal fluid penetration and pharmacokinetic/pharmacodynamic parameters of intravenously administered colistin in a case of multidrug-resistant *Acinetobacter baumannii* meningitis. Eur J Clin Microbiol Infect Dis 2002;21(3):212–14.
7. Segal-Maurer S, Mariano N, Qavi A, Urban C, Rahal JJ Jr. Successful treatment of ceftazidime-resistant *Klebsiella pneumoniae* ventriculitis with intravenous meropenem and intraventricular polymyxin B: case report and review. Clin Infect Dis 1999;28(5):1134–8.
8. Rommes JH, Zandstra DF, van Saene HK. Selectieve darmdecontaminatie voorkomt sterfte bij intensive-carepatienten. [Selective decontamination of the digestive tract reduces mortality in intensive care patients.] Ned Tijdschr Geneeskd 1999;143(12):602–6.
9. Berger RS, Pappert AS, Van Zile PS, Cetnarowski WE. A newly formulated topical triple-antibiotic ointment minimizes scarring. Cutis 2000;65(6):401–4.
10. Koch-Weser J, Sidel VW, Federman EB, Kanarek P, Finer DC, Eaton AE. Adverse effects of sodium colistimethate. Manifestations and specific reaction rates during 317 courses of therapy. Ann Intern Med 1970;72(6):857–68.
11. Lindesmith LA, Baines RD Jr, Bigelow DB, Petty TL. Reversible respiratory paralysis associated with polymyxin therapy. Ann Intern Med 1968;68(2):318–27.
12. Cunningham S, Prasad A, Collyer L, Carr S, Lynn IB, Wallis C. Bronchoconstriction following nebulised colistin in cystic fibrosis. Arch Dis Child 2001;84(5):432–3.
13. Nikolaizik WH, Trociewicz K, Ratjen F. Bronchial reactions to the inhalation of high-dose tobramycin in cystic fibrosis. Eur Respir J 2002;20(1):122–6.
14. Reed MD, Stern RC, O'Riordan MA, Blumer JL. The pharmacokinetics of colistin in patients with cystic fibrosis. J Clin Pharmacol 2001;41(6):645–54.
15. Everett ED, Strausbaugh LJ. Antimicrobial agents and the central nervous system. Neurosurgery 1980;6(6):691–714.
16. Sobek V. Arrest of respiration induced by polypeptide antibiotics. Arzneimittelforschung 1982;32(3):235–7.
17. Linder TE, Zwicky S, Brandle P. Ototoxicity of ear drops: a clinical perspective. Am J Otol 1995;16(5):653–7.
18. O'Regan S, Carson S, Chesney RW, Drummond KN. Electrolyte and acid-base disturbances in the management of leukemia. Blood 1977;49(3):345–53.

19. Rodriguez V, Green S, Bodey GP. Serum electrolyte abnormalities associated with the administration of polymyxin B in febrile leukemic patients. Clin Pharmacol Ther 1970;11(1):106–11.

20. O'Connor DT, Stone RA. Hyperchloremia and negative anion gap associated with polymyxin B administration. Arch Intern Med 1978;138(3):478–80.

21. Stein A, Raoult D. Colistin: an antimicrobial for the 21st century? Clin Infect Dis 2002;35(7):901–2.

22. Hillen U, Geier J, Goos M. Kontaktallergien bei Patienten mit Ekzemen des ausseren Gehorgangs. Ergebnisse des Informationsverbundes Dermatologischer Kliniken und der Deutschen Kontaktallergie-Gruppe. [Contact allergies in patients with eczema of the external ear canal. Results of the Information Network of Dermatological Clinics and the German Contact Allergy Group.] Hautarzt 2000;51(4):239–43.

23. Sasaki S, Mitsuhashi Y, Kondo S. Contact dermatitis due to sodium colistimethate. J Dermatol 1998;25(6):415–17.

24. Zehnder D, Kunzi UP, Maibach R, Zoppi M, Halter F, Neftel KA, Muller U, Galeazzi RL, Hess T, Hoigne R. Die Häufigkeit der Antibiotika-assoziierten Kolitis bei hospitalisierten Patienten der Jahre 1974–1991 im "Comprehensive Hospital Drug Monitoring" Bern/St. Gallen. [Frequency of antibiotics-associated colitis in hospitalized patients in 1974–1991 in "Comprehensive Hospital Drug Monitoring", Bern/St. Gallen.] Schweiz Med Wochenschr 1995;125(14):676–83.

25. Burtnick MN, Woods DE. Isolation of polymyxin B-susceptible mutants of *Burkholderia pseudomallei* and molecular characterization of genetic loci involved in polymyxin B resistance. Antimicrob Agents Chemother 1999;43(11):2648–56.

26. Macfarlane EL, Kwasnicka A, Ochs MM, Hancock RE. PhoP-PhoQ homologues in *Pseudomonas aeruginosa* regulate expression of the outer-membrane protein OprH and polymyxin B resistance. Mol Microbiol 1999;34(2):305–16.

27. Wosten MM, Groisman EA. Molecular characterization of the PmrA regulon. J Biol Chem 1999;274(38):27185–90.

28. Baker SJ, Gunn JS, Morona R. The *Salmonella typhi* melittin resistance gene pqaB affects intracellular growth in PMA-differentiated U937 cells, polymyxin B resistance and lipopolysaccharide. Microbiology 1999;145(Pt 2):367–78.

29. Alavandi SV, Subashini MS, Ananthan S. Occurrence of haemolytic & cytotoxic *Aeromonas* species in domestic water supplies in Chennai. Indian J Med Res 1999;110:50–5.

30. Ghinsberg RC, Dror R, Nitzan Y. Isolation of *Vibrio vulnificus* from sea water and sand along the Dan region coast of the Mediterranean. Microbios 1999;97(386):7–17.

31. Tamm M, Eich C, Frei R, Gilgen S, Breitenbucher A, Mordasini C. Inhalatives Colistin bei zystischer fibrose. [Inhaled colistin in cystic fibrosis.] Schweiz Med Wochenschr 2000;130(39):1366–72.

32. MacAulay MA, Charles D, Burgess FM. Placental transmission of colistimethate. Clin Pharmacol Ther 1967;8(4):578–86.

33. Saito M, Hoshi M, Igarashi A, Ogata H, Edo K. The marked inhibition of the bitter taste of polymyxin B sulfate and trimethoprim × sulfamethoxazole by flavored BMI-60 in pediatric patients. Biol Pharm Bull 1999;22(9):997–8.

34. Conway SP, Etherington C, Munday J, Goldman MH, Strong JJ, Wootton M. Safety and tolerability of bolus intravenous colistin in acute respiratory exacerbations in adults with cystic fibrosis. Ann Pharmacother 2000;34(11):1238–42.

35. Kucers A, Bennett NM. Polymixins. Philadelphia: Lippincott, 1987:905–17.

36. Vasen W, Desmery P, Ilutovich S, Di Martino A. Intrathecal use of colistin. J Clin Microbiol 2000;38(9):3523.

37. Yuasa J, Naya Y, Tanaka M, Amakasu M, Yamaguchi K. [Clinical experiences of endotoxin removal columns in septic shock due to urosepsis: report of three cases.] Hinyokika Kiyo 2000;46(11):819–22.

38. Terawaki H, Kasai K, Kobayashi H, Hirano K, Hamaguchi A, Kase Y, Horiguchi T, Yokoyama K, Yamamoto H, Nakayama M, Kawaguchi Y, Hosoya T. [A study on the mechanism of enhanced diuresis following direct hemoperfusion with polymyxin B-immobilized fiber.] Nippon Jinzo Gakkai Shi 2000;42(5):359–64.

39. Goodwin NJ, Friedman EA. The effects of renal impairment, peritoneal dialysis, and hemodialysis on serum sodium colistimethate levels. Ann Intern Med 1968; 68(5):984–94.

40. Hoeprich PD. The polymyxins. Med Clin North Am 1970;54(5):1257–65.

41. Brown JM, Dorman DC, Roy LP. Acute renal failure due to overdosage of colistin. Med J Aust 1970;2(20):923–4.

42. Cammu G. Interactions of neuromuscular blocking drugs. Acta Anaesthesiol Belg 2001;52(4):357–63.

Polystyrene sulfonates

General Information

Polystyrene sulfonic acid has been used as sodium, potassium, and calcium salts. Sodium polystyrene sulfonate has been used to treat hyperkalemia in patients with renal insufficiency and as an adjuvant during hemodialysis. It can be given orally or rectally in all age groups (1). It has also been added to feeding formulae and nutritional supplements to reduce their potassium contents and so prevent hyperkalemia; however, the reduction in potassium content was more than balanced by a concomitant increase in sodium content, presumably because of exchange of the sodium with calcium and magnesium (2,3). The uses and adverse effects of sodium polystyrene sulfonate have been reviewed (4,5).

Potassium polystyrene sulfonate has been used to treat hypercalciuria and renal calculi. Calcium polystyrene sulfonate has been used to treat hyperkalemia, particularly in patients who cannot tolerate the extra sodium that would be provided by the sodium salt.

A confection containing sodium polystyrene sulfonate resin 5.0 g per piece was used to treat six chronic dialysis patients with predialysis serum potassium concentrations of 5.2 mmol/l or more (6). Over 2 weeks the mean serum potassium fell by 0.7 mmol/l. However, the effectiveness of sodium polystyrene sulfonate in lowering serum potassium concentrations in patients with renal insufficiency has been questioned (7). A cathartic alone (phenolphthalein) in six patients caused an average fecal potassium output of 54 mmol. The addition of sodium polystyrene sulfonate had no further significant effect on total potassium output. With placebo the average serum potassium concentration increased slightly (0.4 mmol/l) during 12 hours. This rise was attenuated by sodium polystyrene sulfonate, perhaps in part because of extracellular volume expansion caused by the absorption of sodium. Phenolphthalein was associated with a slight rise in serum potassium concentration (similar to placebo), perhaps because of extracellular volume contraction produced by a sodium-rich diarrhea and acidosis secondary to bicarbonate loss. None of the regimens reduced the serum potassium concentration, compared with baseline.

Organs and Systems

Respiratory

Pneumonitis has been reported in a woman taking sodium polystyrene sulfonate (8).

Electrolyte balance

Sodium polystyrene sulfonate can cause hypokalemia, hypocalcemia, and hypernatremia (4,5).

Calcium polystyrene sulfonate can cause hypokalemia and hypercalcemia (4,5).

Acid–base balance

Cation-containing antacids and laxatives (for example magnesium hydroxide, calcium carbonate) can reduce the effect of polystyrene sulfonate and metabolic acidosis can develop. This has been reported in both children (9,10) and adults.

- A patient with end-stage renal disease undergoing long-term maintenance hemodialysis developed moderately severe metabolic alkalosis in the absence of vomiting or gastric drainage (10). The cause of the acid–base disorder was the oral administration of exogenous alkali, in the form of "non-absorbable" antacids (aluminium hydroxide and magnesium hydroxide), neutral phosphate, and sodium polystyrene sulfonate.
- In a patient with chronic renal insufficiency, chronic hypocalcemia plus severe metabolic alkalosis due to combined administration of sodium polystyrene sulfonate and magnesium hydroxide caused a generalized tonic-clonic seizure (11).

Hematologic

Thrombocytopenia has been attributed to sodium polystyrene sulfonate (Kayexalate) (12).

- An 84-year-old man with diabetes mellitus and hypertension had gradually worsening renal insufficiency with hyperkalemia and was given oral sodium polystyrene sulfonate (Kayexalate). After 7 days he developed gradually worsening thrombocytopenia, and 12 days later his platelet count, which had initially been $207 \times 10^9/l$, fell to $86 \times 10^9/l$. The thrombocytopenia rapidly improved after withdrawal of the sodium polystyrene sulfonate. At a later date readministration of sodium polystyrene sulfonate for the treatment of hyperkalemia again caused thrombocytopenia. Bone marrow aspiration biopsy showed normal numbers of nucleated cells and megakaryocytes with no increase in blast count. No other disorders which could have caused thrombocytopenia were seen in this patient.

Gastrointestinal

After oral administration the polystyrene sulfonates commonly cause anorexia, nausea, vomiting, and constipation (4,5).

Esophagus, stomach, and duodenum

Upper gastrointestinal damage associated with sodium polystyrene sulfonate in sorbitol is reported far less often than colonic damage. However, endoscopic appearances were markedly abnormal in 11 patients with crystals of sodium polystyrene sulfonate in biopsies from the esophagus ($n = 7$), stomach ($n = 6$), and duodenum ($n = 2$), in some cases closely mimicking other diagnoses, including esophageal carcinoma, *Candida* esophagitis, and gastric bezoar (13). There was histological and/or endoscopic evidence of mucosal injury in the form of an ulcer or erosion in nine patients, and in four patients with mucosal injury, no other cause could be identified.

Esophageal ulceration has occasionally been attributed to sodium polystyrene sulfonate (14).

- An 83-year-old man with septic shock and renal insufficiency after prostatectomy was given sodium polystyrene sulfonate for hyperkalemia and developed a 3 cm esophageal ulcer. Crystals of sodium polystyrene sulfonate were found in a biopsy.

In five infants of extremely low birth weights, who were given either sodium polystyrene sulfonate or calcium polystyrene sulfonate orally for hyperkalemia, masses were palpable in the left upper quadrant of the abdomen and visible radiographically as opaque masses in the stomach (15). At autopsy, the palpable mass was identified as a solid chalk-like concretion and X-ray diffraction showed that the material was Brushite. The authors suggested that oral exchange resins should not be used in critically ill, extremely low birth-weight infants.

Small bowel

In 15 patients who were given sodium polystyrene sulfonate (Kayexalate) in sorbitol as an enema or orally to treat hyperkalemia, sodium polystyrene sulfonate crystals were observed in specimens from gastrointestinal surgical resections ($n = 9$) or endoscopic biopsies ($n = 7$) (16). There was necrosis in seven of eight surgical resection specimens and three of five endoscopic biopsy specimens; four also had necrosis of the small intestine. Four patients with colonic necrosis in the initial resection specimen developed progressive necrosis of the small intestine or rectum, and five died within 1 day to 6 weeks. There were sodium polystyrene sulfonate crystals in upper gastrointestinal tract specimens from four patients, including one with hemorrhagic gastritis.

The incidence of intestinal necrosis has been estimated in 752 hospitalized patients who had received sodium polystyrene sulfonate, of whom 117 were exposed within 1 week of surgery (17). There were two cases of intestinal necrosis, both in patients who had received oral sodium polystyrene sulfonate in sorbitol. Based on these two cases, the postoperative incidence of intestinal necrosis associated with sodium polystyrene sulfonate was 1.8%. In 862 patients, who had undergone hemodialysis, renal transplantation, or cardiac transplantation, but had not received sodium polystyrene sulfonate, there were no cases of idiopathic intestinal necrosis.

With high doses, intestinal impaction can occur and this has been associated with perforation (18).

- A 650-g, 24-week-old neonate with hyperkalemia was given sodium polystyrene sulfonate enemas and developed cecal impaction and perforation. Abdominal radiographs showed radiodense impacted resin outlining the bowel. Pathological examination showed sodium polystyrene sulfonate crystals in a cecal abscess.

Large bowel

After rectal and oral administration, intestinal ulcers and necrosis have occurred (13,19). Several cases affecting the large bowel have been reported and critically ill and uremic patients are at particular risk.

- A 67-year-old man underwent laparotomy for a ruptured abdominal aortic aneurysm (20). Postoperatively he was treated with hemodialysis because of acute renal insufficiency. Hyperkalemia was treated with sodium polystyrene sulfonate, after which he developed ulceration of the colon and required a hemicolectomy because of intractable blood loss.
- Two patients, who had died after cardiac surgery, were in renal insufficiency, and had received sodium polystyrene sulfonate in sorbitol, had colonic luminal crystals of sodium polystyrene sulfonate associated with underlying mucosal necrosis, submucosal edema, and transmural inflammation (21).
- In a patient who developed near-total colonic necrosis shortly after renal transplantation, the onset of symptoms was temporally related to the administration of sodium polystyrene sulfonate plus sorbitol enemas (Kayexalate) for hyperkalemia (22).
- In another case, colonic necrosis presented as an acute abdomen within 24 hours of administration of sodium polystyrene sulfonate in sorbitol (23). After prompt surgical resection of the necrotic transverse colon there was rapid recovery of bowel function.
- A 53-year-old woman took sodium polystyrene sulfonate 15 g twice, 8 days apart, and 15 days later developed colonic necrosis and perforation; there were crystals of sodium polystyrene sulfonate in the inflammatory debris (24).
- An 81-year-old woman with chronic renal insufficiency, who had taken sodium polystyrene sulfonate 2 spoons/day, developed a 3–4 cm ulcer at 45 cm from the anal margin, with crystals of sodium polystyrene sulfonate in the biopsy (25).
- A 74-year-old woman with chronic renal insufficiency, who had taken sodium polystyrene sulfonate 1–2 spoons/day, developed cecal ulceration, with crystals of sodium polystyrene sulfonate in the biopsy (25).
- A giant diverticulum in the sigmoid colon has been attributed to inflammation due to sodium polystyrene sulfonate crystals in a 44-year-old man who had taken 15 mg/day for 2 years (25).

Colonic perforation has been attributed to calcium polystyrene sulfonate in a premature infant (26).

- A boy delivered at 28 weeks was given calcium polystyrene sulfonate 0.2 mg rectally for hyperkalemia (7.1 mmol/l). His abdomen, already distended, became larger with abdominal wall discoloration. An X-ray showed distended loops of bowel and at laparotomy he was found to have a perforation at the rectosigmoid junction.

While crystals of sodium polystyrene sulfonate, which are purple, irregular, and jagged, can be an incidental finding and are not known to cause injury, they are a helpful histological clue to the possibility that sorbitol has been administered (16). Five cases of extensive mucosal necrosis and transmural infarction of the colon have been reported after the use of sodium polystyrene sulfonate (Kayexalate) and sorbitol enemas to treat hyperkalemia in uremic patients (27). The authors also studied the effects of Kayexalate sorbitol enemas in normal and uremic rats and concluded that sorbitol was responsible for colonic damage and that the injury was potentiated in uremic rats. When sorbitol alone or Kayexalate sorbitol was given, extensive transmural necrosis developed in 80% of normal rats and in all the uremic rats. Because uremia and the concomitant use of sorbitol appear to be common denominators in the pathophysiology of this complication, some have suggested that Kayexalate enemas be avoided in renal transplant patients (22). Following reports of colonic necrosis, the Pharmaceutical Affairs Bureau of Japan revised the product information for enemas of polystyrene sulfonate cation exchange resin suspension in sorbitol solution for potassium removal (28).

Two other cases of neonatal bowel opacification secondary to oral and rectal sodium polystyrene sulfonate have been reported (29). Abdominal radiography showed a faint homogeneous increase in density within the bowel lumen.

Hematochezia in a neonate who had been given sodium polystyrene sulfonate enemas prompted a review of the use of such enemas in 20 of 2317 patients (30). Of these 20 patients, four had evidence of hematochezia temporally related to the use of the enemas. There were no episodes of bleeding in infants who were older than 29 weeks or over 1250 g birth weight. In one case, an autopsy performed within 2 days of the enema showed extensive vascular congestion in the mucosa and submucosa, with focal areas of hemorrhage. Sorbitol 20% (1098 mosm/l) was the vehicle for suspension of the sodium polystyrene sulfonate, and the authors thought that the hyperosmolarity of sorbitol had contributed to the colonic damage in these children.

Drug Administration

Drug formulations

Drugs that have similar names are not infrequently confused. The name of Sanofi-Synthelabo's brand of sodium polystyrene sulfonate, Kayexalate, could be confused with the names of proprietary brands of potassium chloride, such as Kay-Cee-L and Kay-Ciel. Furthermore, some formulations of potassium chloride are formulated in packaging that resembles that of Kayexalate. There have been two deaths when potassium chloride was given instead of sodium polystyrene sulfonate for hyperkalemia (31).

Drug–Drug Interactions

Iron

It has been suggested that sodium polystyrene sulfonate might be useful in treating iron overdose, since it binds iron in vitro with high affinity (32). However, in a placebo-controlled crossover study in six healthy adults sodium polystyrene sulfonate 30 g had no significant effect on the kinetics of an oral dose of elemental iron 10 mg/kg (33).

Lithium

Sodium polystyrene sulfonate binds lithium in vitro (34); it is more effective than charcoal, but has a higher affinity for potassium (35). In healthy volunteers who took a single dose of lithium carbonate 600 mg, sodium polystyrene sulfonate 30 g reduced the area under the lithium serum concentration-time curve by 11%, reduced the mean C_{max} by 0.07 mmol/l, and delayed the t_{max} by 2.04 hours (36). In six young healthy volunteers who took lithium carbonate 0.5 mmol/kg (18.5 mg/kg), sodium polystyrene sulfonate 857 mg/kg in 4 ml of water/g taken 1 hour later reduced the mean AUC by 15% and the C_{max} by 0.20 mmol/l (37). There was no significant difference in 24-hour urine lithium excretion or in serum sodium and potassium concentrations. Both of these results suggest that sodium polystyrene sulfonate reduces the absorption of lithium. Furthermore, sodium polystyrene sulfonate increased the clearance of oral lithium in a volunteer when given 30 minutes after each dose of lithium (38). For these reasons it has been used to treat lithium overdose (39,40). However, it can cause hypokalemia and is not currently recommended as routine therapy (41).

Tetracyclines

Since calcium salts can bind tetracyclines, leading to reduced absorption (SED-14, 910), an interaction of this kind might be expected with calcium polystyrene sulfonate, but it does not seem to have been reported.

References

1. Meyer I. Sodium polystyrene sulfonate: a cation exchange resin used in treating hyperkalemia. ANNA J 1993;20(1):93–5.
2. Bunchman TE, Wood EG, Schenck MH, Weaver KA, Klein BL, Lynch RE. Pretreatment of formula with sodium polystyrene sulfonate to reduce dietary potassium intake. Pediatr Nephrol 1991;5(1):29–32.
3. Fassinger N, Dabbagh S, Mukhopadhyay S, Lee DY. Mineral content of infant formula after treatment with sodium polystyrene sulfonate or calcium polystyrene sulfonate. Adv Perit Dial 1998;14:274–7.
4. Takasu T. [Treatment of hyperkalemia associated with renal insufficiency—clinical effects and side reactions of positive-ion-exchange resins, sodium polystyrene sulfonate (Kayexalate).] Nippon Rinsho 1970;28(7):1941–6.
5. Osawa A, Okoshi M, Higuchi J, Yamayoshi W. [Treatment of hyperkalemia in renal insufficiency with cation exchange resin. Experience with use of sodium polystyrene sulfonate.] Hinyokika Kiyo 1969;15(9):645–51.
6. Johnson K, Cazee C, Gutch C, Ogden D. Sodium polystyrene sulfonate resin candy for control of potassium in chronic dialysis patients. Clin Nephrol 1976;5(6):266–8.
7. Gruy-Kapral C, Emmett M, Santa Ana CA, Porter JL, Fordtran JS, Fine KD. Effect of single dose resin-cathartic therapy on serum potassium concentration in patients with end-stage renal disease. J Am Soc Nephrol 1998;9(10):1924–30.
8. Haupt HM, Hutchins GM. Sodium polystyrene sulfonate pneumonitis. Arch Intern Med 1982;142(2):379–81.
9. Nassif F, Sinnassamy P, Bensman A. Une cause d'alcalose chez l'enfant hémodialyse: la coadministration d'hydroxyde de magnesium et de polystyrene sulfonate de sodium. [A cause of alkalosis in children under hemodialysis: combined administration of magnesium hydroxide and polystyrene sodium sulfonate.] Presse Méd 1987;16(20):1003.
10. Madias NE, Levey AS. Metabolic alkalosis due to absorption of "nonabsorbable" antacids. Am J Med 1983;74(1):155–8.
11. Ziessman HA. Alkalosis and seizure due to a cation-exchange resin and magnesium hydroxide. South Med J 1976;69(4):497–9.
12. Mogi Y, Kura T, Takimoto R, Muto F, Maeda T, Muramatsu H, Niitsu Y. [Thrombocytopenia associated with sodium polystyrene sulfonate.] Rinsho Ketsueki 1997;38(11):1224–8.
13. Abraham SC, Bhagavan BS, Lee LA, Rashid A, Wu TT. Upper gastrointestinal tract injury in patients receiving Kayexalate (sodium polystyrene sulfonate) in sorbitol: clinical, endoscopic, and histopathologic findings. Am J Surg Pathol 2001;25(5):637–44.
14. Moguelet P, Houdouin L, Bertheau P, Boudaoud S, Hassani Z, Eurin B, Janin A. Une ulcération oesophagienne. [An esophageal ulcer.] Ann Pathol 2002;22(6):487–8.
15. Ohlsson A, Hosking M. Complications following oral administration of exchange resins in extremely low-birth-weight infants. Eur J Pediatr 1987;146(6):571–4.
16. Rashid A, Hamilton SR. Necrosis of the gastrointestinal tract in uremic patients as a result of sodium polystyrene sulfonate (Kayexalate) in sorbitol: an underrecognized condition. Am J Surg Pathol 1997;21(1):60–9.
17. Gerstman BB, Kirkman R, Platt R. Intestinal necrosis associated with postoperative orally administered sodium polystyrene sulfonate in sorbitol. Am J Kidney Dis 1992;20(2):159–61.
18. Bennett LN, Myers TF, Lambert GH. Cecal perforation associated with sodium polystyrene sulfonate–sorbitol enemas in a 650 gram infant with hyperkalemia. Am J Perinatol 1996;13(3):167–70.
19. Rogers FB, Li SC. Acute colonic necrosis associated with sodium polystyrene sulfonate (Kayexalate) enemas in a critically ill patient: case report and review of the literature. J Trauma 2001;51(2):395–7.
20. Schiere S, Karrenbeld A, Tulleken JE, van der Werf TS, Zijlstra JG. Natriumpolystyreensulfonaat (Resonium A) als mogelijke oorzaak van rectaal bloedverlies. [Sodium polystyrene sulfonate (Resonium A) as possible cause of rectal blood loss.] Ned Tijdschr Geneeskd 1997;141(44):2127–9.
21. Gardiner GW. Kayexalate (sodium polystyrene sulphonate) in sorbitol associated with intestinal necrosis in uremic patients. Can J Gastroenterol 1997;11(7):573–7.
22. Scott TR, Graham SM, Schweitzer EJ, Bartlett ST. Colonic necrosis following sodium polystyrene sulfonate (Kayexalate)-sorbitol enema in a renal transplant patient. Report of a case and review of the literature. Dis Colon Rectum 1993;36(6):607–9.
23. Dardik A, Moesinger RC, Efron G, Barbul A, Harrison MG. Acute abdomen with colonic necrosis induced by Kayexalate–sorbitol. South Med J 2000;93(5):511–3.
24. Cheng ES, Stringer KM, Pegg SP. Colonic necrosis and perforation following oral sodium polystyrene sulfonate (Resonium A/Kayexalate) in a burn patient. Burns 2002;28(2):189–90.
25. Mulder JW, Offerhaus GJ, Drillenburg P, Busch OR. "Giant diverticulum" sigmoid colon. J Am Coll Surg 2002;195(1):130.
26. Grammatikopoulos T, Greenough A, Pallidis C, Davenport M. Benefits and risks of calcium resonium therapy in hyperkalaemic preterm infants. Acta Paediatr 2003;92(1):118–20.

27. Lillemoe KD, Romolo JL, Hamilton SR, Pennington LR, Burdick JF, Williams GM. Intestinal necrosis due to sodium polystyrene (Kayexalate) in sorbitol enemas: clinical and experimental support for the hypothesis. Surgery 1987;101(3):267–72.

28. Anonymous. Sorbitol as a solvent for cation exchange resin enemas composed of polystyrene sulfonate-revised data sheet-colonic necrosis. WHO Newslett 1996;5/6:4.

29. Sherman S, Friedman AP, Berdon WE, Haller JO. Kayexalate: a new cause of neonatal bowel opacification. Radiology 1981;138(1):63–4.

30. Milley JR, Jung AL. Hematochezia associated with the use of hypertonic sodium polystyrene sulfonate enemas in premature infants. J Perinatol 1995;15(2):139–42.

31. Kaplan M, Summerfield MR, Pestaner JP. Mix-up between potassium chloride and sodium polystyrene sulfonate. Am J Health Syst Pharm 2002;59(18):1786–7.

32. O'Connor TA, Gruner BA, Gehrke JC, Watling SM, Gehrke CW. In vitro binding of iron with the cation-exchange resin sodium polystyrene sulfonate. Ann Emerg Med 1996;28(5):504–7.

33. Shepherd G, Klein-Schwartz W, Burstein AH. Efficacy of the cation exchange resin, sodium polystyrene sulfonate, to decrease iron absorption. J Toxicol Clin Toxicol 2000;38(4):389–94.

34. Linakis JG, Savitt DL, Lockhart GR, Trainor B, Lacouture PG, Lewander WJ. In vitro binding of lithium using the cation exchange resin sodium polystyrene sulfonate. Am J Emerg Med 1995;13(6):669–70.

35. Watling SM, Gehrke JC, Gehrke CW, Zumwalt R, Pribble J. In vitro binding of lithium using the cation exchange resin sodium polystyrene sulfonate. Am J Emerg Med 1995;13(3):294–6.

36. Belanger DR, Tierney MG, Dickinson G. Effect of sodium polystyrene sulfonate on lithium bioavailability. Ann Emerg Med 1992;21(11):1312–5.

37. Tomaszewski C, Musso C, Pearson JR, Kulig K, Marx JA. Lithium absorption prevented by sodium polystyrene sulfonate in volunteers. Ann Emerg Med 1992;21(11):1308–11.

38. Gehrke JC, Watling SM, Gehrke CW, Zumwalt R. In-vivo binding of lithium using the cation exchange resin sodium polystyrene sulfonate. Am J Emerg Med 1996;14(1):37–8.

39. Dupuis RE, Cooper AA, Rosamond LJ, Campbell-Bright S. Multiple delayed peak lithium concentrations following acute intoxication with an extended-release product. Ann Pharmacother 1996;30(4):356–60.

40. Roberge RJ, Martin TG, Schneider SM. Use of sodium polystyrene sulfonate in a lithium overdose. Ann Emerg Med 1993;22(12):1911–5.

41. Scharman EJ. Methods used to decrease lithium absorption or enhance elimination. J Toxicol Clin Toxicol 1997; 35(6):601–8.

Polytetrafluoroethylene

General Information

Polytetrafluoroethylene (Polytef) is widely used in industry. "Teflon" is used in household appliances to avoid sticking of food. Polytef paste is used for a variety of medical purposes, including replacement grafts in vascular surgery, vocal cord or fold augmentation, and correction of vesicoureteric reflux and urinary incontinence.

The use of polytetrafluoroethylene has become controversial because of reports of granulomatous reactions and distant migration of the material. Foreign body giant cell responses to the polytetrafluoroethylene implant ("teflonoma") have become a serious complication, and animal models have clearly shown a classic foreign body reaction with multinucleated giant cells, granuloma formation, and migration of Teflon into surrounding muscle after Teflon injection (1). Teflon-related granuloma occurred in 1.3% of a series of 155 patients with trigeminal neuralgia treated by microvascular decompression using Teflon (2). Such granulomas can cause compression syndromes at various locations after varying periods of time.

- A patient who had previously undergone suboccipital microvascular decompression for hemifacial spasm presented 3 years postoperatively with a progressive asymmetric sensorineural hearing loss. At surgery a granuloma was found displacing the structures of the internal auditory canal. Histologically, there was evidence of a Teflon fiber-induced giant cell granuloma (3).

Postoperative failure after Teflon sling repair of a rectal prolapse is probably due to poor technique (4).

Organs and Systems

Cardiovascular

Teflon injected in a young woman for urinary incontinence migrated to the pulmonary vascular system (5).

Particles of Teflon can detach from cardiac valve prostheses, producing embolic complications (6).

Nervous system

Periureteral injection of Teflon has been linked to stroke in a previously healthy child 1 year after the procedure (7).

Urinary tract

Refluxing ureters can be treated endoscopically with suburetic injection of polytetrafluoroethylene paste (Polytef), the "STING" procedure. However, ureteric obstruction has been described as a complication (8). Urinary incontinence has also been treated by periurethral or submucosal injections of Polytef, but reports of urinary obstruction (9,10) and poor long-term success (11,12) have limited the range of indications for this treatment. Other reported complications of Teflon injection for stress urinary incontinence include periurethral abscess, urethral diverticulum, Teflon granuloma with urethral wall prolapse (13), and microembolization (14).

Skin

Skin migration following periurethral polytetrafluoroethylene injection for urinary incontinence has been reported (15).

Musculoskeletal

Interposition of Teflon-Proplast implants for internal derangement of the temporomandibular joint has been used, although cases of osseous destructive changes have been reported (16).

References

1. Flint PW, Corio RL, Cummings CW. Comparison of soft tissue response in rabbits following laryngeal implantation with hydroxylapatite, silicone rubber, and Teflon. Ann Otol Rhinol Laryngol 1997;106(5):399–407.
2. Premsagar IC, Moss T, Coakham HB. Teflon-induced granuloma following treatment of trigeminal neuralgia by microvascular decompression. Report of two cases. J Neurosurg 1997;87(3):454–7.
3. Megerian CA, Busaba NY, McKenna MJ, Ojemann RG. Teflon granuloma presenting as an enlarging, gadolinium enhancing, posterior fossa mass with progressive hearing loss following microvascular decompression. Am J Otol 1995;16(6):783–6.
4. Lescher TJ, Corman ML, Coller JA, Veidenheimer MC. Management of late complications of Teflon sling repair for rectal prolapse. Dis Colon Rectum 1979; 22(7):445–7.
5. Claes H, Stroobants D, Van Meerbeek J, Verbeken E, Knockaert D. Pulmonary migration following periurethral polytetrafluoroethylene injection for urinary incontinence. J Urol 1991;145:839–40.
6. Weingarten J, Kauffman SL. Teflon embolization to pulmonary arteries. Ann Thorac Surg 1977;23(4):371–3.
7. Borgatti R, Tettamanti A, Piccinelli P. Brain injury in a healthy child one year after periureteral injection of Teflon. Pediatrics 1996;98(2 Pt 1):290–1.
8. Davies N, Atwell JD. Primary vesicoureteric reflux: treatment with subureteric injection of Polytef paste. Br J Urol 1991;67(5):536–40.
9. Boykin W, Rodriguez FR, Brizzolara JP, Thompson IM, Zeidman EJ. Complete urinary obstruction following periurethral polytetrafluoroethylene injection for urinary incontinence. J Urol 1989;141(5):1199–200.
10. McKinney CD, Gaffey MJ, Gillenwater JY. Bladder outlet obstruction after multiple periurethral polytetrafluoroethylene injections. J Urol 1995;153(1):149–51.
11. Kiilholma P, Makinen J. Disappointing effect of endoscopic Teflon injection for female stress incontinence. Eur Urol 1991;20(3):197–9.
12. Beckingham IJ, Wemyss-Holden G, Lawrence WT. Long-term follow-up of women treated with perurethral Teflon injections for stress incontinence. Br J Urol 1992; 69(6):580–3.
13. Kiilholma PJ, Chancellor MB, Makinen J, Hirsch IH, Klemi PJ. Complications of Teflon injection for stress urinary incontinence. Neurourol Urodyn 1993;12(2):131–7.
14. Smart RF. Polytef paste for urinary incontinence. Aust NZ J Surg 1991;61(9):663–6.
15. Dewan PA, Fraundorfer M. Skin migration following periurethral polytetrafluoroethylene injection for urinary incontinence. Aust NZ J Surg 1996;66(1):57–9.
16. Kaplan PA, Ruskin JD, Tu HK, Knibbe MA. Erosive arthritis of the temporomandibular joint caused by Teflon-Proplast implants: plain film features. Am J Roentgenol 1988;151(2):337–9.

Polyurethanes

General Information

Polyurethanes are organic polymers that are formed by reacting a polyol (an alcohol with more than two reactive hydroxyl groups per molecule) with a diisocyanate or a polymeric isocyanate in the presence of suitable catalysts and additives. Flexible polyurethane forms are used in upholstery, mattresses, chemical-resistant coatings, adhesives, sealants, and packaging. Rigid foams are used in insulation for buildings, water heaters, refrigerated transport, and commercial and residential refrigerators.

In medical practice, polyurethane is used in implants. Complications of polyurethane implants are not uncommon, mainly due to foreign-body reactions (1), such as with microporous polyurethane (Mitrathane) cardiac patch implants and with breast implants.

Long-Term Effects

Tumorigenicity

In a study of the mortality (1958–98) and cancer morbidity (1971–94) in a cohort of 8288 male and female employees from 11 factories in England and Wales engaged in the manufacture of flexible polyurethane foams, mortality from lung cancer in female employees was significantly increased (standardized mortality ratio 181) (2). There was no excess among male employees (standardized mortality ratio 107). There were no significantly increased cause-specific standardized mortality ratios among the subcohort ($n = 1782$) with some period of isocyanate exposure.

References

1. Mestres CA, Cugat E, Ninot S, Gomez JF, Pomar JL. Severe fibrous epicarditis after microporous polyurethane (Mitrathane) cardiac patch implantation. Thorac Cardiovasc Surg 1986;34(2):137–8.
2. Sorahan T, Nichols L. Mortality and cancer morbidity of production workers in the UK flexible polyurethane foam industry: updated findings, 1958–98. Occup Environ Med 2002;59(11):751–8.

Polyvidone

See also Disinfectants and antiseptics

General Information

Polyvidone (polyvinylpyrrolidone, povidone) is a variable-weight polymer of the monomer *N*-vinylpyrrolidinone. When it enters the body, it causes histologically characteristic reactions in tissues with which it comes into contact (1,2).

Polyvidone co-polymers are used in cosmetics as antimicrobials, antistatics, binding compounds, stabilizers of emulsions, and film-forming, viscosity-controlling, hair-fixing, skin-conditioning, and skin-protective agents. It is used as a component of hair sprays and as a retardant for subcutaneous injections. It was formerly used as a plasma expander (3) and has been inappropriately used for intravenous injection as a "blood tonic," especially in Asian societies. Some products intended for parenteral administration contain polyvidone as an excipient. Polyvidone is widely used as a suspending and coating agent in tablets, for its film-forming properties in eye drops, and as a carrier molecule for iodine in disinfectants. About 20% of all tablets on the market contain polyvidone. It is also used in the cosmetics industry as a dispersing agent and as a lubricant in ointments.

Povidone-iodine

Povidone-iodine is a macromolecular complex (poly-I(I-vinyl-2-pyrrolidinone)) that is used as an iodophor. It is formulated as a 10% applicator solution, a 2% cleansing solution, and in many topical formulations, for example aerosol sprays, aerosol foams, vaginal gels, ointments, and mouthwashes. Because it contains very little free iodine (less than 1 ppm in a 10% solution), its antibacterial effectiveness is only moderate compared with that of a pure solution of iodine.

Systemic absorption
The extent of systemic absorption of povidone-iodine depends on the localization and the conditions of its use (area, skin surface, mucous membranes, wounds, body cavities).

Healthy skin
Repeated surgical skin antisepsis and hand washing did not increase serum iodine concentrations, but produced a small increase in iodine content in the 24-hour urine (4).

Burns
The use of povidone-iodine for the treatment of burns, for peritoneal lavage in the treatment of purulent peritonitis, or as a rinsing solution for body cavities can increase serum iodine concentrations associated with increased urinary excretion of iodine. In people with burns, the extent of iodine absorption depends on the extent of the burned body surface. It is not uncommon for serum iodine concentrations to rise to more than 1000 µg/ml. If renal function is intact, iodine elimination in the urine can be adequate. The serum iodine concentration returns to normal about 1 week after the last application.

The penetration of povidone-iodine has been studied in vivo in rabbits (5). The penetration from third-degree burns on the back was measured autoradiographically in tissues, blood, urine, and bandages. The results showed that about 20% of iodine is absorbed through fresh necrosis, whereas only 5% is absorbed through a clean wound or 24-hour-old necrosis. The passage through burn necrosis was faster than through vital tissue.

In repeated topical use on burns, the extent of absorption seems to decrease with the treatment time.

Wounds
Povidone-iodine inhibits leukocyte migration and fibroblast aggregation in wounds. The effect on the wound healing process has been studied in 294 children undergoing surgery, 283 of whom had undergone appendectomy (6). In a first series using 5% povidone-iodine aerosol for preoperative disinfection, the postoperative wound infection rate was 19% in the test group and only 8% in the controls. When a 1% povidone-iodine solution was used, only 2.6% of the patients were infected (control group 8.5%). Using a drain with a cellulose viscose sponge, 5% povidone-iodine by aerosol inhibited leukocyte migration, but no cell aggregates or fibroblasts were detected. A 5% solution allowed better cellular movement and attachment to the framework, polymorphonuclear leukocytes predominating. The excipients in the aerosol formula must be more toxic to the cell than those in the solution. If a 1% povidone-iodine solution was absorbed by the sponge, the aggregation phenomenon was only slightly averted and cell morphology was similar to that of the saline control.

Povidone-iodine reduced the number of wound infections only in patients with appendicitis in whom neither peritonitis nor a periappendicular abscess had yet developed (SEDA-11, 489).

Mucous membranes
The effect of a povidone-iodine mouthwash on thyroid function has been studied in 16 medically healthy volunteers. After they had used the mouthwash four times daily for a period of 14 days, all thyroid tests were significantly changed, but there was no suppression of thyroid function. However, this was not to be expected, considering the short test period.

Body cavities
When povidone-iodine is used as a rinsing solution in body cavities, absorption of the whole macromolecular complex is possible. The complex has a molecular weight of about 60 000 and cannot be eliminated by the kidneys or metabolically. It is filtered by the reticuloendothelial system (4,7,8).

Although povidone-iodine is no longer used in dialysates, a povidone-iodine-containing cap is used to seal the Tenckhoff catheter during the day. Iodine-induced hypothyroidism occurred in a 3-year-old boy and an 18-month-old girl, in both cases due to the sealing cap (9). The povidone-iodine inside the cap diffused into the catheter and flushed into the peritoneal cavity at the next dialysis session.

Intravaginal administration
Systemic iodine absorption can occur after intravaginal administration of povidone-iodine (10). There were increases in serum iodine, protein-bound iodine, and inorganic iodine, but not serum thyroxine, after a 2-minute vaginal administration of povidone-iodine in nonpregnant women (11).

Guidelines for the safe use of povidone-iodine complexes
In 1985, a working group of the Federal German Medical Association issued a number of recommendations for the

safe use of povidone-iodine complexes (12). They remain valid and can be summarized as follows:

1. The application of povidone-iodine formulations cannot be recommended for surgical hand disinfection, since active iodine-free formulations are available.
2. The activity of povidone-iodine in preoperative skin disinfection in adults is well proven.
3. Povidone-iodine is appropriate for skin disinfection before an incision, a puncture, with use of intravenous or arterial catheters, and for the prophylaxis of iatrogenic *Clostridia* infections.
4. In the case of superficial wounds, povidone-iodine can be applied occasionally or repeatedly in spite of increased iodine absorption through the broken skin surfaces.
5. Lavage of wound and body cavities with povidone-iodine or its instillation is not indicated because of increased iodine absorption.
6. Routine body washing of patients in intensive care units is not cost-beneficial.
7. Vaginal administration of povidone-iodine is not recommended.
8. Povidone-iodine is contraindicated in premature babies and neonates; this also applies to prophylactic disinfection of the umbilical stump.
9. The clinical usefulness of povidone-iodine in the treatment of burns is well proven.
10. Local mouth antiseptics serve no therapeutic purpose; this is also true for povidone-iodine.

Organs and Systems

Nervous system

- A 62-year-old man, treated with continuous mediastinal irrigation with a 1:10 solution of povidone-iodine, developed seizures on the fifth day of drainage (13). After the seizure, his serum iodine concentration was raised (120 µg/ml). Renal insufficiency developed at the same time. The electroencephalogram showed no evidence of epileptic activity or other abnormalities. The povidone-iodine irrigation was replaced by continuous irrigation with a solution of neomycin and polymyxin B. Renal function improved and the creatinine concentration returned to normal 3 days after the seizure.

Endocrine

Extensive iodine absorption can cause transient hypothyroidism, or, in patients with latent hypothyroidism, the risk of destabilization and thyrotoxic crisis (SEDA-20, 226) (SEDA-22, 263). Especially at risk are patients with an autonomous adenoma, localized diffuse autonomy of the thyroid gland, nodular goiter, latent hyperthyroidism of autoimmune origin, or endemic iodine deficiency (4).

Povidone-iodine-induced hyperthyroidism is rarer than hypothyroidism (SEDA-20, 226), but a history of long-term use of iodine-containing medications should be considered when investigating the cause of hyperthyroidism (14).

- A 48-year-old woman developed palpitation and insomnia. The clinical history, physical examination,

and laboratory tests supported hyperthyroidism. Since July 1994, she had been combating constipation by improper use of an iodine-containing antiseptic cream for external use only. She had inserted povidone-iodine into her rectum by means of a cannula. The iodine-containing cream was withdrawn and she was given a beta-blocker. The palpitation resolved within 2 weeks and her plasma thyroid hormone concentrations normalized within 1 month.

Hyperthyroidism in this patient was probably triggered by improper long-term use of an over-the-counter iodine-containing cream.

Thyrotoxicosis related to iodine toxicity in a child with burns occurred after alternate-day povidone-iodine washes (15).

- A 22-month-old boy was admitted to a pediatric intensive care unit after partial and full thickness burns over 80% of his body surface area. After debridement he was given alternate-day povidone-iodine (Betadine) washes. He became increasingly tachycardic, hypertensive, and hyperpyrexic, with sweating, agitation, and diarrhea and developed neutropenia. Daily sepsis screens were negative. Thyroid function tests showed evidence of iodine-induced thyrotoxicosis. He was given propranolol and carbimazole, and chlorhexidine was substituted for povidone-iodine. His tachycardia, hypertension, and diarrhea slowly improved and his neutropenia resolved. By day 42 his free thyroxine concentration was normal and he was given thyroxine. On day 63 the carbimazole, propranolol, and thyroxine were withheld. However thyroid function tests 1 week later showed hypothyroidism, and thyroxine was restarted. Repeat plasma and urine iodine concentrations on day 57 (a month after withdrawal of povidone-iodine) continued to show marked urinary excretion of iodine (urine concentration 65 µmol/l, reference range 0.39–1.97) with high but falling plasma iodine concentrations (5.9 µmol/l, reference range 0.32–0.63).

Hematologic

Severe neutropenia occurred in a patient in whom deep, second-degree burns, involving about 50% of the body surface, were being treated with Betadine Helafoam twice a day (16).

Liver

There have been reports of liver damage from polyvidone (17).

Urinary tract

Povidone-iodine sclerosis has been suggested to be safe and effective in treating lymphoceles after renal transplantation, with only minor complications of the procedure, such as pericatheter cutaneous infections. However, a case of acute renal tubular necrosis has been reported (18).

- In a 23-year-old woman, a kidney allograft recipient with recurrent lymphoceles treated with povidone-iodine irrigations (50 ml of a 1% solution bd for 6 days), a metabolic acidosis occurred and renal function deteriorated. After a few days, despite suspension of irrigation, the patient developed oliguria, and dialysis was needed. A renal biopsy showed acute tubular necrosis.

Iodine-induced renal insufficiency has also been reported after the use of topical povidone-iodine on the skin and after intracavity irrigation.

- A 65-year-old man with second- and third-degree burns covering 26% of his body was given intravenous lactated Ringer solution and topical silver sulfadiazine in addition to debridement and skin grafting (19). However, he developed a wound infection with *Pseudomonas aeruginosa*, which was treated successfully with topical povidone-iodine gel. Persistent nodal bradycardia with hypotension, metabolic acidosis, and renal insufficiency occurred 16 days later. Iodine toxicosis was suspected and the serum iodine concentration was 206 µg/ml (reference range 20–90 µg/ml). The povidone-iodine gel was therefore withdrawn immediately. His family refused hemodialysis and he died 44 days after admission.
- A 57-year-old man developed renal insufficiency after triple coronary bypass grafting, 7 days after povidone-iodine mediastinal irrigation and required 3 days of renal replacement therapy (20). Complete resolution occurred within 8 days and followed a short non-oliguric phase (4 days).

Although other common causes of acute renal insufficiency were present in the second case, the only significant change in management at the time of onset of renal insufficiency was the use of povidone-iodine.

Skin

Povidone-iodine causes concentration-dependent damage to cells and clusters. The effect is most pronounced for isolated cells, but it is also detectable in more complex tissues. Clinical experience with burn victims cannot rule out the possibility that the healing process may be slightly retarded. However, this deficiency may be balanced by an appropriate microbicidal effect on the healing edge (21).

Polyvidone storage disease
Polyvidone molecules that weigh less than 20 kD can be excreted by a normally functioning kidney, whereas larger polymers are phagocytosed and permanently stored in the mononuclear phagocytic system, causing so-called polyvidone storage disease. Polyvidone storage disease occurs in patients who have received polyvidone for prolonged periods of time. The large polymers deposit in the histiocytes and cause them to proliferate and infiltrate histiocytes in the reticuloendothelial system, including osteocytes. There is generally no significant damage to these organs, except that prolonged administration can cause bone destruction, skin lesions, arthritis, and polyneuropathy.

The first cutaneous case of polyvidone storage disease, reported in 1964 (22), was caused by local injection of polyvidone-containing posterior pituitary extracts for the treatment of diabetes insipidus. Similar cases, including those following local injection of porcine polyvidone to treat neuralgia, were documented, mostly in European

reports (23,24). Localized cutaneous polyvidone storage disease was then known as Dupont-Lachapelle disease (25).

Five cases of polyvidone storage disease with cutaneous involvement have been documented (26). Two patients presented with skin eruptions mimicking collagen vascular disease and chronic pigmented purpuric dermatosis. In one, polyvidone was found in a metastatic tumor and in the other in a pemphigus lesion. The fifth case was seen in a blind skin biopsy specimen taken to exclude Niemann-Pick disease after examination of a bone marrow smear. The latter patient and the patient with a collagen vascular-like disease also had severe anemia and serious orthopedic and neurological complications due to massive infiltration of polyvidone-containing cells in the bone marrow, with destruction of the bone.

Polyvidone storage disease can easily be diagnosed by its histopathological features. Skin biopsy specimens show a variable number of characteristic blue–gray vacuolated cells around blood vessels and adnexal structures, and stain positively with mucicarmine, colloidal iron, and alkaline Congo red and negatively with periodic acid Schiff and Alcian blue.

Musculoskeletal

Pathological fractures of several bones and destructive lesions seen radiologically in other bones have been reported in patients who had received repeated intravenous injections of polyvidone for many years (27,28). Biopsies of the fracture sites showed both intracellular deposits of polyvidone and mucoid changes in the affected cells. If of sufficient severity, this may cause a virtual "melt down" of osseous tissue.

Immunologic

Polyvidone has been reported to cause anaphylaxis (29).

- A 32-year-old man took paracetamol (in Doregrippin) for flu-like symptoms and about 10 minutes later developed generalized urticaria, angioedema, hypotonia, and tachycardia, and became semiconscious. His symptoms were rapidly relieved by intravenous antihistamines and steroids. This was the first time he had taken Doregrippin, but he had previously taken paracetamol-containing formulations, which had been well tolerated. He was not taking any regular medications. Subsequent testing of the various constituents of the analgesic tablets identified polyvidone as the cause of the anaphylactic reaction.

This report demonstrates a rare case of a type I allergic reaction toward a commonly used ingredient of tablets and widely used disinfectants.

In principle, all forms of the well-known iodine-induced allergic reactions, such as iododerma tuberosum, dermatitis, petechiae, and sialadenitis are possible with povidone-iodine, but the incidence seems to be very low (SEDA-11, 489) (SEDA-12, 586) (4,30,31).

- A severe anaphylactoid reaction occurred immediately after the instillation of a 10% solution of povidone-iodine into a hydatid cyst cavity during surgery. Severe bronchospasm developed immediately and was followed by a coagulopathy and subsequent liver and renal insufficiency (32).

There have been only a few reports of contact allergy to povidone-iodine, despite its widespread use. In two cases there were positive patch test reactions on days 2, 3, and 7 to povidone-iodine (5% aqueous) and iodine (0.5% in petrolatum), but negative reactions to povidone itself (33).

Second-Generation Effects

Pregnancy

Routine vaginal douching with povidone-iodine during pregnancy causes maternal iodine overload and markedly increases the iodine content in amniotic fluid and of the fetal thyroid, as soon as the trapping mechanism of iodine by the thyroid has started to develop. Vaginal use of povidone-iodine is therefore not recommended during pregnancy (34,35) and labor (36).

The fetal thyroid starts to store iodine between the 10th and 13th weeks of gestation, and to secrete thyroid hormone between the 18th and 24th weeks. Especially after intravaginal administration during pregnancy, povidone-iodine can cause congenital goiter and hypothyroidism in newborn infants. However, hyperthyroidism can also occur.

In 99 of 9320 newborns, TSH concentrations were above the reference range (20 mU/ml) on the fifth day of life, but between the 10th and 21st day, all these infants had normal TSH concentrations and normal thyroid function (37). In 76 of the newborns with hyperthyrotropinemia, urinary iodine excretion was significantly raised (above 16 µg/ml). Most of them were born in obstetric departments where iodophores were routinely used for disinfection during labor.

In 66 mothers and their infants, povidone-iodine was given during labor and delivery as a 1 or 2% solution pumped intravaginally through a plastic catheter until delivery (for 5–30 hours), urinary iodide concentrations on the first and the fifth day, and serum iodine concentrations at birth were significantly raised in the mothers as well as in the neonates (38). At birth, the TSH concentrations in the mothers and infants were no different from those in the controls, but on the third and fifth days they were significantly higher. Thyroxine concentrations were significantly lower in the exposed mothers and infants (at birth and on the third and the fifth days). One-fifth of the infants had high TSH concentrations (above 20 µU/ml) and low thyroxine values (below 7 µg/ml), which is suggestive of hypothyroidism. However, none of the infants developed clinical symptoms, and on the 14th day the values were normal again. In the iodine-exposed mothers and infants, tri-iodothyronine (T3) concentrations were significantly reduced at birth, but not thereafter. The concentrations of reverse T3 did not differ from the controls at birth, but were significantly lower on succeeding days. This reduction in reverse T3 in the iodine-exposed infants was probably due to reduced thyroxine concentrations, causing a lack of substrates for monodeiodination to reverse T3.

Iodine concentrations in breast milk and in random urine in neonates and the serum concentrations of neonatal TSH and free thyroxine on day 5 after delivery were measured after the use of povidone-iodine for disinfection after delivery (36). Iodine concentrations in the breast milk and neonatal TSH were significantly raised.

Perinatal iodine exposure causes transient hypothyroidism in a significant number of neonates, in whom careful monitoring and follow-up of thyroid gland function are needed. It is better to avoid the use of iodine-containing antiseptics in pregnancy and neonates, especially if follow-up cannot be guaranteed.

Susceptibility Factors

Age

Neonates

Hypothyroidism in neonates has been related to the use of small doses of iodine as an antiseptic. The high vulnerability of the neonatal thyroid is a reason for avoiding povidone-iodine for care of the umbilical stump or omphaloceles (SEDA-11, 488) (SEDA-12, 585) (39).

Serum TSH and thyroxine concentrations have been measured 57 days after birth in 365 healthy newborns whose umbilical stump had been treated with 10% povidone-iodine (40). The prevalence of high TSH concentrations was significantly higher in this group than in the general population (3.1 versus 0.4%), as was the rate of transient hypothyroidism (2.7 versus 0.25%). All the children were normal when retested 1 week later.

Transient hypothyroidism due to skin contamination with povidone-iodine occurred in a neonate with an omphalocele (41).

The postnatal iodine overload, measured as urinary iodine concentration, has been studied in ill neonates after the cutaneous application of povidone-iodine (0.96% I_2; Betadine) (SEDA-11, 488) (39). The mean iodine overload was 1297 µg/day in one povidone-iodine group and 1253 µg/day in a second group; in the control group, 64% of the newborns had iodinuria of less than 100 µg/day, and of the 10 others (mean ioduria 1212 has been studied in ill neonates) three were born by cesarean section: in these cases the mothers received an iodine-containing curariform agent. There were 12 cases of hypothyroidism among the neonates exposed to iodine-containing antiseptics, but none in the control group.

Very low birth weight infants admitted to a neonatal intensive care unit who had been given chlorhexidine-containing antiseptics ($n = 29$) were compared with infants in a comparable unit who had been given iodinated antiseptic agents ($n = 54$) (42). The latter had an up to 50-fold higher increase in urinary iodine excretion than the controls. The median serum TSH concentration was significantly higher in the iodine-exposed infants (4.6 mU/ml) than in the control infants (2.4 mU/ml). On day 14, TSH concentrations in nine of the 36 iodine-exposed infants were above 20 mU/ml, their mean thyroxine concentration was significantly lower (44 nmol/1) than the mean thyroxine concentrations (83 nmol/l) in both the exposed infants with normal TSH concentrations and the controls.

Renal disease

Since iodine is eliminated by the kidneys, renal insufficiency increases the risk of toxicity, and the risk may be further increased by metabolic acidosis (43,44).

Drug Administration

Drug contamination

Bacterial contamination of povidone-iodine formulations has been reported. *Pseudomonas cepacia* was discovered in the blood cultures of 52 patients in four hospitals in New York over 7 months, and of 16 patients in a Boston hospital over a 10-week period in 1980 (45). A contaminated povidone-iodine solution produced by one manufacturer was implicated as the source of the bacteria. It is not clear why this solution was contaminated, whereas other marketed povidone-iodine solutions containing equivalent amounts of available or free iodine remained sterile.

Interference with Diagnostic Tests

Povidone-iodine gives a positive reaction with an ortho-toluidine reagent used to detect blood in the urine, for example Hematest reagent tablets or dipsticks (SEDA-11, 488) (46).

Povidone-iodine used for skin disinfection before skin puncture blood was taken altered serum concentrations of potassium, phosphate, and uric acid.

References

1. Bergman M, Flance IJ, Blumenthal HT. Thesaurosis following inhalation of hair spray; a clinical and experimental study. N Engl J Med 1958;258(10):471–6.

2. Bergman M, Flance IJ, Cruz PT, Klam N, Aronson PR, Joshi RA, Blumenthal HT. Thesaurosis due to inhalation of hair spray. Report of twelve new cases, including three autopsies. Nord Hyg Tidskr 1962;266:750–5.

3. Weese HG, Periston H. Ein never Blutluessigkeitsersatz. Münch Med Wochenschr 1943;90:11–15.

4. Gortz G, Haring R. Wirkung und Nebenwirkung von Polyvinylpyrrolidon-Jod (PVP-Jod). Therapiewoche 1981;31:4364.

5. Colcleuth RG. Distribution protein binding of betadine ointment in burn wounds. In: Altemeier WA, editor. II World Congress/Antisepsis Proceedings. New York: HP Publishing Co, 1980:122–3.

6. Viljanto J. Disinfection of surgical wounds without inhibition of normal wound healing. Arch Surg 1980;115(3):253–6.

7. Glick PL, Guglielmo BJ, Tranbaugh RF, Turley K. Iodine toxicity in a patient treated by continuous povidone-iodine mediastinal irrigation. Ann Thorac Surg 1985;39(5):478–80.

8. Campistol JM, Abad C, Nogue S, Bertran A. Acute renal failure in a patient treated by continuous povidone-iodine mediastinal irrigation. J Cardiovasc Surg (Torino) 1988;29(4):410–12.

9. Vulsma T, Menzel D, Abbad FC, Gons MH, de Vijlder JJ. Iodine-induced hypothyroidism in infants treated with continuous cyclic peritoneal dialysis. Lancet 1990;336(8718):812.

10. Jacobson JM, Hankins GV, Murray JM, Young RL. Self-limited hyperthyroidism following intravaginal iodine administration. Am J Obstet Gynecol 1981;140(4):472–3.

11. Vorherr H, Vorherr UF, Mehta P, Ulrich JA, Messer RH. Vaginal absorption of povidone-iodine. JAMA 1980;244(23):2628–9.

12. Wissenschaftlicher Berat der Bundesärztäkammer. Für Anwendung von Polyvinylpyrolidon-Jod Komplexen. Dtsch Ärztebl 1985;82:1434.

13. Zec N, Donovan JW, Aufiero TX, Kincaid RL, Demers LM. Seizures in a patient treated with continuous povidone-iodine mediastinal irrigation. N Engl J Med 1992;326(26):1784.

14. Grant JA, Bilodeau PA, Guernsey BG, Gardner FH. Unsuspected benzyl alcohol hypersensitivity. N Engl J Med 1982;306(2):108.

15. Robertson P, Fraser J, Sheild J, Weir P. Thyrotoxicosis related to iodine toxicity in a paediatric burn patient. Intensive Care Med 2002;28(9):1369.

16. Alvarez E. Neutropenia in a burned patient being treated topically with povidone-iodine foam. Plast Reconstr Surg 1979;63(6):839–40.

17. Golightly LK, Smolinske SS, Bennett ML, Sutherland EW 3rd, Rumack BH. Pharmaceutical excipients. Adverse effects associated with 'inactive' ingredients in drug products (Part II). Med Toxicol Adverse Drug Exp 1988;3(3):209–40.

18. Manfro RC, Comerlato L, Berdichevski RH, Ribeiro AR, Denicol NT, Berger M, Saitovitch D, Koff WJ, Goncalves LF. Nephrotoxic acute renal failure in a renal transplant patient with recurrent lymphocele treated with povidone-iodine irrigation. Am J Kidney Dis 2002;40(3):655–7.

19. Aiba M, Ninomiya J, Furuya K, Arai H, Ishikawa H, Asaumi S, Takagi A, Ohwada S, Morishita Y. Induction of a critical elevation of povidone-iodine absorption in the treatment of a burn patient: report of a case. Surg Today 1999;29(2):157–9.

20. Ryan M, Al-Sammak Z, Phelan D. Povidone-iodine mediastinal irrigation: a cause of acute renal failure. J Cardiothorac Vasc Anesth 1999;13(6):729–31.

21. Kobayashi H. Review of the use of povidone-iodine (PVP-I) in the treatment of burns. Postgrad Med J 1993;69:584–92.

22. Dupont A, Lachapelle JM. Dermite due à un depot medicamenteux au cours du traitement d'un diabète insipide. [Dermatitis due to a medicamentous deposit during the treatment of diabetes insipidus.] Bull Soc Fr Dermatol Syphiligr 1964;71:508–9.

23. Lachapelle JM. Thesaurismose cutanée par polyvinylpyrrolidone. [Cutaneous thesaurismosis due to polyvinylpyrrolidone.] Dermatologica 1966;132(6):476–89.

24. Mensing H, Koster W, Schaeg G, Nasemann T. Zur klinischen Varianz der Polyvinylpyrrolidon-Dermatose. [Clinical variability of polyvinylpyrrolidone dermatosis.] Z Hautkr 1984;59(15):1027–37.

25. Bazex A, Geraud J, Guilhem A, Dupre A, Rascol A, Cantala P. Maladie de Dupont et Lachapelle (thesaurismose cutanée par polyvinylpyrrolidone). [Dupont–Lachapelle disease (cutaneous thesaurismosis due to polyvinylpyrrolidone).] Arch Belg Dermatol Syphiligr 1966;22(4):227–33.

26. Kuo TT, Hu S, Huang CL, Chan HL, Chang MJ, Dunn P, Chen YJ. Cutaneous involvement in polyvinylpyrrolidone storage disease: a clinicopathologic study of five patients, including two patients with severe anemia. Am J Surg Pathol 1997;21(11):1361–7.

27. Kepes JJ, Chen WY, Jim YF. 'Mucoid dissolution' of bones and multiple pathologic fractures in a patient with past history of intravenous administration of polyvinylpyrrolidone (PVP). A case report. Bone Miner 1993;22(1):33–41.

28. Dunn P, Kuo T, Shih LY, Wang PN, Sun CF, Chang MJ. Bone marrow failure and myelofibrosis in a case of PVP storage disease. Am J Hematol 1998;57(1):68–71.

29. Ronnau AC, Wulferink M, Gleichmann E, Unver E, Ruzicka T, Krutmann J, Grewe M. Anaphylaxis to

polyvinylpyrrolidone in an analgesic preparation. Br J Dermatol 2000;143(5):1055–8.

30. Zamora JL. Chemical and microbiologic characteristics and toxicity of povidone-iodine solutions. Am J Surg 1986; 151(3):400–6.

31. Ancona A, Suarez de la Torre R, Macotela E. Allergic contact dermatitis from povidone-iodine. Contact Dermatitis 1985;13(2):66–8.

32. Okten F, Oral M, Canakici N, et al. An anaphylactoid induced with polyvinylpyrrolidone iodine. A case report. Turk Anesteziyol Reanim 1993;21:118–22.

33. Erdmann S, Hertl M, Merk HF. Allergic contact dermatitis from povidone-iodine. Contact Dermatitis 1999; 40(6):331–2.

34. Melvin GR, Aceto T Jr, Barlow J, Munson D, Wierda D. Iatrogenic congenital goiter and hypothyroidism with respiratory distress in a newborn. S D J Med 1978;31(10):15–19.

35. Mahillon I, Peers W, Bourdoux P, Ermans AM, Delange F. Effect of vaginal douching with povidone-iodine during early pregnancy on the iodine supply to mother and fetus. Biol Neonate 1989;56(4):210–17.

36. Koga Y, Sano H, Kikukawa Y, Ishigouoka T, Kawamura M. Effect on neonatal thyroid function of povidone-iodine used on mothers during perinatal period. J Obstet Gynaecol 1995;21(6):581–5.

37. Gruters A, l'Allemand D, Heidemann PH, Schurnbrand P. Incidence of iodine contamination in neonatal transient hyperthyrotropinemia. Eur J Pediatr 1983;140(4):299–300.

38. l'Allemand D, Gruters A, Heidemann P, Schurnbrand P. Iodine-induced alterations of thyroid function in newborn infants after prenatal and perinatal exposure to povidone-iodine. J Pediatr 1983;102(6):935–8.

39. Castaing H, Fournet JP, Leger FA, Kiesgen F, Piette C, Dupard MC, Savoie JC. Thyroide du nouveau-né et surcharge en iode après la naissance. [The thyroid gland of the newborn infant and postnatal iodine overload.] Arch Fr Pediatr 1979;36(4):356–68.

40. Arena J, Eguileor I, Emparanza J. Repercusion sobre la funcion tiroidea del RN a termino de la aplicacion de povidona iodada en el munon umbilical. [Repercussion of the application of povidone-iodine to the umbilical stump on thyroid function of the neonate at term.] An Esp Pediatr 1985;23(8):562–8.

41. Tummers RF, Krul EJ, Bakker HD. Passagere hypothereoidie ten gevolge van huidinfectie met jodium bij een pasgeborene met een omfalocele. [Transient hypothyroidism due to skin contamination with iodine in a newborn infant with an omphalocele.] Ned Tijdschr Geneeskd 1985;129(20):958–9.

42. Smerdely P, Lim A, Boyages SC, Waite K, Wu D, Roberts V, Leslie G, Arnold J, John E, Eastman CJ. Topical iodine-containing antiseptics and neonatal hypothyroidism in very-low-birthweight infants. Lancet 1989;2(8664):661–4.

43. Wilson JP, Solimando DA Jr, Edwards MS. Parenteral benzyl alcohol-induced hypersensitivity reaction. Drug Intell Clin Pharm 1986;20(9):689–91.

44. Shmunes E. Allergic dermatitis to benzyl alcohol in an injectable solution. Arch Dermatol 1984;120(9):1200–1.

45. Craven DE, Moody B, Connolly MG, Kollisch NR, Stottmeier KD, McCabe WR. Pseudobacteremia caused by povidone-iodine solution contaminated with *Pseudomonas cepacia*. N Engl J Med 1981;305(11):621–3.

46. Van Steirteghem AC, Young DS. Povidone-iodine ("Betadine") disinfectant as a source of error. Clin Chem 1977;23(8):1512.

Posaconazole

See also Antifungal azoles

General Information

Posaconazole is similar in structure to itraconazole. It was well tolerated and as effective as fluconazole 100 mg in two large randomized comparisons in HIV-infected patients with oropharyngeal candidiasis. In a salvage study in patients with a variety of invasive fungal infections, there were response rates of 44–80% in patients with aspergillosis, fusariosis, cryptococcosis, candidiasis, and pheohyphomycoses after 4–8 weeks of therapy (1,2).

References

1. Groll AH, Gea-Banacloche JC, Glasmacher A, Just-Nuebling G, Maschmeyer G, Walsh TJ. Clinical pharmacology of antifungal compounds. Infect Dis Clin North Am 2003;17(1):159–91.

2. Hoffman HL, Ernst EJ, Klepser ME. Novel triazole antifungal agents. Expert Opin Investig Drugs 2000;9(3):593–605.

Potassium chloride

General Information

Oral potassium chloride is used to prevent or correct potassium depletion due to diuretic use or other conditions. Potassium chloride is available not only for medicinal purposes but also as a food supplement and salt substitute.

The main adverse effects of oral potassium salts are hyperkalemia, particularly when they are used in combination with potassium-sparing drugs, such as spironolactone and ACE inhibitors, and gastrointestinal ulceration and perforation, particularly with modified-release formulations. The problems surrounding enteric-coated potassium chloride tablets are unresolved. Despite recommendations that they be withdrawn, some are still available. The risks seem to be less with slow-release potassium chloride tablets.

Simple dietary measures provide adequate potassium intake, and it is questionable whether for most patients potassium supplementation in any pharmaceutical form is necessary, as opposed to the use of potassium-sparing drugs.

Organs and Systems

Cardiovascular

When potassium chloride is given by intravenous infusion for the treatment of potassium depletion (for example in diabetic ketoacidosis) there is a risk of cardiac dysrhythmias if the infusion is too rapid. The rate of infusion should be no greater than 20 mmol/hour.

Electrolyte balance

Hyperkalemia is a risk of potassium chloride administration whether medicinal or not. The wide availability of potassium salts can contribute to accidental fatal hyperkalemia. Hyperkalemia has been reported after ingestion of salt substitutes (1,2) and over-the-counter potassium supplements (3).

Gastrointestinal

Potassium chloride is irritating to the gastrointestinal tract, even to the extent of causing perforation (4). In a retrospective study at surgical clinics in Stockholm County there were 22 cases of small-bowel ulceration in which a connection with slow-release potassium chloride tablets was probable (5). Most of the ulcers had caused stenosis of 1–2 cm of gut, and in four cases there was also perforation of the bowel wall. Five patients had perforation without signs of stenosis. Mortality was 27%. The pathology of the ulcers was similar to that described after use of enteric-coated potassium chloride tablets. The frequency of potassium-induced ulceration is low (about 3 cases per 100 000 patient-years of slow-release tablet use), but this complication can be serious.

Susceptibility Factors

Renal disease

The risk of hyperkalemia from potassium chloride is increased in patients with renal insufficiency (6).

Drug Administration

Drug formulations

Microencapsulated potassium chloride tablets have been reported to be less irritating to the gastrointestinal tract than other forms of potassium chloride. In a comparison of a microencapsulated potassium chloride formulation and a wax-matrix formulation in 48 healthy volunteers, the latter were associated with a higher incidence of upper gastrointestinal lesions determined by endoscopy after 1 week (7). The lesions were not accompanied by epigastric symptoms. Glycopyrrolate, given to some volunteers to reduce gastric emptying, aggravated the effects of potassium chloride.

Drug–Drug Interactions

Potassium-sparing drugs

The risk of hyperkalemia with potassium chloride formulations increases when they are given in combination with drugs that are potassium sparing (8), such as ACE inhibitors and angiotensin II receptor antagonists (9), canrenone, spironolactone (10), amiloride, and triamterene (11).

References

1. Schim van der Loeff HJ, Strack van Schijndel RJ, Thijs LG. Cardiac arrest due to oral potassium intake. Intensive Care Med 1988;15(1):58–9.
2. McCaughan D. Hazards of non-prescription potassium supplements. Lancet 1984;1(8375):513–4.
3. Browning JJ, Channer KS. Hyperkalaemic cardiac arrhythmia caused by potassium citrate mixture. BMJ (Clin Res Ed) 1981;283(6303):1366.
4. Des Mesnards G. Un nouveau cas de perforation du grêle après ingestion de comprimés de chlorure de potassium. [A further case of perforation of the small intestine after ingestion of potassium chloride tablets.] Chirurgie 1972;98(7):468–70.
5. Leijonmarck CE, Raf L. Ulceration of the small intestine due to slow-release potassium chloride tablets. Acta Chir Scand 1985;151(3):273–8.
6. Elo H. Spironolaktoni, kaliumkloridi ja hyperkalemia munuaisten vajaatoimintaa potevalla. [Spironolactone, potassium chloride and hyperkalemia in patients with kidney failure.] Duodecim 1992;108(19):1708–10.
7. McMahon FG, Ryan JR, Akdamar K, Ertan A. Upper gastrointestinal lesions after potassium chloride supplements: a controlled clinical trial. Lancet 1982;2(8307):1059–61.
8. Ponce SP, Jennings AE, Madias NE, Harrington JT. Drug-induced hyperkalemia. Medicine (Baltimore) 1985;64(6):357–70.
9. Preston RA, Baltodano NM, Alonso AB, Epstein M. Comparative effects on dynamic renal potassium excretion of ACE inhibition versus angiotensin receptor blockade in hypertensive patients with type II diabetes mellitus. J Clin Pharmacol 2002;42(7):754–61.
10. Simborg DW. Medication prescribing on a university medical service—the incidence of drug combinations with potential adverse interactions. Johns Hopkins Med J 1976;139(1):23–6.
11. Morgan TO. Clinical use of potassium supplements and potassium sparing diuretics. Drugs 1973;6(3):222–9.

Potassium perchlorate

General Information

Potassium perchlorate is a thyrostatic drug that is still used (in a dose of 1000 mg/day or more) as an alternative to the thionamides, especially in cases of allergy. It has also been used to treat the iodine-induced form of thyrotoxicosis, such as type 1 hyperthyroidism due to amiodarone (qv).

Compared with the thionamides, potassium perchlorate has two disadvantages:

1. treatment cannot be directly changed to radioiodine therapy, since perchlorate elimination lasts for some weeks;
2. brief high-dose iodine therapy cannot be used as a preoperative thyrostatic measure.

Potassium perchlorate produces goiter, as do the thionamides, but its effects on the hematological system are the main reason for using it sparingly.

Organs and Systems

Hematologic

Agranulocytosis and aplastic anemia have been described in patients taking potassium perchlorate (SED-8, 897) (1). Deaths have been recorded as a result (2,3).

Skin

Erythema nodosum associated with lupus erythematosus cells has been described as an adverse effect of potassium perchlorate (SED-8, 897) (1).

References

1. Rokke KE, Vogt JH. Combination of potassium perchlorate and propylthiouracil in the treatment of thyrotoxicosis. Acta Endocrinol (Copenh) 1968;57(4):565–77.
2. Johnson RS, Moore WG. Fatal aplastic anaemia after treatment of thyrotoxicosis with potassium perchlorate. BMJ 1961;5236:1369–71.
3. Krevans JR, Asper SP Jr, Rienhoff WF Jr. Fatal aplastic anemia following use of potassium perchlorate in thyrotoxicosis. JAMA 1962;181:162–4.

Practolol

See also Beta-adrenoceptor antagonists

General Information

Practolol is a highly cardioselective beta-adrenoceptor antagonist with partial agonist activity.

Although practolol has long been withdrawn from general oral use (because of the oculomucocutaneous syndrome and sclerosing peritonitis) (1), it is still available for intravenous administration in some countries. The practolol syndrome included a psoriasiform rash, xerophthalmia due to lacrimal gland fibrosis, secretory otitis media, fibrinous peritonitis, and a lupus-like syndrome (SED-8, 444) (SEDA-3, 161) (SEDA-2, 170). The pathogenesis of this adverse effect is unknown, but it appears to be unique to practolol.

Reference

1. Mann RD. A ranked presentation of the MHRA/CSM (Medicines & Health Care Regulatory Agency/Committee on Safety of Medicines) Drug Analysis Print (DAP) data on practolol. Pharmacoepidemiol Drug Saf 2005;14(10):705–10.

Pramipexole

General Information

Pramipexole is a non-ergot dopamine agonist similar to bromocriptine, used in the management of Parkinson's disease as an adjunct to levodopa.

In a systematic review of randomized controlled trials of pramipexole and ropinirole, dizziness, nausea, hypotension, hallucinations, and somnolence were common adverse effects (1). In 306 patients adverse events secondary to pramipexole that occurred in over 10% included dyskinesias, asymptomatic orthostatic hypotension, dizziness, insomnia, and hallucinations (2).

Organs and Systems

Cardiovascular

Orthostatic hypotension is common during oral pramipexole therapy (2).

Peripheral edema has occasionally been described as an adverse effect of dopamine agonist therapy and has been reported in 17 of 300 patients treated with pramipexole (3). The mean dose at onset of edema was 1.7 mg/day and the time after initiation of therapy was 2.6 months. In all cases the edema disappeared after the drug was withdrawn but reappeared on rechallenge. Although the condition was dose-dependent in affected individuals its occurrence was idiosyncratic with no obvious predisposing features. Response to diuretics was minimal.

Nervous system

Drowsiness, dizziness, and insomnia are relatively common adverse nervous system effects of pramipexole in patients with early Parkinson's disease (2).

Worsened dyskinesia is the most common outcome in patients with advanced disease taking concomitant levodopa therapy. In a systematic review of four randomized, placebo-controlled trials of pramipexole in 669 patients with idiopathic Parkinson's disease and long-term complications of levodopa therapy, there were no significant changes in a dyskinesia rating scale, but dyskinesia as an adverse event was reported more often with pramipexole (4).

Eight men aged 54–83 years, who had taken pramipexole 1–4.5 mg/day for Parkinson's disease for an average of 7 months, all fell asleep while driving, resulting in accidents but no injuries (5). They described sudden irresistible sleepiness, with virtually no warning, and four had had similar episodes during other activities. In six patients pramipexole was withdrawn, and in the other two the dose was reduced.

However, doubt has been cast on the existence of sleep attacks, that is acute episodes of sleep that occur without warning, with the newer dopamine receptor agonists (6). In the view of the authors of this review underlying somnolence is always present, even if the patient is not aware of it. They did not attempt to differentiate the risk associated with different agents, but noted that pramipexole doses below 1.5 mg/day are usually adequate and much less likely to cause this problem than higher doses. In general they stressed the importance of keeping doses of all the agents as low as possible and of warning patients about the risk, particularly when driving. They also commented that the possibility of an underlying sleep disorder should be considered in these circumstances.

A study of the effects of pramipexole was generally in agreement with these conclusions (7). In a double-blind study 22 patients were randomized to pramipexole monotherapy (mean 4.4, range 1.5–6, mg/day) and 18 to placebo. Six patients taking pramipexole reported somnolence (one moderate, five mild), compared with two patients taking placebo (one moderate, one mild).

In an open extension of the study, 21 of 37 patients reported somnolence, including 11 with moderate and 3 with severe symptoms. The onset of symptoms occurred at a mean dosage of 4 mg/day and patients had been taking treatment for 10 months on average at the time of the worst symptoms. Of the 14 patients with moderate to severe symptoms, 12 were interviewed in detail; 7 reported falling asleep while driving and 2 had been involved in minor accidents. Most of the patients reported continuous drowsiness as a background, but three said that they experienced sudden waves of irresistible sleepiness, although with some prodromal symptoms. The symptoms resolved on drug withdrawal or dosage reduction (though details of this were not given), and the comments on dosage from the previous paper are surely relevant. In patients taking pramipexole patient education is clearly of vital importance.

The pathophysiology of the restless legs syndrome is poorly understood, but it often responds well to dopaminergic therapy. However, augmentation of symptoms has also been described, especially with levodopa. Of 60 patients (mean age 58 years) with this syndrome who were treated with pramipexole (0.25–1.0 mg/day) 5 had augmentation of symptoms over a period of at least 6 months during continuous treatment and 4 had what was described as a secondary syndrome, in other words with co-existing and possibly causative neurological disease (8). There was no relation to the initial severity of the syndrome or to the dosage of drug, although the authors suggested that the very low dose of 0.25 mg/day is probably optimal.

Psychological, psychiatric

Hallucinations occur in about 10% of patients with Parkinson's disease, regardless of the stage of disease (2).

Fluid balance

Peripheral edema and weight loss have been reported occasionally during pramipexole therapy. Of 300 patients taking pramipexole, 17 had mild to severe peripheral edema attributable to the drug (3). The mean dosage was 1.7 (range 0.75–3.0) mg/day when the edema first appeared and 2.6 (range 1.5–3.0) mg/day when it was at its worst. In all cases, the edema rapidly abated on withdrawal, and rapidly returned on rechallenge.

Gastrointestinal

Gastrointestinal symptoms have tended to be more frequent in patients with early Parkinson's disease compared with those with advanced disease during pramipexole therapy. In patients with early disease, the most common effects have been nausea (up to 20% of patients), dry mouth (up to 10%), and constipation (7%), whereas less frequent ones, such as dyspepsia, anorexia, dysphagia, and flatulence, have been observed (9). In patients with advanced disease, the overall incidence of adverse gastrointestinal effects is usually 5% or less, and includes constipation, dry mouth, and flatulence (10). Abdominal pain and vomiting occasionally occur.

Hair

Hair loss has been attributed to dopamine receptor agonists.

- Two women in New York, aged 66 and 68 years, took pramipexole 15 and 3.5 mg/day (11). Both developed progressive hair loss 2–12 months later. When pramipexole was withdrawn, there was partial regrowth of hair. Ropinirole and levodopa did not provoke hair loss in these women.

The authors noted that this problem appears to be confined to women, at least according to published reports. The mechanism is unknown.

References

1. Etminan M, Gill S, Samii A. Comparison of the risk of adverse events with pramipexole and ropinirole in patients with Parkinson's disease: a meta-analysis. Drug Saf 2003;26(6):439–44.
2. Weiner WJ, Factor SA, Jankovic J, Hauser RA, Tetrud JW, Waters CH, Shulman LM, Glassman PM, Beck B, Paume D, Doyle C. The long-term safety and efficacy of pramipexole in advanced Parkinson's disease. Parkinsonism Relat Disord 2001;7(2):115–20.
3. Tan EK, Ondo W. Clinical characteristics of pramipexole-induced peripheral edema. Arch Neurol 2000;57(5):729–32.
4. Clarke CE, Speller JM, Clarke JA. Pramipexole for levodopa-induced complications in Parkinson's disease. Cochrane. Database Syst Rev 2000;(3):CD002261. http://www.cochrane.org/cochrane/revabstr/ab002261.htm.
5. Frucht S, Rogers JD, Greene PE, Gordon MF, Fahn S. Falling asleep at the wheel: motor vehicle mishaps in persons taking pramipexole and ropinirole. Neurology 1999;52(9):1908–10.
6. Olanow CW, Schapira AH, Roth T. Waking up to sleep episodes in Parkinson's disease. Mov Disord 2000;15(2):212–15.
7. Hauser RA, Gauger L, Anderson WM, Zesiewicz TA. Pramipexole-induced somnolence and episodes of daytime sleep. Mov Disord 2000;15(4):658–63.
8. Ferini-Strambi L. Restless legs syndrome augmentation and pramipexole treatment. Sleep Med 2002;3(Suppl):S23–5.
9. Hubble JP, Koller WC, Cutler NR, Sramek JJ, Friedman J, Goetz C, Ranhosky A, Korts D, Elvin A. Pramipexole in patients with early Parkinson's disease. Clin Neuropharmacol 1995;18(4):338–47.
10. Molho ES, Factor SA, Weiner WJ, Sanchez-Ramos JR, Singer C, Shulman L, Brown D, Sheldon C. The use of pramipexole, a novel dopamine (DA) agonist, in advanced Parkinson's disease. J Neural Transm Suppl 1995;45:225–30.
11. Tabamo RE, Di Rocco A. Alopecia induced by dopamine agonists. Neurology 2002;58(5):829–30.

Pranlukast

See also Leukotriene receptor antagonists

General Information

Pranlukast is a leukotriene receptor antagonist. It was developed primarily for the Japanese market and there is little international experience of it. To date, adverse events have occurred in under 1% of patients and gastrointestinal effects were the most common, accounting for 4.7% of reported adverse events (1).

Organs and Systems

Respiratory

Lung injury with interstitial pneumonitis has been attributed to pranlukast (2).

- A 62-year-old woman with severe asthma took oral pranlukast 450 mg/day and oral prednisolone 80 mg/day for a severe asthmatic attack. After oral prednisolone was tapered and subsequently withdrawn by day 35, she was maintained on pranlukast only and 5 days later had fever, deteriorating pulmonary symptoms, hypoxemia, and bibasal reticulonodular pulmonary infiltrates on chest CT. A transbronchial biopsy was consistent with drug-related interstitial pneumonitis. A lymphocyte stimulation test was positive for pranlukast. Her fever abated and her pulmonary symptoms markedly improved 3 days after withdrawal of pranlukast, and 5 months later the pulmonary infiltrates had completely resolved.

Immunologic

The association of cysteinyl leukotriene receptor antagonists with eosinophilic conditions, especially Churg–Strauss syndrome, has generated widespread interest. However, evaluation of the few data is hampered by poor understanding of the underlying pathophysiology of the syndrome as well as by the limited knowledge of the effect that cysteinyl leukotriene has on the immune response and the possibility of interacting genetic polymorphisms (3).

- A 26-year-old asthmatic woman had severe acute necrotizing eosinophilic endomyocarditis while taking pranlukast, inhaled beclomethasone, and oral theophylline (4). Oral prednisolone had been replaced by pranlukast 9 months before the event. Cardiac injury was accompanied by peripheral eosinophilia, cardiogenic shock, and pulmonary infiltrates, suggesting atypical Churg–Strauss syndrome. She recovered after intensive treatment, steroid pulse therapy, and withdrawal of pranlukast.
- A 53-year-old asthmatic woman developed p-ANCA-positive vasculitis while taking pranlukast 450 mg/day (5). Inhaled beclomethasone dipropionate had previously been tapered from 1200 to 800 µg/day over the previous 17 months. She had a mononeuritis multiplex, eosinophilia, and sinusitis. A lymphocyte stimulation test was negative for pranlukast.

In the second case, because p-ANCA had been positive before the patient started to take pranlukast, the authors suggested that her Churg–Strauss syndrome had occurred either through unmasking of a previously unrecognized forme fruste, through tapering the inhaled corticosteroid, or had been coincidental with the natural course of a pre-existing progressive Churg–Strauss syndrome.

In an NIH workshop summary report on the relation between asthma therapy and Churg–Strauss syndrome, the authors concluded that no one compound or class of antiasthmatic agents was solely implicated. An association was found for pranlukast, montelukast, zafirlukast, the 5-lipoxygenase inhibitor zileuton, inhaled corticosteroids, and salmeterol. As corticosteroids constitute the principal therapy of Churg–Strauss syndrome, tapering of these agents may allow incipient Churg–Strauss syndrome to become manifest. In patients who develop Churg–Strauss syndrome and do not receive corticosteroids (6–8), these various antiasthmatic medications might be used to treat asthmatic symptoms but not the underlying Churg–Strauss syndrome (3).

References

1. Barnes NC, de Jong B, Miyamoto T. Worldwide clinical experience with the first marketed leukotriene receptor antagonist. Chest 1997;111(Suppl 2):S52–60.
2. Hayashi S, Furuya S, Imamura H. Fulminant eosinophilic endomyocarditis in an asthmatic patient treated with pranlukast after corticosteroid withdrawal. Heart 2001;86(3):E7.
3. Hashimoto M, Fujishima T, Tanaka H, Kon H, Saikai T, Suzuki A, Nakatsugawa M, Abe S. Churg–Strauss syndrome after reduction of inhaled corticosteroid in a patient treated with pranlukast for asthma. Intern Med 2001;40(5):432–4.
4. Katz RS, Papernik M. Zafirlukast and Churg–Strauss syndrome. JAMA 1998;279(24):1949.
5. Green RL, Vayonis AG. Churg–Strauss syndrome after zafirlukast in two patients not receiving systemic steroid treatment. Lancet 1999;353(9154):725–6.
6. Tuggey JM, Hosker HS. Churg–Strauss syndrome associated with montelukast therapy. Thorax 2000;55(9):805–6.
7. Reinus JF, Persky S, Burkiewicz JS, Quan D, Bass NM, Davern TJ. Severe liver injury after treatment with the leukotriene receptor antagonist zafirlukast. Ann Intern Med 2000;133(12):964–8.
8. Actis GC, Morgando A, Lagget M, David E, Rizzetto M. Zafirlukast-related hepatitis: report of a further case. J Hepatol 2001;35(4):539–41.

Pranoprofen

See also Non-steroidal anti-inflammatory drugs

General Information

Pranoprofen is an arylalkanoic acid NSAID (1).

Respiratory

Acute eosinophilic pneumonia has been attributed to pranoprofen in a 48-year-old man (2).

Gastrointestinal

Multiple small bowel ulcers and massive bleeding occurred in a patient taking oral pranoprofen and rectal indometacin (SEDA-17, 113).

Urinary tract

Hemolytic urenic syndrome has been reported in a 25-year-old woman on two separate occasions (3).

References

1. Yoshio I, Iwata A, Isobe M, Takamatsu R, Higashi M. [The pharmacokinetics of pranoprofen in humans.] Yakugaku Zasshi 1990;110(7):509–15.
2. Fujimori K, Shimatsu Y, Suzuki E, Gejyo F, Arakawa M. [Pranoprofen-induced lung injury manifesting as acute eosinophilic pneumonia.] Nihon Kokyuki Gakkai Zasshi 1999;37(5):401–5.
3. Okura H, Hino M, Nishiki S, Kono K, Hasegawa T, Nakamae H, Ohta K, Yamane T, Takubo T, Tatsumi N. [Recurrent hemolytic uremic syndrome induced by pranoprofen.] Rinsho Ketsueki 1999;40(8):663–6.

Pravastatin

See also HMG Co-A reductase inhibitors

General Information

In a placebo-controlled study of 1142 hypercholesterolemic patients treated with pravastatin for 8–16 weeks, the numbers of "adverse drug experiences" were similar in the treated and untreated individuals (1). Rash was the only adverse clinical event that was different (4.0 versus 1.1%). However, in the same patients withdrawal of therapy during follow-up was thought to be necessary in 3.2% of those given pravastatin alone. Myopathy was observed in one instance only, and increases in creatine kinase activity in those taking pravastatin did not differ significantly from controls. There were marked persistent increases in transaminases in 1.1%, with no cases of symptomatic hepatitis. Pravastatin is believed to have a particularly low potential for nervous system-related adverse effects, as it has not been shown to enter the cerebrospinal fluid, and clinical experience suggests that muscle toxicity occurs less often with pravastatin than with lovastatin (2).

Organs and Systems

Respiratory

- A 41-year-old man, who had been taking pravastatin for 2 years, developed a hypersensitivity pneumonitis with eosinophilia; the symptoms gradually resolved after withdrawal of pravastatin (3).

Metabolism

- After short-term treatment with pravastatin, a 77-year-old woman transiently developed symptoms diagnosed as porphyria cutanea tarda (4).

Liver

Acute cholestatic hepatitis occurred after 7 weeks of pravastatin 20 mg/day. There was no evidence of allergy (5). It is possible that pravastatin enhances the toxicity of simultaneously administered drugs, for instance, metoprolol in the present case.

- A 64-year-old woman who was twice treated with pravastatin had cholestasis on both occasions with minimal hepatocellular injury (6).

Musculoskeletal

Although myopathy is rarely seen with pravastatin in clinical trials, it does occur.

- Rhabdomyolysis was suspected in a 67-year-old obese man with an acute myocardial infarction (7).
- A 37-year-old man with sarcoidosis developed marked myotonia during several years while he was taking pravastatin 20 mg/day (8). On drug withdrawal his symptoms improved after 2 months.

This association does not prove a causal relation. The authors of the second report pointed to previous observations of myotonia both in sarcoidosis and during the administration of various drugs.

Reproductive system

- A man taking pravastatin 20 mg/day for 3 months reported gynecomastia, which regressed after withdrawal of the drug; he was also taking allopurinol (9).

Drug–Drug Interactions

Fibrate

Rhabdomyolysis can occur when pravastatin is combined with a fibrate (SEDA-21, 460) (10).

Warfarin

With concurrent administration of warfarin and pravastatin there was no evidence of an interaction as assessed by prothrombin time (11).

References

1. Newman TJ, Kassler-Taub KB, Gelarden RT, et al. Safety of pravastatin in long-term clinical trials conducted in the united states. J Drug Dev 1990;3:275–80.
2. Jungnickel PW, Cantral KA, Maloley PA. Pravastatin: a new drug for the treatment of hypercholesterolemia. Clin Pharm 1992;11(8):677–89.
3. Liscoet-Loheac N, Andre N, Couturaud F, Chenu E, Quiot JJ, Leroyer C. Une pneumopathie iatrogénique rapportée a la prise de pravastatine. [Hypersensitivity pneumonitis in a patient taking pravastatin.] Rev Mal Respir 2001;18(4 Pt 1):426–8.
4. Schindl A, Trautinger F, Pernerstorfer-Schon H, Konnaris C, Honigsmann H. Porphyria cutanea tarda induced by the use of pravastatin. Arch Dermatol 1998;134(10):1305–6.
5. Hartleb M, Rymarczyk G, Januszewski K. Acute cholestatic hepatitis associated with pravastatin. Am J Gastroenterol 1999;94(5):1388–90.
6. Batey RG, Harvey M. Cholestasis associated with the use of pravastatin sodium. Med J Aust 2002;176(11):561.
7. Offman EM, Sabawi N, Melendez LJ. Suspected pravastatin-induced rhabdomyolysis in a patient experiencing a myocardial infarction. Can J Hosp Pharm 1998;51:233–5.

8. Riggs JE, Schochet SS Jr. Myotonia associated with sarcoidosis: marked exacerbation with pravastatin. Clin Neuropharmacol 1999;22(3):180–1.

9. Aerts J, Karmochkine M, Raguin G. Gynécomastie attribu-table à la pravastatine. [Gynecomastia due to pravastatin.] Presse Med 1999;28(15):787.

10. Colombo P, Olivetto L, Andreoni P. Rabdiomiolisi acuta in corso di trattamento combinato con pravastatina e bezafi-brato. Considerationi su un caso clinico. G Gerontol 1996;44:399–402.

11. Catalano P. Pravastatin safety: an overview. Round Table Ser 1990;16:26–31.

Praziquantel

General Information

Praziquantel, initially introduced as a veterinary cesticidal drug, was found to have efficacy against all the human species of schistosomes (including cerebral forms), fascio-lopsiasis, cysticercosis, paragonimiasis (lung fluke), *Clonorchis sinensis* (oriental liver fluke), and *Opisthorchis viverrini* infections. It is used in a single oral dose of 40 mg/kg, except in infestations with *Schistosoma japonicum*, *Clonorchis*, and *Paragonimus*, for which more prolonged administration is required, doses varying from 40 to 70 mg/kg/day depending on the infecting species. Evaluation of the result of praziquantel treatment has shown a lower laboratory rate of success than reported for clinical response (SEDA-16, 311).

Praziquantel is effective in human cysticercosis in doses of 10–100 mg/kg for 3–21 days (1). Initially, longer courses of praziquantel were advocated, but even shorter treatment regimens are equally effective: a complete course can be administered in a single day with compar-able efficacy as conventional therapy of 15 days. Praziquantel was originally introduced as a racemic mix-ture; there is evidence that the levorotatory isomer is relatively more effective, but has the same incidence of adverse reactions (2).

Praziquantel is well absorbed and penetrates cyst walls, but it undergoes first-pass metabolism, especially when given together with glucocorticoids and anticonvulsants.

Observational studies

Echinococcosis
The management and operative complications in 70 patients with hydatid disease aged 10–78 years have been studied retrospectively to assess the impact of albendazole and pra-ziquantel compared with surgery (3). In all, 39 patients received albendazole and praziquantel in combination and 19 received albendazole alone; none was treated with praziquantel alone. The combined use of albendazole and praziquantel preoperatively significantly reduced the num-ber of cysts that contained viable protoscolices.

Neurocysticercosis
Praziquantel is generally used to treat neurocysticercosis in an oral dose of 50 mg/kg/day (divided into three doses) for 15 days. Sedation can be marked and driving should be

avoided. Liver enzymes sometimes increase. Ocular cysti-cercosis should not be treated with praziquantel, because destruction of the parasite within the eye can cause irre-parable lesions.

A one-day intensive course of praziquantel has been used experimentally, but results vary, and when there are multiple brain cysts present the outcome is poor (4). When used for this purpose in a dose of 25 mg/kg at 2-hour intervals, adverse effects included mild headache, dizziness, nausea, and vomiting. All the adverse effects remitted with analgesics or dexamethasone 0.2 mg/kg/day and continued for 2 days.

Paragonimiasis
Paragonimiasis is a food-borne parasitic disease common in Southeast Asia, especially in Japan, Korea, The Philippines, Taiwan, and parts of China. In Japan, para-gonimiasis is caused by either *Paragonimus westermani* or *Paragonimus miyazakii*. Traditionally biothionol was used to treat paragonimiasis, a food-borne zoonosis that is endemic in limited areas of the world. However, owing to the need for long-term administration and moderate to severe adverse effects, such as nausea and diarrhea, biothionol has been replaced by praziquantel. At a dose of 75 mg/kg/day for only 2–3 days, praziquantel has the advantage of an easier dosing schedule in combination with excellent therapeutic efficacy. Adverse effects of praziquantel in paragonimiasis, if any, are mild and tran-sient (5). In patients with pleural effusion, pleural fluid must be drained before starting chemotherapy; insuffi-cient drainage often causes complications, such as chronic empyema or insufficient inflation of the lungs. Praziquantel is also effective for cutaneous, cerebral, or any form of extrapulmonary paragonimiasis.

The radiological features and treatment of paragoni-miasis have been described in 13 patients (10 men, three women, aged 25–77 years) (6). All were treated with praziquantel 75 mg/kg/day for 2–3 days. One patient with empyema was also given bithionol. There was mild urticaria in two patients and no serious adverse effects.

Tenia infections
In a report from India the efficacy and safety of treatment of niclosamide-resistant *Tenia saginata* infections with praziquantel 10 mg/kg orally has been confirmed in 185 consecutive patients (7). Follow-up stool examinations at 4 and 12 weeks showed a cure rate of 96%. Eleven patients were lost to follow-up, and eight still produced proglottides at the end of 12 weeks. None passed the worm in their stools, since praziquantel destructs the worm, after which the scolex and worm are digested. Thirty patients (16%) reported minimal adverse effects, such as nausea ($n = 4$), abdominal discomfort ($n = 10$), and giddiness ($n = 16$).

Comparative studies

Praziquantel 100 mg/kg in three divided doses has been compared with albendazole 15 mg/kg/day for 1 week in the treatment of neurocysticercosis in 20 patients (8). In the patients treated with albendazole the number of cysts fell from 64 to 7 and in the patients treated with prazi-quantel it fell from 59 to 24. The difference was not statistically significant. All the patients were concomitantly treated with high doses of glucocorticoids. Nine of the ten patients treated with praziquantel had seizures, headache, and dizziness, and two had hemiparesis before treatment. A few hours after the last dose of praziquantel six patients had adverse reactions, including headache and vomiting in five patients, seizures in one patient, and worsening of the pre-existing motor deficit in one. Analgesics and antiemetics improved the symptoms in four patients. In two patients treatment with mannitol was needed to relief symptoms of increased cranial pressure. The results suggested that single-day treatment with praziquantel of neurocysticercosis may be a useful option. The observed adverse effects were considered to be the result of the inflammatory reaction following the dying of worms and not a toxic effect of the drug itself.

Placebo-controlled studies

In a double-blind, randomized, placebo controlled trial of praziquantel in 42 patients with clonorchiasis and an open study in 32 patients, the adverse effects of praziquantel were transient and included nausea and vomiting (15%), vertigo (12%), hepatomegaly (4.5%), headache (1.5%), rash (1.5%), and hypotension (1.5%) (9). Of 20 patients who received placebo, one developed a transient skin rash, fever, and chills. There were minor and transient, albeit statistically significant, changes in hemoglobin and serum concentrations of total protein, uric acid, cholesterol, and bilirubin.

General adverse effects

Although adverse effects are common they tend to be mild and it is rarely necessary to withdraw praziquantel for this reason; even when used in relatively high doses, as in schistosomiasis, praziquantel has, according to the *British National Formulary* (September 2005), "the most attractive combination of effectiveness, broad-spectrum activity, and low toxicity [of all antihelminthic drugs]." The most common problems relate not so much to direct adverse effects of the drug as to allergic and inflammatory reactions in the host to the presence of dying parasites. Fever, headache, meningism, and exacerbation of neurological symptoms have all been noted; these symptoms tend to be more severe when the pretreatment parasitic infection is widespread and intense (SEDA-20, 282) (SEDA-21, 318). The main direct adverse effects of praziquantel are abdominal discomfort, diarrhea, nausea and vomiting, dizziness, and somnolence (SED-13, 837) (10), (SEDA-16, 310). Among children somnolence was seen in 11%. Headaches, skin rashes, and fever are less common (SED-13, 837). Non-specific effects observed in a minority of patients taking praziquantel include generalized weakness, swelling of the legs, epigastric area, scrotum, or more generally, fatigue (SEDA-16, 354).

Organs and Systems

Respiratory

Acute respiratory failure with exudative polyserositis has been reported in a patient taking praziquantel (11).

Nervous system

An important aspect of drug treatment in neurocysticercosis is the simultaneous use of glucocorticoids with cysticidal drugs (12,13). This combination has been recommended to avoid the secondary effects of treatment due to destruction of parasites within the brain parenchyma. However, these reactions are usually mild and transient and may be ameliorated with analgesics or antiemetics, questioning the need for corticosteroids in every case. Glucocorticoids are currently indicated for patients who develop intracranial hypertension during treatment with cysticidal drugs. This can be anticipated in patients with multiple lesions. However, some forms of neurocysticercosis should not be treated with cysticidal drugs (12,13). Both albendazole and praziquantel can exacerbate the syndrome of intracranial hypertension observed in patients with cysticercotic encephalitis, and are contraindicated during the acute phase of the disease (1). In patients with mixed forms of neurocysticercosis, including hydrocephalus and parenchymal brain cysts, cysticidal drugs should only be used after prior ventricular shunt placement to avoid a further increase in intracranial pressure after treatment. When this precaution is not taken, a further increase in intracranial pressure precipitated by praziquantel can prove fatal (14).

- A 66-year-old man with neurocysticercosis treated with glucocorticoids and praziquantel developed headache and confusion. He did not have a ventricular shunt inserted. A contrast-enhanced CT scan showed multiple focal enhancing lesions with mild edema. An MRI scan of the head was reported as being most consistent with neurocysticercosis. He was given dexamethasone 2 mg bd and praziquantel 50 mg/kg/day. A few days later his headache worsened, with nausea and drowsiness. After 2 weeks he became stuporose and had to be ventilated. A CT scan showed multiple areas of deep subcortical focal edema near the areas of previously enhancing cysts, a striatocapsular stroke, and obstructive hydrocephalus. Two weeks after the last dose of praziquantel and despite a ventriculostomy tube he died.

The authors reported that deaths related to praziquantel in neurocysticercosis are rare. However, this case had characteristics suggestive of a high risk of post-treatment complications. Death was attributed to a sudden increase in intracranial pressure, with multiple foci of edema, meningeal inflammation, and stroke, and occurred despite the concomitant use of glucocorticoids.

In patients with neurocysticercosis treated with praziquantel in increasing doses of 10–50 mg/kg/day for the first week and maintenance therapy during the second week, 27 (60%) presented with adverse effects, three requiring interruption of therapy. Increased intracranial pressure occurred in two cases (one fatal). Exacerbation of CSF pleocytosis was recorded in 26 patients (57%) (SEDA-16, 311).

A delayed reaction, with central nervous system involvement, has been described in patients with cerebral cysticercosis; papilledema, hemorrhages, focal seizures, motor weakness (SEDA-13, 242), and in one case hemiplegia from a vasculitic infarct occurred (SEDA-14, 243). The possibility that this reaction is caused by a massive inflammatory response was discussed (SEDA-14, 243). If this hypothesis is correct, glucocorticoid treatment could be contemplated. A review has suggested that the use of glucocorticoids, although still controversial, is generally accepted as a means of alleviating inflammatory complications; however, simultaneous use of a glucocorticoid seems to reduce the plasma praziquantel concentration significantly. According to one group of investigators, no delayed reaction was seen in patients with cerebral schistosomiasis (SED-13, 837).

Dose-dependent dizziness is a recognized effect in some 14% of cases at higher doses of praziquantel (SEDA-12, 267). Patients predisposed to epilepsy may develop convulsions, probably as a reaction to the death of the parasite (15). Headache (40%) and drowsiness (25–40%) have been common in some studies and the manufacturers warn against driving or operating machinery while taking praziquantel.

Most patients treated for neurocysticercosis with praziquantel develop an early cerebrospinal fluid reaction; a similar late reaction, some 2 weeks after treatment has finished, has also been described (16). In both cases clinical signs and symptoms can include papilledema, headache, nausea, vomiting, neck stiffness, and even focal seizures. Glucocorticoids can usually prevent or relieve both the early and late reactions, but they can also reduce efficacy by lowering plasma concentrations of the drug by some 50% (17).

There is a risk that if patients treated with praziquantel for a disease other than neurocysticercosis do in fact also have neurocysticercosis, serious neurological reactions (notably seizures) can occur as the parasite is killed and toxins are released (18).

Sensory systems

Praziquantel should not be used in ocular cysticercosis, because of the risk of inoperable lesions from destruction of the parasite within the eye (19).

Gastrointestinal

Praziquantel can cause dose-related nausea, vomiting, heartburn, and abdominal pain. For example, at doses of 30 mg/kg in schoolchildren there was stomachache in some 16% (SED-12, 775), while in a study with 40 mg/kg 35% of users had abdominal pain (20).

Bloody diarrhea occurs in some patients, but it can be difficult to distinguish this as an adverse effect from pretreatment symptoms; one Ethiopian study of the use of praziquantel in suspected schistosomiasis found that before treatment there was blood in the stool in 55% of cases, diarrhea in 61%, and abdominal discomfort in 80%, and the figures recorded the next day after treatment were not very different (21).

The efficacy and adverse effects of treatment with a single oral dose of praziquantel 40 mg/kg, in relation to egg counts and morbidity, have been studied in 611 primary schoolchildren infected with *Schistosoma mansoni* in Northeastern Ethiopia (22). Before treatment 40% of the patients had no symptoms and 30–40% complained of nausea, abdominal cramps, and/or bloody diarrhea. The symptoms before treatment were not related to nutritional status, intensity of *S. mansoni* egg excretion, or the presence of concomitant intestinal parasites. In the first 4–6 hours, 90 children (15%) developed severe gastrointestinal symptoms, with vomiting, abdominal cramps, and/or bloody diarrhea. They had higher mean pretreatment egg counts than the children who did not have these symptoms. The day after treatment 529 children (87%) were reviewed. Adverse effects were reported by 92% and consisted of abdominal cramps (87%), bloody diarrhea (50%), dizziness (31%), and vomiting (29%). Skin rashes and edema were observed in four individuals. The combination of abdominal cramps with vomiting, bloody diarrhea, and general weakness was significantly more common in the malnourished children and in the children with higher pretreatment egg counts. The overall cure rate after treatment with praziquantel was 83% after 5 weeks, but this rate fell with increasing pretreatment egg counts. These findings confirm that praziquantel is effective in the treatment of *S. mansoni* infections but that treatment may be associated with severe abdominal adverse effects, which may reduce drug compliance in population chemotherapy.

This point has been further evaluated in a larger double-blind, placebo-controlled study of the concurrent administration of albendazole and praziquantel in over 1500 children with high prevalences of schistosomiasis and other helminthic diseases in China and the Philippines, including two strains of *S. japonicum*, and two different areas of Kenya, one each with *S. mansoni* or *Schistosoma hematobium* (23). There was no difference in the rate of adverse effects after treatment with albendazole compared with placebo, but after treatment with praziquantel the children had significantly more nausea, abdominal pain, and headache. These adverse effects, although considered mild, were more common in children with schistosomiasis, which suggests a reaction to dying schistosomes rather than a toxic effect of the drug itself. There was a very high rate of complaints in Kenya, but both the history and the reactions after placebo suggested that many of the adverse effects reported after treatment reflected complaints before treatment.

Liver

It has been suggested that praziquantel can cause hepatomegaly and splenomegaly in children with schistosomiasis (22), but hepatomegaly and splenomegaly have also been described as complications of the disease in these young patients, and they regress with effective treatment (24).

Immunologic

Allergic reactions to praziquantel can be due to parasite death and include fever, urticaria, pruritic skin rashes, and eosinophilia. In one violent reaction there was marked eosinophilia, pleuritic chest pain, cardiac effusion, and ascites, pointing strongly to an exudative polyserositis (11).

Long-Term Effects

Drug tolerance

Diminished susceptibility to praziquantel of *S. mansoni* was reported in an area in Northern Senegal (25).

Second-Generation Effects

Lactation

Praziquantel is excreted in the breast milk, and mothers should not breastfeed for 72 hours after a dose (26).

Drug–Drug Interactions

Cimetidine

Praziquantel is well absorbed after oral administration and undergoes extensive first-pass metabolism, especially when it is given simultaneously with corticosteroids and anticonvulsants (1). Cimetidine significantly increases praziquantel serum concentrations by inhibiting its first-pass metabolism (27). The concurrent administration of cimetidine with praziquantel in neurocysticercosis allows simplification of the effective praziquantel regimen from 50 mg/kg/day for 2 weeks to a one-day regimen of three doses of 25 mg/kg at 2-hour intervals; this regimen increases the time over which the parasite is exposed to high drug concentrations and produces similar benefits, and also reduces the cost, length of treatment, and total dose used (28). It has also been proposed that simultaneous administration of praziquantel and cimetidine could improve the efficacy of single-day therapy with praziquantel for cysticercosis and other parasitic diseases, such as schistosomiasis (29).

Grapefruit juice

A single dose of grapefruit juice 250 ml significantly increased the AUC and C_{max} of a single dose of praziquantel without changing the t_{max} or half-life, suggesting increased systemic availability (30).

Food–Drug Interactions

Serum praziquantel concentrations increase when a carbohydrate-rich diet is administered (1).

References

1. Garg RK. Medical management of neurocysticercosis. Neurol India 2001;49(4):329–37.
2. Yue-Han L, Xiao-Gen W, Min-Xin Q, et al. A comparative trial of single dose treatment with praziquantel and levopraziquantel in human Schistosomiasis japonica. Jpn J Parasitol 1988;37:331.
3. Ayles HM, Corbett EL, Taylor I, Cowie AG, Bligh J, Walmsley K, Bryceson AD. A combined medical and surgical approach to hydatid disease: 12 years' experience at the Hospital for Tropical Diseases, London. Ann R Coll Surg Engl 2002;84(2):100–5.
4. Pretell EJ, Garcia HH, Gilman RH, Saavedra H, Martinez M. Cysticercosis Working Group in Peru. Failure of one-day praziquantel treatment in patients with multiple neurocysticercosis lesions. Clin Neurol Neurosurg 2001;103(3):175–7.
5. Nakamura-Uchiyama F, Mukae H, Nawa Y. Paragonimiasis: a Japanese perspective. Clin Chest Med 2002;23(2):409–20.
6. Mukae H, Taniguchi H, Matsumoto N, Iiboshi H, Ashitani J, Matsukura S, Nawa Y. Clinicoradiologic features of pleuropulmonary Paragonimus westermani on Kyusyu Island, Japan. Chest 2001;120(2):514–20.
7. Koul PA, Waheed A, Hayat M, Sofi BA. Praziquantel in niclosamide-resistant Taenia saginata infection. Scand J Infect Dis 1999;31(6):603–4.
8. Del Brutto OH, Campos X, Sanchez J, Mosquera A. Single-day praziquantel versus 1-week albendazole for neurocysticercosis. Neurology 1999;52(5):1079–81.
9. Yangco BG, De Lerma C, Lyman GH, Price DL. Clinical study evaluating efficacy of praziquantel in clonorchiasis. Antimicrob Agents Chemother 1987;31(2):135–8.
10. Pungpak S, Bunnag D, Harinasuta T. Studies on the chemotherapy of human opisthorchiasis: effective dose of praziquantel in heavy infection. Southeast Asian J Trop Med Public Health 1985;16(2):248–52.
11. Azher M, el-Kassimi FA, Wright SG, Mofti A. Exudative polyserositis and acute respiratory failure following praziquantel therapy. Chest 1990;98(1):241–3.
12. Di Pentima MC, White AC. Neurocysticercosis: controversies in management. Semin Pediatr Infect Dis 2000;11:261–8.
13. Del Brutto OH. Medical therapy for cysticercosis: indications, risks, and benefits. Rev Ecuat Neurol 2000;9:13–15.
14. Chang GY, Ko DY. Isolated Echinococcus granulosus hydatid cyst in the CNS with severe reaction to treatment Neurology 2000;54(3):778–9.
15. Bada JL, Trevino B, Cabezos J. Convulsive seizures after treatment with praziquantel. BMJ (Clin Res Ed) 1988;296(6622):646.
16. Ciferri F. Delayed CSF reaction to praziquantel. Lancet 1988;1(8586):642–3.
17. Del Brutto OH. Delayed CSF reaction to praziquantel. Lancet 1988;2(8606):341.
18. Torres JR. Use of praziquantel in populations at risk of neurocysticercosis. Rev Inst Med Trop Sao Paulo 1989;31(4):290.
19. Auzemery A, Andriantsimahavandy A, Bernardin P, Queguiner P. La cysticercose intravitréenne. Evolution spontanée. A propos d'un cas. [Intravitreous cysticercosis. Spontaneous course. Apropos of a case.] J Fr Ophtalmol 1996;19(8–9):556–8.
20. Jaoko WG, Muchemi G, Oguya FO. Praziquantel side effects during treatment of Schistosoma mansoni infected pupils in Kibwezi, Kenya. East Afr Med J 1996;73(8):499–501.
21. Fletcher M, Teklehaimanot A. Schistosoma mansoni infection in a new settlement in Metekel district, north-western Ethiopia: morbidity and side effects of treatment with praziquantel in relation to intensity of infection. Trans R Soc Trop Med Hyg 1989;83(6):793–7.
22. Berhe N, Gundersen SG, Abebe F, Birrie H, Medhin G, Gemetchu T. Praziquantel side effects and efficacy related to Schistosoma mansoni egg loads and morbidity in primary school children in north-east Ethiopia. Acta Trop 1999;72(1):53–63.
23. Olds GR, King C, Hewlett J, Olveda R, Wu G, Ouma J, Peters P, McGarvey S, Odhiambo O, Koech D, Liu CY, Aligui G, Gachihi G, Kombe Y, Parraga I, Ramirez B, Whalen C, Horton RJ, Reeve P. Double-blind placebo-controlled study of concurrent administration of albendazole and praziquantel in schoolchildren with schistosomiasis and geohelminths. J Infect Dis 1999;179(4):996–1003.
24. Stephenson LS, Latham MC, Kinoti SN, Oduori ML. Regression of splenomegaly and hepatomegaly in children treated for Schistosoma haematobium infection. Am J Trop Med Hyg 1985;34(1):119–23.
25. Fallon PG, Sturrock RF, Niang AC, Doenhoff MJ. Short report: diminished susceptibility to praziquantel in a Senegal isolate of Schistosoma mansoni. Am J Trop Med Hyg 1995;53(1):61–2.

26. Putter J, Held F. Quantitative studies on the occurrence of praziquantel in milk and plasma of lactating women. Eur J Drug Metab Pharmacokinet 1979;4(4):193–8.
27. Castro N, Gonzalez-Esquivel D, Medina R, Sotelo J, Jung H. The influence of cimetidine on plasma levels of praziquantel after a single day therapeutic regimen. Proc West Pharmacol Soc 1997;40:33–4.
28. Sotelo J, Jung H. Pharmacokinetic optimisation of the treatment of neurocysticercosis. Clin Pharmacokinet 1998;34(6):503–15.
29. Jung H, Medina R, Castro N, Corona T, Sotelo J. Pharmacokinetic study of praziquantel administered alone and in combination with cimetidine in a single-day therapeutic regimen. Antimicrob Agents Chemother 1997;41(6):1256–9.
30. Castro N, Jung H, Medina R, Gonzalez-Esquivel D, Lopez M, Sotelo J. Interaction between grapefruit juice and praziquantel in humans. Antimicrob Agents Chemother 2002;46(5):1614–16.

Prazosin

See also Alpha-adrenoceptor antagonists

General Information

Prazosin is an alpha$_1$-adrenoceptor antagonist.

Organs and Systems

Cardiovascular

Postural hypotension and reflex tachycardia, particularly on standing, are features of the first-dose response to prazosin, but adaptive receptor responses lead to re-setting of the reflex mechanisms within the first few days of treatment, and there are therefore generally no significant changes in heart rate during long-term treatment. An orthostatic component to the hypotensive response persists during long-term treatment, and this may be significant and symptomatic if high dosages are used. It is less frequent with modified-release prazosin.

Metabolism

Prazosin and other quinazolines are associated with small but significant changes in plasma lipid profiles. Generally these are potentially beneficial changes, with reductions in LDL cholesterol, total cholesterol, and triglycerides, and increases in HDL cholesterol.

Urinary tract

Blockade of alpha$_1$-adrenoceptors in the urinary tract leads to smooth muscle relaxation and improvement in urinary flow, and this pharmacological action has been used to ameliorate the urinary symptoms of benign prostatic hyperplasia. Prazosin can occasionally lead to urinary incontinence, particularly stress incontinence in women [1].

Sexual function

There is some evidence that male sexual dysfunction occurs less often with alpha-blockers than with other types of antihypertensive drugs [2]. For example, in a comparison of the effects of prazosin and hydrochlorothiazide on sexual function in 12 hypertensive men, plethysmographic measurements and subjective assessments showed less dysfunction with prazosin than with hydrochlorothiazide [3]. There is no evidence that this effect can be used therapeutically, but cases of priapism have been reported: for example, a 55-year-old man presented with priapism having taken prazosin 7.5 mg tds for 4 months. After a further 3 months, prazosin was discontinued and erectile function became normal [4].

Drug–Drug Interactions

Alcohol

In a well-controlled study in 10 Japanese patients with mild hypertension, the blood pressure reduction caused by alcohol 1 ml/kg was significantly increased by concurrent treatment with prazosin 1 mg tds [5]. At 2–4 hours after ingestion the blood pressure fell by 18/12 mmHg without prazosin and by 24/18 mmHg with prazosin. These results raise the possibility that heavy drinking may cause symptomatic hypotension in patients taking prazosin.

References

1. Wall LL, Addison WA. Prazosin-induced stress incontinence. Obstet Gynecol 1990;75(3 Pt 2):558–60.
2. Neaton JD, Grimm RH Jr, Prineas RJ, Stamler J, Grandits GA, Elmer PJ, Cutler JA, Flack JM, Schoenberger JA, McDonald R, Lewis CE, Liebson PR. Treatment of Mild Hypertension Study. Final results. Treatment of Mild Hypertension Study Research Group. JAMA 1993;270(6):713–24.
3. Scharf MB, Mayleben DW. Comparative effects of prazosin and hydrochlorothiazide on sexual function in hypertensive men. Am J Med 1989;86(1B):110–12.
4. Bullock N. Prazosin-induced priapism. Br J Urol 1988;62(5):487–8.
5. Kawano Y, Abe H, Kojima S, Takishita S, Omae T. Interaction of alcohol and an alpha1-blocker on ambulatory blood pressure in patients with essential hypertension. Am J Hypertens 2000;13(3):307–12.

Prenalterol

General Information

Prenalterol has dobutamine-like positive inotropic effects and has been used in severe heart failure [1]. It can cause cardiac dysrhythmias (SEDA-6, 135).

Reference

1. Kendall MJ, Goodfellow RM, Westerling S. Prenalterol—a new cardioselective inotropic agent. J Clin Hosp Pharm 1982;7(2):107–18.

Prenylamine

See also Calcium channel blockers

General Information

Prenylamine is a coronary vasodilator that depletes myocardial catecholamine stores and has some calcium-channel blocking activity. It has been used in the treatment of angina pectoris, but it often causes ventricular dysrhythmias and has been superseded by less toxic drugs.

Organs and Systems

Cardiovascular

Ventricular tachycardia associated with QT prolongation (torsade de pointes) has often been described with prenylamine (1,2).

Drug–Drug Interactions

Iothalamate

Ventricular tachycardia has been reported after the intravenous administration of sodium iothalamate in a patient taking prenylamine (3). Both drugs can prolong the QT interval.

References

1. Riccioni N, Bartolomei C, Soldani S. Prenylamine-induced ventricular arrhythmias and syncopal attacks with Q-T prolongation. Report of a case and comment on therapeutic use of lignocaine. Cardiology 1980;66(4):199–203.
2. Burri C, Ajdacic K, Michot F. Syndrom der verlangerten QT-Zeit und Kammer-Tachykardie "en torsade de pointe" nach Behandlung mit Prenylamin (Segontin). [Prolonged QT interval and "torsades de pointes" after therapy with prenylamin (Segontin).] Schweiz Rundsch Med Prax 1981;70(16):717–20.
3. Duncan JS, Ramsay LE. Ventricular tachycardia precipitated by sodium iothalamate (Conray 420) injection during prenylamine treatment: a predictable adverse drug interaction. Postgrad Med J 1985;61(715):415–17.

Preservatives

General Information

Preservatives that are often found in cosmetics include formaldehyde, quaternium-15, imidazolidinyl urea, diazolidinyl urea, parabens mix, 5-chloro-2-methyl-4-isothiazolin-3-one + 2-methyl-4-isothiazolin-3-one (MCI/MI, Kathon CG), and methyldibromoglutaronitrile (MDBGN, Euxyl K400). Polyhexamethylenebiguanide, a biocide structurally related to hexamidine, is added to cosmetics as a preservative.

Organs and Systems

Immunologic

Preservatives are important causes of allergic contact dermatitis in cosmetics. In a 10-year analysis in 16 centers in 11 countries, 73 818 consecutive patients were patch-tested for the preservatives listed above. There were several cases of contact allergy to formaldehyde and MCI/MI. These preservatives are currently avoided in cosmetics. However, the frequency of positive reactions to MDBGN has risen, from 0.7% in 1991 to 3.5% in 2000. The authors suggested that the concentration of this preservative should be reduced in leave-on cosmetic products (1).

DMDM hydantoin is a preservative that is used mainly in cosmetics. In 1808 consecutive patients DMDM hydantoin was patch-tested in a concentration of 2% in petroleum, and in a further 34 321 patients it was tested in a concentration of 2% in water. The proportion of positive reactions was 0.39–0.65%, with no evidence of a significant time trend. In the 180 positive cases cosmetics (30%) or topical drugs (22%) were considered causal (2).

Hexamidine (0.15% petrolatum) (SEDA-10, 128) has rarely been reported to cause a contact allergic reaction (3,4). Of 1554 patients tested with polyhexamethylenebiguanide 2.5% in aqua, 6 (0.4%) had a positive reaction, indicating a very low sensitization rate (5).

References

1. Wilkinson JD, Shaw S, Andersen KE, Brandao FM, Bruynzeel DP, Bruze M, Camarasa JM, Diepgen TL, Ducombs G, Frosch PJ, Goossens A, Lachappelle JM, Lahti A, Menne T, Seidenari S, Tosti A, Wahlberg JE. Monitoring levels of preservative sensitivity in Europe. A 10-year overview (1991–2000). Contact Dermatitis 2002;46(4):207–10.
2. Uter W, Frosch PJ; IVDK Study Group and the German Contact Dermatitis Research Group, DKG. Contact allergy from DMDM hydantoin, 1994–2000. Contact Dermatitis 2002;47(1):57–8.
3. Revuz J, Poli F, Wechsler J, Dubertret L. Dermite de contact a l'hexamidine. [Contact dermatitis from hexamidine.] Ann Dermatol Venereol 1984;111(9):805–10.
4. Dooms-Goossens A, Vandaele M, Bedert R, Marien K. Hexamidine isethionate: a sensitizer in topical pharmaceutical products and cosmetics. Contact Dermatitis 1989;21(4):270.
5. Schnuch A, Geier J, Brasch J, Fuchs T, Pirker C, Schulze-Dirks A, Basketter DA. Polyhexamethylenebiguanide: a relevant contact allergen? Contact Dermatitis 2000;42(5):302–3.

Prilocaine and Emla

See also Local anesthetics

General Information

Prilocaine is an aminoamide local anesthetic. It can be used on its own, but it is also included in Emla in a eutectic combination with lidocaine (25 mg/ml each), which is widely used as a local anesthetic in topical administration for, for example, superficial surgery and venepuncture.

Emla cream causes minor local adverse effects, such as itch, burning, and localized purpura (SEDA-19, 131) (SEDA-20, 127) (SEDA-22, 140). A meta-analysis of the use of Emla cream in the elderly (over 65) showed that the technique is generally safe, with only mild transient effects (pallor, redness, and edema) at the application site; there were no systemic effects (1).

However, if large amounts are applied, particularly under occlusion, it can be sufficiently well absorbed to cause systemic effects. Three of 1648 children who received measles vaccination with Emla 1 g had adverse reactions 10–20 minutes later; all required adrenaline for similar symptoms of weakness and dizziness with a cold clammy skin and no pulse or a weak pulse (2). One went on to wheeze markedly and had peripheral cyanosis and shivering, improving with hydrocortisone. The authors proposed that these unusual reactions could have been due to a biphasic local reaction to Emla, with vasodilatation leading to increased absorption and further toxicity.

Organs and Systems

Nervous system

Particular care must be taken with Emla in children, since seizures can occur.

- A 5-year-old child had 35 g of Emla applied under an occlusive dressing to eczematous skin in preparation for cryotherapy for molluscum contagiosum (3). Within 1 hour, the child had a generalized seizure that lasted 10 minutes. The plasma concentrations of lidocaine and prilocaine 30 minutes later were 5.5 and 2.0 μg/ml, respectively, and 6 hours later, the methemoglobin concentration was 19%. The child was given vitamin C 500 mg intravenously, and 2 days later had a methemoglobin concentration of 0.3%.

Errors by pharmacists or parents continue to contribute to severe complications, such as seizures, after overdose of Emla cream in children (4).

- A 21-month-old girl had four generalized tonic-clonic seizures after inadvertent overuse of Emla before curettage of skin lesions of molluscum contagiosum. Because of a pharmacy error, 30 g tubes of Emla were dispensed instead of 5 g tubes. The toddler's mother applied 75 g under occlusive dressing, covering about 350 cm^2 of the child's surface area. This dose significantly exceeds the recommendations for a 14 kg child—maximum 10 g on a maximum area of 100 cm^2. Two doses of intravenous lorazepam (0.1 mg/kg) did not control the seizures, which stopped only after phenobarbital (20 mg/kg) was given. The child then required intubation and ventilation for respiratory depression. The lidocaine concentration 4 hours after the first application of Emla was 2.5 μg/ml and the methemoglobin concentration was 8%.

Seizures have also been reported in adults.

- An 84-year-old woman had three generalized tonic-clonic seizures after repeated applications of Emla (17 applications of 10 g over 23 weeks) (5,6).

Sensory systems

Emla cream can cause severe eye irritation (7).

- Emla cream 30 g was applied to both periorbital and proximal nasal sidewall areas for laser treatment in a 20-year-old woman. Despite the use of a right eye shield for corneal protection, the next day she developed right eye pain and blurred vision and remembered that Emla cream had accidentally entered her right eye before treatment. This caused immediate discomfort, which subsided and then recurred several hours later. She had severe conjunctival injection with loss of epithelium from over 90% of the surface of her cornea, in a pattern more suggestive of chemical than mechanical damage. Treatment with a bandage contact lens and prophylactic antibiotics was effective and her visual acuity returned to baseline.

Hematologic

Methemoglobinemia as an adverse effect of prilocaine (8) has been reported more often than with any other local anesthetic. It is caused by a metabolite and is a particular problem in neonates, who have an immature methemoglobin reductase system and residual fetal hemoglobin, increasing the risk of symptomatic methemoglobinemia.

Neonates and small children who have penile block with prilocaine, for circumcision can develop severe methemoglobinemia (9,10). A report has emphasized the severity of methemoglobinemia in infants especially if premature, when even a small dose of prilocaine is used for infiltration (11).

- A 1.3 kg premature neonate of 30-week gestation, having required ventilation over the first 3 days for respiratory distress syndrome, required reintubation on day 12 of life for recurrent apnea. He developed a pneumothorax requiring an intercostal drain; 0.5 ml of 1% prilocaine was used for infiltration, after which his oxygen requirements overnight went from 28 to 100%; his SpO$_2$ was 90% and he turned pale gray. His PaO$_2$ was 23 kPa (170 mmHg) and his methemoglobin concentration was 15%. He was given methylthioninium chloride, and within 8 hours, his methemoglobin concentration was 0.5% and his SpO$_2$ 96%.

Methemoglobinemia can occur with overdosage of prilocaine (SEDA-20, 129) and after inadvertent intravenous administration, particularly in neonates and children (SEDA-11, 221) (12).

- In a 6-year-old boy, 10 ml of a 2% solution given for bilateral percutaneous nephrostomy produced a degree of cyanosis that demanded methylthioninium chloride treatment (13).

In adults, even those with anemia, the shift in methemoglobin concentrations from prilocaine, while measurable, is not of clinical significance (SEDA-12, 257) (14).

Despite concerns that Emla cream can cause methemoglobinemia in neonates and preterm babies, a French study of 116 infants in neonatal intensive care, who were treated with small amounts of Emla once a day before skin puncture, showed that methemoglobin concentrations never exceeded 5% and were not related to gestational age or duration of application (SEDA-20, 127). Two other studies on the use of Emla as analgesia for neonates and low birth weight infants showed localized pallor, but no evidence of methemoglobinemia (SEDA-22, 140).

However, high doses of Emla have been responsible for two cases of methemoglobinemia in neonates. In one, 3.5 g of Emla was used before circumcision, and in the other 25 g of cream had been applied to a buttock hemangioma by the parents before laser therapy (SEDA-22, 140).

- A 3-year-old girl with multiple lesions of molluscum contagiosum had Emla applied to the lesions before curettage (15). She became lethargic and hypoactive 2 hours later, with periorbital discoloration and cyanosed lips. Her SaO_2 was 85%, systolic blood pressure 185 mmHg, pulse 144/minute, and her methemoglobin concentration 21%. Her caregiver had applied about 25 g of cream to her entire torso, a massive dose of prilocaine (about 625 mg).

This report reinforces previously described problems arising from carers' lack of understanding of instructions when using Emla in children or babies.

- A 4-day-old boy developed methemoglobinemia (16%) after the application of Emla cream to his penis before circumcision (16).
- A 7-month-old girl was ventilated with inhaled nitric oxide 40 ppm and developed methemoglobinemia after the application of Emla to an 8 cm^2 area of skin for 5 hours (17). Shortly after removal she developed cyanosis, with a methemoglobin concentration of 16%, which resolved with two doses of methylthioninium chloride.

In these cases, the prolonged duration of Emla application was thought to be the cause, but concomitant use of inhaled nitric oxide may have contributed.

Skin

The adverse effects of Emla include localized blanching or erythema, burning or itching sensations, irritant and allergic reactions, and purpura (18).

In 29 children with atopic dermatitis who were given Emla cream before curettage of molluscum contagiosum, there were no adverse reactions, apart from mild transient application site reactions, such as pallor, redness, and edema. No systemic reactions were reported, but the authors emphasized that Emla can be rapidly absorbed through atopic skin, and they therefore recommended that when Emla is applied under occlusive dressing, the maximum dose should be 10 g for 30 minutes (19).

The analgesic effects of single and repeated applications of Emla over six consecutive days have been studied in 11 patients with post-herpetic neuralgia (20). There was no evidence of systemic adverse effects, but four patients developed mild erythema at 30 minutes, which may have been due to the occlusive dressing, and one patient had pruritus on day 7.

Two children developed petechial eruptions after the application of Emla for treatment curettage of molluscum contagiosum (21). Neither became systemically unwell, and subsequent reapplication of Emla in one child did not elicit a petechial eruption.

There has been a report of hyperpigmentation following the use of Emla cream (22).

- A 12-year-old black child developed a patch of hyperpigmentation on his forehead where Emla cream had been used for cutaneous anesthesia before local infiltration with lidocaine for removal of a nevus. This persisted, although fading, for at least 4 months. No other cause could be found.

Hypopigmentation has also been reported with Emla (23).

Contact dermatitis was reported in three hemodialysis patients who used Emla cream repeatedly as analgesia for AV fistula cannulation (SEDA-21, 136).

- A 6-year-old boy developed contact dermatitis following the application of Emla for a skin biopsy to diagnose graft-versus-host disease (24). The histopathological features of the contact dermatitis were similar to graft-versus-host disease.

The use of Emla to provide topical anesthesia should be documented in order to avoid misdiagnosis.

References

1. Wahlgren CF, Lillieborg S. Split-skin grafting with lidocaine–prilocaine cream: a meta-analysis of efficacy and safety in geriatric versus nongeriatric patients. Plast Reconstr Surg 2001;107(3):750–6.
2. Dilraj A, Cutts FT, Bennett JV, Coovadia HM, Hopkinson C. Adverse reactions possibly associated with the use of Emla cream. S Afr Med J 1999;89(4):419–20.
3. Capron F, Perry D, Capolaghi B. Crise convulsive et méthémoglobinémie après application de crême anèsthesique. [Convulsive crisis and methemoglobinemia after the application of anesthetic cream.] Arch Pediatr 1998;5(7):812.
4. Rincon E, Baker RL, Iglesias AJ, Duarte AM. CNS toxicity after topical application of EMLA cream on a toddler with molluscum contagiosum. Pediatr Emerg Care 2000;16(4):252–4.
5. Boulinguez S, Sparsa A, Bouyssou-Gauthier ML, Bedane C, Bonnetblanc JM. Adverse effects associated with EMLA cream used as topical anesthetic for the mechanical debridement of leg ulcers. J Am Acad Dermatol 2000;42(1 Pt 1):146–8.
6. Lok C. Adverse effects associated with EMLA cream used as topical anesthetic for the mechanical debridement of leg ulcers. Reply. J Am Acad Dermatol 2000;42(1 Pt 1):147–8.
7. McKinlay JR, Hofmeister E, Ross EV, MacAllister W. EMLA cream-induced eye injury. Arch Dermatol 1999;135(7):855–6.
8. Elsner P, Dummer R. Signs of methaemoglobinaemia after topical application of EMLA cream in an infant with haemangioma. Dermatology 1997;195(2):153–4.
9. Prineas S, Wilkins BH, Halliday RJ. Circumcision blues. Med J Aust 1997;166(11):615.
10. Tse S, Barrington K, Byrne P. Methemoglobinemia associated with prilocaine use in neonatal circumcision. Am J Perinatol 1995;12(5):331–2.
11. Ergenekon E, Atalay Y, Koc E, Turkyilmaz C. Methaemoglobinaemia in a premature infant secondary to prilocaine. Acta Paediatr 1999;88(2):236.
12. Menahem S. Neonatal cyanosis, methaemoglobinaemia and haemolytic anaemia. Acta Paediatr Scand 1988;77(5):755–6.
13. Kilic I, Kalayci O. Methemoglobinemia due to prilocain local anesthesia. Doga Turk J Med Sci 1993;19.

14. Bardoczky GI, Wathieu M, D'Hollander A. Prilocaine-induced methemoglobinemia evidenced by pulse oximetry. Acta Anaesthesiol Scand 1990;34(2):162–4.

15. Touma S, Jackson JB. Lidocaine and prilocaine toxicity in a patient receiving treatment for mollusca contagiosa. J Am Acad Dermatol 2001;44(Suppl 2):399–400.

16. Couper RT. Methaemoglobinaemia secondary to topical lignocaine/prilocaine in a circumcised neonate. J Paediatr Child Health 2000;36(4):406–7.

17. Sinisterra S, Miravet E, Alfonso I, Soliz A, Papazian O. Methemoglobinemia in an infant receiving nitric oxide after the use of eutectic mixture of local anesthetic. J Pediatr 2002;141(2):285–6.

18. de Waard-van der Spek FB, Oranje AP. Purpura caused by Emla is of toxic origin. Contact Dermatitis 1997;36(1):11–13.

19. Ronnerfalt L, Fransson J, Wahlgren CF. EMLA cream provides rapid pain relief for the curettage of molluscum contagiosum in children with atopic dermatitis without causing serious application-site reactions. Pediatr Dermatol 1998;15(4):309–12.

20. Attal N, Brasseur L, Chauvin M, Bouhassira D. Effects of single and repeated applications of a eutectic mixture of local anaesthetics (EMLA) cream on spontaneous and evoked pain in post-herpetic neuralgia. Pain 1999;81(1–2):203–9.

21. Calobrisi SD, Drolet BA, Esterly NB. Petechial eruption after the application of EMLA cream. Pediatrics 1998;101(3 Pt 1):471–3.

22. Godwin Y, Brotherston M. Hyperpigmentation following the use of Emla cream. Br J Plast Surg 2001;54(1):82–3.

23. Santacana E, Aliaga L, Bayo M, Vilanova F, Villar-Landeira JM. Emla cream for 15 or 30 min before venopuncture. Reg Anaesth 1994;19:24.

24. Dong H, Kerl H, Cerroni L. EMLA cream-induced irritant contact dermatitis. J Cutan Pathol 2002;29(3):190–2.

Primaquine

General Information

The 8-aminoquinolines were the first synthetic antimalarial drugs to be introduced into medicine. Pamaquine (Plasmochin) was the first to be marketed in 1926, but primaquine proved to have the highest chemotherapeutic index of the many compounds tested.

Primaquine is rapidly absorbed, extensively distributed, and predominantly cleared by non-renal elimination. Its principal metabolite is carboxyprimaquine. While primaquine itself is rapidly eliminated from the plasma, the drug is effective when given once daily or even once weekly (SEDA-13, 810). The pharmacokinetics in children, pregnant women, and patients with renal or hepatic dysfunction are unknown.

Primaquine is mainly used to eradicate the exoerythrocytic stages of *Plasmodium vivax* and *Plasmodium ovale*, which if untreated cause late relapse (SEDA-18, 287). There is growing concern about primaquine resistance in *P. vivax* (SEDA-21, 296).

Observational studies

Primaquine base 0.5 mg/kg/day in the prophylaxis of *Plasmodium falciparum* and *P. vivax* malaria for a year did not cause noteworthy adverse effects. General complaints were less than in the placebo group but about the same as in those treated with chloroquine. None of the volunteers (smokers or non-smokers) had a methemoglobin concentration greater than 13% (1).

A randomized, placebo-controlled trial of supervised malaria prophylaxis with primaquine (30 mg/day for 20 weeks) in 97 non-immune adults with normal glucose-6-phosphate dehydrogenase (G6PD) concentrations in Papua New Guinea showed 93% protective efficacy of primaquine against malaria (95% CI = 71, 98%) (2). The most common adverse events were headache, abdominal pain, cough, and nausea, but these were not more frequent than with placebo. Transient rises in methemoglobin concentrations (mean 3.4% on the last day of prophylaxis, resolving by day 18) were asymptomatic.

Supervised treatment of *P. vivax* malaria with chloroquine (600 mg on day 1, 450 mg on days 2 and 3) and primaquine (15 mg/day for 14 days) has been studied in 50 patients in a non-endemic area of Brazil in a prospective open trial (3). G6PD status was not checked. The relapse-free cure rate at 6 months was 86%. There were no important adverse events. Risk factors for relapse included lower doses of primaquine. In patients over 60 kg in weight, the dose of primaquine can fall short of recommendations (0.25–0.3 mg/kg/day), and this can contribute to the risk of relapse.

Combination therapy

Primaquine + clindamycin

Primaquine on its own has some effect against *Pneumocystis jiroveci*, but in dosages of 0.25 or 0.5 mg/kg, primaquine alone was ineffective in rats, confirming earlier clinical experience. Clindamycin alone was also ineffective. The combination was effective both in vitro and in animals for treatment and prophylaxis.

Intravenous clindamycin, 900 mg every 8 hours, with oral primaquine 26.3 mg, was effective in a number of patients with active disease. A maintenance oral dose of clindamycin 150 mg four times daily plus primaquine 26.3 mg/day was adequate. The drugs are thought to be synergistic. In a second study, clindamycin 600 mg qds was used intravenously, with a maintenance dose of 300–400 mg orally and primaquine base orally, 15 mg/day. Tolerance was reasonably good; the most frequent adverse effect, in half the patients, was a generalized maculopapular rash after 10–12 days. Rash was accompanied by fever in three cases. Other adverse effects were leukopenia (*n* = 2), nausea (*n* = 2), and diarrhea (*n* = 1) (SEDA-12, 703) (4). In a third study with higher doses of primaquine, methemoglobinemia was a major adverse effect. In a fourth study, clindamycin was given 900 mg tds with primaquine 30 mg/day, except in three of 28 episodes of *P. jiroveci* pneumonia treated in a total in 26 patients, who received primaquine 15 mg/day (two) or 30 mg on alternate days (one). In 11 episodes the patients had been intolerant of standard therapy, in 13 episodes conventional therapy had failed, and in four episodes there had been treatment failure and intolerance. Of the 28 episodes, 24 were successfully treated with clindamycin/primaquine, the most common adverse effect being rash (5). With the use of higher doses of clindamycin, gastrointestinal effects, especially diarrhea and colitis, can be expected. The primaquine component can cause hemolytic anemia and methemoglobinemia. Patients should be screened for G6PD deficiency.

Organs and Systems

Psychological, psychiatric

Severe mental depression and confusion was reported in one patient who had been treated with chloroquine beforehand; all the symptoms disappeared on withdrawal (SEDA-11, 588).

Hematologic

Mild anemia, methemoglobinemia, and leukocytosis have been mentioned occasionally, as well as a very occasional case of agranulocytosis, usually associated with overdosage (6).

Primaquine and its congeners can cause hemolytic anemia in people with G6PD deficiency. The effects are more pronounced in the B type (the Mediterranean type) than in the A type. In a 28-year-old Thai soldier, who developed a hemolytic anemia, G6PD deficiency was not mentioned (SEDA-16, 308), but four patients reported in Vanuatu in 1992 had G6PD deficiency; all developed acute intravascular hemolysis resulting in anemia, hemoglobinuria, and systemic illness after a single dose of the drug (SEDA-17, 328).

Gastrointestinal

The most common adverse effects of primaquine are gastrointestinal: mild to moderate abdominal cramps and occasional gastric distress. In those without G6PD deficiency, primaquine is well tolerated as a prophylactic at doses of 15 mg/day (7), with only 1/106 patients withdrawing because of gastrointestinal upset in one study.

Liver

Primaquine can cause dose-dependent hepatotoxicity, as illustrated by a case of acute liver failure (with spontaneous recovery) caused by accidental overdosage (1260 mg on the second day of treatment for *P. vivax*) (8).

Drug–Drug Interactions

Dapsone

The combination of primaquine with clindamycin is used as second choice in the treatment or prevention of *P. jiroveci* pneumonia. If the patient has been treated immediately beforehand with dapsone, methemoglobinemia can result, especially in patients infected with HIV (SEDA-21, 296).

References

1. Kremsner PG, Radloff P, Metzger W, Wildling E, Mordmuller B, Philipps J, Jenne L, Nkeyi M, Prada J, Bienzle U, et al. Quinine plus clindamycin improves chemotherapy of severe malaria in children. Antimicrob Agents Chemother 1995;39(7):1603–5.

2. Baird JK, Lacy MD, Basri H, Barcus MJ, Maguire JD, Bangs MJ, Gramzinski R, Sismadi P, Krisin, Ling J, Wiady I, Kusumaningsih M, Jones TR, Fryauff DJ, Hoffman SL; United States Naval Medical Research Unit 2 Clinical Trials Team. Randomized, parallel placebo-controlled trial of primaquine for malaria prophylaxis in Papua, Indonesia. Clin Infect Dis 2001;33(12):1990–7.

3. Duarte EC, Pang LW, Ribeiro LC, Fontes CJ. Association of subtherapeutic dosages of a standard drug regimen with failures in preventing relapses of vivax malaria. Am J Trop Med Hyg 2001;65(5):471–6.

4. Ruf B, Pohle HD. Clindamycin/primaquine for *Pneumocystis carinii* pneumonia. Lancet 1989;2(8663):626–7.

5. Noskin GA, Murphy RL, Black JR, Phair JP. Salvage therapy with clindamycin/primaquine for *Pneumocystis carinii* pneumonia. Clin Infect Dis 1992;14(1):183–8.

6. Jaremin B, Felczak-Korzybska I, Myjak P. Przypadek methemoglobinemii i agranulocytozy w przebiegu leczenia malarii (*Pl. ovale*) arechina I primachina. [A case of methemoglobinemia and agranulocytosis during the treatment of malaria (*Pl. ovale*) with arequine and primaquine.] Wiad Lek 1982;35(9):591–4.

7. Schwartz E, Regev-Yochay G. Primaquine as prophylaxis for malaria for nonimmune travelers: A comparison with mefloquine and doxycycline. Clin Infect Dis 1999;29(6):1502–6.

8. Lobel HO, Coyne PE, Rosenthal PJ. Drug overdoses with antimalarial agents: prescribing and dispensing errors. JAMA 1998;280(17):1483.

Primidone

See also Antiepileptic drugs

General Information

Primidone, a deoxybarbiturate, is partly metabolized to phenobarbital, which is responsible for most of its pharmacological effects. During chronic dosing, the adverse effects of primidone are identical to those of phenobarbital. However, at the start of treatment, primidone can cause a transient intolerance reaction with malaise, dizziness, nausea, vomiting, headache, and other symptoms.

Primidone can cause various idiosyncratic reactions, including systemic lupus erythematosus, a syndrome resembling diabetes insipidus, lymphadenopathy, toxic epidermal necrolysis, thyroid enlargement, and edema.

The use and adverse effects of primidone in the treatment of essential tremor has been reviewed (1). Acute reactions include vertigo, nausea, and unsteadiness; chronic reactions include worsening of depression.

At the start of treatment, primidone can cause a transient intolerance reaction with malaise, dizziness, nausea, vomiting, headache, and other symptoms. To minimize this problem, which is more prominent in patients not exposed to other anticonvulsants, primidone should be started in a low dosage (for example 62.5 mg/day) and increased slowly according to response.

Pretreating patients with phenobarbital can reduce the impact of adverse events when primidone is introduced. Of 30 patients with intractable partial epilepsy pretreated with phenobarbital before starting primidone (500 mg/day increasing by 125–250 mg/day every

3 weeks until adverse events or a seizure-free state was reached), 26 tolerated the introduction of primidone with minimal or no adverse events (2). Only one patient had to discontinue primidone during the initial 4 weeks because of severe dizziness. Three other patients had dizziness severe enough to interfere with their activities and this disappeared in two patients after the dose was lowered.

Organs and Systems

Immunologic

Giant cell myocarditis has been reported in a patient taking phenytoin, phenobarbital, and mephobarbital and in one taking primidone (3).

Susceptibility Factors

Like phenobarbital, primidone should not be given to patients with acute intermittent porphyria (4).

Drug Administration

Drug overdose

After overdosage, massive crystalluria can occur, due to overload of the urine with hexagonal primidone crystals (SED-13, 154) (4).

References

1. Koller WC, Hristova A, Brin M. Pharmacologic treatment of essential tremor. Neurology 2000;54(11 Suppl. 4):S30–8.
2. Kanner AM, Parra J, Frey M. The "forgotten" cross-tolerance between phenobarbital and primidone: it can prevent acute primidone-related toxicity. Epilepsia 2000;41(10):1310–14.
3. Daniels PR, Berry GJ, Tazelaar HD, Cooper LT. Giant cell myocarditis as a manifestation of drug hypersensitivity. Cardiovasc Pathol 2000;9(5):287–91.
4. Schmidt D, Seldon L. Adverse effects of antiepileptic drugs. New York: Raven Press, 1982.

Probenecid

General Information

Probenecid is a uricosuric agent. It is generally well tolerated. Soreness of the gums, gastrointestinal irritation, skin rashes, pyrexia, and the nephrotic syndrome have been reported (1).

Drug interactions with probenecid arise, because it is an inhibitor of the renal tubular secretion of acids and bases (2).

Drug–Drug Interactions

Antibiotics

Probenecid inhibits the renal tubular secretion of various penicillins (3–6) and many cephalosporins (6–20). Ceforanide is not affected (21).

Aspirin

In low dosages (up to 2 g/day), aspirin reduces urate excretion and blocks the effects of probenecid and other uricosuric agents (22,23). However, in 11 patients with gout, aspirin 325 mg/day had no effect on the uricosuric action of probenecid (22). In higher dosages (over 5 g/day), salicylates increase urate excretion and inhibit the effects of spironolactone, but it is not clear whether these phenomena are of importance.

Chloroquine

Probenecid may increase the risk of chloroquine-induced retinal damage (24).

Dapsone

Probenecid increases plasma dapsone concentrations by inhibiting its renal clearance (25).

Indometacin

Interactions with indometacin have been documented through inhibition of renal tubular excretion (26,27). In 17 patients with rheumatoid arthritis, probenecid 500 mg bd improved the therapeutic response to indometacin 25 mg tds over 3 weeks (28). There were changes in the pharmacokinetics of indometacin, which the authors attributed to a reduction in the non-renal clearance of indometacin, possibly because of reduced biliary clearance.

Methotrexate

Probenecid reduces the renal tubular secretion of methotrexate, enhancing its effect (29) and may reduce its plasma protein binding (30).

Sulfinpyrazone

Probenecid reduces the renal tubular secretion of sulfinpyrazone but there is no change in the uricosuric effect (31).

Zidovudine

Probenecid reduces the renal tubular secretion of zidovudine (32,33).

References

1. Scott JT, O'Brien PK. Probenecid, nephrotic syndrome, and renal failure. Ann Rheum Dis 1968;27(3):249–52.
2. Cunningham RF, Israili ZH, Dayton PG. Clinical pharmacokinetics of probenecid. Clin Pharmacokinet 1981;6(2):135–51.
3. Waller ES, Sharanevych MA, Yakatan GJ. The effect of probenecid on nafcillin disposition. J Clin Pharmacol 1982;22(10):482–9.

4. Allen MB, Fitzpatrick RW, Barratt A, Cole RB. The use of probenecid to increase the serum amoxycillin levels in patients with bronchiectasis. Respir Med 1990;84(2):143–6.

5. Krogsgaard MR, Hansen BA, Slotsbjerg T, Jensen P. Should probenecid be used to reduce the dicloxacillin dosage in orthopaedic infections? A study of the dicloxacillin-saving effect of probenecid. Pharmacol Toxicol 1994; 74(3):181–4.

6. Tuano SB, Brodie JL, Kirby WM. Cephaloridine versus cephalothin: relation of the kidney to blood level differences after parenteral administration. Antimicrobial Agents Chemother (Bethesda) 1966;6:101–6.

7. Kaplan K, Reisberg BE, Weinstein L. Cephaloridine: antimicrobial activity and pharmacologic behavior. Am J Med Sci 1967;253(6):667–74.

8. Applestein JM, Crosby EB, Johnson WD, Kaye D. In vitro antimicrobial activity and human pharmacology of cephaloglycin. Appl Microbiol 1968;16(7):1006–10.

9. Taylor WA, Holloway WJ. Cephalexin in the treatment of gonorrhea. Int J Clin Pharmacol 1972;6(1):7–9.

10. Duncan WC. Treatment of gonorrhea with cefazolin plus probenecid. J Infect Dis 1974;130(4):398–401.

11. Mischler TW, Sugerman AA, Willard DA, Brannick LJ, Neiss ES. Influence of probenecid and food on the bioavailability of cephradine in normal male subjects. J Clin Pharmacol 1974;14(11–12):604–11.

12. Wise R, Reeves DS. Pharmacological studies on cephacetrile in human volunteers. Curr Med Res Opin 1974;2(5):249–55.

13. Griffith RS, Black HR, Brier GL, Wolny JD. Effects of probenecid on the blood levels and urinary excretion of cefamandole. Antimicrob Agents Chemother 1977; 11(5):809–12.

14. Welling PG, Dean S, Selen A, Kendall MJ, Wise R. Probenecid: an unexplained effect on cephalosporin pharmacology. Br J Clin Pharmacol 1979;8(5):491–5.

15. Reeves DS, Bullock DW, Bywater MJ, Holt HA, White LO, Thornhill DP. The effect of probenecid on the pharmacokinetics and distribution of cefoxitin in healthy volunteers. Br J Clin Pharmacol 1981;11(4):353–9.

16. LeBel M, Paone RP, Lewis GP. Effect of probenecid on the pharmacokinetics of ceftriaxone. J Antimicrob Chemother 1983;12(2):147–55.

17. Stoeckel K, Trueb V, Dubach UC, McNamara PJ. Effect of probenecid on the elimination and protein binding of ceftriaxone. Eur J Clin Pharmacol 1988;34(2):151–6.

18. Ko H, Cathcart KS, Griffith DL, Peters GR, Adams WJ. Pharmacokinetics of intravenously administered cefmetazole and cefoxitin and effects of probenecid on cefmetazole elimination. Antimicrob Agents Chemother 1989; 33(3):356–61.

19. Corvaia L, Li SC, Ioannides-Demos LL, Bowes G, Spicer WJ, Spelman DW, Tong N, McLean AJ. A prospective study of the effects of oral probenecid on the pharmacokinetics of intravenous ticarcillin in patients with cystic fibrosis. J Antimicrob Chemother 1992;30(6):875–8.

20. Shukla UA, Pittman KA, Barbhaiya RH. Pharmacokinetic interactions of cefprozil with food, propantheline, metoclopramide, and probenecid in healthy volunteers. J Clin Pharmacol 1992;32(8):725–31.

21. Jovanovich JF, Saravolatz LD, Burch K, Pohlod DJ. Failure of probenecid to alter the pharmacokinetics of ceforanide. Antimicrob Agents Chemother 1981;20(4):530–2.

22. Harris M, Bryant LR, Danaher P, Alloway J. Effect of low dose daily aspirin on serum urate levels and urinary excretion in patients receiving probenecid for gouty arthritis. J Rheumatol 2000;27(12):2873–6.

23. Brooks CD, Ulrich JE. Effect of ibuprofen or aspirin on probenecid-induced uricosuria. J Int Med Res 1980; 8(4):283–5.

24. Frankel EB. Visual defect from chloroquine phosphate. Arch Dermatol 1975;111(8):1069.

25. Goodwin CS, Sparell G. Inhibition of dapsone excretion by probenecid. Lancet 1969;2(7626):884–5.

26. Brooks PM, Bell MA, Sturrock RD, Famaey JP, Dick WC. The clinical significance of indomethacin–probenecid interaction. Br J Clin Pharmacol 1974;1:287.

27. Sinclair H, Gibson T. Interaction between probenecid and indomethacin. Br J Rheumatol 1986;25(3):316–17.

28. Baber N, Halliday L, Sibeon R, Littler T, Orme ML. The interaction between indomethacin and probenecid. A clinical and pharmacokinetic study. Clin Pharmacol Ther 1978;24(3):298–307.

29. Liegler DG, Henderson ES, Hahn MA, Oliverio VT. The effect of organic acids on renal clearance of methotrexate in man. Clin Pharmacol Ther 1969;10(6):849–57.

30. Evans WE, Christensen ML. Drug interactions with methotrexate. J Rheumatol Suppl 1985;12(Suppl 12):15–20.

31. Perel JM, Dayton PG, Snell MM, Yu TF, Gutman AB. Studies of interactions among drugs in man at the renal level: probenecid and sulfinpyrazone. Clin Pharmacol Ther 1969;10(6):834–40.

32. Hedaya MA, Elmquist WF, Sawchuk RJ. Probenecid inhibits the metabolic and renal clearances of zidovudine (AZT) in human volunteers. Pharm Res 1990;7(4):411–17.

33. Veal GJ, Back DJ. Metabolism of Zidovudine. Gen Pharmacol 1995;26(7):1469–75.

Probucol

General Information

The adverse effects of probucol have been reviewed (1). As the Probucol Quantitative Regression Swedish Trial (PQRST) showed no improvement in lumen volume of the femoral artery in patients given probucol plus colestyramine, as compared with those given colestyramine alone, doubt has been raised about its efficacy (2).

Organs and Systems

Cardiovascular

Prolongation of the QT interval has been seen and 16 cases of tachydysrhythmias, especially torsade de pointes, have been reported in association with probucol, 15 cases in women (SEDSA-13, 1331) (3,4).

Gastrointestinal

According to long-term studies covering 7–9 years, probucol seems to be well tolerated with a reasonably low incidence of adverse effects. All the documented adverse effects were concentrated in the gastrointestinal tract. The incidence of diarrhea fell from 19% in the first year to 5% in the next. Only in some 3% of cases do symptoms such as diarrhea or abdominal pain lead to withdrawal of treatment. Diarrhea and flatulence, which resolve after a few months, are common.

References

1. Zimetbaum P, Eder H, Frishman W. Probucol: pharmacology and clinical application. J Clin Pharmacol 1990;30(1):3–9.
2. Sasich LD, Sukkari SR. Probucol—lack of efficacy and market withdrawals. Saudi Pharm J 1997;5:72–3.
3. Gohn DC, Simmons TW. Polymorphic ventricular tachycardia (torsade de pointes) associated with the use of probucol. N Engl J Med 1992;326(21):1435–6.
4. Matsuhashi H, Onodera S, Kawamura Y, Hasebe N, Kohmura C, Yamashita H, Tobise K. Probucol-induced QT prolongation and torsades de pointes. Jpn J Med 1989;28(5):612–15.

Procainamide

See also Antidysrhythmic drugs

General Information

In a prospective study of 488 inpatients there were adverse reactions in 45 cases (9.2%), thought to have been life-threatening in 7 (1.4%), none of whom died (1). The seven patients all had cardiovascular effects. Common adverse effects included gastrointestinal upsets (19 cases) and fever (8 cases). Reactions were more common at daily dosages of 3 g and more.

Comparative studies

The adverse effects of intravenous procainamide (400 mg up to three times infused over 10 minutes) have been reported in 60 adults with atrial flutter or fibrillation in a comparison with ibutilide (2). The adverse effects were headache in 11%, hypotension in 11%, flushing in 3.1%, dizziness in 3.1%, and hypesthesia in 3.1%. The mean fall in systolic blood pressure was about 20 mmHg and occurred at 30–35 minutes after infusion; the corresponding fall in diastolic blood pressure was 10 mmHg. However, in seven patients there was severe hypotension, with a fall in diastolic blood pressure of up to 67 mmHg; in three cases withdrawal of the infusion was required and these patients were treated with intravenous fluids, dopamine, or both. In the severe cases the hypotension occurred during or immediately after the infusion of procainamide.

A comparison between procainamide and propafenone in 62 patients, who had undergone coronary artery bypass grafting or valvular surgery within 3 weeks and developed sustained atrial fibrillation, showed that both drugs converted the dysrhythmia to sinus rhythm in up to 76% of cases, but that propafenone did it more quickly (3). Symptomatic arterial hypotension occurred more frequently with procainamide (nine of 33 patients) than with propafenone (two of 29 patients). Other adverse effects of procainamide were nausea ($n = 2$) and junctional escape rhythm ($n = 2$).

General adverse effects

The adverse effects of procainamide are predominantly on the heart. It causes reduced myocardial contractility and hypotension, and prolongs the QT interval, with consequent dysrhythmias and conduction defects. The lupus-like syndrome most commonly causes polyarthralgia, myalgia, fever, and pleurisy. Neutropenia has been relatively commonly reported in patients taking modified-release formulations. Other adverse effects are uncommon; these include muscle weakness, ataxia, mental confusion, cholestasis, and skin rashes. Hypersensitivity reactions include fever and hematological reactions, including neutropenia, pancytopenia, and pure red cell aplasia. Tumor-inducing effects have not been reported.

Organs and Systems

Cardiovascular

Procainamide has a negative inotropic effect and can cause hypotension after both intravenous and oral administration (4,5). When given intravenously it should therefore be infused slowly, at no more than 20 mg/minute. In patients with poor cardiac function procainamide can worsen heart failure, and it may reduce survival after myocardial infarction (6).

Procainamide prolongs the QT interval (7) and can cause dysrhythmias. It can also impair cardiac conduction and can cause bradycardia and heart block (1). In the sick sinus syndrome it can alter sinus node recovery time (8), although the clinical significance of this is not clear.

Pericarditis and tamponade have been reported as rare complications of procainamide-induced lupus-like syndrome (9).

Respiratory

Procainamide can cause lung damage in the context of a lupus-like syndrome (SEDA-17, 226).

Nervous system

Procainamide rarely causes nervous system effects. Acute confusion (10), cerebellar ataxia (11), tremor (12), and muscle weakness (13–16) have all been occasionally reported. In high dosages procainamide has anticholinergic effects (17).

Procainamide has been reported to cause a chronic inflammatory demyelinating polyradiculoneuropathy (18).

- A 68-year-old man took procainamide 500 mg qds for 3 years and developed distal paresthesia and dysesthesia in the legs, followed by progressive muscle weakness, mainly affecting the legs. His gait became unsteady and was wide-based. He had antinuclear antibodies directed against histones in a titer of 1:320, but no antibodies to double-stranded DNA. He had a circulating lupus anticoagulant. The serum procainamide concentration was 3.3 µg/ml (target range 4–8). Nerve conduction studies showed a reduction in sensory nerve action potential amplitudes, a mild reduction in sensory nerve conduction velocity, prolongation of distal motor latencies, and reduced conduction velocities, but no conduction block or temporal dispersions. Electromyography was normal. A left sural nerve biopsy showed perivascular inflammation around a single vessel, without evidence of vasculitis. Myelinated nerve fibers were reduced, and scattered nerve fibers showed thin myelin sheaths. About 30% of the fibers showed randomly distributed demyelinated or remyelinated segments. Procainamide was withdrawn and prednisone was given in combination with six plasma exchanges over 2 weeks; after 1 month there was clinical improvement.

This case of polyneuropathy was attributed to a lupus-like effect of procainamide.

Sensory systems

Scleritis has been reported as part of a procainamide-induced, lupus-like syndrome (19).

Psychological, psychiatric

Acute psychosis has been attributed to procainamide (20).

- A 45-year-old woman developed an acute psychosis within 72 hours of starting to take procainamide 75 mg intravenously, followed by a continuous infusion of 2 mg/minute for atrial fibrillation. The plasma procainamide concentration was 8.2 µg/ml and the plasma concentration of the main acetylated metabolite, acecainide, was 4.6 µg/ml. She was then given oral procainamide 500 mg qds, and 2 days later her trough concentrations of procainamide and acecainide were 4.5 and 4.9 µg/ml respectively. The following day she had visual hallucinations and was later found wandering the hospital asking about the babies under her bed. She had no previous history of psychiatric illness and she recovered completely 24 hours after withdrawal of procainamide.

There have been a few previous reports of similar adverse effects with procainamide in therapeutic dosages, and in most cases the plasma concentrations of procainamide and acecainide have been within the usual target ranges, as in this case.

Hematologic

Hematological abnormalities can occur in the absence of a lupus-like syndrome. Hemolytic anemia (21), a circulating anticoagulant (22), thrombocytopenia (23), granulocytopenia (24), and pancytopenia (25) have all been reported occasionally. Thrombocytopenia may be more common in patients taking modified-release formulations (23). Pure red cell aplasia has also been reported (26,27), but it was not clear whether or not there was an associated lupus-like syndrome.

The most common adverse hematological effect of procainamide is neutropenia, which has often been reported, particularly in patients taking modified-release formulations. In one case-control study 4.4% of 114 patients taking modified-release formulations had neutropenia, compared with none in a control group of 509 patients (28). However, a larger subsequent case-control study failed to confirm this association (29). Nevertheless, reports of neutropenia attributed to procainamide continue to appear (30).

There was a positive direct antiglobulin (Coombs') test in about 20% of elderly patients taking procainamide (31). Although a positive Coombs' test can occur in

association with a lupus-like syndrome, there was no relation in these cases between positive tests and the presence of antinuclear antibodies. Three of the patients had an autoimmune hemolytic anemia.

Gastrointestinal

Nausea, vomiting, and diarrhea in response to procainamide are common with dosages of 4 g/day or more (32). Pseudo-obstruction has been attributed to the use of a modified-release formulation of procainamide, perhaps due to its anticholinergic effects (33).

Liver

Procainamide can cause intrahepatic cholestasis, perhaps as part of a hypersensitivity reaction (34).

Skin

Lichen planus has been attributed to procainamide as part of a lupus-like syndrome (35).

Procainamide has been reported to cause urticarial vasculitis, although it was not clear whether or not this was part of a lupus-like syndrome (36).

- A 70-year-old man developed a maculopapular skin rash on the trunk 10 days after starting to take procainamide 1.5 g/day (37). Resolution occurred soon after the withdrawal of procainamide and a similar skin rash occurred on rechallenge. In addition to the maculopapular rash, there was swelling and erythema around the eyes and a purpuric rash on the legs. At the time of rechallenge he also had an eosinophilia.

Musculoskeletal

Procainamide can cause an arthropathy as part of a lupus-like syndrome, and the histological findings are indistinguishable from those in idiopathic SLE (38).

Procainamide has occasionally been reported to cause muscle weakness (SEDA-14, 152) (SEDA-16, 183), and it can also cause or exacerbate myasthenia gravis (39).

Necrotizing myopathy of the diaphragm has been reported, perhaps as part of a lupus-like syndrome (40).

Immunologic

Lupus-like syndrome
DoTS classification (BMJ 2003;327:1222–5)
  Dose-relation: collateral effect
  Time-course: delayed
  Susceptibility factors: genetic (slow acetylators)

Procainamide is one of the common causes of drug-induced lupus-like syndrome (41), which is contrasted with idiopathic lupus erythematosus in Table 1.

Frequency
About 29–35% of patients taking procainamide for at least a year are affected and the effect is dose-related. The average age of onset is 59–68 years and 35–58% of the subjects are women. The syndrome can come on within a few weeks, but has been reported as late as 9 years after starting treatment.

Table 1 The contrast between drug-induced lupus-like syndrome and idiopathic lupus erythematosus

Feature	Idiopathic lupus erythematosus	Drug-induced lupus-like syndrome
Age and sex	Typically young women	Any (depends on use)
Acetylator status	Any	More likely in slow acetylators
Organs involved	Any	Kidneys usually spared
Antinuclear antibody	Usually present	Usually present
Complement	Can be reduced	Usually normal
Anti-DNA antibodies	Usually present (native DNA)	Only to single-stranded DNA

Mechanism

The mechanisms whereby procainamide causes this lupus-like syndrome are not clear. Procainamide is associated with the production of many antibodies, including antihistone, antiguanosine, anti-DNA, and antiphospholipid antibodies (42). The production of autoantibodies may be due to one of two major mechanisms: first, procainamide may act as a hapten, binding to DNA, nuclear protein, or some membrane constituent, the hapten-protein complex stimulating the production of antibodies; secondly, it may alter suppressor cell function (43). There is also evidence that procainamide can combine with ribonucleoprotein from damaged myocardium after myocardial infarction, thus precipitating the production of antibodies to ribonucleoprotein (44).

Thymus function in 10 patients with symptomatic procainamide-induced lupus has been compared with that in 13 asymptomatic patients who only developed drug-induced autoantibodies (45). Newly generated T cells were detected in all the subjects. Although there was no overall quantitative difference between the symptomatic and asymptomatic patients, there was a correlation between the level of T cell receptor rearrangement excision circles in peripheral lymphocytes and serum IgG antichromatin antibody activity in patients with drug-induced lupus. These results support the hypothesis that the thymus is important in the genesis of drug-induced lupus-like syndrome and that the production of autoreactive T cells starts in the thymus when procainamide hydroxylamine alters T cell tolerance.

In procainamide-induced lupus there is an increase in the number of B cells in both blood and pleural fluid to about 80% (normal 10–25%). Concentrations of IL-6 and soluble IL-2R are also increased (46).

IgG antibodies to the (H2A–H2B)-DNA complex are common in patients with immunological reactions to procainamide (SEDA-20, 178). In a prospective study of 62 patients who had taken procainamide for a mean duration of 23 months (range 1 month to 16 years), and excluding patients with pre-existing systemic lupus erythematosus or who were taking other drugs that have been associated with the lupus-like syndrome, nine developed evidence of lupus-like syndrome and were compared with the other 53 (47). The mean dosage in the patients with lupus-like syndrome was 3.7 g/day compared with 3 g/day in the others, and the durations of administration were 8.8 and 38 months respectively. All four patients who had polyarticular arthritis and/or pleural effusions were positive for the IgG antibodies and four of the other five, who had significantly lower IgG concentrations, presented with the more typical manifestations of vasculitic rashes, pericarditis, or

agranulocytosis. In all cases the symptoms and signs either improved markedly or resolved within 3 weeks of withdrawal of procainamide. Seven asymptomatic patients had IgG concentrations comparable with those seen in the patients with lupus-like syndrome, and high concentrations of antibody, although not as high as the two highest in the latter group. Anti-double-stranded DNA antibodies were not detected in any patients. In 33 control subjects there were no detectable antibodies of any kind. The authors therefore suggested that the (H2A-H2B)-DNA IgG antibody is not a useful marker for the occurrence of lupus-like syndrome in patients taking procainamide, although they conceded that the presence of IgG antibody supported the diagnosis of lupus-like syndrome when the main clinical manifestations were arthritis or pleurisy. The significance of the presence of IgG antibodies in asymptomatic patients is not clear, but the authors suggested that it meant that those patients merited careful observation.

The lupus-like syndrome in patients taking procainamide is thought to be due to the procainamide itself, since it has rarely been reported when the main metabolite of procainamide, acecainide, has been administered itself (SEDA-18, 206). Alternatively, the syndrome may be due to a different metabolite of procainamide, and a hydroxylated derivative has been implicated (SEDA-15, 178) (48). CYP2D6 is the major isoform of cytochrome P450 that is involved in the hydroxylation of procainamide, and in the production of some other metabolites (49). It remains to be seen whether extensive CYP2D6 metabolizers are more likely to develop lupus-like syndrome than poor metabolizers.

Susceptibility factors

The lupus-like syndrome is more likely to occur in slow acetylators than in fast acetylators (50), and the rate of development of antinuclear antibody depends on acetylator status (51).

Presentation

The most common feature is arthralgia, in about 77% of cases, with pleural or lung involvement in about 75%. Other common features include myalgia, fever, hepatomegaly, pericarditis, arthritis, and splenomegaly. Skin rashes, adenopathy, and Raynaud's phenomenon occur in 5–10% of cases, and neuropsychiatric and renal involvement are rare. Thrombotic problems can occur because of the properties of anti-DNA and antiphospholipid antibodies (discussed in the next case report). The so-called lupus anticoagulant can be detected in people taking procainamide, even without clinical evidence of lupus

(52). Angioedema has been reported in a patient who had no history of hereditary angioedema (53).

A lupus-like syndrome with an antiphospholipid syndrome has been attributed to procainamide in a patient with pre-existing systemic sclerosis (54).

- A 51-year-old Korean man with systemic sclerosis was given procainamide 2–3 g/day for suppression of ventricular dysrhythmias. About 2 years later he noticed a new skin ulcer on one of his toes. His dorsalis pedis arteries were not palpable and there was tenderness over the proximal interphalangeal and metacarpophalangeal joints. He had a pancytopenia, prolonged coagulation (with prolongation of the activated partial thromboplastin time and prothrombin time and reduced concentrations of factors XI and XII), an increase in the plasma concentration of von Willebrand factor, a raised serum creatinine concentration, a raised serum C-reactive protein concentration, hypergammaglobulinemia, and hypocomplementemia. He had positive circulating immune complexes and mixed-type cryoglobulinemia, antinuclear antibodies, anti-DNA topoisomerase I antibodies, and a positive LE cell preparation. He had anti-DNA antibodies with a high titer of antibodies to single-stranded DNA and a slightly raised titer of antibodies to double-stranded DNA. Anti-U1 ribonuclear protein, anti-Sm, and anti-centromere antibodies were negative. There were high titers of beta$_2$-glycoprotein-I-dependent IgG anti-cardiolipin antibodies and the lupus anticoagulant test was positive. There were antihistone antibodies. Procainamide was withdrawn and prednisolone and azathioprine given. The pancytopenia, coagulopathy, and renal dysfunction resolved, and his general condition improved; serum concentrations of several of the antibodies returned to normal.

The authors suggested that the pre-existence of systemic sclerosis in this case and the presence of allele HIA-DQBP1* 0303 had increased the patient's susceptibility to the lupus-like syndrome and antiphospholipid syndrome.

Diagnosis

The antinuclear antibody is positive in virtually all cases and the ESR is often raised. Antihistone antibodies are also present in most cases. The prevalence of serum auto-antibodies to high-mobility group (HMG) proteins in the serum of patients with drug-induced lupus-like syndrome varies from protein to protein: 67% for HMG-14 and/or HMG-17 compared with 21% for HMG-1 and/or HMG-2. Procainamide-induced lupus is also associated with antibodies to the H2A–H2B dimer (55,56).

Antinuclear antibody is usually present (in 83% of cases), but antibodies to native DNA are not found, although there may be antibodies to single-stranded DNA. Patients taking procainamide can have antinuclear antibodies without developing a lupus-like syndrome.

Management

The syndrome usually regresses rapidly after withdrawal of procainamide, but in a few patients recovery may be

delayed; if there are serious effects oral glucocorticoid therapy may be required.

Body temperature

Fever occasionally occurs in patients taking procainamide (SEDA-1, 155) and has been attributed to an allergic reaction (57).

Susceptibility Factors

Renal disease

Maintenance dosages should be reduced in the presence of renal or hepatic impairment, including hepatic congestion due to cardiac failure (58).

Hepatic disease

Maintenance dosages should also be reduced in the presence of renal or hepatic impairment, including hepatic congestion due to cardiac failure (58).

Other features of the patient

Care must be taken in patients with pre-existing connective tissue disease or heart failure. Loading dosages should be reduced in cardiac failure, because of a lowered apparent volume of distribution (58).

Drug Administration

Drug overdose

Procainamide overdose has been reported.

- A 14-year-old boy took about 21 g of procainamide and developed abdominal pain, weakness, blurred vision, dry mouth, pain on swallowing, and headache (59). His pupils were dilated, his skin dry and pale, and his mucous membranes dry. His blood pressure was 106/49 mmHg, his heart rate 91/minute. Following a tonic-clonic seizure his blood pressure was 125/57 mmHg and his heart rate 136/minute in sinus tachycardia. He became lethargic with slurred speech. He was given repeated doses of activated charcoal and made a full recovery. The serum procainamide and acecainide (*N*-acetylprocainamide) concentrations were 63 and 80 µg/ml respectively.
- A 79-year-old man took about 19 g of procainamide and developed lethargy, vomiting, a wide-complex tachycardia, hypotension, and coma (60). His serum procainamide concentration was 77 µg/ml at 3 hours. He was treated with vasopressors and peritoneal dialysis.
- A 67-year-old woman took about 7 g of procainamide and developed nausea, vomiting, lethargy, a junctional tachycardia, hypotension, and oliguria (61). She was treated with hemodialysis.

Drug–Drug Interactions

Amiodarone

The effects of procainamide on the QT interval may be potentiated by other drugs with this action, for example amiodarone (62).

The pharmacokinetics of procainamide are altered by amiodarone, with a reduction in clearance of about 25% due to changes in both renal and non-renal clearances (62).

Cimetidine

The renal clearance of procainamide is inhibited by cimetidine (63,64).

Class I antidysrhythmic drugs

The effects of procainamide on the QT interval can be potentiated by other drugs with this action, for example other class I antidysrhythmic drugs (62).

Glucose

Procainamide interacts with glucose in vitro to form glucosylamines (63). The reaction was pH-dependent, with a maximum rate of association at a pH of 3.0 and a maximum rate of dissociation at a pH of 1.5. The authors suggested that the loss of procainamide in an intravenous solution of glucose could be marked.

Ofloxacin

The renal clearance of procainamide is inhibited by ofloxacin (66).

Trimethoprim

The renal clearance of procainamide is inhibited by trimethoprim (67).

Monitoring Therapy

The use of serum procainamide concentration measurements in monitoring therapy has been reviewed (58,68). Serum concentrations of 4–10 µg/ml are associated with therapeutic benefit in over 90% of patients with ventricular tachydysrhythmias, and toxicity becomes highly likely over 12 µg/ml. However, the main metabolite of procainamide, acecainide, has antidysrhythmic activity of its own; thus, because metabolism varies widely between individuals, and because acecainide is eliminated by the kidneys, serum concentration measurement of procainamide alone has limited usefulness, particularly in renal insufficiency. There is currently little information on the interpretation of combined measurement of the two compounds.

References

1. Lawson DH, Jick H. Adverse reactions to procainamide. Br J Clin Pharmacol 1977;4(5):507–11.
2. Volgman AS, Carberry PA, Stambler B, Lewis WR, Dunn GH, Perry KT, Vanderlugt JT, Kowey PR. Conversion efficacy and safety of intravenous ibutilide compared with intravenous procainamide in patients with atrial flutter or fibrillation. J Am Coll Cardiol 1998;31(6):1414–19.
3. Geelen P, O'Hara GE, Roy N, Talajic M, Roy D, Plante S, Turgeon J. Comparison of propafenone versus procainamide for the acute treatment of atrial fibrillation after cardiac surgery. Am J Cardiol 1999;84(3):345–7.
4. Koch-Weser J, Klein SW, Foo-Canto LL, Kastor JA, DeSanctis RW. Antiarrhythmic prophylaxis with procainamide in acute myocardial infarction. N Engl J Med 1969;281(23):1253–60.
5. Kosowsky BD, Taylor J, Lown B, Ritchie RF. Long-term use of procaine amide following acute myocardial infarction. Circulation 1973;47(6):1204–10.
6. Hallstrom AP, Cobb LA, Yu BH, Weaver WD, Fahrenbruch CE. An antiarrhythmic drug experience in 941 patients resuscitated from an initial cardiac arrest between 1970 and 1985. Am J Cardiol 1991;68(10):1025–31.
7. Miller RR, Hilliard G, Lies JE, Massumi RA, Zelis R, Mason DT, Amsterdam EA. Hemodynamic effects of procainamide in patients with acute myocardial infarction and comparison with lidocaine. Am J Med 1973;55(2):161–8.
8. Goldberg D, Reiffel JA, Davis JC, Gang E, Livelli F, Bigger JT Jr. Electrophysiologic effects of procainamide on sinus function in patients with and without sinus node disease. Am Heart J 1982;103(1):75–9.
9. Mohindra SK, Udeani GO, Abrahamson D. Cardiac tamponade associated with drug-induced systemic lupus erythematosus. Crit Care Med 1989;17(9):961–2.
10. McCrum ID, Guidry JR. Procainamide-induced psychosis. JAMA 1978;240(12):1265–6.
11. Schwartz AB, Klausner SC, Yee S, Turchyn M. Cerebellar ataxia due to procainamide toxicity. Arch Intern Med 1984;144(11):2260–1.
12. Rubinstein A, Cabili S. Tremor induced by procainamide. Am J Cardiol 1986;57(4):340–1.
13. Miller B, Skupin A, Rubenfire M, Bigman O. Respiratory failure produced by severe procainamide intoxication in a patient with pre-existing peripheral neuropathy caused by amiodarone. Chest 1988;94(3):663–5.
14. Godley PJ, Morton TA, Karboski JA, Tami JA. Procainamide-induced myasthenic crisis. Ther Drug Monit 1990;12(4):411–14.
15. Putnam JB Jr, Bolling SF, Kirsh MM. Procainamide-induced respiratory insufficiency after cardiopulmonary bypass. Ann Thorac Surg 1991;51(3):482–3.
16. Sayler DJ, DeJong DJ. Possible procainamide-induced myopathy. DICP 1991;25(4):436.
17. Prendergast MD, Nasca TJ. Anticholinergic syndrome with procainamide toxicity. JAMA 1984;251(22):2926–7.
18. Erdem S, Freimer ML, O'Dorisio T, Mendell JR. Procainamide-induced chronic inflammatory demyelinating polyradiculoneuropathy. Neurology 1998;50(3):824–5.
19. Turgeon PW, Slamovits TL. Scleritis as the presenting manifestation of procainamide-induced lupus. Ophthalmology 1989;96(1):68–71.
20. Bizjak ED, Nolan PE Jr, Brody EA, Galloway JM. Procainamide-induced psychosis: a case report and review of the literature. Ann Pharmacother 1999;33(9):948–51.
21. Kleinman S, Nelson R, Smith L, Goldfinger D. Positive direct antiglobulin tests and immune hemolytic anemia in patients receiving procainamide. N Engl J Med 1984;311(13):809–12.
22. Galanakis DK, Newman J, Summers D. Circulating thrombin time anticoagulant in a procainamide-induced syndrome. JAMA 1978;239(18):1873–4.
23. Meisner DJ, Carlson RJ, Gottlieb AJ. Thrombocytopenia following sustained-release procainamide. Arch Intern Med 1985;145(4):700–2.
24. Abe H, Suzuka H, Tasaki H, Kuroiwa A. Sustained-release procainamide-induced reversible granulocytopenia after myocardial infarction. Jpn Heart J 1995;36(4):483–7.
25. Bluming AZ, Plotkin D, Rosen P, Thiessen AR. Severe transient pancytopenia associated with procainamide ingestion. JAMA 1976;236(22):2520–1.
26. Giannone L, Kugler JW, Krantz SB. Pure red cell aplasia associated with administration of sustained-release procainamide. Arch Intern Med 1987;147(6):1179–80.

27. Agudelo CA, Wise CM, Lyles MF. Pure red cell aplasia in procainamide induced systemic lupus erythematosus. Report and review of the literature. J Rheumatol 1988; 15(9):1431–2.

28. Ellrodt AG, Murata GH, Riedinger MS, Stewart ME, Mochizuki C, Gray R. Severe neutropenia associated with sustained-release procainamide. Ann Intern Med 1984;100(2):197–201.

29. Meyers DG, Gonzalez ER, Peters LL, Davis RB, Feagler JR, Egan JD, Nair CK. Severe neutropenia associated with procainamide: comparison of sustained release and conventional preparations. Am Heart J 1985; 109(6):1393–5.

30. Hoffman HS. Severe neutropenia with procainamide therapy. Conn Med 1990;54(2):59–61.

31. Kleinman S, Nelson R, Smith L, Goldfinger D. Positive direct antiglobulin tests and immune hemolytic anemia in patients receiving procainamide. N Engl J Med 1984;311(13):809–12.

32. Bigger JT Jr, Heissenbuttel RH. The use of procaine amide and lidocaine in the treatment of cardiac arrhythmias. Prog Cardiovasc Dis 1969;11(6):515–34.

33. Peterson AM, Conrad SD, Bell JM. Procainamide-induced pseudo-obstruction in a diabetic patient. DICP 1991;25(12):1334–5.

34. Chuang LC, Tunier AP, Akhtar N, Levine SM. Possible case of procainamide-induced intrahepatic cholestatic jaundice. Ann Pharmacother 1993;27(4):434–7.

35. Sherertz EF. Lichen planus following procainamide-induced lupus erythematosus. Cutis 1988;42(1):51–3.

36. Knox JP, Welykyj SE, Gradini R, Massa MC. Procainamide-induced urticarial vasculitis. Cutis 1988; 42(5):469–72.

37. Numata T, Abe H, Nakashima Y, Yamamoto O, Kohshi K. [Procainamide-induced skin eruption associated with disseminated intravascular coagulation in a patient with sustained ventricular tachycardia.] J UOEH 1999;21(3):235–40.

38. Vivino FB, Schumacher HR Jr. Synovial fluid characteristics and the lupus erythematosus cell phenomenon in drug-induced lupus. Findings in three patients and review of pertinent literature. Arthritis Rheum 1989;32(5):560–8.

39. Miller CD, Oleshansky MA, Gibson KF, Cantilena LR. Procainamide-induced myasthenia-like weakness and dysphagia. Ther Drug Monit 1993;15(3):251–4.

40. Venkayya RV, Poole RM, Pentz WH. Respiratory failure from procainamide-induced myopathy. Ann Intern Med 1993;119(4):345–6.

41. Yung RL, Richardson BC. Drug-induced lupus. Rheum Dis Clin North Am 1994;20(1):61–86.

42. Smiley JD, Moore SE Jr. Molecular mechanisms of autoimmunity. Am J Med Sci 1988;295(5):478–96.

43. Green BJ, Wyse DG, Duff HJ, Mitchell LB, Matheson DS. Procainamide in vivo modulates suppressor T lymphocyte activity. Clin Invest Med 1988;11(6):425–9.

44. Burlingame RW, Rubin RL. Drug-induced anti-histone autoantibodies display two patterns of reactivity with substructures of chromatin. J Clin Invest 1991;88(2):680–90.

45. Rubin RL, Salomon DR, Guerrero RS. Thymus function in drug-induced lupus. Lupus 2001;10(11):795–801.

46. Winfield JB, Koffler D, Kunkel HG. Development of antibodies to ribonucleoprotein following short-term therapy with procainamide. Arthritis Rheum 1975;18(6):531–4.

47. Lau CC, Clos TD. Anti-[(H2A/2B)-DNA] IgG supports the diagnosis of procainamide-induced arthritis or pleuritis. Arthritis Rheum 1999;42(6):1300–1.

48. Sim E. Drug-induced immune-complex disease. Complement Inflamm 1989;6(2):119–26.

49. Lessard E, Hamelin BA, Labbe L, O'Hara G, Belanger PM, Turgeon J. Involvement of CYP2D6 activity in the N-oxidation of procainamide in man. Pharmacogenetics 1999;9(6):683–96.

50. Uetrecht JP, Woosley RL. Acetylator phenotype and lupus erythematosus. Clin Pharmacokinet 1981;6(2):118–34.

51. Woosley RL, Drayer DE, Reidenberg MM, Nies AS, Carr K, Oates JA. Effect of acetylator phenotype on the rate at which procainamide induces antinuclear antibodies and the lupus syndrome. N Engl J Med 1978; 298(21):1157–9.

52. Heyman MR, Flores RH, Edelman BB, Carliner NH. Procainamide-induced lupus anticoagulant. South Med J 1988;81(7):934–6.

53. Ponte CD, Horner P. Suspected procainamide-induced angioedema. Drug Intell Clin Pharm 1985;19(2):139–40.

54. Kameda H, Mimori T, Kaburaki J, Fujii T, Takahashi T, Akaishi M, Ikeda Y. Systemic sclerosis complicated by procainamide-induced lupus and antiphospholipid syndrome. Br J Rheumatol 1998;37(11):1236–9.

55. Klimas NG, Patarca R, Perez G, Garcia-Morales R, Schultz D, Schabel J, Fletcher MA. Case report: distinctive immune abnormalities in a patient with procainamide-induced lupus and serositis. Am J Med Sci 1992; 303(2):99–104.

56. Rubin RL, Burlingame RW, Arnott JE, Totoritis MC, McNally EM, Johnson AD. IgG but not other classes of anti-[(H2A-H2B)-DNA] is an early sign of procainamide-induced lupus. J Immunol 1995;154(5):2483–93.

57. Murray KD, Vlasnik JJ. Procainamide-induced postoperative pyrexia. Ann Thorac Surg 1999;68(3):1072–4.

58. Kumana CR. Therapeutic drug monitoring-antidysrhythmic drugs. In: Richens A, Marks V, editors. Therapeutic Drug Monitoring. London, Edinburgh: Churchill-Livingstone, 1981:370.

59. White SR, Dy G, Wilson JM. The case of the slandered Halloween cupcake: survival after massive pediatric procainamide overdose. Pediatr Emerg Care 2002;18(3):185–8.

60. Villalba-Pimentel L, Epstein LM, Sellers EM, Foster JR, Bennion LJ, Nadler LM, Bough EW, Koch-Weser J. Survival after massive procainamide ingestion. Am J Cardiol 1973;32(5):727–30.

61. Atkinson AJ Jr, Krumlovsky FA, Huang CM, del Greco F. Hemodialysis for severe procainamide toxicity: clinical and pharmacokinetic observations. Clin Pharmacol Ther 1976;20(5):585–92.

62. Windle J, Prystowsky EN, Miles WM, Heger JJ. Pharmacokinetic and electrophysiologic interactions of amiodarone and procainamide. Clin Pharmacol Ther 1987;41(6):603–10.

63. Somogyi A, McLean A, Heinzow B. Cimetidine–procainamide pharmacokinetic interaction in man: evidence of competition for tubular secretion of basic drugs. Eur J Clin Pharmacol 1983;25(3):339–45.

64. Bauer LA, Black D, Gensler A. Procainamide–cimetidine drug interaction in elderly male patients. J Am Geriatr Soc 1990;38(4):467–9.

65. Sianipar A, Parkin JE, Sunderland VB. The reaction of procainamide with glucose following admixture to glucose infusion. Int J Pharm 1998;176:55–61.

66. Martin DE, Shen J, Griener J, Raasch R, Patterson JH, Cascio W. Effects of ofloxacin on the pharmacokinetics and pharmacodynamics of procainamide. J Clin Pharmacol 1996;36(1):85–91.

67. Kosoglou T, Rocci ML Jr, Vlasses PH. Trimethoprim alters the disposition of procainamide and N-acetylprocainamide. Clin Pharmacol Ther 1988;44(4):467–77.

68. Koch-Weser J. Serum procainamide levels as therapeutic guides. Clin Pharmacokinet 1977;2(6):389–402.

Procaine

See also Local anesthetics

General Information

Procaine is an aminoester local anesthetic. It is most widely used as a component of procaine penicillin.

Organs and Systems

Nervous system

Rare cases of tonic seizures have been reliably attributed to the presence of procaine in procaine penicillin (1).

Skin

The incidence of pruritus has been evaluated in a retrospective study of patients receiving procaine, lidocaine, or bupivacaine in combination with fentanyl for spinal anesthesia for a variety of different surgical procedures (2). Procaine plus fentanyl and bupivacaine plus fentanyl produced a higher incidence of pruritus than lidocaine plus fentanyl. The severity of pruritus was also greater in those given procaine plus fentanyl. The incidence and severity of pruritus was not related to the dose of fentanyl. Although this may represent an interaction between fentanyl and ester local anesthetics that differs from the synergy occurring between fentanyl and amide local anesthetics, this was an observational study and was neither randomized nor blinded. Furthermore, the doses of local anesthetic or fentanyl were not standardized. Further prospective randomized studies are therefore required to confirm or refute these claims.

Drug–Drug Interactions

Acetylcholinesterase inhibitors

Acetylcholinesterase inhibitors inhibit the hydrolysis of procaine and concomitant use can cause procaine toxicity (3).

Suxamethonium

Procaine is hydrolysed by plasma cholinesterase and may therefore competitively enhance the action of suxamethonium (4).

References

1. Malone JD, Lebar RD, Hilder R. Procaine-induced seizures after intramuscular procaine penicillin G. Mil Med 1988;153(4):191–2.
2. Morikawa S, Ishikawa J, Kamatsuki H, Shinzato Y, Watanabe A, Ishikawa H, Chihara H, Nagata T, Kometani K. [Neurobehavior and mental development of newborn infants delivered under epidural analgesia with bupivacaine.] Nippon Sanka Fujinka Gakkai Zasshi 1990;42(11):1495–502.
3. Ellis PP, Littlejohn K. Effects of topical anticholinesterases on procaine hydrolysis. Am J Ophthalmol 1974;77(1):71–5.
4. Matsuo S, Rao DB, Chaudry I, Foldes FF. Interaction of muscle relaxants and local anesthetics at the neuromuscular junction. Anesth Analg 1978;57(5):580–7.

Procarbazine

See also Cytostatic and immunosuppressant drugs

General Information

Procarbazine is an alkylating agent that is used in the treatment of Hodgkin's disease in regimens such as MOPP (chlormethine (mechlorethamine), vincristine (Oncovin), procarbazine, and prednisolone) and BEACOPP (bleomycin, etoposide, doxorubicin (Adriamycin), cyclophosphamide, vincristine, procarbazine, and prednisone) (1). It is also used to treat glioblastoma multiforme.

Organs and Systems

Respiratory

The permanent and acute reversible forms of lung disease attributed to procarbazine have been reviewed (2). Pneumonitis has rarely been reported (3).

Drug–Drug Interactions

Antiepileptic drugs

In a retrospective cohort study in 83 patients with primary brain tumors who were treated with procarbazine, 20 patients had procarbazine hypersensitivity reactions (4). There was a significant association between exposure to antiepileptic drugs and the development of procarbazine hypersensitivity reactions. The authors suggested that this association may have been due to a reactive intermediate generated by induction of CYP3A.

References

1. Massoud M, Armand JP, Ribrag V. Procarbazine in haematology: an old drug with a new life? Eur J Cancer 2004;40(13):1924–7.
2. Millward MJ, Cohney SJ, Byrne MJ, Ryan GF. Pulmonary toxicity following MOPP chemotherapy. Aust NZ J Med 1990;20(3):245–8.
3. Mahmood T, Mudad R. Pulmonary toxicity secondary to procarbazine. Am J Clin Oncol 2002;25(2):187–8.
4. Lehmann DF, Hurteau TE, Newman N, Coyle TE. Anticonvulsant usage is associated with an increased risk of procarbazine hypersensitivity reactions in patients with brain tumors. Clin Pharmacol Ther 1997;62(2):225–9.

Prochlorperazine

See also Neuroleptic drugs

General Information

Prochlorperazine is a phenothiazine derivative.

Organs and Systems

Nervous system

In 192 consecutive patients attending an emergency department for nausea/vomiting or headache, akathisia occurred in 16% of those treated with prochlorperazine (5–10 mg intravenously or intramuscularly); 4% (all of them women) developed dystonias (1).

Slow infusion of prochlorperazine has been used to try to minimize the risk of akathisia in 160 patients randomly assigned to two groups; akathisia developed in 31 of 84 who were given a 2-minute infusion and in 18 of 76 patients who were given a 15-minute infusion (2).

References

1. Olsen JC, Keng JA, Clark JA. Frequency of adverse reactions to prochlorperazine in the ED. Am J Emerg Med 2000;18(5):609–11.
2. Vinson DR, Migala AF, Quesenberry CP Jr. Slow infusion for the prevention of akathisia induced by prochlorperazine: a randomized controlled trial. J Emerg Med 2001;20(2):113–19.

Procyclidine

See also Anticholinergic drugs

General Information

Procyclidine is an anticholinergic drug (1). The usual oral dose, which lies between 20 and 30 mg/day, is likely to produce only mild anticholinergic adverse effects, but involuntary movements, with chewing and sucking, have been described in some patients (SEDA-1, 120). Even small doses have produced toxic confusional states when procyclidine was combined with phenothiazines for schizophrenia. Procyclidine is more likely to produce sedation than stimulation.

Reference

1. Brocks DR. Anticholinergic drugs used in Parkinson's disease: an overlooked class of drugs from a pharmacokinetic perspective. J Pharm Pharmacol Sci 1999; 2(2):39–46.

Progabide

General Information

Progabide is an antispasticity drug that is also used in the treatment of epilepsy (1). Together with its metabolites, it acts as an agonist at both $GABA_A$ and $GABA_B$ receptors.

A high proportion of patients suffer from transient minor adverse effects, such as drowsiness, nausea, weakness, or dizziness.

Organs and Systems

Liver

The most serious adverse effect of progabide is hepatotoxicity. In one study, seven of 30 patients given doses up to 45 mg/kg/day had significant disturbances of liver function tests (which returned to normal on withdrawing the drug) (2). In another study, abnormal liver function tests were reported in 8.4% of 1164 patients; clinical hepatotoxicity occurred in 0.5% and three patients died. Monitoring liver function is recommended and drug withdrawal is indicated if liver transaminases exceed twice normal (SED-13, 155).

References

1. Loiseau P, Duchie B. Prograbide. In: Dam M, Gram L, editors. Comprehensive Epileptology. New York: Raven Press, 1990:641.
2. Rudick RA, Breton D, Krall RL. The GABA-agonist progabide for spasticity in multiple sclerosis. Arch Neurol 1987; 44(10):1033–6.

Progestogens

See also Individual agents

General Information

Most aspects of progestogens are dealt with in the monograph on hormonal contraception. For a complete account of the adverse effects of progestogens, readers should consult the following monographs as well as this one:

- Hormonal contraceptives—intracervical and intravaginal
- Hormonal contraceptives—oral
- Hormonal contraceptives—progestogen implants
- Hormonal contraceptives—progestogen injections
- Hormone replacement therapy—estrogens + progestogens
- Medroxyprogesterone.

While the progestogens have certain characteristic effects of their own, notably on the female menstrual cycle, the spectrum of adverse effects of any particular progestogen (particularly when given in high doses) is likely to depend heavily on the extent to which it also has glucocorticoid, mineralocorticoid, estrogenic, or androgenic properties.

The natural endogenous progestogen is progesterone (rINN), but most progestogens are semisynthetic. Progestogens belong to two main families:

- hydroxyprogesterone derivatives, which include hydroxyprogesterone caproate, dydrogesterone, medroxyprogesterone, chlormadinone, and cyproterone acetate (all rINNs), and which tend to be antiandrogenic
- ethisterone derivatives, which include norethisterone, norgestrel, levonorgestrel, desogestrel, and gestodene (all rINNs), which have some androgenic activity, and norgestimate (rINN), which has some estrogenic activity.

Water retention occasionally occurs and may reflect a degree of deoxycortone acetate (DOCA)-like activity; virilization of a female fetus is more likely to occur with a product that has some androgenic activity, and breast tenderness with a product that has estrogenic activity.

Some individuals taking progestogens for breast cancer will therefore experience, for example, not only painful swelling of the breast and prolonged amenorrhea (which are progestogenic), but also weight gain and hypercalcemia (which are likely to be glucocorticoid effects). Patients who take progestogens during pregnancy are said to be susceptible to prolonged postpartum bleeding, but this probably reflects the pregnancy disorder for which these drugs were at one time given, for example habitual or threatened abortion. Virilization of the female fetus has been described after administration of various progestogens in early pregnancy and is presumably an androgenic effect.

Progestogens given alone for contraceptive purposes can cause a number of adverse effects, some of which may reflect their other hormonal properties while others are non-specific. Headache, nausea and vomiting, breast tenderness, and pain in the back or abdomen can occur.

Animal studies cannot be regarded as providing a reliable indicator of the spectrum of activity of individual compounds; suggestions that derivatives of hydroxyprogesterone (such as megestrol acetate, medroxyprogesterone acetate) are more "natural" (because of their progesterone-like structure) than derivatives of 19-nortestosterone (such as norgestrel, lynestrenol, ethynodiol acetate, norethisterone, and allylestrenol) are not reflected in any biological findings. Experience, too, can be misleading; there is some suggestion that hydroxyprogesterone caproate can have adverse effects on the fetus when used in pregnancy, while similar reports about allylestrenol (used for the same purpose) are lacking, but one must bear in mind the anecdotal nature of such evidence and especially the fact that hydroxyprogesterone caproate appears to have been more widely used than allylestrenol and is hence more likely to have given rise to reports of adverse reactions.

Progestogens belonging to the ethisterone family (norethisterone, levonorgestrel, desogestrel) have some androgenic activity; those in the hydroxyprogesterone family (hydroxyprogesterone caproate, chlormadinone, cyproterone acetate) tend to be antiandrogenic, while norgestimate seems to be somewhat estrogenic. Water retention occasionally occurs and may reflect a degree of DOCA-like activity; virilization of a female fetus is more likely to occur with a product that has some androgenic activity, and breast tenderness with a product that has estrogenic activity.

In a multicenter, prospective, double-blind, randomized, parallel group study undertaken by general practitioners to compare progesterone pessaries with placebo in the relief of symptoms of premenstrual syndrome, spontaneous reports of adverse events were recorded (1). The 41 patients were randomized to treatment or placebo groups. Patients taking active therapy reported more frequent vaginal pruritus, headache, and irregularities of menstruation. However, when cyclical treatment with progestogen alone was given to postmenopausal women, there was no greater degree of endometrial hyperplasia than in untreated women (2).

Semisynthetic progestogens

Desogestrel (rINN)

Desogestrel, one of the so-called third-generation progestogenic steroids intended for use in oral contraceptives, is metabolized to estrogen. It was developed and introduced because of its relatively favorable effect on blood lipids in experimental work; this led to the hope that it might, in the long run, have a relatively favorable effect on the risk of atherogenesis. However, it is not clear that this does in fact happen, and the third-generation progestogens have been associated with an increased risk of thromboembolism.

Gestodene (rINN)

Gestodene is a third-generation progestogen that has been implicated in an increased risk of thromboembolism.

Gestonorone caproate (rINN)

Gestonorone (17-hydroxy-19-norprogesterone) has been used in doses of 200 mg intramuscularly weekly for benign prostatic hyperplasia (3). Mild adverse effects included loss of appetite and mild fever, but more remarkable were significant reductions in erythrocyte count, hemoglobin, and hematocrit, which normalized after drug withdrawal (4).

Hydroxyprogesterone caproate (rINN)

High doses of hydroxyprogesterone and the related norderivative have been used to treat benign prostatic hyperplasia. Very striking is the high incidence of impotence recorded in these studies, which can affect two-thirds of patients and seems to persist in some patients after withdrawal (5).

Levonorgestrel (rINN)

Extensive clinical trials and premarketing studies were conducted before the Norplant (levonorgestrel) implant was registered and approved, in order to elucidate its mode of action, effectiveness, and adverse effects. However, none of these trials included either teenagers under 18 years of age or nulligravid women.

In an 18-month observational study of 136 adolescents (13–18 years) and 542 adults (19–46 years) who were given Norplant levonorgestrel contraceptive implants problems were reported by 110 patients, mostly irregular bleeding (53% of the adolescents and 38% of the adults) (6). Removal of the implant was requested by 11% of both adolescents and adults, most commonly for intolerable menstrual cycle changes, and in 6% of all the adults for irregular bleeding; the time from insertion to removal was 3–15 months for the adolescents and 1–17 months for the adults. Other problems that led to removal (in 5% of adolescents and 7.5% of adults), apart from a desire to become pregnant, included headache, weight gain, and acne.

Lynestrenol (rINN)

Lynestrenol is one of the older progestogens used in oral contraceptives and has been very widely and successfully employed for nearly 40 years; as monotherapy it has been used to treat irregularity of the menstrual cycle.

In a Finnish study analysis of the association between the prolonged use of lynestrenol (to suppress menstruation in mentally retarded women) and arterial disease detected at autopsy, the conclusion was that such treatment, here given for a mean of more than 6 years, increases the risk of arterial disease and that such treatment must be very carefully considered (7).

Medroxyprogesterone acetate (rINNM)

Medroxyprogesterone acetate is the subject of a separate monograph.

Megestrol (rINN)

Megestrol acetate, like medroxyprogesterone acetate, is used for metastatic breast cancer in postmenopausal women. Its commonest adverse effects are typical of the progestogens as a group, but glucocorticoid-like effects are less prominent than with medroxyprogesterone acetate. Typical effects and incidence figures for effective doses in cancer patients (SED-12, 1036) (8,9) have been cited as including weight gain in some 81–88% of cases, mild edema in up to 34%, and hypertension in up to 25%. There are lower but appreciable occurrences of constipation, dyspnea or chest tightness, heartburn, hyperglycemia, and increased urinary frequency; a few cases of phlebitis or thrombosis have been described. Vaginal bleeding, nervousness, sweating, vertigo, gastrointestinal symptoms, skin rash, pruritus, and thrombocytopenia have also been incidentally recorded.

Megestrol acetate has also proved of value in patients with metastatic prostatic cancer, epithelial ovarian cancer, or malignant melanoma and is therefore used in both sexes. The adverse effects are very similar in men to those seen with oncological doses in women; loss of libido and potency is likely to occur in male patients. In one clinical study of 43 men with recurrent and metastatic cancer of the prostate given megestrol acetate 160 mg/day orally, five developed a symptomatic rise in liver enzymes but it resolved during further treatment. In three patients, increasing bone pain occurred, no doubt relating to changes in bony metastases and requiring analgesia. Another patient developed hypercalcemia and one patient developed convulsive epilepsy (10). These latter problems are characteristic of the primary condition as it responds, and not typical for megestrol acetate. The glucocorticoid-induced gain in body weight when it occurs is often linked to improved appetite (11), which can be a positive advantage in cachectic patients with advanced cancers.

When megestrol acetate was used alongside diethylstilbestrol or ethinylestradiol in men with previously untreated metastatic carcinoma of the prostate, there was a high incidence of feminizing adverse effects (70–74%), no doubt attributable to the estrogens; a higher than expected rate of cardiovascular complications (18%) and an unexplained need for cortisone replacement (13%) were also observed (12).

Organs and Systems

Cardiovascular

Progestogens with a degree of mineralocorticoid activity will tend to cause water and salt retention and to increase blood pressure in susceptible subjects. However, effects on blood pressure can be variable; for example, medroxyprogesterone has been variously reported to cause a fall in blood pressure in some initially hypertensive patients while rapidly increasing diastolic pressure in some other women, or to have no effect on blood pressure at all.

Since thromboembolic complications can occur with progestogens, there may be a danger in using them in patients in whom there are other risk factors for thromboembolism. A Spanish group had to deal with patients with AIDS in whom megestrol acetate seems to be helpful in countering AIDS-related anorexia or cachexia. However, advanced HIV infection is itself a risk factor for thromboembolism, as is tuberculosis, which readily occurs in this population. Of 199 patients with AIDS followed for 2 years, 25 took megestrol 320 mg/day. Deep vein thrombosis occurred in seven patients in the entire series, four of them being in the megestrol group and three having tuberculosis. The duration of hormonal therapy up to the moment of thrombosis averaged 98 days. Tuberculosis was an independent risk factor. Statistical analysis led to the conclusion that in this high-risk population the use of megestrol had increased the risk of thrombosis by a factor of 7.6 (13).

Thromboembolism and third-generation progestogens

In October 1995 the UK Committee on Safety of Medicines (CSM) issued a warning that oral contraceptives containing the third-generation progestogens gestodene or desogestrel carry a higher risk of venous thromboembolism, and that women using these should consider changing to another brand (14).

The warning was based on three unpublished studies that had not at the time been formally peer reviewed. All three showed about double the risk of venous thromboembolism with gestodene and desogestrel products compared with oral contraceptives containing other progestogens. The first, a large WHO collaborative case-control study of cardiovascular disease and oral contraceptives was undertaken in 17 countries. It was completed in July 1995, and involved 829 cases of venous thromboembolism and 2641 controls from nine countries in which third-generation oral contraceptives had been used (15). The second, from the Boston Collaborative Drug Surveillance Program, was an analysis of the occurrence of venous thromboembolism in a UK general practice cohort of 238 130 women who had received a prescription for an oral contraceptive containing levonorgestrel, gestodene, or desogestrel (16). The third was a transnational case-control study conducted in five European countries, funded by Schering, the leading manufacturer of gestodene (17).

The WHO study was undertaken because the association between oral contraceptive use and venous thromboembolism had not been examined since the 1970s, when oral contraceptives contained higher doses of estrogen and progestogen than now, and because none of the earlier studies had been done in developing countries. The finding of a higher risk of venous thromboembolism with gestodene and desogestrel came as a surprise, and this, together with publicity in the media, prompted the CSM to commission the UK cohort study. The transnational study was set up at the request of the German regulatory authority to follow up German spontaneous reporting data that in 1990 had strongly suggested higher risks of thromboembolism with gestodene-containing oral contraceptives. This led to much controversy in the press and television. Schering had argued that highly publicized deaths had stimulated selective reporting, and that the claimed higher risk was an artefact.

The sudden announcement by the CSM in October 1995 caught prescribers and users of oral contraceptives completely unprepared. What some General Practitioners described as the "pill panic" in the media (18) drove thousands of women to consult their doctors (18–20), who had not been briefed. A heated debate ensued over whether the CSM's decision was justified, whether its announcement should have been delayed until the data were published, and over the dramatic and confusing way in which it was issued. Before long there was general agreement that the decision was necessary and correct, but that its communication had been handled badly, and the Health Minister said that the Government would review the incident to learn from it. Important suggestions for getting this kind of communication correct have subsequently been made (21–23). Official actions in other countries ranged from the imposition of stronger restrictions (in Germany) to decisions in the Netherlands and Canada to wait and consider the published studies, and in the USA not to advise switching to other products (24). The European Union's Committee on Proprietary Medicinal Products also decided to wait and see.

Although doubts about the relative safety of gestodene emerged in 1990, regulators did not publicly acknowledge them. Nor did they help independent scientists to examine all the relevant data (including prescribing figures, essential to provide denominators for the calculation of risk), perhaps because they were insufficient and might have been wrongly interpreted. In Germany, the regulatory authority privately asked Schering to undertake a case-control study; in the UK the Medicines Control Agency considered the available evidence inadequate and dismissed the doubts. Whether the CSM was consulted at that time or only later remains a minor official secret. The attitude changed early in July 1995, when the CSM saw the early results of the WHO Collaborative Study, and a highly critical UK television programme about gestodene-containing oral contraceptives was broadcast (Granada, "World in Action," 10 July). The CSM asked workers from the transnational case-control

study to "expedite their results," and commissioned the cohort study using data routinely collected from General Practitioners. The analysis of venous thromboembolism in the transnational study was completed on 8 October, and was promptly discussed with members of the Medicines Control Agency and the CSM. The CSM quickly made its decision (17) and announced it on 18 October. The relevant data from the WHO study and the GP cohort study were published on 16 December; those from the transnational study were published on 13 January 1996 (25). A searching independent analysis of these three studies, and of a fourth (26) that the CSM had not considered, supported the decision (27).

In retrospect, what could the CSM and other authorities have done to alert the world to the potential problem during the 5 years of growing doubts about the relative safety of gestodene? To know about the doubts would have helped women and their doctors. They could then have begun to discuss among themselves whether to act on them or not, in order to weigh any real advantages of their gestodene oral contraceptive against the doubt and potential risk. A joint statement by regulators and manufacturers about their plans for further investigations would have made it clear that there was a problem to be resolved, instead of appearing to ignore or deny it. This would have allowed prescribers and independent experts to rethink their prescribing policies, for example deciding in what circumstances gestodene oral contraceptives should no longer be the first choice. That would not have pleased the manufacturers, since it would almost certainly have reduced the sales of their leading product in an uncontrollable way. The position of desogestrel creates additional complications, since its relative safety was not questioned until the data from the WHO study appeared in July 1995. If doubts had been officially expressed about the gestodene-containing products Femodene and Minulet, these oral contraceptives would meanwhile have lost some market share to Marvelon and Mercilon, the desogestrel-containing products. But greater openness from the start could have minimized the alarm and confusion.

Liver

The progestogens as a group have little effect on the liver. However, some progestogens can increase non-conjugated bilirubin (28); norethisterone acetate has been implicated in this effect (29).

Skin

Progestogens have very occasionally been reported to cause hypersensitivity reactions or skin disorders. Pemphigus has been reported (30).

- A 34-year-old woman with a 3-month history of dysphagia, odynophagia, and conjunctivitis with bulbar injection, who had been taking an oral contraceptive containing a progestogen for 7 months, developed typical bullous lesions on her trunk and nose, typical of pemphigus. Ceftriaxone and ampicillin, which can aggravate pemphigus, exacerbated the lesions. There was reason to believe that the patient had a genetic predisposition to the disorder.

The circumstances pointed strongly to a drug association, but the identity of the oral contraceptive was not stated; it is likely to have contained a synthetic progestogen and not progesterone itself.

However progesterone-induced dermatitis certainly does occur.

- A 68-year-old woman who took a formulation containing hydroxyprogesterone acetate + conjugated estrogens had for many years an autoimmune dermatitis (31).

Other complications (acne, alopecia, and pruritus) have been associated with Mirena, an intrauterine system containing levonorgestrel.

- Rosacea accompanied the use of Mirena in a 36-year-old woman for 2 years and disappeared within 6 months of removal (32).

However, one is bound to wonder whether this was a direct reaction to levonorgestrel or a stress reaction to the absence of menstrual periods. Like many other users of Mirena, this woman had amenorrhea associated with facial flushing and pustules; conditions such as urticaria, eczema, pompholyx, and erythema multiforme occur cyclically in some women in the second half of the menstrual cycle, irrespective of contraceptive use.

Long-Term Effects

Tumorigenicity

The effects of adding a progestogen on the carcinogenic effects of estrogens are discussed in the monograph on estrogens.

Second-Generation Effects

Teratogenicity

For a number of years from about 1950 onwards, progestogens were used in cases of threatened and habitual abortion. They were largely abandoned for this purpose because of the general conclusion that they were ineffective. There was no general conclusion as to any adverse effects that might have resulted, although some of the progestogens were suspected of having virilizing effects on the fetus. Subsequently, progestogens (usually natural progesterone) were used to provide "luteal support" for some 4 weeks after in vitro fertilization. In 283 women treated for this reason with injectable progesterone 300 mg/day, oral micronized progesterone 90 mg/day, or a sustained-release transvaginal gel, among the offspring there were incidental cases of facial teratoma associated with a cleft palate, a respiratory distress syndrome, and Pierre–Robin syndrome; there was no clear indication that in this respect one formulation was safer than another or that the effects observed were other than might have been anticipated in untreated controls with a similar history (33). Women who received the injectable progesterone tended to complain of drowsiness, reduced libido, dyspareunia, and vaginal irritability.

With regard to progestogens given alone to prevent threatened or habitual abortion, there is no good evidence that they are beneficial, and much evidence to the contrary; however, effects on the sexual development of the fetus cannot be excluded (34).

Tumors may possibly be induced in the second generation. Neuroblastoma in four infants has been attributed to pregnancy or to gonadotropins, clomiphene citrate, or progestational hormones (35), because these drugs result in increased exposure of the early pregnancy to estrogenic or progestogenic influences. Most of these neuroblastomas regress spontaneously, but when regression does not occur they may become malignant. Children born to women who have taken hormonal preparations in early pregnancy should therefore be screened for urinary vanillylmandelic acid concentrations at the age of 6 months.

Drug Administration

Drug formulations

As with estradiol, a case has been made for using natural progesterone, rather than synthetic analogues, largely because it is assumed that as a physiological substance it will be safer. Progesterone is unsuitable for oral use (unless given in a special micronized form), but it is used by other routes. These include systemic and intra-articular injection (36), an intranasal ointment (37), transdermal formulations (38), and intravaginal formulations (39). Apart from local irritation, the wanted and unwanted effects produced when using these modes of administration are the familiar manifestations of progestogen treatment and are proportional to the amount of the drug that actually enters the circulation.

Micronized oral formulations

The fact that progesterone when given by mouth has poor systemic availability can be largely overcome by micronization, and the first product based on this concept was marketed in France as long ago as 1980. Studies and reviews have appeared, particularly since 1997, suggesting that it is indeed less likely to cause adverse effects than the synthetic progestogens are (40). The most frequently reported adverse reactions are stated to be dizziness or drowsiness, which could be related to the pregnenolone metabolites and do not seem to reflect vasoactive changes. It has been argued theoretically that there might be altered sodium metabolism, but no hypertensive effects have been seen. Unusually high doses of micronized progesterone given in pregnancy (in the hope of avoiding premature labor) have been suspected of causing intrahepatic cholestasis, at least in women with a genetic predisposition, but these doses are much higher that those in normal use. No changes in lipid profile appear to occur.

With these very positive conclusions it is not clear why micronized progesterone has not been more widely used. Commercial factors may well have played a role in maintaining the overwhelming dominance of the patented synthetic progestogens. On the other hand, despite the fact that there are estimated to be 500 000 current users of micronized progesterone in France alone, the worldwide scope of experience is still limited compared with that of the synthetic analogues, and one must be prepared for surprises if this product should ever be used more widely. It is a fact that in the 1970s, when studies in beagle dogs gave rise to much concern regarding progestogens and the induction of mammary tumors, the same effect was also observed with natural progesterone if sufficient doses were administered. Even a natural substance can have unpleasant effects when used in a manner not foreseen in nature.

Intrauterine release systems

The fiber-based ("frameless") FibroPlant delivery system for levonorgestrel has been tested in an open study in 32 women as a means of relieving menorrhagia or for contraceptive purposes (41). The period of exposure was 1–23 months. This system, which releases levonorgestrel 14 micrograms/day, appeared to be effective for both purposes, and there were no cases of infection, expulsion, or perforation.

An alternative intrauterine delivery system (LNG-IUS) consists of an adapted Nova-T device with a silastic reservoir attached to the vertical arm; the reservoir is impregnated with levonorgestrel and is covered with a rate-limiting silastic membrane. The release rate of levonorgestrel is about 20 micrograms/day for at least 5 years. In a 5-year study in which 1821 women used the combined device and 937 others used the plain Nova-T device, the Pearl index (the number of unwanted pregnancies occurring in 100 couples using a given method for a period of one year) was 0.09/100 woman-years for the LNG-IUS and the ectopic pregnancy rate was 0.02/100 woman-years (42). There were fewer withdrawals because of bleeding problems and pelvic inflammatory disease with LNG-IUS compared with Nova-T, but there were more withdrawals because of hormonal adverse effects and absence of bleeding. One of the advantages claimed for LNG-IUS is that there will be less menstrual blood loss. However, all women who used LNG-IUS had some change in their bleeding pattern after the device had been inserted, and some had many days of spotting. Of another 30 women who used the LNG-IUS system to relieve menorrhagia and who were followed for a year, 13 reported one or more pelvic adverse event; there were six complaints of irregular bleeding, four of abdominal pain, three of breast tenderness, and occasional cases of headache, mood changes, or acne (43).

A systematic review of Mirena, an intrauterine progestogen release system (44), has attracted correspondence (45,46). Like other devices, Mirena releases levonorgestrel, in this case 20 micrograms/day. Since it had no greater efficacy than the Copper T device and was very much more costly, the debate has turned on safety. Amenorrhea is common with this device, as with others like it, and correspondents have pointed out that this is regarded by many women as an unwelcome complication.

Transdermal administration

An older 19-norprogesterone (ST 1435, Merck Darmstadt) was used experimentally in a transdermal form as a possible hormonal contraceptive. A dose of 0.8–1 mg/day was needed to inhibit ovulation in all subjects. There was some irregularity of bleeding, and some subjects had breast tenderness (47).

Vaginal gel

To provide luteal support in ovarian stimulation protocols, especially when following the long procedure, progesterone can be administered by various routes. The oral route is relatively ineffective, since progesterone has a low oral systemic availability (below 10%), which may result in adverse effects such as somnolence. Intramuscular administration is painful and inconvenient. Some workers have therefore given progesterone in the form of an 8% vaginal gel, which is effective and better tolerated than alternative approaches. The gel adheres to the vaginal epithelium, and leakage is substantially less than when using capsules or suppositories; there are no local complications (48). No adverse reactions have been reported with the use of a modified-release vaginal gel containing polycarbophil-based progesterone (49).

References

1. Magill PJ. Investigation of the efficacy of progesterone pessaries in the relief of symptoms of premenstrual syndrome. Progesterone Study Group. Br J Gen Pract 1995;45(400):589–93.
2. Rabe T, Mueck AO, Deuringer FU, Vladescu E, Runnebaum B. Spacing-out of progestin—efficacy, tolerability and compliance of two regimens for hormonal replacement in the late postmenopause. Gynecol Endocrinol 1997;11(6):383–92.
3. Iguchi H, Ikeuchi T, Kai Y, Yoshida H. [Influence of antiandrogen therapy for prostatic hypertrophy on lipid metabolism.] Hinyokika Kiyo 1994;40(3):215–19.
4. Okada K, Oishi L, Yoshida O. Effects on the pituitary–gonadal axis in the treatment of benign prostatic hypertrophy with gestoronone caproate. Curr Ther Res 1984;35:139.
5. Palanca E, Juco W. Conservative treatment of benign prostatic hyperplasia. Curr Med Res Opin 1977;4(7):513–20.
6. Cullins VE, Remsburg RE, Blumenthal PD, Huggins GR. Comparison of adolescent and adult experiences with Norplant levonorgestrel contraceptive implants. Obstet Gynecol 1994;83(6):1026–32.
7. Huovinen K, Autio S, Kaprio J. Peroral lynestrenol and arterial disease in mentally retarded women. A case-control study based on autopsy findings. Acta Obstet Gynecol Scand 1988;67(3):211–14.
8. Feliu J, Gonzalez-Baron M, Berrocal A, Artal A, Ordonez A, Garrido P, Zamora P, Garcia de Paredes ML, Montero JM. Usefulness of megestrol acetate in cancer cachexia and anorexia. A placebo-controlled study. Am J Clin Oncol 1992;15(5):436–40.
9. Tchekmedyian NS, Tait N, Aisner J. High-dose megestrol acetate in the treatment of postmenopausal women with advanced breast cancer. Semin Oncol 1986;13(4 Suppl 4):20–5.
10. Crombie C, Raghavan D, Page J, Woods R, Dalley D, Devine R, Rosen M. Phase II study of megestrol acetate for metastatic carcinoma of the prostate. Br J Urol 1987;59(5):443–6.
11. Loeffler TM, Weber FW, Hausamen TU. Einfluss von mittelhoch dosiertem Megestrolacetat auf Appetitstimulation und Gewichtszunahme bei gleichzeitiger zytostatischer Therapie. Tumordiagn Ther 1992;13:72.
12. Johnson DE, Babaian RJ, Swanson DA, von Eschenbach AC, Wishnow KI, Tenney D. Medical castration using megestrol acetate and minidose estrogen. Urology 1988;31(5):371–4.
13. Force L, Barrufet P, Herreras Z, Bolibar I. Deep venous thrombosis and megestrol in patients with HIV infection. AIDS 1999;13(11):1425–6.

14. Carnall D. Controversy rages over new contraceptive data. BMJ 1995;311:1117–18.

15. World Health Organization Collaborative Study of Cardiovascular Disease and Steroid Hormone Contraception. Effect of different progestagens in low oestrogen oral contraceptives on venous thromboembolic disease. Lancet 1995;346(8990):1582–8.

16. Jick H, Jick SS, Gurewich V, Myers MW, Vasilakis C. Risk of idiopathic cardiovascular death and nonfatal venous thromboembolism in women using oral contraceptives with differing progestagen components. Lancet 1995; 346(8990):1589–93.

17. Spitzer WO. Data from transnational study of oral contraceptives have been misused. BMJ 1995;311(7013):1162.

18. Armstrong JL, Reid M, Bigrigg A. Scare over oral contraceptives. Effect on behaviour of women attending a family planning clinic. BMJ 1995;311(7020):1637.

19. Seamark CJ. Scare over oral contraceptives. Effect on women in a general practice in Devon . . . . BMJ 1995;311(7020):1637.

20. Davies AW, York JR, Jones SR. [Scare over oral contraceptives] . . . and south Wales. BMJ 1995;311(7020):1637–8.

21. Ketting E. Third generation oral contraceptives. CSM's advice will harm women's health worldwide. BMJ 1996;312(7030):576.

22. Stewart-Brown S, Pyper C. Third generation oral contraceptives. CSM should rethink its approach for such announcements. BMJ 1996;312(7030):576.

23. Smith C. Third generation oral contraceptives. How one clinic's practice conforms with CSM's advice. BMJ 1996;312(7030):576–7.

24. Carnall D, Karcher H, Lie LG, Sheldon T, Spurgeon D, Josefson D, Zinn C. Third generation oral contraceptives—the controversy BMJ 1995;311(7020):1589–90.

25. Spitzer WO, Lewis MA, Heinemann LA, Thorogood M, MacRae KD. Third generation oral contraceptives and risk of venous thromboembolic disorders: an international case-control study. Transnational Research Group on Oral Contraceptives and the Health of Young Women. BMJ 1996;312(7023):83–8.

26. Bloemenkamp KW, Rosendaal FR, Helmerhorst FM, Buller HR, Vandenbroucke JP. Enhancement by factor V Leiden mutation of risk of deep-vein thrombosis associated with oral contraceptives containing a third-generation progestagen. Lancet 1995;346(8990):1593–6.

27. McPherson K. Third generation oral contraception and venous thromboembolism. BMJ 19967;312(7023):68–9.

28. Boyer JL, Preisig R, Zbinden G, de Kretser DM, Wang C, Paulsen CA. Guidelines for assessment of potential hepatotoxic effects of synthetic androgens, anabolic agents and progestagens in their use in males as antifertility agents. Contraception 1976;13(4):461–8.

29. Werner T. Ikterus mit Worschluss-syndrom nach Behandlung mit Norethisteronazetat. Z Gastroenterol 1969;7:186.

30. Lo Schiavo A, D'Avino M. Progesterone, an unsuspected pemphigus inductor. G Ital Dermatol Venereol 1999;134:331–4.

31. Ingber A, Trattner A, David M. Hypersensitivity to an oestrogen–progesterone preparation and possible relationship to autoimmune progesterone dermatitis and corticosteroid hypersensitivity. J Dermatol Treat 1999; 10:139–40.

32. Choudry K, Humphreys F, Menage J. Rosacea in association with the progesterone-releasing intrauterine contraceptive device. Clin Exp Dermatol 2001;26(1):102.

33. Pouly JL, Bassil S, Frydman R, Hedon B, Nicollet B, Prada Y, Antoine JM, Zambrano R, Donnez J. Luteal support after in-vitro fertilization: Crinone 8%, a sustained release vaginal progesterone gel, versus Utrogestan, an oral micronized progesterone. Hum Reprod 1996;11(10): 2085–9.

34. World Health Organization. Treatment of threatened or habitual abortion. In: Drugs in Pregnancy and Delivery. 11th European Symposium on Clinical Pharmacological Evaluation in Drug Control. Copenhagen: WHO Regional Office for Europe, 1984:6.

35. Mandel M, Toren A, Rechavi G, Dor J, Ben-Bassat I, Neumann Y. Hormonal treatment in pregnancy: a possible risk factor for neuroblastoma. Med Pediatr Oncol 1994;23(2):133–5.

36. Cuchacovich M, Tchernitchin A, Gatica H, Wurgaft R, Valenzuela C, Cornejo E. Intraarticular progesterone: effects of a local treatment for rheumatoid arthritis. J Rheumatol 1988;15(4):561–5.

37. Dalton ME, Bromham DR, Ambrose CL, Osborne J, Dalton KD. Nasal absorption of progesterone in women. Br J Obstet Gynaecol 1987;94(1):84–8.

38. Persico N, Mancini F, Artini PG, Regnani G, Volpe A, de Aloysio D, Battaglia C. Transdermal hormone replacement therapy and Doppler findings in normal and overweight postmenopausal patients. Gynecol Endocrinol 2004; 19(5):274–81.

39. Lightman A, Kol S, Itskovitz-Eldor J. A prospective randomized study comparing intramuscular with intravaginal natural progesterone in programmed thaw cycles. Hum Reprod 1999;14(10):2596–9.

40. de Lignieres B. Oral micronized progesterone. Clin Ther 1999;21(1):41–60.

41. Wildemeersch D, Schacht E. Treatment of menorrhagia with a novel "frameless" intrauterine levonorgestrel-releasing drug delivery system: a pilot study. Eur J Contracept Reprod Health Care 2001;6(2):93–101.

42. Andersson K, Guillebaud J. The levonorgestrel intrauterine system: more than a contraceptive. Eur J Contracept Reprod Health Care 2001;6(Suppl 1):15–22.

43. Istre O, Trolle B. Treatment of menorrhagia with the levonorgestrel intrauterine system versus endometrial resection. Fertil Steril 2001;76(2):304–9.

44. French RS, Cowan FM, Mansour D, Higgins JP, Robinson A, Procter T, Morris S, Guillebaud J. Levonorgestrel-releasing (20 microgram/day) intrauterine systems (Mirena) compared with other methods of reversible contraceptives. BJOG 2000;107(10):1218–25.

45. Gerber B, Reimer T, Krause A, Friese K, Muller H. Levonorgestrel-releasing intrauterine devices. Lancet 2001;357(9258):801.

46. Onyeka BA, French R, Mansour D, Robinson A, Guillebaud J. Levonorgestrel-releasing (20 mcg/day) intrauterine systems (Mirena) compared with other methods of reversible contraceptives. BJOG 2001; 108(7):770–1.

47. Laurikka-Routti M, Haukkamaa M, Lahteenmaki P. Suppression of ovarian function with the transdermally given synthetic progestin ST 1435. Fertil Steril 1992;58(4):680–4.

48. Ludwig M, Diedrich K. Evaluation of an optimal luteal phase support protocol in IVF. Acta Obstet Gynecol Scand 2001;80(5):452–66.

49. Warren MP, Biller BM, Shangold MM. A new clinical option for hormone replacement therapy in women with secondary amenorrhea: effects of cyclic administration of progesterone from the sustained-release vaginal gel Crinone (4% and 8%) on endometrial morphologic features and withdrawal bleeding. Am J Obstet Gynecol 1999;180(1 Pt 1):42–8.

Proglumetacin

See also Non-steroidal anti-inflammatory drugs

General Information

Proglumetacin, an indoleacetic acid derivative, is particularly associated with gastrointestinal adverse effects: in different trials 18–41% of patients had adverse effects, but not to the extent that they interfered with treatment. Comparisons of proglumetacin with indometacin and oxyphenbutazone showed that it is equally effective and usually better tolerated (SEDA-5, 103). In an uncontrolled, open, multicenter, short-term study in patients with cervical or low back pain treated with proglumetacin, the most frequent adverse effects were gastrointestinal, while adverse effects on the nervous system were rare (1).

Reference

1. Ginsberg F, Lefebvre D. A large, open-label study of proglumetacin in the treatment of patients with cervical and low-back pain. Curr Ther Res Clin Exp 1995;56:1237–46.

Proguanil and chlorproguanil

General Information

Proguanil is one of the antimalarial drugs most widely used for prophylactic purposes, usually in combination with chloroquine or atovaquone in malaria prophylaxis, and with atovaquone in malaria treatment (SEDA-21, 297). A biguanide, it is rapidly absorbed in standard doses and mainly excreted by the kidneys. Its antimalarial effect is due to its metabolite cycloguanil. However, its metabolism varies individually, and this is reflected in a variable degree of efficacy (SEDA-17, 328).

A derivative, chlorproguanil, is similarly effective in chemoprophylaxis of malaria tropica (SEDA-20, 260).

No serious adverse effects of proguanil have been reported in otherwise healthy patients (SEDA-13, 811) (SEDA-17, 328). Skin rashes and hair loss can occur. Mouth ulcers have been mentioned, as have abdominal discomfort and vomiting. The incidence of mouth ulcers in a group of soldiers was 24% in those taking proguanil only and 37% in those taking proguanil 200 mg plus chloroquine either 300 or 150 mg weekly (SEDA-13, 811). With the use of large doses hematuria has been seen.

Organs and Systems

Hematologic

Since chlorproguanil + dapsone exerts lower resistance pressure on *Plasmodium falciparum* than does pyrimethamine + sulfadoxine, a randomized trial in outpatients with uncomplicated falciparum malaria was conducted in Africa in 910 children (1). Treatment failure was more common

with pyrimethamine + sulfadoxine. Despite the rapid elimination of chlorproguanil + dapsone, children treated with this combination did not have more episodes of malaria than those who were treated with pyrimethamine + sulfadoxine. However, there was a higher incidence of anemia.

Liver

Hepatitis with mild jaundice has been attributed to proguanil (2).

Susceptibility Factors

Genetic factors

The major limitation of proguanil is that in most ethnic groups there are individuals who have limited ability to metabolize proguanil to the active metabolite cycloguanil. Consequently, poor proguanil metabolizers treated with combination drugs are effectively taking monotherapy. Poor metabolizers also have an increased incidence of adverse effects with proguanil, especially gastrointestinal effects (3).

Renal disease

The urinary excretion of proguanil may mean that caution is advisable when treating patients with renal disorders. Two patients with renal insufficiency became severely ill while taking standard doses of proguanil (SEDA-12, 694) (4). One developed anorexia, dizziness, vomiting, diarrhea, mouth ulcers, a low white cell count, and a low platelet count. The other developed extensive purpura, epistaxis, and vomiting. Bone marrow studies showed hypoplasia and gross megaloblastic changes. The relation of these findings to proguanil therapy is nevertheless questionable, and whether the drug was or was not causative is not known. While it is tempting to seek an explanation in the fact that these biguanides interfere with (plasmodial) folate synthesis, the serum folate and vitamin B_{12} concentrations were normal in both patients.

Drug–Drug Interactions

Cimetidine

Cimetidine co-administration increased the C_{max} of proguanil, and significantly reduced the C_{max} and AUC of cycloguanil, presumably by inhibiting the metabolism of proguanil; co-administration is probably inadvisable (5).

Coumarin

Proguanil potentiates the response to warfarin (6), perhaps by inhibiting CYP2C19 (7).

Levothyroxine

A rise in serum TSH has been described after antimalarial prophylaxis with chloroquine and proguanil in patients taking levothyroxine (SEDA-22, 469). In one case there was a marked increase in serum TSH in the same patient on two occasions after several weeks of antimalarial prophylaxis with chloroquine and proguanil, the likely mechanism being enzyme catabolism (8).

References

1. Sulo J, Chimpeni P, Hatcher J, Kublin JG, Plowe CV, Molyneux ME, Marsh K, Taylor TE, Watkins WM, Winstanley PA. Chlorproguanil–dapsone versus sulfadoxine–pyrimethamine for sequential episodes of uncomplicated falciparum malaria in Kenya and Malawi: a randomised clinical trial. Lancet 2002;360(9340):1136–43.
2. Oostweegel LM, Beijnen JH, Mulder JW. Hepatitis during chloroguanide prophylaxis. Ann Pharmacother 1998;32(10):1023–5.
3. Kaneko A, Bergqvist Y, Taleo G, Kobayakawa T, Ishizaki T, Bjorkman A. Proguanil disposition and toxicity in malaria patients from Vanuatu with high frequencies of CYP2C19 mutations. Pharmacogenetics 1999;9(3):317–26.
4. White NJ. Clinical pharmacokinetics of antimalarial drugs. Clin Pharmacokinet 1985;10(3):187–215.
5. Kolawole JA, Mustapha A, Abdul-Aguye I, Ochekpe N, Taylor RB. Effects of cimetidine on the pharmacokinetics of proguanil in healthy subjects and in peptic ulcer patients. J Pharm Biomed Anal 1999;20(5):737–43.
6. Jassal SV. Warfarin potentiated by proguanil. BMJ 1991;303(6805):789.
7. Goldstein JA. Clinical relevance of genetic polymorphisms in the human CYP2C subfamily. Br J Clin Pharmacol 2001;52(4):349–55.
8. Hassan Alin M, Ashton M, Kihamia CM, Mtey GJ, Bjorkman A. Multiple dose pharmacokinetics of oral artemisinin and comparison of its efficacy with that of oral artesunate in falciparum malaria patients. Trans R Soc Trop Med Hyg 1996;90(1):61–5.

Prolintane

General Information

Prolintane, an amfetamine-related substance, is a central nervous system stimulant with similar structure and properties to dexamfetamine. Prolintane hydrochloride is available mainly in many formulations with multivitamin supplements in many European countries, Australia, and South Africa.

Organs and Systems

Nervous system

The adverse effects of prolintane include insomnia, nervousness, irritability, euphoria, headache, dizziness, and psychotic reactions (1).

Psychological, psychiatric

Prolintane can cause visual hallucinations (2).

Drug Administration

Drug overdose

Acute overdose can produce cardiorespiratory arrest and death (SEDA-22, 7).

Drug–Drug Interactions

Diphenhydramine

An interaction of prolintane with diphenhydramine has been reported (2).

- A young man developed visual hallucinations after taking prolintane and diphenhydramine. He had started to take prolintane 20 mg/day before 2 months, in order to enhance his intellectual performance and academic grades. Soon afterward he had sleep disturbance and resorted to a hypnotic containing diphenhydramine 25 mg. Despite this, insomnia preceded the acute psychotic episode. Prolintane and diphenhydramine were withdrawn, and he was given oral haloperidol and clorazepate. The symptoms gradually abated.

Pharmacological kindling resulting from increased dopaminergic activity could have explained this psychotic episode (3).

References

1 Martinez-Mir I, Catalan C, Palop V. Prolintane: a "masked" amphetamine. Ann Pharmacother 1997;31(1):256.
2 Paya B, Guisado JA, Vaz FJ, Crespo-Facorro B. Visual hallucinations induced by the combination of prolintane and diphenhydramine. Pharmacopsychiatry 2002;35(1):24–5.
3 Moskovitz C, Moses H 3rd, Klawans HL. Levodopa-induced psychosis: a kindling phenomenon. Am J Psychiatry 1978;135(6):669–75.

Promethazine

See also Antihistamines

General Information

Promethazine is a first-generation antihistamine (SEDA-15, 158) (SEDA-21, 176). In vitro studies suggest that CYP2D6 is a key enzyme for the metabolism for promethazine, which could lead to interaction problems (SEDA-21, 176).

Organs and Systems

Nervous system

Neuroleptic malignant syndrome has been associated with promethazine (1).

- A 42-year-old man took promethazine 50 mg every 4–6 hours for 2 days and developed hyperthermia (42.4°C). He died 3 days later despite intensive care and treatment with bromocriptine.

Promethazine intoxication from topical application has been observed in children (2) and adults (3). Symptoms include disorientation, hallucinations, hyperactivity, convulsions, and coma.

References

1. Chan-Tack KM. Neuroleptic malignant syndrome due to promethazine. South Med J 1999;92(10):1017–18.
2. Shawn DH, McGuigan MA. Poisoning from dermal absorption of promethazine. Can Med Assoc J 1984;130(11):1460–1.
3. Vidal Pan C, Gonzalez Quintela A, Galdos Anuncibay P, Mateo Vic J. Topical promethazine intoxication. DICP 1989;23(1):89.

Propafenone

See also Antidysrhythmic drugs

General Information

Propafenone is both a class I antidysrhythmic drug and a beta-adrenoceptor antagonist. Its pharmacological effects, clinical pharmacology, therapeutic uses, adverse effects, and interactions have been reviewed (1–5).

The main adverse effects of propafenone are cardiovascular (27%), central nervous (21%), and gastrointestinal (20%) (6). Other adverse effects occur in under 6% of cases. The overall risk of non-cardiac effects is around 14%. These adverse effects are dose-related: the incidence is 11% at 300 mg/day, 22% at 450 mg/day, 33% at 600 mg/day, and 48% at 900 mg/day (6).

Observational studies

In 87 patients with atrial fibrillation who were given propafenone 2 mg/kg intravenously over 10 minutes, four had hypotension at 8–45 minutes after the start of infusion (7). In two cases this was accompanied by sinus bradycardia, nausea, and slight malaise. In all cases the hypotension resolved rapidly with saline infusion; the drug was withdrawn in only one case. In two cases atrial fibrillation was transformed to asymptomatic atrial flutter with 2:1 atrioventricular conduction.

Quinidine has been added to propafenone with the intention of inhibiting propafenone metabolism via CYP2D6 in the hope of improving outcome (8). Of 60 patients with paroxysmal atrial fibrillation given propafenone 300–450 mg/day for 8 weeks there were 19 refractory cases, who were then randomized double-blind to receive either a higher dose of propafenone (450–675 mg/day) or the standard dose of propafenone with extra low-dose quinidine (150 mg/day), each for 8 weeks, with subsequent crossover to the alternative. Patients who even then were not adequately controlled were given the standard dose of propafenone plus a standard dose of quinidine (600 mg/day) for a further 8 weeks. The plasma propafenone concentrations during the four phases were as follows:

1. standard-dose propafenone alone 128 ng/ml;
2. standard-dose propafenone plus low-dose quinidine 259 ng/ml;
3. high-dose propafenone alone 336 ng/ml;
4. standard-dose propafenone plus standard-dose quinidine 490 ng/ml.

The beneficial effects were related to these plasma concentrations, as were the time to the first bout of atrial fibrillation, the frequency of bouts of atrial fibrillation, and the time between episodes. However, when atrial fibrillation occurred there was no difference in the ventricular rate in the different groups. Adverse effects necessitated drug withdrawal in four patients; one had heart failure and two had gastrointestinal symptoms. These effects were not dose-related, although there were too few occurrences for a definitive conclusion. The authors suggested that this stepwise approach, with increasing doses of propafenone and increasing doses of quinidine could be beneficial in the treatment of paroxysmal atrial fibrillation.

Comparative studies

Amiodarone

Amiodarone 30 mg/kg orally for the first 24 hours plus, if necessary, 15 mg/kg over 24 hours has been compared with propafenone 600 mg in the first 24 hours plus, if necessary, 300 mg in the next 24 hours in 86 patients with recent onset atrial fibrillation (9). Conversion to sinus rhythm occurred faster with propafenone (2.4 hours) than amiodarone (6.9 hours). However, by 24 hours and 48 hours the same proportions of patients were in sinus rhythm; one patient given amiodarone had a supraventricular tachycardia and one a non-sustained ventricular tachycardia.

Of 136 patients with atrial fibrillation treated with either amiodarone ($n = 96$) or propafenone ($n = 40$), 15 developed subsequent persistent atrial flutter, nine of those taking amiodarone and six of those taking propafenone (10). In all cases radiofrequency ablation was effective. It is not clear to what extent these cases of atrial flutter were due to the drugs, although the frequencies of atrial flutter in previous studies with propafenone have been similar. Atrial enlargement was significantly related to the occurrence of persistent atrial flutter in these patients.

Procainamide

A comparison between procainamide and propafenone in 62 patients, who had undergone coronary artery bypass grafting or valvular surgery within 3 weeks and developed sustained atrial fibrillation, showed that both drugs converted the dysrhythmia to sinus rhythm in up to 76% of cases, but that propafenone did it more quickly (11). Symptomatic arterial hypotension occurred more frequently with procainamide (nine of 33 patients) than propafenone (two of 29 patients). Other adverse effects of procainamide were nausea ($n = 2$) and junctional escape rhythm ($n = 2$). Other adverse effects of propafenone were hot flushes ($n = 1$), nausea ($n = 3$), bronchospasm ($n = 1$), and junctional escape rhythm ($n = 2$).

Quinidine

A placebo-controlled study of the use of propafenone 450–600 mg orally, either alone or in combination with digoxin, has been carried out in 176 patients with atrial fibrillation; a further 70 patients were given digitalis plus quinidine (12). There were no significant differences across the groups in terms of percentage conversion to sinus rhythm, although conversion occurred more quickly in those given digoxin plus propafenone; this catch-up of the other treatments was attributed to spontaneous conversion in those groups. There were no serious adverse effects in this study. The QT_c interval was slightly prolonged by digitalis plus quinidine and not by the other treatments. In six patients taking propafenone alone there were mild non-cardiac effects, including sickness in two, headache in one, gastrointestinal disturbances in two, and paresthesia in one. Four patients taking propafenone plus digitalis had either sickness or dizziness, and nine patients taking digitalis plus quinidine had gastrointestinal disturbances, sickness, dizziness, or headache. There were no major dysrhythmias; four of the patients who took digitalis plus propafenone had asymptomatic ventricular extra beats, as did one patient who took digitalis plus quinidine. In nine patients who took digitalis plus quinidine there were asymptomatic short-lasting episodes of atrial flutter with atrial ventricular conduction of at least 2:1 immediately before the restoration of sinus rhythm; this happened in 13 patients who took propafenone, 12 patients who took digitalis plus propafenone, and three patients who took placebo. There were two cases of complete left bundle branch block in patients who took digitalis plus quinidine, in three patients who took propafenone, and in two who took digitalis plus propafenone. In two patients who took digitalis plus quinidine and two who took propafenone there was reversible asymptomatic sinoatrial block of Wenckebach type II. Transient mild hypotension occurred in one patient taking digitalis plus quinidine, five taking propafenone, one taking digitalis plus propafenone, and one taking placebo, but the hypotension was transient and not severe. The authors concluded that the addition of digitalis to propafenone hastened cardioversion from atrial fibrillation, although they conceded that the balance of other evidence suggests that digitalis is not effective in restoring sinus rhythm and were unable to explain the efficacy of the combination of digitalis with propafenone.

Sotalol

In a randomized, double-blind, placebo-controlled comparison of propafenone (mean dose 13 mg/kg/day; $n = 102$) and sotalol (mean dose 3 mg/kg/day; $n = 106$) in maintaining sinus rhythm after conversion of recurrent symptomatic atrial fibrillation in 300 patients, efficacy was comparable (13). Tolerable adverse effects in those who took propafenone were gastrointestinal discomfort ($n = 15$), neurological disturbances ($n = 9$), a metallic taste ($n = 4$), and generalized weakness ($n = 1$); nine patients withdrew owing to adverse effects, four with gastrointestinal disorders, three with dizziness, and two with headache; there were no prodysrhythmias.

Propafenone 450 mg/day and sotalol 240 mg/day have been compared in a placebo-controlled study of 300 patients with atrial fibrillation (14). The two drugs had similar efficacy. There were adverse events in 38 of the patients who took propafenone, compared with 12 of those who took placebo. These included gastrointestinal discomfort, neurological disturbances, asymptomatic bradycardia, a metallic taste, and general weakness. In nine patients the adverse effects were sufficient to cause withdrawal of propafenone.

Placebo-controlled studies

In controlled trials in patients with recent-onset atrial fibrillation without heart failure, oral propafenone (450–600 mg as a single dose) had a relatively quick effect (within 3–4 hours) and a high rate of efficacy (72–78% within 8 hours) (15).

The adverse effects of propafenone in placebo-controlled trials in patients with atrial tachydysrhythmias have been reviewed (16). The following effects were reported after single intravenous oral doses to produce conversion of atrial fibrillation to sinus rhythm. Non-cardiac adverse effects included mild dizziness. Mild hypotension was also noted, but only required withdrawal of propafenone in one of 29 patients in one study. There have been prodysrhythmic effects in several studies, including atrial flutter with a broad QRS complex, which can occur in up to 5% of cases; in some cases atrial flutter can have a rapid ventricular response due to 1:1 atrioventricular conduction, which has been attributed to slowing of atrial conduction and reduced refractoriness of the atrioventricular node. Other prodysrhythmic effects in a few patients included sinus bradycardia with sinus pauses and effects on atrioventricular conduction.

In patients taking long-term propafenone for supraventricular dysrhythmias adverse effects were more common and have been reported in 14–60% of cases. Cardiac adverse effects were more common in patients with structural heart disease. The non-cardiac effects were either gastrointestinal (nausea, vomiting, taste disturbances) or neurological (dizziness). Adverse effects are dose-related. In one large study there was no difference between propafenone and placebo in the risk of death.

The use of propafenone in atrial fibrillation (SEDA-23, 202) has been studied in a randomized, double-blind, placebo-controlled trial in 55 patients (17). The dose of propafenone was chosen according to body weight: 450, 600, and 750 mg for those weighing 50–64, 65–80, and over 80 kg respectively. Propafenone converted atrial fibrillation to sinus rhythm significantly more quickly than placebo, and most patients given propafenone had converted by 6 hours. However, by 24 hours there was no significant difference between the two groups. Four patients had hypotension after propafenone, in three cases transiently. The patient with sustained hypotension had poor left ventricular systolic function, but it responded promptly to the administration of fluids and electrical cardioversion. In one patient with transient hypotension there was a brief episode of sinus bradycardia and in another an isolated sinus pause.

Organs and Systems

Cardiovascular

Cardiovascular adverse effects have been reported in 13–27% of patients taking propafenone and ventricular dysrhythmias in 8–19% in small studies. However, in large studies the risk has been reported to be about 5%.

Conduction disturbances are common with propafenone and can result in sinus bradycardia, sinoatrial block, sinus arrest, any degree of atrioventricular block, and right or left bundle-branch block (SEDA-10, 151) (SEDA-15, 179).

The adverse effects of a single oral dose of propafenone for cardioversion of recent-onset atrial fibrillation have been evaluated in a systematic review (18). The adverse effects were transient dysrhythmias (atrial flutter, bradycardia, pauses, and junctional rhythm), reversible widening of the QRS complex, transient hypotension, and mild non-cardiac effects (nausea, headache, gastrointestinal disturbances, dizziness, and paresthesia).

Dysrhythmias can occur; these include ventricular tachycardia, ventricular flutter, and atrial fibrillation (19–21). Hypotension and worsening of heart failure have occasionally been reported (SEDA-10, 151) (22).

- Wide-complex tachycardias occurred in two elderly patients (a 74-year-old man and an 80-year-old woman) who had taken propafenone for atrial fibrillation (23). In the first case the dysrhythmia was due to atrial flutter with 1:1 conduction.

Although drugs of class Ic, such as propafenone, can slow atrial and atrioventricular nodal conduction in patients with atrial fibrillation or atrial flutter, they do not alter the refractoriness of the atrioventricular node, and this allows 1:1 atrioventricular conduction as the atrial rate slows. This happens despite prolongation of the PR interval.

Class Ic drugs can also convert atrial fibrillation to atrial flutter, reportedly in 3.5–5% of patients. Of 187 patients with paroxysmal atrial fibrillation who were treated with flecainide or propafenone, 24 developed atrial flutter, which was typical in 20 cases (24). These patients underwent radiofrequency ablation, which failed in only one case. All the patients continued to take their pre-existing drugs, and during a mean follow-up period of 11 months, the incidence of atrial fibrillation was higher in patients who were taking combined therapy than in those taking monotherapy. The authors suggested that in patients with atrial fibrillation who developed typical atrial flutter due to class Ic antidysrhythmic drugs, combined catheter ablation and continued drug treatment is highly effective in reducing the occurrence and duration of atrial tachydysrhythmias. They did not report adverse effects.

In controlled trials of oral propafenone (450–600 mg as a single dose) in patients with recent-onset atrial fibrillation without heart failure, atrial flutter with 1:1 atrioventricular conduction occurred in only two of 709 patients (0.3%) who received propafenone (15).

Respiratory

Since propafenone is a beta-adrenoceptor antagonist it can cause shortness of breath or worsening of asthma (25).

Nervous system

Adverse effects on the nervous system are common with propafenone and include somnolence, weakness and disorientation, global amnesia (26), dizziness and vertigo, tremor, visual disturbances, and convulsions (SEDA-10, 151).

- Peripheral neuropathy has been reported in a 41-year-old man who took propafenone 450 mg/day for about a year (27).

Ataxia has been reported in patients taking propafenone (28).

- An 80-year-old man taking propafenone 150 mg tds for paroxysmal atrial fibrillation developed progressive generalized ataxia and weakness 4 days after starting treatment. He had a bilateral symmetrical ataxia, unclear speech, impairment of gait, altered hand coordination, and tremor. The ataxia resolved completely within 3 days of withdrawal.

- A 73-year-old woman taking propafenone 150 mg tds for paroxysmal atrial tachycardia underwent cardioversion during an attack, and the dose of propafenone was increased to 300 mg tds. After 5 days she developed severe ataxia and progressive weakness. The ataxia was symmetrical and there was severe impairment of gait, altered hand coordination, and tremor. The dose of propafenone was reduced to 600 mg/day and the ataxia resolved completely within 6 days. A year later, when the dose of propafenone was increased to 900 mg/day, progressive ataxia again developed after 2 days and became severe within 1 week. Propafenone was withdrawn and the ataxia resolved within a few days.

- An 85-year-old woman took propafenone 150 mg tds for paroxysmal atrial fibrillation and 2 months later developed a progressive ataxia and recurrent falls. The ataxia was symmetrical and there was altered hand coordination, impairment of gait, and tremor. The propafenone was withdrawn and the ataxia resolved completely within 4 days.

Endocrine

Propafenone can cause hyponatremia due to inappropriate secretion of ADH (29).

Hematologic

Propafenone can occasionally cause neutropenia, with a calculated incidence of about one in 10 000 prescriptions per year (30).

Gastrointestinal

Unwanted gastrointestinal effects are the most common adverse effects of propafenone, occurring in up to 30% of cases. They include anorexia, nausea and vomiting, dry mouth, a metallic or bitter taste in the mouth, abdominal discomfort, and constipation (SEDA-10, 151).

Liver

Propafenone can increase the serum activities of transaminases and other enzymes associated with liver function (31). There have also been reports of cholestatic jaundice (32).

Skin

Skin rashes have been reported occasionally (29); these include an acneiform rash and urticaria.

Sexual function

Impotence has occasionally been reported, in one case with a reduced sperm count (33,34).

Immunologic

Propafenone can cause a rise in antinuclear antibody titers (34) and has once been reported to have caused a lupus-like syndrome (35).

Body temperature

Drug fever without agranulocytosis has been attributed to propafenone (36).

Second-Generation Effects

Pregnancy

When a pregnant woman was given propafenone from the fifth month to term in a dosage of 300 mg tds her dysrhythmias responded satisfactorily and the neonate was healthy (37).

Susceptibility Factors

Genetic factors

Poor and extensive oxidation phenotypes for CYP2D6, which metabolizes propafenone, have been studied in 42 patients, aged 36–75 years, with paroxysmal atrial fibrillation (38). Efficacy was 100% in poor metabolizers, 61% in extensive metabolizers, and 0% in very extensive metabolizers. There was a significant correlation between oxidation phenotype and the ability to maintain sinus rhythm.

Age

The incidence of adverse effects of propafenone in children has varied from study to study, but has sometimes been as high as 25%, requiring withdrawal in 6% of cases (39). Elderly people are at increased risk of adverse effects.

The safety of oral propafenone in the treatment of dysrhythmias has been studied retrospectively in infants and children (40). There were significant electrophysiological adverse effects and prodysrhythmia in 15 of 772 patients (1.9%). These included sinus node dysfunction in four, complete atrioventricular block in two, aggravation of supraventricular tachycardia in two, acceleration of ventricular rate during atrial flutter in one, ventricular prodysrhythmia in five, and unexplained syncope in one. Cardiac arrest or sudden death occurred in five patients (0.6%); two had a supraventricular tachycardia due to Wolff–Parkinson–White syndrome; the other three had structural heart disease. Adverse cardiac events were more common in the presence of structural heart disease and there was no difference between patients with supraventricular and ventricular dysrhythmias.

Drug Administration

Drug dosage regimens

Three different regimens of oral propafenone have been compared in patients with paroxysmal atrial fibrillation (41). In 48 patients who took 600 mg followed 8 hours later by 150 mg there was a higher rate of early successful cardioversion with a lower incidence of adverse effects than in two other groups who took either 300 mg three times over 8 hours ($n = 82$) or four doses of 150 mg over 9 hours ($n = 58$). The rates of conversion were around 80%, similar to those found in other studies. There was QRS prolongation in all three groups, and four of those who took a total of 900 mg developed a broad complex tachycardia.

Drug overdose

About 60 cases of propafenone poisoning have been reported. Even low doses can lead to serious poisoning. Some symptoms, such as gastrointestinal or neurological symptoms, are misleading. Cardiovascular abnormalities include bradycardia, atrioventricular block, abnormal intraventricular conduction, shock, and electromechanical dissociation. The simultaneous presence of neurological symptoms (especially seizures) and abnormal cardiac conduction suggests serious poisoning.

The mortality from propafenone overdose is 23%, according to a retrospective series of 120 patients in Germany over 14 years (42). Severity was related to cardiac conduction disorders and cardiac hyperexcitability.

Seizures have been reported in cases of overdose.

- A 24-year-old woman who took an overdose of propafenone 2.7 g had a convulsion and complete heart block (43). The plasma propafenone concentration 4 hours after ingestion was 2930 ng/ml (target range 400–1600 ng/ml). She was given activated charcoal 50 g, mannitol 200 ml, and clonazepam 1 mg intravenously. By 19 hours after ingestion the electrocardiogram was normal and the plasma propafenone concentration was 858 ng/ml.
- A 22-year-old woman took an overdose of propafenone (amount unknown) and developed tetany and then generalized convulsions requiring intravenous clonazepam (44). She had a low blood pressure and first-degree atrioventricular block associated with prolonged intraventricular conduction. She was intubated and given intravenous fluids, equimolar sodium lactate, dopamine, and adrenaline. Her cardiac conduction returned to normal.

Treatment is symptomatic. Sodium lactate may be required for abnormal intraventricular conduction. Plasma exchange has been successfully used to treat propafenone overdose (45).

- An 18-year-old woman took 35 tablets of propafenone, 300 mg each. She had dilated, non-reactive pupils and greatly increased activity of neuron-specific enolase. She had atrioventricular and intraventricular conduction disorders, and repeated resuscitation was necessary. Propafenone was eliminated by plasma exchange, and the conduction disturbances disappeared rapidly during treatment.

Drug–Drug Interactions

Metoprolol

Propafenone reduces the apparent oral clearance of metoprolol, but it is not clear whether the mechanism is by reduction of true clearance or an increase in systemic availability (46). In addition the beta-blocking action of metoprolol is increased by propafenone; this could be due either to reduced clearance of metoprolol or to a true pharmacodynamic interaction between the two drugs, since propafenone has beta-blocking activity.

Monitoring Therapy

Therapeutic benefit is most likely when the plasma propafenone concentration is in the range 0.5–2.0 mg/ml, although the correlation is poor (47), and there is a large overlap between therapeutic and toxic concentrations (32). The therapeutic effect of propafenone correlates better with prolongation of the PR and QRS intervals (48).

References

1. Birgersdotter-Green U. Propafenone for cardiac arrhythmias. Am J Med Sci 1992;303(2):123–8.
2. Bryson HM, Palmer KJ, Langtry HD, Fitton A. Propafenone. A reappraisal of its pharmacology, pharmacokinetics and therapeutic use in cardiac arrhythmias. Drugs 1993;45(1):85–130.
3. Cobbe SM. Drug therapy of supraventricular tachyarrhythmias—based on efficacy or futility? Eur Heart J 1994;15(Suppl A):22–6.
4. Paul T, Janousek J. New antiarrhythmic drugs in pediatric use: propafenone. Pediatr Cardiol 1994;15(4):190–7.
5. Valderrabano M, Singh BN. Electrophysiologic and Antiarrhythmic Effects of Propafenone: Focus on Atrial Fibrillation. J Cardiovasc Pharmacol Ther 1999;4(3):183–98.
6. Ravid S, Podrid PJ, Novrit B. Safety of long-term propafenone therapy for cardiac arrhythmia—experience with 774 patients. J Electrophysiol 1987;1:580–90.
7. Bianconi L, Mennuni M. Comparison between propafenone and digoxin administered intravenously to patients with acute atrial fibrillation. PAFIT-3 Investigators. The Propafenone in Atrial Fibrillation Italian Trial. Am J Cardiol 1998;82(5):584–8.
8. Lau CP, Chow MS, Tse HF, Tang MO, Fan C. Control of paroxysmal atrial fibrillation recurrence using combined administration of propafenone and quinidine. Am J Cardiol 2000;86(12):1327–32.
9. Blanc JJ, Voinov C, Maarek M. Comparison of oral loading dose of propafenone and amiodarone for converting recent-onset atrial fibrillation. PARSIFAL Study Group. Am J Cardiol 1999;84(9):1029–32.
10. Tai CT, Chiang CE, Lee SH, Chen YJ, Yu WC, Feng AN, Ding YA, Chang MS, Chen SA. Persistent atrial flutter in patients treated for atrial fibrillation with amiodarone and propafenone: electrophysiologic characteristics, radiofrequency catheter ablation, and risk prediction. J Cardiovasc Electrophysiol 1999;10(9):1180–7.
11. Geelen P, O'Hara GE, Roy N, Talajic M, Roy D, Plante S, Turgeon J. Comparison of propafenone versus procainamide for the acute treatment of atrial fibrillation after cardiac surgery. Am J Cardiol 1999;84(3):345–7.
12. Capucci A, Villani GQ, Aschieri D, Piepoli M. Safety of oral propafenone in the conversion of recent onset atrial fibrillation to sinus rhythm: a prospective parallel placebo-controlled multicentre study. Int J Cardiol 1999; 68(2):187–96.
13. Bellandi F, Simonetti I, Leoncini M, Frascarelli F, Giovannini T, Maioli M, Dabizzi RP. Long-term efficacy and safety of propafenone and sotalol for the maintenance of sinus rhythm after conversion of recurrent symptomatic atrial fibrillation. Am J Cardiol 2001; 88(6):640–5.
14. Bellandi F, Leoncini M, Maioli M, Gallopin M, Dabizzi RP. Comparing agents for prevention of atrial fibrillation recurrence. Cardiol Rev 2002;19:18–21.
15. Chopra IJ, Baber K. Use of oral cholecystographic agents in the treatment of amiodarone-induced hyperthyroidism. J Clin Endocrinol Metab 2001;86(10):4707–10.
16. Rae AP, Camm J, Winters S, Page R. Placebo-controlled evaluations of propafenone for atrial tachyarrhythmias. Am J Cardiol 1998;82(8A):N59–65.
17. Azpitarte J, Alvarez M, Baun O, Garcia R, Moreno E, Navarrete A, Fernandez R. Using propafenone to convert recent-onset atrial fibrillation. Cardiol Rev 2000;17:37–43.
18. Khan IA. Single oral loading dose of propafenone for pharmacological cardioversion of recent-onset atrial fibrillation. J Am Coll Cardiol 2001;37(2):542–7.
19. Antman EM, Beamer AD, Cantillon C, McGowan N, Friedman PL. Therapy of refractory symptomatic atrial fibrillation and atrial flutter: a staged care approach with new antiarrhythmic drugs. J Am Coll Cardiol 1990; 15(3):698–707.
20. Escande M, Diadema B, Maarek-Charbit M. Étude a long terme de la propafénone dans l'extrasystolie ventriculaire grave du sujet agé. [Long-term study of propafenone in severe ventricular extrasystole in elderly subjects.] Ann Cardiol Angeiol (Paris) 1989;38(9): 555–60.
21. Colas A, Maarek-Charbit M. Propafenone per os dans les troubles du rythme ventriculaire. [Propafenone per os in ventricular arrhythmia.] Cah Anesthesiol 1989; 37(4):241–4.
22. Cobbe SM, Rae AP, Poloniecki JD. A randomized, placebo-controlled trial of propafenone in the prophylaxis of paroxysmal supraventricular tachycardia and paroxysmal atrial fibrillation. UK Propafenone PSVT Study Group. Circulation 1995;92(9):2550–7.
23. Mackstaller LL, Marcus FI. Rapid ventricular response due to treatment of atrial flutter or fibrillation with Class I antiarrhythmic drugs. Ann Noninvasive Electrocardiol 2000;5:101–4.
24. Schumacher B, Jung W, Lewalter T, Vahlhaus C, Wolpert C, Luderitz B. Radiofrequency ablation of atrial flutter due to administration of class IC antiarrhythmic drugs for atrial fibrillation. Am J Cardiol 1999;83(5):710–13.
25. Veale D, McComb JM, Gibson GJ. Propafenone. Lancet 1990;335(8695):979.
26. Jones RJ, Brace SR, Vander Tuin EL. Probable propafenone-induced transient global amnesia. Ann Pharmacother 1995;29(6):586–90.
27. Galasso PJ, Stanton MS, Vogel H. Propafenone-induced peripheral neuropathy. Mayo Clin Proc 1995;70(5):469–72.
28. Odeh M, Seligmann H, Oliven A. Propafenone-induced ataxia: report of three cases. Am J Med Sci 2000; 320(2):151–3.
29. Hammill SC, Sorenson PB, Wood DL, Sugrue DD, Osborn MJ, Gersh BJ, Holmes DR Jr. Propafenone for the treatment of refractory complex ventricular ectopic activity. Mayo Clin Proc 1986;61(2):98–103.
30. Miwa LJ, Jolson HM. Propafenone associated agranulocytosis. Pacing Clin Electrophysiol 1992;15(4 Pt 1): 387–90.
31. Connolly SJ, Kates RE, Lebsack CS, Harrison DC, Winkle RA. Clinical pharmacology of propafenone. Circulation 1983;68(3):589–96.

32. Mondardini A, Pasquino P, Bernardi P, Aluffi E, Tartaglino B, Mazzucco G, Bonino F, Verme G, Negro F. Propafenone-induced liver injury: report of a case and review of the literature. Gastroenterology 1993;104(5): 1524–6.

33. Korst HA, Brandes JW, Littmann KP. Potenz- und Spermiogenesestorungen durch Propafenon. [Disturbances of potency and spermiogenesis due to propafenon.] Dtsch Med Wochenschr 1980;105(34):1187–9.

34. Gaita F, Richiardi E, Bocchiardo M, Asteggiano R, Pinnavaia A, Di Leo M, Rosettani E, Brusca A. Short- and long-term effects of propafenone in ventricular arrhythmias. Int J Cardiol 1986;13(2):163–70.

35. Guindo J, Rodriguez de la Serna A, Borja J, Oter R, Jane F, Bayes de Luna A. Propafenone and a syndrome of the lupus erythematosus type. Ann Intern Med 1986; 104(4):589.

36. O'Rourke DJ, Palac RT, Holzberger PT, Gerling BR, Greenberg ML. Propafenone-induced drug fever in the absence of agranulocytosis. Clin Cardiol 1997;20(7): 662–4.

37. Brunozzi LT, Meniconi L, Chiocchi P, Liberati R, Zuanetti G, Latini R. Propafenone in the treatment of chronic ventricular arrhythmias in a pregnant patient. Br J Clin Pharmacol 1988;26(4):489–90.

38. Jazwinska-Tarnawska E, Orzechowska-Juzwenko K, Niewinski P, Rzemislawska Z, Loboz-Grudzien K, Dmochowska-Perz M, Slawin J. The influence of CYP2D6 polymorphism on the antiarrhythmic efficacy of propafenone in patients with paroxysmal atrial fibrillation during 3 months propafenone prophylactic treatment. Int J Clin Pharmacol Ther 2001;39(7):288–92.

39. Vignati G, Mauri L, Figini A. The use of propafenone in the treatment of tachyarrhythmias in children. Eur Heart J 1993;14(4):546–50.

40. Janousek J, Paul T. Safety of oral propafenone in the treatment of arrhythmias in infants and children (European Retrospective Multicenter Study). Working Group on Pediatric Arrhythmias and Electrophysiology of the Association of European Pediatric Cardiologists. Am J Cardiol 1998;81(9):1121–4.

41. Antonelli D, Darawsha A, Rimbrot S, Freedberg NA, Rosenfeld T. [Propafenone dose for emergency room conversion of paroxysmal atrial fibrillation.] Harefuah 1999;136(11):857–9, 915.

42. Koppel C, Oberdisse U, Heinemeyer G. Clinical course and outcome in class IC antiarrhythmic overdose. J Toxicol Clin Toxicol 1990;28(4):433–44.

43. Rambourg-Schepens MO, Grossenbacher F, Buffet M, Lamiable D. Recurrent convulsions and cardiac conduction disturbances after propafenone overdose. Vet Hum Toxicol 1999;41(3):153–4.

44. Genty A, De Brabant F, Pibarot N, Busseuil C, Dubien PY, Ducluze R. Seizure disclosing acute propafenone poisoning. Jeur 2001;14:248–54.

45. Schwenger V. Plasma separation in severe propafenone intoxication. Intensivmed Notf Med 2001;38:124–7.

46. Wagner F, Kalusche D, Trenk D, Jahnchen E, Roskamm H. Drug interaction between propafenone and metoprolol. Br J Clin Pharmacol 1987;24(2):213–20.

47. Dinh H, Murphy ML, Baker BJ, De Soyza N. Propafenone:a new antiarrhythmic for treatment of chronic ventricular arrhythmias. Clin Progr Electrophysiol Pacing 1986;4:535–45.

48. De Soyza N, Murphy M, Sakhaii M, Treat L. The safety and efficacy of propafenone in suppressing ventricular ectopy. In: Shlepper M, Olsen B, editors. Cardiac Arrhythmias. Berlin: Springer Verlag, 1983:221.

Propanidid

See also General anesthetics

General Information

Propanidid was used as an intravenous anesthetic for rapid induction and for maintenance of general anesthesia of short duration. However, it was withdrawn because of safety considerations regarding the solvent used, polyethoxylated castor oil (Cremophor EL) (SED-11, 211) (1).

Reference

1. Dye D, Watkins J. Suspected anaphylactic reaction to Cremophor EL. BMJ 1980;280(6228):1353.

Propantheline

See also Anticholinergic drugs

General Information

Propantheline is an anticholinergic drug. Oral doses are 7.5–30 mg, the latter being used at bedtime; injections of 15 mg have been used in radiology. The persisting doubt as to the incidence of adverse reactions probably reflects the poor and variable systemic availability of the oral form, which also seems to account for conflicting reports about its efficacy. All typical anticholinergic effects can occur if effective doses are given, but central nervous and ocular effects are relatively slight. Propantheline, like others of this type, is not contraindicated in glaucoma or prostatic hyperplasia, but it can influence the response of these conditions to other treatment and hence should be used with some caution.

Drug–Drug Interactions

Digoxin

The interactions of propantheline are similar to those of atropine; for example it increases the rate of absorption of digoxin (1).

Nitrofurantoin

Propantheline increases the rate of absorption of nitrofurantoin (2).

Paracetamol

Propantheline reduces the rate of absorption of paracetamol (3).

References

1. Manninen V, Apajalahti A, Simonen H, Reissell P. Effect of propantheline and metoclopramide on absorption of digoxin. Lancet 1973;1(7812):1118–19.
2. Jaffe JM. Effect of propantheline on nitrofurantoin absorption. J Pharm Sci 1975;64(10):1729–30.
3. Nimmo J, Heading RC, Tothill P, Prescott LF. Pharmacological modification of gastric emptying: effects of propantheline and metoclopromide on paracetamol absorption. BMJ 1973;1(5853):587–9.

Propiram

General Information

Propiram is an orally active opioid analgesic with weak antagonist activity and effects typical of its class (SED-11, 150) (1,2).

References

1. Desjardins PJ, Cooper SA, Gallegos TL, Allwein JB, Reynolds DC, Kruger GO, Beaver WT. The relative analgesic efficacy of propiram fumarate, codeine, aspirin, and placebo in post-impaction dental pain. J Clin Pharmacol 1984;24(1):35–42.
2. Goa KL, Brogden RN. Propiram. A review of its pharmacodynamic and pharmacokinetic properties, and clinical use as an analgesic. Drugs 1993;46(3):428–45.

Propiverine

See also Adrenoceptor agonists

General Information

Propiverine is an anticholinergic drug, used mainly for its effects on the bladder. It is effective in detrusor hyperreflexia and in patients with symptoms of an overactive bladder. Adverse effects occur in about 13% of patients (1).

Organs and Systems

Nervous system

A report of parkinsonism due to propiverine combines a clinical observation with basic pharmacology (2).

- A 72-year-old man had taken propiverine 20 mg/day for nocturia. The exact symptoms are difficult to define, because of the rather curious terminology used in the report, but it appears that he rapidly developed parkinsonian symptoms soon after the start of treatment and was given levodopa 3 months later, with a limited response. After 1 month it was decided to withdraw propiverine and his symptoms disappeared within 2 weeks.

The authors then studied the effect of propiverine on the induction of catalepsy in mice, comparing it with oxybutynin, pentoxyverine, and etafenone, using haloperidol as a reference. They also examined dopamine receptor binding in the striatum. They concluded that any of these agents could cause catalepsy in mice, and that propiverine had greater potency than oxybutynin but less than the others. It was also noted that all the drugs had sub-micromolar affinity for striatal dopamine D_2 receptors. The authors suggested that any drug, such as these, that has a diethylaminomethyl moiety has the potential for extrapyramidal effects, because of interaction with dopamine receptors in the basal ganglia.

Sensory systems

The effect of propiverine on the eye has been investigated in normal and glaucomatous eyes. There was considerable reduction in accommodation in younger individuals in both groups. The drug should therefore be given to younger patients only on very strict indications (3).

References

1. Madersbacher H, Murtz G. Efficacy, tolerability and safety profile of propiverine in the treatment of the overactive bladder (non-neurogenic and neurogenic). World J Urol 2001;19(5):324–35.
2. Matsuo H, Matsui A, Nasu R, Takanaga H, Inoue N, Hattori F, Ohtani H, Sawada Y. Propiverine-induced Parkinsonism: a case report and a pharmacokinetic/pharmacodynamic study in mice. Pharm Res 2000;17(5):565–71.
3. Priz U. Die Nebenwirkungen des Urologikums Mictonorm auf das Auge. Fol Ophthalmol 1985;10:105.

Propofol

See also General anesthetics

General Information

Propofol is a short-acting intravenous induction agent, which is dissolved in a mixture of long-chain triglycerides and soya bean emulsion. It is now in general use in daycare anesthesia and is being increasingly used in infusions in intensive care units. Recovery from anesthetic doses compares favorably with that after enflurane and isoflurane (1).

It has been claimed that propofol produces good recovery after anesthesia. A review of the literature has shown that, for operations that last under 30 minutes, propofol seems to give the best recovery, but for longer operations isoflurane gave better quality recovery (2).

Comparative studies

Propofol versus midazolam

A combination of midazolam plus propofol has been compared with midazolam only for sedation in colonoscopy (3). Midazolam alone produced less profound amnesia, and patients took longer to recover. There were no differences in cardiovascular or respiratory parameters. Oxygen saturation was poor in both groups, with saturations less than 85% in 22% of patients given midazolam and in 19% of patients given propofol, although the patients did not initially receive supplementary oxygen. In a similar comparison of midazolam and propofol as sedative agents for diagnostic endoscopy in 80 patients, endoscopy was judged successful in 98% of patients given propofol (mean total dose 354 mg) and 80% of patients given midazolam (mean total dose 8 mg) (4). Patients in the propofol group recovered consciousness more quickly and had complete amnesia. One patient in the propofol group suffered an apneic phase with impaired circulation, requiring manual ventilation and drug therapy.

In a Canadian multicenter, open, randomized trial in 156 patients to determine whether sedation with propofol would lead to shorter times to tracheal extubation and length of stay in ICU than sedation with midazolam, the patients who received propofol spent longer at the target sedation level than those who received midazolam (60 versus 44% respectively) (5). Propofol allowed clinically significantly earlier tracheal extubation than midazolam (6.7 versus 25 hours). However, this did not result in earlier discharge from the ICU.

Anesthetist-administered midazolam and patient-controlled propofol have been compared for sedation during vitreoretinal surgery (6). The patients received propofol 15–18 mg according to age, with a 1-minute lockout, or 0.25–0.5 mg of midazolam as judged necessary by the anesthetist. Few patients were amnesic for the procedure and both techniques produced satisfactory sedation and comfort. Non-anesthetists need to be extremely wary if using propofol for sedation, since propofol has a low therapeutic index and commonly causes unconsciousness, respiratory depression, and cardiovascular collapse, particularly when it is used in combination with either midazolam or alfentanil (7). Adequate staff, training, and facilities for resuscitation of patients must be available before considering propofol sedation. Propofol can cause deep sedation, and the episode reported in one of these studies is not surprising. Extreme caution must be exercised in recommending these techniques to non-anesthetists.

Organs and Systems

Cardiovascular

Propofol is a cardiodepressant and resets the baroreflex set-point, with a tendency to bradycardia (which occurs in some 5% of cases), hypotension (16%), or both (1.3%) (8). The hypotension may be brought about by peripheral vasodilatation, reduced myocardial contractility, and inhibition of sympathetic nervous system outflow (9). Four deaths due to cardiovascular collapse during induction have been reported in patients aged 78–92 years given propofol 1.1–1.8 mg/kg (10). The patients were of ASA classes 3 or 4.

Total intravenous anesthesia with propofol resulted in a reduced heart rate and a higher frequency of oculocardiac reflex bradycardia than thiopental/isoflurane anesthesia, with a higher sensitivity of children younger than 6 years in all groups (11).

Hemodynamic effects

The cardiovascular effects of propofol have been examined in a randomized trial in 40 healthy subjects using transthoracic echocardiography (12). Propofol was given to the same total dose (2.5 mg/kg) at two different rates, 2 mg/second or 10 mg/second. In both groups, global and segmental ventricular function was unchanged, but propofol caused a markedly reduced end-systolic quotient, presumably related to reduced afterload. With the higher infusion rate, there was a significant reduction in fractional shortening, thought to be related principally to reduced preload.

There has been a prospective, double-blind, controlled comparison of propofol, midazolam, and propofol + midazolam for postoperative sedation in 75 patients who received low-dose opioid-based anesthesia for coronary bypass grafting (13). Mean induction doses of propofol and midazolam used alone were 2.5 times higher than when both were used together. The single agents caused significant reductions in blood pressure, left atrial filling pressure, and heart rate after induction. These hemodynamic changes returned to normal after 15 minutes with midazolam and after 30 minutes with propofol, except for the bradycardia, which remained for the duration of the sedation. The combination of propofol + midazolam had no significant hemodynamic effects, but was also associated with bradycardia lasting the duration of the sedation. There was a greater than 68% reduction in maintenance doses with the combination. Propofol and propofol + midazolam were associated with comparable times to awakening and extubation, while with midazolam alone recovery was slower. This study clearly showed a reduction in adverse effects from exploiting the sedative synergism between propofol and midazolam.

In a placebo-controlled study of induction of anesthesia with a combination of propofol + fentanyl in 90 patients aged over 60 years, prophylactic intravenous ephedrine 0.1 or 0.2 mg/kg given 1 minute before induction of anesthesia significantly attenuated the fall in blood pressure and heart rate that is usually observed (14). Prophylactic use of ephedrine may be useful in preventing the occasional instances of cardiovascular collapse recorded after induction of anesthesia using these agents in elderly people.

The hemodynamic effects of combining ephedrine with propofol in an effort to prevent hypotension and bradycardia have been investigated in 40 elderly patients of ASA grades III and IV, who received ephedrine 15, 20, or 25 mg added to propofol 200 mg (15). The hypotensive response to propofol was effectively prevented, but marked tachycardia in the majority of patients meant that the technique may not be beneficial, given the high incidence of ischemic heart disease in this age group.

The effects of giving calcium chloride 10 mg/kg after induction of anesthesia with propofol, fentanyl, and pancuronium have been investigated in 58 patients undergoing elective coronary artery bypass grafting (16). Calcium chloride reduced the fall in arterial blood pressure and prevented the reductions in heart rate, stroke volume index, cardiac index, and cardiac output, compared with placebo. Propofol reduces the availability of calcium to the myocardial cells, and calcium chloride effectively minimizes the hemodynamic effects of propofol. However, given that intravenous calcium can be locally toxic when given via peripheral veins, the technique may have limited applicability.

Cardiac dysrhythmias
Propofol causes bradydysrhythmias by reducing sympathetic nervous system activity.

- A four-year-old patient developed a nodal bradycardia while receiving propofol 6 mg/kg/hour + remifentanil 0.25 microgram/kg/minute (17). The bradycardia responded to atropine 0.3 mg.
- Complete atrioventricular heart block occurred in a 9-year-old boy with Ondine's curse who received a single bolus injection of propofol (18).

The authors questioned the safe use of propofol in congenital central hypoventilation syndrome, which is a generalized disorder of autonomic function.

- Propofol caused marked prolongation of the QT_c interval in a 71-year-old woman with an acute myocardial infarction who required ventilatory support (19). Substituting midazolam for propofol was associated with normalization of the QT_c interval. Rechallenge with propofol was associated with further prolongation. There were no malignant ventricular dysrhythmias.

Pain on injection
Propofol can cause severe pain on injection, especially when injected into a small vein (20); the incidence is 25–74% (21). Administration of the lipid solvent in which propofol dissolved has confirmed that the solvent is responsible for this adverse effect (22).

- Severe pain on injection of propofol occurred in a 36-year-old man with severe Raynaud's phenomenon, including a history of skin ulceration when he was given a 2% propofol + lidocaine mixture into a vein on the back of his hand (23).

The author suggested that selecting a larger antecubital vein might be a wiser choice in these patients.

The effectiveness of lidocaine in preventing pain on injection has been confirmed, and a concentration of 0.1% was optimal (24). The kallikrein inhibitor nafamostat mesilate was as effective as lidocaine.

A controlled study in 100 women showed that pretreatment with intravenous ketamine 10 mg reduced the incidence of injection pain from 84 to 26% of patients (25).

Warming propofol to 37°C had no effect on the incidence of pain (26,27).

The effects of different doses of ketorolac, with or without venous occlusion, on the incidence and severity of pain after propofol injection have been studied in a randomized, double-blind study in 180 patients (28). Pretreatment with intravenous ketorolac 15 mg and 30 mg reduced the pain after propofol injection. A lower dose of ketorolac 10 mg with venous occlusion for 120 seconds achieved the same effect.

Ondansetron, tramadol, and metoclopramide were less effective than lidocaine in preventing pain on injection (29–31). Ondansetron and tramadol have been compared in patients being given propofol in a randomized, double-blind study in 100 patients (32). Tramadol 50 mg

intravenously was as effective as ondansetron 4 mg intravenously with 15 seconds of venous occlusion at preventing propofol injection pain. However, there was significantly less nausea and vomiting in those given ondansetron.

Respiratory

Respiratory depression due to propofol is well recognized; apnea can result, especially with rapid injection (33).

Pulmonary fat embolism after the use of propofol has been attributed to the milky emulsion in which the propofol was dissolved (34).

Two cases of propofol-induced bronchoconstriction have been reported (35). Both patients had allergic rhinitis and had taken antihistamines during the hay fever season, but were otherwise healthy.

Nervous system

Dystonias
Dystonic movements induced by propofol occurred in a patient undergoing elective cardioversion (36). Benzatropine 2 mg intravenously terminated the abnormal movements. The authors also reviewed all other reports of abnormal movements after propofol.

- Acute dystonia has been reported in a 14-year-old girl after the administration of propofol 150 mg + fentanyl 50 mg for dental anesthesia (37). The intraoperative course was uneventful, but she developed non-rhythmic and non-symmetrical shaking in her upper limbs, unresponsive to diazepam and paraldehyde. A CT scan of the brain was normal. Her symptoms were eventually relieved by procyclidine 2.5 mg.

This adverse effect has been reported many times with propofol in adults, but rarely in children.

Seizures
Myoclonus and opisthotonos, especially in children (38), and choreoathetosis (39) have been attributed to propofol. However, in experimental studies propofol has been shown to be effective against drug-induced seizures (40,41). It has been suggested that propofol inhibits efferent inhibitory neurons in the midbrain and reticular activating system, producing movements that originate subcortically and in the spinal cord (42).

- An otherwise healthy 63-year-old man was anesthetized with propofol 2 mg/kg + fentanyl 1 micrograms/kg followed by an infusion of propofol 6 mg/kg/hour (43). Three minutes after induction he developed myoclonus in his legs. This continued for 10 minutes and the anesthetic was abandoned. When he awoke 10 minutes later, the myoclonus stopped. A repeat anesthetic with propofol soon after caused the same response. When the procedure was performed 12 days later under regional block with propofol infusion for sedation, the myoclonus recurred, and lasted for 2 hours. The patient was alert after each anesthetic and did not appear to be post-ictal. An MRI scan of the spinal cord was normal.

Myoclonus after propofol does not appear to be associated with an adverse outcome.

Convulsions have been reported in two patients with no history of epilepsy after induction of anesthesia with propofol (44). However, in a crossover comparison in 20 epileptic patients undergoing cortical resection, in which the effects on the electrocorticogram of either propofol or thiopental during isoflurane + nitrous oxide anesthesia were studied, propofol caused no greater proconvulsive effect than thiopental, which is used to treat status epilepticus (45). In spite of occasional reports, a true epileptogenic effect of propofol remains to be proven.

A generalized tonic–clonic seizure has been attributed to propofol in a patient with tonic–clonic seizures after surgery for subarachnoid hemorrhage (46).

Psychological, psychiatric

The association of propofol with a range of excitatory events is well recognized. Behavioral disturbances with repeated propofol sedation have been reported in a 30-month-old child (47). Propofol was well tolerated initially, but the child then became increasing irritable, aggressive, and uncooperative during awakening from subsequent sedations, including screaming, kicking, hitting, and biting. The next two sedations were performed using methohexital and were not followed by any behavioral disturbances.

Prolonged delirium after emergence from propofol anesthesia has also been reported (48).

A psychotic reaction has been reported (49).

- A 37-year-old man who had abused metamfetamine, paint thinner, psychotomimetic drugs, and alcohol for 20 years was given chlorpromazine, haloperidol, and flunitrazepam just before surgery. After spinal anesthesia he was given propofol 5 mg/kg/hour intravenously. However, euphoria and excitement occurred 10 minutes after the start of the infusion and he had excitement, hallucinations, and delirium. His symptoms were suppressed by intravenous haloperidol 5 mg.

The authors speculated that propofol may produce psychotic symptoms when it is used in patients with a history of drug abuse.

Metabolism

Hyperlipidemia
Five cases of hyperlipidemia have been reported in 12 patients who received propofol infusions 3–8 mg/kg/hour for 10–187 hours for sedation in an intensive care unit (50). Propofol was their only source of lipids.

Propofol 2% has been compared with midazolam for sedation in 63 ventilated patients in intensive care (51). They were randomly assigned to either propofol 1.5–6.0 mg/kg/hour or midazolam 0.10–0.35 mg/kg/hour. Sedation was considered a failure if greater rates were required or if triglyceride concentrations were over 5.7 mmol/l (500 mg/dl) on one occasion or greater than 4.0 mmol/l (350 mg/dl) on two occasions. Hemodynamic, respiratory, and neurological variables were similar. Sedation failure occurred in 15 patients given propofol, three with increased triglyceride concentrations and 12 with poor sedation. In comparison, sedation failed in only one of the patients given midazolam. Average serum triglyceride concentrations were higher in the propofol group. In a separate retrospective comparison, triglyceride concentrations were lower than in similar patients treated with 1% propofol, and the sedation failure rate was lower using 2% propofol (9 versus 36%). The authors concluded that 2% propofol is safe but may be less efficient than midazolam. It should be noted that the dose ranges that they used may not have been comparable, leading to an artificially high rate of failure to provide adequate sedation in the propofol group.

Lactic acidosis
There have been several reports of lactic acidosis with and without rhabdomyolysis after propofol infusion, and two fatal cases have been reported (52).

- Two men, aged 7 and 17 years, presented with refractory status epilepticus. Both were treated with high-dose propofol infusions to achieve burst suppression on the electroencephalogram. During the second day of propofol infusion there was progressive severe lactic acidosis, hypoxia, pyrexia, and rhabdomyolysis, followed by hypotension, bradydysrhythmias, and renal dysfunction, leading to death. The total doses of propofol were 1275 mg/kg over 2.7 days and 482 mg/kg over 2 days.

Lactic acidosis and rhabdomyolysis have been reported in a child receiving an infusion of propofol for sedation in an intensive care unit (53).

- A previously healthy 10-month-old boy with an esophageal foreign body was given endotracheal intubation to protect his airway. Midazolam and morphine did not produce satisfactory sedation and he was given propofol by infusion, increased from 3.5 to 7 mg/kg/hour over 2 hours to a total dose of about 500 mg/kg over the next 2 days. Other drugs given included cefotaxime, flucloxacillin, and ranitidine. He developed green urine, triglyceridemia of 907 mg/dl (10 mmol/l), and lactic acidosis, with a peak lactate concentration of 18 mmol/l. He also developed hypotension, with first-degree atrioventricular block and right bundle branch block, unresponsive to atropine, external cardiac pacing, or isoprenaline. Continuous venovenous hemofiltration was instituted. He slowly improved over the next 2 days, but developed a raised creatine kinase activity (over 30 000 U/l) and myoglobinuria. A liver biopsy showed 10% necrosis of zone 3, with fatty infiltration characteristic of a toxic effect. A muscle biopsy showed large areas of muscle necrosis. Extensive investigations showed no underlying infectious or metabolic causes. He slowly recovered over 10 days and appeared to have completely recovered at 3 months.

Lactic acidosis without rhabdomyolysis has been reported in another case (54).

- A 61-year-old woman undergoing mitral valve surgery received fentanyl, midazolam, nitrous oxide, and propofol infusion 3 mg/kg/hour during a 5-hour anesthetic. She developed lactic acidosis soon after the completion of surgery and required reintubation and ventilation. The peak lactate concentration, which occurred 1 day later, was 14.3 mmol/l. There was also mild disturbance of liver function. She eventually recovered.

These cases are important because, unlike previous reports of metabolic acidosis after propofol infusion, the patients had no documented infections and, in at least one case, extensive investigation showed no other causes of the acidosis. The role of propofol in causing the metabolic problems appears to have been more likely in these than in previous reports. In the first three cases the doses of propofol used, both per hour and in all, were extremely high compared with normal therapeutic practice. The subject has also been reviewed, and it was pointed out that, although suggestive, the association of fatal metabolic acidosis with propofol infusion in sick patients is as yet unproven and to date hinges on 11 case reports of patients who had multiple problems (55).

Porphyria

An acute attack of porphyria has been reported in association with propofol (56).

- A 23-year-old man, with a past history of Fallot's tetralogy repaired at age 2, had catheter ablation of an aberrant conduction pathway causing right ventricular tachycardia, a procedure that took 16 hours. He was sedated with propofol at an average rate of 100 micrograms/kg/minute, and required intubation for respiratory insufficiency half way through the procedure. He also received caffeine and isoprenaline during the procedure to induce ventricular tachycardia. After the procedure he could not be roused or extubated for a further 10 hours and remained drowsy for a further day. He had weakness of an arm and a leg and had lancinating abdominal and shoulder pains. Urinary concentrations of porphyrins, aminolevulinic acid, porphobilinogen, and coproporphyrin III were markedly raised. He made a good recovery after administration of dextrose.

Propofol is regarded as being safe in patients with different types of porphyria. This is the first reported case in which propofol had a possible role in causing raised porphyrin concentrations perioperatively. However, severe illness can also precipitate porphyria, so the association with propofol may have been incidental.

Hematologic

In 10 patients, propofol, but not intralipos, its solvent, inhibited platelet aggregation both in vivo and in vitro (57). This defect was not associated with a change in bleeding time, and it was assumed that the effect is not clinically significant. The cause was probably suppression of calcium influx and release from platelets.

Fat emulsions affect coagulation and fibrinolysis (58). In a study of 36 patients undergoing aortocoronary bypass operations with midazolam + fentanyl or propofol + alfentanil anesthesia, factor XIIa concentrations and kallikrein-like activity were about 30% higher in the propofol group. The authors suggested that there had been stronger activation of the contact phase at the start of recirculation and stronger fibrinolysis in the propofol group. They also found more hypotension in the propofol group, which they assumed to be due to release of

kallikrein, resulting in release of bradykinin. Propofol has not been shown to cause increased perioperative bleeding.

Gastrointestinal

Propofol in subhypnotic doses is a potent antiemetic. In a double-blind, randomized study, a small dose of propofol (0.5 mg/kg) was compared with droperidol (20 micrograms/kg) or metoclopramide (0.2 mg/kg) given at the completion of surgery performed in 90 patients under standard anesthesia with thiopental, fentanyl, and sevoflurane (59). Follow-up was to 24 hours. The incidence of emesis at 24 hours was significantly lower in those who received propofol (10 versus 33% and 40% for droperidol and metoclopramide respectively).

Liver

Hepatocellular injury has been reported after the sole use of propofol for outpatient anesthesia (60).

- A young woman with multiple allergies underwent femoral hernia repair and the next day developed acute hepatitis, with severe nausea and vomiting and diffuse abdominal tenderness. She had very high transaminase activities and the prothrombin time was slightly raised. No viral cause could be demonstrated. Antinuclear antibody and smooth muscle antibody titers were not raised and the ceruloplasmin concentration was normal. Abdominal ultrasound did not show gallstones or any other abnormality. The urine was normal and did not contain porphyrins or porphobilinogen. She recovered spontaneously and refused liver biopsy.

Pancreas

There have been several reports of postoperative pancreatitis in association with propofol-induced anesthesia (61–63). In view of the very widespread use of propofol for induction of anesthesia, the very rare reports, and the complexity of establishing the cause of acute pancreatitis, a causal relation between propofol and pancreatitis has not been clearly established.

- A healthy 35-year-old man developed acute pancreatitis a few hours after receiving a 15-minute propofol anesthetic for laser treatment of a urethral stricture (64). He spent 3 weeks in an intensive care unit, requiring both respiratory and renal support. There was no evidence of gallstones on abdominal imaging. There was no defect of lipid metabolism.
- A 51-year-old woman with a past medical history of a seizure disorder, schizophrenia, and asthma, who had been admitted with pneumonia, was sedated using a propofol infusion to assist mechanical ventilation (65). Over 7 days she received a total of 26.5 g of propofol at a maximum rate of 0.2 mg/kg/minute. When pancreatitis, which was associated with hypertriglyceridemia, was diagnosed, the propofol infusion was stopped. In addition to raised amylase activity, serum triglyceride concentrations peaked at 17 mmol/l and lipase activity at 564 U/l. She recovered over the next 7 days. On day 17 she underwent tracheostomy revision, during which

she received propofol 200 mg. The subsequent post-operative period was complicated by another episode of pancreatitis, this time without associated hypertriglyceridemia. She recovered over the next several days. An ultrasound examination ruled out gallstone pancreatitis, despite the presence of cholelithiasis.

- A healthy 21-year-old woman developed acute pancreatitis a day after an anesthetic that lasted 138 minutes, with propofol for induction (66). She recovered after supportive therapy for 6 days. There was no evidence of gallstones on abdominal imaging and there was no defect in lipid metabolism.

The association between propofol and pancreatitis has been listed as "probable" in 25 reports of pancreatitis associated with propofol to the FDA registry. However, the features of this case, which included resolution of pancreatitis on drug withdrawal and recurrence on rechallenge, suggested that the association should be upgraded to "definitely causal."

Skin

A fixed drug eruption has been attributed to propofol (67).

Musculoskeletal

In an in vitro experiment using uterine muscle strips from 10 consenting parturients undergoing cesarean section, therapeutic concentrations of propofol had no effect on isometric tension developed during contraction of the muscle (68). However, higher than therapeutic concentrations did reduce the peak muscle tension that developed. These results confirm that propofol is free of this adverse effect, which is a known cause of postpartum bleeding after the use of volatile anesthetic drugs.

Rhabdomyolysis

Rhabdomyolysis has been reported in two patients receiving propofol for sedation while being ventilated for severe asthma (69).

- A 47-year-old woman had an infusion of propofol 200 micrograms/kg/minute for 4 days. On day 2 she developed hematuria, and laboratory investigations showed renal insufficiency with hyperkalemic metabolic acidosis. She died as a result of rhabdomyolysis with cardiac involvement.
- A 41-year-old man, who received propofol at rates of up to 222 micrograms/kg/minute for 2 days, developed oliguria, and the propofol was withdrawn. He was also receiving fentanyl and low molecular weight heparin for prophylaxis of deep vein thrombosis. He subsequently developed a very high creatine kinase activity (over 170 000 IU/l). Echocardiography showed globally depressed myocardial dysfunction. He subsequently recovered. The rates of propofol infusion were high and this was thought to be a contributing factor.

A similar death, possibly relating to propofol, has been reported.

- An 18-year-old man suffered multiple trauma (70). He was sedated for 98 hours with propofol 530–700 mg/hour. On day 5 he developed a metabolic acidosis with hyperkalemia and his serum was lipemic. An

echocardiogram showed global hypokinesia. He deteriorated and died shortly afterwards.

Although in none of these cases was a definitive link between propofol and the pathology established, the authors pointed out that several other cases have been reported, especially in children. Clinicians should be more aware that propofol may cause rhabdomyolysis, which appears to occur particularly at high doses.

Rhabdomyolysis and the propofol infusion syndrome

The propofol-infusion syndrome consists of a metabolic acidosis, rhabdomyolysis, and cardiovascular collapse. It occurs after prolonged infusion of propofol (over 48 hours) and has generally been reported in children, but also occasionally in adults.

Propofol infusion syndrome mimics the mitochondrial myopathies, in which there are specific defects in the mitochondrial respiratory chain. The clinical features of mitochondrial myopathy result from a disturbance in lipid metabolism in cardiac and skeletal muscle. These patients generally remain well until stressed by infection or starvation, although subclinical biochemical abnormalities of mitochondrial transport can be demonstrated. It has been suggested that early management of critically ill children may not include adequate calorific intake to balance the increase in metabolic demands, and that in susceptible children the diversion of metabolism to fat substrates may cause the propofol infusion syndrome. It is unclear if the dose or duration of propofol infusion alters this effect. As adults have larger carbohydrate stores and require lower doses of propofol for sedation, this may account for the relative rarity of the syndrome in adults. The authors suggested that adequate early carbohydrate intake may prevent the propofol infusion syndrome (71).

- Five adults with head injuries inexplicably had fatal cardiac arrests in a neurosurgical intensive care unit after the introduction of a sedation formulation containing an increased concentration of propofol (72). There were striking similarities with the previously reported syndrome of myocardial failure, metabolic acidosis, and rhabdomyolysis in children who received high-dose propofol infusions for more than 48 hours.

In a subsequent retrospective cohort analysis the odds ratio for the propofol infusion syndrome was 1.93 (95% CI = 1.12, 3.32) for every 1 mg/kg/hour increase in mean propofol dose above 5 mg/kg/hour. The authors suggested that propofol infusion at rates over 5 mg/kg/hour should be discouraged for long-term sedation.

- A 13-year-old girl with a head injury, who received a high-dose infusion of propofol for 4 days, developed the propofol infusion syndrome (73).

In an accompanying editorial, aspects of the propofol infusion syndrome were reviewed, and the author suggested that prolonged high-dose propofol infusions (over 4.8–6.0 mg/kg/hour for over 48–72 hours) should be avoided and that if high-dose metabolic suppression is required for more than 3 days in head injury, the alternative of a barbiturate should be considered (74). However, these long-acting agents have well-known potent myocardial depressant effects of their own, which are difficult to manage.

- A 2-year-old boy with a gunshot head injury developed the propofol infusion syndrome after receiving propofol in an average dosage of 5.2 mg/kg/hour for 72 hours (71). On the fourth day he became oliguric, with raised potassium, urea, and creatinine concentrations, and then developed a nodal bradycardia (28 minute). Propofol was withdrawn and an isoprenaline infusion was started, but only emergency transvenous pacing restored his heart rate. Hemofiltration was begun, on the basis of another case report, and the acidosis cleared and cardiovascular function was restored. In a blood sample taken before hemofiltration malonylcarnitine, C5-acylcarnitine, creatine kinase, troponin T, and myoglobinemia were raised. The child made a complete recovery and 9 months later all markers of fatty-acid oxidation were normal.

These findings are consistent with impaired fatty-acid oxidation: reduced mitochondrial entry of long-chain acylcarnitine esters due to inhibition of the transport protein (carnitine palmityl transferase 1) and failure of the respiratory chain at complex II. Another previously reported abnormality of the respiratory chain in propofol-infusion syndrome is a reduction in cytochrome C oxidase activity, with reduced complex IV activity and a reduced cytochrome oxidase ratio of 0.004. Propofol can also impair the mitochondrial electron transport system in isolated heart preparations.

Sexual function

Sexual illusions and disinhibition were a problem in two women (aged 20 and 47 years) after sedation with propofol (75).

Immunologic

True anaphylaxis to propofol has been observed (76).

Infection risk

Soon after the introduction of propofol in 1989, clusters of infections related to its use were reported, and there have since been several reports (77,78). The complications include hypotension, tachycardia, septic shock, convulsions, and death. Ethylenediaminetetra-acetic acid (EDTA) was added to the formulation to retard microbial growth. However, there have been concerns over the effects of this additive on trace element homeostasis, particularly when it is used in intensive care units for long-term sedation. Five randomized controlled trials have been reviewed, and minimal or no effects have been found on zinc, magnesium, or calcium homeostasis. However, there is no evidence to suggest that cluster infection has been or will be reduced with this formulation and there is still a need for care with sterility when using this product.

Long-Term Effects

Drug withdrawal

Excitation, including generalized tonic–clonic seizures, has been observed on withdrawal of a propofol infusion in intensive care (79).

Susceptibility Factors

Age

Propofol has previously been associated with death after prolonged infusion in seriously ill children. An in vitro study of the effects of propofol on GABA neurons in a cell culture showed evidence of toxicity after exposure for 8 hours (80). The authors proposed that this toxicity could be the cause of the problems observed in children.

In 21 critically ill children aged 1 week to 12 years, who were also receiving morphine by infusion, propofol kinetics were altered in very small babies and in children of all ages recovering from cardiac surgery (81). Increased volume of distribution and reduced metabolic clearance caused a prolonged half-life. The combination of morphine 20–40 micrograms/kg and 2% propofol 4–6 mg/kg/hour for up to 28 hours appears to be safe.

Drug Administration

Drug formulations

Propofol is formulated as a 1% solution in Intralipid 10% (82). This formulation has been associated with hyperlipidemia, especially raised triglycerides, when given by prolonged infusion to the critically ill, particularly children or patients with liver disease. A formulation of propofol 6% in lipofundin (medium-chain + long-chain triglycerides 10%) has been developed to reduce the risk of hyperlipidemia. In 24 patients who received an induction dose of propofol 2.5 mg/kg over 60 seconds of either the new formulation in 6% or 1% solution and of the original 1% formulation, the pharmacokinetics, induction time, dosage requirements, and safety profile of the three agents were similar. Pain on injection was reported by 17% of the patients, and did not vary between formulations. The 6% solution may be safer for long-term infusion, when reducing the fat load is important.

References

1. Millar JM, Jewkes CF. Recovery and morbidity after daycase anaesthesia. A comparison of propofol with thiopentone–enflurane with and without alfentanil. Anaesthesia 1988;43(9):738–43.
2. Carpentier JP, Riou O, Petrognani R, Seignot P, Aubert M. Étude comparée du reveil après entretien de l'anesthésie par propofol ou isoflurane. Essai de synthese des données actuelles. [A comparative study of recovery following maintenance of anesthesia with propofol or isoflurane. An attempt to synthesize current data.] Cah Anesthesiol 1993;41(4):327–30.
3. Reimann FM, Samson U, Derad I, Fuchs M, Schiefer B, Stange EF. Synergistic sedation with low-dose midazolam and propofol for colonoscopies. Endoscopy 2000;32(3):239–44.
4. Jung M, Hofmann C, Kiesslich R, Brackertz A. Improved sedation in diagnostic and therapeutic ERCP: propofol is an alternative to midazolam. Endoscopy 2000;32(3):233–8.
5. Hall RI, Sandham D, Cardinal P, Tweeddale M, Moher D, Wang X, Anis AH. Study Investigators. Propofol vs midazolam for ICU sedation: a Canadian multicenter randomized trial. Chest 2001;119(4):1151–9.

6. Morley HR, Karagiannis A, Schultz DJ, Walker JC, Newland HS. Sedation for vitreoretinal surgery: a comparison of anaesthetist-administered midazolam and patient-controlled sedation with propofol. Anaesth Intensive Care 2000;28(1):37–42.

7. Bell GD, Charlton JE. Colonoscopy—is sedation necessary and is there any role for intravenous propofol? Endoscopy 2000;32(3):264–7.

8. Hug CC Jr, McLeskey CH, Nahrwold ML, Roizen MF, Stanley TH, Thisted RA, Walawander CA, White PF, Apfelbaum JL, Grasela TH, et al. Hemodynamic effects of propofol: data from over 25,000 patients. Anesth Analg 1993;77(Suppl 4):S21–9.

9. Searle NR, Sahab P. Propofol in patients with cardiac disease. Can J Anaesth 1993;40(8):730–47.

10. Warden JC, Pickford DR. Fatal cardiovascular collapse following propofol induction in high-risk patients and dilemmas in the selection of a short-acting induction agent. Anaesth Intensive Care 1995;23(4):485–7.

11. Wilhelm S, Standl T. Bietet Propofol Vorteile gegeniiber Isofluran für die sufentanil-supplementierte Auästhesie bei kindern in des strabismuschirurgie? [Does propofol have advantages over isoflurane for sufentanil supplemented anesthesia in children for strabismus surgery?] Anasthesiol Intensivmed Notfallmed Schmerzther 1996;31(7):414–19.

12. Bilotta F, Fiorani L, La Rosa I, Spinelli F, Rosa G. Cardiovascular effects of intravenous propofol administered at two infusion rates: a transthoracic echocardiographic study. Anaesthesia 2001;56(3):266–71.

13. Carrasco G, Cabre L, Sobrepere G, Costa J, Molina R, Cruspinera A, Lacasa C. Synergistic sedation with propofol and midazolam in intensive care patients after coronary artery bypass grafting. Crit Care Med 1998;26(5):844–51.

14. Michelsen I, Helbo-Hansen HS, Kohler F, Lorenzen AG, Rydlund E, Bentzon MW. Prophylactic ephedrine attenuates the hemodynamic response to propofol in elderly female patients. Anesth Analg 1998;86(3):477–81.

15. Gamlin F, Freeman J, Winslow L, Berridge J, Vucevic M. The haemodynamic effects of propofol in combination with ephedrine in elderly patients (ASA groups 3 and 4). Anaesth Intensive Care 1999;27(5):477–80.

16. Tritapepe L, Voci P, Marino P, Cogliati AA, Rossi A, Bottari B, Di Marco P, Menichetti A. Calcium chloride minimizes the hemodynamic effects of propofol in patients undergoing coronary artery bypass grafting. J Cardiothorac Vasc Anesth 1999;13(2):150–3.

17. Bagshaw O. TIVA with propofol and remifentanil. Anaesthesia 1999;54(5):501–2.

18. Sochala C, Deenen D, Ville A, Govaerts MJ. Heart block following propofol in a child. Paediatr Anaesth 1999;9(4):349–51.

19. Sakabe M, Fujiki A, Inoue H. Propofol induced marked prolongation of QT interval in a patient with acute myocardial infarction. Anesthesiology 2002;97(1):265–6.

20. Tan CH, Onsiong MK. Pain on injection of propofol. Anaesthesia 1998;53(5):468–76.

21. Sear JW, Jewkes C, Wanigasekera V. Hemodynamic effects during induction, laryngoscopy, and intubation with eltanolone (5 beta-pregnanolone) or propofol. A study in ASA I and II patients. J Clin Anesth 1995;7(2):126–31.

22. Nakane M, Iwama H. A potential mechanism of propofol-induced pain on injection based on studies using nafamostat mesilate. Br J Anaesth 1999;83(3):397–404.

23. Gilston A. Raynaud's phenomenon and propofol. Anaesthesia 1999;54(3):307.

24. Ho CM, Tsou MY, Sun MS, Chu CC, Lee TY. The optimal effective concentration of lidocaine to reduce pain on injection of propofol. J Clin Anesth 1999;11(4):296–300.

25. Tan CH, Onsiong MK, Kua SW. The effect of ketamine pretreatment on propofol injection pain in 100 women. Anaesthesia 1998;53(3):302–5.

26. Uda R, Kadono N, Otsuka M, Shimizu S, Mori H. Strict temperature control has no effect on injection pain with propofol. Anesthesiology 1999;91(2):591–2.

27. Ozturk E, Izdes S, Babacan A, Kaya K. Temperature of propofol does not reduce the incidence of injection pain. Anesthesiology 1998;89(4):1041.

28. Huang YW, Buerkle H, Lee TH, Lu CY, Lin CR, Lin SH, Chou AK, Muhammad R, Yang LC. Effect of pretreatment with ketorolac on propofol injection pain. Acta Anaesthesiol Scand 2002;46(8):1021–4.

29. Ambesh SP, Dubey PK, Sinha PK. Ondansetron pretreatment to alleviate pain on propofol injection: a randomized, controlled, double-blinded study. Anesth Analg 1999;89(1):197–9.

30. Pang WW, Huang PY, Chang DP, Huang MH. The peripheral analgesic effect of tramadol in reducing propofol injection pain: a comparison with lidocaine. Reg Anesth Pain Med 1999;24(3):246–9.

31. Mok MS, Pang WW, Hwang MH. The analgesic effect of tramadol, metoclopramide, meperidine and lidocaine in ameliorating propofol injection pain: a comparative study. J Anaesthesiol Clin Pharmacol 1999;15:37–42.

32. Memis D, Turan A, Karamanlioglu B, Kaya G, Pamukcu Z. The prevention of propofol injection pain by tramadol or ondansetron. Eur J Anaesthesiol 2002;19(1):47–51.

33. Gillies GW, Lees NW. The effects of speed of injection on induction with propofol. A comparison with etomidate. Anaesthesia 1989;44(5):386–8.

34. el-Ebiary M, Torres A, Ramirez J, Xaubet A, Rodriguez-Roisin R. Lipid deposition during the long-term infusion of propofol. Crit Care Med 1995;23(11):1928–30.

35. Nishiyama T, Hanaoka K. Propofol-induced bronchoconstriction: two case reports. Anesth Analg 2001;93(3):645–6.

36. Schramm BM, Orser BA. Dystonic reaction to propofol attenuated by benztropine (Cogentin). Anesth Analg 2002;94(5):1237–40.

37. Bragonier R, Bartle D, Langton-Hewer S. Acute dystonia in a 14-yr-old following propofol and fentanyl anaesthesia. Br J Anaesth 2000;84(6):828–9.

38. Saunders PR, Harris MN. Opisthotonus and other unusual neurological sequelae after outpatient anaesthesia. Anaesthesia 1990;45(7):552–7.

39. McHugh P. Acute choreoathetoid reaction to propofol. Anaesthesia 1991;46(5):425.

40. Hasan MM, Hasan ZA, al-Hader AF, Takrouri MS. The anticonvulsant effects of propofol, diazepam, and thiopental, against picrotoxin-induced seizure in the rat. Middle East J Anesthesiol 1993;12(2):113–21.

41. Heavner JE, Arthur J, Zou J, McDaniel K, Tyman-Szram B, Rosenberg PH. Comparison of propofol with thiopentone for treatment of bupivacaine-induced seizures in rats. Br J Anaesth 1993;71(5):715–19.

42. Borgeat A, Dessibourg C, Popovic V, Meier D, Blanchard M, Schwander D. Propofol and spontaneous movements: an EEG study. Anesthesiology 1991;74(1):24–7.

43. Kiyama S, Yoshikawa T. Persistent intraoperative myoclonus during propofol–fentanyl anaesthesia. Can J Anaesth 1998;45(3):283–4.

44. Yasukawa M, Yasukawa K. [Convulsion in two non-epileptic patients following induction of anesthesia with propofol.] Masui 1999;48(3):271–4.

45. Sneyd JR. Propofol and epilepsy. Br J Anaesth 1999;82(2):168–9.

46. Iwasaki F, Mimura M, Yamazaki Y, Hazama K, Sato Y, Namiki A. [Generalized tonic-clonic seizure induced by propofol in a patient with epilepsy.] Masui 2001;50(2):168–70.

47. Gozal D, Gozal Y. Behavior disturbances with repeated propofol sedation in a child. J Clin Anesth 1999;11(6):499.

48. Seppelt IM. Neurotoxicity from overuse of nitrous oxide. Med J Aust 1995;163(5):280.

49. Yamaguchi S, Mishio M, Okuda Y, Kitajima T. [A patient with drug abuse who developed multiple psychotic symptoms during sedation with propofol.] Masui 1998;47(5):589–92.

50. Mateu J, Barrachina F. Hypertriglyceridaemia associated with propofol sedation in critically ill patients. Intensive Care Med 1996;22(8):834–5.

51. Sandiumenge Camps A, Sanchez-Izquierdo Riera JA, Toral Vazquez D, Sa Borges M, Peinado Rodriguez J, Alted Lopez E. Midazolam and 2% propofol in long-term sedation of traumatized critically ill patients: efficacy and safety comparison. Crit Care Med 2000;28(11):3612–19.

52. Hanna JP, Ramundo ML. Rhabdomyolysis and hypoxia associated with prolonged propofol infusion in children. Neurology 1998;50(1):301–3.

53. Cray SH, Robinson BH, Cox PN. Lactic acidemia and bradyarrhythmia in a child sedated with propofol. Crit Care Med 1998;26(12):2087–92.

54. Watanabe Y. Lactic acidosis associated with propofol in an adult patient after cardiovascular surgery. J Cardiothorac Vasc Anesth 1998;12:611–12.

55. Susla GM. Propofol toxicity in critically ill pediatric patients: show us the proof. Crit Care Med 1998;26(12):1959–60.

56. Asirvatham SJ, Johnson TW, Oberoi MP, Jackman WM. Prolonged loss of consciousness and elevated porphyrins following propofol administrations. Anesthesiology 1998;89(4):1029–31.

57. Aoki H, Mizobe T, Nozuchi S, Hiramatsu N. In vivo and in vitro studies of the inhibitory effect of propofol on human platelet aggregation. Anesthesiology 1998;88(2):362–70.

58. Schulze HJ, Wendel HP, Kleinhans M, Oehmichen S, Heller W, Elert O. Effects of the propofol combination anesthesia on the intrinsic blood-clotting system. Immunopharmacology 1999;43(2–3):141–4.

59. Fujii Y, Tanaka H, Kobayashi N. Prevention of postoperative nausea and vomiting with antiemetics in patients undergoing middle ear surgery: comparison of a small dose of propofol with droperidol or metoclopramide. Arch Otolaryngol Head Neck Surg 2001;127(1):25–8.

60. Anand K, Ramsay MA, Crippin JS. Hepatocellular injury following the administration of propofol. Anesthesiology 2001;95(6):1523–4.

61. Leisure GS, O'Flaherty J, Green L, Jones DR. Propofol and postoperative pancreatitis. Anesthesiology 1996;84(1):224–7.

62. Wingfield TW. Pancreatitis after propofol administration: is there a relationship? Anesthesiology 1996;84(1):236.

63. Goodale DB, Suljaga-Petchel K. Pancreatitis after propofol administration: is there a relationship? In reply. Anesthesiology 1996;84(1):236–7.

64. Betrosian AP, Balla M, Papanikolaou M, Kofinas G, Georgiadis G. Post-operative pancreatitis after propofol administration. Acta Anaesthesiol Scand 2001;45(8):1052.

65. Kumar AN, Schwartz DE, Lim KG. Propofol-induced pancreatitis: recurrence of pancreatitis after rechallenge. Chest 1999;115(4):1198–9.

66. Jawaid Q, Presti ME, Neuschwander-Tetri BA, Burton FR. Acute pancreatitis after single-dose exposure to propofol: a case report and review of literature. Dig Dis Sci 2002;47(3):614–18.

67. Jamieson V, Mackenzie J. Allergy to propofol? Anaesthesia 1988;43(1):70.

68. Shin YK, Kim YD, Collea JV. The effect of propofol on isolated human pregnant uterine muscle. Anesthesiology 1998;89(1):105–9.

69. Stelow EB, Johari VP, Smith SA, Crosson JT, Apple FS. Propofol-associated rhabdomyolysis with cardiac involvement in adults: chemical and anatomic findings. Clin Chem 2000;46(4):577–81.

70. Perrier ND, Baerga-Varela Y, Murray MJ. Death related to propofol use in an adult patient. Crit Care Med 2000;28(8):3071–4.

71. Wolf A, Weir P, Segar P, Stone J, Shield J. Impaired fatty acid oxidation in propofol infusion syndrome. Lancet 2001;357(9256):606–7.

72. Cremer OL, Moons KG, Bouman EA, Kruijswijk JE, de Smet AM, Kalkman CJ. Long-term propofol infusion and cardiac failure in adult head-injured patients. Lancet 2001;357(9250):117–18.

73. Cannon ML, Glazier SS, Bauman LA. Metabolic acidosis, rhabdomyolysis, and cardiovascular collapse after prolonged propofol infusion. J Neurosurg 2001;95(6):1053–6.

74. Kelly DF. Propofol-infusion syndrome. J Neurosurg 2001;95(6):925–6.

75. Kent EA, Bacon DR, Harrison P, Lema MJ. Sexual illusions and propofol sedation. Anesthesiology 1992;77(5):1037–8.

76. Laxenaire MC, Gueant JL, Bermejo E, Mouton C, Navez MT. Anaphylactic shock due to propofol. Lancet 1988;2(8613):739–40.

77. Zaloga GP, Teres D. The safety and efficacy of propofol containing EDTA: a randomised clinical trial programme focusing on cation and trace metal homeostasis in critically ill patients. Intensive Care Med 2000;26(Suppl 4):S398–9.

78. Mehta U, Gunston GD, O'Connor N. Serious consequences to misuse of propofol anaesthetic. S Afr Med J 2000;90(3):240.

79. Shearer ES. Convulsions and propofol. Anaesthesia 1990;45(3):255–6.

80. Matthieu JM, Honegger P. Le propofol est toxique pour les neurones GABAergiques immatures. [Propofol is toxic for immature GABAergic neurons.] Rev Med Suisse Romande 1996;116(12):971–3.

81. Rigby-Jones AE, Nolan JA, Priston MJ, Wright PM, Sneyd JR, Wolf AR. Pharmacokinetics of propofol infusions in critically ill neonates, infants, and children in an intensive care unit. Anesthesiology 2002;97(6):1393–400.

82. Knibbe CA, Voortman HJ, Aarts LP, Kuks PF, Lange R, Langemeijer HJ, Danhof M. Pharmacokinetics, induction of anaesthesia and safety characteristics of propofol 6% SAZN vs propofol 1% SAZN and Diprivan-10 after bolus injection. Br J Clin Pharmacol 1999;47(6):653–60.

Propranolol

See also Beta-adrenoceptor antagonists

General Information

Propranolol is a lipophilic, non-selective, pure antagonist at beta-adrenoceptors, with membrane-stabilizing action.

Organs and Systems

Cardiovascular

An unusual dysrhythmia has been attributed to propranolol: alternating sinus rhythm with intermittent sinoatrial block. The authors suggested that this was accounted for by the existence of sinoatrial conduction via two pathways, the first with 2:1 block and the second with a slightly longer conduction time and intermittent 2:1 block (1).

Immunologic

Propranolol has been implicated in hypersensitivity pneumonitis (2,3), although other beta-blockers have also been associated with this complication.

References

1. Ozturk M, Demiroglu C. Alternating sinus rhythm and intermittent sinoatrial block induced by propranolol. Eur Heart J 1984;5(11):890–5.
2. Aellig WH, Clark BJ. Is the ISA of pindolol beta 2-adrenoceptor selective? Br J Clin Pharmacol 1987;24(Suppl 1):S21–8.
3. Gauthier-Rahman S, Akoun GM, Milleron BJ, Mayaud CM. Leukocyte migration inhibition in propranolol-induced pneumonitis. Evidence for an immunologic cell-mediated mechanism. Chest 1990;97(1):238–41.

Propylhexedrine

General Information

In the form of the volatile base, propylhexedrine is used in nasal inhalers; it is also a component of some liquid decongestant mixtures. When inhaled, and especially if over-used, it can cause nasal irritation, rebound congestion, and chronic rhinitis.

Long-Term Effects

Drug abuse

There have been several reports of abuse of propylhexedrine by addicts, who extract the contents of the cotton wad (250 mg propylhexedrine with added aromatics) and take them either orally or intravenously (1). In a few reported cases, deaths have occurred in abusers because of myocardial infarction or pulmonary hypertension, and psychoses of the amphetamine type have been induced (SED-9, 216).

- A 25-year-old white man tried to inject his right internal jugular vein with "home-made crank" [propylhexedrine] (2). After injection, he developed right-sided neck pain, followed by fever, chills, inspiratory stridor, and respiratory distress. He had edema extending from his anterior chest to the right parotid. Neck radiography showed extensive paracervical swelling with displacement of the trachea. At surgery his neck contained extensive necrotic tissue that was debrided. In spite of treatment with antibiotics, he developed progressive renal insufficiency and hypotension unresponsive to fluid therapy, followed by cardiopulmonary arrest and death.

There have been cases of definite brainstem dysfunction and five of transient diplopia secondary to intravenous abuse of Benzedrex, a nasal decongestant that contains propylhexedrine (3). All seven had transient diplopia within seconds after injection. One had a right-internuclear ophthalmoplegia and another had a depressed right gag reflex and paralysis of the right half of the tongue. The deficits in these two patients persisted for many months.

References

1. Smith DE, Wesson DR, Sees KL, Morgan JP. An epidemiological and clinical analysis of propylhexedrine abuse in the United States. J Psychoactive Drugs 1988;20(4):441–2.
2. Perez J, Burton BT, McGirr JG. Airway compromise and delayed death following attempted central vein injection of propylhexedrine. J Emerg Med 1994;12(6):795–7.
3. Fornazzari L, Carlen PL, Kapur BM. Intravenous abuse of propylhexedrine (Benzedrex) and the risk of brainstem dysfunction in young adults. Can J Neurol Sci 1986;13(4):337–9.

Propyphenazone

General Information

Propyphenazone is a pyrazolone derivative that has been incorporated into many over-the-counter analgesic combinations in many countries. There is no evidence that it has a lower incidence of adverse effects than phenazone (antipyrine), as was originally supposed, since neither compound has been widely studied alone.

In a systematic review of comparisons of Saridon (propyphenazone 150 mg + paracetamol 250 mg + caffeine 50 mg), paracetamol 500 mg + aspirin 500 mg + ibuprofen 200 mg, and placebo in 500 healthy adults, of whom 329 (66%) had moderate and 171 (34%) severe acute dentoalveolar pain, more of the patients who received Saridon reported "pain gone/partly gone" and fewer reported "pain unchanged or worse" at 30 and 60 minutes (1). There were adverse events in 20 patients (4.0%), with no significant differences between the groups. The most common adverse events were gastrointestinal disorders, followed by nervous system, skin, subcutaneous tissue, respiratory, cardiac, and general disorders.

Organs and Systems

Immunologic

Severe type I hypersensitivity reactions have been reported (SEDA-16, 108). Serious generalized urticaria with angioedema has occurred (2). Rechallenge with oral propyphenazone caused a severe anaphylactic reaction in a patient with a negative skin test. Although the report stressed the importance of oral challenge, it also drew attention to its risks (SEDA-12, 83).

In 44 of 53 patients, all of whom developed symptoms suggestive of IgE-mediated anaphylaxis within 30 minutes of taking propyphenazone, skin tests showed typical wheal and flare reactions and significant amounts of propyphenazone-specific serum IgE was detected in 31 (3). In seven of nine patients with negative skin tests, propyphenazone-specific IgE was detected.

Drug Administration

Drug overdose

In overdose, propyphenazone, like other pyrazolones, mainly affects the central nervous system, causing coma and convulsions, and the liver; dysrhythmias and cardiogenic shock can occur; hemoperfusion has been recommended for patients with severe pyrazolone intoxication (4).

References

1. Kiersch TA, Minic MR. The onset of action and the analgesic efficacy of Saridon (a propyphenazone/paracetamol/caffeine combination) in comparison with paracetamol, ibuprofen, aspirin and placebo (pooled statistical analysis). Curr Med Res Opin 2002;18(1):18–25.
2. Kienlein-Kletschka B, Baurle G. Epicutane sofort Reaktion. Aktuelle Derm 1981;7:88.
3. Himly M, Jahn-Schmid B, Pittertschatscher K, Bohle B, Grubmayr K, Ferreira F, Ebner H, Ebner C. IgE-mediated immediate-type hypersensitivity to the pyrazolone drug propyphenazone. J Allergy Clin Immunol 2003;111(4):882–8.
4. Okonek S, Reinecke HJ. Acute toxicity of pyrazolones. JAMA 1983;75(5A):94–8.

Prostaglandins

See also Individual agents

General Information

Eicosanoids are the oxygenated metabolites of 20-carbon unsaturated fatty acids found in the phospholipids of cell membranes (Greek eikosi = 20). The eicosanoids include the prostaglandins, thromboxanes, and leukotrienes. Precursor fatty acids include arachidonic acid C20:4n–6 (for 2-series prostaglandins and thromboxane and 4-series leukotrienes), dihomogammalinolenic acid C20:3n–6 (for PGE$_1$), and eicosapentaenoic acid C20:5n–3 (for 3-series prostaglandins and 5-series leukotrienes). Naturally occurring eicosanoids are predominantly metabolites of arachidonic acid, reflecting the dominance of n–6 fatty acids in the terrestrial food chain.

The principal biologically active, naturally occurring prostaglandins are prostaglandin E$_1$ (PGE$_1$), prostaglandin E$_2$ (PGE$_2$), prostaglandin F$_{2\alpha}$ (PGF$_{2\alpha}$), prostacyclin (PGI$_2$), and thromboxane (TXA$_2$). These agents have various, sometimes opposed, biological actions (1). Their half-lives are short, owing to their rapid breakdown (a few minutes for PGE$_2$ and PGF$_{2\alpha}$, a few seconds for PGI$_2$) (2). Prostaglandins thus have principally local biological actions. Analogues (mostly methyl derivatives) have been synthesized and are more slowly inactivated. The adverse

Table 1 Indications for prostaglandin therapy

In obstetrics
First- and second-trimester abortion
Cervical reopening
Induction of labor
Augmentation of labor
Postpartum hemorrhage
Ectopic pregnancy
Lactation suppression

In gastrointestinal disease
Peptic ulceration
Liver transplantation
Chemotherapy-induced mucosal lesions

In cardiovascular disease
Congenital cardiac malformations
Raynaud's syndrome
Chronic obstructive pulmonary disease
Adult respiratory distress syndrome
Pulmonary hypertension
Arterial occlusive disease
Extracorporeal circulation

In urology
Erectile dysfunction
Cystitis after radiation or chemotherapy

In ophthalmology
Glaucoma

reactions encountered when prostaglandins are used therapeutically will depend on the indications (see Table 1), since these will determine the dose and route of administration and hence the type of reaction likely to occur. Many of the problems experienced are attributable to their main pharmacological effects (Table 2).

Nomenclature

The names of prostaglandins are generally abbreviated to a three-letter abbreviation with a subscripted number. The first two letters are always PG; the third is E, F, or I. The recommended International Non-proprietary Names (rINNs) of various prostaglandins are given in Table 3. The convention is that, for example, PGE$_1$ is the name given to the endogenous prostaglandin and alprostadil is the name given to the same compound available for exogenous administration.

Synthetic analogues of PGE$_1$, PGE$_2$, PGF$_1$, PGF$_{2\alpha}$, and PGI$_2$

Synthetic analogues of prostaglandins are listed in Table 4. Their use allows reduction of dosages and adverse effects. In general, they cause fewer adverse effects than their naturally occurring counterparts, although this depends on the method of administration. Newer analogues (3) and oral forms (4) are in development.

General adverse effects

The most prominent and frequent adverse effects of prostaglandins are those on the gastrointestinal tract. However, the most dangerous are likely to be the cardiovascular effects, which in predisposed patients can sometimes cause life-threatening collapse and heart failure. Hyperthermia and headache are frequent nervous

Table 2 Actions of prostaglandins

Prostaglandin E series
Increased hormone secretion
  Growth hormone, corticotropin, thyrotropin, luteinizing
  hormone, thyroid hormone, insulin, glucocorticoids,
  progesterone, erythropoietin, renin
Increased body temperature
Sensitization of pain-mediating nerve fibers
Increased force of myocardial contraction
Increased blood flow in gastric mucosa, liver, kidney, and placenta
Increased renal secretion of sodium, potassium, and water
Antagonistic action against antidiuretic hormone
Increased intraocular pressure
Increased permeability of blood capillaries
Increased gastrointestinal motility
Reduced gastrointestinal secretions
Reduced blood pressure
Bronchodilatation
Inhibition of bronchial secretions
Sedation
Contraction of the non-pregnant uterus
Induction of abortion and labor

Prostaglandin F series
Bronchial constriction, especially in patients with asthma
Reduced pulmonary blood flow and increased pulmonary blood
  pressure
Increased erythropoietin secretion
Increased neurotransmission at sympathetic nerve endings
Increased gastrointestinal motility
Reduced blood pressure
Sedation (effects on the central nervous system)
Luteolytic effects in mammalian species (except man)
Induction of abortion and labor

Prostaglandin I series
Reduced platelet aggregation
Reduced mean arterial pressure
Reduced total peripheral and pulmonary resistances
Increased heart rate
Increased renal secretion of sodium (tubular effect)

congenital cardiac malformations (6,7). The most frequent adverse effects during prolonged treatment are diarrhea, necrotizing enterocolitis, cortical hyperostosis (8–10), fever, respiratory depression and apnea, and seizure-like activity (11). The frequency of adverse effects is not necessarily reduced with low-dose intravenous or oral administration (12). Maternal/fetal hyperglycemia due to reduced insulin secretion is rare, except in the infants of diabetic mothers (13). Less common adverse effects include gastric outlet obstruction due to antral hyperplasia (14).

Raynaud's phenomenon and digital ischemia
Studies of PGE_1 infusion for treatment of Raynaud's syndrome have shown variable changes in frequency of attacks and of healing ischemic digital ulcers (15–18). Prostacyclin

Table 4 Synthetic analogues of prostaglandins (rINNs except where stated)

PGE₁ analogues
Enisoprost
Limaprost
Mexiprostil
Misoprostol
Ornoprostil
Rioprostil
Rosaprostol

PGE₂ analogues
Arbaprostil
Enprostil
Gemeprost
Meteneprost
Nocloprost
Sulprostone
Trimoprostol
Viprostol

PGF₁ analogues
Prostalene (pINN)

PGF₂ₐ analogues
Alfaprostol
Bimatoprost
Carboprost
Cloprostenol
Fenprostalene
Fluprostenol
Latanoprost
Luprostiol
Tiaprost
Travoprost
Unoprostone

PGI₂ analogues
Beraprost
Cicaprost
Ciprostene
Iloprost

system effects. Epileptiform convulsions occur rarely. When used for termination of pregnancy, uterine hyperstimulation and, less often, uterine rupture can occur (5). Hypersensitivity to prostaglandins can cause skin reactions, bronchospasm (also seen as a direct pharmacological effect), and occasionally anaphylaxis. Tumor-inducing effects have not been reported. There have been a few reports of infants with limb deformities with and without Möbius sequence after exposure to misoprostol (a PGE_1 analogue) in the first trimester.

Prostaglandins in cardiovascular disease

Maintenance of the ductus arteriosus
PGE_1 and PGE_2 are effective in maintaining the patency of the ductus arteriosus in the initial management of

Table 3 Recommended International Non-proprietary Names (rINNs) and chemical names of the major prostaglandins

Prostaglandin	rINN	Chemical name (omitting stereochemical information)
PGE_1	Alprostadil	11,15-dihydroxy-9-oxoprosta-13-en-1-oic acid
PGE_2	Dinoprostone	11,15-dihydroxy-9-oxoprosta-5,13-dien-1-oic acid
$PGF_{2\alpha}$	Dinoprost	9,11,15-trihydroxyprosta-5,13-dien-1-oic acid
PGI_2 (PGX, prostacyclin)	Epoprostenol	6,9-epoxy-11,15-dihydroxyprosta-5,13-dien-1-oic acid

infusion (using PGI_2 or its synthetic analogue iloprost) appears to have beneficial effects, both in reducing the severity and frequency of attacks and healing ischemic digital ulcers. Adverse effects are common and include headache, flushing, jaw pain, nausea, vomiting, diarrhea, and inflammation and pain at the injection site (19,20). Iloprost has also been used effectively in the treatment of local gangrene secondary to chemotherapy (21). Application of a PGE_2 analogue to the skin produced both subjective and objective improvement in patients with Raynaud's syndrome and produced only minor self-limiting adverse effects (headache, flushing, and diarrhea) (22).

Peripheral vascular disease

Synthetic PGI_2 has been used in arterial occlusive disease as an anti-aggregatory drug (23–28). Adverse effects are common (85%). Headache, fever, nausea, anorexia, diarrhea, pain at the infusion site, and arthralgia are the most prominent. A single study has suggested an increased risk of thromboembolism after the use of iloprost in peripheral vascular disease (29).

Beraprost, an epoprostenol (PGI_2) analogue, has been studied in intermittent claudication. Adverse events include gastrointestinal disorders, headaches, skin disorders, and fever (30).

Primary pulmonary hypertension

Initial studies of continuous intravenous prostacyclin infusion in patients with primary pulmonary hypertension have shown sustained improvement in pulmonary artery pressure, exercise capacity, and survival compared with historical controls (31,32). Minor complications (diarrhea, jaw pain, flushing, photosensitivity, and headache) were dose-related. Serious complications were related to problems with the drug delivery system, including catheter thrombosis, sepsis, and temporary interruption of the infusion, resulting in abrupt deterioration (31).

Regulation of pulmonary vascular perfusion in advanced respiratory disease

PGE_1 significantly reduces right ventricular pulmonary after-load in patients with pulmonary hypertension due to chronic obstructive airways disease (33). PGE_1 can also be useful in the treatment of adult respiratory distress syndrome (34). Preliminary studies using aerosolized prostacyclin showed a reduction in pulmonary artery pressure and improved arterial oxygenation with reduction in intrapulmonary shunt in ventilated patients with adult respiratory distress syndrome (35) and severe community-acquired pneumonia (36). However, ventilated patients with severe community-acquired pneumonia and pre-existing fibrosis required much higher doses, with a reduction in systemic vascular resistance and an increase in intrapulmonary shunting (36). A single report described improved oxygenation, mainly due to reduction of intrapulmonary shunting, in two neonates with pulmonary hypertension treated with aerosolized prostacyclin (37).

Other uses

PGI_2 has been used to reduce the re-stenosis rate during transluminal coronary angioplasty (38).

Prostacyclin infusion (using PGI_2 or its synthetic analogue, iloprost) has been used during extracorporeal circulation to prevent blood clotting in the dialyser coil (39). The risk of severe hypotension can be avoided by carefully controlling the infusion rate.

Prostaglandins in gastrointestinal disease

Peptic ulceration and NSAID-induced gastropathy

Prostaglandins of the E series (misoprostol, enprostil) have antiulcer activity in the upper gastrointestinal tract (40). They inhibit gastric acid secretion at modest doses and provide mucosal protection against noxious agents, including non-steroidal anti-inflammatory drugs, smoking, alcohol, and chemotherapy. They have been used to prevent NSAID-induced gastroduodenal lesions (41,42). They may also be effective in preventing NSAID-induced renal impairment (43).

The cure rate for gastric and duodenal ulcers is comparable to the results with H_2-receptor antagonists (44–46). Relapses appear to be fewer with prostaglandin therapy (44,45). Healing of duodenal ulcers refractory to H_2-receptor antagonists has been described.

Diarrhea (4–38%), abdominal pain or cramp, flatulence, and nausea or vomiting account for most of the adverse effects reported. No biochemical or hematological adverse effects have been noted.

These agents are contraindicated in women of childbearing age, unless they are using adequate contraceptive measures, because of uncertain abortifacient effects. They have been used as illegal abortifacients in some countries (47).

Prostaglandins in liver disease

Liver failure and transplant dysfunction

Prostaglandins of the E series (both intravenous and oral formulations) have been used to treat fulminant hepatic failure, primary non-function following orthotopic liver transplantation, and recurrent hepatitis B infection after orthotopic liver transplantation in open trials (48–50). Adverse effects are almost universal. They include gastrointestinal symptoms (abdominal pain and cramping, watery diarrhea), which affect 33–100% and are more common with oral formulations and possibly amongst those with raised blood glucose concentrations. Cardiovascular effects, which affect about 33%, include migraine, hypotension, peripheral edema, and myocardial infarction (in those with pre-existing risk factors). Painful clubbing and cortical hyperostosis (92–100%) developed 10–60 days after the start of intravenous or oral therapy. Arthritis/arthralgia developed in 8% of those receiving intravenous and 92% of those taking oral PGE_1 or PGE_2. All adverse reactions appear to be dose-related and resolve with reductions in dose. Two patients developed calcium oxalate stones after 1 year of oral therapy (51).

Prostaglandins in urology

Prostacyclin infusion in men with persistent pain associated with Peyronie's disease was of little value but produced marked adverse effects (bradycardia, hypotension, nausea, flushing) (52).

A single dose of PGE_1 into the corpus cavernosum is highly effective in inducing artificial penile erection in cases of erectile dysfunction. The reported adverse effects include pain and a burning sensation, prolonged penile erection, and local fibrosis. The incidence of pain was high (75%) in older studies (53), while later data improved to 13–44% (54–57). Pain is cited as a prominent factor in non-adherence to therapy and in the dropout rate of patients from self-injection programs, although the incidence may fall with time (57). An alprostadil sterile powder formulation had a lower incidence of pain after penile injection (6.6%), attributed to lower doses and the lack of alcohol in the formulation (58). Burning and pain can be reduced by using a lower initial dose, with incremental increases until a satisfactory erection is produced (59).

Although the incidence of priapism varies in different studies, depending on its definition (erection lasting anywhere from 2 to 11 hours), an analysis of 48 studies in 8090 patients showed an overall incidence of 1% (55).

Prolonged erections induced by PGE_1 usually require drainage and phenylephrine irrigation, although a small percentage can be managed with oral terbutaline or oral pseudoephedrine if treated within 3 hours of PGE_1 injection (56). Local fibrosis is infrequent, occurring in 2% at 6 months and in 8% at 18 months (60). A single case of Peyronie's-like plaque and penile curvature deformity has been reported after repeated PGE_1 use (61).

Complications of alprostadil injections include hematoma and ecchymoses (8%) and systemic effects (6%), which mostly occur in the urogenital system (testicular pain and swelling, scrotal pain and edema, changes in urinary frequency, hematuria, and pelvic pain) (62). In 1% there were symptoms related to hypotension.

Massive diffuse hemorrhage due to cyclophosphamide-induced or radiation cystitis has been treated successfully with intravesicular PGE_1, PGE_2, and carboprost. Febrile reactions and severe bladder spasm are dose-dependent (63–65).

Prostaglandins in ophthalmology

Topical PGE_2 and $PGF_{2\alpha}$ significantly reduce intraocular pressure for at least 24 hours and are used in the treatment of glaucoma. Derivatives of the isopropyl ester of $PGF_{2\alpha}$ appear to be the most effective. Transient ocular adverse effects include conjunctival hyperemia, local irritation, intermittent photophobia, and pain in the eye (66–68). Newer derivatives, such as latanoprost, travoprost, and bimatoprost, appear to be better tolerated, with less severe and less frequent adverse effects (69). They reduce intraocular pressure by increasing uveoscleral outflow. The ocular pressure-lowering effect of latanoprost appears to be additive with timolol, with mild transient hyperemia in 50% of those treated with latanoprost alone (70).

Latanoprost, travoprost, and bimatoprost cause increased pigmentation of the iris in some patients after prolonged treatment (3.0–4.5 months) (71). Most data have been obtained with latanoprost, and it appears that there is a predisposition to iris pigmentation in patients with eyes of hazel or heterochromic color. As latanoprost and travoprost are selective agonists at $PGF_{2\alpha}$ receptors, it is likely that the phenomenon is mediated by these receptors. Latanoprost stimulates melanogenesis in iris

melanocytes, and transcription of the tyrosinase gene is upregulated. No evidence of harmful consequences of this adverse effect has been found, and the only disadvantage appears to be potential heterochromia between the eyes in unilaterally treated patients: the heterochromia is likely to be permanent, or very slowly reversible (72–74).

The adverse effects of travoprost include gradual darkening of the color of the iris and the eyelid skin, increased thickness, number, and darkness of the eyelashes, conjunctival hyperemia, and ocular pruritus (75).

Cystoid macular edema, iritis, *Herpes simplex* keratitis, periocular skin darkening, and headaches have been described in patients treated with prostaglandin analogues. These adverse effects occur rarely, and cystoid macular edema, iritis and *H. simplex* keratitis occur in eyes with risk factors. Repeated rechallenge with masked controls is required to establish a causal relation. However, even without firm establishment of a causal relation, caution is advised with the use of prostaglandin analogues in the eyes of patients with risk factors for macular edema, iritis, and *H. simplex* keratitis (76).

The ocular adverse effects of latanoprost include conjunctival hyperemia, iris pigmentation, periocular skin color changes, anterior uveitis, and cystoid macular edema in pseudophakic patients (77,78). *H. simplex* dendritic keratitis has been reported after treatment with latanoprost (79). In patients with uveitic glaucoma, latanoprost can cause increased intraocular pressure and recurrence of inflammation (80).

Exacerbation of angina pectoris has been described in association with latanoprost (81). $PGF_{2\alpha}$ is a vasoconstrictor, and systemic absorption of topical latanoprost can cause vasoconstriction in coronary arteries.

Three patients had new-onset migraine after using latanoprost, perhaps through activation of the trigeminal vascular system (82).

Prostaglandins in obstetrics

Prostaglandins of the E and F series are widely used in obstetrics for ripening the uterine cervix and stimulating uterine contraction at any stage of pregnancy. They are used in first- and second-trimester abortions, cervical priming, the induction and augmentation of labor, and postpartum hemorrhage (83–89). The route of administration can be vaginal, cervical, extra-amniotic, intra-amniotic, oral, intramuscular, or intravenous, and varies according to indication. Mifepristone (RU 486), a synthetic 19-norsteroid and progesterone antagonist, has been used in combination with synthetic prostaglandins in the induction of abortion.

A less well-established use involves intratubal injection of $PGF_{2\alpha}$ for ectopic pregnancy (90,91). Oral PGE_2 can be used to suppress lactation, for which it is as effective as bromocriptine, and causes less breast tenderness (92).

Organs and Systems

Cardiovascular

Both PGE_2 and $PGF_{2\alpha}$ commonly cause a fall in blood pressure and a degree of bradycardia (1,93). PGE_2 can cause vasodilatation of small vessels and $PGF_{2\alpha}$ can cause vasoconstriction (94). These changes are common but often mild. However, angina pectoris and myocardial infarction have been reported with prostaglandins of all types, particularly after inadvertent intramyometrial injection (95–98). A single case of pulmonary edema after the infusion of PGE_1 has been reported (99). In patients with pre-existing cardiovascular disease, the risk of serious aggravation is very real, and both pre-existing hypertension and states of shock can be worsened. A severe rise in maternal blood pressure occurred in a few cases in which fetal death was associated with unresolved pre-eclampsia.

Respiratory

People with asthma are more sensitive than healthy subjects to bronchoconstriction induced by $PGF_{2\alpha}$ (100,101).

Nervous system

Increased body temperature, pyrexia (both intra- and postpartum), and chills are thought to result from central stimulation of temperature regulatory centers by prostaglandins (102,103). Headache and migraine are the most common adverse effects on the central nervous system (5,104).

Prostaglandin therapy can cause electroencephalographic abnormalities (105). Convulsions, which occur occasionally, are a particular risk in epileptic patients (5,104,105). The combination of prostaglandins and oxytocin can be complicated by tonic-clonic seizures (106).

Enhancement of the pain sensation may reflect a direct effect on nerve fibers. The presence of pain correlates well with the effect on the uterus.

Sensory systems

Increased intraocular pressure and miosis have been reported (5,104).

Mouth and teeth

Gingivitis has been associated with obstetric prostaglandins (5).

Gastrointestinal

Nausea, vomiting, diarrhea, and abdominal pain (107) occur in about 90% of all patients given prostaglandins systemically. The frequency and duration of these adverse effects depend on the mode of application, the dosage, and the molecule used, and are very variable (108).

Reproductive system

Uterine hypertonia and hyperstimulation are well-recognized adverse effects of induction of abortion and labor with prostaglandins. Cervical rupture and uterine rupture have been reported with every prostaglandin and analogue, even in previously unscarred uteri (5,109–116). The risks can be minimized by using lower doses (0.5 mg intracervically or 3 mg intravaginally), by allowing longer intervals between re-applications, and by avoiding combination with oxytocin, which has a potentiating effect. However, there is a single case report of uterine rupture in a multiparous woman with unscarred uterus

following low-dose (1.5 mg) intravaginal PGE_2 (117). In the event of uterine hyperstimulation, beta$_2$-adrenoceptor agonists may reduce uterine contractility. Intensive monitoring of uterine activity and fetal condition is mandatory, since the rate of absorption of PGE_2 after intravaginal or cervical administration is unpredictable.

Second-Generation Effects

Teratogenicity

Seven Brazilian infants were born with limb deficiencies both with and without Möbius sequence after exposure to misoprostol in the first trimester during unsuccessful abortion attempts (118).

Fetotoxicity

Like oxytocin, prostaglandins have been responsible rarely for fetal distress and even fetal death (119,120). The risk of fetal death underlines the importance of cardiotocography during prostaglandin (pre)induction. Prostaglandins should be used with extreme caution if there is a risk of placental insufficiency (120).

The incidence of neonatal jaundice was not increased after induction of labor with prostaglandins (47).

Susceptibility Factors

When PGE_2 and $PGF_{2\alpha}$ are used for induction of labor and abortion, the following contraindications must be respected and (until proven otherwise) also apply to the methyl analogues of these two prostaglandins:

- previous cesarean section or hysterotomy (because of the risk of rupture) (110);
- previous major abdominal surgery;
- prior abnormal delivery;
- a history of severe abdominal inflammation and/or infection;
- a predisposition to uterine cramps or tetanus uteri.

However, uneventful vaginal deliveries have been reported in patients with two previous cesarean sections in whom labor was induced with vaginal PGE_2 (121). Women with a history of six or more deliveries and anomalies of the fetus (for example hydrocephalus causing cephalopelvic disproportion) must also be excluded.

Predispositions to glaucoma, epilepsy, pre-eclampsia, hypertension, asthma, and ischemic heart disease are relative contraindications.

Drug Administration

Drug administration route

Intrauterine infusion

Intrauterine infusion (intra-amniotic or extra-amniotic) has been reported to be associated with fewer gastrointestinal symptoms and less fever than parenteral or intravaginal administration (122). In intra-amniotic use, the puncture must be guided by ultrasonography, and before injection a control aspiration of some amniotic fluid is required in order to avoid intrauterine or intravascular injection. Uterine rupture has been described with intra-amniotic treatment.

Intramuscular or intradermal injection

Inflammation and pain are common at the site of injection when prostaglandins are given intramuscularly or intradermally (123,124).

Intravenous injection

Prostaglandins have been used intravenously, both for induction of mid-trimester abortion and for induction of labor in cases of intrauterine death. The same adverse effects as described above occur, and are usually very pronounced. Routine premedication with an antiemetic and an antidiarrheal agent significantly reduces gastrointestinal adverse effects.

Inhalation

Intravenous epoprostenol increases exercise tolerance, improves pulmonary hemodynamics, and improves survival in patients with primary pulmonary hypertension. However, there are limitations to intravenous administration, and a significant proportion of patients develop catheter-related problems, such as thrombosis, pump failure, and catheter-related sepsis. In an attempt to improve delivery, several trials of aerosolized prostacyclin have been undertaken, primarily in patients with primary pulmonary hypertension.

There has been a sequential comparison of inhaled nitric oxide 40 ppm with aerosolized iloprost 14–17 micrograms in 35 adults with primary pulmonary hypertension (125). Five of the patients had minor headache and facial flushing during inhalation of iloprost, but these symptoms were short-lived and abated a few minutes after the inhalation ended. One patient had mild jaw pain after aerosolized iloprost, but again this was short-lived. There was an unexpected increase in pulmonary artery pressure in 10 patients and vascular resistance in six patients who received nitric oxide. The authors were uncertain of the cause of this increase, as nitric oxide generally behaves as a vasodilator, but they noted that nitric oxide is a vasoconstrictor in certain conditions, such as the presence of hemolysate (126).

There has been a trial of aerosolized iloprost in 24 patients with primary pulmonary hypertension and New York Heart Association class III or IV disability, who were refractory to conventional medical treatment (127). They were given aerosolized iloprost in a total daily dose of 100–150 micrograms (in 6–8 divided doses, given every 2–3 hours while awake) over 12 months. The treatment was generally well tolerated, except for coughing during inhalation, which was common initially but resolved spontaneously in all patients within the first 4 weeks. Five patients reported symptoms of flushing, headache, and jaw pain at the end of inhalation, but all rated the symptoms as mild and none discontinued treatment because of adverse effects. There was an asymptomatic but significant fall in systemic arterial pressure (from 98 to 90 mmHg) and vascular resistance at 3 and 12 months compared with baseline.

The effects of aerosolized iloprost have been reported in three patients with severe pulmonary hypertension (mean pulmonary artery pressure 50 mmHg or more) who were already being treated with intravenous epoprostenol (10–16 micrograms/kg/minute) (128). The aim of the study was to replace continuous intravenous epoprostenol with intermittent aerosolized iloprost (150–300 micrograms/day in 6–18 divided doses). All three patients had gradual weaning of intravenous epoprostenol (1 micrograms/kg/minute every 3–10 hours) under close supervision and hemodynamic monitoring in intensive care. All three had initial falls in pulmonary arterial pressure and improved right ventricular function with inhaled iloprost. The first could not be fully weaned from epoprostenol, because of right ventricular failure with dyspnea and hypoxemia, accompanied by a three-fold increase in serum bilirubin and lactate dehydrogenase and echocardiographically demonstrated right ventricular failure. The second and third patients both tolerated complete withdrawal of epoprostenol. However, one developed right ventricular failure within 2 hours of withdrawal. The third was successfully discharged from hospital taking aerosolized therapy, but presented 2 weeks later with severe right ventricular failure. Thus, caution should be taken in patients who have been previously maintained on intravenous prostacyclin when trying to convert to aerosolized therapy, as there appears to be a high chance of treatment failure, which can occur abruptly.

Platelet function after inhaled prostacyclin has been measured in a randomized, double-blind study in 28 patients undergoing elective cardiothoracic surgery (129). They were given aerosolized prostacyclin (5 or 10 micrograms) for 6 hours postoperatively. All the patients, regardless of dose, had a lower rate of platelet aggregation in response to adenosine diphosphate (ADP) than controls. There were no differences in clinically significant indices, such as chest tube drainage or bleeding time. This study has shown that prostacyclin, given as an aerosol, can cause measurable alterations in platelet function, with a possibly higher risk of bleeding.

References

1. Dusting GJ, Moncada S, Vane JR. Prostaglandins, their intermediates and precursors: cardiovascular actions and regulatory roles in normal and abnormal circulatory systems. Prog Cardiovasc Dis 1979;21(6):405–30.
2. Nakano J. General pharmacology of prostaglandins. In: Cuthbert MF, editor. The Prostaglandins: Pharmacological and Therapeutic Advances. Philadelphia: JB Lippincott, 1973:23–124.
3. Hattori R, Yui Y, Shirotani M, Kawai C. A stable prostacyclin analogue, 9B methylcarbacyclin (U-61, 431F). Cardiovasc Drug Rev 1992;10:233–42.
4. Hildebrand M, Pfeffer M, Mahler M, Staks T, Windt-Hanke F, Schutt A. Oral iloprost in healthy volunteers. Eicosanoids 1991;4(3):149–54.
5. Karim SMM. Prostaglandin—physiological basis of practical applications. In: Proceedings 6th Asia and Oceania Congress in Endocrinology 1978.
6. Momma K, Takao A, Sone K, Tashiro M. Prostaglandin E1 treatment of ductus-dependent infants with congenital heart disease. Int Angiol 1984;3:33.
7. van der Sijp JR, Rohmer J. Prostaglandinetherapie bij pasgeborenen met een ductus Botalli-afhankeliijke circulatie. [Prostaglandin therapy in newborn infants with a Botalli

duct-dependent circulation.] Tijdschr Kindergeneeskd 1985;53(1):20–5.

8. Woo K, Emery J, Peabody J. Cortical hyperostosis: a complication of prolonged prostaglandin infusion in infants awaiting cardiac transplantation. Pediatrics 1994; 93(3):417–20.

9. Letts M, Pang E, Simons J. Prostaglandin-induced neonatal periostitis. J Pediatr Orthop 1994;14(6):809–13.

10. Kaufman MB, El-Chaar GM. Bone and tissue changes following prostaglandin therapy in neonates. Ann Pharmacother 1996;30(3):269–77.

11. Lewis AB, Freed MD, Heymann MA, Roehl SL, Kensey RC. Side effects of therapy with prostaglandin E1 in infants with critical congenital heart disease. Circulation 1981;64(5):893–8.

12. Singh GK, Fong LV, Salmon AP, Keeton BR. Study of low dosage prostaglandin—usages and complications. Eur Heart J 1994;15(3):377–81.

13. Cohen MH, Nihill MR. Postoperative ketotic hyperglycemia during prostaglandin E1 infusion in infancy. Pediatrics 1983;71(5):842–4.

14. Peled N, Dagan O, Babyn P, Silver MM, Barker G, Hellmann J, Scolnik D, Koren G. Gastric-outlet obstruction induced by prostaglandin therapy in neonates. N Engl J Med 1992;327(8):505–10.

15. Gryglewski RJ. Prostacyclin: pharmacology and clinical trials. Int Angiol 1984;3:89.

16. Katoh K, Kawai T, Narita M, Uemura J, Tani K, Okubo T. Use of prostaglandin E1 (lipo-PGE1) to treat Raynaud's phenomenon associated with connective tissue disease: thermographic and subjective assessment. J Pharm Pharmacol 1992;44(5):442–4.

17. Langevitz P, Buskila D, Lee P, Urowitz MB. Treatment of refractory ischemic skin ulcers in patients with Raynaud's phenomenon with PGE1 infusions. J Rheumatol 1989;16(11):1433–5.

18. Mohrland JS, Porter JM, Smith EA, Belch J, Simms MH. A multiclinic, placebo-controlled, double-blind study of prostaglandin E1 in Raynaud's syndrome. Ann Rheum Dis 1985;44(11):754–60.

19. Wigley FM, Wise RA, Seibold JR, McCloskey DA, Kujala G, Medsger TA Jr, Steen VD, Varga J, Jimenez S, Mayes M, Clements PJ, Weiner SR, Porter J, Ellman M, Wise C, Kaufman LD, Williams J, Dole W. Intravenous iloprost infusion in patients with Raynaud phenomenon secondary to systemic sclerosis. A multicenter, placebo-controlled, double-blind study. Ann Intern Med 1994;120(3):199–206.

20. Belch JJ, Newman P, Drury JK, McKenzie F, Capell H, Leiberman P, Forbes CD, Prentice CR. Intermittent epoprostenol (prostacyclin) infusion in patients with Raynaud's syndrome. A double-blind controlled trial. Lancet 1983;1(8320):313–15.

21. Vowden P, Wilkinson D, Kester RC. Treatment of digital ischaemia associated with chemotherapy using the prostacyclin analogue iloprost. Eur J Vasc Surg 1991;5(5):593–5.

22. Belch JJ, Madhok R, Shaw B, Leiberman P, Sturrock RD, Forbes CD. Double-blind trial of CL115,347, a transdermally absorbed prostaglandin E2 analogue, in treatment of Raynaud's phenomenon. Lancet 1985;1(8439):1180–3.

23. Gruss JD, Vargas-Montano H, Bartels D, et al. Use of prostaglandins in arterial occlusion diseases. Int Angiol 1984;3:7.

24. Shionoya S. Clinical experience with prostaglandin E1 in occlusive arterial disease. Int Angiol 1984;3:99.

25. Tanabe T, Mishima Y, Shionoya Y, Katsumara T, Kusaba A. Effect of intravenous drip infusion of prostaglandin E1 on peripheral vascular reconstruction. Int Angiol 1984;3(Suppl):63.

26. Nizankowski R, Krolikowski W, Bielatowicz J, Szczeklik A. Prostacyclin for ischemic ulcers in peripheral arterial disease. A random assignment, placebo controlled study. Thromb Res 1985;37(1):21–8.

27. Telles GS, Campbell WB, Wood RF, Collin J, Baird RN, Morris PJ. Prostaglandin E1 in severe lower limb ischaemia: a double-blind controlled trial. Br J Surg 1984;71(7):506–8.

28. Staben P, Albring M. Treatment of patients with peripheral arterial occlusive disease Fontaine stage III and IV with intravenous iloprost: an open study in 900 patients. Prostaglandins Leukot Essent Fatty Acids 1996;54(5):327–33.

29. Kovacs IB, Mayou SC, Kirby JD. Infusion of a stable prostacyclin analogue, iloprost, to patients with peripheral vascular disease: lack of antiplatelet effect but risk of thromboembolism. Am J Med 1991;90(1):41–6.

30. Lievre M, Azoulay S, Lion L, Morand S, Girre JP, Boissel JP. A dose-effect study of beraprost sodium in intermittent claudication. J Cardiovasc Pharmacol 1996;27(6):788–93.

31. Barst RJ, Rubin LJ, McGoon MD, Caldwell EJ, Long WA, Levy PS. Survival in primary pulmonary hypertension with long-term continuous intravenous prostacyclin. Ann Intern Med 1994;121(6):409–15.

32. Higenbottam TW, Spiegelhalter D, Scott JP, Fuster V, Dinh-Xuan AT, Caine N, Wallwork J. Prostacyclin (epoprostenol) and heart-lung transplantation as treatments for severe pulmonary hypertension. Br Heart J 1993;70(4):366–70.

33. Gassner A, Sommer G, Fridrich L, Magometschnigg D, Priol A. Der Einfluss von Prostaglandin E1 (Alprostadil) auf die pulmonale Hypertonie bei Patienten mit chronisch obstructiven Atemwegserkrankungen (COPD). [Effect of prostaglandin El (alprostadil) on pulmonary hypertension in patients with chronic obstructive respiratory tract diseases (COPD).] Prax Klin Pneumol 1988;42(7):521–4.

34. Sinzinger H, Fitscha P. Leberfunktionsparameter und Fibrinogen bei i.a. und i.v. PGE1-infusion. [Liver function parameters and fibrinogen in intra-arterial and intravenous PGE1 infusion.] Wien Klin Wochenschr 1988;100(14):488–90.

35. Walmrath D, Schneider T, Pilch J, Grimminger F, Seeger W. Aerosolised prostacyclin in adult respiratory distress syndrome. Lancet 1993;342(8877):961–2.

36. Walmrath D, Schneider T, Pilch J, Schermuly R, Grimminger F, Seeger W. Effects of aerosolized prostacyclin in severe pneumonia. Impact of fibrosis. Am J Respir Crit Care Med 1995;151(3 Pt 1):724–30.

37. Bindl L, Fahnenstich H, Peukert U. Aerosolised prostacyclin for pulmonary hypertension in neonates. Arch Dis Child Fetal Neonatal Ed 1994;71(3):F214–16.

38. Darius H, Nixdorff U, Zander J, Rupprecht HJ, Erbel R, Meyer J. Effects of ciprostene on restenosis rate during therapeutic transluminal coronary angioplasty. Agents Actions Suppl 1992;37:305–11.

39. Zusman RM, Rubin RH, Cato AE, Cocchetto DM, Crow JW, Tolkoff-Rubin N. Hemodialysis using prostacyclin instead of heparin as the sole antithrombotic agent. N Engl J Med 1981;304(16):934–9.

40. O'Keefe SJ, Spitaels JM, Mannion G, Naiker N. Misoprostol, a synthetic prostaglandin E1 analogue, in the treatment of duodenal ulcers. A double-blind, cimetidine-controlled trial. S Afr Med J 1985;67(9):321–4.

41. Graham DY, White RH, Moreland LW, Schubert TT, Katz R, Jaszewski R, Tindall E, Triadafilopoulos G, Stromatt SC, Teoh LS. Duodenal and gastric ulcer prevention with misoprostol in arthritis patients taking NSAIDs. Misoprostol Study Group. Ann Intern Med 1993;119(4):257–62.

42. Grazioli I, Avossa M, Bogliolo A, Broggini M, Carcassi A, Carcassi U, Cecconami L, Ligniere GC, Colombo B, Consoli G, et al. Multicenter study of the safety/efficacy of misoprostol in the prevention and treatment of NSAID-induced gastroduodenal lesions. Clin Exp Rheumatol 1993;11(3):289–94.

43. Wilkie ME, Davies GR, Marsh FP, Rampton DS. Effects of indomethacin and misoprostol on renal function in healthy volunteers. Clin Nephrol 1992;38(6):334–7.

44. Goldin E, Fich A, Eliakim R, Zimmerman J, Ligumsky M, Rachmilewitz D. Comparison of misoprostol and ranitidine in the treatment of duodenal ulcer. Isr J Med Sci 1988;24(6):282–5.

45. Wilson DE. Misoprostol and gastroduodenal mucosal protection (cytoprotection). Postgrad Med J 1988;64 (Suppl 1): 7–11.

46. Watkinson G, Hopkins A, Akbar FA. The therapeutic efficacy of misoprostol in peptic ulcer disease. Postgrad Med J 1988;64(Suppl 1):60–77.

47. Lange AP, Secher NJ, Westergaard JG, Skovgard I. Neonatal jaundice after labour induced or stimulated by prostaglandin E2 or oxytocin. Lancet 1982;1(8279):991–4.

48. Greig PD, Woolf GM, Sinclair SB, Abecassis M, Strasberg SM, Taylor BR, Blendis LM, Superina RA, Glynn MF, Langer B, Levy GA. Treatment of primary liver graft nonfunction with prostaglandin E1. Transplantation 1989;48(3):447–53.

49. Flowers M, Sherker A, Sinclair SB, Greig PD, Cameron R, Phillips MJ, Blendis L, Chung SW, Levy GA. Prostaglandin E in the treatment of recurrent hepatitis B infection after orthotopic liver transplantation. Transplantation 1994;58(2):183–92.

50. Tancharoen S, Jones RM, Angus PW, Michell ID, McNicol L, Hardy KJ. Prostaglandin E1 therapy in orthotopic liver transplantation recipients: indications and outcome. Transplant Proc 1992;24(5):2248–9.

51. Cattral MS, Altraif I, Greig PD, Blendis L, Levy GA. Toxic effects of intravenous and oral prostaglandin E therapy in patients with liver disease. Am J Med 1994;97(4):369–73.

52. Strachan JR, Pryor JP. Prostacyclin in the treatment of painful Peyronie's disease. Br J Urol 1988;61(6):516–17.

53. Waldhauser M, Schramek P. Efficiency and side effects of prostaglandin E1 in the treatment of erectile dysfunction. J Urol 1988;140(3):525–7.

54. Derouet H, Weirauch A, Bewermeier H. Prostaglandin E1 (PGE1) in der Diagnostik und Langzeittherapie der erektilen Dysfunktion. [Prostaglandin E1 (PGE1) in diagnosis and long-term therapy of erectile dysfunction.] Urologe A 1996;35(1):62–7.

55. Lea AP, Bryson HM, Balfour JA. Intracavernous alprostadil. A review of its pharmacodynamic and pharmacokinetic properties and therapeutic potential in erectile dysfunction. Drugs Aging 1996;8(1):56–74.

56. Canale D, Giorgi PM, Lencioni R, Morelli G, Gasperi M, Macchia E. Long-term intracavernous self-injection with prostaglandin E1 for the treatment of erectile dysfunction. Int J Androl 1996;19(1):28–32.

57. The European Alprostadil Study Group. The long-term safety of alprostadil (prostaglandin-E1) in patients with erectile dysfunction. Br J Urol 1998;82(4):538–43.

58. Colli E, Calabro A, Gentile V, Mirone V, Soli M. Alprostadil sterile powder formulation for intracavernous treatment of erectile dysfunction. Eur Urol 1996;29(1):59–62.

59. Chen J, Godschalk M, Katz PG, Mulligan T. The lowest effective dose of prostaglandin E1 as treatment for erectile dysfunction. J Urol 1995;153(1):80–1.

60. Lowe FC, Jarow JP. Placebo-controlled study of oral terbutaline and pseudoephedrine in management of prostaglandin E1-induced prolonged erections. Urology 1993;42(1):51–4.

61. Chen J, Godschalk M, Katz PG, Mulligan T. Peyronie's-like plaque after penile injection of prostaglandin E1. J Urol 1994;152(3):961–2.

62. Linet OI, Ogrinc FG. Efficacy and safety of intracavernosal alprostadil in men with erectile dysfunction. The Alprostadil Study Group. N Engl J Med 1996; 334(14):873–7.

63. Hemal AK, Vaidyanathan S, Sankaranarayanan A, Ayyagari S, Sharma PL. Control of massive vesical hemorrhage due to radiation cystitis with intravesical instillation of 15 (s) 15-methyl prostaglandin F2-alpha. Int J Clin Pharmacol Ther Toxicol 1988;26(10):477–8.

64. Levine LA, Jarrard DF. Treatment of cyclophosphamide-induced hemorrhagic cystitis with intravesical carboprost tromethamine. J Urol 1993;149(4):719–23.

65. Trigg ME, O'Reilly J, Rumelhart S, Morgan D, Holida M, de Alarcon P. Prostaglandin E1 bladder instillations to control severe hemorrhagic cystitis. J Urol 1990; 143(1):92–4.

66. Flach AJ, Eliason JA. Topical prostaglandin E2 effects on normal human intraocular pressure. J Ocul Pharmacol 1988;4(1):13–8.

67. Lee PY, Shao H, Xu LA, Qu CK. The effect of prostaglandin F2 alpha on intraocular pressure in normotensive human subjects. Invest Ophthalmol Vis Sci 1988;29(10):1474–7.

68. Patel SS, Spencer CM. Latanoprost. A review of its pharmacological properties, clinical efficacy and tolerability in the management of primary open-angle glaucoma and ocular hypertension. Drugs Aging 1996;9(5):363–78.

69. Serle JB. Pharmacological advances in the treatment of glaucoma. Drugs Aging 1994;5(3):156–70.

70. Rulo AH, Greve EL, Hoyng PF. Additive effect of latanoprost, a prostaglandin F2 alpha analogue, and timolol in patients with elevated intraocular pressure. Br J Ophthalmol 1994;78(12):899–902.

71. Stjernschantz JW, Albert DM, Hu DN, Drago F, Wistrand PJ. Mechanism and clinical significance of prostaglandin-induced iris pigmentation. Surv Ophthalmol 2002;47(Suppl 1):S162–75.

72. Fristrom B. A 6-month, randomized, double-masked comparison of latanoprost with timolol in patients with open angle glaucoma or ocular hypertension. Acta Ophthalmol Scand 1996;74(2):140–4.

73. Watson P, Stjernschantz J. A six-month, randomized, double-masked study comparing latanoprost with timolol in open-angle glaucoma and ocular hypertension. The Latanoprost Study Group. Ophthalmology 1996;103(1): 126–37.

74. Camras CB. Comparison of latanoprost and timolol in patients with ocular hypertension and glaucoma: a six-month masked, multicenter trial in the United States. The United States Latanoprost Study Group. Ophthalmology 1996;103(1):138–47.

75. Chernin T. The eyes have it. FDA clears several ophthalmic drops for glaucoma in a row. Drug Topics 2001;145:20.

76. Schumer RA, Camras CB, Mandahl AK. Putative side effects of prostaglandin analogues. Surv Ophthalmol 2002;47(Suppl 1):S219.

77. Linden C. Therapeutic potential of prostaglandin analogues in glaucoma. Expert Opin Investig Drugs 2001;10(4):679–94.

78. Wand M, Ritch R, Isbey EK Jr, Zimmerman TJ. Latanoprost and periocular skin color changes. Arch Ophthalmol 2001;119(4):614–15.

79. Ekatomatis P. Herpes simplex dendritic keratitis after treatment with latanoprost for primary open angle glaucoma. Br J Ophthalmol 2001;85(8):1008–9.

80. Sacca S, Pascotto A, Siniscalchi C, Rolando M. Ocular complications of latanoprost in uveitic glaucoma: three case reports. J Ocul Pharmacol Ther 2001;17(2):107–13.

81. Mitra M, Chang B, James T. Drug points. Exacerbation of angina associated with latanoprost. BMJ 2001; 323(7316):783.

82. Weston BC. Migraine headache associated with latanoprost. Arch Ophthalmol 2001;119(2):300–1.

83. Hayashi RH, Castillo MS, Noah ML. Management of severe postpartum hemorrhage due to uterine atony using an analogue of prostaglandin F2 alpha. Obstet Gynecol 1981;58(4):426–9.

84. Pulkkinen MO, Kajanoja P, Kivikoski A, Saastamoinen J, Selander K, Tuimala R. Abortion with sulprostone, a prostaglandin E2 derivative. Int J Gynaecol Obstet 1980;18(1):40–3.

85. Robins J, Surrago EJ. Alternatives in midtrimester abortion induction. Obstet Gynecol 1980;56(6):716–22.

86. Thong KJ, Robertson AJ, Baird DT. A retrospective study of 932 second trimester terminations using gemeprost (16,16 dimethyl-trans delta 2 PGE1 methyl ester). Prostaglandins 1992;44(1):65–74.

87. Hill NCW, Selinger M, Ferguson J, MacKenzie IZ. Management of intra-uterine fetal death with vaginal administration of gemeprost or prostaglandin E2: a random allocation controlled trial. J Obstet Gynaecol 1991;11:422–6.

88. Poulsen HK, Moller LK, Westergaard JG, Thomsen SG, Giersson RT, Arngrimsson R. Open randomized comparison of prostaglandin E2 given by intracervical gel or vagitory for preinduction cervical ripening and induction of labor. Acta Obstet Gynecol Scand 1991;70(7–8):549–53.

89. Jaschevatzky OE, Dascalu S, Noy Y, Rosenberg RP, Anderman S, Ballas S. Intrauterine PGF2 alpha infusion for termination of pregnancies with second-trimester rupture of membranes. Obstet Gynecol 1992;79(1):32–4.

90. Egarter C, Husslein P. Treatment of tubal pregnancy by prostaglandins. Lancet 1988;1(8594):1104–5.

91. Eckford S, Fox R. Intratubal injection of prostaglandin in ectopic pregnancy. Lancet 1993;342(8874):803.

92. England MJ, Tjallinks A, Hofmeyr J, Harber J. Suppression of lactation. A comparison of bromocriptine and prostaglandin E2. J Reprod Med 1988;33(7):630–2.

93. Lee JB. Cardiovascular–renal effects of prostaglandins: the antihypertensive, natriuretic renal "endocrine" function. Arch Intern Med 1974;133(1):56–76.

94. Olsson AG, Carlson LA. Clinical, hemodynamic and metabolic effects of intraarterial infusions of prostaglandin E1 in patients with peripheral vascular disease. Adv Prostaglandin Thromboxane Res 1976;1:429–32.

95. Bugiardini R, Galvani M, Ferrini D, Gridelli C, Tollemeto D, Mari L, Puddu P, Lenzi S. Myocardial ischemia induced by prostacyclin and iloprost. Clin Pharmacol Ther 1985;38(1):101–8.

96. Fliers E, Duren DR, van Zwieten PA. A prostaglandin analogue as a probable cause of myocardial infarction in a young woman. BMJ 1991;302(6773):416.

97. Lennox CE, Martin J. Cardiac arrest following intramyometrial prostaglandin E2. J Obstet Gynaecol 1991;11:263–4.

98. Meyer WJ, Benton SL, Hoon TJ, Gauthier DW, Whiteman VE. Acute myocardial infarction associated with prostaglandin E2. Am J Obstet Gynecol 1991;165(2):359–60.

99. White JL, Fleming NW, Burke TA, Katz NM, Moront MG, Kim YD. Pulmonary edema after PGE1 infusion. J Cardiothorac Anesth 1990;4(6):744–7.

100. Smith AP, Cuthbert MF. The response of normal and asthmatic subjects to prostaglandins E2 and F2alpha by different routes, and their significance in asthma. Adv Prostaglandin Thromboxane Res 1976;1:449–59.

101. Fishburne JI Jr, Brenner WE, Braaksma JT, Hendricks CH. Bronchospasm complicating intravenous prostaglandin F 2a for therapeutic abortion. Obstet Gynecol 1972;39(6):892–6.

102. Milton AS. Modern views on the pathogenesis of fever and the mode of action of antipyretic drugs. J Pharm Pharmacol 1976;28(Suppl 4):393–9.

103. Callen PJ, de Louvois J, Hurley R, Trudinger BJ. Intrapartum and postpartum pyrexia and infection after induction with extra-amniotic prostaglandin E2 in tylose. Br J Obstet Gynaecol 1980;87(6):513–18.

104. Haller U, Kubli R. Klinische Nebenwirkungen und Komplikationen der Prostaglandine bei Abortinduktion. Gynekologie 1978;11:39.

105. Lyneham RC, Low PA, McLeod JC, Shearman RP, Smith ID, Korda AR. Convulsions and electroencephalogram abnormalities after intra-amniotic prostaglandin F2a. Lancet 1973;2(7836):1003–5.

106. Sederberg-Olsen J, Olsen CE. Prostaglandin–oxytocin induction of mid-trimester abortion complicated by grand mal-like seizures. Acta Obstet Gynecol Scand 1983; 62(1):79–81.

107. Rachmilewitz D. Prostaglandins and diarrhea. Dig Dis Sci 1980;25(12):897–9.

108. Kirton KT, Kimball FA, Porteus SE. Reproductive physiology: prostaglandin-associated events. Adv Prostaglandin Thromboxane Res 1976;2:621–5.

109. Cederqvist LL, Birnbaum SJ. Rupture of the uterus after midtrimester prostaglandin abortion. J Reprod Med 1980;25(3):136–8.

110. Bromham DR, Anderson RS. Uterine scar rupture in labour induced with vaginal prostaglandin E2. Lancet 1980;2(8192):485–6.

111. El-Etriby EK, Daw E. Rupture of the cervix during prostaglandin termination of pregnancy. Postgrad Med J 1981;57(666):265–6.

112. Sawyer MM, Lipshitz J, Anderson GD, Dilts PV Jr. Third-trimester uterine rupture associated with vaginal prostaglandin E2. Am J Obstet Gynecol 1981;140(6):710–11.

113. Geirsson RT. Uterine rupture following induction of labour with prostaglandin E2 pessaries, an oxytocin infusion and epidural analgesia. J Obstet Gynecol 1981;2:76.

114. Thavarasah AS, Achanna KS. Uterine rupture with the use of Cervagem (prostaglandin E1) for induction of labour on account of intrauterine death. Singapore Med J 1988;29(4):351–2.

115. Maymon R, Shulman A, Pomeranz M, Holtzinger M, Haimovich L, Bahary C. Uterine rupture at term pregnancy with the use of intracervical prostaglandin E2 gel for induction of labor. Am J Obstet Gynecol 1991;165(2):368–70.

116. Maymon R, Haimovich L, Shulman A, Pomeranz M, Holtzinger M, Bahary C. Third-trimester uterine rupture after prostaglandin E2 use for labor induction. J Reprod Med 1992;37(5):449–52.

117. Azem F, Jaffa A, Lessing JB, Peyser MR. Uterine rupture with the use of a low-dose vaginal PGE2 tablet. Acta Obstet Gynecol Scand 1993;72(4):316–17.

118. Gonzalez CH, Vargas FR, Perez AB, Kim CA, Brunoni D, Marques-Dias MJ, Leone CR, Correa Neto J, Llerena Junior JC, de Almeida JC. Limb deficiency with or without Mobius sequence in seven Brazilian children associated with misoprostol use in the first trimester of pregnancy. Am J Med Genet 1993;47(1):59–64.

119. Quinn MA, Murphy AJ. Fetal death following extra-amniotic prostaglandin gel. Report of two cases. Br J Obstet Gynaecol 1981;88(6):650–1.

120. Beck I, Clayton JK. Hazards of prostaglandin pessaries in postmaturity. Lancet 1982;2(8290):161.

121. Chattopadhyay SK, Sherbeeni MM, Anokute CC. Planned vaginal delivery after two previous caesarean sections. Br J Obstet Gynaecol 1994;101(6):498–500.

122. Quinn MA, Shekleton PA, Wein R, Kloss M. Single dose extra-amniotic prostaglandin gel for midtrimester termination of pregnancy. Aust NZ J Obstet Gynaecol 1980;20(2):77–9.

123. Moncada S, Ferreira SH, Vane JR. Sensitization of pain receptors of dog knee joint by prostaglandins. In: Robinson HJ, Vane JR, editors. Prostaglandin Synthetase Inhibitors. New York: Raven Press, 1974:189.

124. Ferreira SH, Moncada S, Vane JR. Prostaglandins and signs and symptoms of inflammation. In: Robinson HJ, Vane JR, editors. Prostaglandin Synthetase Inhibitors. New York: Raven Press, 1974:175.

125. Hoeper MM, Olschewski H, Ghofrani HA, Wilkens H, Winkler J, Borst MM, Niedermeyer J, Fabel H, Seeger W, Grimminger F, et al. A comparison of the acute hemodynamic effects of inhaled nitric oxide and aerosolized iloprost in primary pulmonary hypertension. German PPH study group. J Am Coll Cardiol 2000;35(1):176–82.

126. Voelkel NF, Lobel K, Westcott JY, Burke TJ. Nitric oxide-related vasoconstriction in lungs perfused with red cell lysate. FASEB J 1995;9(5):379–86.

127. Hoeper MM, Schwarze M, Ehlerding S, Adler-Schuermeyer A, Spiekerkoetter E, Niedermeyer J, Hamm M, Fabel H. Long-term treatment of primary pulmonary hypertension with aerosolized iloprost, a prostacyclin analogue. N Engl J Med 2000;342(25):1866–70.

128. Schenk P, Petkov V, Madl C, Kramer L, Kneussl M, Ziesche R, Lang I. Aerosolized iloprost therapy could not replace long-term IV epoprostenol (prostacyclin) administration in severe pulmonary hypertension. Chest 2001;119(1):296–300.

129. Haraldsson A, Kieler-Jensen N, Wadenvik H, Ricksten SE. Inhaled prostacyclin and platelet function after cardiac surgery and cardiopulmonary bypass. Intensive Care Med 2000;26(2):188–94.

Protamine

General Information

Protamine, derived from salmon sperm, combines with and neutralizes heparin through an acid-base interaction. It is most commonly used as the sulfate, but chloride and hydrochloride salts are also occasionally used.

The relative insolubility of protamine–insulin suspension in water slows the subcutaneous resorption of the hormone, and consequently prolongs its biological activity.

In a prospective study of patients undergoing cardiopulmonary bypass, 10.7% of patients receiving protamine sulfate had adverse reactions of varying types (1).

Protamine sulfate regularly induces hypotension, bradycardia, transient flushing, and a feeling of warmth when administered too rapidly. These non-allergic effects are not severe, provided the injection is given slowly (50 mg, the maximum recommended dose, over 10 minutes).

Comparative studies

In a double-blind, randomized trial, 167 patients undergoing aortocoronary bypass graft surgery received

either heparinase I (maximum 35 µg/kg) or protamine (maximum 650 mg) for heparin reversal (2). Although the two treatments had similar efficacy, protamine had a better safety profile. Those given heparinase I had longer hospital stays, were more likely to have a serious adverse event, and were less likely to avoid transfusion. A composite morbidity score was not different, and there were similar rates of hemodynamic instability.

Organs and Systems

Cardiovascular

Severe acute pulmonary vasoconstriction with cardiovascular collapse was identified in 1983 and subsequent studies showed that the incidence of protamine-induced pulmonary artery vasoconstriction was about 1.5% after cardiac surgery (3). Protamine-induced pulmonary artery vasoconstriction is accompanied by generation of large quantities of thromboxane A_2, a potent vasoconstrictor (3).

The precise mechanisms that explain protamine-mediated systemic hypotension are unknown, but there is evidence that it may be mediated by the endothelium and dependent on nitric oxide/cyclic guanosine monophosphate; it has been suggested that methylthioninium chloride (methylene blue) may be of use in treating hemodynamic complications caused by the use of protamine after cardiopulmonary bypass (4).

Immunologic

Although protamine itself was for a long time not generally considered allergenic, allergic reactions can occur in susceptible individuals. Attributed to residual fish antigens that remained after purification, they are characterized by flushing, urticaria, wheezing, angioedema, and hypotension, and they can occur even after slow intravenous administration. True anaphylaxis with bronchospasm and/or anaphylactic shock is very rare (5).

It now seems to be widely believed that, exceptionally, protamine itself can act as an allergen. There were positive skin tests with protamine in patients who had anaphylaxis and who had all previously received protamine (5). Cases of anaphylactic shock after slow intravenous administration of protamine sulfate to patients with diabetes mellitus suggested cross-allergy to protamine present in protamine zinc insulin (6–8), especially in patients with serum antiprotamine IgE or IgG antibodies (9). Insulin-dependent patients with diabetes who use protamine insulin may be at greater risk of adverse effects when they receive protamine sulfate. A retrospective study in patients who received protamine sulfate to reverse the effects of heparin during catheterization procedures or cardiac surgery showed a relative risk of anaphylaxis four times higher in patients with diabetes who had used protamine insulin than in non-diabetic controls (10). In these patients, the risk of anaphylaxis on administration of protamine sulfate is about 1%.

References

1. Weiler JM, Gellhaus MA, Carter JG, Meng RL, Benson PM, Hottel RA, Schillig KB, Vegh AB, Clarke WR. A prospective study of the risk of an immediate adverse reaction to protamine sulfate during cardiopulmonary bypass surgery. J Allergy Clin Immunol 1990;85(4):713–19.
2. Stafford-Smith M, Lefrak EA, Qazi AG, Welsby IJ, Barber L, Hoeft A, Dorenbaum A, Mathias J, Rochon JJ, Newman MF; Members of the Global Perioperative Research Organization. Efficacy and safety of heparinase I versus protamine in patients undergoing coronary artery bypass grafting with and without cardiopulmonary bypass. Anesthesiology 2005;103(2):229–40.
3. Lowenstein E, Zapol WM. Protamine reactions, explosive mediator release, and pulmonary vasoconstriction. Anesthesiology 1990;73(3):373–5.
4. Viaro F, Dalio MB, Evora PR. Catastrophic cardiovascular adverse reactions to protamine are nitric oxide/cyclic guanosine monophosphate dependent and endothelium mediated: should methylene blue be the treatment of choice? Chest 2002;122(3):1061–6.
5. Doolan L, McKenzie I, Krafchek J, Parsons B, Buxton B. Protamine sulphate hypersensitivity. Anaesth Intensive Care 1981;9(2):147–9.
6. Gottschlich GM, Gravlee GP, Georgitis JW. Adverse reactions to protamine sulfate during cardiac surgery in diabetic and non-diabetic patients. Ann Allergy 1988;61(4):277–81.
7. Gupta SK, Veith FJ, Ascer E, Wengerter KR, Franco C, Amar D, el-Gaweet ES, Gupta A. Anaphylactoid reactions to protamine: an often lethal complication in insulin-dependent diabetic patients undergoing vascular surgery. J Vasc Surg 1989;9(2):342–50.
8. Stewart WJ, McSweeney SM, Kellett MA, Faxon DP, Ryan TJ. Increased risk of severe protamine reactions in NPH insulin-dependent diabetics undergoing cardiac catheterization. Circulation 1984;70(5):788–92.
9. Weiss ME, Nyhan D, Peng ZK, Horrow JC, Lowenstein E, Hirshman C, Adkinson NF Jr. Association of protamine IgE and IgG antibodies with life-threatening reactions to intravenous protamine. N Engl J Med 1989;320(14):886–92.
10. Vincent GM, Janowski M, Menlove R. Protamine allergy reactions during cardiac catheterization and cardiac surgery: risk in patients taking protamine–insulin preparations. Cathet Cardiovasc Diagn 1991;23(3):164–8.

Protease inhibitors

See also Individual agents

General Information

All the HIV protease inhibitors have in common a specific effect against the aspartic HIV protease that cleaves viral proteins to yield structural proteins. Competitive inhibition of this process by the protease inhibitors results in the production of immature, non-infectious virus particles. These drugs are also characterized by their high specificity, being more than a thousand-fold more active against viral than human aspartic proteases.

Combination therapy including a protease inhibitor resulted in the first breakthrough of antiviral treatment in the mid-1990s, since when several protease inhibitors have been developed. However, results from in vitro and clinical studies clearly showed that these drugs share a cross-resistance pattern, probably due to secondary conformational changes of the protease outside the active binding site of the protease inhibitor. Nevertheless, some patients may benefit from a second protease inhibitor if therapy is promptly switched before multiple mutations have accumulated.

Drug interactions with protease inhibitors

Drug interactions with protease inhibitors, which are potent inhibitors of CYP3A4 and CYP2D6, have been comprehensively reviewed (1), and an updated summary of interactions is presented on the World Wide Web by the University of Liverpool (http://www.hiv-druginteractions.org); the drugs that should not be co-administered with protease inhibitors are summarized in Table 1.

Interactions between protease inhibitors

Evidence suggests that some protease inhibitors can inhibit the metabolism of others. For example, ritonavir inhibits CYP3A4 and CYP2D6 and has been used to enhance the actions of other protease inhibitors, by inhibiting their clearance (2).

In an open, randomized study of amprenavir combined with indinavir, nelfinavir, and saquinavir (3), saquinavir lowered the amprenavir AUC by 32%; amprenavir did not alter the pharmacokinetics of saquinavir. The amprenavir AUC increased by 35% when it was combined with indinavir, and indinavir concentrations also fell, suggesting that this protease inhibitor combination should be avoided. There was no significant interaction of amprenavir with nelfinavir.

In attempts to lower the amprenavir capsule burden, low-dose ritonavir has been used as a pharmacokinetic booster. When ritonavir was added to amprenavir, the amprenavir AUC increased 3–4 times (4), which should allow the total daily capsule burden to be reduced. Adverse effects included diarrhea, nausea, paresthesia, rash, increased cholesterol, and increased triglycerides. The frequency of adverse events correlated with the dose of ritonavir.

In nine patients who received amprenavir 750 mg bd for at least 3 weeks plus one of two doses of lopinavir + ritonavir, the trough concentration of amprenavir was 0.35–2.54 with lopinavir + ritonavir 400/100 mg bd ($n = 5$) and 1.92–2.83 with lopinavir + ritonavir 532/133 mg bd ($n = 4$); the corresponding trough concentrations of lopinavir were 0.35–2.54 and 4.74–6.71 (5).

A pharmacokinetic model has been developed to describe the interaction of amprenavir with ritonavir (6). A two-compartment linear model with first-order absorption fitted the amprenavir data best, while a one-compartment model best described the ritonavir data. Inhibition of the elimination of amprenavir by ritonavir was modelled with an E_{max} inhibition model. Simulation of drug regimens based on the model suggested that in patients who fail to respond to a traditional amprenavir regimen, amprenavir 600 mg plus ritonavir 100 mg bd would produce similar C_{min}:IC_{50} ratios to amprenavir 1200 mg bd alone.

Using ritonavir as a booster allows indinavir to be given twice daily and with food. In a cohort survey of 100

Table 1   Drugs that should not be co-administered with protease inhibitors

Drug	APV	ATV	IDV	LPV	NFV	RTV	SQV
Alprazolam			x				
Amiodarone			x	x	x	x	x
Astemizole	x	x	x	x	x	x	x
Atazanavir			x				
Bepridil		x				x	x
Cisapride	x	x	x	x	x	x	x
Clorazepate						x	
Diazepam	x					x	
Ergot derivatives	x	x	x	x	x	x	x
Estazolam						x	
Flecainide	x	x	x	x		x	x
Flurazepam	x					x	
Halofantrine	x	x	x	x	x	x	x
Indinavir		x					
Lovastatin	x	x	x	x	x	x	x
Lumefantrine	x	x	x	x	x	x	x
Midazolam	x	x	x	x	x	x	x
Pethidine						x	
Pimozide	x	x	x	x	x	x	x
Piroxicam						x	
Propafenone	x	x				x	x
Quinidine		x			x	x	x
Rifabutin							x
Rifampicin	x	x	x	x			x
Simvastatin	x	x	x	x	x	x	x
St John's wort	x	x	x	x	x	x	x
Terfenadine	x	x	x	x	x	x	x
Triazolam	x	x	x	x	x	x	x
Vardenafil			x			x	
Vitamin E	x						
Voriconazole						x	
Zolpidem						x	

APV = amprenavir and fosamprenavir
ATV = atazanavir
IDV = indinavir
LPV = lopinavir
NFV = nelfinavir
RTV = ritonavir
SQV = saquinavir

patients the combination of indinavir plus ritonavir (400 mg/400 mg or 800 mg/100 mg bd) was a safe and effective option to reduce the tablet burden and improve adherence (7).

Observational studies

Combinations of NRTIs and protease inhibitors
A variable-dose plasma concentration-controlled approach to combination antiretroviral therapy (zidovudine, lamivudine, and indinavir) has been compared with conventional fixed-dose therapy in 40 patients in a randomized, 52-week, open trial (8). Significantly more concentration-controlled recipients achieved the desired concentrations for all three drugs: there was a good response in 15 of 16 concentration-controlled recipients compared with nine of 17 conventional regimen recipients. However, there was no difference in the occurrence of drug-related clinical events or laboratory abnormalities between the two regimens. Three patients withdrew because of gastrointestinal adverse effects, one because

of a peripheral neuropathy, and one with headache and anemia. There was nephrolithiasis in four cases.

The combination of indinavir + ritonavir 400/400 mg bd plus two NRTIs has been studied in 93 patients in an open, uncontrolled, multicenter trial (9). Raised triglycerides ($n = 78$) and cholesterol ($n = 63$) were the commonest adverse effects, followed by nausea ($n = 22$) and circumoral paresthesia ($n = 9$). Withdrawal was required in four cases of nausea, four of lipodystrophy, one of diarrhea, and one of osteonecrosis.

Combinations of NRTIs, NNRTIs, and protease inhibitors
In an open, 48-week, single-arm, multicenter phase II study in 99 patients abacavir 300 mg bd, amprenavir 1200 mg bd, and efavirenz 600 mg/day were associated with rashes in 50 patients, possibly because of abacavir hypersensitivity; 17 permanently discontinued one or more drugs as a result (10). Other adverse effects included nausea ($n = 41$), diarrhea ($n = 27$), sleep disorders ($n = 27$), dizziness ($n = 25$), fatigue ($n = 23$),

Table 2 Numbers (%) of infants and children with moderate or severe adverse events in a study of one or two NRTIs plus an NNRTI and/or a protease inhibitor

System affected by the adverse event	Regimen			
	Stavudine + nevirapine + ritonavir ($n = 41$)	Stavudine + nevirapine + nelfinavir ($n = 44$)	Stavudine + lamivudine + nevirapine + nelfinavir ($n = 44$)	Stavudine + lamivudine + nelfinavir ($n = 52$)
Respiratory	12 (29)	18 (41)	23 (52)	50 (96)
Hematologic (neutropenia)	17 (41)	9 (20)	14 (32)	23 (44)
Gastrointestinal				
Nausea/vomiting	29 (71)	32 (73)	18 (41)	15 (29)
Other	10 (24)	25 (27)	18 (41)	19 (37)
Liver	12 (29)	14 (32)	18 (41)	23 (44)
Skin	27 (66)	41 (93)*	32 (73)	17 (33)*
Body temperature (fever)	24 (59)	30 (68)*	20 (45)	10 (19)*

*Significantly different from the other groups

hypertriglyceridemia ($n = 18$), neutropenia ($n = 8$), hyperamylasemia ($n = 4$), leukopenia ($n = 3$), hypercholesterolemia ($n = 2$), raised alkaline phosphatase ($n = 1$), and raised aspartate transaminase ($n = 1$).

In infants and children assigned to different combinations of one or two NRTIs plus an NNRTI and/or a protease inhibitor, the numbers of patients with moderate or severe adverse events were as shown in Table 2 (11). In cases of rash, the rash was worse in those who were taking nevirapine-containing regimens.

Organs and Systems

Nervous system

In a randomized comparison of a protease inhibitor-containing regimen and an efavirenz-containing regimen, nervous system adverse effects were specifically sought (12). Patients were randomized to two NRTIs plus one or more protease inhibitors ($n = 49$) or two NRTIs plus efavirenz ($n = 51$). The patients who took the protease inhibitors reported the following at week 4: light-headedness (8%), dizziness (5%), difficulty in sleeping (4%), nervousness (4%), and headaches (3%). They reported the following at week 48: difficulty in sleeping (4%), nervousness (3%), headaches (3%), and light-headedness (2%). Three patients withdrew because of adverse events: diarrhea ($n = 2$) and nephrolithiasis ($n = 1$).

Sensory systems

- Lipemia retinalis and pancreatitis have been reported in a 39-year-old man with HIV infection associated with protease inhibitor therapy (13). He developed lipemia retinalis after switching to an antiretroviral regimen including ritonavir and saquinavir (together with zalcitabine and delavirdine). He had previously been taking zidovudine, lamivudine, and indinavir.

The ophthalmoscopic changes of lipemia retinalis include a milky-white discoloration of the retinal vessels, beginning at the periphery but progressing to involve the posterior pole as the triglyceride concentration rises. The fundus can appear salmon-colored, owing to the effect

of triglycerides on the choroidal circulation. Experience from HIV-negative patients with hyperlipidemia has shown that plasma triglyceride concentrations must be at least 28 mmol/l (2500 mg/dl) for lipemia retinalis to occur (reference value below 1.52 mmol/l). This patient had a plasma triglyceride concentration of 53 mmol/l. On withdrawal of ritonavir and saquinavir the appearance of his retinal vessels returned to normal in parallel with a fall in his plasma triglycerides.

Endocrine

Two case reports have suggested that when a protease inhibitor is used with a glucocorticoid the tendency to adverse corticosteroid effects is potentiated (14,15). Two HIV-positive patients developed severely disfiguring skin striae within 3 months of starting indinavir therapy (16).

Metabolism

Metabolic changes that protease inhibitors can cause after prolonged therapy include raised serum lactate, hypogonadism, hypertension and accelerated cardiovascular disease, reduced bone density, and avascular necrosis of the hip. Two large prospective studies in 1207 patients (17) and 3191 patients (18) have clarified the spectrum and incidence of metabolic changes in HAART and have explored the relative importance of protease inhibitors. In addition, data on fat redistribution from a postmarketing review of HIV-infected individuals taking indinavir have been published (19).

Blood glucose concentration

Protease inhibitors can cause a rise in blood glucose concentration, although only a few cases have been reported. Patients with a family history of diabetes mellitus may be at a greater risk, and they demand especially close monitoring, for example with both baseline and quarterly glucose determinations, at least during the first 6–12 months of treatment (20,21).

Dyslipidemias

While abnormal concentrations of circulating lipids are common in patients with HIV infection (usually hypercholesterolemia and moderate hypertriglyceridemia), there is no doubt that some members of this group of drugs can cause much more marked changes. The possible differences between the effects of various protease inhibitors on the lipid spectrum have been characterized in 93 HIV-infected adults taking ritonavir, indinavir, or nelfinavir, alone or in combination with saquinavir (22). There was a rise in plasma cholesterol concentration in all those who took a protease inhibitor, but it was more pronounced with ritonavir than with indinavir or nelfinavir. Plasma HDL cholesterol was unchanged. Ritonavir, but not indinavir or nelfinavir, was associated with a marked rise in plasma triglyceride concentrations. The combination of ritonavir or nelfinavir with saquinavir did not further alter plasma lipid concentrations. There was a 48% increase in plasma concentrations of lipoprotein(a) in those taking a protease inhibitor, with pretreatment values exceeding 200 µg/ml. There were similar changes in plasma lipid concentrations in six children taking ritonavir. The risk of pancreatitis and premature atherosclerosis as a consequence of such dyslipidemia remains to be established.

- A 35-year-old HIV-positive man developed a serum cholesterol concentration of 38 mmol/l and a fasting serum triglyceride concentration of 98 mmol/l after he started to take ritonavir, saquinavir, nevirapine, and didanosine (23). All other medications had been stable during this time; the condition resolved with antiretroviral drug withdrawal and lipid-lowering therapy. It was striking that the raised cholesterol and triglyceride concentrations did not recur when therapy was restarted in modified form with nelfinavir, saquinavir, nevirapine, and didanosine; the hyperlipidemia was therefore attributed to ritonavir.

In 19 consecutive HIV-positive men examined before and during treatment with a protease inhibitor (nelfinavir, ritonavir, or indinavir) and two nucleoside analogue reverse transcriptase inhibitors (NRTI), median treatment duration 22 (range 7–40) weeks, the predominant feature of dyslipidemia was an increase in triglyceride-containing lipoproteins (24). This observation is in accordance with the hypothesis of increased apoptosis of peripheral adipocytes, release of free fatty acids, and subsequent increased synthesis of VLDL cholesterol. The lipid profile, based on the ratio of total cholesterol to HDL cholesterol and the ratio HDL2 to HDL3, is significantly more atherogenic than normal.

Lipodystrophy

Soon after the introduction of highly active antiretroviral combination treatments (HAART), lipodystrophy was associated with the use of protease inhibitors, and several reports have confirmed that a syndrome of peripheral lipodystrophy, central adiposity, breast hypertrophy in women, hyperlipidemia, and insulin resistance with hyperglycemia is an adverse event associated with the use of potent combination antiretroviral therapy, particularly including HIV-1 protease inhibitors (25–30).

Peripheral lipodystrophy in patients is characterized by fat wasting of the face, limbs, buttocks, and upper trunk, while central adiposity can cause an increase in belly size ("Crix-belly" or "protease pouch") and an increase in the dorsocervical fat pad, creating the appearance of a

"buffalo hump" (31–33). These effects may be related to a glucocorticoid-like action. The increase in belly size is often associated with symptoms of abdominal fullness, distension, and bloating. This is probably due to a change in body fat distribution, with selective accumulation of fat intra-abdominally (34).

Lipodystrophy is not limited to patients taking protease inhibitors (35,36). Nevertheless, protease inhibitors are strongly associated with metabolic alterations and with lipodystrophy, while NRTIs are associated with low-grade lactic acidosis and less markedly with lipodystrophy. Some reports have speculated a link between mitochondrial dysfunction and lipodystrophy. It is clear, however, that the syndrome is related to total duration of antiviral therapy and inversely related to viral load.

In a longitudinal study from an Aquitaine cohort of more than 1400 subjects, hypertriglyceridemia was significantly associated with age, low viral load, and protease inhibitors, but not NRTIs or NNRTIs. However, lipodystrophy also occurred in patients naive to protease inhibitors (37).

- "Buffalo neck" was described in a middle-aged man taking indinavir who developed a lipomatous formation in the retrocervical area; abdominal fat also increased in volume, while the subcutaneous fat on the lower limbs decreased (38).

Of 494 patients during median follow-up of 18 months, 17% developed lipodystrophy (39). Study limitations included the short time of follow-up and the lack of a standardized and accepted definition of lipodystrophy.

Hematologic

There is still no clear explanation for a series of seven patients in whom treatment with various protease inhibitors was associated with early thrombosis (40). Hematological or vascular effects conducive to thrombosis are not recognized as a complication with this group of compounds; the only previous similar cases were associated with prolonged therapy.

In contrast, a detailed report on a large series of patients has provided impressive evidence that the use of protease inhibitors in HIV-infected patients with hereditary bleeding disorders can lead to an increased bleeding tendency (41). This effect, which is most likely to occur when ritonavir is used, is also unexplained.

Liver

In a retrospective study of patients taking one protease inhibitor ($n = 39$) or two ($n = 27$) who discontinued protease inhibitor therapy as a result of hepatotoxicity, the proportions of patients with raised alanine transaminase activity to at least five times the upper limit of the reference range (26 versus 19%) and hyperbilirubinemia (38 versus 30%) were similar (42). Rates of withdrawal due to hepatotoxicity were also similar.

Pancreas

- Lipemia retinalis and pancreatitis have been reported in a 39-year-old man with HIV infection associated with protease inhibitor therapy (13). His plasma triglyceride concentration was 53 mmol/l.

Urinary tract

In a randomized comparison of a protease inhibitor-containing regimen and an efavirenz-containing regimen in 100 patients, six patients taking protease inhibitors developed nephrolithiasis; one withdrew as a result (12).

Musculoskeletal

The results of a questionnaire survey of 878 people with HIV infection treated with antiretroviral drugs also suggested that other protease inhibitors can cause arthralgia; indinavir and the combination of ritonavir + saquinavir were particularly implicated (43).

Immunologic

A man developed several erythematous plaques on his face due to borderline tuberculoid leprosy with a reversal reaction (44). He had severe CD4 T cell lymphocytopenia due to HIV infection and had been given highly active antiretroviral therapy (HAART). A fall in viral load and an increase in CD4 count preceded the development of the skin lesions, suggesting immune reconstitution as the underlying mechanism for the reversal reaction. Paradoxical reactions are often observed in patients with pulmonary and extra-pulmonary tuberculosis being treated with HAART. Clinicians need to distinguish these from other adverse reactions related to drug therapy. Reversal reactions in leprosy are increasingly likely as more patients with HIV infection are treated with HAART in developing countries.

Drug–Drug Interactions

See also General information and Table 1.

Ecstasy

A patient infected with HIV-1 who was taking ritonavir and saquinavir had a prolonged effect from a small dose of methylenedioxymetamfetamine (MDMA, ecstasy) and a near-fatal reaction from a small dose of gammahydroxybutyrate (45).

Gammahydroxybutyrate

A patient infected with HIV-1 who was taking ritonavir and saquinavir had a prolonged effect from a small dose of MDMA and a near-fatal reaction from a small dose of gammahydroxybutyrate (45).

Statins

There has been a study of the effects of ritonavir 400 mg bd plus saquinavir soft-gel capsules 400 mg bd on the pharmacokinetics of pravastatin, simvastatin, and atorvastatin (40 mg/day each), and of the effect of pravastatin on the pharmacokinetics of nelfinavir in a randomized, open study in 56 healthy HIV-negative adults (46). Ritonavir + saquinavir reduced the steady-state AUC of pravastatin, markedly increased the AUC of simvastatin, and slightly increased the AUC of total active atorvastatin. The AUCs of nelfinavir and its active M8 metabolite were not altered by pravastatin. The authors concluded that simvastatin (and by implication lovastatin, which in

common with simvastatin inhibits CYP3A4) should be avoided and atorvastatin should be used with caution in people taking ritonavir and saquinavir, that dosage adjustment of pravastatin may be necessary with concomitant use of ritonavir + saquinavir, and that concomitant use of pravastatin with nelfinavir appears to be safe.

References

1. Malaty LI, Kuper JJ. Drug interactions of HIV protease inhibitors. Drug Saf 1999;20(2):147–69.
2. Rathbun RC, Rossi DR, Nazario M, Edouard B. Low-dose ritonavir for protease inhibitor pharmacokinetic enhancement. Ann Pharmacother 2002;36(4):702–6.
3. Sadler BM, Gillotin C, Lou Y, Eron JJ, Lang W, Haubrich R, Stein DS. Pharmacokinetic study of human immunodeficiency virus protease inhibitors used in combination with amprenavir. Antimicrob Agents Chemother 2001;45(12):3663–8.
4. Sadler BM, Gillotin C, Lou Y, Stein DS. Pharmacokinetic and pharmacodynamic study of the human immunodeficiency virus protease inhibitor amprenavir after multiple oral dosing. Antimicrob Agents Chemother 2001;45(1):30–7.
5. Khanlou H, Graham E, Brill M, Farthing C. Drug interaction between amprenavir and lopinavir/ritonavir in salvage therapy. AIDS 2002;16(5):797–8.
6. Sale M, Sadler BM, Stein DS. Pharmacokinetic modeling and simulations of interaction of amprenavir and ritonavir. Antimicrob Agents Chemother 2002;46(3):746–54.
7. Burger DM, Hugen PW, Aarnoutse RE, Dieleman JP, Prins JM, van der Poll T, ten Veen JH, Mulder JW, Meenhorst PL, Blok WL, van der Meer JT, Reiss P, Lange JM. A retrospective, cohort-based survey of patients using twice-daily indinavir + ritonavir combinations: pharmacokinetics, safety, and efficacy. J Acquir Immune Defic Syndr 2001;26(3):218–24.
8. Fletcher CV, Anderson PL, Kakuda TN, Schacker TW, Henry K, Gross CR, Brundage RC. Concentration-controlled compared with conventional antiretroviral therapy for HIV infection. AIDS 2002;16(4):551–60.
9. Lichterfeld M, Nischalke HD, Bergmann F, Wiesel W, Rieke A, Theisen A, Fatkenheuer G, Oette M, Carls H, Fenske S, Nadler M, Knechten H, Wasmuth JC, Rockstroh JK. Long-term efficacy and safety of ritonavir/indinavir at 400/400 mg twice a day in combination with two nucleoside reverse transcriptase inhibitors as first line antiretroviral therapy. HIV Med 2002;3(1):37–43.
10. Falloon J, Ait-Khaled M, Thomas DA, Brosgart CL, Eron JJ Jr, Feinberg J, Flanigan TP, Hammer SM, Kraus PW, Murphy R, Torres R, Masur H, Manion DJ, Rogers M, Wolfram J, Amphlett GE, Rakik A, Tisdale M; CNA2007 Study Team. HIV-1 genotype and phenotype correlate with virological response to abacavir, amprenavir and efavirenz in treatment-experienced patients. AIDS 2002;16(3):387–96.
11. Krogstad P, Lee S, Johnson G, Stanley K, McNamara J, Moye J, Jackson JB, Aguayo R, Dieudonne A, Khoury M, Mendez H, Nachman S, Wiznia A, Ballow A, Aweeka F, Rosenblatt HM, Perdue L, Frasia A, Jeremy R, Anderson M, Japour A, Fields C, Farnsworth A, Lewis R, Schnittman S, Gigliotti M, Maldonaldo S, Lane B, Hernandez JE, et al; Pediatric AIDS Clinical Trials Group 377 Study Team. Nucleoside-analogue reverse-transcriptase inhibitors plus nevirapine, nelfinavir, or ritonavir for pretreated children infected with human immunodeficiency virus type 1. Clin Infect Dis 2002;34(7):991–1001.
12. Fumaz CR, Tuldra A, Ferrer MJ, Paredes R, Bonjoch A, Jou T, Negredo E, Romeu J, Sirera G, Tural C, Clotet B.

Quality of life, emotional status, and adherence of HIV-1-infected patients treated with efavirenz versus protease inhibitor-containing regimens. J Acquir Immune Defic Syndr 2002;29(3):244–53.

13. Eng KT, Liu ES, Silverman MS, Berger AR. Lipemia retinalis in acquired immunodeficiency syndrome treated with protease inhibitors. Arch Ophthalmol 2000;118(3):425–6.

14. Chen F, Kearney T, Robinson S, Daley-Yates PT, Waldron S, Churchill DR. Cushing's syndrome and severe adrenal suppression in patients treated with ritonavir and inhaled nasal fluticasone. Sex Transm Infect 1999;75(4):274.

15. Hillebrand-Haverkort ME, Prummel MF, ten Veen JH. Ritonavir-induced Cushing's syndrome in a patient treated with nasal fluticasone. AIDS 1999;13(13):1803.

16. Darvay A, Acland K, Lynn W, Russell-Jones R. Striae formation in two HIV-positive persons receiving protease inhibitors. J Am Acad Dermatol 1999;41(3 Pt 1):467–9.

17. Bonfanti P, Valsecchi L, Parazzini F, Carradori S, Pusterla L, Fortuna P, Timillero L, Alessi F, Ghiselli G, Gabbuti A, Di Cintio E, Martinelli C, Faggion I, Landonio S, Quirino T. Incidence of adverse reactions in HIV patients treated with protease inhibitors: a cohort study. Coordinamento Italiano Studio Allergia e Infezione da HIV (CISAI) Group. J Acquir Immune Defic Syndr 2000;23(3):236–45.

18. Thiebaut R, Dabis F, Malvy D, Jacqmin-Gadda H, Mercie P, Valentin VD. Serum triglycerides, HIV infection, and highly active antiretroviral therapy, Aquitaine Cohort, France, 1996 to 1998. Groupe d'Epidemiologie Clinique du Sida en Aquitaine (GECSA). J Acquir Immune Defic Syndr 2000;23(3):261–5.

19. Benson JO, McGhee K, Coplan P, Grunfeld C, Robertson M, Brodovicz KG, Slater E. Fat redistribution in indinavir-treated patients with HIV infection: a review of postmarketing cases. J Acquir Immune Defic Syndr 2000;25(2):130–9.

20. Kaufman MB, Simionatto C. A review of protease inhibitor-induced hyperglycemia. Pharmacotherapy 1999;19(1):114–17.

21. Rodriguez-Rosado R, Soriano V, Blanco F, Dona C, Gonzalez-Lahoz J. Diabetes mellitus associated with protease inhibitor use. Eur J Clin Microbiol Infect Dis 1999;18(9):675–7.

22. Periard D, Telenti A, Sudre P, Cheseaux JJ, Halfon P, Reymond MJ, Marcovina SM, Glauser MP, Nicod P, Darioli R, Mooser V. Atherogenic dyslipidemia in HIV-infected individuals treated with protease inhibitors. The Swiss HIV Cohort Study. Circulation 1999;100(7):700–5.

23. Echevarria KL, Hardin TC, Smith JA. Hyperlipidemia associated with protease inhibitor therapy. Ann Pharmacother 1999;33(7–8):859–63.

24. Berthold HK, Parhofer KG, Ritter MM, Addo M, Wasmuth JC, Schliefer K, Spengler U, Rockstroh JK. Influence of protease inhibitor therapy on lipoprotein metabolism. J Intern Med 1999;246(6):567–75.

25. Roth VR, Kravcik S, Angel JB. Development of cervical fat pads following therapy with human immunodeficiency virus type 1 protease inhibitors. Clin Infect Dis 1998;27(1):65–7.

26. Striker R, Conlin D, Marx M, Wiviott L. Localized adipose tissue hypertrophy in patients receiving human immunodeficiency virus protease inhibitors. Clin Infect Dis 1998;27(1):218–20.

27. Viraben R, Aquilina C. Indinavir-associated lipodystrophy. AIDS 1998;12(6):F37–9.

28. Toma E, Therrien R. Gynecomastia during indinavir antiretroviral therapy in HIV infection. AIDS 1998;12(6):681–2.

29. Lui A, Karter D, Turett G. Another case of breast hypertrophy in a patient treated with indinavir. Clin Infect Dis 1998;26(6):1482.

30. Walli R, Herfort O, Michl GM, Demant T, Jager H, Dieterle C, Bogner JR, Landgraf R, Goebel FD. Treatment with protease inhibitors associated with peripheral insulin resistance and impaired oral glucose tolerance in HIV-1-infected patients. AIDS 1998;12(15):F167–73.

31. Carr A, Cooper DA. Images in clinical medicine. Lipodystrophy associated with an HIV-protease inhibitor. N Engl J Med 1998;339(18):1296.

32. Carr A, Samaras K, Burton S, Law M, Freund J, Chisholm DJ, Cooper DA. A syndrome of peripheral lipodystrophy, hyperlipidaemia and insulin resistance in patients receiving HIV protease inhibitors. AIDS 1998;12(7):F51–8.

33. Lo JC, Mulligan K, Tai VW, Algren H, Schambelan M. "Buffalo hump" in men with HIV-1 infection. Lancet 1998;351(9106):867–70.

34. Miller KD, Jones E, Yanovski JA, Shankar R, Feuerstein I, Falloon J. Visceral abdominal-fat accumulation associated with use of indinavir. Lancet 1998;351(9106):871–5.

35. Carr A, Samaras K, Thorisdottir A, Kaufmann GR, Chisholm DJ, Cooper DA. Diagnosis, prediction, and natural course of HIV-1 protease-inhibitor-associated lipodystrophy, hyperlipidaemia, and diabetes mellitus: a cohort study. Lancet 1999;353(9170):2093–9.

36. Saint-Marc T, Touraine JL. Effects of metformin on insulin resistance and central adiposity in patients receiving effective protease inhibitor therapy. AIDS 1999;13(8):1000–2.

37. Thiebaut R, Daucourt V, Malvy D. Lipodystrophy, glucose and lipid metabolism dysfunctions. Aquitaine Cohort. First International Workshop on Adverse Drug Reactions and Lipodystrophy in HIV, San Diego, 1999: Abstract 17.

38. Milpied-Homsi B, Krempf M, Gueglio B, Raffi F, Stalder JF. "Bosse de bison": un effet secondaire inattendu des traitements parinhibiteurs de protéases anti-VIH. ["Buffalo neck": an unintended secondary effect of treatment with anti-HIV protease inhibitors.] Ann Dermatol Venereol 1999;126(3):254–6.

39. Martinez E, Mocroft A, Garcia-Viejo MA, Perez-Cuevas JB, Blanco JL, Mallolas J, Bianchi L, Conget I, Blanch J, Phillips A, Gatell JM. Risk of lipodystrophy in HIV-1-infected patients treated with protease inhibitors: a prospective cohort study. Lancet 2001;357(9256):592–8.

40. George SL, Swindells S, Knudson R, Stapleton JT. Unexplained thrombosis in HIV-infected patients receiving protease inhibitors: report of seven cases. Am J Med 1999;107(6):624–30.

41. Wilde JT, Lee C, Collins P, Giangrande PL, Winter M, Shiach CR. Increased bleeding associated with protease inhibitor therapy in HIV-positive patients with bleeding disorders. Br J Haematol 1999;107(3):556–9.

42. Lawn SD, Wood C, Lockwood DN. Borderline tuberculoid leprosy: an immune reconstitution phenomenon in a human immunodeficiency virus-infected person. Clin Infect Dis 2003;36(1):e5–6.

43. Cooper CL, Parbhakar MA, Angel JB. Hepatotoxicity associated with antiretroviral therapy containing dual versus single protease inhibitors in individuals coinfected with hepatitis C virus and human immunodeficiency virus. Clin Infect Dis 2002;34(9):1259–63.

44. Florence E, Schrooten W, Verdonck K, Dreezen C, Colebunders R. Rheumatological complications associated with the use of indinavir and other protease inhibitors. Ann Rheum Dis 2002;61(1):82–4.

45. Harrington RD, Woodward JA, Hooton TM, Horn JR. Life-threatening interactions between HIV-1 protease inhibitors and the illicit drugs MDMA and gamma-hydroxybutyrate. Arch Intern Med 1999;159(18):2221–4.

46. Fichtenbaum CJ, Gerber JG, Rosenkranz SL, Segal Y, Aberg JA, Blaschke T, Alston B, Fang F, Kosel B, Aweeka F; NIAID AIDS Clinical Trials Group. Pharmacokinetic interactions between protease inhibitors and statins in HIV seronegative volunteers: ACTG Study A5047. AIDS 2002;16(4):569–77.

Protein hydrolysates

General Information

Protein hydrolysates are added to hair-care products, such as shampoos and conditioners, and are supposed to "repair" damaged hair. Hydrolysed proteins are also used in other body-care products, for example soaps, bath gels, and creams.

Organs and Systems

Immunologic

Occasionally single reports of contact urticaria and of allergic contact dermatitis due to hair conditioner and skin cleanser have been published (SEDA-21, 166) (1). Protein hydrolysates used in hair-care products have been tested in 11 hairdressers with hand dermatitis, in 2160 consecutive adults with suspected respiratory disease, and in 28 adults with chronic atopic dermatitis (2). The hairdressers underwent both scratch tests (1% aqueous) and patch tests (5% aqueous) with 22 protein hydrolysates (collagen, keratin, elastin, milk, wheat, almond, silk). Skin prick tests with one to three hydrolysates (1% aqueous) were conducted in the other patients. All 2199 patients were tested with hydroxypropyl trimonium hydrolysed collagen (Crotein Q). There were positive scratch/prick test reactions in 12 patients to three protein hydrolysates. Remarkably, all were women with atopic dermatitis. They reacted at least to hydroxypropyl trimonium-hydrolysed collagen (Crotein Q) and 11 had positive reactions to one or more allergens in a standard prick series. In three patients, clinical relevance could be confirmed by open tests with both undiluted and diluted hair conditioner containing Crotein Q (one hairdresser with contact urticaria on the hands, two cases of contact urticaria on the head, face, and upper body from a hair conditioner containing Crotein Q). Furthermore, in seven of eight sera studied, specific IgE to Crotein Q was detected, while 11 control sera were negative. These results show that protein hydrolysates in hair-care products may be underestimated causes of contact urticaria, particularly in patients with atopy.

References

1. van der Walle HB, Brunsveld VM. Dermatitis in hairdressers. (I). The experience of the past 4 years. Contact Dermatitis 1994;30(4):217–21.
2. Niinimaki A, Niinimaki M, Makinen-Kiljunen S, Hannuksela M. Contact urticaria from protein hydrolysates in hair conditioners. Allergy 1998;53(11):1078–82.

Prothrombin complex concentrate

See also Coagulation proteins

General Information

Prothrombin complex products contain constant amounts of clotting factors II, VII, IX, and X, bypassing the need for factor VIII in the clotting cascade. They are used to reverse the effects of oral anticoagulants (for example during surgery or bleeding episodes) (1) and to treat bleeding episodes in hemophiliacs with inhibitors of factor VIII (2). Prothrombin complex achieves more rapid and effective reversal of acquired coagulation defects than fresh frozen plasma. However, a potential disadvantage is the risk of thromboembolism.

Organs and Systems

Cardiovascular

Thromboembolic events in relation to activated prothrombin complex products include deep venous thrombosis and pulmonary embolism (3–5). So far, the exact mechanism of how thromboembolic events are stimulated by prothrombin complex products is not known. It has been postulated that the presence of activated clotting factors VII, IX, and X, as well as procoagulatory phospholipids in prothrombin complex products, are responsible (6).

In 42 patients who required immediate reversal of oral anticoagulant therapy by prothrombin complex concentrate, no laboratory and clinical evidence for coagulation activation was found (7). The authors suggested that the concentration of protein C within the prothrombin complex concentrate is an important factor for preventing thrombosis. The activated form of protein C is an important natural anticoagulant.

Myocardial necrosis has been described after the administration of a prothrombin complex products, probably because of excessive kininogen in the product.

Hematologic

The administration of prothrombin complex concentrate to reverse anticoagulant treatment has been associated with thrombotic complications, such as disseminated intravascular coagulation (8). However, such complications have typically occurred in patients with liver failure or after repeated treatment, such as in patients with hemophilia B treated with prothrombin complex concentrate (9).

Hypofibrinogenemia has been observed immediately after infusion of one of the activated prothrombin complex products (such as Autoplex). It has been advised that antifibrinolytic substances should be avoided in conjunction with Autoplex.

Skin

An erythematous pruritic eruption has been described after infusion of Autoplex (3).

Immunologic

In about 5% of patients with hemophilia A with antibodies to factor VIII treated with an activated prothrombin complex product (Autoplex), there was a significant increase in antibody titer (10).

Susceptibility Factors

Relative contraindications for prothrombin complex concentrate are liver disease, coronary heart disease, and factors that predispose to thrombosis (11). It is contra-indicated in disseminated intravascular coagulopathy and hyperfibrinolysis.

References

1. Cartmill M, Dolan G, Byrne JL, Byrne PO. Prothrombin complex concentrate for oral anticoagulant reversal in neurosurgical emergencies. Br J Neurosurg 2000; 14(5):458–61.
2. DellaCroce FJ, Kountakis S, Aguilar EF 3rd. Manifestations of factor VIII inhibitor in the head and neck. Arch Otolaryngol Head Neck Surg 1999;125(11):1258–61.
3. Penner JA. Management of haemophilia in patients with high-titre inhibitors: focus on the evolution of activated prothrombin complex concentrate AUTOPLEX T. Haemophilia 1999;5(Suppl 3):1–9.
4. Roberts HR. The use of agents that by-pass factor VIII inhibitors in patients with haemophilia. Vox Sang 1999;77(Suppl 1):38–41.
5. Shapiro AD. Recombinant factor VIIa: A viewpoint. BioDrugs 1999;12:78.
6. Barthels M. Clinical efficacy of prothrombin complex concentrates and recombinant factor VIIa in the treatment of bleeding episodes in patients with factor VII and IX inhibitors. Thromb Res 1999;95(4 Suppl 1):S31–8.
7. Preston FE, Laidlaw ST, Sampson B, Kitchen S. Rapid reversal of oral anticoagulation with warfarin by a prothrombin complex concentrate (Beriplex): efficacy and safety in 42 patients. Br J Haematol 2002;116(3):619–24.
8. Roddie PH, Stirling C, Mayne EE, Ludlam CA. Thrombosis and disseminated intravascular coagulation following treatment with the prothrombin complex concentrate, DEFIX. Thromb Haemost 1999;81(4):667.
9. Evans G, Luddington R, Baglin T. Beriplex P/N reverses severe warfarin-induced overanticoagulation immediately and completely in patients presenting with major bleeding. Br J Haematol 2001;115(4):998–1001.
10. White GC 2nd. Seventeen years' experience with Autoplex/Autoplex T: evaluation of inpatients with severe haemophilia A and factor VIII inhibitors at a major haemophilia centre. Haemophilia 2000;6(5):508–12.
11. Butler AC, Tait RC. Management of oral anticoagulant-induced intracranial haemorrhage. Blood Rev 1998;12(1):35–44.

Protirelin

General Information

Protirelin is a synthetic tripeptide that stimulates the hypophyseal secretion of thyrotrophin (thyroid-stimulating hormone, TSH). It is used mainly for diagnostic purposes in dynamic tests of pituitary and hypothalamic function, but its use in the assessment of hyperthyroidism has been superseded by sensitive assays of thyrotrophin

(SED-13, 1311) (1). Protirelin has neurotransmitter properties and has been used to treat a variety of neurological disorders, including intractable epilepsy (2). Some experiments have also been performed to evaluate its effects in mental disorders.

Protirelin is generally given intravenously (as a bolus of 200 micrograms), as absorption after oral and intranasal administration is unpredictable.

Comparative studies

Protirelin has been given antenatally in combination with a glucocorticoid, to accelerate fetal lung maturation in an attempt to reduce the incidence of infant respiratory distress syndrome. However, there was no improvement in outcome and the mothers experienced more adverse effects (particularly flushing, headache, nausea, and vomiting) in the protirelin group in two large prospective studies (3,4). The infants were reported to have mild developmental delay at 12 months of age (5): this finding was initially criticized because of methodological problems and there was no consensus that protirelin induces harmful effects in these infants (6).

Subsequently, the addition of protirelin to glucocorticoid therapy was the subject of a meta-analysis (7). In 1134 premature infants the serum TSH concentration was increased for the first 6 hours after the last maternal dose of protirelin, then suppressed for 36 hours before returning to control values (8). The largest controlled trial (in 1368 infants) reported a small delay in development at 12 months (5). However, developmental assessment was by questionnaire, with incomplete ascertainment, and these findings have been questioned (6). In the mothers, there was a three-fold increase in nausea, vomiting, or flushing and a two-fold increase in hypertension compared with glucocorticoid therapy alone.

General adverse effects

The adverse effects of protirelin are usually mild. These include facial flushing, urinary urgency, vaginal sensations, nausea, chest pain, and altered taste sensation (9).

Organs and Systems

Cardiovascular

A transient rise in blood pressure occurs immediately after the administration of protirelin (10). In very rare cases, transient amaurosis and bronchospasm have been reported, thought to be due to either vasopressor syncope or cardiac arrhythmias (11–13).

Nervous system

The most serious adverse effect of protirelin is pituitary apoplexy (pituitary hemorrhage or infarction, characterized by severe headache, visual loss, and often by pituitary failure, hypotension, and coma). This complication has been described in 15 cases after pituitary function testing with protirelin. Pituitary macroadenoma was present in all cases. Although insulin and gonadorelin were also used in these patients, protirelin was considered to be the most likely agent responsible, owing to its vasoactive properties (SED-13, 1311) (14).

- A woman developed severe bifrontal headache and visual blurring 5 minutes after the intravenous administration of protirelin 200 micrograms to investigate her pituitary macroadenoma (15). The symptoms resolved in less than 2 hours without sequelae.
- A patient developed a severe headache, nausea and vomiting, visual disturbance, and altered mental function 88 hours after a protirelin/gonadorelin stimulation test to investigate a pituitary macroadenoma (16). Bleeding into the tumor was seen on CT scan. The patient died 9 days later of pneumonia.

Loss of consciousness or convulsions occurred in a few patients who received high doses (400 micrograms) of protirelin intravenously.

References

1. Surks MI, Chopra IJ, Mariash CN, Nicoloff JT, Solomon DH. American Thyroid Association guidelines for use of laboratory tests in thyroid disorders. JAMA 1990;263(11):1529–32.
2. Takeuci Y. Thyrotropin-releasing hormone (protirelin). Role in the treatment of epilepsy. CNS Drugs 1996;6:341–50.
3. Australian Collaborative Trial of Antenatal Thyrotropin-releasing Hormone (ACTOBAT) for prevention of neonatal respiratory disease. Lancet 1995;345(8954):877–82.
4. Ballard RA, Ballard PL, Cnaan A, Pinto-Martin J, Davis DJ, Padbury JF, Phibbs RH, Parer JT, Hart MC, Mannino FL, Sawai SK. Antenatal thyrotropin-releasing hormone to prevent lung disease in preterm infants. North American Thyrotropin-Releasing Hormone Study Group. N Engl J Med 1998;338(8):493–8.
5. Crowther CA, Hiller JE, Haslam RR, Robinson JS. Australian Collaborative Trial of Antenatal Thyrotropin-Releasing Hormone: adverse effects at 12-month follow-up. ACTOBAT Study Group. Pediatrics 1997;99(3):311–17.
6. McCormick MC. The credibility of the ACTOBAT follow-up study. Pediatrics 1997;99(3):476–8.
7. Gross I, Moya FR. Is there a role for antenatal TRH therapy for the prevention of neonatal lung disease? Semin Perinatol 2001;25(6):406–16.
8. Ballard PL, Ballard RA, Ning Y, Cnann A, Boardman C, Pinto-Martin J, Polk D, Phibbs RH, Davis DJ, Mannino FL, Hart M. Plasma thyroid hormones in premature infants: effect of gestational age and antenatal thyrotropin-releasing hormone treatment. TRH Collaborative Trial Participants. Pediatr Res 1998;44(5):642–9.
9. Dolva LO, Riddervold F, Thorsen RK. Side effects of thyrotrophin releasing hormone. BMJ (Clin Res Ed) 1983;287(6391):532.
10. Devlieger R, Vanderlinden S, de Zegher F, Van Assche FA, Spitz B. Effect of antenatal thyrotropin-releasing hormone on uterine contractility, blood pressure, and maternal heart rate. Am J Obstet Gynecol 1997;177(2):431–3.
11. McFadden RG, McCourtie DR, Rodger NW. TRH and bronchospasm. Lancet 1981;2(8249):758–9.
12. Drury PL, Belchetz PE, McDonald WI, Thomas DG, Besser GM. Transient amaurosis and headache after thyrotropin releasing hormone. Lancet 1982;1(8265):218–19.
13. Cimino A, Corsini R, Radaeli E, Bollati A, Giustina G. Transient amaurosis in patient with pituitary macroadenoma after intravenous gonadotropin and thyrotropin releasing hormones. Lancet 1981;2(8237):95.
14. Masago A, Ueda Y, Kanai H, Nagai H, Umemura S. Pituitary apoplexy after pituitary function test: a report of two cases and review of the literature. Surg Neurol 1995;43(2):158–64.
15. Sachmechi I, Bitton RN, Patel D, Schneider BS. Transient headache and impaired vision after intravenous thyrotropin-releasing hormone in a patient with pituitary macroadenoma. Mt Sinai J Med 1999;66(5–6):330–3.
16. Dokmetas HS, Selcuklu A, Colak R, Unluhizarci K, Bayram F, Kelestimur F. Pituitary apoplexy probably due to TRH and GnRH stimulation tests in a patient with acromegaly. J Endocrinol Invest 1999;22(9):698–700.

Proton pump inhibitors

See also Individual agents

General Information

Proton pump inhibitors inhibit the H/K-ATPase (proton pump) in oxyntic cells of the stomach, the final common pathway in the secretion of gastric acid in response to a variety of stimuli, such as gastrin and histamine. Their use in acid-related disorders has been extensively reviewed (1–3).

Comparative studies

Comparisons between proton pump inhibitors
Lansoprazole 15 mg/day and omeprazole 10 mg/day for 4 weeks have been compared in the relief of heartburn and epigastric pain in a randomized, double-blind, parallel-group study in 609 patients with acid-related dyspepsia (4). Low-dose lansoprazole was more effective in controlling symptoms. There were no significant differences in adverse events between the two groups, although there was a trend toward a higher incidence of more severe adverse events with omeprazole. Most of the reported adverse events were difficult to relate to the treatments.

An unblinded questionnaire survey has been carried out to determine patients' perceptions of differences in the efficacy, adverse effects, and value of omeprazole versus lansoprazole for gastro-esophageal reflux disease maintenance therapy (5). The patients had been taking omeprazole for at least 2 months and then switched to lansoprazole for a minimum of 2 months. There was no significant difference between median symptom scores with the two drugs, but 64% of patients preferred omeprazole to lansoprazole. The most commonly reported adverse effects with both drugs were flatulence, headache, and diarrhea. Significantly more patients reported adverse effects with lansoprazole than with omeprazole.

Rabeprazole 20 mg/day has been compared with omeprazole 20 mg/day in a randomized, double-blind, multicenter study in 205 patients with active duodenal ulcers (6). Rabeprazole produced healing rates equivalent to omeprazole at 2 and 4 weeks of treatment (69 versus 61% and 98 versus 93% respectively) and greater improvement in day-time pain. Both drugs were well tolerated; adverse effects were similar, and included headache, infections, diarrhea, gastritis, stomatitis, rash, and sweating. Serum gastrin concentrations increased over time in both groups. There was a statistically significant difference between the groups in the mean change in fasting serum gastrin from baseline to end-point; +40 pg/ml with rabeprazole and +19 pg/ml with omeprazole. However, mean values at the end of the study were in the reference range in both groups.

Rabeprazole 20 mg/day and omeprazole 20 mg/day have been compared in the treatment of erosive or ulcerative esophagitis in a double-blind, multicenter study in 202 patients (7). Overall healing rates for rabeprazole and omeprazole at 4 and 8 weeks of treatment were equivalent (81 versus 81% and 92 versus 94% respectively), as was symptom relief. Both drugs were well tolerated, and there was no significant difference in reported adverse events, except for flatulence, which was only reported by patients taking omeprazole (4%). Other adverse effects included headache, diarrhea, rash, flu-like syndrome, gastroenteritis, raised aspartate transaminase and gamma-glutamyltransferase, weakness, myalgia, somnolence, and hypertension. Serum gastrin concentrations increased over time in both groups; however, there was no significant difference between the treatment groups in the mean change in fasting serum gastrin concentrations from baseline to end-point.

The proton pump inhibitors produce a higher intragastric pH in the presence of *Helicobacter pylori* than after eradication. The mechanism of this effect is unclear, but possible explanations are reduced production of ammonia or other neutralizing substances after eradication of the infection or the development of gastritis during omeprazole therapy in the presence of *H. pylori*, leading to reduced acid secretion. In a double-blind, crossover study in 13 subjects with *H. pylori*, pumaprazole (BY841) 100 mg bd, a reversible proton pump inhibitor, which (unlike omeprazole) does not require activation in the acid compartment of the parietal cell, produced a similar rise in intragastric pH to that produced by omeprazole before and after eradication of *H. pylori* (8). Adverse events during the study were mild and assessed as probably not related to the drugs. They included headache, abdominal pain, and diarrhea. Serum gastrin concentrations rose during pumaprazole therapy and were higher than during omeprazole therapy, both before and after eradication of *H. pylori*.

The common adverse events during treatment with proton pump inhibitors used in general practice in England have been reviewed in a prescription event monitoring study in 16 205 patients taking omeprazole, 17 329 taking lansoprazole, and 11 541 taking pantoprazole (9). The commonest adverse events in all three groups were diarrhea, nausea/vomiting, abdominal pain, and headache. There was little difference in the adverse event rates between the three groups. However, diarrhea was more commonly associated with lansoprazole compared with omeprazole, particularly in elderly people.

To assess acid control, esomeprazole 20 or 40 mg/day has been compared with omeprazole 20 mg/day for 5 days in a double-blind, crossover study in 38 patients with symptoms of gastro-esophageal reflux disease (10). Pharmacokinetic variables and 24-hour intragastric pH were measured on day 5 of each dosing period.

Esomeprazole provided more effective acid control than omeprazole. Both dosages of esomeprazole were well tolerated, and the profile and incidence of adverse events were similar to that observed with omeprazole. The most common were abdominal pain, nausea, diarrhea, respiratory infection, and headache.

Esomeprazole 20 or 40 mg/day and omeprazole 20 mg/day for 8 weeks have been compared in the treatment of gastro-esophageal reflux disease in a multicenter, randomized, double-blind trial in 1960 patients (11). Symptom control and healing rates were significantly better with either dose of esomeprazole than with omeprazole. There was no significant difference in reported adverse events between the treatment groups. The most commonly reported were headache, abdominal pain, and diarrhea.

The results of a therapeutic interchange program, in which 78 patients with acid peptic disease requiring proton pump inhibitor therapy (both newly diagnosed patients and those previously stabilized on omeprazole) were treated with lansoprazole, have been retrospectively analysed (12). Although the switch was associated with considerable pharmaceutical savings, there was an overall lansoprazole-associated failure rate of 28%. Reported lack of efficacy required withdrawal of lansoprazole in 15%, while adverse effects required withdrawal of lansoprazole in 13% of patients (versus none with omeprazole). The main adverse effect was diarrhea.

The clinical and fiscal impact of replacing omeprazole with lansoprazole as the only proton pump inhibitor has been assessed by reviewing the medical records of 3833 patients requiring long-term proton pump inhibitor therapy (2224 were started on lansoprazole and 1479 were converted from omeprazole to lansoprazole) (13). There were considerable pharmaceutical savings. The true lansoprazole failure rate (requiring conversion to omeprazole) was 5.3%. Withdrawal of lansoprazole was due to poor symptom control (in 69%) and/or adverse effects (in 22%). The most common adverse effects were diarrhea (10%), abdominal pain (5%), and urticaria (1%).

Omeprazole 40 mg/day for 6 weeks and lansoprazole 30 mg bd have been compared for symptom control in a randomized study in 96 patients with gastro-esophageal reflux disease who had earlier failed to respond to lansoprazole 30 mg/day (14). The two drugs were equally effective in symptom control. There were no significant differences in adverse events between the two groups. The most frequent adverse events reported were diarrhea, abdominal pain/discomfort, bloating/gas, vomiting, and headache.

Omeprazole multiple unit pellet system (MUPS) 20 mg/day and pantoprazole 40 mg/day for 8 weeks were more effective than lansoprazole 30 mg/day in relieving heartburn in a randomized, double-blind trial in 461 patients with symptomatic reflux esophagitis (15). Patient satisfaction and adverse effects were similar in the three groups. The most common adverse effects were diarrhea, headache, and nausea.

In a multicenter, double-blind, crossover study in primary care in 240 patients with acid-related disorders, omeprazole 20 mg/day and rabeprazole 40 mg/day for 4 weeks provided similar symptom control (16). The adverse effect profiles were also similar in the two groups. However, more patients preferred rabeprazole to omeprazole.

Omeprazole 40 mg/day and rabeprazole 20 mg/day for 4 weeks have been compared in a randomized, double-blind trial in 251 patients with erosive esophagitis (17). The two treatments had similar efficacy in relieving symptoms on day 4 and healing esophageal lesions, but rabeprazole had a faster onset of action in patients with severe heartburn. Both drugs were well tolerated and gave rise to similar frequencies of adverse effects, commonly involving the gastrointestinal tract (10%) and nervous system (4.4%).

Rabeprazole 10 or 20 mg bd and omeprazole 20 mg/day have been compared in the healing of erosive gastro-esophageal reflux disease in a double-blind, multicenter study in 310 patients (18). Overall healing rates for rabeprazole (both dosage regimens) and omeprazole at 4 and 8 weeks of treatment were equivalent. The drugs were equally well tolerated, and there was no significant difference in reported adverse events. The more frequent were abdominal pain, pharyngitis, bronchitis, headache, and diarrhea.

Esomeprazole 40 mg/day and omeprazole 20 mg/day for 8 weeks have been compared in the treatment of erosive esophagitis in a multicenter, randomized, double-blind trial in 2425 patients (19). Significantly more patients were healed with esomeprazole. There was no significant difference in reported adverse events between the treatment groups. The most commonly reported were headache, diarrhea, and nausea.

The effects of omeprazole 40 mg/day and esomeprazole 40 mg/day for 5 days on intragastric acidity have been compared in an open, crossover study in 130 patients with symptoms of gastro-esophageal reflux (20). Esomeprazole provided more effective acid control than twice the standard dose of omeprazole. Adverse effects were similar with the two drugs, and the most commonly reported were headache, nausea, and abdominal pain.

Pantoprazole 20 mg/day and omeprazole 20 mg/day for 8 weeks have been compared in the treatment of grade I reflux esophagitis in a multicenter, randomized, open trial in 328 patients (21). Symptom relief and healing rates were similar and both treatments were well tolerated. There was no significant difference in reported adverse events between the groups. The most commonly reported were nausea, diarrhea, and headache.

Lansoprazole 30 mg/day and omeprazole 20 mg/day for 8 weeks have been compared in the relief of heartburn in a multicenter, randomized, double-blind trial in 3510 patients with erosive esophagitis (22). Symptom control was significantly more effective and faster with lansoprazole than omeprazole. Both drugs were well tolerated. The most common adverse effect was diarrhea.

Rabeprazole 10 mg bd or 20 mg/day, omeprazole 20 mg/day, and placebo for 7 days in reducing esophageal acid exposure have been compared in a multicenter, randomized, double-blind trial in 82 patients with symptomatic gastro-esophageal reflux disease (23). Esophageal pH was monitored for 24 hours before treatment and on day 7. Esophageal acid exposure was significantly reduced in all the treatment groups compared with placebo, with no significant difference in efficacy. Both rabeprazole and omeprazole were well tolerated. The most commonly reported adverse effects were diarrhea, abdominal pain, nausea, and headache.

Comparisons between proton pump inhibitors and H₂ receptor antagonists

The effects of famotidine 20 mg bd and omeprazole 20 mg/day for 8 weeks have been compared in the treatment of reflux esophagitis in a randomized trial in 56 patients (24). Omeprazole was more effective in healing esophagitis and providing symptom relief. Adverse events, which were rare, were similar in the two groups, and consisted of nausea, palpitation, abdominal pain, and mild abnormalities of liver function tests.

Lansoprazole 30 mg/day, lansoprazole 15 mg/day, and ranitidine 150 mg/day have been compared in a randomized, double-blind, multicenter trial in the prevention of relapse of duodenal ulcer and symptom control over 12 months in 359 patients (25). Both doses of lansoprazole were superior to ranitidine. There was no significant difference between the two lansoprazole groups, although there was a trend in favor of lansoprazole 30 mg/day. There were no differences in adverse effects profiles in the three groups. The adverse effects included diarrhea, abdominal pain, viral infections, headache, and vomiting.

Lansoprazole 30 mg/day, lansoprazole 15 mg/day, and ranitidine 150 mg bd for 8 weeks have been compared in a randomized, double-blind, multicenter trial in the healing of NSAID-associated gastric ulceration in 353 patients (26). Both doses of lansoprazole were superior to ranitidine in healing gastric ulcers. Healing rates were similar between *H. pylori* infected and non-infected patients, again with significantly better healing rates with lansoprazole than ranitidine. There were no differences in adverse effects profiles in the three groups. The most commonly reported adverse effect was diarrhea.

Lansoprazole 15 or 30 mg/day and ranitidine 150 mg bd for 8 weeks have been compared in the treatment of non-erosive gastro-esophageal reflux disease in two double-blind, multicenter trials in 901 patients (27). Overall symptom control was significantly better with either dose of lansoprazole than with ranitidine or placebo. There was no significant difference in reported adverse events between the treatment groups. The more commonly reported were abdominal pain and diarrhea.

Pantoprazole 20 mg/day (low dose) and ranitidine 300 mg/day (standard dose) have been compared in the treatment of mild gastro-esophageal reflux disease in a double-blind, multicenter trial in 201 patients (28). Overall symptom control and healing rates were significantly better with pantoprazole. There was no significant difference in reported adverse events between the treatment groups. The more commonly reported were diarrhea, headache, and abdominal pain.

General adverse effects

The adverse effects profile of the proton pump inhibitors during short-term administration (under 12 weeks) is similar to that reported with short-term use of histamine receptor antagonists. The type and frequency of adverse effects reported with lansoprazole, omeprazole, pantoprazole, and rabeprazole are comparable. The most common adverse effects include headache, diarrhea, nausea, abdominal pain, constipation, dizziness, and skin rashes.

Proton pump inhibitors can interact with other drugs by increasing gastric pH, inhibiting hepatic cytochrome

P450, or inducing specific isoforms of this enzyme system. However, drug interactions involving these isoenzymes and omeprazole or lansoprazole are uncommon and generally appear to be clinically unimportant. Pantoprazole seems to have a lower drug interaction potential than either omeprazole or lansoprazole.

Organs and Systems

Cardiovascular

Reversible peripheral edema has been reported in five women taking the proton pump inhibitors omeprazole, lansoprazole, or pantoprazole for 7–15 days for peptic disorders in recommended standard doses (29). Edema disappeared within 2–3 days of withdrawal and reappeared in all five patients after re-exposure. High-dose intravenous infusions of omeprazole and pantoprazole (8 mg/hour) caused peripheral edema in three of six young female volunteers and two of six female volunteers respectively. The edema disappeared within 24 hours of stopping the infusion. Similar high doses of omeprazole did not produce edema in male volunteers. Subsequent studies performed on 10 female volunteers to elucidate the cause of the edema did not show any changes in concentrations of serum hormones or C1 esterase inhibitor.

Long-Term Effects

Tumorigenicity

There has been concern about the potential for proton pump inhibitors to cause enterochromaffin-like cell hyperplasia, gastric carcinoid tumors and gastric cancers, colorectal polyps and adenocarcinoma, atrophic gastritis, and intestinal metaplasia in patients with *H. pylori* infection, and bacterial overgrowth.

Carcinoid nodules were detected in the stomach of rats given large doses of omeprazole over prolonged periods. A variety of evidence, however, suggests that these findings were neither specific to omeprazole nor likely to indicate material risks to man (30), and that other arguments for a tumor-inducing effect of proton pump inhibitors are equally unconvincing. Firstly, similar carcinoid change has been detected with secretory antagonists and the fibrates, which are anti-secretory in rats. Secondly carcinoidogenesis can be inhibited by antrectomy, presumably by removing an antral gastrin drive, and it can be enhanced by partial fundectomy, when relative anacidity increases antral gastrin release. Thirdly, although omeprazole treatment can raise serum gastrin levels quite markedly in man, they do so by a level of magnitude less than in pernicious anemia, in which carcinoid tumors are recorded, albeit rarely. Fourthly, despite close searching, carcinoids have not been detected complicating ordinary ulcer treatment in man. Others have claimed on the basis of tissue work in vitro that omeprazole may itself be a mitogen or mutagen; it has been counter-claimed that the technique used in the studies concerned is inherently unreliable and that other standard techniques have failed to reveal mutagenic potential (SED-12, 943). Finally, selective and important actions on a cytochrome which would activate carcinogens have been claimed, but seem unlikely experimentally. This is one of the situations in which there is inherent difficulty in disproving a postulated relationship. Currently it seems very unlikely that an appreciable risk exists, but most experts would now recommend that any patient requiring long-term treatment with a proton pump inhibitor should take treatment to eradicate *H. pylori* infection (SEDA-20, 318).

Therapeutic doses of proton pump inhibitors usually produce somewhat higher serum gastrin concentrations than histamine receptor antagonists. However, except for small intestinal bacterial overgrowth, there is no convincing evidence yet to implicate proton pump inhibitors in the development of malignant or premalignant lesions in the human gastrointestinal tract. Nevertheless, although omeprazole has been used for more than 14 years and lansoprazole for more than 10 years, longer-term data are required to completely rule out the possibility of increased risk of gastric tumor formation.

An increasing number of gastric polyps is being reported in patients taking proton pump inhibitors. Although these may be coincidental and may only account for a minority of sporadic cases (31), it is too early to disregard the possibility that they are treatment induced (32). Long-term prospective controlled trials including investigation of the effects of stopping and restarting proton pump inhibitors on the evolution of gastric polyps will have to be done before a firm causal relation can be established.

An uncontrolled retrospective study of patients who had taken proton pump inhibitors for an average of 33 months found gastric polyps in 17 of 231 patients who underwent two or more endoscopies for complicated gastro-esophageal reflux disease (33). The polyps were generally small (under 1 cm), sessile, and multiple, and were present in the proximal or mid gastric body. Of the 15 polyps removed endoscopically, nine were fundic gland type, four were hyperplastic, and two were inflammatory. None had any dysplasia or carcinoma.

A gastric carcinoid tumor, detected during long-term anti-ulcer therapy with a histamine receptor antagonist and proton pump inhibitors, has been reported (34).

- A 31 year old Japanese man with recurrent duodenal ulcer was treated with famotidine, omeprazole, and lansoprazole at different times over 3 years. Gastroscopy showed a small carcinoid tumor in the upper cardia after 35 months. The lesion became larger while the patient was taking lansoprazole.

References

1. Berardi RR, Welage LS. Proton-pump inhibitors in acid-related diseases. Am J Health Syst Pharm 1998; 55(21):2289–98.
2. Garnett WR. Considerations for long-term use of proton-pump inhibitors. Am J Health Syst Pharm 1998; 55(21):2268–79.
3. Israel DM, Hassall E. Omerprazole and other proton pump inhibitors: pharmacology, efficacy, and safety, with special reference to use in children. J Pediatr Gastroenterol Nutr 1998;27(5):568–79.

4. Jones R, Crouch SL. Low-dose lansoprazole provides greater relief of heartburn and epigastric pain than low-dose omeprazole in patients with acid-related dyspepsia. Aliment Pharmacol Ther 1999;13(3):413–19.

5. Condra LJ, Morreale AP, Stolley SN, Marcus D. Assessment of patient satisfaction with a formulary switch from omeprazole to lansoprazole in gastroesophageal reflux disease maintenance therapy. Am J Manag Care 1999;5(5):631–8.

6. Dekkers CP, Beker JA, Thjodleifsson B, Gabryelewicz A, Bell NE, Humphries TJ. Comparison of rabeprazole 20 mg versus omeprazole 20 mg in the treatment of active duodenal ulcer: a European multicentre study. Aliment Pharmacol Ther 1999;13(2):179–86.

7. Dekkers CP, Beker JA, Thjodleifsson B, Gabryelewicz A, Bell NE, Humphries TJ. Double-blind comparison [correction of double-blind, placebo-controlled comparison] of rabeprazole 20 mg vs. omeprazole 20 mg in the treatment of erosive or ulcerative gastro-oesophageal reflux disease. The European Rabeprazole Study Group. Aliment Pharmacol Ther 1999;13(1):49–57.

8. Martinek J, Blum AL, Stolte M, Hartmann M, Verdu EF, Luhmann R, Dorta G, Wiesel P. Effects of pumaprazole (BY841), a novel reversible proton pump antagonist, and of omeprazole, on intragastric acidity before and after cure of *Helicobacter pylori* infection. Aliment Pharmacol Ther 1999;13(1):27–34.

9. Martin RM, Dunn NR, Freemantle S, Shakir S. The rates of common adverse events reported during treatment with proton pump inhibitors used in general practice in England: cohort studies. Br J Clin Pharmacol 2000;50(4):366–72.

10. Lind T, Rydberg L, Kyleback A, Jonsson A, Andersson T, Hasselgren G, Holmberg J, Rohss K. Esomeprazole provides improved acid control vs. omeprazole in patients with symptoms of gastro-oesophageal reflux disease. Aliment Pharmacol Ther 2000;14(7):861–7.

11. Kahrilas PJ, Falk GW, Johnson DA, Schmitt C, Collins DW, Whipple J, D'Amico D, Hamelin B, Joelsson B. Esomeprazole improves healing and symptom resolution as compared with omeprazole in reflux oesophagitis patients: a randomized controlled trial. The Esomeprazole Study Investigators. Aliment Pharmacol Ther 2000;14(10):1249–58.

12. Amidon PB, Jankovich R, Stoukides CA, Kaul AF. Proton pump inhibitor therapy: preliminary results of a therapeutic interchange program. Am J Manag Care 2000;6(5):593–601.

13. Gerson LB, Hatton BN, Ryono R, Jones W, Pulliam G, Sampliner RE, Triadafilopoulos G, Fass R. Clinical and fiscal impact of lansoprazole intolerance in veterans with gastro-oesophageal reflux disease. Aliment Pharmacol Ther 2000;14(4):397–406.

14. Fass R, Murthy U, Hayden CW, Malagon IB, Pulliam G, Wendel C, Kovacs TO. Omeprazole 40 mg once a day is equally effective as lansoprazole 30 mg twice a day in symptom control of patients with gastro-oesophageal reflux disease (GERD) who are resistant to conventional-dose lansoprazole therapy—a prospective, randomized, multi-centre study. Aliment Pharmacol Ther 2000;14(12):1595–603.

15. Mulder CJ, Westerveld BD, Smit JM, Oudkerk Pool M, Otten MH, Tan TG, van Milligen de Wit AW, de Groot GH, Dutch omeprazole MUPS study group. A double-blind, randomized comparison of omeprazole Multiple Unit Pellet System (MUPS) 20 mg, lansoprazole 30 mg and pantoprazole 40 mg in symptomatic reflux oesophagitis followed by 3 months of omeprazole MUPS maintenance treatment: a Dutch multicentre trial. Eur J Gastroenterol Hepatol 2002;14(6):649–56.

16. Johnson M, Guilford S, Libretto SE, Collaborative GP Research Group. Patients have treatment preferences: a multicentre, double-blind, crossover study comparing rabeprazole and omeprazole. Curr Med Res Opin 2002;18(5):303–10.

17. Holtmann G, Bytzer P, Metz M, Loeffler V, Blum AL. A randomized, double-blind, comparative study of standard-dose rabeprazole and high-dose omeprazole in gastro-oesophageal reflux disease. Aliment Pharmacol Ther 2002;16(3):479–85.

18. Delchier JC, Cohen G, Humphries TJ. Rabeprazole, 20 mg once daily or 10 mg twice daily, is equivalent to omeprazole, 20 mg once daily, in the healing of erosive gastrooesophageal reflux disease Scand J Gastroenterol 2000;35(12):1245–50.

19. Richter JE, Kahrilas PJ, Johanson J, Maton P, Breiter JR, Hwang C, Marino V, Hamelin B, Levine JG, Esomeprazole Study Investigators. Efficacy and safety of esomeprazole compared with omeprazole in GERD patients with erosive esophagitis: a randomized controlled trial. Am J Gastroenterol 2001;96(3):656–65.

20. Rohss K, Hasselgren G, Hedenstrom H. Effect of esomeprazole 40 mg vs omeprazole 40 mg on 24-hour intragastric pH in patients with symptoms of gastroesophageal reflux disease. Dig Dis Sci 2002;47(5):954–8.

21. Bardhan KD, Van Rensburg C. Comparable clinical efficacy and tolerability of 20 mg pantoprazole and 20 mg omeprazole in patients with grade I reflux oesophagitis. Aliment Pharmacol Ther 2001;15(10):1585–91.

22. Richter JE, Kahrilas PJ, Sontag SJ, Kovacs TO, Huang B, Pencyla JL. Comparing lansoprazole and omeprazole in onset of heartburn relief: results of a randomized, controlled trial in erosive esophagitis patients. Am J Gastroenterol 2001;96(11):3089–98.

23. Galmiche JP, Zerbib F, Ducrotte P, Fournet J, Rampal P, Avasthy N, Humphries TJ. Decreasing oesophageal acid exposure in patients with GERD: a comparison of rabeprazole and omeprazole. Aliment Pharmacol Ther 2001;15(9):1343–50.

24. Kawano S, Murata H, Tsuji S, Kubo M, Tatsuta M, Iishi H, Kanda T, Sato T, Yoshihara H, Masuda E, Noguchi M, Kashio S, Ikeda M, Kaneko A. Randomized comparative study of omeprazole and famotidine in reflux esophagitis. J Gastroenterol Hepatol 2002;17(9):955–9.

25. Bardhan KD, Crowe J, Thompson RP, Trewby PN, Keeling PN, Weir D, Crouch SL. Lansoprazole is superior to ranitidine as maintenance treatment for the prevention of duodenal ulcer relapse. Aliment Pharmacol Ther 1999;13(6):827–32.

26. Agrawal NM, Campbell DR, Safdi MA, Lukasik NL, Huang B, Haber MM. Superiority of lansoprazole vs ranitidine in healing nonsteroidal anti-inflammatory drug-associated gastric ulcers: results of a double-blind, randomized, multicenter study. NSAID-Associated Gastric Ulcer Study Group. Arch Intern Med 2000;160(10):1455–61.

27. Richter JE, Campbell DR, Kahrilas PJ, Huang B, Fludas C. Lansoprazole compared with ranitidine for the treatment of nonerosive gastroesophageal reflux disease. Arch Intern Med 2000;160(12):1803–9.

28. van Zyl JH, de K Grundling H, van Rensburg CJ, Retief FJ, O'Keefe SJ, Theron I, Fischer R, Bethke T. Efficacy and tolerability of 20 mg pantoprazole versus 300 mg ranitidine in patients with mild reflux-oesophagitis: a randomized, double-blind, parallel, and multicentre study. Eur J Gastroenterol Hepatol 2000;12(2):197–202.

29. Brunner G, Athmann C, Boldt JH. Reversible pheripheral edema in female patients taking proton pump inhibitors for peptic acid diseases. Dig Dis Sci 2001;46(5):993–6.

30. Langman MJ. Omeprazole. BMJ 1991;303(6801):481–2.

31. Declich P, Ferrara A, Galati F, Caruso S, Baldacci MP, Ambrosiani L. Do fundic gland polyps develop under long-term omeprazole therapy? Am J Gastroenterol 1998;93(8):1393.

32. Naegels S, Urbain D. Omeprazole and fundic gland polyps. Am J Gastroenterol 1998;93(5):855.

33. Choudhry U, Boyce HW Jr, Coppola D. Proton pump inhibitor-associated gastric polyps: a retrospective analysis of their frequency, and endoscopic, histologic, and ultra-structural characteristics. Am J Clin Pathol 1998;110(5):615–21.

34. Haga Y, Nakatsura T, Shibata Y, Sameshima H, Nakamura Y, Tanimura M, Ogawa M. Human gastric carcinoid detected during long-term antiulcer therapy of H2 receptor antagonist and proton pump inhibitor. Dig Dis Sci 1998;43(2):253–7.

Proxymetacaine

See also Local anesthetics

General Information

Proxymetacaine is an ester of meta-aminobenzoic acid. It is often used in ophthalmology.

Organs and Systems

Skin

Proparacaine has been reported to cause contact dermatitis.

- A 49-year-old ophthalmologist developed fissuring and bleeding of his finger-tips (1). Skin patch tests using a series of standard and preservative allergens showed only mild reactions to some. Various treatments were attempted, with minimal success, and skin patch testing was repeated using 32 specific formulations that he had contact with in his practice; he had a severe reaction to proxymetacaine hydrochloride 0.5%. Subsequent removal of proparacaine from his practice resulted in resolution over 6 months.

- An ophthalmologist developed chronic finger pad dermatitis with fissuring and scaling, which mainly affected his thumbs for 3 years (2). Patch testing confirmed that "ophthetic solution" (proxymetacaine hydrochloride 0.5%, glycerine, and benzalkonium chloride 0.01%) was the sensitizing agent. He was instructed to change to tetracaine, to which he had had a negative patch test. However, 2 years later his symptoms recurred and a repeat patch testing was carried out. This was now positive to both tetracaine 1% and proxymetacaine 0.5%.

Cross-sensitization between proxymetacaine and tetracaine is thought to be rare. Moreover, the chemical structure of proxymetacaine is sufficiently different from tetracaine to make cross-reactivity unlikely. This case suggests, however, that some degree of cross-sensitization can occur.

References

1. Liesegang TJ, Perniciaro C. Fingertip dermatitis in an ophthalmologist caused by proparacaine. Am J Ophthalmol 1999;127(2):240–1.

2. Dannaker CJ, Maibach HI, Austin E. Allergic contact dermatitis to proparacaine with subsequent cross-sensitization to tetracaine from ophthalmic preparations. Am J Contact Dermatitis 2001;12(3):177–9.

Proxyphylline

General Information

Proxyphylline is a theophylline derivative used as a bronchodilator. It is readily absorbed from the gastro-intestinal tract and is not converted to theophylline.

In 12 patients with chronic obstructive pulmonary disease, intravenous proxyphylline 16 mg/kg lowered airway resistance by 30% in 9 patients and by 40% in 7 (1). There were no serious adverse effects and, in particular, no adverse cardiovascular effects or muscle tremor.

In a short-term, double-blind, crossover study in 10 adult asthmatics, a modified-release formulation of proxyphylline (2400 mg/day) was compared with theophylline (800 mg/day) and placebo (2). There were no significant differences between the treatments with regard to relief of asthma symptoms, the need for additional medication, or the incidence and intensity of adverse effects. The adverse reactions included loss of appetite, palpitation, headache, nausea, stomach ache, muscle tremor, and sleep disturbances.

References

1 Geisler LS, Thiel H, Forster OB, Rohner HG. Proxyphyllinwirkung bei chronisch-obstruktiven Atemweg-serkrankungen. [Effectiveness of proxyphylline in chronic obstructive pulmonary disease.] Dtsch Med Wochenschr 1980;105(25):894–7.

2 Mosbech H, Paulsen H, Soborg M. Controlled-release theophylline and proxyphylline in asthmatics: a comparative study. Pharmatherapeutica 1984;3(9):626–30.

Pyrantel

General Information

Pyrantel is an antihelminthic drug that is effective against intestinal nematodes, including roundworms (*Ascaris lumbricoides*), threadworms (*Enterobius vermicularis*), *Trichostrongylus* species, and the tissue nematode *Trichinella spiralis*. Although it is effective against hookworms, it is less effective against *Necator americanus* than against *Ancylostoma duodenale*.

Pyrantel is usually given as the embonate or pamoate in a single dose of 10 mg/kg, and adverse reactions rarely impede treatment. They include gastrointestinal disturbance (nausea, anorexia, abdominal pain, diarrhea), headache, and vomiting, which are usually mild but can occur in up to 20% of patients.

Organs and Systems

Nervous system

Myasthenia gravis has reportedly been aggravated by pyrantel pamoate (1).

Liver

In children aged 5–10 years pyrantel caused mild transient changes in liver function tests (2).

Drug–Drug Interactions

Theophylline

An interaction of pyrantel with theophylline has been reported (3).

- An 8-year-old boy with status asthmaticus was given intravenous aminophylline and then switched to modified-release oral theophylline on day 3, when his serum theophylline concentration was 15 µg/ml. On day 4 he was given a single dose of pyrantel 160 mg (for *A. lumbricoides* infection) at the same time as his second oral dose of theophylline. About 2.5 hours later his serum theophylline concentration was 24 µg/ml, and a further 1.5 hours later it had risen to 30 µg/ml. No further theophylline was given and no theophylline toxicity occurred.

References

1. Bescansa E, Nicolas M, Aguado C, Toledano M, Vinals M. Myasthenia gravis aggravated by pyrantel pamoate. J Neurol Neurosurg Psychiatry 1991;54(6):563.
2. Dotsenko VA, Ordyntseva AP, Makarova TA, Shirinian AA, Lysakova LA. [Experience with the use of nemocide (pyrantel pamoate) in nematodiases.] Med Parazitol (Mosk) 1989;(5):36–9.
3. Hecht L, Mssurray WE. Theophylline–pyrantel pamoate interaction. DICP 1989;23(3):258.

Pyrazinamide

See also Antituberculosis drugs

General Information

Pyrazinamide is a pyrazine analogue of nicotinamide. It is bactericidal for *Mycobacterium tuberculosis* in an acid environment and within macrophages (1). Regimens that include pyrazinamide produce significantly more rapid rates of sputum conversion than any other combination. Pyrazinamide is therefore especially appropriate in the initial phase of treatment. In the 6-month regimen of the American Thoracic Society, pyrazinamide was used together with isoniazid and rifampicin for the first 2 months (2).

Pyrazinamide is distributed throughout the body. Peak plasma concentrations are reached 2 hours after oral administration. Excretion is primarily by glomerular filtration. Serum concentrations are generally 30–50 µg/ml with daily doses of 20–25 mg/kg. The maximum daily dose should not exceed 3 g, regardless of weight. At a pH of 5.5, the minimal inhibitory concentration of pyrazinamide for *Mycobacterium tuberculosis* is 20 µg/ml (1).

Observational studies

The combination of pyrazinamide plus levofloxacin is first-line treatment for multidrug-resistant latent tuberculosis. In 17 Canadian patients there were important adverse reactions affecting the musculoskeletal and central nervous systems; hyperuricemia, gastrointestinal effects, and dermatological effects were also common (3). This combination may be used with careful monitoring for adverse effects.

General adverse effects

Most of the adverse effects of pyrazinamide are toxic effects. Reactions involving the liver, hyperuricemia with and without gout, and symptoms of pellagra have particularly been recognized. Fever and urticaria are described. Sideroblastic anemia, thrombocytopenia, anorexia, nausea and vomiting, dysuria, malaise, and aggravation of peptic ulcer can occur (SEDA-13, 261). Allergic reactions and tumor-inducing effects have not been reported.

Organs and Systems

Cardiovascular

Acute symptomatic hypertension consistently followed the administration of pyrazinamide to a 65-year-old woman with pulmonary tuberculosis (4).

Metabolism

Pyrazinamide interferes with the renal excretion of urate, resulting in hyperuricemia. Acute episodes of gout or arthralgia have occurred. Arthralgia responds better to NSAIDs than to uricosuric drugs (5).

Pyrazinamide can aggravate porphyria (1).

Liver

Liver damage is the most common adverse effect of pyrazinamide (6). It varies from asymptomatic alteration of liver function detectable only by laboratory tests, through a mild syndrome characterized by fever, anorexia, malaise, liver tenderness, hepatomegaly, and splenomegaly, to more serious reactions with clinical jaundice, and finally the rare form with progressive acute yellow atrophy and death. As most patients take a combined regimen of pyrazinamide with isoniazid and rifampicin, it is difficult to determine which of the three drugs causes the hepatotoxicity; it could be due to a combined effect (7). As with isoniazid and rifampicin, hepatic function should initially be monitored every few weeks.

Skin

Pyrazinamide can cause pellagra. However, prophylactic nicotinamide is not generally recommended. In cases of pellagra, a dosage of 300 mg/day should be given (8).

In one case, erythema multiforme and urticaria occurred together after administration of pyrazinamide, and there were circulating immune complexes (9).

Photosensitization has been rarely described in patients taking pyrazinamide (10).

Susceptibility Factors

Age

00Although pyrazinamide is a part of conventional combination therapy for children with tuberculosis, as in adults (11), there is little published information on its safety. In those with raised transaminases before the start of therapy there was no increase during therapy, and the activities normalized in all patients after its conclusion.

Hepatic disease

Pyrazinamide should be avoided in patients with liver disease and porphyria (1). Liver function tests should be repeated at frequent intervals during the entire period of treatment.

Other features of the patient

Pyrazinamide should be used with extreme caution in patients with a history of gout, especially in elderly people, in whom urinary urate stones can cause renal insufficiency.

In patients with hemoptysis, the possibility that pyrazinamide may have an adverse effect on blood clotting time or vascular integrity should be borne in mind (12,13).

References

1. Mandell GL, Sande MA. Antimicrobial agents: drugs used in the chemotherapy of tuberculosis and leprosy. In: Goodman Gilman A, Rall TW, Nies AS, Taylor P, editors. Goodman and Gilman's The Pharmacological Basis of Therapeutics. 8th ed. Chapter 49. New York: Pergamon Press, 1990:1146.
2. Bass JB Jr, Farer LS, Hopewell PC, O'Brien R, Jacobs RF, Ruben F, Snider DE Jr, Thornton G. Treatment of tuberculosis and tuberculosis infection in adults and children. American Thoracic Society and The Centers for Disease Control and Prevention. Am J Respir Crit Care Med 1994;149(5):1359–74.
3. Papastavros T, Dolovich LR, Holbrook A, Whitehead L, Loeb M. Adverse events associated with pyrazinamide and levofloxacin in the treatment of latent multidrug-resistant tuberculosis. CMAJ 2002;167(2):131–6.
4. Goldberg J, Moreno F, Barbara J. Acute hypertension as an adverse effect of pyrazinamide. JAMA 1997;277(17):1356.
5. Patel AM, McKeon J. Avoidance and management of adverse reactions to antituberculosis drugs. Drug Saf 1995;12(1):1–25.
6. Danan G, Pessayre D, Larrey D, Benhamou JP. Pyrazinamide fulminant hepatitis: an old hepatotoxin strikes again. Lancet 1981;2(8254):1056–7.
7. Pretet S, Perdrizet S. La toxicité du pyrazinamide dans les traitements antituberculeux. [Toxicity of pyrazinamide in antituberculous treatments.] Rev Fr Mal Respir 1980;8(4):307–30.
8. Jorgensen J. Pellagra probably due to pyrazinamide: development during combined chemotherapy of tuberculosis. Int J Dermatol 1983;22(1):44–5.
9. Perdu D, Lavaud F, Prevost A, Deschamps F, Cambie MP, Bongrain E, Barhoum K, Kalis B. Erythema multiforme due to pyrazinamide. Allergy 1996;51(5):340–2.
10. Chan SL. Chemotherapy of tuberculosis. In: Davies PDO, editor. Clinical Tuberculosis. London: Chapman and Hall, 1994:141.
11. Britsch Medical Association and Royal Pharmaceutical Society of Great Britain. Antituberculous drugs. Br Natl Formulary 1998;35:160.
12. Jenner PJ, Ellard GA, Allan WG, Singh D, Girling DJ, Nunn AJ. Serum uric acid concentrations and arthralgia among patients treated with pyrazinamide-containing regimens in Hong Kong and Singapore. Tubercle 1981;62(3):175–9.
13. Lukaszczyk E, Radecki A, Ignasiak J. Wplyw pobierania pyrazinamidu na uklad krzepniecia krwi i fibrynolize. [Effect of pyrazinamide on the blood coagulation system and fibrinolysis.] Gruzlica 1970;38(3):229–37.

Pyridoxine

See also Vitamins

General Information

Pyridoxine (vitamin B_6) requirements vary with protein intake: the daily Average Requirement is 13 micrograms/g protein intake and the Population Reference Intake is 15 micrograms/g protein intake. In adults this translates into a daily Average Requirement of 1.3 mg/day for men and 1.0 mg/day for women, and a Population Reference Intake of 1.5 mg/day for men and 1.1 mg/day for women.

Uses

Pyridoxine is used to prevent the adverse nervous system effects of isoniazid (1). Adherence to therapy is improved by prescribing combined tablets containing 20 mg of pyridoxine per 100 mg of isoniazid.

Megadoses of pyridoxine are commonly used to treat homocystinuria, cystathioninuria, and primary oxalosis type I (2,3). In some diseases pyridoxine is used empirically, including rheumatic diseases, degenerative joint diseases, carpal tunnel syndrome, Chinese restaurant syndrome, and premenstrual syndrome. A rare form of neonatal seizures, reported as early as 1954, seems to respond only to large doses of pyridoxine (4,5). Occasionally, the condition can appear up to 2 years after birth. Affected patients can have abrupt seizure cessation and dramatic improvement in the electroencephalogram after receiving an intravenous dose of pyridoxine 50–100 mg. The mechanism of this rare condition is unclear. It has been suggested that in these infants there is a shift in the balance of glutamate and GABA in the central nervous system; giving pyridoxine increases the co-enzyme pool, offsetting the adverse kinetics that result from altered glutamate decarboxylase binding. One adverse consequence of the large dose of pyridoxine required is a diffuse inhibitory state, with effects ranging from excessive drowsiness to coma and electrocerebral silence. Resuscitation equipment should be on hand if this treatment is used.

Extremely high doses of pyridoxine, even up to 6000 mg/day, have also sometimes been used therapeutically. While few problems arise from controlled application of high doses of pyridoxine under medical supervision, self-medication in doses exceeding 300–500 mg/day can lead to adverse effects, especially when continued over a long period of time. Many patients have self-medicated with more than 2000 mg/day for long periods of time (SEDA-10, 334) (6,7).

In many countries, pyridoxine is a component of "vitamin B complex" products, administered orally or parenterally as "tonics," commonly because of their supposedly beneficial effects on the nervous system.

General adverse effects

Under the headline "Still time for rational debate about vitamin B_6" the controversial debate on the safety of pyridoxine has been revived (8). Pyridoxine is marketed for stress in general, for depression associated with premenstrual syndrome and oral contraceptives, and for carpal tunnel syndrome, although it is doubtful that it has more than a placebo effect. It is legitimately prescribed in general deficiency states in doses starting at 150 mg/day. Adverse events include sensory neuropathy at oral doses about 2–3 g/day or more.

The editorial refers to the attempts of the UK Government's Committee on Toxicity to find the safe level of daily consumption of pyridoxine. In July 1997 the committee recommended that the sale of pyridoxine in, for instance, health-food shops would be restricted to doses of 10 mg/day. Doses between 10 and 50 mg would be restricted to sale at pharmacies; and doses of 50 mg and above would be available only on prescription. Contrary to these UK recommendations the Committee of the US National Academy of Science concluded that there were no convincing reports of adverse events at doses of up to 200 mg/day. Paying attention to the fact that recommendations tend to be more cautious than might seem necessary from the available evidence, the US experts halved the 200 mg/day dose to define their limit as 100 mg/day.

The author of the editorial found fault with the fact that the US experts have based their recommendations on the slimmest of evidence. The main human study was a self-recall series of 172 patients presenting to a private practice in London (9). In a letter to the editor, Beckett (10) pointed out that daily doses of 200 mg or less have been taken by millions of people worldwide for several decades without evident toxicity and that testimonials from clinicians expert in the use of pyridoxine have attested to its safety in these doses (11). Referring to the editorial, the author of the study in question stated that their study referred to 172 women with raised blood concentrations of pyridoxine that reverted to normal within 4 days of stopping pyridoxine, and was not a "self-recall series." In a recent follow-up of these women who had raised blood concentrations, compared with controls from the same practice who had had a blood test in 1985–86 and whose record showed that they were not taking pyridoxine or multivitamins at that time or since, 16 of 50 respondents had subsequently had autoimmune disease, compared with one of the 38 controls. The autoimmune diseases included thyroid disease ($n = 5$), rheumatoid arthritis ($n = 3$), diabetes ($n = 2$), Sjögren's syndrome ($n = 2$), primary biliary cirrhosis ($n = 1$), polymyalgia rheumatica ($n = 1$), and polyarteritis nodosum ($n = 1$). In the controls there was one case of diabetes.

In another letter to the editor (12) it was mentioned that the suspicion of partiality about the Committee on Toxicity becomes more plausible when one considers the issue of homocysteine. This intermediate metabolite may well turn out to be of greater importance as a risk factor for cardiovascular disease than cholesterol and blood pressure. Raised homocysteine concentrations appear to be accessible to treatment with pyridoxine (100 mg/day) together with vitamin B_{12} and folic acid (13). Furthermore, the statement that there is no good evidence for the efficacy of pyridoxine in any disease, apart from depression, was criticized, because this ignores important studies in autism, pregnancy outcome, asthma, and sickle-cell anemia (12).

In a systematic review on the efficacy of pyridoxine in the treatment of premenstrual syndrome, adverse effects were reported in 63 patients (6.7%) (see Table 1) (14). In another study of 940 women one had a neuropathy associated with pyridoxine toxicity (15).

Table 1 Adverse effects of pyridoxine in the treatment of premenstrual syndrome

Number taking		Dosage and duration	Adverse effects	Number with adverse effects	
Pyridoxine	Placebo			Pyridoxine	Placebo
204	230	10–200 mg/day	Tingling in the fingers	11	8
49	70	200 mg/day*, four cycles		5	1
46	59	100 mg/day*, four cycles		5	2
14	8	600 mg/day, three cycles		1	0
31	–	150–600 mg/day*	Gastrointestinal	5	–
630	–	4–200 mg/day	Indigestion (7), nausea (5), breast soreness (3)	15	–
336	–	Over 200 mg/day	Nausea (8), dizziness (5), mild tingling or numbness (6)	21	–

*In a multivitamin formulation

Organs and Systems

Nervous system

Pyridoxine has both dopamine-enhancing and dopamine-blocking properties: on the one hand pyridoxine (like dopamine) depresses the release of prolactin from the pituitary gland; on the other hand, in oral doses of 10–20 mg it rapidly reverses the therapeutic effect of dopamine (16). This should be borne in mind if pyridoxine is prescribed for nursing mothers or for patients treated with levodopa for Parkinson's disease or syndrome, although the problem does not seem to arise when using the combination of levodopa with decarboxylase inhibitors.

Reviews of sensory neuropathies and pyridoxine toxicity have been published (17–19). Sensory neuropathy has been described in certain individuals taking high daily doses of pyridoxine on a long-term basis. Although it is generally reversible, a chronic painful neuropathy can occur. Besides individual patient susceptibility, the risk of neurotoxic effects of pyridoxine is related to both the daily dose and the duration of administration. Peripheral neuropathy did not develop in individuals taking 500 mg/day for up to 2 years, whereas it did develop almost universally in patients who took more than 1000 mg/day for variable periods (17). In an adult, a daily dose of 500 mg/day is about 7.1 mg/kg/day. Therefore a child with pyridoxine-dependency taking 5 mg/kg/day may not be at risk of neuropathy. Only one patient with pyridoxine-dependent seizures in whom a sensory neuropathy developed has been described (20). It is recommended that patients with this disorder who will require life-long pharmacological doses of pyridoxine should be assessed for signs of a sensory peripheral neuropathy.

Sensory neuropathy was reported as an adverse effect in eight patients with homocystinuria who took 600–1200 mg/day of pyridoxine for 4–22 years. Nerve conduction studies of the sural nerve in five affected patients showed abnormalities in four (21). Neuropathies have been observed in women taking doses as low as 50–500 mg/day for one to several months (22,23).

Neurotoxicity can be associated with pyridoxine megavitamin therapy (24), the main symptom being a peripheral sensory neuropathy (see Table 2) (25,26).

Table 2 Peripheral sensory neuropathy during pyridoxine megatherapy

Authors	Cases	Daily dose	Duration of treatment
Schaumburg et al. (1983)	7	2–6 g	2–40 months
Berger and Schaumburg (1974)	1	500 mg	1 year
Vasile et al. (1984)	1	3 g	6 months
De Zegher et al. (1985)	1	1 g	Not specified
Dalton (1985)	23	50–300 mg	Not specified
Parry and Bredesen (1985)	16	200–5000 mg	1–36 months
Podell (1985)	1	500 mg	8 years
Baer and Stillman (1984)	1	4 g	4 years (dermatosis)
Friedman et al. (1986)	1	2 g	1 year (dermatosis)

Hematologic

Reduced serum folate concentrations have been demonstrated in patients with homocystinuria taking pyridoxine. The mechanism of this effect may involve removal of substrate inhibition of the enzyme, $N5$-methyltetrahydrofolate homocysteine methyltransferase, due to pyridoxine-induced reduction of the substrate, homocysteine (27).

Skin

Pyridoxine-induced photosensitivity has been reported in a patient with hypophosphatasia (28).

- A 30-year-old woman, a heterozygote for hypophosphatasia, who had been taking two tablets of a multivitamin formulation (pyridoxine hydrochloride 100 mg, riboflavin butyrate 30 mg, nicotinamide 40 mg, biotin 0.05 mg, ascorbic acid 100 mg) once daily for 6 years, had severe skin eruptions and pruritus on exposure to the sun. The minimum erythema doses for UVB (20 mJ/cm^2) and UVA (4 J/cm^2) were lower than normal only for UVB (reference ranges 60–100 mJ/cm^2 for UVB and below 10 J/cm^2 for UVA). Patch and photopatch tests with the constituents of the tablets produced reactions to pyridoxine and pyridoxal phosphate only.

The authors suggested that photosensitivity in this patient may have been caused by abnormal metabolism of pyridoxine because of hypophosphatasia. Pyridoxine (given alone or in combination with vitamin B_{12}) can aggravate acne vulgaris or eruption of an acneiform exanthema (29). Excessive doses of pyridoxine appear to cause a metabolic defect that impairs the structural integrity of the skin, especially during the summer months (30). There are some case reports of photosensitive dermatitis caused by pyridoxine hydrochloride (31–33). Vesicular skin lesions on the hands and feet have also been reported, possibly as a symptom secondary to the neurological disturbances (34).

Contact hypersensitivity to pyridoxine is rare. Only three cases of allergy to pyridoxine have been reported: in hair lotion (35), a glucocorticoid cream (36), and a skin cream (Iruxol) (37). There have also been a few reports of photosensitivity due to pyridoxine hydrochloride (30,31,33).

Occupational systemic contact dermatitis with photosensitivity has been attributed to pyridoxine (38).

- A 45-year-old man developed eczema over the back of his hands, the back and sides of his fingers (sparing the little fingers), the forearms, and the face. This lasted for 6 years, with recurrences and remissions. He was tested with allergens, supplemented with a drop each of various injectable medicaments (streptomycin, benzylpenicillin, ampicillin–cloxacillin, oxytetracycline, vitamins B_1, B_2, and B_{12}, gentamicin, amikacin, and analgesics). Patch tests were positive to nitrofurazane and three different B vitamins. Reactivation of lesions on the hands, face, and neck was noted during patch-testing, and subsided within 1 week. After a further 6 weeks he was tested on the forearms with B_1, B_6, and B_{12}, each in 10% propylene glycol, resulting in a ++ reaction for B_6. Prick testing with B_1, B_2, and B_6 gave negative results. Another 2 months later oral provocation with two tablets each containing B_6 100 mg was performed. Before taking the second tablet he started to itch, and 18 hours later he developed itching and severe erythema over the face, neck, back of the hands, forearms, and the distal half of the upper arms (sun-exposed areas). Reactivation of previous positive patch test sites (on the back and forearms) and a negative prick test site were also observed.

Rosacea fulminans is a rare variant of rosacea conglobata and is seen almost exclusively in postadolescent women. It is characterized by the sudden appearance of abscess-forming nodules and draining sinuses. The lesions are usually limited to the center of the face and are precipitated by marked seborrhea. The cause is unknown. Rosacea fulminans temporally associated with the ingestion of high-dose vitamin B supplements has been reported (39).

- A 17-year-old woman with a 5-week history of a facial rash took minocycline (100 mg/day for 14 days) without effect. She had been taking vitamin B supplements (pyridoxine 80 mg, which is over 40 times the recommended daily allowance) and vitamin B_{12} (20 micrograms, which is 20 times the recommended daily allowance) for 2 weeks before the onset of the eruption. She had had low-grade acne vulgaris since puberty and a tendency to facial flushing after drinking alcohol and eating spicy food. There were numerous confluent nodules and pustules on a livid erythematous background on the cheeks and chin, and a few pustules on the neck. There was seborrhea on the affected skin areas. There was an indolent lymphadenopathy in the submandibular region. Histology showed a superficial and deep inflammatory infiltrate with perifollicular distribution, from the upper dermis down to the septa of the subcutaneous fat. Routine laboratory tests showed no abnormalities. There were no pathogenic organisms in bacteriological or mycological cultures from the pustules on the face. She stopped taking the nutritional supplement and was given warm compresses and clobetasol propionate cream twice daily for 2 weeks, methylprednisolone 60 mg/day for 2 weeks, followed by isotretinoin 60 mg/day. Her skin changes resolved within 4 months, with no residual scarring.

Second-Generation Effects

Teratogenicity

- A malformed infant was born to a mother who had taken daily doses of pyridoxine during pregnancy (50 mg for the first 7 months) and unknown doses of lecithin and vitamin B_{12}. The girl was born with near-total amelia of her left leg at the knee (40).

Although this case may have been coincidental, as a precaution, megadoses of pyridoxine should be avoided during pregnancy.

References

1. Mandell GL, Sande MA. Antimicrobial agents: drugs used in the chemotherapy of tuberculosis and leprosy. In: Goodman Gilman A, Rall TW, Nies AS, Taylor P, editors. Goodman and Gilman's The Pharmacological Basis of Therapeutics. 8th ed, chapter 49. New York: Pergamon Press, 1990:1146.

2. Bremer HJ, Endres W. Primary cystathioninuria. Methionine load tests and response to pyridoxine. Helv Paediatr Acta 1972;27(5):525–36.

3. Marangella M. Transplantation strategies in type 1 primary hyperoxaluria: the issue of pyridoxine responsiveness. Nephrol Dial Transplant 1999;14(2):301–3.

4. Hunt AD Jr, Stokes J Jr, McCrory WW, Stroud HH. Pyridoxine dependency: report of a case of intractable convulsions in an infant controlled by pyridoxine. Pediatrics 1954;13(2):140–5.

5. Bass NE, Wyllie E, Cohen B, Joseph SA. Pyridoxine-dependent epilepsy: the need for repeated pyridoxine trials and the risk of severe electrocerebral suppression with intravenous pyridoxine infusion. J Child Neurol 1996;11(5):422–4.

6. Dalton K. Pyridoxine overdose in premenstrual syndrome. Lancet 1985;1(8438):1168–9.

7. Parry GJ, Bredesen DE. Sensory neuropathy with low-dose pyridoxine. Neurology 1985;35(10):1466–8.

8. Anonymous. Still time for rational debate about vitamin B6. Lancet 1998;351(9115):1523.

9. Dalton K, Dalton MJ. Characteristics of pyridoxine overdose neuropathy syndrome. Acta Neurol Scand 1987;76(1):8–11.

10. Beckett A. Debate continues on vitamin B6. Lancet 1998;352(9121):62.

11. IPCS International Programme on Chemical Safety in cooperation with the joint FAO/WHO Expert Committee on Food Additives (JECFA). Environmental Health Criteria 70. Geneva: WHO, 1987.

12. Downing D. Debate continues on vitamin B6. Lancet 1998;352(9121):63.

13. Selhub J, Jacques PF, Wilson PW, Rush D, Rosenberg IH. Vitamin status and intake as primary determinants of homocysteinemia in an elderly population. JAMA 1993; 270(22):2693–8.

14. Wyatt KM, Dimmock PW, Jones PW, Shaughn O'Brien PM. Efficacy of vitamin B-6 in the treatment of premenstrual syndrome: systematic review. BMJ 1999;318(7195):1375–81.

15. London RS, Bradley L, Chiamori NY. Effect of a nutritional supplement on premenstrual symptomatology in women with premenstrual syndrome: a double-blind longitudinal study. J Am Coll Nutr 1991;10(5):494–9.

16. Greentree LB. Dangers of vitamin B6 in nursing mothers. N Engl J Med 1979;300(3):141–2.

17. Bendich A, Cohen M. Vitamin B6 safety issues. Ann NY Acad Sci 1990;585:321–30.

18. Bernstein AL. Vitamin B6 in clinical neurology. Ann NY Acad Sci 1990;585:250–60.

19. Gospe SM Jr. Current perspectives on pyridoxine-dependent seizures. J Pediatr 1998;132(6):919–23.

20. McLachlan RS, Brown WF. Pyridoxine dependent epilepsy with iatrogenic sensory neuronopathy. Can J Neurol Sci 1995;22(1):50–1.

21. Ludolph AC, Masur H, Oberwittler C, Koch HG, Ullrich K. Sensory neuropathy and vitamin B6 treatment in homocystinuria. Eur J Pediatr 1993;152(3):271.

22. Dalton K. Toxicity of vitamins. BMJ 1986;292:903.

23. Reimann, Rothenberger. Neuro- und embryotoxische Nebenwirkungen von Vitamin B6. [Neuro- and embryotoxic side effects of vitamin B6.] Med Monatsschr Pharm 1989;12(12):392–6.

24. Schaumburg H, Kaplan J, Windebank A, Vick N, Rasmus S, Pleasure D, Brown MJ. Sensory neuropathy from pyridoxine abuse. A new megavitamin syndrome. N Engl J Med 1983;309(8):445–8.

25. Camarasa JG, Serra-Baldrich E, Lluch M. Hipersensibilidad de contacto a la vitamina B6. Acta Dermo-Sif 8339–340.

26. Bässler KH. Nutzen und Gefahren einer Megavitamintherapie mit Vitamin B6. Dtsch Apoth Ztg 1990;130:1964–6.

27. Meyers DG, Maloley PA, Weeks D. Safety of antioxidant vitamins. Arch Intern Med 1996;156(9):925–35.

28. Kawada A, Kashima A, Shiraishi H, Gomi H, Matsuo I, Yasuda K, Sasaki G, Sato S, Orimo H. Pyridoxine-induced photosensitivity and hypophosphatasia. Dermatology 2000;201(4):356–60.

29. Braun-Falco O, Lincke H. Zur Frage der Vitamin B6/B12-Akne: ein Beitrag zur Acne medicamentosa. [The problem of vitamin B6/B12 acne. A contribution on acne medicamentosa.] MMW Munch Med Wochenschr 1976;118(6):155–60.

30. Baer RL. Cutaneous skin changes probably due to pyridoxine abuse. J Am Acad Dermatol 1984;10(3):527–8.

31. Murata Y, Kumano K, Ueda T, Araki N, Nakamura T, Tani M. Photosensitive dermatitis caused by pyridoxine hydrochloride. J Am Acad Dermatol 1998;39(2 Pt 2):314–17.

32. Tanaka M, Niizeki H, Shimizu S, Miyakawa S. Photoallergic drug eruption due to pyridoxine hydrochloride. J Dermatol 1996;23(10):708–9.

33. Morimoto K, Kawada A, Hiruma M, Ishibashi A. Photosensitivity from pyridoxine hydrochloride (vitamin B6). J Am Acad Dermatol 1996;35(2 Pt 2):304–5.

34. Friedman MA, Resnick JS, Baer RL. Subepidermal vesicular dermatosis and sensory peripheral neuropathy caused by pyridoxine abuse. J Am Acad Dermatol 1986;14(5 Pt 2):915–17.

35. Fujita M, Aoki T. Allergic contact dermatitis to pyridoxine ester and hinokitiol. Contact Dermatitis 1983;9(1):61–5.

36. Yoshikawa K, Watanabe K, Mizuno N. Contact allergy to hydrocortisone 17-butyrate and pyridoxine hydrochloride. Contact Dermatitis 1985;12(1):55–6.

37. Camarasa JG, Serra-Baldrich E, Lluch M. Contact allergy to vitamin B6. Contact Dermatitis 1990;23(2):115.

38. Bajaj AK, Rastogi S, Misra A, Misra K, Bajaj S. Occupational and systemic contact dermatitis with photosensitivity due to vitamin B6. Contact Dermatitis 2001;44(3):184.

39. Jansen T, Romiti R, Kreuter A, Altmeyer P. Rosacea fulminans triggered by high-dose vitamins B6 and B12. J Eur Acad Dermatol Venereol 2001;15(5):484–5.

40. Stephensen CB, Franchi LM, Hernandez H, Campos M, Gilman RH, Alvarez JO. Adverse effects of high-dose vitamin A supplements in children hospitalized with pneumonia. Pediatrics 1998;101(5):E3.

Pyrimethamine

General Information

Pyrimethamine

Pyrimethamine is the most active antimalarial of the 2–4-diaminopyrimidines, its effect being due to inhibition of the conversion of folic acid to its active form, folinic acid. It is also effective in toxoplasmosis. Its antiprotozoal and antimalarial activity is enhanced by the addition of sulfonamides.

Pyrimethamine is well absorbed in healthy subjects; the half-life is 80–95 hours (SEDA-13, 811). Absorption after intramuscular injection is slower; this may be of importance in patients with reduced muscle blood flow (SEDA-17, 328). Pyrimethamine penetrates the cerebrospinal fluid.

With the usual antimalarial prophylactic dosage of 25 mg/week, adverse reactions are generally slight or absent. With intensive treatment in high cumulative doses, as used in the treatment of toxoplasmosis, gastrointestinal intolerance, neurological symptoms, and depression of hemopoiesis can occur. Allergic reactions have not been reported. Tumor-inducing effects have also not been reported.

Pyrimethamine + azithromycin

Azithromycin is efficacious in animal models of toxoplasmic encephalitis. In a Phase I/II dose-escalation study of pyrimethamine (50 mg/day) plus azithromycin (900, 1200, or 1500 mg/day) for induction and maintenance treatment in 30 patients with AIDS and definite or suspected *Toxoplasma* encephalitis, the overall response rate was 67% after 6 weeks of induction therapy (1). However, maintenance therapy for 24 weeks with this combination was associated with a high relapse rate (47%); only six patients successfully completed induction and maintenance therapy. Adverse events were common (particularly in those taking azithromycin 1500 mg) and included hepatotoxicity, bone marrow suppression, ototoxicity, and gastrointestinal disturbances, which led 20% of patients to withdraw. All adverse events resolved on withdrawal.

In a prospective, randomized, open, multicenter trial of pyrimethamine + azithromycin versus pyrimethamine + sulfadiazine for the treatment of ocular toxoplasmosis in 46 patients with sight-threatening ocular toxoplasmosis, the two regimens had similar efficacy; however, the adverse effects were significantly less common and severe with pyrimethamine + azithromycin (2).

Pyrimethamine + clarithromycin

Clarithromycin, a macrolide, and other macrolide and lincosamine antibiotics (azithromycin, clindamycin, spiramycin, and roxithromycin) have been used in combination with pyrimethamine in the treatment of *Toxoplasma gondii* infections, especially cases of *Toxoplasma* encephalitis.

Clarithromycin 2 g plus pyrimethamine 75 mg/day has been given for 6 weeks to a few AIDS patients with encephalitis (SEDA-13, 814). The adverse effects were many and severe: severe thrombocytopenia, anemia, neutropenia, liver toxicity of varying degree, nausea, vomiting, skin rashes, and hearing loss were found in two of three patients tested in a group of 13. The dose of clarithromycin in this study was the maximum dosage used in an earlier investigation of the treatment of mycobacterial infections in HIV-infected patients.

Pyrimethamine + clindamycin

Pyrimethamine 50 mg/day has been used in combination with clindamycin for the treatment of *Toxoplasma* encephalitis in AIDS. Adverse effects were common (rash, diarrhea, nausea), but the incidence of hematological reactions was lower than with the combination of sulfadiazine and pyrimethamine (SEDA-16, 309).

Pyrimethamine + dapsone

Pyrimethamine and dapsone are available in two fixed combinations:

1. 12.5 mg of pyrimethamine + 100 mg of dapsone = Maloprim.
2. 25 mg of pyrimethamine + 100 mg of dapsone = Deltaprim.

A "dapsone syndrome" was reported in a 30-year-old woman after 4 weeks of treatment with Maloprim and chloroquine base 300 mg/weekly. The symptoms comprised fever, joint and muscle pains, dry cough, and a diffuse red urticarial rash, followed by generalized lymphadenopathy, a painful exudative tonsillitis, and a prominent atypical lymphocytosis.

In Britain, the retrospective reported rate for serious reactions with Maloprim was one in 9100, the incidence of blood dyscrasias being one in 20 000. These figures are lower than those reported with Fansidar (pyrimethamine + sulfadoxine) (SEDA-16, 309).

Pyrimethamine + sulfadoxine

Pyrimethamine 25 mg plus sulfadoxine 500 mg is available in the combination formulation known as Fansidar. This combination, while effective in the prevention and treatment of *Plasmodium falciparum* malaria, carries a high frequency of adverse effects; hematological and serious skin reactions occur, but there are also reports of polyneuritis, vasculitis, and hepatotoxicity. Most of the severe skin reactions and the cases of vasculitis developed within under a month (SEDA-13, 812). The use of Fansidar for malaria prophylaxis has therefore been virtually abandoned (SEDA-21, 297). However, Fansidar is being increasingly used for the treatment of *P. falciparum* malaria in Africa. With the higher dosage used for that purpose, an increase in adverse effects, particularly hematological, can be expected. In Britain the retrospective reported rate for all serious reactions to Fansidar was one in 2100 prescriptions and for skin reactions one in 4900 prescriptions, the death rate being one in 11 100 (SEDA-16, 309).

Observational studies

In a single-arm, open, prospective study between 1990 and 1995 (before HAART) the prophylactic efficacy of Fansidar was evaluated in 95 HIV-infected patients with successfully treated *Pneumocystis jiroveci* pneumonia and no history of *Toxoplasma* encephalitis (3). Patients took Fansidar with folinic acid (15 mg) twice weekly and were followed for a median of 19 (range 1–72) months. Five patients had a *Pneumocystis* relapse, but three had not taken their therapy. Of the 69 patients positive for anti-*Toxoplasma* IgG antibodies, only one developed toxoplasma encephalitis after 50 months. A rash developed in 16 patients after a median of 3 weeks, and required withdrawal in six. Two developed Stevens–Johnson syndrome after three or four doses. There was no significantly increased risk of adverse reactions to Fansidar in patients with previous hypersensitivity reactions to co-trimoxazole. The results of this study are of particular relevance to areas in which HAART is unavailable and where the antimalarial activity of Fansidar may confer additional benefit.

Placebo-controlled studies

In a placebo-controlled study of chemoprophylaxis for malaria, 701 Tanzanian infants were assigned to intermittent pyrimethamine + sulfadoxine (under 5 kg, a quarter of a tablet; 5–10 kg, half a tablet; over 10 kg, one tablet; each tablet contained pyrimethamine 25 mg plus sulfadoxine 500 mg) alongside routine childhood immunizations and iron supplementation at 2, 3, and 9 months of age (4). The combination was well tolerated, with no reported adverse events. Episodes of clinical malaria fell by 59% (95% CI = 41, 72) and the incidence of severe anemia by 50% (95% CI = 8, 73%) in the first year of life. Contrary to previous studies involving continuous prophylaxis in infants, there was no increase in the frequency of rebound episodes of malaria up to 18 months of age, suggesting that the development of malaria-specific immunity was unimpaired. Responses to vaccines were unaffected.

Pyrimethamine + sulfadoxine + mefloquine

Pyrimethamine (25 mg), sulfadoxine (500 mg), and mefloquine (250 mg) are available in the combination formulation known as Fansimef. The adverse effects characteristic of all three components can be expected.

Pyrimethamine + trimethoprim

With the combination of pyrimethamine plus trimethoprim the risk of megaloblastic anemia is higher than with pyrimethamine alone, which on theoretical grounds might be expected. Concomitant administration of folic acid has been recommended (SEDA-11, 590), but the effect of folic acid on efficacy is not known.

Organs and Systems

Respiratory

Pyrimethamine

Non-cardiogenic pulmonary edema has been reported with pyrimethamine alone (SEDA-13, 811).

Pyrimethamine + sulfadoxine

Dyspnea and pleurisy have been described. Of 52 travellers with adverse reactions to Fansidar in Sweden, six had pulmonary infiltrates accompanied by fever (SEDA-13, 241). Such infiltrates have also been described in the past, and in one case a diagnosis of eosinophilic infiltration was made (SEDA-11, 590). A case of non-cardiogenic pulmonary edema was reported in 1989 (SEDA-13, 813).

Nervous system

High doses of pyrimethamine can cause rapid development of neurological symptoms such as ataxia, tremor, and convulsions, probably by a direct toxic effect (SEDA-11, 588).

Hematologic

Pyrimethamine

Leukopenia, agranulocytosis, and thrombocytopenia have been reported and, as might be expected in view of folate antagonism, megaloblastic anemia. The latter is more common when high doses are used or when pyrimethamine is given in combination with a drug such as trimethoprim. The bone marrow depression can be reversed using folic acid (SEDA-18, 287).

Pancytopenia has been reported after the use of pyrimethamine alone, but is more often the result of its use in combination with dapsone or sulfonamides (SEDA-11, 589) (SEDA-14, 241) (SEDA-17, 328).

Although the hematological complications of pyrimethamine are generally a consequence of therapeutic use, long-term prophylactic treatment with pyrimethamine and dapsone in malaria could well involve an increased risk of megaloblastic anemia in patients whose nutritional state is not optimal (SEDA-13, 812).

Pyrimethamine + dapsone

The combination of pyrimethamine plus dapsone causes a higher incidence of blood dyscrasias than pyrimethamine alone; in particular, the occurrence of agranulocytosis increases and even deaths have been reported (SEDA-13, 812) (SEDA-18, 287).

Dapsone (alone or in combination with pyrimethamine) can cause methemoglobinemia and hemolytic anemia. These complications tend to be dose-related and are more often encountered in G6PD-deficient subjects (SEDA-18, 287).

When the pyrimethamine + dapsone combination was used in the prophylaxis of *Pneumocystis jiroveci* pneumonia in 173 patients with AIDS, there was anemia in about 20, and in all 117 cases for which data were available, serum haptoglobin concentrations had fallen (SEDA-18, 287).

Pyrimethamine + sulfadoxine

The hematological adverse effects of the combination of pyrimethamine plus sulfadoxine are largely those known from pyrimethamine, that is leukopenia, agranulocytosis, thrombocytopenia, and pancytopenia, but the literature gives the impression that when using this combination these effects are more marked, with lower cell counts (5).

Intermittent iron supplementation with pyrimethamine + sulfadoxine has been investigated in 328 anemic but symptom-free Kenyan children, who were randomly given either iron (ferrous fumarate suspension 6.25 g/l twice a week) or placebo and pyrimethamine + sulfadoxine (25 mg and 1.25 mg/kg once every 4 weeks) or placebo (82 in each group) (6). After 12 weeks, those who took iron and pyrimethamine + sulfadoxine, iron alone, or pyrimethamine + sulfadoxine alone had higher hemoglobin concentrations than those who took the double placebo. No adverse effects were reported.

Severe megaloblastic anemia has also been described (7).

- Hemolytic–uremic syndrome was reported in a 24-year-old man with glucose-6-phosphate dehydrogenase (G6PD) deficiency (SEDA-18, 288).

Gastrointestinal

Gastric disturbances due to pyrimethamine are dose-related; the high doses used in the treatment of toxoplasmosis caused abdominal pains, vomiting, and dizziness (8). Gastrointestinal bleeding related to thrombocytopenia has also been reported (SEDA-11, 589).

Liver

Pyrimethamine + sulfadoxine

Liver function abnormalities with Fansidar (pyrimethamine + sulfadoxine) vary from raised serum transaminase activities to more marked disturbances, with jaundice and granulomatous hepatitis. An occasional case of fatal hepatic failure has been reported; this was the case in a young white American woman who had taken three doses of Fansidar with chloroquine (SEDA-12, 242). Hepatic symptoms may be part of a vasculitis syndrome or can be seen in association with skin reactions (SEDA-13, 241).

Skin

Pyrimethamine

Photosensitivity has been attributed to pyrimethamine (9).

Hyperpigmentation is a very rare adverse effect of pyrimethamine.

- A 29-year-old woman (HIV-negative) developed hyperpigmentation after taking pyrimethamine 25 mg bd for 40 days (10). The hyperpigmentation regressed 15 days after withdrawal of pyrimethamine.

Pyrimethamine + dapsone

Skin rashes are uncommon with the combination of pyrimethamine + dapsone. A lichen planus type of skin reaction has been described (11).

Pyrimethamine + sulfadoxine

Severe skin reactions have been reported with the combination of pyrimethamine + sulfadoxine (Fansidar) from various countries. These include erythema exudativum multiforme, Stevens–Johnson syndrome, toxic epidermal necrolysis, cutaneous vasculitis, lichen planus, a single case of ectodermosis pluriorificialis, and some cases of photosensitivity.

The incidence of skin reactions seems to vary regionally: there is a low incidence in Switzerland (12), but a high incidence has been reported by the US Centers for Disease Control. The latter reported skin reactions in 1:5000 to 1:8000 cases, with fatal reactions in 1:10 000 to 1:25 000 users (SEDA-12, 242). In Britain the retrospective reporting rate for all serious reactions was 1:2100 and for cutaneous reactions one in 4900 prescriptions, with a fatality rate of one in 11 100 (SEDA-16, 309).

In a spontaneous reporting system of individuals who had been exposed to Fansidar in 27 countries, an estimated 117 million users, there were 126 reports: 87 cases of erythema multiforme or Stevens–Johnson syndrome and 39 cases of toxic epidermal necrolysis; 86% of the cases were reported in Europe or North America (13). The fatality rates were 36% for toxic epidermal necrolysis (95% CI = 21, 53) and 9% for erythema multiforme/Stevens–Johnson syndrome (4, 18). The overall SCAR risk was 1.1 (0.9, 1.3) per million. For developing countries with mainly single-dose use, the risk was estimated at 0.1 (0.0, 0.1) per million. For Europe and North America, with mainly prophylactic use, the risks were 10 (8, 12) and 36 (23, 48) per million respectively.

The prevalence of oral lichenoid reactions was 4.8% in 186 Malay army personnel who used Fansidar for 9 weeks, 0.5% in 186 army personnel who had stopped using Fansidar for 2 months, and 0% in 143 army personnel (control group) who had not used Fansidar for at least 4 months (14).

- Exudative erythema multiforme with chronic proliferation of the conjunctiva causing blindness was described in a 24-year-old man who had taken one tablet of Fansidar at 6-day intervals on three occasions (SEDA-16, 309).

Immunologic

Pyrimethamine + dapsone

Maloprim given for antimalarial prophylaxis was associated with immunosuppression: in military personnel in Singapore (15). The incidence of upper respiratory tract infections was 64% higher than in the non-treated group.

Three patients developed a hypersensitivity syndrome after taking pyrimethamine 12.5 mg + dapsone 100 mg weekly as malaria prophylaxis (16). The diagnosis was based on the presence of fever, lymphadenopathy, a maculopapular rash, and hepatitis. A mild Coombs'-positive hemolytic anemia was also observed in one of the patients. All the clinical, hematological, and biochemical abnormalities normalized within 3 months of tapering regimens of moderate-dose prednisolone.

Pyrimethamine + sulfadoxine

Generalized vasculitis was reported in two cases in Sweden; one developed fever, jaundice, orchitis, and gastrointestinal bleeding after 2 weeks, the other cutaneous vasculitis and rapid progressive nephritis after 3 weeks (SEDA-13, 241).

An illness resembling Sézary syndrome was seen after combined treatment with chloroquine 150 mg every third day (total seven tablets) plus Fansidar one tablet weekly (total six tablets); the symptoms comprised fever, diarrhea, erythroderma, jaundice, lymphadenopathy, and hepatosplenomegaly (SEDA-12, 696).

The safety and efficacy of a fixed combination of pyrimethamine 25 mg + sulfadoxine 500 mg, supplemented with folinic acid 15 mg, both twice a week, as primary prophylaxis of *Pneumocystis* pneumonia and *Toxoplasma* encephalitis has been evaluated in 106 patients infected with HIV in a single-arm, open, prospective study (17). There were allergic reactions in 18 patients and permanent withdrawal was required in seven. One patient who took continued prophylaxis despite progressive hypersensitivity reactions developed a serious adverse reaction (Stevens–Johnson syndrome).

Long-Term Effects

Drug tolerance

Resistance to pyrimethamine has been reported from the Amazon region and Southeast Asia (SEDA-21, 297).

Second-Generation Effects

Pregnancy

Pyrimethamine + dapsone

A stillborn male child with a severe defect of the abdominal and thoracic wall and a missing left arm was delivered at 26 weeks to a woman who had used Maloprim on days

10, 20, and 30 after conception (SEDA-11, 589). The case was anecdotal and the relation to medication uncertain.

Teratogenicity

Pyrimethamine

Pyrimethamine is an inhibitor of dihydrofolate reductase and causes tetrahydrofolate deficiency. It is teratogenic in animals: in rats it produces limb defects, cleft palate, and brachygnathia, and in chick embryos micromelia. Fetal death has been seen in rats and hamsters. However, in toxoplasmosis, pyrimethamine, with or without a sulfonamide, has been given to pregnant women without evidence of subsequent abnormalities. Supplementation with folic acid has been advocated to prevent or reduce adverse effects (SEDA-13, 812), but it is not known if this could impair efficacy.

Pyrimethamine + sulfadoxine

Malaria during pregnancy is associated with an increased risk of severe anemia and babies of low birth weight. Effective intermittent therapy with pyrimethamine + sulfadoxine reduces parasitemia and severe anemia and improves birth weight in areas in which *P. falciparum* is sensitive to this combination. In an open, prospective trial in 287 pregnant women in the Gambia who were exposed to a single dose of a combination of artesunate and pyrimethamine + sulfadoxine there was no evidence of a teratogenic or otherwise harmful effect (18).

Susceptibility Factors

Pyrimethamine

Pyrimethamine should not be given to patients with depleted folic acid reserves (19).

Pyrimethamine + sulfadoxine

Sulfonamide and/or pyrimethamine sensitivity, pregnancy, and G6PD deficiency are contraindications. Use in young infants is considered inadvisable; the history of an 8-month-old infant with *P. falciparum* malaria who developed high fever, tachycardia, hypotension, chills, jaundice, and splenomegaly 48 hours after a single parenteral dose of Fansidar (pyrimethamine + sulfadoxine) (SEDA-16, 309) seems to confirm the wisdom of this advice. It has been advocated that Fansidar should not be used prophylactically if exposure to malaria will last less then 3 weeks, in view of the incidence of severe skin reactions during the first month.

Drug–Drug Interactions

Chloroquine

Pyrimethamine + sulfadoxine

The combined use of Fansidar (sulfadoxine + pyrimethamine) with chloroquine has been reported to result in more severe adverse reactions (20). However, an increased risk has not been reported in recent studies (21).

Liver metabolized drugs

Pyrimethamine + sulfadoxine

Both pyrimethamine and sulfonamides are liver enzyme inhibitors, and can cause interactions with drugs that are normally metabolized in the liver.

References

1. Jacobson JM, Hafner R, Remington J, Farthing C, Holden-Wiltse J, Bosler EM, Harris C, Jayaweera DT, Roque C, Luft BJ; ACTG 156 Study Team. Dose-escalation, phase I/II study of azithromycin and pyrimethamine for the treatment of toxoplasmic encephalitis in AIDS. AIDS 2001;15(5):583–9.
2. Bosch-Driessen LH, Verbraak FD, Suttorp-Schulten MS, van Ruyven RL, Klok AM, Hoyng CB, Rothova A. A prospective, randomized trial of pyrimethamine and azithromycin vs pyrimethamine and sulfadiazine for the treatment of ocular toxoplasmosis. Am J Ophthalmol 2002;134(1):34–40.
3. Schurmann D, Bergmann F, Albrecht H, Padberg J, Grunewald T, Behnsch M, Grobusch M, Vallee M, Wunsche T, Ruf B, Suttorp N. Twice-weekly pyrimethamine–sulfadoxine effectively prevents *Pneumocystis carinii* pneumonia relapse and toxoplasmic encephalitis in patients with AIDS. J Infect 2001;42(1):8–15.
4. Schellenberg D, Menendez C, Kahigwa E, Aponte J, Vidal J, Tanner M, Mshinda H, Alonso P. Intermittent treatment for malaria and anaemia control at time of routine vaccinations in Tanzanian infants: a randomised, placebo-controlled trial. Lancet 2001;357(9267):1471–7.
5. Hellgren U, Rombo L, Berg B, Carlson J, Wiholm BE. Adverse reactions to sulphadoxine–pyrimethamine in Swedish travellers: implications for prophylaxis. BMJ (Clin Res Ed) 1987;295(6594):365–6.
6. Verhoef H, West CE, Nzyuko SM, de Vogel S, van der Valk R, Wanga MA, Kuijsten A, Veenemans J, Kok FJ. Intermittent administration of iron and sulfadoxine–pyrimethamine to control anaemia in Kenyan children: a randomised controlled trial. Lancet 2002;360(9337):908–14.
7. Chute JP, Decker CF, Cotelingam J. Severe megaloblastic anemia complicating pyrimethamine therapy. Ann Intern Med 1995;122(11):884–5.
8. Deron Z, Jablkowski M. Objawy uboczne w przebiegu leczenia toksoplazmozy. [Side effects of toxoplasmosis treatment.] Pol Tyg Lek 1980;35(23):857–9.
9. Craven SA. Letter: Photosensitivity to pyrimethamine? BMJ 1974;2(918):556.
10. Ozturk R, Engin A, Ozaras R, Mert A, Tabak F, Aktuglu Y. Hyperpigmentation due to pyrimethamine use. J Dermatol 2002;29(7):443–5.
11. Cutler TP. Lichen planus caused by pyrimethamine. Clin Exp Dermatol 1980;5(2):253–6.
12. Steffen R, Somaini B. Severe cutaneous adverse reactions to sulfadoxine–pyrimethamine in Switzerland. Lancet 1986;1(8481):610.
13. Sturchler D, Mittelholzer ML, Kerr L. How frequent are notified severe cutaneous adverse reactions to Fansidar? Drug Saf 1993;8(2):160–8.
14. Zain RB. Oral lichenoid reactions during antimalarial prophylaxis with sulphadoxine–pyrimethamine combination. Southeast Asian J Trop Med Public Health 1989;20(2):253–6.
15. Lee PS, Lau EY. Risk of acute non-specific upper respiratory tract infections in healthy men taking dapsone–pyrimethamine for prophylaxis against malaria. BMJ (Clin Res Ed) 1988;296(6626):893–5.
16. Thong BY, Leong KP, Chng HH. Hypersensitivity syndrome associated with dapsone/pyrimethamine (Maloprim) antimalaria chemoprophylaxis. Ann Allergy Asthma Immunol 2002;88(5):527–9.
17. Schurmann D, Bergmann F, Albrecht H, Padberg J, Wunsche T, Grunewald T, Schurmann M, Grobusch M, Vallee M, Ruf B, Suttorp N. Effectiveness of twice-weekly pyrimethamine–sulfadoxine as primary prophylaxis of Pneumocystis carinii pneumonia and toxoplasmic encephalitis in patients with advanced HIV infection. Eur J Clin Microbiol Infect Dis 2002;21(5):353–61.
18. Fishman JA. Prevention of infection caused by Pneumocystis carinii in transplant recipients. Clin Infect Dis 2001;33(8):1397–405.
19. Akinyanju O, Goddell JC, Ahmed I. Pyrimethamine poisoning. BMJ 1973;4(5885):147–8.
20. Rombo L, Stenbeck J, Lobel HO, Campbell CC, Papaioanou M, Miller KD. Does chloroquine contribute to the risk of serious adverse reactions to Fansidar? Lancet 1985;2(8467):1298–9.
21. Rahman M, Rahman R, Bangali M, Das S, Talukder MR, Ringwald P. Efficacy of combined chloroquine and sulfadoxine–pyrimethamine in uncomplicated *Plasmodium falciparum* malaria in Bangladesh. Trans R Soc Trop Med Hyg 2004;98(7):438–41.

Pyritinol

General Information

Pyritinol is a sulfhydryl-containing compound, a dimer of 5-thiopyridoxine. It was used from 1961 onwards as a psychostimulant of doubtful efficacy, but apparently without adverse effects, and then largely abandoned. When it was re-introduced in some countries for rheumatoid arthritis, adverse effects were registered in 25% of patients.

Cross-allergy with D-penicillamine has been hypothesized to explain the apparently higher frequency of adverse effects of pyritinol in patients with rheumatoid arthritis (1).

In usual doses, 600–800 mg/day, pyritinol has a profile of adverse reactions reminiscent of that of penicillamine (2,3). Some 40% of users have adverse reactions, leading to withdrawal in about 23% of the total. The most common are non-specific rashes and stomatitis; in addition, pemphigus, lichen planus, and photosensitivity have occurred. Gastrointestinal symptoms (diarrhea, gastralgia, nausea, loss of taste) can occur, but are less frequent than with penicillamine. Thrombocytopenia, reversible extramembranous glomerulonephritis with nephrotic syndrome (4), a myasthenia-like picture, and acute polymyositis with positive rechallenge have also been described (5).

In a collaborative study of the French Pharmacovigilance Centers there were 23 reports of suspected reactions to pyritinol, including four cases of pemphigus, three of agranulocytosis (but other drugs taken were oxyphenbutazone or clomipramine), two of nephrosis, and two of a lupus-like syndrome (6).

Comparative studies

In a multicenter, double-blind study, patients with rheumatoid arthritis took pyritinol 600 mg/day or auranofin 6 mg/day for 1 year (7). Of 139 patients randomized to pyritinol, 61 (44%) dropped out because of adverse events or response failure compared with 44 (31%) of the 142 patients randomized to auranofin. Among the rest, adverse events occurred in 64% of patients taking pyritinol and in 58% of patients taking auranofin: the main events were mucocutaneous symptoms (pyritinol 36%, auranofin 23%) and gastrointestinal complaints (pyritinol 30%, auranofin 37%). There were single cases of proteinuria, hepatic abnormalities, and hematological abnormalities in both groups.

Organs and Systems

Metabolism

Autoimmune hypoglycemia with detectable anti-insulin antibodies, probably caused by pyritinol, has been described in one patient (8). This syndrome has previously been reported in connection with other thiol compounds, (penicillamine, methimazole, and tiopronin).

Liver

Pyritinol-induced acute hepatitis has been described (9).

Pancreas

Pancreatitis has been attributed to pyritinol.

- A 23-year-old student had three episodes of acute pancreatitis after the occasional ingestion of pyritinol for better performance in examinations. Immunological investigations pointed to a probable T cell-mediated hypersensitivity reaction (10).

Immunologic

A high titer of antinuclear antibodies and anti-double-stranded native DNA antibodies occurred during treatment with pyritinol 400 mg/day in a woman with rheumatoid arthritis (11). A clear temporal relation and a reduction in antinuclear antibody titers and disappearance of anti-DNA antibodies after drug withdrawal strongly suggested a causal relation.

References

1. Meraud JP, Geniaux M, Tamisier JM, Delaunay MM, Texier L. Eruption squamocrouteuse à type histologique de lichen plan au cours d'un traitement par le pyritinol. [Squamous eruption of the lichen planus histological type during treatment with pyritinol.] Ann Dermatol Venereol 1980;107(6):561–4.
2. Jaffe IA. Adverse effects profile of sulfhydryl compounds in man. Am J Med 1986;80(3):471–6.
3. Crouzet J, Beraneck L. Pyrithioxine et polyarthrite rhumatoïde. [Pyrithioxin and rheumatoid polyarthritis.] Rev Rhum Mal Osteoartic 1986;53(1):45–8.
4. Segond P, Dellas JA, Massias P, Delfraissy JF. Syndrome nephrotique en cours d'une polyarthrite rheumatoïde traitée par la pyrithioxine. [Nephrotic syndrome during rheumatoid polyarthritis treated with pyrithioxin.] Rev Rhum Mal Osteoartic 1979;46(7–9):509–10.
5. Treves R, Tabaraud F, Arnaud M, Jacob P, Hugon J, Lubeau M, Burki F, Desproges-Gotteron R. Polymyosite aiguë compliquant une polyarthrite rheumatoïde traitée a la pyrithioxinë. [Acute polymyositis complicating rheumatoid arthritis treated with pyrithioxin.] Rev Rhum Mal Osteoartic 1984;51(5):283–5.
6. Netter P, Trechôt P, Bannwarth B, Faure G, Royer RJ. Effets secondaires de la D-pénicillamine et du pyritinol. Etude cooperative des centers de pharmacovigilance hospitaliers français. [Side effects of D-penicillamine and pyritinol. Cooperative study among French hospital drug surveillance centers.] Therapie 1985;40(6):475–9.
7. Lemmel EM. Comparison of pyritinol and auranofin in the treatment of rheumatoid arthritis. The European Multicentre Study Group. Br J Rheumatol 1993;32(5):375–382.
8. Faguer de Moustier B, Burgard M, Boitard C, Desplanque N, Fanjoux J, Tchobroutsky G. Syndrome hypoglycémique auto-immune induit par le pyritinol. [Auto-immune hypoglycemic syndrome induced by pyritinol.] Diabete Metab 1988;14(4):423–9.
9. Macedo G, Sarmento JA, Allegro S. Acute hepatitis due to pyritinol. Gastroenterol Clin Biol 1992;16(2):186–7.
10. Straumann A, Bauer M, Pichler WJ, Pirovino M. Acute pancreatitis due to pyritinol: an immune-mediated phenomenon. Gastroenterology 1998;115(2):452–4.
11. Larbre JP, Perret P, Collet P, Llorca G. Antinuclear antibodies during pyrithioxine treatment. Br J Rheumatol 1990;29(6):496–7.

Pyrrolizidine alkaloids

General Information

Pyrrolizidine alkaloids occur in a large number of plants, notably the genera *Crotalaria* (Fabaceae), *Cynoglossum* (Boraginaceae), *Eupatorium* (Asteraceae), *Heliotropium* (Boraginaceae), *Petasites* (Asteraceae), *Senecio* (Asteraceae), and *Symphytum* (Boraginaceae) (Table 1). Certain representatives of this class and the plants in which they occur are hepatotoxic as well as mutagenic and hepatocarcinogenic. They can produce veno-occlusive disease of the liver with clinical features like abdominal pain with ascites, hepatomegaly and splenomegaly, anorexia with nausea, vomiting, and diarrhea. Sometimes there is also damage to the pulmonary region.

The German Federal Health Office has restricted the availability of botanical medicines containing unsaturated pyrrolizidine alkaloids (1,2). Herbal medicines that provide over 1 mg/day internally or over 100 mg/day externally are not permitted; herbal medicines that provide 0.1–1 mg/day internally or 10–100 mg/day externally may be applied for only a maximum of 6 weeks per year, and they should not be used during pregnancy or lactation.

Table 1 Pyrrolizidine alkaloids in various genera

Genus	Pyrrolizidine alkaloids
Crotalaria albida	Croalbidine
Crotalaria anagyroides	Anacrotine, methylpyrrolizidine
Crotalaria aridicola	Various dehydropyrrolizidines
Crotalaria axillaris	Axillaridine, axillarine
Crotalaria barbata	Crobarbatine
Crotalaria burha	Croburhine, crotalarine
Crotalaria candicans	Crocandine, cropodine
Crotalaria crassipes	Retusamine
Crotalaria crispata	Crispatine, fulvine
Crotalaria dura	Crotaline
Crotalaria fulva	Fulvine
Crotalaria globifer	Crotaline, globiferine
Crotalaria goreensis	Hydroxymethylenepyrrolizidine
Crotalaria grahamiana	Grahamine
Crotalaria grantiana	Grantianine
Crotalaria incana	Anacrotine
Crotalaria intermedia	Integerrimine, usaramine
Crotalaria laburnifolia	Crotalaburnine, hydroxysenkirkine
Crotalaria madurensis	Crotafoline, madurensine
Crotalaria mitchelii	Retusamine
Crotalaria mucronata	Mucronitine, mucronitinine
Crotalaria nana	Crotaburnine, crotananine
Crotalaria novae-hollandiae	Retusamine
Crotalaria retusa	Retusamine
Crotalaria semperflorus	Crosemperine
Crotalaria spectabilis	Retronecanol
Crotalaria stricta	Crotastrictine
Crotalaria trifoliastrum	Various alkylpyrrolizidines
Crotalaria usaramoensis	Usaramine, usaramoensine
Crotalaria virgulata	Grantaline, grantianine
Crotalaria walkeri	Acetylcrotaverrine, crotaverrine
Cynoglossum amabile	Amabiline, echinatine
Cynoglossum glochidiatum	Amabiline
Cynoglossum lanceolatum	Cynaustine, cynaustraline
Cynoglossum latifolium	Latifoline
Cynoglossum officinale	Heliosupine
Cynoglossum pictum	Echinatine, heliosupine
Cynoglossum viridiflorum	Heliosupine, viridiflorine
Eupatorium cannabinum	Echinatine, supinine
Eupatorium maculatum	Echinatine, trachelantimidine
Heliotropium acutiflorum	Heliotrine
Heliotropium arguzoides	Trichodesmine
Heliotropium curassavicum	Angelylheliotridine
Heliotropium dasycarpum	Heliotrine
Heliotropium eichwaldii	Angelylheliotrine
Heliotropium europeum	Acetyl-lasiocarpine, helioitrine
Heliotropium indicum	Acetylindicine, indicine, indicinine
Heliotropium lasiocarpum	Heliotrine, lasiocarpine
Heliotropium olgae	Heliotrine, incanine, lasiocarpine
Heliotropium ovalifolium	Heliofoline
Heliotropium ramosissimum	Heliotrine
Heliotropium strigosum	Strigosine
Heliotropium supinum	Heliosupine, supinine
Heliotropium transoxanum	Heliotrine
Petasites japonicus	Fukinotoxin, petasinine, petasinoside
Senecio adnatus	Platyphylline
Senecio alpinus	Seneciphylline
Senecio amphibolus	Macrophylline
Senecio angulatus	Angulatine
Senecio aquaticus	Aquaticine

Genus	Pyrrolizidine alkaloids
Senecio argentino	Retrorsine, senecionine
Senecio aureus	Floridanine, florosenine, otosenine
Senecio auricula	Neosenkirkine
Senecio borysthenicus	Seneciphylline
Senecio brasiliensis	Brasilinecine
Senecio campestris	Campestrine
Senecio cannabifolius	Senecicannabine
Senecio carthamoides	Carthamoidine
Senecio cineraria	Jacobine, seneciphylline
Senecio cissampelinum	Senampelines
Senecio crucifolia	Jacobine
Senecio doronicum	Doronine
Senecio erraticus	Erucifoline, floridanine
Senecio filaginoides	Retrorsine, ionine
Senecio franchetti	Franchetine, sarracine
Senecio fuchsii	Fuchsisenecionine
Senecio gillesiano	Retrorsine, senecionine
Senecio glabellum	Integerrimine, senecionine
Senecio glandulosus	Retrorsine, senecionine
Senecio glastifolius	Graminifoline
Senecio hygrophylus	Hygrophylline, platyphylline
Senecio ilicifolius	Pterophine, senecionine
Senecio illinitus	Acetylsenkirkine, senecionine
Senecio incanus	Seneciphylline
Senecio integerrimus	Integerrimine, senecionine
Senecio isatideus	Isatidine, retrorsine
Senecio jacobaea	Jacobine, jacoline, jaconine, jacozine, otosenine, renardine
Senecio kirkii	Acetylsenkirkine, senkirkine
Senecio kubensis	Seneciphylline
Senecio latifolius	Senecifolidine, senecifoline
Senecio leucostachys	Retrorsine, senecionine
Senecio longibolus	Integerrimine, longiboline, retronecanol, retrorsine, riddelline, senecionine, seneciphylline
Senecio macrophyllus	Macrophylline
Senecio mikanoides	Mikanoidine
Senecio nemorensis	Nemorensine, oxynemorensine
Senecio othonnae	Floridnine, onetine, otosenine
Senecio othonniformis	Bisline, isoline
Senecio palmatus	Seneciphylline
Senecio paucicalyculatus	Paucicaline
Senecio petasis	Bisline
Senecio phillipicus	Retrorsine, seneciphylline
Senecio platyphylloides	Neoplatyphylline, platyphylline, sarracine, seneciphylline
Senecio platyphyllus	Platyphylline, seneciphylline
Senecio pojarkovae	Sarracine, seneciphylline
Senecio procerus	Procerine
Senecio propinquus	Seneciphylline
Senecio pseudoarnica	Senecionine
Senecio pterophorus	Pterophine
Senecio ragonesi	Retrorsine, senecionine, uspallatine
Senecio renardi	Renardine, seneciphylline
Senecio retrorsus	Senkirkine
Senecio rhombifolius	Isatidine, retrorsine, neoplatyphylline, platyphylline sarracine, seneciphylline
Senecio Riddellii	Riddelline
Senecio rivularis	Angeloyloxyheliotrine
Senecio rosmarinifolius	Rosmarinine

Genus	Pyrrolizidine alkaloids
Senecio ruwenzoriensis	Ruwenine, ruzorine
Senecio sarracenicus	Sarracine
Senecio scleratus	Isatidine, scleratine
Senecio seratophiloides	Senecivernine
Senecio spartioides	Seneciphylline, spartoidine
Senecio squalidus	Senecionine, squalidine
Senecio stenocephalus	Seneciphylline
Senecio subalpinus	Seneciphylline
Senecio subulatus	Retrorsine, senecionine
Senecio swaziensis	Swazine
Senecio triangularis	Triangularine
Senecio uspallatensis	Senecionine, uspallatine
Senecio vernalis	Senecivernine
Senecio vira-vira	Anacrotine, neoplatyphylline
Senecio viscosus	Senecionine
Senecio vulgaris	Senecionine
Symphytum asperum	Asperumine, echinatine
Symphytum caucasicum	Heliosupine, echinatine
Symphytum officinalis	Lasiocarpine, symphytine, viridiflorine
Symphytum orientale	Echinatine, heliosupine
Symphytum tuberosum	Lasiocarpine, symphytine
Symphytum uplandicum	Viridflorine, anadoline, heneicisane, tricosane, acetylintermedine, acetyl-lycopsamine, uplandicine

Organs and Systems

Liver

In a South African study 20 children were identified as suffering from hepatic veno-occlusive disease thought to be caused by the administration of traditional remedies (3). The predominant clinical presentation was ascites and hepatomegaly. Nine children died. The surviving patients progressed to cirrhosis and portal hypertension. In four cases early urine specimens were available, and in all of these the presence of pyrrolizidine alkaloids was confirmed.

Second-Generation Effects

Fetotoxicity

It is prudent to avoid exposing unborn or suckling children to herbal remedies containing pyrrolizidine alkaloids. Animal studies have shown that transplacental passage and transfer to breast milk are possible, and there is a human case on record of fatal neonatal liver injury, in which the mother had used a herbal cough tea containing pyrrolizidine alkaloids throughout her pregnancy.

References

1. Anonymous. Vorinformation Pyrrolizidinalkaloidhaltige human Arzneimittel. Pharm Ztg 1990;135:2532–3; 1990; 135:2623–4.
2. Anonymous. Aufbereitungsmonographien Kommission E. Pharm Ztg 990;135:2081–2.
3. Steenkamp V, Stewart MJ, Zuckerman M. Clinical and analytical aspects of pyrrolizidine poisoning caused by South African traditional medicines. Ther Drug Monit 2000;22(3):302–6.

Pyrvinium embonate

General Information

Pyrvinium is a deep-red insoluble dye used as an antihelminthic drug. It is well tolerated in doses up to 5 mg/kg. Nausea, vomiting, diarrhea, and cramping abdominal pain are more frequent at higher doses. Feces and vomit are stained red. Isolated cases of severe allergy (1), transient photosensitivity, and Stevens–Johnson syndrome (2) have been reported.

References

1. Desser KB, Baden M. Allergic reaction to pyrvinium pamoate. Am J Dis Child 1969;117(5):589.
2. Coursin DB. Stevens–Johnson syndrome: nonspecific parasensitivity reaction? JAMA 1966;198(2):113–16.

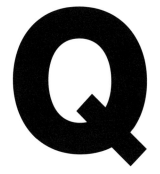

Quazepam

See also Benzodiazepines

General Information

Quazepam is a long-acting benzodiazepine with effects similar to those of diazepam.

Food–Drug Interactions

The disposition of quazepam 20 mg, in the fasting state and 30 minutes after the consumption of meals containing different amounts of dietary fat, has been studied in a three-arm, randomized, crossover study in nine healthy men (1). Plasma concentrations of quazepam and its metabolite, 2-oxoquazepam, were measured for up to 48 hours after dosing. The peak concentrations of quazepam 30 minutes after low-fat and high-fat meals were 243% and 272%, respectively, of those in the fasted state. The AUCs of quazepam from 0 to 8 hours and from 0 to 48 hours were increased by both the low-fat and high-fat meals by 1.4–2 times. Quazepam was well tolerated, with no significant difference in the Stanford Sleepiness Scale between fasted and fed conditions. Thus, food significantly increased the absorption of quazepam but did not prolong the half-life. Quazepam is lipophilic; it would therefore be more highly dissolved in a fatty meal and more available for absorption.

Reference

1. Yasui-Furukori N, Kondo T, Takahata T, Mihara K, Ono S, Kaneko S, Tateishi T. Effect of dietary fat content in meals on pharmacokinetics of quazepam. J Clin Pharmacol 2002;42(12):1335–40.

Quetiapine

See also Neuroleptic drugs

General Information

The pharmacology, efficacy, and safety of quetiapine, an atypical neuroleptic drug, have been extensively reviewed (1). Quetiapine interacts with a broad range of neurotransmitter receptors and has a higher affinity for serotonin ($5-HT_{2A}$) receptors than dopamine (D_2) receptors in the brain. In a meta-analysis, quetiapine was as effective as haloperidol with fewer extrapyramidal adverse effects (2).

Data from short-term clinical trials (6 weeks) suggest that quetiapine may be useful for the management of psychotic disorders in patients who do not tolerate the adverse effects of the typical antipsychotic drugs or clozapine (3). The most common adverse effects of quetiapine were dizziness, hypotension, somnolence, and weight gain. Raised hepatic enzymes have also been reported. In addition, two patients with idiopathic Parkinson's disease and psychosis were treated with quetiapine for 52 weeks (4). Psychotic symptoms were successfully controlled without worsening of motor disability.

Organs and Systems

Nervous system

Although quetiapine seems to cause a lower incidence of extrapyramidal symptoms, a case of neuroleptic malignant syndrome has been described (5).

- A 40-year-old man with chronic schizophrenia and borderline intelligence presented with acute psychotic decompensation. He had previously taken several different neuroleptic drugs and had had significant extrapyramidal symptoms but never neuroleptic malignant syndrome. He was given quetiapine 25 mg bd, increasing to 250 mg bd by day 13. He then had increasing symptoms of restlessness, agitation, and episodic sweating. Loxapine 25 mg and lorazepam 2 mg were added. On day 14 he developed confusion, lead-pipe muscle rigidity, a temperature of 38.2°C, a labile blood pressure, tachypnea, and tachycardia; creatine kinase activity was 18 354 IU/l and he had myoglobinuria. Quetiapine was withdrawn and supportive treatment was instituted. He recovered 5 days after withdrawal.

Endocrine

The effects of haloperidol and quetiapine on serum prolactin concentrations have been compared in 35 patients with schizophrenia during a drug-free period of at least 2 weeks in a randomized study (6). There was no significant difference in prolactin concentration between the groups at the start of the study, and control prolactin concentrations were significantly lower with quetiapine than haloperidol. No patients taking quetiapine had galactorrhea.

Dose-dependent decreases in total T3 and T4 and free T4, without an increase in TSH, have been reported (7,8). Such changes have not been observed with other neuroleptic drugs.

References

1. Goldstein JM. Quetiapine fumarate (Seroquel): a new atypical antipsychotic. Drugs Today (Barc) 1999;35(3):193–210.
2. Leucht S, Pitschel-Walz G, Abraham D, Kissling W. Efficacy and extrapyramidal side-effects of the new antipsychotics olanzapine, quetiapine, risperidone, and sertindole compared to conventional antipsychotics and placebo. A meta-analysis of randomized controlled trials. Schizophr Res 1999;35(1):51–68.
3. Misra LK, Erpenbach JE, Hamlyn H, Fuller WC. Quetiapine: a new atypical antipsychotic. S D J Med 1998;51(6):189–93.
4. Parsa MA, Bastani B. Quetiapine (Seroquel) in the treatment of psychosis in patients with Parkinson's disease. J Neuropsychiatry Clin Neurosci 1998;10(2):216–19.
5. al-Waneen R. Neuroleptic malignant syndrome associated with quetiapine. Can J Psychiatry 2000;45(8):764–5.

6. Atmaca M, Kuloglu M, Tezcan E, Canatan H, Gecici O. Quetiapine is not associated with increase in prolactin secretion in contrast to haloperidol. Arch Med Res 2002;33(6):562–5.
7. Henderson DC, Nasrallah RA, Goff DC. Switching from clozapine to olanzapine in treatment-refractory schizophrenia: safety, clinical efficacy, and predictors of response. J Clin Psychiatry 1998;59(11):585–8.
8. Sacristan JA, Gomez JC, Martin J, Garcia-Bernardo E, Peralta V, Alvarez E, Gurpegui M, Mateo I, Morinigo A, Noval D, Soler R, Palomo T, Cuesta M, Perez-Blanco F, Massip C. Pharmacoeconomic assessment of olanzapine in the treatment of refractory schizophrenia based on a pilot clinical study. Clin Drug Invest 1998;15:29–35.

Quinagolide

General Information

Quinagolide is a non-ergot benzoquinoline dopamine D_2 receptor agonist. Reported adverse effects include gastrointestinal upsets, anorexia, weight loss, and episodes of fainting (1).

Reference

1. Khalfallah Y, Claustrat B, Grochowicki M, Flocard F, Horlait S, Serusclat P, Sassolas G. Effects of a new prolactin inhibitor, CV 205-502, in the treatment of human macroprolactinomas. J Clin Endocrinol Metab 1990;71(2):354–9.

Quinapril

See also Angiotensin converting enzyme inhibitors

General Information

The pharmacology, therapeutic uses, and safety of the ACE inhibitor quinapril have been reviewed (1).

Organs and Systems

Psychological, psychiatric

Depression has been attributed to quinapril (2).

- A 90-year-old man with a history of peripheral arterial disease and mild heart failure presented with reduced appetite, insomnia, anhedonia, reduced energy, and suicidal ideation. His symptoms had started a month before, when he had begun to take quinapril 10 mg/day. He was also taking furosemide 20 mg/day and digoxin. He was alert, coherent, and cognitively intact, but depressed with a flat affect. He had no psychotic symptoms. Quinapril was withdrawn. He improved within 48 hours and recovered fully in 5 days.

The authors cited several reports of depression, mania, and psychosis with various ACE inhibitors.

Acute psychosis has been attributed to quinapril (3).

- A 93-year-old woman with heart failure was given quinapril 2.5 mg bd. Two hours after the first dose she became confused, disoriented, and anxious. During the night, she made many frantic telephone calls to her daughter and other family members complaining that she was being assaulted. Her anxiety, disorientation, and visual hallucinations continued for 5 days. She had had an episode of hallucinations 2 years before, while taking a beta-blocker. Quinapril was withdrawn. She recovered over the next day.

The authors commented on three previous cases of visual hallucination with other ACE inhibitors.

Pancreas

A possible association between quinapril and pancreatitis has been reported in an 85-year-old woman, very similar to other previously reported cases with other ACE inhibitors (4).

References

1. Plosker GL, Sorkin EM. Quinapril. A reappraisal of its pharmacology and therapeutic efficacy in cardiovascular disorders. Drugs 1994;48(2):227–52.
2. Gunduz H, Georges JL, Fleishman S. Quinapril and depression. Am J Psychiatry 1999;156(7):1114–15.
3. Tarlow MM, Sakaris A, Scoyni R, Wolf-Klein G. Quinapril-associated acute psychosis in an older woman. J Am Geriatr Soc 2000;48(11):1533.
4. Arjomand H, Kemp DG. Quinapril and pancreatitis. Am J Gastroenterol 1999;94(1):290–1.

Quinethazone

See also Diuretics

General Information

Quinethazone is chemically related to the thiazides; early work suggested that it was in all essential respects identical (SED-8, 488), and there is no newer evidence that it has any special characteristics.

Quinfamide

General Information

Quinfamide acts on the trophozoites of *Entamoeba histolytica*, making the trophozoite incapable of propagation. It is not active against amebic cysts. In doses of 100–1200 mg adverse effects have been frequent but mild, mainly comprising headaches and nausea (SEDA-12, 705) (1).

Reference

1. Robinson CP. Quinfamide. Drugs Today 1984;20:479.

Quinidine

See also Antidysrhythmic drugs

General Information

Quinidine is a class I antidysrhythmic drug. Its actions, clinical use, interactions, and adverse effects have been reviewed (1).

In 652 consecutive inpatients 91 adverse reactions to quinidine occurred in as many patients (14%); of these, 51 were gastrointestinal, 16 dysrhythmic, 11 febrile, six dermatological, and one hematological; there were six cases of cinchonism (2). Although there were four cases of potentially fatal dysrhythmias, there were no deaths.

In a study of 245 patients, the most common adverse effects were diarrhea (35%), upper gastrointestinal distress (22%), and light-headedness (15%). Other common adverse effects included fatigue (7%), palpitation (7%), headache (7%), angina-like pain (6%), weakness (5%), and rash (5%) (3).

Comparative studies

Quinidine and sotalol have been compared in a prospective multicenter trial of 121 patients after conversion of atrial fibrillation (4). Patients with low left ventricular ejection fractions (below 0.4) or high left atrial diameters (over 5.2 cm) were excluded. After 6 months the percentages of patients remaining in sinus rhythm were similar in the two groups (around 70%), but when the dysrhythmia recurred it occurred later with sotalol than with quinidine (69 versus 10 days). There was also a difference between patients who had been converted from recent-onset atrial fibrillation, in whom sotalol was more effective than quinidine, and in patients who had had chronic atrial fibrillation for more than 3 days, in whom quinidine was more effective. There were significant adverse effects requiring withdrawal of therapy in 17 patients, of whom nine were taking quinidine; three patients had gastrointestinal symptoms, two had central nervous symptoms, two had allergic reactions, one had undefined palpitation, and one had QT interval prolongation. One patient taking quinidine, a 65-year-old man, had frequent episodes of non-sustained ventricular tachycardia.

General adverse reactions

Gastrointestinal symptoms, including anorexia, nausea, and vomiting, are common. Quinidine has a negative inotropic effect on the heart and can cause heart failure and hypotension. It prolongs the QRS complex and QT interval and can cause cardiac dysrhythmias, which can result in syncope (so-called "quinidine syncope").

"Cinchonism" is the term used to describe a cluster of adverse effects that occur at high dosages, including nausea, vomiting, diarrhea, tinnitus, dizziness, and blurred vision; in severe cases there may be deafness and toxic amblyopia in addition to cardiac abnormalities. Other adverse effects that have been described include dementia, psychosis, esophagitis, sometimes resulting in stricture, and exacerbation of myasthenia.

Various hypersusceptibility reactions have been attributed to quinidine, including fever, skin rashes, various types of hematological abnormalities (particularly thrombocytopenia), hepatitis, asthma, and anaphylactic shock. Quinidine has rarely been reported to cause a lupus-like syndrome. Tumor inducing effects have not been reported.

Organs and Systems

Cardiovascular

Quinidine prolongs the QRS complex and QT interval, the effect being related to plasma quinidine concentrations (5) and being greater in women (6). As a result, torsade de pointes or other ventricular tachydysrhythmias can occur and may lead to syncope ("quinidine syncope"). The minimum risk of torsade de pointes has been estimated at 1.5% per year (7).

The relation between serum quinidine concentrations and QT interval dispersion has been studied in 11 patients with atrial dysrhythmias and subtherapeutic or therapeutic serum quinidine concentrations (1.48 and 3.78 µg/ml respectively) (8). The baseline QT_c interval was 430 ms. At subtherapeutic and therapeutic serum quinidine concentrations, mean QT_c intervals were 451 and 472 ms respectively. Mean QT dispersion was 47 ms at baseline, 98 ms at subtherapeutic concentrations, and 71 ms at therapeutic concentrations. Despite QT interval lengthening with increasing serum quinidine concentrations, QT dispersion was greatest at subtherapeutic concentrations.

Quinidine has also been incriminated in cases of sinoatrial block and sinus arrest, but it was not clearly established that quinidine was responsible (9,10). The anticholinergic effects of quinidine can increase the risk of dysrhythmias (11).

Treatment of tachydysrhythmias secondary to quinidine is problematic. Other class I antidysrhythmic drugs are theoretically contraindicated. Some success has been reported with bretylium and with a combination of a beta-adrenoceptor antagonist and phenytoin (12,13). Overdrive pacing has also been reported to be of value (14).

Quinidine has a negative inotropic effect on the heart and causes peripheral vasodilatation. Hypotension can occur secondary to these effects (15).

Nervous system

Quinidine rarely causes effects on the nervous system when used in therapeutic dosages, although there have been occasional reports of dementia (16–18). However, in toxicity it can cause vertigo and tinnitus (19).

Sensory systems

Quinidine rarely affects vision, but can cause scotomata, impaired color vision, and toxic amblyopia (20), altered vision (21), sicca syndrome (22), keratopathy (23), and granulomatous uveitis (24).

Hematologic

Hypersusceptibility reactions to quinidine include thrombocytopenia, hemolytic anemia, and neutropenia.

The overall annual incidence of acute thrombocytopenia has been estimated at 18 cases per million (25), and two possible mechanisms have been invoked:

1. direct combination of quinidine with platelets, causing the production of antibodies, which then cause platelet lysis;
2. formation of quinidine-antibody complexes, which are then deposited on the platelet (the so-called "innocent bystander" mechanism).

There is evidence in favor of both of these mechanisms (26). Other hematological effects are much less common, and include hemolytic anemia (26,27), neutropenia (28,29), and eosinophilia (30).

Withdrawal of quinidine and the administration of corticosteroids is the usual treatment for thrombocytopenia (31), although intravenous immune globulin has also been used (32).

In a review of all English-language reports on drug-induced thrombocytopenia, excluding heparin, 561 case articles reporting on 774 patients were analysed (33). A definite or probable causal role for the drug used was attributed in 247 case reports, and of the 98 that were implicated quinidine was mentioned in 38 cases. The next most common drugs involved were gold salts (11 cases) and co-trimoxazole (10 cases).

Mouth and teeth

A blue–black pigmentation of the oral mucosa has been reported with quinidine (34).

Gastrointestinal

Anorexia, nausea, vomiting, and diarrhea are common adverse effects of quinidine and occur in up to 30% of patients (2,35). These effects can be minimized by the use of modified-release formulations (36).

In one series diarrhea was reported commonly (37), and it can occur late in treatment (38).

Quinidine sometimes causes esophagitis (39,40), especially when there is some abnormality of the esophagus or cardiomegaly. This sometimes results in esophageal stricture (41).

The quinidine derivative hydroquinidine had some beneficial effects in 10 patients with myotonic dystrophy with slow saccadic eye movements, apathy, and hypersomnia (42,43). However, two patients had nausea and epigastric pain and withdrew while taking the active treatment. Although there were no cases of cardiac abnormalities, the authors raised the concern that in patients with myotonic dystrophy, who have a high frequency of cardiac disturbances, the risk of cardiac

dysrhythmias with quinidine derivatives may be too high to take.

Liver

Hypersusceptibility reactions to quinidine include granulomatous hepatitis. In one retrospective series of 487 patients, 32 had evidence of hypersusceptibility, 10 of whom had hepatotoxicity (44). In another series of 1500 patients, quinidine-induced hepatitis was identified in 33 (2.2%) (45); these represented one-third of all cases of drug-induced hepatitis in those patients. In all cases the liver damage resolved on withdrawal.

Urinary tract

Glomerulonephritis has been reported in association with Henoch–Schönlein purpura (46) and nephrotic syndrome, possibly as part of a lupus-like syndrome (47).

Skin

Skin rashes are uncommon (48), but can occur as part of a hypersusceptibility reaction. In a review of drug-induced skin disorders, from a list of 26 drugs or groups of drugs, only quinidine was mentioned of all antidysrhythmic drugs (49). The reaction rate was quoted as 12 per 1000 recipients. Several different kinds of rash have been reported, including photosensitivity (50), which can result in a variety of types of rash, contact dermatitis (51), pigmentation (52), urticaria (53), exfoliative dermatitis (54,55), granuloma annulare (56), and exacerbation of psoriasis.

Musculoskeletal

Quinidine is a neuromuscular blocking drug and can exacerbate myasthenia gravis (57). It can also cause an increase in the serum activity of the muscle-specific isozyme of creatine phosphokinase (58–60).

- A 56-year-old man who took quinidine 324 mg five times daily for prevention of paroxysmal atrial fibrillation developed a syndrome similar to polymyalgia rheumatica which settled on drug withdrawal (60).

Quinidine can cause polyarthropathy (61), both in association with and independent of a lupus-like syndrome.

Immunologic

A variety of immune syndromes have occasionally been reported with quinidine, including a lupus-like syndrome, polymyalgia rheumatica, and vasculitis (SEDA-20, 179) (SEDA-23, 202).

Life-threatening vasculitis has been attributed to quinidine in a healthy volunteer taking part in a clinical trial (62).

- A 58-year-old man took quinidine 200 mg tds for 7 days as part of an interaction study with a new alpha-blocker. He developed widespread maculopapular purpuric lesions on the limbs, trunk, and ears. His temperature rose to 38.4°C and some of the lesions on his fingers, toes, ears, and nose became necrotic. He had peripheral edema with a bluish purpuric discoloration of the hands and feet. There was mucous membrane involvement with purpuric, partially necrotic lesions on the tongue and palate. A skin biopsy showed necrotizing vasculitis with focal leukocytoclasia. Direct immunofluorescence showed microgranular deposits of IgA, IgM, and C3 around the superficial skin vessels. Quinidine was withdrawn and he was given intravenous methyl prednisolone followed by oral prednisone for one month. He recovered completely within 3 weeks.

There has been a report of a dermatomyositis-like illness in a man taking quinidine (63).

- A previously healthy 63-year-old man, who had taken quinidine gluconate 972 mg/day for 9 months, developed diffuse edematous erythema on the extensive surfaces of the hands, arms, and face, with marked accentuation over the joints. His nail-fold capillaries were dilated and the shoulder abductors were slightly weak. His erythrocyte sedimentation rate was slightly raised (29 mm/hour) and there was a positive ANA titer (1:640) with a speckled pattern. There were no antibodies to Sm, ribonucleoprotein, SSA or SSB antigens, or histones. There was no evidence of inflammatory myopathy on electromyography, and a skin biopsy showed a mild, superficial, perivascular, lymphocytic inflammation with positive direct immunofluorescence for IgG and IgM at the dermoepidermal junction. There was no evidence of malignancy. All these abnormalities resolved rapidly after quinidine withdrawal.

Lupus-like syndrome
A lupus-like syndrome has occasionally been reported in patients taking quinidine (60,61,64). It usually presents with polyarthralgia, a raised erythrocyte sedimentation rate, and a raised antinuclear antibody titer. It can occasionally be associated with antihistone antibodies and a circulating coagulant. In two cases (65) the syndrome was associated with quinidine and not with procainamide. Lupus anticoagulant has been reported with the use of quinine and quinidine, and an associated antiphospholipid syndrome has been described (66).

Susceptibility Factors

Age

Maintenance dosages should be reduced in elderly people (67).

Sex

The effect of quinidine on the QT interval is greater in women than in men at equivalent serum concentrations (6). In 12 men and 12 women who received a single intravenous dose of quinidine (4 mg/kg) in a randomized, single-blind, placebo-controlled, crossover study, total and unbound serum concentrations of quinidine and 3-hydroxyquinidine were measured and QT intervals were corrected for differences in heart rate using Bazett's method. The QT interval at baseline was longer in women than in men (407 versus 395 ms). The slope of the relation between the serum concentration of quinidine and the change in the QT_c interval from baseline was 44% greater in the women than in the men. However,

there were no significant differences between the men and the women in the disposition of quinidine, apart from a small reduction in the unbound fraction of 3-hydroxyquinidine in the men (0.47 versus 0.53). The authors proposed that estrogens and androgens differentially affect the expression and activity of potassium channels in the heart, and that a lower density of potassium channels could contribute to a larger effect of quinidine in the women. They suggested that women are at greater risk of quinidine-induced cardiac dysrhythmias and that altering dosages according to weight would not correct for this difference. They also pointed to the fact that in the SWORD study the risk of excess mortality in those taking D-sotalol was greater in the women than in the men.

Hepatic disease

Maintenance dosages should be reduced if hepatic metabolism is reduced, for example in congestive cardiac failure and hepatic disease and in elderly people (67).

Other features of the patient

Care must be taken in patients with pre-existing conduction tissue disease or heart failure. Loading doses should be reduced in cardiac failure, because of a lowered apparent volume of distribution (67).

Drug Administration

Drug overdose

In acute overdosage the chief effect of quinidine is profound hypotension, due to the combination of peripheral vasodilatation, and a negative inotropic effect on the heart (68,69). Charcoal hemoperfusion has been successfully used in the treatment of quinidine overdose (70).

Drug–Drug Interactions

Amiloride

Quinidine has a pharmacodynamic interaction with amiloride, further prolonging the duration of the QRS complex, but not the QT interval (71).

Amiodarone

Quinidine prolongs the QT interval and will therefore potentiate the effects of other antidysrhythmic drugs that have the same effect (for example amiodarone) (72).

Antacids

The interactions of quinidine with antacids have been reviewed (73). Although the data are inconclusive, it has been suggested that at least 2 hours should elapse between quinidine and antacid doses.

Class I antidysrhythmimc drugs

Quinidine prolongs the QT interval and will therefore potentiate the effects of other antidysrhythmic drugs that have the same effect (for example Class I antidysrhythmic drugs). Specific interactions of this kind have been reported with tocainide (74) and mexiletine (75); in these cases the interactions were reported to be beneficial in terms of antidysrhythmic effects.

Diclofenac

In human liver microsomes, diclofenac inhibited testosterone 6-beta-hydroxylation with characteristics that suggested that it inactivated CYP3A4 (76). Quinidine, which stimulates CYP3A4-mediated diclofenac 5-hydroxylation, did not affect the inactivation of CYP3A4 assessed by testosterone 6-beta-hydroxylation activity but accelerated the inactivation assessed by diazepam 3-hydroxylation activity.

In 30 healthy young men the pharmacokinetics of a single oral dose of quinidine 200 mg were studied before and during the daily administration of diclofenac 100 mg (a substrate of CYP2C9) (63). The clearance of quinidine by N-oxidation was reduced by diclofenac, but only by 27%. This small effect of diclofenac suggests a minor role for CYP2C9 in the metabolism of quinidine.

Digoxin

Quinidine reduces the renal and non-renal clearance of digoxin and reduces its apparent volume of distribution. The combination should be avoided. This interaction is discussed fully in the monograph on cardiac glycosides.

Enzyme-inducing drugs

The metabolism of quinidine is enhanced by drugs that induce hepatic microsomal drug-metabolizing enzymes (67), such as rifampicin (77) and phenytoin and phenobarbital (78). This leads to an increase in the first-pass metabolism of quinidine, and thus increased requirements of oral quinidine but little change in intravenous dosages.

Inhibitors of CYP3A4

There is in vitro evidence that the oxidation of quinidine to 3-hydroxyquinidine is catalysed by CYP3A4. However, the extent to which other cytochrome P450 isoforms, such as CYP2C9 and CYP2E1, are involved in the oxidation of quinidine is not clear. In 30 healthy young men the pharmacokinetics of a single oral dose of quinidine 200 mg were studied before and during the daily administration of diclofenac 100 mg (a substrate of CYP2C9), disulfiram 200 mg (an inhibitor of CYP2E1), three inhibitors of CYP3A4 (grapefruit juice, itraconazole, and erythromycin), and probes of other enzyme activities, namely caffeine (CYPA2), sparteine (CYP2D6), mephenytoin (CYP2C19), and tolbutamide (CTP2C9) (63). The clearance of quinidine by N-oxidation was reduced by 27% by diclofenac. Itraconazole, grapefruit juice, and erythromycin all reduced the clearance of quinidine, including its partial clearance by 3-hydroxylation and N-oxidation, by up to 84%, confirming the involvement of CYP3A4 in the in vivo oxidation of quinidine. Specifically, itraconazole reduced quinidine total clearance, partial clearance by 3-hydroxylation, and partial clearance by N-oxidation by 61, 84, and 73% respectively. Thus, it is likely that inhibitors of CYP3A4 will cause significant drug interactions with quinidine.

Metoprolol

Quinidine inhibits drug hydroxylation and can thus convert extensive hydroxylators to poor hydroxylators, as in the case of metoprolol (79). Inhibition of hydroxylation does not occur in poor hydroxylators.

Neuromuscular blocking drugs

Quinidine is a non-depolarizing muscle blocker and potentiates the effects of neuromuscular blocking drugs (80).

Timolol

The combination of quinidine with timolol causes an increased risk of bradycardia (81).

Warfarin

Quinidine potentiates the effects of warfarin by a pharmacodynamic effect (82).

However, it has also been reported that quinidine increased the 4'-hydroxylation of S-warfarin and the 10-hydroxylation of R-warfarin in human liver microsomes and intact hepatocytes by stimulation of CYP3A4 (83). The increases were concentration-dependent and respectively maximized at about three and five times control values. In contrast, warfarin did not affect the 3-hydroxylation of quinidine. These results are consistent with previous findings suggesting that there is more than one binding site on CYP3A4 through which interactions can occur.

References

1. Malcolm AD, David GK. Quinidine in cardiology. Acta Leiden 1987;55:87–98.
2. Cohen IS, Jick H, Cohen SI. Adverse reactions to quinidine in hospitalized patients: findings based on data from the Boston Collaborative Drug Surveillance Program. Prog Cardiovasc Dis 1977;20(2):151–63.
3. Roos JC, Paalman DC, Dunning AJ. Electrophysiological effects of mexiletine in man. Postgrad Med J 1977;53(Suppl 1):92–6.
4. de Paola AA, Veloso HH. Efficacy and safety of sotalol versus quinidine for the maintenance of sinus rhythm after conversion of atrial fibrillation. SOCESP Investigators. The Cardiology Society of Sao Paulo. Am J Cardiol 1999;84(9):1033–7.
5. White NJ, Looareesuwan S, Warrell DA, Chongsuphajaisiddhi T, Bunnag D, Harinasuta T. Quinidine in falciparum malaria. Lancet 1981;2(8255):1069–71.
6. Benton RE, Sale M, Flockhart DA, Woosley RL. Greater quinidine-induced QTc interval prolongation in women. Clin Pharmacol Ther 2000;67(4):413–18.
7. Roden DM, Woosley RL, Primm RK. Incidence and clinical features of the quinidine-associated long QT syndrome: implications for patient care. Am Heart J 1986;111(6):1088–93.
8. Mathis AS, Gandhi AJ. Serum quinidine concentrations and effect on QT dispersion and interval. Ann Pharmacother 2002;36(7–8):1156–61.
9. Grayzel J, Angeles J. Sino-atrial block in man provoked by quinidine. J Electrocardiol 1972;5(3):289–94.
10. Jeresaty RM, Kahn AH, Landry AB Jr. Sinoatrial arrest due to lidocaine in a patient receiving guinidine. Chest 1972;61(7):683–5.

11. Cappato R, Alboni P, Codeca L, Guardigli G, Toselli T, Antonioli GE. Direct and autonomically mediated effects of oral quinidine on RR/QT relation after an abrupt increase in heart rate. J Am Coll Cardiol 1993;22(1):99–105.

12. VanderArk CR, Reynolds EW, Kahn DR, Tullett G. Quinidine syncope. A report of successful treatment with bretylium tosylate. J Thorac Cardiovasc Surg 1976;72(3):464–7.

13. Koster RW, Wellens HJ. Quinidine-induced ventricular flutter and fibrillation without digitalis therapy. Am J Cardiol 1976;38(4):519–23.

14. DiSegni E, Klein HO, David D, Libhaber C, Kaplinsky E. Overdrive pacing in quinidine syncope and other long QT-interval syndromes. Arch Intern Med 1980;140(8):1036–40.

15. Luchi RJ, Helwig J Jr, Conn HL Jr. Quinidine toxicity and its treatment. An Experimental study. Am Heart J 1963;65:340–8.

16. Gilbert GJ. Quinidine dementia. JAMA 1977;237(19):2093–4.

17. Billig N, Buongiorno P. Quinidine-induced organic mental disorders. J Am Geriatr Soc 1985;33(7):504–6.

18. Deleu D, Schmedding E. Acute psychosis as idiosyncratic reaction to quinidine: report of two cases. BMJ (Clin Res Ed) 1987;294(6578):1001–2.

19. Abrams J. Quinidine toxicity: a review. Rocky Mt Med J 1973;70(5):31–4.

20. Bolton FG. Thrombocytopenic purpura due to quinidine. II. Serologic mechanisms. Blood 1956;11(6):547–64.

21. Fisher CM. Visual disturbances associated with quinidine and quinine. Neurology 1981;31(12):1569–71.

22. Naschitz JE, Yeshurun D. Quinidine induced sicca syndrome. J Toxicol Clin Toxicol 1983;20(4):367–71.

23. Zaidman GW. Quinidine keratopathy. Am J Ophthalmol 1984;97(2):247–9.

24. Hustead JD. Granulomatous uveitis and quinidine hypersensitivity. Am J Ophthalmol 1991;112(4):461–2.

25. Kaufman DW, Kelly JP, Johannes CB, Sandler A, Harmon D, Stolley PD, Shapiro S. Acute thrombocytopenic purpura in relation to the use of drugs. Blood 1993;82(9):2714–18.

26. Garratty G. Review: Immune hemolytic anemia and/or positive direct antiglobulin tests caused by drugs. Immunohematol 1994;10(2):41–50.

27. Barzel US. Quinidine-sulfate-induced hypoplastic anemia and agranulocytosis. JAMA 1967;201(5):325–7.

28. Castro O, Nash I. Quinidine leukopenia and thrombocytopenia with a drug-dependent leukoagglutinin. N Engl J Med 1977;296(10):572.

29. Eisner EV, Carr RM, MacKinney AR. Quinidine-induced agranulocytosis. JAMA 1977;238(8):884–6.

30. Religa H, Rozniecki J, Szmidt M. Eozynofilia w przebiegu leczenia lanatozydem C i siarczanem chinidyny jako jedyny przejaw nadwrazliwoski polekowej. [Eosinophilia in the course of lanatoside C and quinidine treatment as the sole sign of drug hypersensitivity.] Pol Tyg Lek 1972;27(44):1727–9.

31. Saleh MN, Dhodaphar N, Allen K, LoBuglio AF. Quinidine-induced immune thrombocytopenia. Henry Ford Hosp Med J 1989;37(1):28–32.

32. Redell MA, Moore BR, Fass L. Use of i.v. immune globulin for presumed quinidine-induced thrombocytopenia. Clin Pharm 1989;8(2):89.

33. George JN, Raskob GE, Shah SR, Rizvi MA, Hamilton SA, Osborne S, Vondracek T. Drug-induced thrombocytopenia: a systematic review of published case reports. Ann Intern Med 1998;129(11):886–90.

34. Birek C, Main JH. Two cases of oral pigmentation associated with quinidine therapy. Oral Surg Oral Med Oral Pathol 1988;66(1):59–61.

35. Rokseth R, Storstein O. Quinidine therapy of chronic auricular fibrillation. The occurrence and mechanism of syncope. Arch Intern Med 1963;111:184–9.

36. Mahon WA, Mayersohn M, Inaba T. Disposition kinetics of two oral forms of quinidine. Clin Pharmacol Ther 1976;19(5 Pt 1):566–75.

37. Kennedy HL, DeMaria AN, Sprague MK, Wiens RD, Redd RM, Janosik DL, Buckingham TA. Comparative efficacy of moricizine and quinidine for benign and potentially lethal ventricular arrhythmias. Am J Noninvas Cardiol 1988;2:98–105.

38. Zahger D, Gilon D, Gotsman MS. Delayed quinidine-induced diarrhea after five years of treatment. Chest 1992;101(1):296.

39. Bott SJ, McCallum RW. Medication-induced oesophageal injury. Survey of the literature. Med Toxicol 1986;1(6):449–57.

40. Wong RK, Kikendall JW, Dachman AH. Quinaglute-induced esophagitis mimicking an esophageal mass. Ann Intern Med 1986;105(1):62–3.

41. Bonavina L, DeMeester TR, McChesney L, Schwizer W, Albertucci M, Bailey RT. Drug-induced esophageal strictures. Ann Surg 1987;206(2):173–83.

42. Di Costanzo A, Mottola A, Toriello A, Di Iorio G, Tedeschi G, Bonavita V. Does abnormal neuronal excitability exist in myotonic dystrophy? I. Effects of the antiarrhythmic drug hydroquinidine on slow saccadic eye movements. Neurol Sci 2000;21(2):73–80.

43. Di Costanzo A, Mottola A, Toriello A, Di Iorio G, Tedeschi G, Bonavita V. Does abnormal neuronal excitability exist in myotonic dystrophy? II. Effects of the antiarrhythmic drug hydroquinidine on apathy and hypersomnia. Neurol Sci 2000;21(2):81–6.

44. Geltner D, Chajek T, Rubinger D, Levij IS. Quinidine hypersensitivity and liver involvement. A survey of 32 patients. Gastroenterology 1976;70(5 Pt 1):650–2.

45. Knobler H, Levij IS, Gavish D, Chajek-Shaul T. Quinidine-induced hepatitis. A common and reversible hypersensitivity reaction. Arch Intern Med 1986;146(3):526–8.

46. Aviram A. Henoch-Schonlein syndrome associated with quinidine. JAMA 1980;243(5):432–3.

47. Chisholm JC Jr. Quinidine-induced nephrotic syndrome. J Natl Med Assoc 1985;77(11):920–2.

48. Pariser DM, Taylor JR. Quinidine photosensitivity. Arch Dermatol 1975;111(11):1440–3.

49. Duncan KO. Severe cutaneous adverse reactions to medications. Prim Care Case Rev 2001;4:171–85.

50. Lang PG Jr. Quinidine-induced photodermatitis confirmed by photopatch testing. J Am Acad Dermatol 1983;9(1):124–8.

51. Fowler JF. Allergic contact dermatitis to quinidine. Contact Dermatitis 1985;13(4):280–1.

52. Mahler R, Sissons W, Watters K. Pigmentation induced by quinidine therapy. Arch Dermatol 1986;122(9):1062–4.

53. Shaftel N, Halpern A. The quinidine problem. Angiology 1958;9(1):34–46.

54. Taylor DR, Potashnick R. Quinidine-induced exfoliative dermatitis; with a brief review of quinidine idiosyncrasies. JAMA 1951;145(9):641–2.

55. Gouffault J, Pawlotsky Y, Morel H, Bourel M. Erythrodermie d'origine quinidinique. [Erythrodermia of quinidine origin.] Sem Hop 1965;41(22):1350–3.

56. Ross V, Cobb M. Generalized granuloma annulare associated with quinidine therapy. J Assoc Military Dermatol 1991;17:16–17.

57. Stoffer SS, Chandler JH. Quinidine-induced exacerbation of myasthenia gravis in patient with Graves' disease. Arch Intern Med 1980;140(2):283–4.

58. Weiss M, Hassin D, Eisenstein Z, Bank H. Elevated skeletal muscle enzymes during quinidine therapy. N Engl J Med 1979;300(21):1218.

59. Ramsey R, Higbee M, Wood JS. Quinidine-induced creatine phosphokinase elevations:case report and

prospective case survey in the elderly. J Geriatr Drug Ther 1989;3:97.

60. Alloway JA, Salata MP. Quinidine-induced rheumatic syndromes. Semin Arthritis Rheum 1995;24(5):315–22.

61. Yagiela JA, Benoit PW. Skeletal-muscle damage from quinidine. N Engl J Med 1979;301(8):437.

62. Lipsker D, Walther S, Schulz R, Nave S, Cribier B. Life-threatening vasculitis related to quinidine occurring in a healthy volunteer during a clinical trial. Eur J Clin Pharmacol 1998;54(9–10):815.

63. Gilliland WR. Quinidine-induced dermatomyositis-like illness. J Clin Rheumatol 1999;5:39.

64. Tebas P, Lozano I, de la Fuente J, Ortigosa J, Perez Maestu R, Masa C, de Letona JM. Lupus inducido por quinidina. [Lupus induced by quinidine.] Rev Clin Esp 1991;189(3):123–4.

65. Amadio P Jr, Cummings DM, Dashow L. Procainamide, quinidine, and lupus erythematosus. Ann Intern Med 1985;102(3):419.

66. Bird MR, O'Neill AI, Buchanan RR, Ibrahim KM, Des Parkin J. Lupus anticoagulant in the elderly may be associated with both quinine and quinidine usage. Pathology 1995;27(2):136–9.

67. Kumana CR. Therapeutic drug monitoring—antidysrhythmic drugs. In: Richens A, Marks V, editors. Therapeutic Drug Monitoring. London, Edinburgh: Churchill-Livingstone; 1981:370.

68. Kerr F, Kenoyer G, Bilitch M. Quinidine overdose. Neurological and cardiovascular toxicity in a normal person. Br Heart J 1971;33(4):629–31.

69. Woie L, Oyri A. Quinidine intoxication treated with hemodialysis. Acta Med Scand 1974;195(3):237–9.

70. Haapanen EJ, Pellinen TJ. Hemoperfusion in quinidine intoxication. Acta Med Scand 1981;210(6):515–16.

71. Wang L, Sheldon RS, Mitchell LB, Wyse DG, Gillis AM, Chiamvimonvat N, Duff HJ. Amiloride–quinidine interaction: adverse outcomes. Clin Pharmacol Ther 1994;56(6 Pt 1):659–67.

72. Tartini R, Kappenberger L, Steinbrunn W. Gefahrliche Interaktionen zwischen Amiodaron und Antiarrhythmika der Klasse I. [Harmful interactions of amiodarone and class I anti-arrhythmia agents.] Schweiz Med Wochenschr 1982;112(45):1585–7.

73. Sadowski DC. Drug interactions with antacids. Mechanisms and clinical significance. Drug Saf 1994;11(6):395–407.

74. Barbey JT, Thompson KA, Echt DS, Woosley RL, Roden DM. Tocainide plus quinidine for treatment of ventricular arrhythmias. Am J Cardiol 1988;61(8):570–3.

75. Giardina EG, Wechsler ME. Low dose quinidine–mexiletine combination therapy versus quinidine monotherapy for treatment of ventricular arrhythmias. J Am Coll Cardiol 1990;15(5):1138–45.

76. Masubuchi Y, Ose A, Horie T. Diclofenac-induced inactivation of CYP3A4 and its stimulation by quinidine. Drug Metab Dispos 2002;30(10):1143–8.

77. Twum-Barima Y, Carruthers SG. Quinidine–rifampin interaction. N Engl J Med 1981;304(24):1466–9.

78. Data JL, Wilkinson GR, Nies AS. Interaction of quinidine with anticonvulsant drugs. N Engl J Med 1976; 294(13):699–702.

79. Leemann T, Dayer P, Meyer UA. Single-dose quinidine treatment inhibits metoprolol oxidation in extensive metabolizers. Eur J Clin Pharmacol 1986;29(6):739–41.

80. Hartshorn EA. Interactions of cardiac drugs. Drug Intell Clin Pharm 1970;4:272.

81. Dinai Y, Sharir M, Naveh N, Halkin H. Bradycardia induced by interaction between quinidine and ophthalmic timolol. Ann Intern Med 1985;103(6 Pt 1):890–1.

82. Koch-Weser J. Quinidine-induced hypoprothrombinemic hemorrhage in patients on chronic warfarin therapy. Ann Intern Med 1968;68(3):511–17.

83. Ngui JS, Chen Q, Shou M, Wang RW, Stearns RA, Baillie TA, Tang W. In vitro stimulation of warfarin metabolism by quinidine: increases in the formation of 4'- and 10-hydroxywarfarin. Drug Metab Dispos 2001;29(6):877–86.

Quinine

General Information

Quinine was originally extracted from the bark of the *Cinchona* tree (Peruvian bark or Jesuits' bark) and was used to treat ague, that is fever, usually due to malaria. It fell out of fashion with the advent of other antimalarial drugs, but has once again become the drug of first choice for malaria originating in areas with multiresistant *Plasmodium falciparum*. To be effective, quinine plasma concentrations greater than the minimal inhibitory concentration must be achieved and maintained.

Pharmacokinetics

Quinine given orally is well absorbed; the half-life is 11 hours. Clearance is predominantly by hepatic metabolism; urinary clearance accounts for only 20%. Information on pharmacokinetics in healthy volunteers can be misleading, since plasma quinine concentrations are higher in the presence of malaria infection than in healthy subjects given the same dose (SEDA-13, 814). The dosage regimen therefore needs to be adapted to the severity of the illness and amended as improvement occurs.

A population pharmacokinetic study of intramuscular quinine (loading dose 20 mg/kg salt diluted 1:1 in water) in 120 Ghanaian children with severe malaria showed predictable profiles, which were within the target range for quinine (15–20 µg/ml) and independent of clinical and laboratory variables (1). Adverse events included skin induration or abscesses at the injection site (12%), all of which resolved without surgical intervention, and hypoglycemia (10%), a special risk in children who were hypoglycemic at presentation.

Adverse effects of quinine are common at plasma concentrations over 10 µg/ml. The dose often recommended, 10 mg/kg intravenously over 10–20 minutes, may be too high in patients with cerebral malaria (SEDA-14, 240). In the USA, intravenous quinine has been discontinued in favor of quinidine (SEDA-17, 329). In some areas, a high rate of recrudescence is seen after short-term treatment with quinine. The addition of specific antibiotics may improve the cure rate.

Placebo-controlled studies

A double-blind, placebo-controlled trial of a 3-day combination regimen of quinine (8 mg/kg tds) and clindamycin (5 mg/kg tds) ($n = 53$) versus 7-day quinine (8 mg/kg tds intravenously for 3 days, then orally; $n = 55$) to treat uncomplicated imported falciparum malaria showed no significant differences in the parasite and fever clearance times or the 28-day cure rate (100 versus 96%) (2). The frequencies of mild adverse events (tinnitus and nausea) were similar in the two groups. There were two serious adverse events that necessitated treatment withdrawal: one patient taking quinine alone had a hemolytic episode and another a "severe toxic rash."

General adverse effects

Quinine is not pleasant to take, and adverse effects, including nausea, tinnitus, dizziness, and hypoglycemia, are well recognized and common compared with other antimalarial drugs (3) in the doses used to treat malaria, although not in the smaller doses used to prevent leg cramps, when classical allergic reactions can still occur (4). Most serious adverse effects are due to the prodysrhythmic properties of quinine, and its effects as a hypoglycemic agent, especially in pregnant women with severe malaria. The prolonged use of normal or low doses of quinine can lead to "cinchonism" in sensitive individuals; this in mild form consists of tinnitus, headache, nausea, and visual disturbances (SEDA-13, 814). Overdosage can cause marked gastrointestinal intolerance, central nervous system disturbances (especially vertigo), visual disorders (very occasionally involving sudden blindness), and cardiovascular problems related to impaired intracardiac conduction. A major risk with quinine is that of direct intravenous injection given too fast. Allergic reactions are not uncommon. They are usually limited to fever and rashes, but angioedema and asthma have been seen. Thrombocytopenic purpura and thrombocytopenia are, at least in some cases, caused by an allergic reaction, and the amounts of quinine present in some "tonics" are sufficient to trigger thrombocytopenia in such patients. Anaphylactic shock has been reported in rare cases (SEDA-13, 814).

Organs and Systems

Cardiovascular

Quinine can cause atrioventricular conduction disturbances. In sensitive patients, such changes can occur with normal dosages given over a prolonged period; however, in most cases cardiac effects are due to overdosage.

Electrocardiographic changes, such as prolongation of the QT interval, widening of the QRS complex, and T wave flattening, can be seen with plasma concentrations above 15 µg/ml (SEDA-11, 590) (SEDA-14, 239).

Quinine, and more profoundly quinidine, its diastereomer, can cause ventricular tachycardia, torsade de pointes, and ventricular fibrillation by prolonging the QT interval (SEDA-20, 261).

- An 8-year-old child given an incorrect dose of quinine had ventricular tachycardia and status epilepticus after 48 hours; the plasma quinine concentration was 20 µg/ml (SEDA-18, 288), compared with the target range of 1.9–4.9 µg/ml.

Respiratory

Quinine can cause allergic asthmatic reactions.

- A 45-year-old woman with long-standing rheumatoid arthritis developed wheeze, severe anxiety, breathlessness, cough, orthopnea, mild fever, chills, and pleuritic chest discomfort after taking a single dose of quinine for nocturnal leg cramps (5). A chest X-ray showed diffuse, bilateral pulmonary infiltrates suggestive of pulmonary edema. No cause other than acute quinine ingestion was identified despite thorough cardiac and infectious disease evaluation.

Quinine poisoning can cause respiratory depression.

Nervous system

Tinnitus and vertigo are not uncommon with quinine, especially at higher dosages (6,7).

Headache and tinnitus occur in chronic toxicity (cinchonism) (8).

Acute intoxication can be followed by convulsions and coma (9).

- A general organic brain syndrome was observed in a 24-year-old woman with tropical malaria after the third day of treatment with quinine sulfate 500 mg tds; her symptoms were headache, blurred vision, vertigo, tinnitus, impaired hearing, increasing apathy, disorientation, speech changes, incoherent thinking, and disorientation with respect to time and place; recovery followed withdrawal (SEDA-16, 305).

A quinidine-induced myopathy has been reported (10).

Sensory systems

Eyes

Amaurosis connected with damage to the retina is most common with high plasma concentrations, and thus follows high dosages and especially overdosage. The outdated, but still practiced, use of quinine to induce abortion is probably the most common cause. Quinine initially affects the photoreceptor and ganglion cell layers; retinal vascular changes are secondary. The first sign may be widely dilated pupils that still respond to light; later, visual field contraction and loss of vision can occur. In milder cases, vision can return, but possibly with a residual disturbance of dark adaptation and/or restricted visual fields. However, loss of vision can be permanent. In cases of permanent damage, the classic late appearance of the fundus after quinine intoxication, with marked pallor and vascular narrowing, appears after some months (SEDA-13, 815). Loss of vision occurs mainly at serum concentrations over 10 µg/ml. Such concentrations are thought not to be toxic in patients with malaria, who have high circulating concentrations of alpha$_1$-acid glycoprotein, resulting in a lower fraction of unbound drug in the plasma (SEDA-17, 329).

Ocular toxicity with vasospasm has been described after poisoning with 4.5 g of quinine 24–36 hours before (11). Therapy for vasospasm using nimodipine, hemodilution, and hypervolemia was instituted, with subsequent resolution of the symptoms.

Blindness has been attributed to quinine (12).

- A 43-year-old Ghanaian man with a mild attack of malaria due to *P. falciparum* received quinine 750 mg intravenously over 5 hours and another identical infusion 3.5 hours after the end of the first infusion. Half an hour after the start of the second infusion he wakened and reported complete blindness. The infusion was immediately stopped, and ocular examination showed fixed, dilated pupils, complete blindness, and normal fundi. A CT scan of the brain, electroencephalography, and retinal fluorescein angiography were all normal. Serum quinine concentrations continued to rise after the end of the infusion, but this effect was mitigated by an increase in the serum concentration of alpha$_1$-acid glycoprotein, to which quinine binds. Six hours after the end of the infusion of quinine his sight began to improve.

In a case of quinine poisoning, stellate ganglion block was performed immediately on the basis of the clinical history of visual disturbance without waiting for physical signs to develop. There was no residual field defect despite the presence of toxic concentrations of the drug. The authors suggested that stellate ganglion block may prevent development of visual field defects due to quinine toxicity (13). However, in other cases it was ineffective (14,15). The effectiveness of this treatment may be a function of the speed with which it is instituted.

Ears

Tinnitus is a fairly frequent complaint and is not only seen after quinine overdosage. Permanent impairment of hearing has long been thought to be a possible consequence of long-term use of quinine, but this belief has recently been challenged, and the original description of it is questionable (SEDA-13, 816); the complication is certainly rare (16).

Serial audiometry in 10 patients receiving quinine for acute falciparum malaria showed a reduction in high-tone auditory acuity in all patients, resulting in flattening of the audiogram. The onset of the effect was rapid and it resolved completely after the end of treatment; only seven of these patients reported tinnitus. Hearing impairment was investigated in six volunteers after single doses of quinine at 5, 10, and 15 mg/kg. A clear effect on hearing was found, but with high variability (SEDA-17, 306).

Metabolism

Clinical signs and symptoms of hypoglycemia are reported occasionally; most cases are subclinical, but severe cases have been described (SEDA-13, 815). A study of the effect of quinidine on glucose homeostasis in Thai patients with malaria showed a near doubling of plasma insulin concentrations and a corresponding fall in serum glucose concentrations. An additional factor may have been impaired nutritional status and the effects of parenteral quinine in severely ill patients not taking food (SEDA-13, 815) (SEDA-14, 240) (SEDA-18, 288).

Hematologic

Thrombocytopenia is often reported with quinine. It is probably due to hypersusceptibility rather than a toxic effect, since even the ingestion of minimal amounts of quinine, such as those present in commercial tonic waters, can cause it. A drug–antibody complex has been demonstrated (SEDA-11, 591). In some cases of quinine-induced thrombocytopenia, there was autoantibody-binding to glycoprotein Ib-IX, IIb, and IIIa complexes. In three published cases, quinine-dependent autoantibodies to glycoproteins Ib-IX and IIb/IIIa were associated with both thrombocytopenia and a hemolytic–uremic syndrome (SEDA-16, 305) (SEDA-17, 329). Two other patients had recurrent febrile illnesses characterized by hypotension, pancytopenia, coagulopathy, and renal insufficiency, and both had high titers of quinine-dependent antibodies, which showed cross-sensitivity with quinidine. In one case there was a link with tonic water, while the other had taken quinine sulfate for leg cramps before each episode (17). A list of nine earlier published cases with antibody findings was added to these two case histories.

Isolated thrombocytopenia after the use of quinine for malaria or leg cramps has been described in isolated cases. The FDA's Center for Drug Evaluation and Research received 141 reports of isolated thrombocytopenia in association with quinine from 1974 to December 2000 (18). After elimination of cases that were confounded by acute or chronic disease or concomitant drug therapy, 64 reports of quinine-associated thrombocytopenia were analysed. Thrombocytopenia occurred soon after the start of therapy (median 7 days) and was often severe (hospitalization reported in 55 of the 64 cases).

Since 1972, the Australian Adverse Drug Reactions Advisory Committee has received 198 reports of thrombocytopenia associated with quinine, four of which had a fatal outcome (19). In 17 of the 20 reports received since the beginning of 2000, patients had platelet counts of 0–14×10^9/l; most of them required hospitalization and treatment with platelet transfusions, glucocorticoids, or immunoglobulin. In most cases the platelet count normalized within 1 week of quinine withdrawal. As quinine-induced thrombocytopenia has an immune-based mechanism, the Committee suggested that patients who develop this reaction should subsequently avoid all products that contain quinine, including drinks such as tonic water. They also reminded prescribers that quinine is no longer recommended for the treatment of nocturnal cramps; the FDA withdrew nocturnal cramps as an indication for all quinine products in 1995 because of lack of evidence of efficacy, and the Australian Medicines Handbook advises against its use for this indication.

Glycoprotein epitopes involved in quinine-induced thrombocytopenia have been characterized (20).

Acute intravascular hemolysis with renal involvement and even renal insufficiency can occur with quinine and can follow relatively small doses. Quinine-induced hemolysis has probably played a role in the clinical syndrome of blackwater fever in the past.

- The combination of renal insufficiency with cortical necrosis, thrombocytopenia, intravascular coagulation, and deposition of fibrin was seen in a 63-year-old woman who had drunk tonic water. She had had two previous episodes of acute renal insufficiency also associated with quinine-containing drinks; this most certainly reflected a hypersensitivity reaction (SEDA-13, 815).

- A 65-year-old man, who had taken a single dose of quinine 300 mg for leg cramps, developed both acral necrosis and hemolytic–uremic syndrome, which resolved promptly after treatment with glucocorticoids (21).

Lupus anticoagulant has been reported with the use of quinine and quinidine, and an associated antiphospholipid syndrome has been described (22).

Disseminated intravascular coagulation has been attributed to quinine (23).

- A 79-year-old woman developed disseminated intravascular coagulation. She had taken a dose of quinine for leg cramps 3 months before and on the day before admission. Her only other medication was bendroflumethiazide. Investigations showed a platelet-associated immunoglobulin with positive immunofluorescence on exposure to quinine sulfate.
- Quinine-induced disseminated intravascular coagulation and hemolytic–uremic syndrome occurred in a 78-year-old woman who took quinine 150 mg for leg cramps; this is the first report of the two diseases occurring simultaneously after quinine (24).

In a retrospective survey of thrombotic thrombocytopenic purpura with hemolytic–uremic syndrome reported to the Oklahoma TTP/HUS Registry, 17 of 225 cases were associated with quinine (doses not stated) taken long-term for leg cramps (25). Patients typically presented with an acute onset of fever, chills, nausea, vomiting, diarrhea, and abdominal pain within hours of quinine ingestion. Laboratory findings included thrombocytopenia, microangiopathic hemolytic anemia, and liver and renal dysfunction. This is an immune-mediated reaction associated with quinine-dependent antiplatelet antibodies and a high mortality (three of the 17 patients). It can be triggered by small amounts of quinine, such as those present in tonic water.

Gastrointestinal

Nausea and abdominal pain can occur with quinine (26). With high doses, diarrhea has been seen (26).

Liver

Granulomatous hepatitis has been reported in a patient taking quinine sulfate for night cramps (27). Cholestatic jaundice was reported in another patient who had taken quinine for night cramps (SEDA-13, 815). Except for the occasional anecdotal case, there is no evidence that true hepatotoxicity occurs with quinine.

Urinary tract

Renal damage accompanies acute hemolysis due to quinine. Renal insufficiency in cases of quinine poisoning is probably due to circulatory collapse. Allergic reactions underlie at least some cases. The picture can be complex, with the renal insufficiency coming in association with cortical necrosis, thrombocytopenia, intravascular coagulation, and deposition of fibrin.

Skin

Rashes are common in allergic reactions. Photosensitivity induced by quinine has been reported; some of the cases occurred in elderly persons taking quinine for night cramps (28). Another form of hypersensitivity to quinine is cutaneous neutrophilic vasculitis, which is a form of photosensitivity (SEDA-16, 305). Local pigmentation has been described after intramuscular injection (SEDA-13, 815).

Immunologic

Quinine can cause a variety of immune-mediated syndromes, most commonly isolated thrombocytopenia, but rarely microangiopathic hemolytic anemia with thrombocytopenia and acute renal insufficiency (hemolytic–uremic syndrome). Two reports of immune-mediated syndromes following the use of quinine for leg cramps have helped to provide an immunopathological explanation for the diversity of such presentations (29,30).

- One patient presented with thrombocytopenic purpura, presumed to be idiopathic (which responded to glucocorticoids and intravenous immunoglobulin) and subsequently presented again with hemolytic–uremic syndrome, and required intensive renal replacement and immunosuppressive therapy. Analysis of serum samples from the isolated thrombocytopenic stage of the presentation showed the presence of quinine-dependent antibodies specific for platelet surface glycoprotein GPIb/IX. Quinine-dependent antibody targets widened to include glycoprotein IIb/IIIa during the hemolytic–uremic phase of the illness, with additional binding to neutrophils and lymphocytes.
- In another case of acute systemic allergy to quinine, which mimicked septic shock, with little hemolysis or renal involvement, the patient presented twice with a virtually identical clinical picture: sudden fever, rigors, and back pain, followed by hypotension, metabolic acidosis, granulocytopenia, and disseminated intravascular coagulation. On each occasion clinical and laboratory indices recovered spontaneously within 36 hours. A retrospective analysis of the patient's serum showed the presence of neutrophil-specific, quinine-dependent antibodies.

A quinine-induced lupus-like syndrome, including pericarditis and polyarthralgia, and positive antinuclear and anti-cardiolipin antibodies, and a polymyalgia rheumatica-like syndrome have been described with quinine or quinidine (SEDA-20, 261) (SEDA-21, 298).

Second-Generation Effects

Teratogenicity

Quinine crosses the placenta and can be found in relatively high concentrations in cord blood; it is also excreted in the breast milk. Data about possible teratogenicity related to the therapeutic use of malaria are scanty (SEDA-14, 239). Hypoplasia of the optic nerve and deafness have been reliably described in children born after failure to induce abortion with the drug.

35. Weser JK, Sellers E. Drug interactions with coumarin anticoagulants. 2. N Engl J Med 1971;285(10):547–58.

36. Amabeoku GJ, Chikuni O, Akino C, Mutetwa S. Pharmacokinetic interaction of single doses of quinine and carbamazepine, phenobarbitone and phenytoin in healthy volunteers. East Afr Med J 1993;70(2):90–3.

37. Ajana F, Fortier B, Martinot A, et al. Mefloquine prophylaxis and neurotoxicity. Report of a case. Sem Hop 1990;66:918.

38. Shmuklarsky MJ, Klayman DL, Milhous WK, Kyle DE, Rossan RN, Ager AL Jr, Tang DB, Heiffer MH, Canfield CJ, Schuster BG. Comparison of beta-artemether and beta-arteether against malaria parasites in vitro and in vivo. Am J Trop Med Hyg 1993;48(3):377–84.

39. Meshnick SR. The mode of action of antimalarial endoperoxides. Trans R Soc Trop Med Hyg 1994;88(Suppl 1):S31–2.

40. Kirkwood LC, Nation RL, Somogyi AA. Characterization of the human cytochrome P450 enzymes involved in the metabolism of dihydrocodeine. Br J Clin Pharmacol 1997;44(6):549–55.

41. Hedman A, Angelin B, Arvidsson A, Dahlqvist R, Nilsson B. Interactions in the renal and biliary elimination of digoxin: stereoselective difference between quinine and quinidine. Clin Pharmacol Ther 1990;47(1):20–6.

42. Aronson JK, Carver JG. Interaction of digoxin with quinine. Lancet 1981;1(8235):1418.

43. Zhao XJ, Ishizaki T. A further interaction study of quinine with clinically important drugs by human liver microsomes: determinations of inhibition constant (Ki) and type of inhibition. Eur J Drug Metab Pharmacokinet 1999;24(3):272–8.

44. Pukrittayakamee S, Prakongpan S, Wanwimolruk S, Clemens R, Looareesuwan S, White NJ. Adverse effect of rifampin on quinine efficacy in uncomplicated falciparum malaria. Antimicrob Agents Chemother 2003;47(5):1509–13.

45. Gibson JR, Saunders NA, Burke B, Owen RJ. Novel method for rapid determination of clarithromycin sensitivity in *Helicobacter pylori*. J Clin Microbiol 1999;37(11):3746–8.

46. Munafo A, Reymond-Michel G, Biollaz J. Altered flecainide disposition in healthy volunteers taking quinine. Eur J Clin Pharmacol 1990;38(3):269–73.

47. Baune B, Furlan V, Taburet AM, Farinotti R. Effect of selected antimalarial drugs and inhibitors of cytochrome P-450 3A4 on halofantrine metabolism by human liver microsomes. Drug Metab Dispos 1999;27(5):565–8.

48. Shane R. Potential toxicity of theophylline in combination with Quinamm. Am J Hosp Pharm 1982;39(1):40.

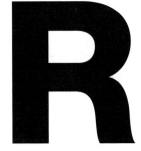

Rabeprazole

See also Proton pump inhibitors

General Information

The benefits and risk profile of rabeprazole, a proton pump inhibitor, have been reviewed (1,2). It has been well tolerated in both short-term and long-term studies. The overall rate of drug withdrawal because of adverse effects was 3%. Common adverse effects included diarrhea, headache, and rash.

Observational studies

Rabeprazole 10 and 20 mg/day in the morning were effective in erosive or ulcerative gastro-esophageal reflux disease, gastric and duodenal ulcers, and long-term maintenance of gastro-esophageal reflux disease healing (1). Healing rates were equivalent to those with omeprazole and superior (gastro-esophageal reflux disease healing and duodenal ulcer healing) or equal (gastric ulcer healing) to ranitidine.

In an open study in 189 patients rabeprazole 20 mg/day for 4 weeks was effective in functional dyspepsia (3). The incidence of adverse events was 8%, and included dysgeusia, diarrhea, constipation, and headache.

In a crossover study in 24 healthy volunteers, rabeprazole 10, 20, and 40 mg produced significant dose-related reductions in intragastric acidity associated with a significant rise in serum gastrin concentration (4). There were no serious adverse effects. After taking into account increases in serum gastrin concentrations and interindividual variation in the antisecretory response, 20 mg appears to be the preferred dose for routine clinical use. Similar potent dose-related gastric acid inhibition and rises in serum gastrin were found with rabeprazole 5–40 mg/day in the morning for 7 days in 38 subjects infected with *Helicobacter pylori* (5). There was less than 50% recovery of acid by 48 hours after the seventh dose. In this study the optimal acid inhibitory dose appeared to be 20 mg/day, and there were no serious adverse effects.

The safety and efficacy of rabeprazole have been evaluated in 124 patients aged 65 years and over being treated for a variety of acid-related disorders (6). Rabeprazole controlled symptoms and healed mucosal lesions. The incidence of adverse effects was 4.9%, and adverse effects were more common in the presence of hepatic dysfunction and with increasing duration of treatment.

The efficacy and tolerability of rabeprazole 10 mg/day for 8 weeks in the treatment of reflux esophagitis has been assessed in an open, postmarketing surveillance investigation in 61 patients (7). Rabeprazole was well tolerated and was effective in relieving symptoms and healing esophagitis. Two patients developed slight rises in liver enzymes, which resolved after treatment.

In an open, multicenter trial in 2579 patients with erosive gastro-esophageal reflux disease, rabeprazole 20 mg/day for 8 weeks relieved symptoms in most patients (in over 60% by day 1 and over 80% by day 7) (8). Rabeprazole was well tolerated, and the most common adverse effects were headache, diarrhea, abdominal pain, and nausea, each reported by under 2% of the patients.

In another open, multicenter study in 92 patients with erosive esophagitis, rabeprazole 20 mg/day was effective in healing esophageal lesions and relieving heartburn (9). Adverse effects (diarrhea, headache, and nausea) were attributed to the medication in four cases.

Placebo-controlled studies

In a double-blind, placebo-controlled study in 288 patients with previously treated erosive or ulcerative gastro-esophageal reflux disease rabeprazole 10 or 20 mg/day was significantly more effective than placebo in preventing relapse of erosive or ulcerative gastro-esophageal reflux disease and was well tolerated (10). Commonly reported adverse events were abdominal pain, nausea, diarrhea, rhinitis, pharyngitis, a flu-like syndrome, and back pain. Rabeprazole had no clinically significant effects on laboratory values, thyroid function tests, the electrocardiogram, vital signs, or body weight.

General adverse effects

Rabeprazole was generally well tolerated in both short-term and long-term studies of up to 2 years. Headache was the most important reported adverse effect. Other commonly reported adverse effects were diarrhea, rhinitis, nausea, pharyngitis, abdominal pain, and flatulence. The changes in serum gastrin concentrations were consistent with proton pump inhibitor pharmacology, and no study has reported mean values at end-point that were outside the reference range. In controlled trials, the frequency of abnormalities of hepatic aminotransferases was similar to that of placebo. Scoring of enterochromaffin-like cells in gastric biopsies taken prospectively from patients in studies of up to 2 years have shown some hyperplastic changes, but no evidence of adenomatous, dysplastic, or neoplastic changes.

Organs and Systems

Liver

- Acute fulminant hepatitis occurred in a previously healthy 46-year-old man who took rabeprazole and terbinafine (11). His condition improved gradually after withdrawal of both drugs.

References

1. Johnson D, Perdomo C, Barth J, Jokubaitis L. The benefit/risk profile of rabeprazole, a new proton-pump inhibitor. Eur J Gastroenterol Hepatol 2000;12(7):799–806.
2. Carswell CI, Goa KL. Rabeprazole: an update of its use in acid-related disorders. Drugs 2001;61(15):2327–56.
3. Mundo-Gallardo F, De Mezerville-Cantillo L, Burgos-Quiroz H, Izquierdo E, Chang-Mayorga J, Azteguieta L, Passarrelli-Sandhoff LF. Latin American open-label study with rabeprazole in patients with functional dyspepsia. Mexican Rabeprazole Investigators Group. Adv Ther 2000;17(4):190–4.
4. Williams MP, Blanshard C, Millson C, Sercombe J, Pounder RE. A placebo-controlled study to assess the effects of 7-day dosing with 10, 20 and 40 mg rabeprazole on 24-h intragastric acidity and plasma gastrin in healthy male subjects. Aliment Pharmacol Ther 2000;14(6):691–9.

5. Ohning GV, Barbuti RC, Kovacs TO, Sytnik B, Humphries TJ, Walsh JH. Rabeprazole produces rapid, potent, and long-acting inhibition of gastric acid secretion in subjects with *Helicobacter pylori* infection. Aliment Pharmacol Ther 2000;14(6):701–8.

6. Fujita R, Takahashi H, Iwashige M, Kamiyama T, Hara H, Koyoma T. Clinical evaluation of proton pump inhibitor, rabeprazole—special surveillance in patients of advanced age with peptic ulcer diseases. Jpn Pharmacol Ther 2002;30:539–49.

7. Kinoshita Y, Hirayama M, Hamada S, Yoshida T, Ishii N, Nakata R, Chishima J, Handa Y, Saito K, Takayama T, Tatsumi S, Iishi H, Kohll Y, Fujita S, Tanaka H, Ookuchi S, Suzuki S, Koyama T, Yoshida Y, Kabemura T, Matsumoto K. Efficacy of rabeprazole in patients with reflux esophagitis: a single-center, open-label, practice-based, postmarketing surveillance investigation. Curr Ther Res Clin Exp 2002;63:810–20.

8. Robinson M, Fitzgerald S, Hegedus R, Murthy A, Jokubaitis L; FAST Trial Investigators. Onset of symptom relief with rabeprazole: a community-based, open-label assessment of patients with erosive oesophagitis. Aliment Pharmacol Ther 2002;16(3):445–54.

9. de Freitas JA. Effectiveness and tolerability of rabeprazole 20 mg as once-daily monotherapy in treatment of erosive or ulcerative gastro-oesophageal disease. Clin Drug Invest 2002;22:279–89.

10. Birbara C, Breiter J, Perdomo C, Hahne W. Rabeprazole for the prevention of recurrent erosive or ulcerative gastro-oesophageal reflux disease. Rabeprazole Study Group. Eur J Gastroenterol Hepatol 2000;12(8):889–97.

11. Johnstone D, Berger C, Fleckman P. Acute fulminant hepatitis after treatment with rabeprazole and terbinafine. Arch Intern Med 2001;161(13):1677–8.

Rabies vaccine

See also Vaccines

General Information

Rabies vaccine was for a long time prepared from infected brain tissue, and neurological complications were likely to occur in as many as one in 300 cases. A second-generation vaccine prepared from duck embryo tissue has been found to be better tolerated in this respect, and third-generation vaccines prepared in non-neural tissue cultures or in human diploid cell (HDC) vaccines with a progressive improvement in safety have now become the vaccines of choice where they are available.

Any rabies vaccine can apparently cause mild local discomfort and swelling, and either of the animal preparations can result in hypersensitivity reactions, for example pyrexia, serum sickness, or urticaria; sensitization can occur.

Third-generation rabies vaccines include a purified vero-cell rabies vaccine (PVRV) and HDC vaccine purified by zonal centrifugation. In clinical trials (SEDA-12, 284) (SEDA-15, 357) the improved vaccines were well tolerated. In 1988, Rabies Vaccine Adsorbed (RVA), a new cell culture-derived rabies vaccine (Kissling strain of rabies virus adapted to a diploid cell line of the fetal rhesus lung cells in medium-free of human albumin and adsorbed on aluminium phosphate) for human use was licensed in the USA. Reactions after primary immunization are similar to those observed with HDC. Systemic allergic reactions have been reported at a rate <1% (HDC 6%) (1).

Organs and Systems

Nervous system

Brain tissue rabies vaccine

There are many countries that still use first-generation brain tissue rabies vaccine because of limited financial resources and where neurological complications after immunization still occur. The neurological effects produced by this type of vaccine are very variable. Sometimes a peripheral neuropathy occurs, while other vaccinees develop encephalomyelitis, dorsolumbar myelitis, ascending myelitis, hemiplegia, or general subjective neurological symptoms, such as stiffness of the neck or physical weakness.

It has been argued that there may be a risk of transmitting scrapie (spongiform encephalopathy of sheep, similar to bovine spongiform encephalopathy of cattle) through blood donation from individuals who have been immunized against rabies with sheep brain rabies vaccine still used in developing countries (2).

Duck embryo rabies vaccine (DEV)

Nervous system complications after administration of DEV occurred, but in much lower frequency than after brain tissue rabies vaccines. Reports of transverse myelitis and other neurological complications have been published (SEDA-8, 300). There have been some efforts to develop a more purified version of DEV, but improvements in third-generation vaccines have made these the vaccines of choice when they can be afforded, much reducing the motivation to develop duck embryo vaccines further.

Human diploid cell (HDC) vaccines

The major advantage of third-generation rabies vaccines prepared in non-neural tissue cultures or in human diploid cells is the greatly reduced risk of neurological complications. Millions of doses of these vaccines have been administered worldwide since 1974, and only a few neurological complications have been reported. The overall risk of neurological complications is estimated to be less than 1 per 150 000 (SEDA-15, 356), and complications after the administration of third-generation rabies vaccines cultured in non-neural tissues have been very rarely reported. However, those that have been published are of various types.

Isolated case reports of Guillain–Barré syndrome after HDC vaccine have been published (SED-11, 684) (SEDA-15, 356) (3). Polyneuropathy and oculomotor nerve impairment have been reported after Russian cell-culture vaccine (SEDA-12, 284).

- Two weeks after the second injection of HDC vaccine a 45-year-old farmer developed meningoradiculitis. The symptoms regressed spontaneously (4).
- A 25-year-old veterinary practitioner developed an inflammatory demyelinating process affecting the

central nervous system 8 days after the second HDC vaccine immunization (5).

- Acute disseminated encephalomyelitis developed in a 15-year-old boy after HDC vaccine immunization (SEDA-21, 337).
- A 14-year-old boy had a seizure after the administration of human diploid rabies cell vaccine simultaneously with rabies immune globulin. The symptoms developed within minutes after injection. After treatment and about 2 hours later, his mental status returned to normal (6).

Immunologic

In recipients given primary courses of third-generation rabies vaccines, only mild local and systemic reactions were reported by about 20%. Systemic allergic reactions have occurred in 11 per 10 000 vaccinees (7). However, 2–21 days after the administration of HDC vaccine, about 5% of patients receiving booster injections for pre-exposure prophylaxis and a few receiving postexposure primary immunization develop an immune complex (serum sickness-like) reaction, including urticaria, fever, malaise, arthralgias, arthritis, nausea, and vomiting. This syndrome may prove to be less common with RVA, but direct comparisons are lacking.

Anaphylaxis has been reported rarely after HDC vaccine prophylaxis (3).

References

1. Anonymous. Human rabies prophylaxis, 1987. Wkly Epidemiol Rec 1988;13:357.
2. Arya SC. Blood donated after vaccination with rabies vaccine derived from sheep brain cells might transmit CJD. BMJ 1996;13(7069):1405.
3. Anonymous. Rabies vaccine. Med Lett 1991;117–18.
4. Moulignier A, Richer A, Fritzell C, Foulon D, Khoubesserian P, de Recondo J. Méningo-radiculite secondaire à une vaccination antirabique. [Meningoradiculitis after injection of an antirabies vaccine. A vaccine from human diploid cell culture.] Presse Méd 1991;20(24):1121–3.
5. Tornatore CS, Richert JR. CNS demyelination associated with diploid cell rabies vaccine. Lancet 1990;335(8701):1346–7.
6. Mortiere MD, Falcone AL, Plotkin SA, Loupi E, Lang J. An acute neurologic syndrome temporally associated with postexposure treatment of rabies. Pediatrics 1997;100(4):718–21.
7. Committee on Immunization. Guide for Adult Immunization. Philadelphia: American College of Physicians, 1985.

Racecadotril

General Information

Racecadotril is an orally active potent inhibitor of enkephalinase, which has an antihypersecretory effect without increasing intestinal transit time.

Racecadotril 100 mg tds has been compared with loperamide 2 mg tds in a single-blind study in 945 outpatients with acute diarrhea in 21 centers in 14 countries (1).

Racecadotril resolved acute diarrhea as rapidly and as effectively as loperamide and produced more rapid resolution of abdominal symptoms and less constipation. The incidence of adverse effects attributable to medication was less in the racecadotril group (9 versus 18%). Common adverse effects were constipation, abdominal distension, anorexia, headache, and abdominal pain.

Reference

1. Prado D; Global Adult Racecadotril Study Group. A multinational comparison of racecadotril and loperamide in the treatment of acute watery diarrhoea in adults. Scand J Gastroenterol 2002;37(6):656–61.

Radioactive iodine

General Information

Three radioactive isotopes of ^{127}I are currently used in clinical medicine:

1. ^{131}I (radioactive half-life of 8 days and a high-energy emitter), used mainly in the therapy of hyperthyroidism and thyroid cancer.
2. ^{123}I (radioactive half-life 13 hours) has replaced ^{131}I for diagnostic purposes; however, for in vivo imaging meta-stable technetium-99 (^{99m}Tc) is often preferred, because of its lower radiation dose, availability, and cost.
3. ^{125}I (radioactive half-life of 60 days and a low energy emitter), previously used in the treatment of hyperthyroidism, but now replaced by ^{131}I because of disappointing therapeutic results (1,2).

Radioactive isotopes of iodine are handled by the thyroid in the same way as stable iodine and are therefore actively concentrated, incorporated into thyroglobulin, stored, metabolized, and secreted as thyroid hormones. Small amounts of radioactive iodine are therefore ideal probes to analyse the uptake of iodine, the distribution of iodine in the gland, and possibly even its turnover and incorporation into thyroid hormones. Larger amounts of radioactive iodine selectively radiate the thyroid gland and therefore selectively impair the function of the follicular thyroid cells and eventually destroy them.

Doses

Three dosage ranges for radioactive forms of iodine are used:

1. For diagnostic purposes usually much less than 1 mCi (37 MBq) is given with thyroid radiation doses of a few rads of ^{123}I up to 50–200 rads (0.5–2.0 Gray) (^{131}I).
2. In the treatment of hyperthyroidism the dose of ^{131}I is usually a few millicuries and is either roughly estimated or calculated according to the size of the thyroid gland, the uptake of a tracer dose of iodine, and the type of thyroid disorder (diffuse or nodular), with

doses ranging from 80 to 150 microCi (3.0–5.5 MBq) per gram of thyroid tissue (3,4).

3. In thyroid cancer, ^{131}I can be used to eliminate tumor tissue that cannot be removed surgically but still captures iodine; in such circumstances, amounts of 100 mCi (4000 MBq) of ^{131}I or more are not unusual; with such high amounts, other tissues besides the thyroid gland can also receive substantial amounts of radiation.

The administration of ^{131}I requires safety measurements to reduce to a minimum the irradiation of medical personnel and to avoid contamination of rooms and relatives of patients. Capsules containing ^{131}I are therefore to be preferred to liquid iodine. At doses above 25 mCi (555 MBq), usually intended only for treatment of patients with thyroid cancer, isolation in a specially constructed room of a service for nuclear medicine is necessary. Waste disposal should also be carefully managed so as to avoid overall contamination (5,6).

General adverse effects

Radiation thyroiditis is an infrequent complication resulting in swelling and localized pain over the thyroid gland which subsides spontaneously or with anti-inflammatory or corticosteroid therapy (SEDA-1, 314).

Acute exacerbation of hyperthyroidism, resulting particularly in cardiac complications (arrhythmias or decompensation) or even "thyroid storm," has been reported several times (SEDA-1, 314) and should be avoided by treating very severely hyperthyroid patients with antithyroid drugs prior to the administration of [131]I. A temporary increase in serum triiodothyronine and l-thyroxine without clinical symptoms of exacerbation of hyperthyroidism, however, occurs much more frequently (SEDA-1, 314). In 71 patients given ^{131}I for differentiated thyroid carcinoma, short-term adverse effects included gastrointestinal complaints, salivary gland swelling with pain, change in taste and headache (7).

Organs and Systems

Cardiovascular

In a series of thyrocardiac patients, of those dying primarily from thyrotoxicosis more than 21% did so within 3 weeks of ^{131}I treatment (8), presumably reflecting too sudden a change in metabolic activity for patients with existing cardiac complications.

Respiratory

Acute respiratory embarrassment due to thyroid swelling or subsequently due to cicatrization occurs only rarely.

Nervous system

Although aseptic meningitis has been associated with the use of radioactive iodine, the products used were albumin complexes (^{131}I-RISA); this complication is almost certainly attributable to the protein content or to pyrogens rather than to the radioactive iodine itself (8).

Sensory systems

Several papers have reported that radioiodine therapy can lead to worsening of ophthalmopathy, possibly because of the release of thyroid antigens during the inflammatory reaction after ^{131}I therapy. The worsening can be prevented by glucocorticoid therapy (9).

Endocrine

The calcitonin-producing cells of the thyroid are usually destroyed by [131]I (SEDA-14, 369).

Both hyperfunction (10) and hypofunction of the parathyroid glands have been described after the use of [131]I (11).

Hypothyroidism

There is an increased incidence of late hypothyroidism in patients with autoimmune hyperthyroidism, but the risk increases markedly after extensive thyroid surgery and especially after ^{131}I treatment. Analysis of the cumulative incidence of hypothyroidism shows two phases: an early phase of radiation death of thyroid cells, depending on the ^{131}I dosage and occurring during the first 1–2 years after treatment; a second period of a lower (0.5–3.5% per year) but life-long risk of developing hypothyroidism for a variety of reasons (natural history of the disease, autoimmune processes) (see Table 1) (12–14).

The total incidence of hypothyroidism can therefore be reduced by lowering the therapeutic dose, but at the expense of a higher incidence of more prolonged or recurrent hyperthyroidism. Calculation of the therapeutic dose according to thyroid gland size, iodine uptake, or biological half-life and type of thyroid disorder can help to reduce the total incidence of hypothyroidism, although this is less well documented than many believe (15,16). Moreover, the occurrence of hypothyroidism after the use of ^{131}I should not be dramatized, since treatment is much

Table 1 The risk of hypothyroidism after [131]I

N	[131]I dose (mCi)	Total follow-up period (years)	Incidence of hypothyroidism (%)				Total annual cumulative incidence (% per year)	Reference
			One-year follow-up		End of follow-up			
			Diffuse goiter	Nodular goiter	Diffuse goiter	Nodular goiter		
4473	8–20	26	8	3	77	64	3	(12)
1369	9	17	6	3	26	14	3.5	(13)
248	6–10	10	38	11	70	18	0.5	(14)

simpler than abandoning the patient first to the prolonged risk of recurrent hyperthyroidism and thereafter to life-long follow-up for hypothyroidism. Hypothyroidism after ^{131}I can also be transient, and replacement therapy should not be started too early (17).

Hematologic

Leukemia does not occur more often in patients treated with ^{131}I for hyperthyroidism than in similar patients treated by surgery. After use of the high doses used in the treatment of thyroid cancer there was a definite increase in the incidence of leukemia (18).

Salivary glands

In 71 patients given ^{131}I for differentiated thyroid carcinoma, salivary gland swelling with pain occurred in 50% (7); women had a significantly higher incidence than men.

Gastrointestinal

Of 71 patients given ^{131}I for differentiated thyroid carcinoma, 65% had gastrointestinal complaints: appetite loss, nausea, and vomiting occurred in 61, 40, and 7.6% respectively and increased significantly in the patients who received doses above 55.5 MBq/kg and with rises in TSH (7).

Reproductive system

Large amounts of ^{131}I, as used in thyroid cancer therapy, can cause testicular damage as documented from hormonal and sperm analysis (19), but long-term results are nevertheless reassuringly normal (20).

Long-Term Effects

Mutagenicity

Mutagenic effects on the sexual organs are difficult to determine in practice. However, while the radiation dose to the ovary and testes is rather small after ^{131}I treatment for hyperthyroidism (maximum 5 roentgens) it can be substantial after the higher amounts of ^{131}I that are used for thyroid cancer. In any case, children born to mothers previously treated with ^{131}I did not have an increased incidence of congenital malformations. The number of such observations is too small, however, to allow definite conclusions about its safety (21). In patients treated for thyroid carcinoma there was no differences in fertility rate, birth weight, prematurity, or congenital malformations compared with healthy subjects, providing reassurance about the use of radioiodine to treat hyperthyroidism in women of child-bearing age (SEDA-20, 394).

Tumorigenicity

The total number of case reports of thyroid cancer after ^{131}I is very small (under 30 cases) (22) in relation to the estimated number of patients treated with ^{131}I since 1941 (over 1 000 000 patients). Moreover, systematic follow-up or retrospective studies did not show an increased risk of thyroid carcinoma in patients treated with ^{131}I for hyperthyroidism. The results of two such studies are shown in more detail in Table 2 (23) and Table 3 (24).

Table 2 ^{131}I treatment and thyroid cancer: a comparison with thyroidectomy and antithyroid drugs

Incidence of thyroid cancer	Thyroidectomy ($n = 11\ 732$)	[131]I ($n = 21\ 714$)	Antithyroid drugs ($n = 1238$)
Within 1 year of treatment	50	9	0
After 1 year of treatment	4	19	4
Total	54 (4.6%)	28 (11.3%)	4 (3.2%)
Number of deaths from thyroid cancer	4	6	0

Table 3 ^{131}I treatment and thyroid cancer

Number of patients treated with [131]I	3000
Mean age	57 years
Mean dose of [131]I	13.3 mCi
Mean observation period	13 years
Thyroid cancer	
Observed incidence	4%
Expected incidence	3.2%
Thyroid cancer more than 5 years after [131]I	
Observed incidence	2.1%
Expected incidence	3%

In another follow-up study of 1005 women treated with ^{131}I there was no increase in total morbidity or in the incidence of thyroid cancer (20).

In 10 552 Swedish patients (mean age 57 years) who received ^{131}I for hyperthyroidism (mean follow-up 15 years) there were increases in overall cancer mortality and deaths due to carcinoma of the stomach, lung, and kidney. While the findings for stomach cancer may be of significance, for tumors at other sites, because of an association with time after ^{131}I treatment (58 cases at 10 years or more of follow-up against the expected 44 cases), the lack of a relation between cancer mortality and either the time from radioiodine treatment or the dose administered argues against a carcinogenic effect of radioiodine (SEDA-17, 475) (25).

The use of very high amounts of ^{131}I for thyroid cancer imposes special care and risks: the frequency of radiation thyroiditis is much higher (more than 20%) and similar symptoms of pain and swelling can also be observed in the salivary glands. Nausea and vomiting may also occur. The incidence of leukemia is increased: 15 cases being reported in 5000 patients treated with ^{131}I for thyroid cancer (18); it therefore seems wise to limit the total dose of ^{131}I in a single patient to 500 mCi unless the thyroid disease activity permits higher long-term risks. It is also important to keep such patients well hydrated to allow rapid elimination of ^{131}I not retained by thyroid tissue. The radiation dose to the ovaries is not negligible, being approximately 200 roentgens after 500 mCi of ^{131}I, a dose sufficient to increase slightly the subsequent risk of miscarriage or congenital abnormalities. However, no apparent increase in the rate of abnormalities has been observed in the outcome of pregnancies among women previously treated for thyroid cancer.

The use of ^{131}I in children is different from its use in adults. Experience worldwide is much more limited as regards both the number of children treated and the total number of years of observation (SEDA-20, 394). The risk of eventual tumor-inducing effects in the thyroid or other tissues is real. The young thyroid is very sensitive to external radiation or to nuclear fall-out: 66% of young adults developed thyroid lesions 25 years after such exposure (26). One report on a high prevalence of hypothyroidism after ^{131}I showed no cases of thyroid or other malignancies after a mean follow-up period of almost 15 years (27). However, others found an increased frequency of thyroid nodules: among case reports on thyroid cancer after ^{131}I in the world literature the younger age group is largely over-represented, owing to the frequency of ^{131}I use in this age group (22). In view of the small number of long-term results in a young population with probably higher susceptibility for thyroid tumors it seems unwise to use ^{131}I as preferred treatment for adolescents or young adults with hyperthyroidism. Much longer follow-up periods will be necessary, preferably with central registration to allow a definite conclusion about treatment (21,18). However, many experts consider the current follow-up period sufficiently long to extend the use of ^{131}I to all patients with Graves' disease above the age of 25 (SEDA-14, 368) (28). There are, however, large discrepancies in treatment strategies globally.

Second-Generation Effects

Pregnancy

Radioactive iodine passes the placenta and accumulates in the fetal thyroid where the concentration probably exceeds that in the maternal thyroid. Detailed studies show that the fetal dose of iodine is virtually nil before the 90th day of gestation but sharply increases thereafter (29). This alone is sufficient reason to avoid the use of ^{131}I in pregnancy, but there is also some controversial evidence that various congenital deformities have been produced by the isotope (30).

Teratogenicity

Concern about possible second-generation effects of ^{131}I is difficult to allay but has not been substantiated, since there is an absence of obvious birth defects or genetic changes in the offspring of patients treated with ^{131}I (20,22,24,31,32). Moreover, the radiation dose to the ovaries in ^{131}I therapy for hyperthyroidism is usually below three roentgens and thus comparable to the radiation due to common radiographic abdominal examinations. If ^{131}I is given during pregnancy, fetal hypothyroidism and chromosomal aberrations can occur (33).

Lactation

^{131}I is transferred in the milk and should not be given during lactation. Even the diagnostic use of radioisotopes of iodine should be avoided (34).

Interference with Diagnostic Tests

Detection of pulmonary embolism

Injections of ^{131}I given to detect pulmonary embolism can result in false-negative results in the ^{125}I-labeled fibrinogen test for venous thrombosis.

References

1. Glanzmann C, Kaestner F, Horst W. Therapie der Hyperthyreose mit Radioisotopen des Jods: Erfahrungen bei über 2000 Patienten. [Radio-iodine treatment of hyperthyroidism. Experience in more than 2000 patients.] Klin Wochenschr 1975;53(14):669–78.
2. Glanzmann C, Horst W. Iodine-125 and iodine-131 in the treatment of hyperthyroidism. Clin Nucl Med 1980;5(7):325–33.
3. Holm LE, Lundell G, Dahlqvist I, Israelsson A. Cure rate after ^{131}I therapy for hyperthyroidism. Acta Radiol Oncol 1981;20(3):161–6.
4. Bliddal H, Hansen JM, Rogowski P, Johansen K, Friis T, Siersbaek-Nielsen K. ^{131}I treatment of diffuse and nodular toxic goitre with or without antithyroid agents. Acta Endocrinol (Copenh) 1982;99(4):517–21.
5. Thomas SR, Maxon HR, Fritz KM, Kereiakes JG, Connell WD. A comparison of methods for assessing patient body burden following ^{131}I therapy for thyroid cancer. Radiology 1980;137(3):839–42.
6. Radioprotection Committee. Radioprotection in radioactive iodine therapy. Belg Tijdschr Radiol 1980;63:39.
7. Kita T, Yokoyama K, Higuchi T, Kinuya S, Taki J, Nakajima K, Michigishi T, Tonami N. Multifactorial analysis on the short-term side effects occurring within 96 hours after radioiodine-131 therapy for differentiated thyroid carcinoma. Ann Nucl Med 2004;18(4):345–9.
8. Shani J, Atkins HL, Wolf W. Adverse reactions to radiopharmaceuticals. Semin Nucl Med 1976;6(3):305–28.
9. Bartalena L, Marcocci C, Bogazzi F, Panicucci M, Lepri A, Pinchera A. Use of corticosteroids to prevent progression of Graves' ophthalmopathy after radioiodine therapy for hyperthyroidism. N Engl J Med 1989;321(20):1349–52.
10. Triggs SM, Williams ED. Irradiation of the thyroid as a cause of parathyroid adenoma. Lancet 1977;1(8011):593–4.
11. Jialal I, Pillay NL, Asmal AC. Radio-iodine-induced hypoparathyroidism. A case report. S Afr Med J 1980;58(23):939–40.
12. Holm LE, Lundell G, Israelsson A, Dahlqvist I. Incidence of hypothyroidism occurring long after iodine-131 therapy for hyperthyroidism. J Nucl Med 1982;23(2):103–7.
13. Best JD, Chan V, Khoo R, Teng CS, Wang C, Yeung RT. Incidence of hypothyroidism after radioactive iodine therapy for thyrotoxicosis in Hong Kong Chinese. Clin Radiol 1981;32(1):57–61.
14. Kamphuis JJ. Behandeling van hyperthyreoïdie met ^{131}I: een retrospectief onderzoek. [Treatment of hyperthyroidism using ^{131}I: a retrospective study.] Ned Tijdschr Geneeskd 1980;124(26):1045–9.
15. Hayes MT. Hypothyroidism following iodine-131 therapy. J Nucl Med 1982;23(2):176–9.
16. Watson AB, Brownlie BE, Frampton CM, Turner JG, Rogers TG. Outcome following standardized 185 MBq dose ^{131}I therapy for Graves' disease. Clin Endocrinol (Oxf) 1988;28(5):487–96.
17. MacFarlane IA, Shalet SM, Beardwell CG, Khara JS. Transient hypothyroidism after iodine-131 treatment for thyrotoxicosis. BMJ 1979;2(6187):421.
18. Blahd WH. Treatment of malignant thyroid disease. Semin Nucl Med 1979;9(2):95–99.

19. Handelsman DJ, Conway AJ, Donnelly PE, Turtle JR. Azoospermia after iodine-131 treatment for thyroid carcinoma. BMJ 1980;281(6254):1527.

20. Hoffman DA, McConahey WM, Diamond EL, Kurland LT. Mortality in women treated for hyperthyroidism. Am J Epidemiol 1982;115(2):243–54.

21. Maxon HR, Thomas SR, Chen IW. The role of nuclear medicine in the treatment of hyperthyroidism and well-differentiated thyroid adenocarcinoma. Clin Nucl Med 1981;6(10S):P87–98.

22. McDougall IR, Nelsen TS, Kempson RL. Papillary carcinoma of the thyroid seven years after I-131 therapy for Graves' disease. Clin Nucl Med 1981;6(8):368–71.

23. Wolff J. Risks for stable and radioactive iodine in radiation protection of the thyroid. In: Hall R, Kobberling J, editors. Thyroid Disorders Associated with Iodine Deficiency and Excess. Serono Symposia Publications. New York: Raven Press, 1985;22:111.

24. Holm LE, Dahlqvist I, Israelsson A, Lundell G. Malignant thyroid tumors after iodine-131 therapy: a retrospective cohort study. N Engl J Med 1980;303(4):188–91.

25. Holm LE, Hall P, Wiklund K, Lundell G, Berg G, Bjelkengren G, Cederquist E, Ericsson UB, Hallquist A, Larsson LG, et al. Cancer risk after iodine-131 therapy for hyperthyroidism. J Natl Cancer Inst 1991;83(15):1072–7.

26. Larsen PR, Conard RA, Knudsen K. Thyroid hypofunction appearing as a delayed manifestation of accidental exposure to radioactive fallout in a Marshallese population. In: Biological Effects of Ionizing Radiation. Vienna: International Atomic Energy Agency, 1978;1:101.

27. Freitas JE, Swanson DP, Gross MD, Sisson JC. Iodine-131: optimal therapy for hyperthyroidism in children and adolescents? J Nucl Med 1979;20(8):847–50.

28. Graham GD, Burman KD. Radioiodine treatment of Graves' disease. An assessment of its potential risks. Ann Intern Med 1986;105(6):900–5.

29. Johnson JR. Fetal thyroid dose from intakes of radioiodine by the mother. Health Phys 1982;43(4):573–82.

30. Nishimura H, Tanimura T. Clinical Aspects of Teratogenicity of Drugs. Amsterdam: Excerpta Medica, 1976.

31. Dobyns BM, Sheline GE, Workman JB, Tompkins EA, McConahey WM, Becker DV. Malignant and benign neoplasms of the thyroid in patients treated for hyperthyroidism: a report of the cooperative thyrotoxicosis therapy follow-up study. J Clin Endocrinol Metab 1974;38(6): 976–98.

32. Sarkar SD, Beierwaltes WH, Gill SP, Cowley BJ. Subsequent fertility and birth histories of children and adolescents treated with ^{131}I for thyroid cancer. J Nucl Med 1976;17(6):460–4.

33. Goh KO. Radioiodine treatment during pregnancy: chromosomal aberrations and cretinism associated with maternal iodine-131 treatment. J Am Med Womens Assoc 1981;36(8):262–5.

34. Dydek GJ, Blue PW. Human breast milk excretion of iodine-131 following diagnostic and therapeutic administration to a lactating patient with Graves' disease. J Nucl Med 1988;29(3):407–10.

Radiopharmaceuticals

General Information

Radioactive substances may be used in medicine as tracers, the quantities used in this case being merely sufficient to enable them to be detected, or as therapeutic agents, in which case the quantities employed and the amount of radiation emitted may be considerable. Risks resulting from the radiation itself fall outside the scope of this volume.

Radio-iodine is covered in a separate monograph.

General adverse effects

Radiopharmaceuticals have a good safety record. The prevalence of adverse reactions is approximately 1000-fold than less than that occurring with iodinated contrast media and drugs. The Society of Nuclear Medicine has maintained a register of adverse reactions to radiopharmaceuticals occurring in USA since 1976. The frequency of reactions appears to be falling because of improved quality control of radiopharmaceuticals. Many of the earlier adverse reactions were attributed to iron-containing formulations, gelatin-stabilized formulations, materials such as albumin contaminated with pyrogens, and other products no longer in use. The overall incidence of reactions for the year 1978 was estimated to be 1–6 per 100 000 examinations (1).

In order to determine the prevalence of adverse reactions to radiopharmaceuticals, a 5-year prospective study (1989–94) was performed in 18 institutions in the USA (2). The reported incidence rate was 0.0023%. No adverse reaction required hospitalization or had significant sequelae. The adverse reactions and types of radiopharmaceuticals are shown in Table 1.

Another study was undertaken to determine the prevalence of adverse reactions to positron-emitting radiopharmaceuticals through a prospective 4-year study in 22 institutions. PET radiopharmaceuticals have an excellent safety record because no adverse reactions were reported in over 80 000 administered doses in this study (3).

In a review of UK reports of adverse reactions to radiopharmaceuticals from 1977 to 1983, there was a changing distribution pattern with time (Table 2) (4). This was partly due to elimination of some of the earlier, more toxic formulations and partly due to changing usage, more particularly the increased use of phosphonate formulations. The authors estimated that only 10% of reactions were reported and that the probable

Table 1 Adverse reactions to 783 525 radiopharmaceutical doses in 1989–94 in the USA

Radiopharmaceutical	Adverse reaction	Number
[67]Gallium citrate	Rash	1
[^{131}I] Iobenguane (MIBG)	Chest discomfort, light-headedness	1
[99m]Tc-macroaggregated albumin	Rash	1
[99m]Tc-medronate (MDP)	Rash/nausea/mild anaphylaxis	2/1/1
[99m]Tc-oxidronate (HDP)	Rash/sweating	4/1
[99m]Tc-pentetate (DTPA)	Rash	1
[99m]Tc-sestamibi	Rash	1
[99m]Tc-sulfur colloid	Nausea, vomiting, rash, headache	1
Stannous pyrophosphate (non-radioactive)*	Mild anaphylaxis/ light-headedness	2/1
Total		18

*Given intravenously to allow in vivo radiolabeling of erythrocytes and considered part of the final radiopharmaceutical.

Table 2 Major groupings of adverse reactions to radiopharmaceuticals reported in the UK from January 1977 to December 1983

Period	Colloids	Phosphonates	Albumin particulates	Others
1977 to mid-1980	12 (48%)	2 (8%)	5[*] (16%)	8[*] (28%)
Mid-1980 to 1983	8[†] (21%)	15[†] (45%)	3 (10%)	8[*] (24%)
Total	20[†] (33%)	17[†] (28%)	8[*] (13%)	16[*] (26%)

[*]1 case or [†]2 cases considered to be "unlikely to be due to the radiopharmaceutical".

incidence rate was between one in 1000 and one in 10 000. There was one death associated with a hypotensive reaction to colloid in a severely ill patient. One elderly patient had a cardiac arrest after injection of macro-aggregated albumin but was resuscitated. In a European prospective survey during 1996, there was a prevalence of 11 events per 105 administrations of radiopharmaceuticals. No serious or life-threatening events were reported (5).

^{99m}Technetium

The widespread use of ^{99m}Tc-DTPA (diethylaminetriaminepenta-acetate), mostly used for renal imaging, has brought with it a number of reported DTPA adverse reactions. Typical symptoms include low pressure, loss of consciousness, feeling faint and occasionally skin rash and bronchospasm. In Europe, a patient with a history of asthma developed severe bronchospasm and died within a matter of minutes (6). A series of very serious problem developed following intrathecal injection of ^{99m}Tc-DTPA in what turned out to be, strictly speaking, a misformulation incident. Almost all currently used DTPA formulations contain the mixed calcium/sodium salt of DTPA. However, one particular manufacturer used the trisodium salt. This form is capable of chelation of cerebrospinal fluid calcium and magnesium and causing gradual onset of severe neurological signs and severe paresthesia (7).

^{99m}Tc-labeled serum albumin microspheres have in one case caused collapse, apparently because the patient in question had earlier been sensitized by blood transfusions (SEDA-2, 376).

A case of anaphylaxis occurred after the injection of a leukocyte suspension labeled with ^{99m}Tc-hexamethyl propylene amine oxime (8).

Inhalation of Technigas (an ultrafine suspension of ^{99m}Tc-labeled carbon particles) for ventilation scintigraphy, in a series of patients led to a temporary reduction in oxygenation in 87% of cases, often in sufficient degree to cause some discomfort (SEDA-17, 539) (9). Injection of ^{99m}Tc-MAA for perfusion scintigraphy similarly tended to cause a decrease in oxygenation, but insufficient to cause symptoms.

Others

Aseptic meningitis has been reported after isotope cisternography with indium diethylenetriaminopentaacetic acid (SEDA-2, 376).

Dipyridamole-^{201}thallium imaging has been used to assess cases of suspected coronary disease (SEDA-15, 506) (SEDA-16, 537) (SEDA-17, 539). It is difficult to distinguish the adverse effects of dipyridamole from those of the pharmaceutical agent (dipyridamole-^{201}thallium), since dipyridamole can cause bronchospasm. In one series of 400 examinations, there was severe chest pain due to myocardial ischemia in 9% of cases, milder chest pain (probably not associated with cardiac events) in 21%, and severe hypotension in 2.5% (10). Others have reported instances of cardiovascular collapse (SEDA-15, 506).

Second-Generation Effects

Lactation

Many radiopharmaceuticals are excreted in breast milk, and two reviews have discussed the implications of nuclear medicine examinations in the nursing mother (11,12).

Iodides are excreted in high concentrations in breast milk. The use of the short half-life ^{123}I in preference to ^{131}I partly overcomes this problem, but iodide or perchlorate, which is used to block thyroid uptake in the mother can be excreted in the milk. Likewise, furosemide or cholecystokinin, which can be used to alter the distribution of radiopharmaceuticals, can be excreted in breast milk.

Technetium compounds are the most widely used radiopharmaceuticals; the highest excretion in breast milk occurs with sodium pertechnetate and the lowest with technetium diethylenetriaminepenta-acetic acid, which is rapidly excreted by the kidneys. Depending on the type of examination and the dose of radiopharmaceutical, the mother should be advised to withhold breast-feeding for 12–24 hours. Advice may also be required concerning external radiation when the mother holds the child.

Before deciding to perform nuclear medicine tests in young women, it is important to consider the possibility of future lactation. Only essential investigations should be performed: the most appropriate radiopharmaceutical should be selected, and the dose reduced to the minimum compatible with obtaining a diagnostic result. According to the radiopharmaceutical in question, interruption of breastfeeding may be necessary. Breastfeeding is contra-indicated for ^{201}thallium chloride, ^{67}gallium citrate, ^{131}iodide, ^{75}selenomethionine, and ^{125}I fibrinogen (13).

Drug–Drug Interactions

Heparin

The use of heparinized catheters for in vivo erythrocyte labelling with ^{99m}Tc-pyrophosphate occasionally produces adverse reports, such as diminution of cardiac activity and increase of renal activity due to the formation of a technetium-heparin complex which localizes avidly in the kidneys. A few cases reported the possibility of reaction of radiopharmaceuticals with the components of a syringe or needle.

Drugs that interfere with the radiolabeling of blood cells

There is evidence that some drugs can adversely affect the radiolabeling of leukocytes. In a survey for the years 1981–97 of instances of unusually low labelling efficiencies of leukocytes labelled with ^{111}In-tropolone and ^{99m}Tc-HMPAO, respondents were asked to ascertain which drugs were being taken on the day of the test (14). Fifty adverse reports were received during that period. Many patients were taking drugs that are known to affect leukocyte function, including azathioprine, cephalosporins, cyclophosphamide, heparin, iron salts, nifedipine, prednisolone, and sulfasalazine. The author used Bradford–Hill's criteria (15) to assess whether the association between two variables was also one of causation, and thought that there was a high probability that these drugs had caused the low labeling efficiency.

References

1. Rhodes BA, Cordova MA. Adverse reactions to radiopharmaceuticals: incidence in 1978, and associated symptoms. Report of the Adverse Reactions Subcommittee of the Society of Nuclear Medicine. J Nucl Med 1980;21(11):1107–10.
2. Silberstein EB, Ryan J. Prevalence of adverse reactions in nuclear medicine. Pharmacopeia Committee of the Society of Nuclear Medicine. J Nucl Med 1996;37(1):185–92.
3. Silberstein EB. Prevalence of adverse reactions to positron emitting radiopharmaceuticals in nuclear medicine. Pharmacopeia Committee of the Society of Nuclear Medicine. J Nucl Med 1998;39(12):2190–2.
4. Keeling DH, Sampson CB. Adverse reactions to radiopharmaceuticals. United Kingdom 1977–1983. Br J Radiol 1984;57(684):1091–6.
5. Hesslewood SR, Keeling DH. Frequency of adverse reactions to radiopharmaceuticals in Europe. Eur J Nucl Med 1997;24(9):1179–82.
6. Sampson CB. Adverse reactions and drug interactions with radiopharmaceuticals. Drug Saf 1993;8(4):280–94.
7. Verbruggen A. Complications after intrathecal administration of 99mTc DTPA. In: Cox P, editor. Progress in Radiopharmacology, Part III. The Hague: Martinus Nijhoff, 1982:223–35.
8. Giaffer MH, Tindale WB, Senior S, Holdsworth CD. Anaphylactoid reaction associated with the use of 99cmT hexamethyl propylene amine oxime as a leukocyte labelling agent. Br J Radiol 1991;64(763):625–6.
9. James JM, Lloyd JJ, Leahy BC, Shields RA, Prescott MC, Testa HJ. The incidence and severity of hypoxia associated with 99Tmc Technegas ventilation scintigraphy and 99cmT MAA perfusion scintigraphy. Br J Radiol 1992;65(773):403–8.
10. Perper EJ, Segall GM. Safety of dipyridamole–thallium imaging in high risk patients with known or suspected coronary artery disease. J Nucl Med 1991;32(11):2107–14.
11. Coakley AJ, Mountford PJ. Nuclear medicine and the nursing mother. BMJ (Clin Res Ed) 1985;291(6489):159–60.
12. Rubow S, Klopper J, Wasserman H, Baard B, van Niekerk M. The excretion of radiopharmaceuticals in human breast milk: additional data and dosimetry. Eur J Nucl Med 1994;21(2):144–53.
13. Harding LK, Bossuyt A, Pellet C, Talbot JN. Recommendations for nuclear medicine physicians regarding breastfeeding mothers. Eur J Nucl Med 1995;22:BP17.
14. Sampson CB. Interference of patient medication in the radiolabelling of white blood cells: an update. Nucl Med Commun 1998;19(6):529–33.
15. Aronson JK. Biomarkers and surrogate endpoints. Br J Clin Pharmacol 2005;59(5):491–4.

Raloxifene

General Information

Raloxifene is a non-steroidal so-called "selective estrogen receptor modulator" (SERM), that is it binds to estrogen receptors, but this binding produces agonist effects at some sites and antagonist effects at others (1). It has estrogen agonist effects on bone and lipid metabolism but estrogen antagonist effects on the breast and endometrium; it is also claimed by its protagonists to have cardioprotective effects, perhaps through an effect on endothelial cells and a reduction in homocysteine concentrations (2).

Reports of adverse reactions to raloxifene should be considered alongside those reported for tamoxifen and other anti-estrogens. However, earlier reports have pointed to a considerable increase in thromboembolism, as has some recent large-scale work (3), and it would be premature to draw final conclusions about the conditions in which it can safely be used.

Raloxifene has been studied for its ability to reduce bone loss in postmenopausal women (4). Some specialized SERMs could reduce the risk of osteoporosis after the menopause without having other troublesome hormonal effects (5), but much more work is needed to determine whether they will fulfill this hope.

In a critical review of raloxifene, published in France, it was concluded that the compound has no advantages compared with a traditional estrogen, and that in view of certain findings in animal studies there is a possibility that it might increase the risk of ovarian cancer; there is also a need to determine whether it is sufficiently safe in women with a history of (or predisposition to) breast cancer (6).

One also finds a critical view expressed in the USA, where a survey of the literature up to the end of 1999 concluded that while raloxifene might carry a lesser risk of breast cancer than estrogen replacement therapy, it was also less effective in maintaining bone density, and that as regards cardiovascular risk the estrogenic treatment produced a more favorable outcome (7).

The use and adverse effects of raloxifene have been reviewed (8–10). Many centers continue to examine this and other SERMs, for example in countering menopausal bone loss (11), in the hope that they can take the place of tamoxifen and provide a means of avoiding the risks of such complications as endometrial cancer, cataract, and stroke (12–14).

Organs and Systems

Cardiovascular

In one published study there was a two- to three-fold rise in the incidence of thromboembolism, similar to that seen with estrogen treatment. There were also some cases of leg cramps and hot flushes (15).

There have been conflicting reports on the incidence and severity of symptoms such as hot flushes (also known as hot flashes) during long-term treatment with raloxifene for the prevention of osteoporosis. In fact the difference between raloxifene and placebo does not seem to be very great. In a review of three identical randomized trials in which raloxifene 60 mg was given for long periods to healthy postmenopausal women of various ages it was concluded that after 30 months the cumulative incidence of hot flushes was 21% for placebo and 28% for raloxifene, but the difference in frequency was confined to the first 6 months of therapy (16). There was no difference between placebo and raloxifene in the maximum severity of symptoms or the rate of early discontinuation, while the period during which hot flushes continued was only a little shorter in the raloxifene group. In a US study in more than 1100 postmenopausal women who took raloxifene 30–150 mg/day the only significant adverse effect of therapy was hot flushes (25% with 60 mg/day and 18% in the placebo group) (17).

Metabolism

LDL cholesterol and total cholesterol concentrations fell significantly in women taking raloxifene compared with placebo, but there was no change in HDL cholesterol or triglyceride concentrations, nor was endometrial thickness affected; the incidence of vaginal bleeding was not increased (18).

Reproductive system

Several sources have suggested that raloxifene can on occasion either cause uterine endometrial polyps or cause pre-existent polyps to enlarge considerably (19).

Drug–Drug Interactions

Warfarin

To assess the potential for an interaction between raloxifene and warfarin, 15 healthy postmenopausal women each received single doses of warfarin 20 mg before and during 2 weeks of dosing with raloxifene 120 mg/day (20). Raloxifene reduced the oral clearance of *R*- and *S*-warfarin respectively by 7.1 and 14% and the oral volume of distribution by 7.4 and 9.8%. Raloxifene reduced the maximum prothrombin time by 10% and the area under the prothrombin versus time curve from 0–120 hours by an average of 8%. The authors concluded that raloxifene may produce a small increase in systemic warfarin exposure but a reduced pharmacodynamic effect. Since the effects are slight this interaction is unlikely to have clinical consequences.

References

1. Young RL. An introduciosn to SERMs and their gynecologic effects. Am J Managed Care 1999;5(Suppl):S146–55.
2. Saitta A, Morabito N, Frisina N, Cucinotte D, Corrado F, D'Anna R, Altavilla D, Squadrito G, Minutoli L, Arcoraci V, Cancellieri F, Squadrito F. Cardiovascular effects of raloxifene hydrochloride. Cardiovasc Drug Rev 2001;19(1):57–74.
3. Cauley JA, Norton L, Lippman ME, Eckert S, Krueger KA, Purdie DW, Farrerons J, Karasik A, Mellstrom D, Ng KW, Stepan JJ, Powles TJ, Morrow M, Costa A, Silfen SL, Walls EL, Schmitt H, Muchmore DB, Jordan VC, Ste-Marie LG. Continued breast cancer risk reduction in postmenopausal women treated with raloxifene: 4-year results from the MORE trial. Multiple outcomes of raloxifene evaluation. Breast Cancer Res Treat 2001;65(2):125–34.
4. Vignot E, Meunier PJ. Effets du raloxifène sur la perte osseuse et le risque fracturaire chez la femme menopausée. [Effects of raloxifene on bone loss and fracture risk in the menopausal woman.] Contracept Fertil Sex 1999;27(12):858–60.
5. Albertazzi P, Purdie DW. Oestrogen and selective oestrogen receptor modulators (SERMs): current roles in the prevention and treatment of osteoporosis. Best Pract Res Clin Rheumatol 2001;15(3):451–68.
6. Anonymous. Raloxifene: new preparation. Not better than oestrogen. Prescrire Int 1999;8(44):165–7.
7. Umland EM, Rinaldi C, Parks SM, Boyce EG. The impact of estrogen replacement therapy and raloxifene on osteoporosis, cardiovascular disease, and gynecologic cancers. Ann Pharmacother 1999;33(12):1315–28.
8. Snyder KR, Sparano N, Malinowski JM. Raloxifene hydrochloride. Am J Health Syst Pharm 2000;57(18):1669–78.
9. Sismondi P, Biglia N, Roagna R, Ponzone R, Ambroggio S, Sgro L, Cozzarella M. How to manage the menopause following therapy for breast cancer is raloxifene a safe alternative? Eur J Cancer 2000;36(Suppl 4):S74–6.
10. Body JJ, Sternon J. Raloxifène (Celvista, Evista). Rev Med Brux 2000;21(1):35–41.
11. Brandi ML. Raloxifene reduces vertebral fracture risk in postmenopausal women with osteoporosis. Clin Exp Rheumatol 2000;18(3):309–10.
12. Rosenbaum Smith SM, Osborne MP. Breast cancer chemoprevention. Am J Surg 2000;180(4):249–51.
13. Dardes RC, Jordan VC. Future directions in endocrine therapy for the treatment and prevention of breast cancer. Sem Breast Dis 2000;3:119–30.
14. Goldstein SR, Siddhanti S, Ciaccia AV, Plouffe L Jr. A pharmacological review of selective oestrogen receptor modulators. Hum Reprod Update 2000;6(3):212–24.
15. Compston JE. Selective oestrogen receptor modulators: potential therapeutic applications. Clin Endocrinol (Oxf) 1998;48(4):389–91.
16. Cohen FJ, Lu Y. Characterization of hot flashes reported by healthy postmenopausal women receiving raloxifene or placebo during osteoporosis prevention trials. Maturitas 2000;34(1):65–73.
17. Johnston CC Jr, Bjarnason NH, Cohen FJ, Shah A, Lindsay R, Mitlak BH, Huster W, Draper MW, Harper KD, Heath H 3rd, Gennari C, Christiansen C, Arnaud CD, Delmas PD. Long-term effects of raloxifene on bone mineral density, bone turnover, and serum lipid levels in early postmenopausal women: three-year data from 2 double-blind, randomized, placebo-controlled trials. Arch Intern Med 2000;160(22):3444–50.
18. Delmas PD, Bjarnason NH, Mitlak BH, Ravoux AC, Shah AS, Huster WJ, Draper M, Christiansen C. Effects of raloxifene on bone mineral density, serum cholesterol concentrations, and uterine endometrium in postmenopausal women. N Engl J Med 1997;337(23):1641–7.
19. Maia H Jr, Maltez A, Oliveira M, Almeida M, Coutinho EM. Growth of an endometrial polyp in a postmenopausal patient using raloxifene. Gynaecol Endosc 2000;9:117–21.

20. Miller JW, Skerjanec A, Knadler MP, Ghosh A, Allerheiligen SR. Divergent effects of raloxifene HCl on the pharmacokinetics and pharmacodynamics of warfarin. Pharm Res 2001;18(7):1024–8.

Raltitrexed

See also Cytostatic and immunosuppressant drugs

General Information

Raltitrexed is a specific inhibitor of thymidylate synthase. It is used to treat colorectal cancers.

In about 1000 patients with advanced colorectal cancer, the dose-limiting toxic effects in phase 1 studies were gastrointestinal toxicity, myelosuppression, and weakness; adverse events during phase 2 and 3 studies were similar to those seen during phase 1 (1). In all comparative studies, mucositis and leukopenia were markedly less common and less severe in patients treated with raltitrexed than with bolus fluorouracil + leucovorin. Thrombocytopenia was more common with raltitrexed but it was not associated with an increase in clinically significant hemorrhage. In contrast, raltitrexed-related myelosuppression was more severe than with fluorouracil + leucovorin when the antimetabolite was given by continuous infusion. Raised transaminases were common with raltitrexed but were usually reversible with continued dosing and were not associated with clinical sequelae.

Organs and Systems

Hematologic

In 21 patients with advanced colorectal cancer, intravenous raltitrexed 3 mg/m^2 plus mitomycin 6 mg/m^2 was associated with WHO grade 3/4 anemia in 2, and neutropenia and thrombocytopenia in one each (2).

Liver

Raltitrexed-induced hepatotoxicity is usually characterized by a transient and self-limiting increase in transaminases. However, it can occasionally be fatal.

- A woman aged 76 years and a man aged 56 years were given raltitrexed as adjuvant treatment of colorectal carcinoma and as palliative therapy for advanced biliary carcinoma respectively (3). Both developed fulminant liver failure with rapid deterioration after the second and sixth cycles of chemotherapy respectively, and both died within 24 hours. Autopsy showed signs of acute necrosis involving roughly 50% of the liver without signs of subacute liver damage.

In 130 patients treated with raltitrexed 3 mg/m^2 ($n = 52$) or raltitrexed plus oxaliplatin ($n = 78$), of whom 78 had liver metastases and 25 had raised transaminases, hepatotoxicity caused delays of a week or more in 60 of 584 chemotherapy cycles and was the reason for withdrawal of chemotherapy in eight patients (4). Raised baseline transaminases, the number of chemotherapy cycles, the cumulative dose of raltitrexed, short intervals between courses, and the addition of oxaliplatin predicted hepatotoxicity, while sex, age, creatinine clearance, previous chemotherapy, and the presence of liver metastases did not. Whether glutathione and ademethionine are hepatoprotective is unclear.

Skin

Two patients, aged 75 and 65 years, were given raltitrexed for colorectal cancers. After 5 and 7 days they developed erythematous, edematous, and purpuric skin reactions associated with weakness, diarrhea, and moderate fever (5). The lesions were painful and pseudocellulitic. They were generalized in the first case and localized to the legs in the second. They subsided 15 days after drug withdrawal.

Immunologic

Of 52 patients with colorectal cancer treated with a median of six 3-weekly cycles of raltitrexed 1.5–3.0 mg/m^2 combined with oral carmofur 300–400 mg/m^2 on cycle days 2–14, 39 had a fever on days 2–9 after receiving raltitrexed, 49 had fatigue, and 49 had a raised serum C-reactive protein concentration without a documented infection (6). Median concentrations of C-reactive protein, interleukin-6, interleukin-8, and tumor necrosis factor-alfa were higher 7 days after raltitrexed or raltitrexed + carmofur than at baseline. The authors suggested that patients with colorectal cancer treated with raltitrexed may develop drug-related systemic inflammation, which may be difficult to distinguish from infection.

Susceptibility Factors

Age

Of 90 patients treated with raltitrexed 3 mg/m^2 every 3 weeks, of whom 50 were aged over 70 years, 437 cycles of chemotherapy were administered and grade 3–4 toxicity was reported in under 10% (7). There were no significant differences between younger and older patients, apart from grade 3–4 weakness, which was reported by three of the older patients and none of the younger. This was despite a significantly lower calculated mean creatinine clearance in the older patients.

Renal disease

The pharmacokinetics of raltitrexed, and hence its toxic effects, particularly on the bone marrow and gut, are directly related to creatinine clearance (8). It is recommended that the dose be reduced and dosage interval increased in patients with mild to moderate renal impairment, based on the fact that raltitrexed is mainly excreted unchanged in the urine.

References

1. Zalcberg J. Overview of the tolerability of "Tomudex" (raltitrexed): collective clinical experience in advanced colorectal cancer. Anticancer Drugs 1997;8(Suppl 2):S17–22.

2. Rosati G, Rossi A, Germano D, Reggiardo G, Manzione L. Raltitrexed and mitomycin-C as third-line chemotherapy for colorectal cancer after combination regimens including 5-fluorouracil, irinotecan and oxaliplatin: a phase II study. Anticancer Res 2003;23(3C):2981–5.
3. Raderer M, Fiebiger W, Wrba F, Scheithauer W. Fatal liver failure after the administration of raltitrexed for cancer chemotherapy: a report of two cases. Cancer 2000;89(4):890–2.
4. Massacesi C, Santini D, Rocchi MB, La Cesa A, Marcucci F, Vincenzi B, Delprete S, Tonini G, Bonsignori M. Raltitrexed-induced hepatotoxicity: multivariate analysis of predictive factors. Anticancer Drugs 2003;14(7):533–41.
5. Topard D, Hellier I, Ychou M, Guillot B. Toxidermie au raltitrexed: 2 cas. [Raltitrexed-induced skin reaction.] Ann Dermatol Venereol 2000;127(12):1080–2.
6. Osterlund P, Orpana A, Elomaa I, Repo H, Joensuu H. Raltitrexed treatment promotes systemic inflammatory reaction in patients with colorectal carcinoma. Br J Cancer 2002;87(6):591–9.
7. Romiti A, Tonini G, Santini D, Di Seri M, Masciangelo R, Mezi S, Veri A, Santuari L, Vincenzi B, Brescia A, Marchei P, Frati L, Tomao S. Tolerability of raltitrexed ("Tomudex") in elderly patients with colorectal cancer. Anticancer Res 2002;22(5):3071–6.
8. Judson I, Maughan T, Beale P, Primrose J, Hoskin P, Hanwell J, Berry C, Walker M, Sutcliffe F. Effects of impaired renal function on the pharmacokinetics of raltitrexed (Tomudex ZD1694). Br J Cancer 1998;78(9):1188–93.

Ramipril

See also Angiotensin converting enzyme inhibitors

General Information

Ramipril is an ACE inhibitor, a prodrug that is rapidly hydrolysed after absorption to its active metabolite ramiprilat. It has been used in patients with hypertension, heart failure, and myocardial infraction.

Organs and Systems

Metabolism

Hypoglycemia has been attributed to several drugs in a complicated sequence of effects (1).

- A 64-year-old man with type II diabetes, hypertension, and bilateral renal artery stenosis presented with confusion and dysarthria related to profound hypoglycemia (2.2 mmol/l). He was taking naproxen 500 mg bd, ramipril 2.5 mg/day, glibenclamide 2.5 mg bd, metformin 850 mg bd, a thiazide diuretic, terazosin, ranitidine, paracetamol, and codeine. His plasma creatinine concentration, previously 185 µmol/l, was 362 µmol/l and it fell to 210 µmol/l after the withdrawal of ramipril and naproxen.

The authors discussed the possible role of renal insufficiency, resulting from co-prescription of naproxen and ramipril in the presence of volume depletion, which may have increased the risk of hypoglycemia related to glibenclamide plus metformin.

Gastrointestinal

Two cases of severe vomiting, dyspepsia, and headache, with falls in body weight and plasma albumin, have been reported in patients on chronic peritoneal dialysis (2). Both occurred a few days after they started to take ramipril (dose not reported) and totally resolved after withdrawal. Both patients subsequently took losartan, which was well tolerated. This led the authors to suggest that the mechanism was mediated by bradykinin and/or prostaglandins, through an interaction with gastrointestinal motility, which may also be affected by peritoneal dialysis.

Diarrhea is a recognized infrequent adverse effect of ACE inhibitors. A convincing case of diarrhea associated with ramipril has been reported (3).

References

1. Collin M, Mucklow JC. Drug interactions, renal impairment and hypoglycaemia in a patient with Type II diabetes. Br J Clin Pharmacol 1999;48(2):134–7.
2. Riley S, Rutherford PA. Gastrointestinal side effects of ramipril in peritoneal dialysis patients. Perit Dial Int 1998;18(1):83–4.
3. Tosetti C. Angiotensin-converting enzyme inhibitors and diarrhea. J Clin Gastroenterol 2002;35(1):105–6.

Ranitidine

See also Histamine H$_2$-receptor antagonists

General Information

Ranitidine is a histamine H$_2$ receptor antagonist. Compared with cimetidine, it inhibits hepatic metabolism of other substances only to a very slight extent and is not anti-androgenic. In most other respects it is similar to cimetidine.

Comparative studies

Effervescent ranitidine 150 mg bd has been compared with as-needed calcium carbonate antacids 750 mg in a randomized study in 115 subjects who frequently self-treated heartburn (1). Effervescent ranitidine was significantly more effective than antacids in reducing heartburn, healing erosive esophagitis, alleviating pain, and improving quality of life. The overall incidences of adverse events were not significantly different in the two groups; 12% in the antacid group and 3% in the ranitidine group had adverse events related to the gastrointestinal system: nausea, vomiting, diarrhea, constipation, gas, fecal incontinence; and 1% in the antacid group and 4% in the ranitidine group had adverse events related to the central nervous system: headache, dizziness, insomnia, malaise, fatigue, weakness, nervousness.

Placebo-controlled studies

The efficacy of low-dose ranitidine for the relief of heartburn has been studied in a double-blind, placebo-controlled trial (2). Subjects with heartburn were randomized to ranitidine 75 mg ($n = 491$), ranitidine 25 mg ($n = 504$), or placebo ($n = 494$), to be taken as needed up to four times a day for 2 weeks. Ranitidine 75 mg was significantly more effective than placebo and provided prompt relief of heartburn lasting up to 12 hours. The most common adverse effects were nausea, diarrhea, and headache, which occurred in under 2% of patients in each group.

In a randomized, placebo-controlled, four-way, crossover study of the effects of low-dose ranitidine and an antacid on meal-induced heartburn and acidity in 26 subjects, ranitidine 75 mg significantly reduced gastric but not esophageal acidity, calcium carbonate 420 mg significantly reduced esophageal but not gastric acidity, and ranitidine plus calcium carbonate reduced both esophageal and gastric acidity (3). Both drugs given alone reduced heartburn severity compared with placebo.

Organs and Systems

Cardiovascular

Atrioventricular block has been attributed to ranitidine (4).

- A 20-year-old man taking ranitidine 300 mg/day had a brief episode of syncope. The only abnormal finding was first-degree atrioventricular block, which disappeared after withdrawal of ranitidine. Rechallenges on two separate occasions produced recurrence of asymptomatic first-degree atrioventricular block, but cimetidine 400–800 mg/day and famotidine 40–80 mg/day caused no electrocardiographic abnormalities.

The authors hypothesized that this patient may have been abnormally susceptible to the cholinergic or cholinergic-like effect of ranitidine, unrelated to its histamine H_2 blocking action. However, the ability of ranitidine to release histamine may also have contributed.

Bradycardia occurred in a 4-day-old full-term male neonate 2 hours after the intravenous injection of ranitidine and resolved over 24 hours (5).

Respiratory

H_2 receptor antagonists can increase the risk of respiratory infections, and the possible significance of this effect has been studied best with ranitidine; there seems to be no reason for concern in most patients, but the risk can be considerable in some older patients with pre-existing health problems rendering them unduly susceptible to infection (SEDA-18, 372).

Nervous system

Chorea has been reported occasionally with ranitidine (6). Headache and lethargy have been described in a neonate (SEDA-18, 372).

Psychological, psychiatric

Depression has been estimated to occur in 1–5% of patients taking ranitidine (SEDA-17, 418) (7).

Occasional confusion and behavioral disturbances have been attributed to ranitidine (8–10).

Hematologic

Pancytopenia and agranulocytosis have been documented with ranitidine (11).

Liver

There seem to be individuals with a metabolic idiosyncrasy who develop serious but probably fully reversible liver damage when exposed to ranitidine. The Netherlands Centre for Monitoring of Adverse Reactions has published data on six cases, in most of which other causal factors could be excluded (12), and a fatal case of liver injury has been reported from France (SEDA-16, 422).

Cholestatic liver damage due to ranitidine has been reported (13).

- A 29-year-old man developed cholestasis (confirmed histologically) having taken ranitidine 150 mg bd for about 2 weeks. The drug was withdrawn and he was treated with glucocorticoids and ursodeoxycholic acid. Three months later he had recovered completely. Rechallenge was not attempted.
- Cholestatic jaundice has been reported in a 73-year-old woman who had taken ranitidine 150 mg bd (14). She developed pruritus 4 days after starting to take the drug and jaundice after 3 weeks. Her liver function tests returned to normal 50 days after ranitidine was withdrawn.

Hepatitis associated with ranitidine is rare.

- Drug hypersensitivity hepatitis with progression to fulminant hepatic failure and death has been reported in a previously healthy 66-year-old woman who had taken ranitidine for 14 days before the onset of jaundice and for 5 days after hepatitis was diagnosed (15).
- A 45-year-old woman with multiple sclerosis developed severe liver injury after taking ranitidine 300 mg/day (16).

Pancreas

In one case where pancreatitis occurred without identifiable cause other than ranitidine, it was confirmed by rechallenge on two occasions (SEDA-16, 422).

Urinary tract

As with cimetidine, acute interstitial nephritis has been documented in a few cases (17).

- Acute interstitial nephritis in a cadaveric renal allograft occurred in a 44-year-old man who had taken ranitidine 150 mg bd for 2 days (18). Allograft function improved rapidly and returned to normal after ranitidine was withdrawn.

Skin

- Stevens–Johnson syndrome has been reported in two patients, a 62-year-old woman and a 58-year-old man, with severe liver disease and jaundice, who had taken ranitidine 150 mg bd; both recovered on withdrawal (19).

Persistent UVB photosensitivity due to ranitidine (300 mg/day) has been reported (20).

Sexual function

Several cases of impotence have been described in patients taking ranitidine, strongly suggesting that this is an effect that all H_2 receptor antagonists can have on occasion (21).

Long-Term Effects

Tumorigenicity

- A gastric carcinoid tumor was found in a man of 62 taking ranitidine (22). The dosage had been unusually high and there was pre-existing chronic renal insufficiency as well as diabetes, but the tumor was similar in type to that seen in animals; it was successfully removed by partial gastrectomy and did not recur.

Susceptibility Factors

Age

The pharmacokinetics and pharmacodynamics of a single dose of ranitidine 75 mg have been evaluated in a randomized, double-blind, placebo-controlled trial in 29 children aged 4–11 years with gastro-esophageal reflux disease (23). Ranitidine significantly increased the intragastric pH in children, and the pharmacokinetics and pharmacodynamics were similar to those in adults. The drug was effective in the control of intragastric acidity for 5–6 hours. Adverse effects were reported only in children taking ranitidine, and included nausea, vomiting, abdominal pain, dizziness, intermittent headache, and lightheadedness.

Renal disease

In renal impairment, the risk of adverse reactions with intravenous ranitidine is doubled (SEDA-18, 371).

Drug Administration

Drug dosage regimens

Different doses of ranitidine (150 mg bd and 300 mg bd for 8 weeks) have been compared in resolving heartburn in 271 patients with gastro-esophageal reflux disease who had been symptomatic after 6 weeks of therapy with ranitidine 150 mg bd (24). Less than 20% of the patients in either group had complete resolution of heartburn at 4 and 8 weeks; there was no significant difference in the efficacy between the two treatment groups. At least one adverse event was reported by 38% of the patients in each group. They included sinusitis, nausea, abdominal pain, dyspepsia, constipation, and increased liver enzymes.

References

1. Earnest D, Robinson M, Rodriguez-Stanley S, Ciociola AA, Jaffe P, Silver MT, Kleoudis CS, Murdock RH. Managing heartburn at the "base" of the GERD "iceberg": effervescent ranitidine 150 mg b.d. provides faster and better heartburn relief than antacids. Aliment Pharmacol Ther 2000;14(7):911–18.
2. Pappa KA, Gooch WM, Buaron K, Payne JE, Giefer EE, Sirgo MA, Ciociola AA. Low-dose ranitidine for the relief of heartburn. Aliment Pharmacol Ther 1999;13(4):459–65.
3. Robinson M, Rodriguez-Stanley S, Ciociola AA, Filinto J, Zubaidi S, Miner PB Jr, Gardner JD. Synergy between low-dose ranitidine and antacid in decreasing gastric and oesophageal acidity and relieving meal-induced heartburn. Aliment Pharmacol Ther 2001;15(9):1365–74.
4. Allegri G, Pellegrini K, Dobrilla G. First-degree atrioventricular block in a young duodenal ulcer patient treated with a standard oral dose of ranitidine. Agents Actions 1988;24(3-4):237–42.
5. Nahum E, Reish O, Naor N, Merlob P. Ranitidine-induced bradycardia in a neonate—a first report. Eur J Pediatr 1993;152(11):933–4.
6. Lehmann AB. Reversible chorea due to ranitidine and cimetidine. Lancet 1988;2(8603):158.
7. Stocky A. Ranitidine and depression. Aust NZ J Psychiatry 1991;25(3):415–18.
8. Delerue O, Muller JP, Destee A, Warot P. Mania-like episodes associated with ranitidine. Am J Psychiatry 1988;145(2):271.
9. Tamarin F, Brandstetter RD, Price W. Mental confusion and ranitidine. Crit Care Med 1988;16(8):819.
10. Sonnenblick M, Yinnon A. Mental confusion as a side effect of ranitidine. Am J Psychiatry 1986;143(2):257.
11. Bader A, Carrigan T, Gopalswamy N, Trulzsch DV. Reversible hematologic suppression during ranitidine treatment. DICP 1989;23(6):508–9.
12. van Bommel EF, Meyboom RH. Leverbeschadiging door ranitidine. [Liver damage caused by ranitidine.] Ned Tijdschr Geneeskd 1992;136(9):435–7.
13. Ramrakhiani S, Brunt EM, Bacon BR. Possible cholestatic injury from ranitidine with a review of the literature. Am J Gastroenterol 1998;93(5):822–6.
14. Liberopoulos EN, Nonni AB, Tsianos EV, Elisaf MS. Possible ranitidine-induced cholestatic jaundice. Ann Pharmacother 2002;36(1):172.
15. Ribeiro JM, Lucas M, Baptista A, Victorino RM. Fatal hepatitis associated with ranitidine. Am J Gastroenterol 2000;95(2):559–60.
16. Luparini RL, Rotundo A, Mattace R, Marigliano V. Verosimile epatite autoimmune da ranitidina. [Possibly ranitidine-induced autoimmune hepatitis.] Ann Ital Med Int 2000;15(3):214–17.
17. Gaughan WJ, Sheth VR, Francos GC, Michael HJ, Burke JF. Ranitidine-induced acute interstitial nephritis with epithelial cell foot process fusion. Am J Kidney Dis 1993;22(2):337–40.
18. Emovon OE, King JA, Holt CO, Browne BJ. Ranitidine-induced acute interstitial nephritis in a cadaveric renal allograft. Am J Kidney Dis 2001;38(1):169–72.
19. Lin CC, Wu JC, Huang DF, Huang YS, Huang YH, Huo TI, Chang FY, Lee SD. Ranitidine-related Stevens–Johnson syndrome in patients with severe liver diseases: a report of two cases. J Gastroenterol Hepatol 2001;16(4):481–3.
20. Kondo S, Kagaya M, Yamada Y, Matsusaka H, Jimbow K. UVB photosensitivity due to ranitidine. Dermatology 2000;201(1):71–3.
21. Bera F, Jonville-Bera AP, Doustin F, Autret E. Impuissance et gynécomastie secondaires a une hyperprolactinémie induite par la ranitidine. [Impotence and gynecomastia secondary to hyperprolactinemia induced by ranitidine.] Therapie 1994;49(4):361–2.
22. Rao SS, Nayak KS, Swarnalata G, Goyal DN, Rao KP, Mitros FA. Gastric carcinoid associated with ranitidine in

a patient with renal failure. Am J Gastroenterol 1993;88(8):1273–4.

23. Orenstein SR, Blumer JL, Faessel HM, McGuire JA, Fung K, Li BU, Lavine JE, Grunow JE, Treem WR, Ciociola AA. Ranitidine, 75 mg, over-the-counter dose: pharmacokinetic and pharmacodynamic effects in children with symptoms of gastro-oesophageal reflux. Aliment Pharmacol Ther 2002;16(5):899–907.

24. Kahrilas PJ, Fennerty MB, Joelsson B. High- versus standard-dose ranitidine for control of heartburn in poorly responsive acid reflux disease: a prospective, controlled trial. Am J Gastroenterol 1999;94(1):92–7.

Ranunculaceae

See also Herbal medicines

General Information

The genera in the family of Ranunculaceae (Table 1) include anemone, buttercup, columbine, hellebore, larkspur, marsh marigold, and pasque flower.

Aconitum species

Species of aconite contain a variety of diterpene alkaloids; *Aconitum napellus* (monkshood) contains isonapelline, luciculine, and napelline.

Adverse effects

Aconite roots can produce serious heart failure. Among the other symptoms of aconite poisoning are numbing of mouth and tongue, gastrointestinal disturbances,

Table 1 The genera of Ranunculaceae

Aconitum (monkshood)
Actaea (baneberry)
Adonis (pheasant's eye)
Anemone (anemone)
Aquilegia (columbine)
Caltha (marsh marigold)
Ceratocephala (curveseed butterwort)
Cimicifuga (bugbane)
Clematis (leather flower)
Consolida (knight's-spur)
Coptis (gold thread)
Delphinium (larkspur)
Enemion (false rue anemone)
Eranthis (eranthis)
Helleborus (hellebore)
Hepatica (hepatica)
Hydrastis (hydrastis)
Kumlienia (false buttercup)
Myosurus (mousetail)
Nigella (nigella)
Pulsatilla (pasque flower)
Ranunculus (buttercup)
Thalictrum (meadow rue)
Trautvetteria (bugbane)
Trollius (globe flower)
Xanthorhiza (yellow root)

muscular weakness, incoordination, and vertigo (1). A review from Hong Kong reported 17 cases of aconite poisoning after the administration of Chinese herbal mixtures. The toxicity of raw aconite can be reduced substantially by decoction, as this process leads to a change in alkaloid composition (2).

Cimicifuga racemosa

Cimicifuga racemosa (black bugbane, black cohosh, black snakeroot, rattleroot, rattletop, rattleweed) contains a variety of cycloartane triterpene glycosides, some of which have cytotoxic effects (3).

Cimicifuga racemosa has been used to relieve symptoms of menopause, although with little evidence of efficacy (4).

Adverse effects

Liver damage has been attributed to black cohosh, which contains diterpenoids that cause liver damage in animals, either via reactive metabolites or by an autoimmune mechanism. However, causality was not demonstrated beyond reasonable doubt.

- A 47-year-old woman took an extract of *C. racemosa* for 1 week to treat menopausal symptoms; she developed jaundice and raised liver enzymes (5). No other causes of liver damage were found. She required liver transplantation.

Delphinium species

Delphinium species contain complex diterpenoid alkaloids that cause acute intoxication and death in cattle (6). The alkaloids and their concentrations vary with the species and plant part involved, which causes variability in toxicity. In *Delphinium consolida* (larkspur) there are toxic alkaloids in the non-medicinal plant parts (root, seed, herb), but they are purportedly absent in the medicinal part (the flower).

Hydrastis canadensis

The root of *Hydrastis canadensis* (golden seal) contains isoquinoline alkaloids, including the quaternary base berberine and the tertiary base hydrastine. As the latter can stimulate uterine contractions, it is prudent to avoid golden seal root during pregnancy, even though the actual risk of premature labor still has to be verified.

Adverse effects

In man berberine has positive inotropic, negative chronotropic, antidysrhythmic, and vasodilator properties (7).

Cardiovascular

There is experimental evidence that berberine can cause arterial hypotension (8,9).

Nervous system

Berberine displaces bilirubin from albumin and there is therefore a risk of kernicterus in jaundiced neonates (10).

Gastrointestinal

In a study of the effect of berberine in acute watery diarrhea, oral doses of 400 mg were well tolerated, except for complaints about its bitter taste and a few instances of transient nausea and abdominal discomfort. However, patients with cholera given tetracycline plus berberine were more ill, suffered longer from diarrhea, and required larger volumes of intravenous fluid than those given tetracycline alone (11).

Skin

- A 32-year-old woman had a phototoxic reaction after taking a dietary supplement containing ginseng, golden seal, bee pollen, and other ingredients (12). She had a pruritic, erythematous rash, localized to the sun-exposed surfaces of her neck and limbs. She had no significant past medical history and was not taking any other medications. The skin rash slowly resolved after withdrawal of the supplement and treatment with subcutaneous and topical glucocorticoids.

Although the individual ingredients in this dietary supplement have not been associated with cases of photosensitivity, it is possible that the combination of ingredients may have interacted to cause this effect.

Drug interactions

Golden seal root inhibits various isoforms of cytochrome P450, including CYP3A4 (13). However, in a crossover study, goldenseal root (1140 mg bd for 14 days) had no effect on the pharmacokinetics of a single oral dose of indinavir 800 mg (14).

Pulsatilla species

Pulsatilla (pasque flower) species are widely used in homeopathic medicine. Some of them contain podophyllotoxins. High doses of *Pulsatilla vulgaris* (meadow windflower) can irritate the kidneys and urinary tract. Pregnancy is a contraindication.

Ranunculus damascenus

Ranunculus damascenus (buttercup) is used topically for abscess drainage, hemorrhoids, and burns.

Adverse effects

Ranunculus damascenus has been reported to cause skin damage (15).

- A 45-year-old Turkish woman developed open wounds on the abdomen, right knee, and neck. She had used buttercup topically and orally for pain relief. She was treated with antibiotics and adequate wound care. Complete healing was achieved within 10 days.

The authors argued that protoanemonin, a constituent of *R. damascenus*, which inhibits mitosis in plants, had caused this severe reaction.

References

1. Kelly SP. Aconite poisoning. Med J Aust 1990;153(8):499.
2. Hikino H, Yamada C, Nakamura K, Sato H, Ohizumi Y. [Change of alkaloid composition and acute toxicity of *Aconitum* roots during processing.] Yakugaku Zasshi 1977;97(4):359–66.
3. Watanabe K, Mimaki Y, Sakagami H, Sashida Y. Cycloartane glycosides from the rhizomes of *Cimicifuga racemosa* and their cytotoxic activities. Chem Pharm Bull (Tokyo) 2002;50(1):121–5.
4. Borrelli F, Ernst E. *Cimicifuga racemosa*: a systematic review of its clinical efficacy. Eur J Clin Pharmacol 2002;58(4):235–41.
5. Whiting PW, Clouston A, Kerlin P. Black cohosh and other herbal remedies associated with acute hepatitis. Med J Aust 2002;177(8):440–3.
6. Puschner B, Booth MC, Tor ER, Odermatt A. Diterpenoid alkaloid toxicosis in cattle in the Swiss Alps. Vet Hum Toxicol 2002;44(1):8–10.
7. Lau CW, Yao XQ, Chen ZY, Ko WH, Huang Y. Cardiovascular actions of berberine. Cardiovasc Drug Rev 2001;19(3):234–44.
8. Sabir M, Bhide NK. Study of some pharmacological actions of berberine. Indian J Physiol Pharmacol 1971;15(3):111–32.
9. Chun YT, Yip TT, Lau KL, Kong YC, Sankawa U. A biochemical study on the hypotensive effect of berberine in rats. Gen Pharmacol 1979;10(3):177–82.
10. Chan E. Displacement of bilirubin from albumin by berberine. Biol Neonate 1993;63(4):201–8.
11. Khin-Maung-U, Myo-Khin, Nyunt-Nyunt-Wai, Aye-Kyaw, Tin-U. Clinical trial of berberine in acute watery diarrhoea. BMJ (Clin Res Ed) 1985;291(6509):1601–5.
12. Palanisamy A, Haller C, Olson KR. Photosensitivity reaction in a woman using an herbal supplement containing ginseng, goldenseal, and bee pollen. J Toxicol Clin Toxicol 2003;41(6):865–7.
13. Foster BC, Vandenhoek S, Hana J, Krantis A, Akhtar MH, Bryan M, Budzinski JW, Ramputh A, Arnason JT. In vitro inhibition of human cytochrome P450-mediated metabolism of marker substrates by natural products. Phytomedicine 2003;10(4):334–42.
14. Sandhu RS, Prescilla RP, Simonelli TM, Edwards DJ. Influence of goldenseal root on the pharmacokinetics of indinavir. J Clin Pharmacol 2003;43(11):1283–8.
15. Metin A, Calka O, Behcet L, Yildirim E. Phytodermatitis from *Ranunculus damascenus* Contact Dermatitis 2001; 44(3):183.

Rapacuronium

See also Neuromuscular blocking drugs

General Information

Rapacuronium, an aminosteroid non-depolarizing neuromuscular blocking agent with a rapid onset and a comparatively short duration of action (1,2), was withdrawn from the US market in March 2001 and subsequently worldwide. The manufacturers informed the FDA in an open letter about postmarketing reports of severe bronchospasm and some deaths of unknown origin associated with rapacuronium. The severity of the incidents recently reported to the manufacturers was impressive enough to cause fears about patient safety. This event highlights the need for continued surveillance, not only during clinical trials but also during the routine use of approved drugs.

Organs and Systems

Cardiovascular

A major adverse effect of rapacuronium is an increase in heart rate (3). Plasma histamine concentrations may increase after rapacuronium injection, but this was not correlated with changes in blood pressure or heart rate (4).

Respiratory

In a study of the effects of rapacuronium on respiratory function, performed while rapacuronium was still on the market in the USA, the authors observed statistically significant reductions in peak inspiratory flow rate, peak expiratory flow rate, and dynamic compliance, and increases in peak inflating pressure when rapacuronium 1.5 mg/kg was given under steady-state conditions to patients who were already anesthetized, intubated, and ventilated (5). In five of the 10 patients these changes amounted to more than 25% from baseline and were considered clinically relevant. As rapacuronium is no longer available this has no direct clinical impact. However, while discussing the mechanisms of rapacuronium-induced bronchospasm the authors speculated that differential effects of the drug on several subtypes of muscarinic acetylcholine receptors might be responsible. As raised histamine concentrations were not found in seven patients with rapacuronium-induced bronchospasm in another study (4), they reckoned that histamine release was an unlikely explanation. Referring to the observation that pipecuronium, another non-steroidal muscle relaxant, blocked pilocarpine-stimulated prejunctional M_2 receptors in vitro (6), they suggested that a similar effect might result in rapacuronium-induced bronchospasm. Prejunctional M_2 receptors are thought to have a role in negative feedback and inhibition of further acetylcholine release, thereby reducing smooth muscle relaxation. These aspects will need to be taken into account when new substances are considered for clinical use.

Second-Generation Effects

Pregnancy

Some controversy has been raised by the use of rapacuronium for rapid sequence induction in elective cesarean section (7). The authors reported that intubating conditions 60 seconds after rapacuronium 2.5 mg/kg were comparable with those after suxamethonium 1.5 mg. The percentage of the drug that crossed the placenta to the fetus was low (umbilical/maternal vein concentration ratio 0.088) compared with other non-depolarizing agents, and there were no adverse effects on the fetus. Others, however, would not use rapacuronium or other non-depolarizing agents for cesarean section, referring to the longer duration of action, which might be a problem in cases of failed intubation (8). Rapid sequence induction with thiopental plus suxamethonium is still standard for cesarean section. Rapacuronium should be considered for cesarean section only in patients in whom suxamethonium is contraindicated. In such cases, induction with propofol plus alfentanil without a neuromuscular blocking agent may be an alternative, which still awaits evaluation with regard to maternal and fetal safety.

Susceptibility Factors

Renal disease

Rapacuronium plasma clearance was reduced in patients with renal insufficiency, but this did not result in an increased duration of action (9).

Hepatic disease

Although not completely understood, hepatic uptake is assumed to be the reason for the short duration of action of rapacuronium. However, neither recovery time nor drug half-life after a single bolus of rapacuronium was prolonged in patients with liver cirrhosis compared with healthy controls (10).

References

1. Fleming NW, Chung F, Glass PS, Kitts JB, Kirkegaard-Nielsen H, Gronert GA, Chan V, Gan TJ, Cicutti N, Caldwell JE. Comparison of the intubation conditions provided by rapacuronium (ORG 9487) or succinylcholine in humans during anesthesia with fentanyl and propofol. Anesthesiology 1999;91(5):1311–17.
2. Sparr HJ, Mellinghoff H, Blobner M, Noldge-Schomburg G. Comparison of intubating conditions after rapacuronium (Org 9487) and succinylcholine following rapid sequence induction in adult patients. Br J Anaesth 1999;82(4):537–41.
3. Osmer C, Wulf K, Vogele C, Zickmann B, Hempelmann G. Cardiovascular effects of Org 9487 under isoflurane anaesthesia in man. Eur J Anaesthesiol 1998;15(5):585–9.
4. Levy JH, Pitts M, Thanopoulos A, Szlam F, Bastian R, Kim J. The effects of rapacuronium on histamine release and hemodynamics in adult patients undergoing general anesthesia. Anesth Analg 1999;89(2):290–5.
5. Tobias JD, Johnson JO, Sprague K, Johnson G. Effects of rapacuronium on respiratory function during general anesthesia: a comparison with cis-atracurium. Anesthesiology 2001;95(4):908–12.
6. Zappi L, Song P, Nicosia S, Nicosia F, Rehder K. Do pipecuronium and rocuronium affect human bronchial smooth muscle? Anesthesiology 1999;91(6):1616–21.
7. Abouleish EI, Abboud TK, Bikhazi G, Kenaan CA, Mroz L, Zhu J, Lee J, Abboud TS. Rapacuronium for modified rapid sequence induction in elective caesarean section: neuromuscular blocking effects and safety compared with succinylcholine, and placental transfer. Br J Anaesth 1999;83(6):862–7.
8. Young SJ, Kilpatrick A. Alternatives to succinylcholine at caesarean section. Br J Anaesth 2000;84(5):695–6.
9. Szenohradszky J, Caldwell JE, Wright PM, Brown R, Lau M, Luks AM, Fisher DM. Influence of renal failure on the pharmacokinetics and neuromuscular effects of a single dose of rapacuronium bromide. Anesthesiology 1999;90(1):24–35.
10. Duvaldestin P, Slavov V, Rebufat Y. Pharmacokinetics and pharmacodynamics of rapacuronium in patients with cirrhosis. Anesthesiology 1999;91(5):1305–10.

Ravuconazole

See also Antifungal azoles

General Information

Ravuconazole is similar in structure to fluconazole. It has a long half-life suitable for once-daily dosing.

The safety and efficacy of ravuconazole have been studied in a randomized, double-blind comparison with fluconazole in 71 patients with esophageal candidiasis; ravuconazole was as effective as fluconazole and there were no apparent differences in adverse effects (1,2).

References

1. Groll AH, Gea-Banacloche JC, Glasmacher A, Just-Nuebling G, Maschmeyer G, Walsh TJ. Clinical pharmacology of antifungal compounds. Infect Dis Clin North Am 2003;17(1):159–91.
2. Hoffman HL, Ernst EJ, Klepser ME. Novel triazole antifungal agents. Expert Opin Investig Drugs 2000;9(3):593–605.

Reboxetine

See also Antidepressants, second-generation

General Information

Reboxetine is a selective noradrenaline re-uptake inhibitor with low affinity for α-adrenoceptors and muscarinic receptors. In controlled trials the following adverse events occurred significantly more often with reboxetine than with placebo: dry mouth (27%), constipation (17%), increased sweating (14%), insomnia (14%), urinary hesitancy (5%), impotence (5%), tachycardia (5%), and vertigo (2%) (SEDA-21, 13).

Organs and Systems

Electrolyte balance

Hyponatremia has been reported with reboxetine (1,2).

- A 72-year-old man with diabetes mellitus and cardiovascular disease developed major depression. He was taking aspirin (100 mg/day), enalapril (20 mg/day), and glibenclamide (5 mg/day). His serum sodium was 133 mmol/l (reference range 134–146 mmol/l). He started to take reboxetine (4 mg/day) and after 8 days experienced malaise and nausea, at which time his serum sodium had fallen to 118 mmol/l. The reboxetine was withdrawn, and both his symptoms and the low serum sodium remitted over the next 6 days. Rechallenge with reboxetine produced a recurrence of both the low sodium and the accompanying symptoms.

It appears that, like SSRIs, reboxetine can cause sodium depletion in elderly people. However, in this case the contributions of concomitant general medical illness and its treatment were uncertain.

Urinary tract

One of the adverse effects of reboxetine is difficulty in passing urine (SEDA-21, 13). Eight patients taking reboxetine (4–8 mg/day) had troublesome urinary hesitancy (3). They were successfully treated with tamsulosin (0.4 mg/day), and in two patients tamsulosin was withdrawn after 2 weeks without recurrence of the urinary symptoms. Reboxetine is a selective noradrenaline re-uptake inhibitor and may therefore produce urinary symptoms by activating α_1-adrenoceptors in the bladder, which tamsulosin would be expected to reverse. However, tamsulosin is also effective for urinary symptoms caused by other mechanisms, for example benign prostatic hyperplasia. Whether its apparent effectiveness in reboxetine-induced dysuria represents specific pharmacological antagonism is therefore uncertain.

Drug–Drug Interactions

Fluoxetine

In the pharmacological management of patients with treatment-resistant depression, it is a common strategy to combine a drug that selectively inhibits noradrenaline re-uptake (for example reboxetine) with one that selectively inhibits the re-uptake of serotonin (for example an SSRI). As well as the hoped-for pharmacodynamic interaction, a kinetic interaction can also occur, because of the effect of SSRIs on CYP450 enzymes. The effect of combined treatment with reboxetine (8 mg/day) and fluoxetine (20 mg/day) has been compared with each treatment given alone for 8 days in 30 healthy volunteers in a parallel design (4). There was no potentiation of adverse effects by the combination. Fluoxetine increased the plasma AUC of reboxetine by 20%, but this was not statistically significant. The authors suggested that the combination of fluoxetine and reboxetine should have minimal adverse impact in depressed patients. However, the major metabolite of fluoxetine, norfluoxetine, is also an inhibitor of CYP3A4 and would not have reached steady-state concentrations during the time of the study. This suggests that caution might still be needed during longer-term use of this combination in depressed patients.

Ketoconazole

Reboxetine is metabolized by CYP3A4. In 11 healthy volunteers ketoconazole, an inhibitor of CYP3A4, increased the plasma AUC of reboxetine by about 50% and prolonged the half-life (5). The adverse effects profile of reboxetine was not altered by ketoconazole, but the finding suggests that reboxetine should be used with caution in combination with drugs that inhibit CYP3A4, for example nefazodone and fluvoxamine.

References

1. Ranieri P, Franzoni S, Trabucchi M. Reboxetine and hyponatremia. N Engl J Med 2000;342(3):215–16.

2. Schwartz GE, Veith J. Reboxetine and hyponatremia. N Engl J Med 2000;342:216.
3. Kasper S, Wolf R. Successful treatment of reboxetine-induced urinary hesitancy with tamsulosin. Eur Neuropsychopharmacol 2002;12(2):119–22.
4. Fleishaker JC, Herman BD, Pearson LK, Ionita A, Mucci M. Evaluation of the potential pharmacokinetic/pharmacodynamic interaction between fluoxetine and reboxetine in healthy volunteers. Clin Drug Invest 1999;18:141–50.
5. Herman BD, Fleishaker JC, Brown MT. Ketoconazole inhibits the clearance of the enantiomers of the antidepressant reboxetine in humans. Clin Pharmacol Ther 1999;66(4):374–9.

Remacemide

See also Antiepileptic drugs

General Information

Remacemide hydrochloride is a low-affinity, non-competitive *N*-methyl-D-aspartate (NMDA) channel blocker that has been used in epilepsy, Parkinson's disease, Huntington's chorea, and neuroprotection after stroke. Its pharmacology, clinical pharmacology, uses, and adverse effects and interactions have been reviewed (1,2).

The adverse effects of remacemide have been studied in 40 patients with refractory epilepsy randomized to placebo or ascending weekly doses of remacemide in a twice or four times a day regimen for up to 1 month (3). There were adverse events in 38 patients; the most common were dizziness, abdominal pain, headache, diplopia, fatigue, dyspepsia, and abnormal vision.

Observational studies

The efficacy of adjunctive therapy with remacemide has been evaluated in 11 children (4). Remacemide was well tolerated in doses up to 13.5 mg/kg/day. The most common adverse events were dizziness, ataxia, and gastrointestinal events. One patient died after a suspected seizure, which was unlikely to have been related to remacemide.

Placebo-controlled studies

The efficacy, safety, and pharmacokinetics of adjunctive remacemide have been investigated in a randomized, double-blind, placebo-controlled, crossover study in 28 adult patients with refractory epilepsy (5). The mean plasma carbamazepine concentration increased by about 15%. Three patients withdrew owing to adverse events (two remacemide, one placebo). Adverse events that occurred more often with remacemide than placebo included dyspepsia, dizziness, abnormal gait, diplopia, abnormal vision, somnolence, chest pain, and fatigue.

In a randomized, double-blind, placebo-controlled study of remacemide in 200 patients with early Parkinson's disease who were not yet taking levodopa or dopamine agonists, remacemide did not produce improvement in signs or symptoms (6). Significantly fewer patients taking remacemide 600 mg/day were able

to tolerate 5 weeks of their assigned treatment on a twice-daily schedule compared with patients taking placebo (64 versus 94%). However, most patients who had intolerable adverse effects with the twice-daily schedule could tolerate the same daily dosage given in four parts during the day. The most common adverse events were dizziness and nausea. There were no serious adverse events or clinically significant treatment-related changes in vital signs, laboratory values, or electrocardiograms.

In a double-blind, randomized study of remacemide in 262 patients with partial seizures there was a trend for efficacy, but not significantly different from placebo (7). The most frequent adverse events were headache, fatigue, dizziness, diplopia, and somnolence. There were no significant changes in vital signs, electrocardiograms, or biochemistry. In another double-blind, placebo-controlled study in patients with refractory epilepsy undergoing in-patient video-electroencephalographic monitoring, the pattern of adverse events was similar (8).

Drug–Drug Interactions

Levodopa

Remacemide delays the absorption of levodopa and increases the concentrations of drugs that are metabolized by CYP3A4 (2).

References

1. Willmore LJ. Clinical pharmacology of new antiepileptic drugs. Neurology 2000;55(11 Suppl. 3):S17–24.
2. Schachter SC, Tarsy D. Remacemide: current status and clinical applications. Expert Opin Investig Drugs 2000;9(4):871–83.
3. Chadwick D, Smith D, Crawford P, Harrison B. Remacemide hydrochloride: a placebo-controlled, one month, double-blind assessment of its safety, tolerability and pharmacokinetics as adjunctive therapy in patients with epilepsy. Seizure 2000;9(8):544–50.
4. Besag FM, Newton RE, Blakey GE, Dean AD. Safety, tolerability, and pharmacokinetics of remacemide in children. Pediatr Neurol 2001;24(5):352–6.
5. Richens A, Mawer G, Crawford P, Harrison B. A placebo-controlled, double-blind cross-over trial of adjunctive one month remacemide hydrochloride treatment in patients with refractory epilepsy. Seizure 2000;9(8):537–43.
6. Shoulson I, Greenamyre T, Kieburtz K, Schwid S, McDermott M, Kayson E, Chase T, Fahn S, Lang A, Penney J. A multicenter randomized controlled trial of remacemide hydrochloride as monotherapy for PD. Parkinson Study Group. Neurology 2000;54(8):1583–8.
7. Chadwick DW, Betts TA, Boddie HG, Crawford PM, Lindstrom P, Newman PK, Soryal I, Wroe S, Holdich TA, Clegg LS. Remacemide hydrochloride as an add-on therapy in epilepsy: a randomized, placebo-controlled trial of three dose levels (300, 600 and 1200 mg/day) in a Q.I.D. regimen. Seizure 2002;11(2):114–23.
8. Devinsky O, Vazquez B, Faught E, Leppik IE, Pellock JM, Schachter S, Alderfer V, Holdich TA. A double-blind, placebo-controlled study of remacemide hydrochloride in patients with refractory epilepsy following pre-surgical assessment. Seizure 2002;11(6):371–6.

Remifentanil

General Information

Remifentanil is a pure OP₃ (µ) opioid receptor agonist with a very short duration of action. It therefore has to be given by continuous intravenous infusion and is used as a supplement to general anesthesia during induction and as an analgesic during maintenance of anesthesia. It has the familiar adverse effects of opioids: respiratory depression, sedation, nausea and vomiting, muscle rigidity, bradycardia, and pruritus. These are short-lived and are antagonized by naloxone. The onset of muscle rigidity and apnea can be alarmingly rapid. Bradycardia occurred more often with remifentanil than alfentanil in patients undergoing abdominal surgery and in children undergoing strabismus surgery; the oculocardiac response was more marked with remifentanil than alfentanil (1).

Drug studies

Pain relief

Three studies have focused on the analgesic use of remifentanil (2–4). In a double-blind, crossover, randomized study 20 healthy volunteers received an infusion of either remifentanil or saline (2). Thermal sensory testing of the heat pain threshold was performed every 5 minutes and the dose of remifentanil was increased by 0.01 micrograms/kg/minute every 5 minutes. Remifentanil produced a dose-dependent increase in the heat pain threshold, and a dose of 0.05 micrograms/kg/minute was suggested as an effective and safe increment in healthy volunteers. The rate of adverse effects (nausea, vomiting, and pruritus) was comparable with previous reports; there were no cardiovascular adverse effects.

General surgery

Mixtures of remifentanil and sevoflurane have been used in two prospective, open, randomized studies (5,6), which showed that adding remifentanil results in a reduced requirement for sevoflurane for maintenance of anesthesia, leading to faster and easier recovery.

In a double-blind, randomized study a continuous infusion of remifentanil (1 microgram/kg followed by 0.5 micrograms/kg/minute) was compared with alfentanil (25 micrograms/kg followed by 1 microgram/kg/minute) during anesthesia in patients undergoing major abdominal surgery (7). Both systolic pressure and heart rate were significantly lower with remifentanil, with a higher incidence of hypotension (53 versus 39%) and bradycardia (10 versus 3%).

Bronchoscopy

In a randomized study, remifentanil 0.5 micrograms/kg/minute was compared with fentanyl 2 micrograms/kg in 22 patients undergoing rigid bronchoscopy (8). The results suggested that remifentanil attenuated the hemodynamic response to bronchoscopy without significantly increasing the incidences of hypotension or bradycardia. Four patients given remifentanil developed ST segment depression compared with eight patients given fentanyl.

Colonoscopy

Remifentanil by infusion (n = 49) has been compared with titrated boluses of pethidine (n = 51) in a randomized, double-blind study in 100 patients undergoing outpatient colonoscopy (9). The incidences of tachycardia, hypotension, and nausea were significantly less with remifentanil than with pethidine, but there were higher anxiety and pain scores with remifentanil. However, the study was a comparison of two opioids with different pharmacokinetic profiles, which makes it very difficult to achieve equipotent doses for the purpose of comparison.

Lithotripsy

In two randomized, double-blind, controlled comparisons of anesthetic techniques for extracorporeal shock wave lithotripsy remifentanil infusion had no advantage over the combination of fentanyl bolus plus propofol infusion, but caused more adverse effects (nausea and vomiting) (10). In another study remifentanil infusion provided comparable analgesia and caused less respiratory depression and fewer gastrointestinal symptoms than intravenous boluses of sufentanil (11).

Cardiac surgery

In a prospective multicenter, double-blind, randomized study in 297 patients undergoing elective coronary artery bypass surgery, remifentanil infusion 1 microgram/kg/minute was compared with a loading dose of fentanyl 15 micrograms/kg (12). The most common adverse effects were nausea and vomiting, which occurred equally often in the two groups. Hypertension and shivering were significantly more common with remifentanil (12).

Obstetrics and gynecology

The role of remifentanil-based anesthesia in gynecological and obstetric procedures has been reviewed (13).

In a double-blind, randomized comparison of remifentanil (0.25/0.5 micrograms/kg/minute) and alfentanil (50 micrograms and 0.5 micrograms/kg/minute) in 35 patients undergoing total abdominal hysterectomy, remifentanil provided more stable analgesia during anesthesia but caused significantly more hypotension (14).

Orthopedic surgery

Intravenous remifentanil 0.3 micrograms/kg with propofol 2 micrograms/ml has been compared with propofol 2 micrograms/ml alone in a double-blind, randomized study in 86 day-case adults undergoing elective orthopedic surgery (15). The study was designed to assess whether remifentanil improves conditions for laryngeal mask airway insertion. Those given remifentanil had a better quality of airway patency, with minimal cardiorespiratory changes.

Orthopedic and urological surgery

The respiratory depressant and gastrointestinal adverse effects of remifentanil have been observed in a randomized, single-blind study of 125 patients undergoing elective orthopedic and urological surgery under spinal or brachial plexus anesthesia (16). They were randomized to either remifentanil (a bolus of 0.5 micrograms/kg plus an infusion of 0.1 micrograms/kg/minute) or propofol (a bolus of 500 micrograms/kg plus an infusion of 50 micrograms/kg/minute). Owing to a significantly higher rate of respiratory depression with remifentanil (46%) than with propofol (19%), the mean remifentanil infusion rate was reduced to 0.078 ± 0.028 micrograms/kg/minute. The incidence of intraoperative nausea and vomiting with remifentanil was 27% compared with 2% with propofol. Postoperatively there was no significant difference in the incidence of gastrointestinal symptoms. Remifentanil may be considered as an alternative if propofol is contraindicated (for example because of amnesic episodes).

Vascular surgery

In a double-blind, randomized, placebo-controlled study in 28 adults undergoing carotid endarterectomy, remifentanil provided adequate analgesia, and supplementary local anesthetics were not needed (17). The remifentanil infusion rate was as low as 0.04 micrograms/kg/minute and there were no episodes of respiratory depression or hemodynamic instability.

In 60 patients receiving cervical plexus block during carotid endarterectomy who were given either remifentanil 3 micrograms/kg/hour or propofol 1 mg/kg/hour there was a higher incidence of adverse respiratory effects with remifentanil and a similar sedative effect (18). The authors suggested that when using remifentanil for sedation in patients undergoing carotid endarterectomy, the initial dose of remifentanil should be reduced to 1.5–2 micrograms/kg/hour to minimize cardiovascular and respiratory adverse effects.

Ophthalmological surgery

The analgesic effects of remifentanil and alfentanil have been compared during ophthalmological nerve block in a randomized, double-blind, parallel-group study in 79 patients (19). Remifentanil (as a single dose of 1 microgram/kg or as a loading dose of 1 microgram/kg followed by an infusion of 0.2 micrograms/kg/minute) was more effective than alfentanil (as a single dose of 7 micrograms/kg). Of the patients given remifentanil, three had mild nausea and three had transient muscle rigidity that resolved spontaneously within 1 minute. There were no adverse effects of alfentanil. The authors suggested that remifentanil 1 microgram/kg given over 30 seconds is a useful alternative to alfentanil 7 micrograms/kg as an analgesic before ophthalmological nerve block.

Anesthesia in ischemic heart disease

In a prospective randomized comparison of combined sevoflurane plus remifentanil with combined fentanyl plus etomidate for induction of anesthesia in 10 patients with ischemic heart disease, 3 of the 20 patients given sevoflurane plus remifentanil developed severe bradycardia (heart rate less than 40) and one developed asystole, but the difference between the two groups did not reach statistical significance (20). Therefore, in patients with ischemic heart disease remifentanil should be used with caution, and concurrent administration of glycopyrrolate 0.2 mg is advisable to reduce the incidence of bradycardia, hypotension, or both, without increasing the heart rate.

Organs and Systems

Cardiovascular

Three groups of 20 women due to undergo elective surgery were recruited into a randomized, double-blind study (21). Group 1 received a bolus dose of remifentanil 1 microgram/kg and an infusion of remifentanil (0.5 micrograms/kg/minute); groups 2 and 3 received remifentanil 0.5 micrograms/kg and an infusion of 0.25 micrograms/kg/minute. Groups 1 and 2 received pretreatment with glycopyrrolate 200 micrograms whilst group 3 did not. Cardiovascular responses to laryngoscopy and orotracheal intubation were measured. There were no significant differences in the three groups, except that there was a significantly lower heart rate in group 3 after induction of anesthesia and after intubation.

The hemodynamic effects of bolus intravenous remifentanil 0.2, 0.33, and 1 microgram/kg/minute have been studied in patients scheduled for coronary artery bypass grafting (22). The study was terminated after only eight patients had been recruited, because of severe hypotension, bradycardia, and/or evidence of myocardial ischemia. The authors concluded that remifentanil should not be given as a bolus dose of 1 microgram/kg but as an infusion at a low rate. An editorial response to this article suggested that the hemodynamic instability reported may have resulted from other contributing factors, such as hypovolemia, impairment of venous return, or excessive anesthesia due to remifentanil toxicity (23).

In a prospective study in 12 men undergoing elective coronary artery bypass grafting, remifentanil 0.5 and 2.0 micrograms/kg/minute combined with propofol preserved hemodynamic stability and reduced myocardial blood flow and metabolism to a similar extent (24).

Asystole has been attributed to remifentanil (25).

- A 78-year-old man with laryngeal cancer developed asystole 1 minute after an intravenous bolus of remifentanil 0.5 micrograms/kg followed by a continuous infusion of 0.5 micrograms/kg/hour. The asystole was unresponsive to intravenous atropine 1 mg. The remifentanil infusion was stopped and cardiac sinus rhythm resumed after two precordial thumps.

The authors postulated that rapid-sequence induction of anesthesia with sevoflurane had blunted sympathetic tone and allowed uncompensated parasympathetic activation by remifentanil.

Remifentanil-induced bradycardia and asystole may be useful as a protective effect in patients with atrial fibrillation (26).

- A 90-year-old woman with atrial fibrillation was given digoxin for 3 days before surgery for a pelvic mass. Following anesthesia, induced with thiopental and atracurium, her heart rate rose to 105/minute and her electrocardiogram showed fast atrial fibrillation and ST segment depression. She was given remifentanil 0.25 micrograms/kg/minute and her heart rate fell to 95/minute.

Nervous system

Seizures have been attributed to remifentanil (27).

- A 42-year-old woman asked for an intravenous opioid as analgesia during paracervical block and was given an intravenous infusion of remifentanil 1.0 microgram/kg/minute. After 3 minutes she became unresponsive, with upward deviation of gaze and tonic-clonic contractions of the arms. The infusion was discontinued and after another 3 minutes of generalized seizure activity she was given intravenous propofol 80 mg and intravenous suxamethonium 60 mg; she recovered completely 15 minutes later.

Psychological, psychiatric

In 201 patients scheduled for day-case surgery, those who received remifentanil had significantly fewer responses to surgical stimulation and had better psychomotor and psychometric function during the recovery period, although there was no significant difference in time to recovery room or hospital discharge (28).

Second-Generation Effects

Pregnancy

Six patients admitted at 36 weeks pregnancy with pre-eclampsia received patient-controlled intravenous analgesia with remifentanil for labor (3). Remifentanil was delivered as continuous background infusion of 0.05 micrograms/kg/minute and boluses of 25 micrograms with a 5-minute lockout period. The procedure did not cause adverse maternal or neonatal adverse effects and this small uncontrolled study suggests that patient-controlled intravenous analgesia with remifentanil might be an effective alternative when epidural analgesia is contraindicated.

In a dose-finding study in 17 healthy pregnant women in the first stage of labor, the PCA bolus of remifentanil was increased from 0.2 micrograms/kg in 0.2 micrograms/kg increments during 60 minutes until analgesia was considered adequate (29). The median effective dose of remifentanil was 0.4 (range 0.2–0.8) micrograms/kg and consumption was 0.066 (range 0.027–0.207) micrograms/kg/minute. All the women reported slight sedation; five had slight to moderate nausea throughout the study. Supplementary oxygen 2 l/minute via nasal cannula was given to three women who had repeated episodes of oxygen desaturation. Two women reported difficulties in reading and visual focusing and one woman had difficulty in swallowing toward the end of remifentanil administration. In five cases there were changes in fetal heart rate indices within 30 minutes of the first dose. The neonates had Apgar scores of 8–10. The authors concluded that remifentanil is a potentially effective obstetric analgesic but that adverse effects will limit its use.

A similar observation was made in an open pilot study in 36 women randomized during the early stages of labor to either intramuscular pethidine 100 mg or remifentanil given as patient-controlled analgesia (20-microgram bolus over 20 seconds) (30). Remifentanil provided better pain relief but a higher risk of lower oxygen saturation compared with pethidine. Remifentanil was given only a cautious welcome by the authors, owing to its respiratory depressant effects.

Susceptibility Factors

Age

In maintenance of anesthesia in 62 children vomiting occurred in 31% (31). However, the dose of remifentanil was twice the ED_{50} in adults and may have been much larger than required.

The effects of remifentanil on vomiting and the quality of emergence from anesthesia have been studied in children undergoing dental restoration and extraction (32). The children received desflurane with or without remifentanil 0.2 micrograms/kg/minute. The two groups did not differ in adverse effects profile or quality of recovery.

Seven randomized controlled trials and one descriptive trial using infused remifentanil as part of an anesthetic technique in children between 1997 and 2000 have been reviewed (33). The general consensus is that a bolus dose of remifentanil 0.5–1 microgram/kg appears to be well tolerated when it is given over at least 60 seconds. However, a loading dose is not required if the infusion can be started at least 10 minutes before the skin incision is made. Infusion rates of 0.25–0.5 micrograms/kg/minute provide hemodynamic stability when propofol or a volatile agent is also given. The authors advised that infants who receive remifentanil should be paralysed and mechanically ventilated, because of the possible risk of respiratory depression due to chest wall rigidity in non-paralysed patients.

Remifentanil is liable to cause respiratory depression in children (33,34), as well as muscle rigidity, hypotension, and bradycardia, without increasing the incidence of gastrointestinal symptoms (35).

The adverse effects profiles of remifentanil in neonates and infants undergoing pyloromyotomy have been investigated (36,37).

The hemodynamic responses, recovery profiles, and perioperative and postoperative respiratory patterns in 38 children given remifentanil plus nitrous oxide and 22 given halothane plus nitrous oxide have been studied in a multicenter, open, randomized comparison (36). There were no cases of bradycardia or dysrhythmias. There were hypertensive responses at the time of incision in 24% of those given remifentanil and 18% of those given halothane and vomiting in 34 and 45% respectively. None of those who were given remifentanil developed new-onset postoperative apnea compared with three of those who were given halothane. All other adverse effects had similar incidences in the two groups.

Remifentanil 0.1 micrograms/kg/minute by infusion was safe and efficacious in 55 patients (aged 2 months to 12 years) undergoing cardiac catheterization (38).

Drug Administration

Drug dosage regimens

In a double-blind, randomized study of 178 patients scheduled for major thoracic, intra-abdominal, and orthopedic surgery, a high dose of remifentanil (bolus dose of 1 microgram/kg followed by 1 microgram/kg/minute) was compared with a low dose (bolus dose 1 microgram/kg followed by 0.5 micrograms/kg/minute) (39). In this study, intraoperative hypotension (30% and 27% respectively) and bradycardia (9% and 7% respectively) were equally frequent in the two groups. The authors proposed that infusion rates of remifentanil over 0.4 micrograms/kg/minute provide satisfactory analgesia throughout surgery but can cause significant hypotension. Prolonged infusion of remifentanil for several hours of surgery does not delay recovery or cause respiratory depression.

The postoperative analgesic efficacy and safety of two continuous constant-dose intravenous remifentanil infusions have been investigated in a double-blind, randomized study in 30 patients scheduled to undergo elective abdominal or thoracic surgery (4). The patients were randomly assigned to intravenous remifentanil 0.05 micrograms/kg/minute or 0.1 micrograms/kg/minute. There were no cases of respiratory depression, and nausea and vomiting occurred in one patient in each group. There was adequate analgesia in 75% and 78% of the patients in the low-dose and high-dose groups respectively and pethidine rescue analgesia was required in 26% and 6% respectively. Remifentanil 0.1 micrograms/kg/minute was therefore effective and safe for postoperative pain.

Drug overdose

A nurse was found dead at home with a syringe and empty vials of remifentanil (2 mg) and midazolam (1 mg/ml); toxicological studies showed that she had not been a chronic user of remifentanil (40).

Drug–Drug Interactions

Propofol

In eight subjects the concentration of remifentanil was significantly increased when therapeutic concentrations of propofol were present in the body (41). The combination of propofol and remifentanil can cause cardiovascular depression. As with other opioids, remifentanil competes with propofol for hydrophobic binding in the lungs and heart.

References

1. Duthie DJ. Remifentanil and tramadol. Br J Anaesth 1998;81(1):51–7.
2. Gustorff B, Felleiter P, Nahlik G, Brannath W, Hoerauf KH, Spacek A, Kress HG. The effect of remifentanil on the heat pain threshold in volunteers. Anesth Analg 2001;92(2):369–74.
3. Roelants F, De Franceschi E, Veyckemans F, Lavand'homme P. Patient-controlled intravenous analgesia using remifentanil in the parturient. Can J Anaesth 2001;48(2):175–8.
4. Calderon E, Pernia A, De Antonio P, Calderon-Pla E, Torres LM. A comparison of two constant-dose continuous infusions of remifentanil for severe postoperative pain. Anesth Analg 2001;92(3):715–19.
5. Breslin DS, Reid JE, Mirakhur RK, Hayes AH, McBrien ME. Sevoflurane–nitrous oxide anaesthesia supplemented with remifentanil: effect on recovery and cognitive function. Anaesthesia 2001;56(2):114–19.
6. Joo HS, Perks WJ, Belo SE. Sevoflurane with remifentanil allows rapid tracheal intubation without neuromuscular blocking agents. Can J Anaesth 2001;48(7):646–50.
7. Camu F, Royston D. Inpatient experience with remifentanil. Anesth Analg 1999;89(Suppl 4):S15–21.
8. Prakash N, McLeod T, Gao Smith F. The effects of remifentanil on haemodynamic stability during rigid bronchoscopy. Anaesthesia 2001;56(6):576–80.
9. Greilich PE, Virella CD, Rich JM, Kurada M, Roberts K, Warren JF, Harford WV. Remifentanil versus meperidine for monitored anesthesia care: a comparison study in older patients undergoing ambulatory colonoscopy. Anesth Analg 2001;92(1):80–4.
10. Burmeister MA, Brauer P, Wintruff M, Graefen M, Blanc I, Standl TG. A comparison of anaesthetic techniques for shock wave lithotripsy: the use of a remifentanil infusion alone compared to intermittent fentanyl boluses combined with a low dose propofol infusion. Anaesthesia 2002;57(9):877–81.
11. Beloeil H, Corsia G, Coriat P, Riou B. Remifentanil compared with sufentanil during extra-corporeal shock wave lithotripsy with spontaneous ventilation: a double-blind, randomized study. Br J Anaesth 2002;89(4):567–70.
12. Mollhoff T, Herregods L, Moerman A, Blake D, MacAdams C, Demeyere R, Kirno K, Dybvik T, Shaikh S; Remifentanil Study Group. Comparative efficacy and safety of remifentanil and fentanyl in 'fast track' coronary artery bypass graft surgery: a randomized, double-blind study. Br J Anaesth 2001;87(5):718–26.
13. Buerkle H, Wilhelm W. Remifentanil for gynaecological and obstetric procedures. Curr Opin Anaesthesiol 2000;13:271–5.
14. Kovac AL, Azad SS, Steer P, Witkowski T, Batenhorst R, McNeal S. Remifentanil versus alfentanil in a balanced anesthetic technique for total abdominal hysterectomy. J Clin Anesth 1997;9(7):532–41.
15. Grewal K, Samsoon G. Facilitation of laryngeal mask airway insertion: effects of remifentanil administered before induction with target-controlled propofol infusion. Anaesthesia 2001;56(9):897–901.
16. Servin FS, Raeder JC, Merle JC, Wattwil M, Hanson AL, Lauwers MH, Aitkenhead A, Marty J, Reite K, Martisson S, Wostyn L. Remifentanil sedation compared with propofol during regional anaesthesia. Acta Anaesthesiol Scand 2002;46(3):309–15.
17. Marrocco-Trischitta MM, Bandiera G, Camilli S, Stillo F, Cirielli C, Guerrini P. Remifentanil conscious sedation during regional anaesthesia for carotid endarterectomy: rationale and safety. Eur J Vasc Endovasc Surg 2001;22(5):405–9.
18. Krenn H, Deusch E, Jellinek H, Oczenski W, Fitzgerald RD. Remifentanil or propofol for sedation during carotid endarterectomy under cervical plexus block. Br J Anaesth 2002;89(4):637–40.
19. Ahmad S, Leavell ME, Fragen RJ, Jenkins W, Roland CL. Remifentanil versus alfentanil as analgesic adjuncts during placement of ophthalmologic nerve blocks. Reg Anesth Pain Med 1999;24(4):331–6.
20. Wang JY, Winship SM, Thomas SD, Gin T, Russell GN. Induction of anaesthesia in patients with coronary artery disease: a comparison between sevoflurane-remifentanil and fentanyl–etomidate Anaesth Intensive Care 1999;27(4):363–8.
21. Hall AP, Thompson JP, Leslie NA, Fox AJ, Kumar N, Rowbotham DJ. Comparison of different doses of remifentanil on the cardiovascular response to laryngoscopy and tracheal intubation. Br J Anaesth 2000;84(1):100–2.
22. Elliott P, O'Hare R, Bill KM, Phillips AS, Gibson FM, Mirakhur RK. Severe cardiovascular depression with remifentanil. Anesth Analg 2000;91(1):58–61.
23. Michelsen LG. Hemodynamic effects of remifentanil in patients undergoing cardiac surgery. Anesth Analg 2000;91(6):1563.
24. Kazmaier S, Hanekop GG, Buhre W, Weyland A, Busch T, Radke OC, Zoelffel R, Sonntag H. Myocardial consequences of remifentanil in patients with coronary artery disease. Br J Anaesth 2000;84(5):578–83.

25. Kurdi O, Deleuze A, Marret E, Bonnet F. Asystole during anaesthetic induction with remifentanil and sevoflurane. Br J Anaesth 2001;87(6):943.

26. Williams H, Spoelstra C. Use of remifentanil in fast atrial fibrillation. Br J Anaesth 2002;88(4):614.

27. Haber GW, Litman RS. Generalized tonic-clonic activity after remifentanil administration. Anesth Analg 2001;93(6):1532–3.

28. Cartwright DP, Kvalsvik O, Cassuto J, Jansen JP, Wall C, Remy B, Knape JT, Noronha D, Upadhyaya BK. A randomized, blind comparison of remifentanil and alfentanil during anesthesia for outpatient surgery. Anesth Analg 1997;85(5):1014–19.

29. Volmanen P, Akural EI, Raudaskoski T, Alahuhta S. Remifentanil in obstetric analgesia: a dose-finding study. Anesth Analg 2002;94(4):913–17.

30. Thurlow JA, Laxton CH, Dick A, Waterhouse P, Sherman L, Goodman NW. Remifentanil by patient-controlled analgesia compared with intramuscular meperidine for pain relief in labour. Br J Anaesth 2002;88(3):374–8.

31. Davis PJ, Lerman J, Suresh S, McGowan FX, Cote CJ, Landsman I, Henson LG. A randomized multicenter study of remifentanil compared with alfentanil, isoflurane, or propofol in anesthetized pediatric patients undergoing elective strabismus surgery. Anesth Analg 1997;84(5):982–9.

32. Pinsker MC, Carroll NV. Quality of emergence from anesthesia and incidence of vomiting with remifentanil in a pediatric population. Anesth Analg 1999;89(1):71–4.

33. Booker PD, Whyte SD. Paediatric applications of concentration-oriented anaesthesia. Best Pract Res Clin Anaesthesiol 2001;15:97–111.

34. Keidan I, Berkenstadt H, Sidi A, Perel A. Propofol/remifentanil versus propofol alone for bone marrow aspiration in paediatric haemato-oncological patients. Paediatr Anaesth 2001;11(3):297–301.

35. Thees Ch, Frenkel Ch, Hoeft A. Remifentanil in der Neuroanästhesie—eine multizentrische Anwendungsbeobachtung. [Remifentanil in neuroanesthesia – a multicenter study.] Anästhesiol Intensivmed 2001;42:205–11.

36. Davis PJ, Galinkin J, McGowan FX, Lynn AM, Yaster M, Rabb MF, Krane EJ, Kurth CD, Blum RH, Maxwell L, Orr R, Szmuk P, Hechtman D, Edwards S, Henson LG. A randomized multicenter study of remifentanil compared with halothane in neonates and infants undergoing pyloromyotomy. I. Emergence and recovery profiles. Anesth Analg 2001;93(6):1380–6.

37. Galinkin JL, Davis PJ, McGowan FX, Lynn AM, Rabb MF, Yaster M, Henson LG, Blum R, Hechtman D, Maxwell L, Szmuk P, Orr R, Krane EJ, Edwards S, Kurth CD. A randomized multicenter study of remifentanil compared with halothane in neonates and infants undergoing pyloromyotomy. II. Perioperative breathing patterns in neonates and infants with pyloric stenosis. Anesth Analg 2001;93(6):1387–92.

38. Donmez A, Kizilkan A, Berksun H, Varan B, Tokel K. One center's experience with remifentanil infusions for pediatric cardiac catheterization. J Cardiothorac Vasc Anesth 2001;15(6):736–9.

39. Hogue CW Jr, Bowdle TA, O'Leary C, Duncalf D, Miguel R, Pitts M, Streisand J, Kirvassilis G, Jamerson B, McNeal S, Batenhorst R. A multicenter evaluation of total intravenous anesthesia with remifentanil and propofol for elective inpatient surgery. Anesth Analg 1996;83(2):279–85.

40. Asselborn G, Yegles M, Wennig R. Suicide with remifentanil and midazolam: a case report. Acta Clin Belg Suppl 2002;(1):54–7.

41. Crankshaw DP, Chan C, Leslie K, Bjorksten AR. Remifentanil concentration during target-controlled infusion of propofol. Anaesth Intensive Care 2002;30(5):578–83.

Repirinast

General Information

Repirinast is an antiallergic prodrug whose active metabolite has a stabilizing action on mast cells that resembles that of sodium cromoglicate (1).

When repirinast was given to 56 asthmatic patients for 6 months, it was effective in 47% and moderately effective in 81%. Two patients complained of sleepiness, but repirinast was continued with or without dosage reduction (SEDA-17, 205).

Organs and Systems

Skin

Solar urticaria has been attributed to repirinast in a 72-year-old woman who had taken it for 20 months (2). She developed urticaria immediately after irradiation with 1.5 J/cm² of UVA, and a provocation test confirmed that repirinast was responsible for the urticarial reaction, with a spectrum of 320–350 nm.

References

1. Takei M, Endo K, Takahashi K. Mechanism of action of MY-1250, an active metabolite of repirinast, in inhibiting histamine release from rat mast cells. Br J Pharmacol 1992;105(3):587–90.

2. Kurumaji Y, Shomo M. Drug-induced solar urticaria due to repirinast. Dermatology 1994;188(2):117–21.

Reserpine

General Information

The Rauwolfia alkaloids, including reserpine, are now little used. They act by depleting neurotransmitter stores of catecholamines and reducing sympathetic nervous activity, but their effects are non-specific, and nervous system adverse effects (depression, drowsiness, tiredness, confusion) are prominent. There is also a troublesome incidence of diarrhea, hyperprolactinemia, gynecomastia, and a possible withdrawal syndrome.

Organs and Systems

Psychological, psychiatric

Depression is a very common adverse effect of reserpine (SED-9, 328) (1).

- A 66-year-old woman was admitted to hospital suffering from an agitated depressive psychosis. This settled with standard antipsychotic therapy. It was subsequently found that she had been taking reserpine in an over-the-counter formulation and had stopped this a week before her admission (2). Her doctor felt that the syndrome had occurred as a result of nervous system hypersensitivity after reserpine withdrawal.

Endocrine

In women reserpine causes a small increase in circulating concentrations of prolactin (3), which could be related to the small increase in the risk of breast cancer. In 27 hypertensive men reserpine 0.25 mg/day for 3 months had no effect on testosterone, dihydrotestosterone, estradiol, luteinizing hormone, or prolactin (4).

Long-Term Effects

Drug withdrawal

Acute psychosis has been reported after the withdrawal of reserpine (2,5). During long-term therapy in animals reserpine causes denervation sensitivity to dopamine in the basal ganglia and chemotactic trigger zone in man and to catecholaminergic agents in the basal ganglia and mesolimbic system; withdrawal could lead to rebound supersensitivity of these systems to endogenous catecholamines, causing the reported symptoms.

Tumorigenicity

Early retrospective studies suggested that reserpine was associated with breast cancer, but prospective studies and meta-analyses of case-control studies have shown only a weak association (6). In vitro studies have shown that rauwolfia alkaloids are not genotoxic or mutagenic (7).

References

1. Riddiough MA. Preventing, detecting and managing adverse reactions of antihypertensive agents in the ambulant patient with essential hypertension. Am J Hosp Pharm 1977;34(5):465–79.
2. Samuels AH, Taylor AJ. Reserpine withdrawal psychosis. Aust N Z J Psychiatry 1989;23(1):129–30.
3. Ross RK, Paganini-Hill A, Krailo MD, Gerkins VR, Henderson BE, Pike MC. Effects of reserpine on prolactin levels and incidence of breast cancer in postmenopausal women. Cancer Res 1984;44(7):3106–8.
4. Boyden TW, Nugent CA, Ogihara T, Maeda T. Reserpine, hydrochlorothiazide and pituitary–gonadal hormones in hypertensive patients. Eur J Clin Pharmacol 1980;17(5):329–32.
5. Kent TA, Wilber RD. Reserpine withdrawal psychosis: the possible role of denervation supersensitivity of receptors. J Nerv Ment Dis 1982;170(8):502–4.
6. Grossman E, Messerli FH, Goldbourt U. Carcinogenicity of antihypertensive therapy. Curr Hypertens Rep 2002;4(3):195–201.
7. von Poser G, Andrade HH, da Silva KV, Henriques AT, Henriques JA. Genotoxic, mutagenic and recombinogenic effects of rauwolfia alkaloids. Mutat Res 1990;232(1):37–43.

Resorcinol

General Information

Resorcinol, which was formerly used to treat leg ulcers, is nowadays mainly used in the treatment of acne vulgaris as a peeling agent. In the older literature (1), several cases of systemic toxicity from percutaneous absorption were reported and there were deaths (2). The use of resorcinol in the treatment of acne is considered safe (SEDA-9, 142).

Signs and symptoms of resorcinol intoxication (1,2) include:

- pallor, dizziness, cold sweat, collapse, cyanosis;
- tremor;
- hypothyroidism;
- methemoglobinemia, hemolytic anemia;
- hemoglobinuria, violet-black urine;
- maculopapular eruptions;
- ochronosis.

Organs and Systems

Immunologic

Systemic allergic reactions have been reported in eight patients after topical application of a wart formulation containing resorcinol (3). All developed a marked eczematous, sometimes bullous reaction, localized to the site of application; in four cases there were generalized urticaria and angioedema, in one pompholyx eczema, and in three generalized eczema with pompholyx. In all cases there were positive patch tests with resorcinol.

References

1. Bontemps H, Mallaret M, Besson G, Bochaton H, Carpentier F. Confusion after topical use of resorcinol. Arch Dermatol 1995;131(1):112.
2. Cunningham AA. Resorcin poisoning. Arch Dis Child 1956;31(157):173–6.
3. Barbaud A, Modiano P, Cocciale M, Reichert S, Schmutz JL. The topical application of resorcinol can provoke a systemic allergic reaction. Br J Dermatol 1996;135(6):1014–15.

Rhamnaceae

See also Herbal medicines

General Information

The genera in the family of Rhamnaceae (Table 1) include buckthorn and jujube.

Rhamnus purshianus

The bark of *Rhamnus purshiana* (cascara sagrada) contains laxative anthranoid derivatives, which occur primarily in various laxative herbs (such as aloe, cascara sagrada,

Table 1 The genera of Rhamnaceae

Adolphia (prickbush)
Alphitonia (alphitonia)
Auerodendron (auerodendron)
Berchemia (supplejack)
Ceanothus (ceanothus)
Colubrina (nakedwood)
Condalia (snakewood)
Frangula (buckthorn)
Gouania (chewstick)
Hovenia (hovenia)
Karwinskia (karwinskia)
Krugiodendron (krugiodendron)
Maesopsis (umbrella-tree)
Paliurus (Jeruselem thorn)
Reynosia (darlingplum)
Rhamnus (buckthorn)
Sageretia (mock buckthorn)
Smythea
Ziziphus (jujube)

medicinal rhubarb, and senna) in the form of free anthraquinones, anthrones, dianthrones, and/or *O*- and *C*-glycosides derived from these substances.

Adverse effects

The anthranoids produce harmless discoloration of the urine. Depending on intrinsic activity and dose, they can also produce abdominal discomfort and cramps, nausea, violent purgation, and dehydration. They can be distributed into breast milk, but not always in sufficient amounts to affect the suckling infant. Long-term use can result in electrolyte disturbances and in atony and dilatation of the colon.

Respiratory
Cascara sagrada can cause IgE-mediated occupational asthma and rhinitis (1).

Liver
Cascara sagrada has been reported to cause liver damage (2).

- A 48-year-old man developed cholestatic hepatitis and hypertension shortly after he started to use the herbal laxative cascara sagrada. He took one capsule (425 mg of aged cascara sagrada bark) tds for 3 days and subsequently developed right upper quadrant pain, nausea, abdominal bloating, anorexia, and jaundice. The cascara was withdrawn, but his symptoms persisted and his liver function tests were abnormal. One week later, he developed ascites and jaundice and underwent liver biopsy, which showed moderately severe portal inflammation, intracanalicular bile stasis, portal bridging fibrosis, and mild steatosis. He gradually improved without specific treatment and 3 months later his ascites and jaundice had resolved.

Tumorigenicity
Several anthranoid derivatives (notably the aglycones aloe-emodin, chrysophanol, emodin, and physicon) are genotoxic in bacterial and/or mammalian test systems

(SEDA-12, 409), and two anthranoid compounds (the synthetic laxative dantron and the naturally occurring l-hydroxyanthraquinone) have carcinogenic activity in rodents. In an epidemiological study, chronic abusers of anthranoid laxatives (identified by the presence of pseudomelanosis coli) had an increased relative risk of 3.04 (95% CI = 1.18, 4.90) for colorectal cancer (3). The German health authorities therefore restricted the indication of herbal anthranoid laxatives to constipation which has not responded to bulk-forming therapy (which rules out their inclusion in slimming aids). In addition, they imposed restrictions on the laxative use of anthranoid-containing herbs (for example not to be used for more than 1–2 weeks without medical advice, not to be used in children under 12 years of age, and not to be used during pregnancy and lactation) (3,4).

Zizyphus jujuba

The fruit of *Zizyphus jujuba* (dazao) is often consumed in Eastern Asia as food or as a tonic and sedative.

Adverse effects
Angioedema has been described after the oral ingestion of dazao (5).

References

1. Giavina-Bianchi PF Jr, Castro FF, Machado ML, Duarte AJ. Occupational respiratory allergic disease induced by *Passiflora alata* and *Rhamnus purshiana*. Ann Allergy Asthma Immunol 1997;79(5):449–54.
2. Nadir A, Reddy D, Van Thiel DH. *Cascara sagrada*-induced intrahepatic cholestasis causing portal hypertension: case report and review of herbal hepatotoxicity. Am J Gastroenterol 2000;95(12):3634–7.
3. Siegers CP, von Hertzberg-Lottin E, Otte M, Schneider B. Anthranoid laxative abuse—a risk for colorectal cancer? Gut 1993;34(8):1099–101.
4. Kommission E. Aufbereitungsmonographien. Dtsch Apoth Ztg 1993;133:2791–4.
5. Chan TY, Chan AY, Critchley JA. Hospital admissions due to adverse reactions to Chinese herbal medicines. J Trop Med Hyg 1992;95(4):296–8.

Ribavirin

General Information

The synthetic triazole nucleoside, ribavirin (1-beta-D-ribofuranosyl-1,2,4-triazole-3-carboxamide, tribavirin, virazole), has a broad spectrum of antiviral activity, including DNA as well as RNA viruses (1). Ribavirin closely resembles guanosine and is converted intracellularly to mono-, di-, and triphosphate derivatives, which inhibit the virally induced enzymes involved in viral nucleic acid synthesis by different mechanisms that are not fully understood (2). Of the DNA viruses, ribavirin is active against *Herpes simplex* virus and hepatitis B virus; among the RNA viruses, good activity has been observed against hepatitis C virus, orthomyxoviruses, paramyxoviruses, arenaviruses, and bunyaviruses. Although active against HIV in vitro and in vivo (3), ribavirin is not widely used in the treatment of HIV infection. So far, drug resistance has not been described.

Oral ribavirin has been successfully used in the treatment of Lassa fever (4), Crimean Congo hemorrhagic fever (5), and in combination therapy with interferon alfa for hepatitis C infection (6,7). Several publications have suggested enhanced efficacy of the combination of interferon alfa with ribavirin when compared with monotherapy with interferon alfa. There is also evidence that re-treatment with the combination may succeed in controlling or eliminating viremia when monotherapy has failed. Although the combination may lead to some increase in the adverse effects normally associated with interferon alfa (dyspnea, pharyngitis, pruritus, nausea, insomnia, and anorexia) (SEDA-23, 315), there is no doubt that oral ribavirin adds to the overall toxicity of the combination by causing hemolytic anemia, which is usually mild.

Ribavirin is well absorbed orally, but it can be given in aerosol form for the treatment of respiratory syncytial virus (RSV) infections in immunocompromised patients, and in those with cardiopulmonary abnormalities, or in infants receiving mechanical ventilation (8,9).

The adverse effects and other safety aspects of interferon and ribavirin in the treatment of hepatitis C infection have been reviewed (10).

Comparative studies

Two, large, randomized, placebo-controlled comparisons of interferon alfa-2b alone with the combination of interferon alfa-2b plus ribavirin have been published. In the initial treatment of chronic hepatitis C, 912 patients were randomly assigned to receive standard-dose interferon alfa-2b alone or in combination with ribavirin (1000 or 1200 mg/day orally, depending on body weight) for 24 or 48 weeks (7). As expected, dosage reduction for anemia was necessary in 8% of patients taking the combination therapy and in none of those treated with interferon alone. Dyspnea, pharyngitis, pruritus, rash, nausea, insomnia, and anorexia were adverse effects that were reported more often during combination therapy with ribavirin (7). In patients whose chronic hepatitis had relapsed after therapy with interferon alfa-2b alone, 345 patients were randomized to receive standard-dose interferon alfa-2b alone or in combination with ribavirin (1000 or 1200 mg/day orally, depending on body weight) for 6 months (6). Dosage reduction for anemia was required in 12/173 patients assigned to combination therapy and in none assigned to interferon alone. As was the case in the initial therapy study, dyspnea, nausea, and rash were significantly more common in patients treated with the combination of interferon and ribavirin (6).

Ribavirin 15 mg/kg/day plus interferon alfa in 12 teenagers has been compared with interferon alone in 10 (11). There was no difference in dropout rate, but viral clearance was achieved in 50% of the patients who took the combination treatment versus 30% of those who took monotherapy. Adverse events were similar in the two groups. There was mild hemolytic anemia at the end of the first month in most of the children who took ribavirin,

but four had moderate to severe hemolysis and two had to stop taking ribavirin. Severe hemolysis in a patient with thalassemia warranted withdrawal of ribavirin within 3 months.

Organs and Systems

Hematologic

Ribavirin accumulates in erythrocytes, resulting in hemolysis by an unknown mechanism, perhaps related to oxidative damage to the erythrocyte membrane. Time-dependent and dose-dependent hemolytic anemia (eventually associated with hyperbilirubinemia and a high reticulocyte count) is the only major toxic effect associated with oral or intravenous ribavirin and is reversible on withdrawal. There was a fall in hemoglobin concentrations below 10.0 g/dl in 9% of patients with hepatitis C treated with ribavirin and interferon alfa (6,7).

In 140 patients with Nipah virus infection there was no difference in the incidence of adverse effects between those who elected to have ribavirin treatment and those who refused (12). Dosing was based on recommendations used to achieve the same approximate concentrations as those seen with 100–1200 mg/day in the treatment of hepatitis C. Anemia occurred in 37% of the ribavirin-treated patients and in the same number of controls, suggesting that ribavirin was equally well tolerated in the two groups.

In patients taking ribavirin plus interferon alfa-2b the average fall in hemoglobin is 2–3 g/dl. Of 57 patients taking ribavirin 800 mg/day 28 were randomized to a high dose of peginterferon alfa-2b once a week (3 micrograms/kg for 1 week, 1.5 micrograms/kg for 3 weeks, and 1.0 microgram/kg for 44 weeks) and 27 patients were randomized to receive a low dose (0.5 micrograms/kg) for 48 weeks; three patients required reduced doses of ribavirin because of anemia (13).

In a randomized controlled trial of high-dose interferon alfa-2b plus oral ribavirin for 6 or 12 months in 50 patients with chronic hepatitis C, the sequential effects of treatment on hemoglobin, leukocytes, and platelets were recorded (14). There was a fall in hemoglobin, and the lowest concentrations were recorded after 6 months of treatment in both groups. All hematological measurements returned to normal after the end of treatment.

Detailed studies of the effects of ribavirin on erythrocyte ATP content and on the hexose monophosphate shunt have been conducted in vitro. ATP concentrations were significantly reduced and the hexose monophosphate shunt increased, suggesting erythrocyte susceptibility to oxidation. In vivo, ribavirin, alone or in combination with interferon, was associated with significant reductions in hemoglobin concentrations and a marked increase in absolute reticulocyte counts. Erythrocyte Na/K pump activity was significantly reduced, whereas K/Cl co-transport and its dithiothreitol-sensitive fraction and malondialdehyde and methemoglobin concentrations increased significantly. Ribavirin-treated patients showed an increase in aggregated band 3, which was associated with significantly increased binding of autologous antibodies and complement C3 fragments, suggesting erythrophagocytic removal by the reticuloendothelial system (15).

A low pretreatment platelet count, the dose of interferon alfa, and the haptoglobin phenotype are risk factors for ribavirin-induced anemia, and the fall in hemoglobin is independent of dose in the therapeutic range (16). In five patients with chronic hepatitis C on hemodialysis who received subcutaneous interferon alfa-2b and oral ribavirin for 40 weeks, the dose of ribavirin was titrated based on hemoglobin, with bone marrow support by erythropoietin (17). There was significant bone marrow toxicity in all five. A dose of 200 mg/day produced a steady-state AUC comparable to that obtained with 1000–1200 mg/day in historical controls with normal renal function. More severe anemia was possibly due to chronic renal insufficiency in addition to the prolonged effects of ribavirin.

Treatment of ribavirin-induced hemolytic anemia with recombinant human erythropoietin has been described in 13 patients (18). The hemoglobin concentration increased from a nadir of 10.2 g/dl to a median of 11.5 g/dl and ribavirin treatment did not have to be withdrawn.

Liver

As part of a multicenter, randomized, double-blind, placebo-controlled trial of ribavirin in 59 patients with hepatitis C virus infection, liver biopsies were studied for iron deposition (19). Increased total iron deposition, preferentially in hepatocytes, occurred during a 9-month course of ribavirin. The deposition had no apparent effect on the biochemical or histological response to ribavirin therapy.

Skin

Photosensitivity after administration of ribavirin has been described (20). A well-documented photoallergic reaction in a woman who was taking both ribavirin and interferon alfa provided evidence that ribavirin is a potential photosensitizer for UVB, a problem that may become increasingly relevant in patients with chronic hepatitis C taking combination therapy for 6–12 months with interferon alfa and ribavirin (20).

Transient acantholytic dermatosis (Grover's disease) was first described by Grover in 1970 as a pruritic, self-limiting, popular, or papulovesicular eruption, mainly distributed on the trunk of white middle-aged men. The histopathological hallmark is suprabasal acantholysis at different levels of the epidermis. Its origin is uncertain; most cases are related to sunlight, heat, or sweating. Grover's disease has been attributed to ribavirin (21).

- A 55-year-old man with chronic hepatitis C presented with a pruritic papular eruption on the trunk lasting 2 weeks. He had multiple, erythematous, excoriated papules on the neck, trunk, upper arms, and thighs. The lesions appeared 2 weeks after combination therapy with oral ribavirin and subcutaneous interferon alfa-2b. He had previously been treated with interferon alfa alone (in the same dosage). On withdrawal of ribavirin the lesions gradually faded, but they returned 1 week after reintroduction.

Second-Generation Effects

Teratogenicity

Ribavirin is teratogenic and embryotoxic in laboratory animals and should not be given to pregnant women. Concern has been expressed about the safety of people in the same room as patients being treated with ribavirin by aerosol, particularly women of child-bearing age. However, no ribavirin was detected in the urine, plasma, or erythrocytes of 19 nurses exposed to ribavirin administered via ventilator, oxygen tent, or oxygen hood over 3 days (22).

Drug–Drug Interactions

Didanosine

Multisystem organ dysfunction and lactic acidemia occurred in two of 15 patients with HIV and hepatitis C infections who received interferon alfa, didanosine, and ribavirin (23). Co-administration of didanosine with ribavirin can lead to increased toxicity secondary to raised intracellular concentrations of phosphorylated didanosine (ddA-TP) (24,25). Thus, the evidence suggests that the combination of didanosine plus ribavirin increases the risk of lactic acidosis.

Warfarin

An interaction of warfarin with ribavirin has been reported (26).

- In a 61-year-old white man with chronic hepatitis C, who took interferon plus ribavirin, the dosage of warfarin had to be increased by about 40% (from 45 to 63 mg/week) in order to maintain the desired degree of anticoagulation. This effect was reproduced on rechallenge with ribavirin.

The mechanism of this supposed interaction is not known. For example, ribavirin is cleared by intracellular phosphorylation and its metabolites by the kidneys, warfarin by cytochrome P450 isozymes in the liver; warfarin is highly protein bound, ribavirin is not. However, an effect on warfarin absorption or its action on clotting factor synthesis is possible.

References

1. Stapleton T, et al. Studies with a Broad Spectrum Antiviral Agent. International Congress and Symposium Series. London/New York: Royal Society of Medicine Services, 1986.
2. Couch RB. Respiratory disease. In: Galasso GJ, Whitley RJ, Merigan TC, editors. Antiviral Agents and Viral Diseases of Man. New York: Raven Press, 1990:327.
3. Japour AJ, Lertora JJ, Meehan PM, Erice A, Connor JD, Griffith BP, Clax PA, Holden-Wiltse J, Hussey S, Walesky M, Cooney E, Pollard R, Timpone J, McLaren C, Johanneson N, Wood K, Booth D, Bassiakos Y, Crumpacker CS. A phase-I study of the safety, pharmacokinetics, and antiviral activity of combination didanosine and ribavirin in patients with HIV-1 disease. AIDS Clinical Trials Group 231 Protocol Team. J Acquir Immune Defic Syndr Hum Retrovirol 1996;13(3):235–46.

4. McCormick JB, King IJ, Webb PA, Scribner CL, Craven RB, Johnson KM, Elliott LH, Belmont-Williams R. Lassa fever. Effective therapy with ribavirin. N Engl J Med 1986;314(1):20–6.

5. Fisher-Hoch SP, Khan JA, Rehman S, Mirza S, Khurshid M, McCormick JB. Crimean Congo–haemorrhagic fever treated with oral ribavirin. Lancet 1995;346(8973):472–5.

6. Davis GL, Esteban-Mur R, Rustgi V, Hoefs J, Gordon SC, Trepo C, Shiffman ML, Zeuzem S, Craxi A, Ling MH, Albrecht J. Interferon alfa-2b alone or in combination with ribavirin for the treatment of relapse of chronic hepatitis C. International Hepatitis Interventional Therapy Group. N Engl J Med 1998;339(21):1493–9.

7. McHutchison JG, Gordon SC, Schiff ER, Shiffman ML, Lee WM, Rustgi VK, Goodman ZD, Ling MH, Cort S, Albrecht JK. Interferon alfa-2b alone or in combination with ribavirin as initial treatment for chronic hepatitis C. Hepatitis Interventional Therapy Group. N Engl J Med 1998;339(21):1485–92.

8. Hall CB, McBride JT, Walsh EE, Bell DM, Gala CL, Hildreth S, Ten Eyck LG, Hall WJ. Aerosolized ribavirin treatment of infants with respiratory syncytial viral infection. A randomized double-blind study. N Engl J Med 1983;308(24):1443–7.

9. Smith DW, Frankel LR, Mathers LH, Tang AT, Ariagno RL, Prober CG. A controlled trial of aerosolized ribavirin in infants receiving mechanical ventilation for severe respiratory syncytial virus infection. N Engl J Med 1991;325(1):24–9.

10. Chutaputti A. Adverse effects and other safety aspects of the hepatitis C antivirals. J Gastroenterol Hepatol 2000;15(Suppl):E156–63.

11. Suoglu D OD, Elkabes B, Sokucu S, Saner G. Does interferon and ribavirin combination therapy increase the rate of treatment response in children with hepatitis C? J Pediatr Gastroenterol Nutr 2002;34(2):199–206.

12. Chong HT, Kamarulzaman A, Tan CT, Goh KJ, Thayaparan T, Kunjapan SR, Chew NK, Chua KB, Lam SK. Treatment of acute Nipah encephalitis with ribavirin. Ann Neurol 2001;49(6):810–3.

13. Buti M, Sanchez-Avila F, Lurie Y, Stalgis C, Valdes A, Martell M, Esteban R. Viral kinetics in genotype 1 chronic hepatitis C patients during therapy with 2 different doses of peginterferon alfa-2b plus ribavirin. Hepatology 2002;35(4):930–6.

14. Marco VD, Almasio P, Vaccaro A, Ferraro D, Parisi P, Cataldo MG, Di Stefano R, Craxi A. Combined treatment of relapse of chronic hepatitis C with high-dose alpha2b interferon plus ribavirin for 6 or 12 months. J Hepatol 2000;33(3):456–62.

15. De Franceschi L, Fattovich G, Turrini F, Ayi K, Brugnara C, Manzato F, Noventa F, Stanzial AM, Solero P, Corrocher R. Hemolytic anemia induced by ribavirin therapy in patients with chronic hepatitis C virus infection: role of membrane oxidative damage. Hepatology 2000;31(4):997–1004.

16. Van Vlierbergh H, Delanghe JR, De Vos M, Leroux-Roel G. BASL Steering Committee. Factors influencing ribavirin-induced hemolysis. J Hepatol 2001;34(6):911–16.

17. Tan AC, Brouwer JT, Glue P, van Leusen R, Kauffmann RH, Schalm SW, de Vries RA, Vroom B. Safety of interferon and ribavirin therapy in haemodialysis patients with chronic hepatitis C: results of a pilot study. Nephrol Dial Transplant 2001;16(1):193–5.

18. Gergely AE, Lafarge P, Fouchard-Hubert I, Lunel-Fabiani F. Treatment of ribavirin/interferon-induced anemia with erythropoietin in patients with hepatitis C. Hepatology 2002;35(5):1281–2.

19. Fiel MI, Schiano TD, Guido M, Thung SN, Lindsay KL, Davis GL, Lewis JH, Seeff LB, Bodenheimer HC Jr. Increased hepatic iron deposition resulting from treatment of chronic hepatitis C with ribavirin. Am J Clin Pathol 2000;113(1):35–9.

20. Stryjek-Kaminska D, Ochsendorf F, Roder C, Wolter M, Zeuzem S. Photoallergic skin reaction to ribavirin. Am J Gastroenterol 1999;94(6):1686–8.

21. Antunes I, Azevedo F, Mesquita-Guimaraes J, Resende C, Fernandes N, MacEdo G. Grover's disease secondary to ribavirin. Br J Dermatol 2000;142(6):1257–8.

22. Rodriguez WJ, Bui RH, Connor JD, Kim HW, Brandt CD, Parrott RH, Burch B, Mace J. Environmental exposure of primary care personnel to ribavirin aerosol when supervising treatment of infants with respiratory syncytial virus infections. Antimicrob Agents Chemother 1987;31(7):1143–6.

23. Lafeuillade A, Hittinger G, Chadapaud S. Increased mitochondrial toxicity with ribavirin in HIV/HCV coinfection. Lancet 2001;357(9252):280–1.

24. Kakuda TN, Brinkman K. Mitochondrial toxic effects and ribavirin. Lancet 2001;357(9270):1802–3.

25. Salmon-Ceron D, Chauvelot-Moachon L, Abad S, Silbermann B, Sogni P. Mitochondrial toxic effects and ribavirin. Lancet 2001;357(9270):1803–4.

26. Schulman S. Inhibition of warfarin activity by ribavirin. Ann Pharmacother 2002;36(1):72–4.

Riboflavin

See also Vitamins

General Information

The Average Requirement of riboflavin is 1.3 mg/day for men and 1.1 mg/day for women, the Population Reference Intake 1.6 and 1.3 mg/day respectively, and the Lowest Threshold Intake 0.6 mg/day for both.

Riboflavin is poorly absorbed and adverse reactions are almost unknown.

Because it can be detected fluorimetrically in the urine it has been used as a tracer to mark adherence to therapy (1,2).

Organs and Systems

Immunologic

Anaphylaxis has been reported in a boy who took a multivitamin tablet containing riboflavin (3).

- A 15-year-old boy developed flushing and a generalized papular rash after taking one multivitamin tablet, followed by dizziness, dyspnea, nausea, and severe angioedema of the face 40 minutes later. He became drowsy and developed hypotension (67/48 mmHg) and tachycardia (131/minute). He was given subcutaneous adrenaline, intravenous isotonic saline, and diphenhydramine and hydrocortisone, and after 30 minutes his vital signs became stable; he recovered consciousness shortly after. He had no history of atopic diseases or adverse drug reactions, but reported that he had had dizziness many times after drinking one particular yellow-colored brand of soft drink and that he had lost consciousness twice after drinking it about 5 years before. Intradermal skin tests with the vitamins and determination of in vitro histamine release showed a strong positive response to riboflavin. He was advised to exclude riboflavin-containing products from his diet and to carry adrenaline for self-administration. During the next 13 months he had no further adverse reactions.

The multivitamin tablet that this boy took contained 100 mg of vitamins B_1, B_2, and B_6, cyanocobalamin concentrate 500 micrograms, and vitamin C 500 mg. The soft drink contained vitamin B_1 (0.6 ppm), vitamin B_2 (8.9 ppm), and vitamin C 200 micrograms/ml.

References

1. Dubbert PM, King A, Rapp SR, Brief D, Martin JE, Lake M. Riboflavin as a tracer of medication compliance. J Behav Med 1985;8(3):287–99.
2. Babiker IE, Cooke PR, Gillett MG. How useful is riboflavin as a tracer of medication compliance? J Behav Med 1989;12(1):25–38.
3. Ou LS, Kuo ML, Huang JL. Anaphylaxis to riboflavin (vitamin B2). Ann Allergy Asthma Immunol 2001;87(5):430–3.

Ribonucleic acid

General Information

Ribonucleic acid has been used to enhance immune function in patients with cancer. Of 83 patients who received subcutaneous injections of ribonucleic acid (10 mg every other day) for various skin diseases, three developed an erythematous edematous reaction around the injection sites after the 7th to 15th injections (1). Although patch tests were negative in all three patients, lesions were reproduced after intradermal injection in one patient.

Reference

1. Li LF. Erythematous skin reaction to subcutaneous injection of ribonucleic acid. Contact Dermatitis 1999;41(4):239.

Rifamycins

See also Antituberculosis drugs

General Information

The rifamycins are a group of macrocyclic antibiotics that were originally derived from a culture of *Streptomyces mediterranei*, the products of which were named after the French film "Rififi chez les hommes" (director Jules Dassin).

Rifampicin

Rifampicin (rINN) is a semisynthetic derivative of rifamycin B. By suppressing the initiation of chain formation in RNA synthesis, it inhibits the DNA-dependent RNA polymerase of mycobacteria and other microorganisms (1). It inhibits the growth of most Gram-positive and many Gram-negative bacteria: *Escherichia coli*, some strains of *Pseudomonas*, *Proteus*, *Klebsiella*, *Staphylococcus aureus*, *Neisseria meningitidis*, *Hemophilus influenzae*, and *Legionella* species. *Mycobacterium tuberculosis*, *Mycobacterium kansasii*, *Mycobacterium scrofulaceum*, and *Mycobacterium intracellulare* are suppressed with increasing concentrations between 0.005 and 4 µg/ml. Rifampicin is bactericidal for *Mycobacterium leprae* in a concentration of less than 1 µg/ml. *Mycobacterium fortuitum* is not susceptible. Primary resistance is very rare, but secondary resistance among mycobacteria and meningococci develops very rapidly when rifampicin is used as a single drug (1).

In a prospective, randomized trial in 12 high-risk adult patients, the use of polyurethane, triple-lumen, central venous catheters impregnated with minocycline and rifampicin (on both the luminal and external surfaces) is associated with a lower rate of infection than the use of catheters impregnated with chlorhexidine and silver sulfadiazine (on the external surface only) (2). There were low rates of catheter-related bloodstream infection (0.3%) and catheter colonization (7.9%) with the use of catheters impregnated with minocycline and rifampicin. This favorable result may be explained either by differences in the coating of the catheters (internal and external surfaces versus external surface only), by microbiological advantages of minocycline and rifampicin over chlorhexidine and silver sulfadiazine, or even by an effect unrelated to the antibacterial activity. The additional costs of preventing an infection and a death would be about $3125 and $12 500 respectively (3).

Pharmacokinetics

Rifampicin is distributed to nearly all organs and body fluids in adequate antibacterial concentrations. The rifamycins are concentrated several-fold in alveolar macrophages (4). This explains their efficacy against intracellular bacteria. Peak concentrations of up to 7 µg/ml are reached within 2–4 hours after a dose of 600 mg before a meal. After gastrointestinal absorption, rifampicin is quickly eliminated in the bile, following enterohepatic circulation. It is also excreted in various fluids, and causes orange–red discoloration of the urine, feces, saliva, tears, sputum, and sweat (SED-10, 576) (5). Rifampicin is progressively deacetylated. Its half-life varies between 2.5 and 5 hours and is prolonged to various degrees by isoniazid and hepatic disorders (1). There is a progressive shortening of the half-life of rifampicin by about 40% during the first 14 days of treatment, owing to self-induction of the hepatic microsomal enzymes that metabolize it (6).

Because rifampicin is a potent inducer of hepatic microsomal drug-metabolizing enzymes, it has been implicated in reducing the effectiveness of many drugs that are metabolized in the liver (SEDA-21, 313). Interactions continue to be recognized, reflecting the extension of the use of rifampicin from an antituberculosis agent to an antistaphylococcal drug, particularly useful in the treatment of methicillin-resistant *Staphylococcus aureus* (MRSA) and when prostheses are infected.

General adverse effects

Rifampicin given in usual doses (for example 10 mg/kg/day) is well tolerated and causes adverse effects in only about 4% of patients. Adverse reactions are predominantly hepatic and allergic. Gastrointestinal symptoms are generally transient. Risk factors are age, alcoholism, and hepatic disorders (1). As a potent microsomal enzyme inducer, rifampicin shortens the half-lives of many other drugs (1). This effect occurs after about 7 days and persists for a few days after withdrawal. Allergic reactions can cause rashes (in 0.8%), fever, a flu-like illness (malaise, headache), eosinophilia, and much less often hemolytic anemia, hemoglobinuria, and kidney damage with acute renal insufficiency. These reactions occur especially during intermittent treatment (less than twice weekly) or after re-introduction of rifampicin. Anaphylactoid reactions to rifampicin have been described in HIV-positive patients (7). Light-chain proteinuria and concomitant kidney damage are attributed to an immunological process (SEDA-10, 273). Rifampicin antibodies have been found using an antiglobulin test (8). Hemolysis as an adverse effect seems to be mainly of the immune-complex type, exceptionally of the IgG-antibody type (9). The drug-induced lupus-like syndrome has been linked to rifampicin in a few cases. Tumor-inducing effects and chromosome aberrations have not been noted with rifampicin or during the combined use of isoniazid and rifampicin (SEDA-9, 276).

A flu-like illness, with fever, headache, malaise, and bone pain, can occur shortly after the administration of rifampicin, and was observed in a man who had taken rifampicin 600 mg monthly for multibacillary leprosy (10). However, the reaction usually occurs with higher doses given weekly or twice weekly. The usual procedure is to reduce the dose or increase the frequency of treatment. Antipyretic drugs can be used to provide symptomatic relief.

Intermittent rifampicin therapy introduces risks of hematological and renal adverse reactions, probably through immunological mechanisms. Restarting rifampicin after a drug-free interval has to be carefully guided using small initial dosages of about 75 mg/day and increasing to a final dosage of about 500–600 mg/day. It is essential to monitor blood counts, coagulation factors, and kidney function. The authors of a comprehensive review of the adverse effects of rifampicin (11) have made the point that these are likely to increase, because reactions such as hemolysis, thrombocytopenia, and flu-like syndromes are more likely in patients who take rifampicin intermittently, a pattern of treatment that is becoming recognized as the best way to manage tuberculosis in developing countries and in patients everywhere whose compliance cannot be relied upon, since it is impractical to administer directly observed therapy (DOTS) more often than two or three times a week.

Some drug interactions with rifampicin have been reviewed (SEDA-21, 313) (SEDA-24, 354).

Rifabutin

Rifabutin (rINN), a spiropiperidyl derivative of rifamycin, is more effective in vitro against *M. tuberculosis* than rifampicin. It has a longer half-life, better tissue penetration, and causes less enzyme induction than rifampicin. Rifabutin is well absorbed from the gastrointestinal tract and reaches a peak serum concentration of about 0.5 μg/ml 4 hours after a single dose of 300 mg.

A 300 mg dose of rifabutin is usually well tolerated. Adverse effects include neutropenia, thrombocytopenia, rash, and gastrointestinal disturbances (nausea, flatulence). Myositis (12) and uveitis (13) are rarely observed. The drug-induced lupus-like syndrome has been linked in a few cases with rifampicin and rifabutin.

In a multicenter study from the National Institute of Allergy and Infectious Diseases in the USA, azithromycin (600 mg/day) plus rifabutin (300 mg/day) was poorly tolerated by 31 patients with or without HIV infection (14). Gastrointestinal symptoms and neutropenia were the major adverse effects. There was no significant pharmacokinetic interaction between the two drugs.

Rifamycin SV

Rifamycin SV (rINN), a semisynthetic macrocyclic antibiotic derived from natural rifamycin B, has been used in the therapy of tuberculosis and in some European countries as a topical antibiotic. Anaphylaxis has been reported after systemic administration, and rarely after topical application.

Organs and Systems

Cardiovascular

Shock and a flu-like illness (fever, chills, and myalgia) have been observed most often in patients taking intermittent rifampicin, dosages over 1000 mg/day, or on restarting treatment (1,15). Shock and cerebral infarction have been reported in an HIV-positive patient after re-exposure to rifampicin (16).

Local thrombophlebitis can occur during prolonged intravenous administration (17).

Respiratory

Respiratory symptoms from rifampicin are very rare. They can be part of a flu-like illness with bronchial obstruction (18,19).

Rifampicin-induced pneumonitis is rare.

- An 81-year-old man with smear- and culture-positive pulmonary tuberculosis developed clinical and radiological features of localized interstitial pneumonitis 1 week after starting to take rifampicin, isoniazid, and ethambutol (20). The bronchoalveolar lavage fluid contained 83% lymphocytes with a CD4/CD8 ratio of 10.5. Antituberculosis treatment was withheld and he was treated with methylprednisolone for 3 days because of progressive respiratory failure. A drug lymphocyte stimulation test showed a high stimulation index with rifampicin (370%). He was subsequently treated with streptomycin instead of rifampicin. Re-challenge with rifampicin was not undertaken.

Sudden clinical and radiological worsening during treatment for pulmonary tuberculosis may be due to bronchogenic spread of infection, immune reconstitution producing a paradoxical reaction, drug-induced hypersensitivity pneumonitis, or other unrelated causes, such as pulmonary embolism. Allergic pneumonitis with rifampicin is most unusual, as is the high CD4/CD8 ratio observed in the bronchoalveolar lavage fluid.

Nervous system

Rifampicin is widely used in tuberculous and meningococcal meningitis, since it passes into the cerebrospinal fluid (21). Rifampicin-induced neurological effects include drowsiness, headache, dizziness, ataxia, generalized numbness, pain in the extremities, muscular weakness, confusion, inability to concentrate, delusions, disorientation, hallucinations, and agitation (1,22).

Sensory systems

Drug-induced uveitis is rare. Antibiotics that have been implicated include rifabutin and sulfonamides. Furthermore, nearly all antibiotics injected intracamerally have been reported to produce uveitis (23).

In one study, the most important adverse effect of rifabutin was uveitis, which occurred in 24 of 63 patients taking rifabutin 600 mg/day and three of 53 patients taking 300 mg/day (24). No patients taking quadruple therapy developed uveitis (25). Initially, uveitis was thought to occur only with dosages of rifabutin over 1200 mg/day. However, a review of 54 cases has shown that it can occur at dosages of 300–600 mg/day and is more likely to occur in patients with a low body mass (26). The patients presented with uveitis 2 weeks to 7 months after starting therapy. In all cases they were also taking fluconazole and clarithromycin, drugs that inhibit cytochrome P450 drug metabolism, leading to increased blood concentrations of rifabutin. Rifabutin is less likely to cause uveitis when it is used in combination with azithromycin 500 mg/day than with clarithromycin. If rifabutin is combined with clarithromycin 1 g/day the dose of rifabutin should be limited to 300 mg/day—advice which has been endorsed by the UK Medicines Control Agency (27).

Topical administration of a glucocorticoid and a cycloplegic drug (such as atropine) is suitable as initial treatment. Withdrawal of causative drugs is not always necessary (28).

Endocrine

In patients taking glucocorticoids for Addison's disease, rifampicin may necessitate an increase in glucocorticoid dosage. Thus, incipient adrenal insufficiency can be unmasked by rifampicin (SEDA-13, 261). The phenomenon is due to liver enzyme induction (29).

A significantly raised concentration of TSH during therapy with rifampicin has been reported in a man taking levothyroxine; TSH concentrations returned to baseline 9 days after withdrawal of rifampicin (30).

Metabolism

The combination of rifampicin and isoniazid reduces serum concentrations of 25-hydroxycholecalciferol. Rifampicin acts by induction of an enzyme that promotes conversion of 25-hydroxycholecalciferol to an inactive metabolite, and isoniazid acts by inhibiting 25-hydroxylation and 1-hydroxylation (SEDA-14, 258). Children or pregnant women with tuberculosis have increased calcium requirements independent of rifampicin administration (31). In 132 children of Afro-Asian origin there was a significant increase in serum alkaline phosphatase activity. This was more pronounced in patients taking both isoniazid and rifampicin than with isoniazid alone (32). The rise in alkaline phosphatase could reflect an effect on either liver or bone. The possibility of a link between this effect and osteomalacia is unclear.

Rifampicin-induced porphyria cutanea tarda has been described in one case, combined with altered liver function (33).

Hematologic

Hemolysis (34,35), agranulocytosis (36), leukopenia (37), and thrombocytopenia (38) have been reported in patients taking rifampicin (SED-10, 578) and constitute contraindications to continuation of therapy.

Hemorrhagic states have been induced by rifampicin in pregnant women and their offspring because of drug-induced hepatic breakdown of vitamin K (39).

Disseminated intravascular coagulation has been attributed to rifampicin (40).

- A 46-year-old woman died of severe disseminated intravascular coagulation after her third monthly dose of rifampicin, given with daily dapsone for the treatment of leprosy (41).

Erythrocytes

Isolated cases of massive hemolysis, with or without renal insufficiency, have been observed in patients taking rifampicin (42–44). Whereas rifampicin given repeatedly and in the usual dose is quite safe, it can cause intravascular hemolysis when given intermittently (45).

Antibodies to rifampicin have been found in several studies, with a positive Coombs' test in the presence of the drug (SEDA-5, 291), more often of the immunocomplex type (46,47) than with IgG or IgM antibodies (43,44).

- In one case, hemolysis started after the second dose of rifampicin, and the patient's blood contained rifampicin-dependent IgG and IgM antibodies, which caused erythrocyte lysis through an interaction with the I antigen on the erythrocyte surface (35). This antigen is also expressed on renal tubular epithelium and the hemolysis was accompanied by acute renal insufficiency.

Intermittent or interrupted treatment appears to predispose to this complication.

Leukocytes

There were four cases of agranulocytosis due to antituberculosis drugs (rifampicin, isoniazid, ethambutol, streptomycin, or pyrazinamide) among about 6400 patients who underwent chemotherapy from 1981 to 2002; the incidence rate of agranulocytosis was estimated at 0.06% (36).

In 140 patients who took Rimapen (Orion, Finland) there were 11 cases of leukopenia, while in 132 patients who took Rimactan (Ciba-Geigy, Switzerland) there was only one case, a statistically significant difference (37).

Platelets

Reports of drug-induced thrombocytopenia have been systematically reviewed (48). Among the 98 different drugs described in 561 articles, the following antibiotics were found with level I (definite) evidence: co-trimoxazole, rifampicin, vancomycin, sulfisoxazole, cefalothin, piperacillin, methicillin, novobiocin. Drugs with level II (probable) evidence were oxytetracycline and ampicillin. There is an increased frequency of thrombocytopenia with intermittent therapy (40).

Immune thrombocytopenia during rifampicin therapy has been attributed to drug-dependent binding of an IgG antibody to platelets; the binding epitope of the antibody was found in the glycoprotein Ib/IX complex (38).

Gastrointestinal

Nausea, vomiting, epigastric pain, diarrhea, loss of appetite, abdominal cramps, and meteorism are often restricted to the beginning of rifampicin therapy. However, gastric burning can oblige some patients to take the drug after meals. Hemorrhage from gastric erosions is a rare complication (49).

- Tablet-associated esophagitis has been reported in a 70-year-old white man on the fourth day of antibiotic therapy with vancomycin, gentamicin, and oral rifampicin for *Staphylococcus epidermidis* prosthetic valve endocarditis (50).

The authors noted that age, bedridden state, gastroesophageal reflux disease, simultaneous administration of several medications, and nasopharyngeal obstruction may have increased the risk of esophagitis. They found a second case of tablet-associated esophagitis caused by rifampicin in their review of the published literature.

Histologically confirmed pseudomembranous colitis has been reported in patients taking rifampicin. Bacteriology showed mainly *Clostridium difficile* resistant to rifampicin and several other antibiotics. Withdrawal of rifampicin and the use of vancomycin has been helpful (SEDA-6, 275) (SEDA-7, 310) (51).

Liver

Rifampicin is rarely used as monotherapy. The risk of hepatotoxicity appears to be very low in patients with normal liver function, especially if rifampicin is given continuously. When given with isoniazid, rifampicin can cause a fulminant liver reaction. This may be attributable to enhancement of isoniazid hepatotoxicity as a result of enzyme induction by rifampicin. In some cases, jaundice occurred within 6–10 days after beginning isoniazid plus rifampicin (52). High serum transaminase activities, disturbances of consciousness, and centrilobular necrosis were found. All the patients recovered.

Hepatotoxicity of combined therapy for leprosy has been reported in 39 patients treated with dapsone, protionamide, and rifampicin. There were similar findings in 50 patients treated with dapsone, clofazimine, rifampicin, and protionamide. Deaths probably related to the drugs occurred in both groups after 3–4 months of treatment

(53). The drug responsible for liver injury may have been protionamide, although rifampicin administered simultaneously could also have contributed (53).

Among 50 000 patients treated prophylactically with rifampicin, there were 16 deaths associated with jaundice (0.03%) (SED-10, 578) (54,55).

Raised transaminases in children commonly cause withdrawal of therapy (56).

Transaminase activities and other liver function tests should be measured weekly in cases with liver dysfunction and every 4 weeks in patients with no known liver disease.

Severe itching is often a distressing symptom in patients with primary biliary cirrhosis and in cholestatic jaundice due to other causes. Rifampicin has been recommended for controlling this symptom, even though it is known to be hepatotoxic. Rifampicin-induced hepatitis has been reported in three of 41 patients with primary biliary cirrhosis (7.3%; 95% CI = 2.5, 19) (57). This risk is greater than the risk of hepatitis during rifampicin monotherapy for latent tuberculosis. Pre-existing liver disease is a recognized risk factor for drug-induced hepatitis, and these patients need to be monitored carefully during rifampicin therapy.

Biliary tract

Total serum bile acid concentrations were raised in 72% of 61 patients treated with rifampicin and isoniazid; in some patients, the concentrations were as much as 40 times above normal, but in only four was the serum bilirubin raised (58).

Skin

Pruritus, rashes, and urticaria have been reported. Rifampicin-induced rashes often resolve spontaneously, even without drug withdrawal, although in others they can be severe and can be accompanied by systemic symptoms, in some cases amounting to anaphylaxis (11).

Acne occurs more often in patients taking rifampicin and isoniazid combinations than those without rifampicin (SEDA-9, 270).

- A patient developed pemphigus foliaceus induced by rifampicin and improved after withdrawal (72).
- Another patient developed an exacerbation of pemphigus vulgaris during rifampicin therapy, which improved after withdrawal (73).

Severe bullous reactions have been associated with subepidermal detachment typical of toxic epidermal necrolysis (74).

After intravenous rifampicin, a severe cutaneous hypersensitivity reaction has been described, similar to the pattern known as the red man syndrome seen after rapid infusion of vancomycin. The reaction responded to a histamine H_1 receptor antagonist (75).

Rifampicin can cause a fixed drug eruption (76).

Musculoskeletal

Of 26 patients who received rifabutin 600 mg/day in combination with ethambutol, streptomycin, and either clarithromycin (500 mg bd; $n = 15$) or azithromycin (600 mg/day; $n = 11$), there were rifabutin-related adverse events in 20; these included a diffuse polyarthralgia syndrome in 5 (77).

Immunologic

There is no evidence that rifampicin causes clinically significant deleterious effects on the immune system in humans (78), whereas it can cause immunosuppression in animals (79). Rifampicin partially suppresses cutaneous hypersensitivity to tuberculin and T cell function (80). In 33 patients with leprosy treated with a rifampicin drug combination, a flu-like illness or antibodies to rifampicin-conjugated proteins were not observed (81).

A possible explanation of the association of allergic reactions with intermittent therapy is that during daily regimens the antigen–antibody complexes are continuously cleared from the plasma without reaching a critical concentration, whereas in intermittent regimens, antibody titers can increase markedly during the drug-free days. This is supported by the observation that anti-rifampicin antibodies, measured by the indirect Coombs' test, developed more commonly during intermittent than during daily therapy and that antibodies may disappear from the serum when patients change from intermittent to daily regimens.

Severe anaphylaxis has been reported in two patients with infected wounds that had been treated with topical rifamycin for several months (82). There was urticaria, angioedema, and hypotension in one case, and urticaria, wheezing, dyspnea, and hypotensive shock in the other. In both cases, prick tests with 10% rifamycin solution were positive, while there were no positive reactions in 20 controls.

- A 36-year-old woman developed generalized urticaria during a second course of treatment with rifamycin eye-drops within a month and a 49-year-old man had systemic urticaria, bronchospasm, and hypotension shortly after his surgical wound had been washed with a solution of rifamycin (83). Both patients had positive skin prick tests to rifamycin (1 mg/ml) when tested several weeks after the acute episode, while 10 healthy volunteers had negative tests. The woman also had a positive skin prick test to rifampicin 2 mg/ml, although she had never taken it before.

An HIV-infected patient who developed an anaphylactic reaction to rifampicin tolerated treatment with rifabutin without any adverse event.

The lupus-like syndrome has been reported in seven patients, six of them women who were taking rifampicin ($n = 4$) or rifabutin ($n = 3$) in standard dosages for mycobacterial infections (84). None was HIV-1 positive, none was also taking isoniazid, and although they were taking other antimycobacterial drugs, their symptoms disappeared after withdrawal of the rifamycin alone. All had two or more episodes of fever, malaise, myalgia, and arthralgia, and all had positive antinuclear antibodies. All were also taking either ciprofloxacin or clarithromycin, and the authors speculated that these drugs, which are cytochrome P_{450} enzyme inhibitors, could have increased the serum concentrations of the rifamycins.

Desensitization protocols can be helpful in patients who have had anaphylactic reactions, and the detection of IgE

antibodies to rifampicin may be helpful in clarifying pathogenesis. A switch to a daily regimen, when administration was previously intermittent, may allow resumption of rifampicin without further problems. In 35 HIV-positive patients with previous allergic reactions to rifampicin, oral desensitization was safe and allowed the reintroduction of rifampicin in 60% of cases (85). However, the flu-like syndrome, hemolytic and thrombocytopenic crises, and acute renal insufficiency are not IgE-mediated, and when rifampicin is thought to be indispensable, a course of treatment may be completed under glucocorticoid cover. Four patients with reactions to rifampicin, one with rash, fever, and lymphadenopathy and one with hepatitis, completed courses of antituberculosis therapy for nervous system infections under glucocorticoid cover (86).

Second-Generation Effects

Pregnancy

Rifampicin is currently recommended by the WHO for the treatment of tuberculosis during pregnancy. On the other hand, drug companies advise against the use of rifampicin during the first 3 months of pregnancy, even though deleterious effects on the fetus have not been confirmed in man.

Induction of hepatic microsomal enzymes by rifampicin is believed to be the cause of vitamin K deficiency in pregnancy, leading to hemorrhagic disturbances in pregnant women and their neonates. Prophylactic vitamin K should therefore be given to all mothers and their offspring when the mother has taken rifampicin during late pregnancy. Blood coagulation tests should be done on both (SEDA-8, 288).

Teratogenicity

Rifampicin crosses the placenta, and although teratogenicity is uncertain, it may not be as innocuous during pregnancy as isoniazid or ethambutol (SEDA-6, 277) (87).

Lactation

Lactation is not a contraindication to rifampicin; only small amounts pass into the milk with no relevant effects on the newborn (88).

Susceptibility Factors

Renal disease

Impaired renal function has to be taken into consideration when calculating the dosage of rifampicin (89).

Hepatic disease

Pre-existing liver damage has to be taken into consideration when calculating the dosage of rifampicin (90).

Other features of the patient

Chronic alcoholism is an important risk factor for adverse effects of the rifamycins. In 79 consecutive patients taking rifampicin in combination with isoniazid and another drug, there was a high incidence of acute clinical liver disease; about half of the patients were advanced alcoholics and almost all the cases of hepatitis came from this group (91). Most of those with pretreatment abnormalities of liver function had abnormalities in liver biopsies, not attributable to alcohol. In one patient, active chronic hepatitis was attributed to rifampicin.

However, in 531 eligible patients enrolled in a US Public Health Service Cooperative Trial of Short-Course Chemotherapy of Pulmonary Tuberculosis, of whom 58% were classified as alcoholic, although the alcoholics had more abnormal concentrations of aspartate transaminase before and during therapy, there was no significant difference between the alcoholics and non-alcoholics in the incidence of adverse reactions, including hepatotoxic reactions (92). The authors concluded that in the absence of clinically significant and persistent pretreatment abnormalities of hepatic function tests, rifampicin and isoniazid are not contraindicated in patients categorized as alcoholic.

In patients with suspected disorders of vitamin D and calcium metabolism, caution has to be taken (SEDA-9, 269).

Drug Administration

Drug overdose

Severe overdosage has been observed in inadvertent administration of an excessive dose of rifampicin in children (93) and also in suicide attempts (94,95). It can also occur when there is impaired hepatic function or severe renal insufficiency. Symptoms are nausea, vomiting, headache, abdominal pain, diarrhea, and pruritus.

Drug–Drug Interactions

Amiodarone

Rifampicin has been reported to reduce the effects of amiodarone (96).

- A 33-year-old woman was given rifampicin to suppress an MRSA infection of a pacing system that could not be removed. She was already taking amiodarone which, with the pacing system, was intended to manage her complex dysrhythmias. The introduction of antibiotic therapy was followed by an increase in bouts of palpitation and in shocks from her defibrillator. Her amiodarone concentrations had fallen and returned to the target range, with disappearance of her symptoms, when the rifampicin was withdrawn.

The authors discussed the possible reasons for this interaction, including a reduction in systemic availability of amiodarone or induction of metabolism by rifampicin.

Antacids

Antacids, particularly aluminium hydroxide gel, magnesium trisilicate, and sodium bicarbonate, reduce the systemic availability of rifampicin (97).

Antiretroviral drugs

The recommendations of the Center for Disease Control and Prevention in Atlanta regarding the use of antituberculosis drugs in combination with antiretroviral drugs have been published (98). In general, the use of rifampicin in patients taking protease inhibitors is contraindicated, except in the following circumstances:

- patients taking the NNRTI efavirenz and two NRTIs;
- patients taking the protease inhibitor ritonavir and one or more NRTIs;
- patients taking a combination of the two protease inhibitors ritonavir and saquinavir.

However, Roche Pharma have recommended that rifampicin should not be used in patients who are taking ritonavir + saquinavir, because of the results of a study in which 11 of 28 patients who took rifampicin 300 mg/day with ritonavir 100 mg bd + saquiniavir 1000 mg bd developed severe hepatotoxicity [http://www.fda.gov/medwatch/safety/2005/Saquinavir-Rifampin_deardoc_Feb05].

The use of rifampicin with the protease inhibitors indinavir, nelfinavir, and amprenavir is contraindicated. However, these agents can be used with rifabutin after appropriate dosage reduction. Failure to reduce the dosage of rifabutin can result in toxic manifestations, such arthralgia and uveitis.

Rifamycins can be used with the NNRTIs nevirapine or efavirenz, but not with delavirdine.

Data on drug pharmacokinetics and drug interactions in patients taking treatment for HIV infection and tuberculosis are scanty, and the current recommendations are almost certain to be modified in the near future. Furthermore, it may be prudent to monitor rifampicin concentrations in the event of intolerance or adverse drug reactions.

Barbiturates

Barbiturates, which induce liver drug-metabolizing enzymes, increase the rate of metabolism of rifampicin (99).

Cardiac glycosides

In eight healthy volunteers rifampicin reduced digoxin plasma concentrations (100), mirroring clinical experience. The authors hypothesized that this effect may be brought about by induction of P-glycoprotein, which increases excretion of digoxin into the gut lumen; however, renal digoxin clearance, which is also mediated by P-glycoprotein, was not affected. In these healthy volunteers, rifampicin reduced digoxin concentrations by about 50%, so the interaction is likely to be clinically important.

Digitoxin plasma concentrations can be reduced by rifampicin, and the dosage should be adjusted according to the serum concentration (SEDA-10, 272).

Ciclosporin

Increased dosages of ciclosporin are recommended when patients take rifampicin (SEDA-21, 314). In one study it was necessary to increase the dosage of ciclosporin from 225 to 800 mg/day during treatment with rifampicin and for 7 days afterwards in order to maintain therapeutic concentrations (101). Low ciclosporin blood concentrations and acute graft rejection have been observed in a renal transplant recipient during prophylactic rifampicin therapy (102).

Clarithromycin

Severe interactions have been observed when rifabutin and clarithromycin were given simultaneously (103). The mean concentrations of rifabutin and 25-*O*-desacetyl-rifabutin in healthy subjects who took clarithromycin and rifabutin concomitantly were respectively more than 4 times and 37 times greater than the concentrations recorded when rifabutin was administered alone. Neutropenia was detected in 14 of 18 subjects taking rifabutin. Myalgia and high fever were also common. In another study, clarithromycin increased the AUC of rifabutin by 76% (104). Physicians should be aware that recommended prophylactic doses of rifabutin can be associated with severe neutropenia within 2 weeks after the start of therapy, and all patients taking rifabutin, especially with clarithromycin, should be monitored carefully for neutropenia.

Clofibrate

The interaction of rifampicin with clofibrate has been reviewed (105). Rifampicin induces the metabolism of clofibrate, and in five subjects rifampicin 600 mg/day caused a 35% fall in steady-state serum clofibrate concentrations (106).

Clonidine

Rifampicin 600 mg/day had no effect on the pharmacokinetics of clonidine 0.4 mg/day in six healthy subjects (105,107).

Clozapine

Rifampicin can reduce plasma concentrations of clozapine and exacerbate psychotic symptoms (108).

Contrast media

Excretion of contrast media through the bile can be impaired by rifampicin (1,82).

Corticosteroids

Rifampicin enhances the catabolism of many glucocorticoids. For example, it increases the plasma clearance of prednisolone by 45% and may reduce the amount of drug available to the tissues by as much as 66% (SEDA-8, 288). Glucocorticoid therapy for concomitant diseases should therefore be adjusted in the light of plasma concentrations and clinical effects during rifampicin treatment (SEDA-10, 272). For example, rejection of a kidney transplant occurred after 7 weeks of rifampicin therapy (109).

Co-trimoxazole

In patients taking co-trimoxazole, rifampicin in a standard oral antituberculosis regimen (600 mg/day plus isoniazid 300 mg/day and pyrazinamide 30 mg/kg for more than 12 days) reduced the steady-state AUC of trimethoprim and sulfamethoxazole by 47 and 23% respectively (110). The same authors had previously reported reduced efficacy of co-trimoxazole in the prevention of toxoplasmosis in HIV-infected subjects (111). The reduction in prophylactic efficiency was more pronounced in subjects who took a single double-strength tablet.

There have been no reports on the risk of *Pneumocystis jiroveci* pneumonia in patients taking rifampicin plus co-trimoxazole prophylaxis. Until such time as more data are available, it is prudent to use double-strength co-trimoxazole tablets twice daily for prophylaxis of toxoplasmosis and *P. jiroveci* pneumonia in patients taking concomitant rifampicin.

Coumarin anticoagulants

Coumarin anticoagulants undergo accelerated metabolism in patients taking rifampicin (112). Rifampicin greatly increases the clearance of warfarin by inducing hepatic enzymes, and difficulty in achieving an optimal INR despite an increase in the dose of warfarin has been highlighted (113). In patients taking rifampicin, warfarin should be started in dosages of 20–30 mg/day for two days, subsequently adjusting the dose according to the prothrombin time; a daily maintenance dose of 20 mg may be required (114) and close monitoring is required during the initial weeks to achieve a therapeutic INR (115). Offset of the interaction when rifampicin is withdrawn can take as long as 4–5 weeks, during which time the dose of warfarin should be reduced gradually to avoid a high INR and bleeding complications.

Dapsone

The interaction of rifampicin with dapsone has been reviewed (105). In seven patients with leprosy, rifampicin shortened the half-life of dapsone by 50% (116).

Diazepam

The interaction of rifampicin with diazepam has been reviewed (105). The mean half-life of diazepam fell from 58 to 14 hours in seven patients who took isoniazid, rifampicin, and ethambutol (117).

Fluconazole

Fluconazole increased the AUC of rifabutin by 76% (104).

Haloperidol

Blood concentrations of haloperidol are reduced during rifampicin administration, owing to shortening of the half-life of haloperidol (SEDA-12, 258) (118).

Ketoconazole

Ketoconazole interacts with rifampicin, and the serum concentrations of both drugs are reduced (SEDA-9, 269).

Methadone

Methadone metabolism is increased and a withdrawal syndrome has been reported (1).

Mexiletine

The interaction of rifampicin with mexiletine has been reviewed (105). The mean half-life of a single dose of mexiletine 400 mg fell from 8.5 to 5 hours in eight healthy subjects who took rifampicin 600 mg/day for 10 days (119).

Nifedipine

The elimination of nifedipine is enhanced by rifampicin (SEDA-14, 259).

Oral contraceptives

The serum concentrations of ethinylestradiol and similar steroids used as contraceptives are reduced during rifampicin therapy; it is therefore not surprising that unexpected pregnancies have occurred (120). The effects of rifampicin have been compared with those of rifabutin (increasingly used for the treatment of atypical mycobacterial infections) in a double-blind, crossover study in 12 women who were taking a stable oral contraceptive regimen containing ethinylestradiol and norethindrone (121). Rifampicin had the greater effect in reducing the mean AUC, but none of the subjects ovulated during the cycle in which either of the rifamycins was administered.

Oral hypoglycemic agents

Oral hypoglycemic agents (glibenclamide, gliclazide, repaglinide, and rosiglitazone) undergo accelerated metabolism in patients taking rifampicin (112).

The addition of rifampicin to glimepiride (metabolized by CYP2C9) produced only a modest reduction in AUC and no significant effect on blood glucose (122).

Phenazone

Rifampicin significantly reduces the half-life of phenazone (antipyrine) (123).

Probenecid

Probenecid can increase the serum concentration of rifampicin; this can reduce costs and hepatotoxicity in long-term therapy (124). Interactions of rifampicin with probenecid have been reviewed (105).

Propranolol

The metabolism of propranolol is enhanced by rifampicin (SEDA-9, 269).

Quinidine

Quinidine plasma concentrations can be lowered by rifampicin because of enzyme induction (125).

Repaglinide

Co-administration of rifampicin with repaglinide considerably lowers the concentration of repaglinide and alters its therapeutic effect in diabetes mellitus (126). In nine healthy volunteers, the maximum reduction in blood glucose after a single 0.5 mg dose of repaglinide fell from 1.6 to 1.0 mmol/l after pretreatment with rifampicin for 5 days. This presumably occurred by induction of CYP3A4.

Statins

In healthy subjects taking rifampicin the C_{max} and AUC of simvastatin were greatly reduced (127), presumably by enzyme induction. It is likely that other HMG-CoA reductase inhibitors, including lovastatin and atorvastatin, also have clinically significant interactions with rifampicin.

Tacrolimus

An interaction of rifampicin with tacrolimus has been documented (128,129).

- A 61-year-old Chinese renal transplant recipient, who had taken tacrolimus for 1 year after an episode of rejection had failed to respond to ciclosporin, took rifampicin and 12 days later had an episode of biopsy-proven graft rejection, associated with very low serum tacrolimus concentrations.
- A 50-year-old woman, a renal transplant recipient, developed a brain abscess due to *Nocardia otitidiscaviarum* after craniotomy and was given meropenem and rifampicin. The dose of tacrolimus had to be increased three-fold to maintain adequate trough concentrations.

Theophylline

Rifampicin increases the metabolic clearance of theophylline by 45%, especially after intravenous use (130,131).

Thyroxine

Induction of cytochrome P_{450} may be the explanation for a modest increase in the clearance of levothyroxine (10–15%) which may necessitate an increase in dosage. In two cases, rifampicin led to significant increases in TSH concentrations in patients being treated for hypothyroidism (30).

Trimethoprim

The interaction of rifampicin with trimethoprim has been reviewed (105). Rifampicin has a small effect on the clearance of trimethoprim but it is not clinically significant (132,133).

Interference with Diagnostic Tests

von Jaksch test

Rifampicin metabolites in urine can cause a false positive test for melanin when assessed with the von Jaksch test (134).

References

1. Mandell GL, Sande MA. Antimicrobial agents: drugs used in the chemotherapy of tuberculosis and leprosy. In: Goodman Gilman A, Rall TW, Nies AS, Taylor P, editors. Goodman and Gilman's The Pharmacological Basis of Therapeutics. 8th ed. Chapter 49. New York: Pergamon Press, 1990:1146.
2. Darouiche RO, Raad II, Heard SO, Thornby JI, Wenker OC, Gabrielli A, Berg J, Khardori N, Hanna H, Hachem R, Harris RL, Mayhall G. A comparison of two antimicrobial-impregnated central venous catheters. Catheter Study Group. N Engl J Med 1999;340(1):1–8.
3. Wenzel RP, Edmond MB. The evolving technology of venous access. N Engl J Med 1999;340(1):48–50.
4. Hand WL, Boozer RM, King-Thompson NL. Antibiotic uptake by alveolar macrophages of smokers. Antimicrob Agents Chemother 1985;27(1):42–5.

5. Newton RW, Forrest AR. Rifampicin overdosage—"the red man syndrome". Scott Med J 1975;20(2):55–6.

6. Immanuel C, Jayasankar K, Narayana AS, Santha T, Sundaram V, Sarma GR. Induction of rifampicin metabolism during treatment of tuberculous patients with daily and fully intermittent regimens containing the drug. Indian J Chest Dis Allied Sci 1989;31(4):251–7.

7. Wurtz RM, Abrams D, Becker S, Jacobson MA, Mass MM, Marks SH. Anaphylactoid drug reactions to ciprofloxacin and rifampicin in HIV-infected patients. Lancet 1989;1(8644):955–6.

8. Pujet JC, Homberg JC, Decroix G. Sensitivity to rifampicin: incidence, mechanism, and prevention. BMJ 1974;2(916):415–18.

9. Stevens E, Bloemmen F, Mbuyi JM, Gyselen A, Mattson K, Hellström H, Riska N. Aspects immunologiques des reactions secondaires a la rifampicine. [Immunological aspects of reactions caused by rifampicin (proceedings).] Bull Int Union Tuberc 1979;54(2):179–80.

10. Vaz M, Jacob AJ, Rajendran A. "Flu" syndrome on once monthly rifampicin: a case report. Lepr Rev 1989;60(4):300–2.

11. Martinez E, Collazos J, Mayo J. Hypersensitivity reactions to rifampin. Pathogenetic mechanisms, clinical manifestations, management strategies, and review of the anaphylactic-like reactions. Medicine (Baltimore) 1999;78(6):361–9.

12. Masur H. Recommendations on prophylaxis and therapy for disseminated *Mycobacterium avium* complex disease in patients infected with the human immunodeficiency virus. Public Health Service Task Force on Prophylaxis and Therapy for Mycobacterium avium Complex. N Engl J Med 1993;329(12):898–904.

13. Havlir D, Torriani F, Dube M. Uveitis associated with rifabutin prophylaxis. Ann Intern Med 1994;121(7):510–12.

14. Hafner R, Bethel J, Standiford HC, Follansbee S, Cohn DL, Polk RE, Mole L, Raasch R, Kumar P, Mushatt D, Drusano G; DATRI 001B Study Group. Tolerance and pharmacokinetic interactions of rifabutin and azithromycin. Antimicrob Agents Chemother 2001;45(5):1572–7.

15. Ramachandran A, Bhatia VN. Rifampicin induced shock—a case report. Indian J Lepr 1990;62(2):228–9.

16. Martinez E, Collazos J, Mayo J. Shock and cerebral infarct after rifampin re-exposure in a patient infected with human immunodeficiency virus. Clin Infect Dis 1998;27(5):1329–30.

17. Kissling M, Xilinas M. Rimactan parenteral formulation in clinical use. J Int Med Res 1981;9(6):459–69.

18. Singapore Tuberculosis Service and British Medical Research Council. Controlled trial of intermittent regimens of rifampicin plus isoniazid for pulmonary tuberculosis in Singapore. Lancet 1975;2(7945):1105–9.

19. Anastasatu C, Bungeteanu G, Sibila S. The intermittent chemotherapy of tuberculosis with rifampicin regimens on ambulatory basis. Scand J Respir Dis Suppl 1973;84:136–9.

20. Kunichika N, Miyahara N, Kotani K, Takeyama H, Harada M, Tanimoto M. Pneumonitis induced by rifampicin. Thorax 2002;57(11):1000–1.

21. Artaza A, Gallofre M, Arboix M, Laporte JR. Niveles de la rifampicina en liquido cefalorraquideo en cuadros de inflammacion meningea. [Rifampicin levels in cerebrospinal fluid in meningeal inflammation.] Arch Farmacol Toxicol 1983;9(1):121–4.

22. Pratt TH. Rifampin-induced organic brain syndrome. JAMA 1979;241(22):2421–2.

23. Moorthy RS, Valluri S, Jampol LM. Drug-induced uveitis. Surv Ophthalmol 1998;42(6):557–70.

24. Kelleher P, Helbert M, Sweeney J, Anderson J, Parkin J, Pinching A. Uveitis associated with rifabutin and macrolide therapy for *Mycobacterium avium* intracellulare infection in AIDS patients. Genitourin Med 1996;72(6):419–21.

25. Shafran SD, Singer J, Zarowny DP, Phillips P, Salit I, Walmsley SL, Fong IW, Gill MJ, Rachlis AR, Lalonde RG, Fanning MM, Tsoukas CM. A comparison of two regimens for the treatment of *Mycobacterium avium* complex bacteremia in AIDS: rifabutin, ethambutol, and clarithromycin versus rifampin, ethambutol, clofazimine, and ciprofloxacin. Canadian HIV Trials Network Protocol 010 Study Group. N Engl J Med 1996;335(6):377–83.

26. Tseng AL, Walmsley SL. Rifabutin-associated uveitis. Ann Pharmacother 1995;29(11):1149–55.

27. Committee on Safety of Medicines and the Medicines Control Agency. Revised indication and drug interaction of rifabutin. Curr Prob Pharmacovig 1997;23:14.

28. Anonymous. Drug-induced uveitis can usually be easily managed. Drugs Ther Perspect 1998;11:11–14.

29. Kyriazopoulou V, Parparousi O, Vagenakis AG. Rifampicin-induced adrenal crisis in Addisonian patients receiving corticosteroid replacement therapy. J Clin Endocrinol Metab 1984;59(6):1204–6.

30. Nolan SR, Self TH, Norwood JM. Interaction between rifampin and levothyroxine. South Med J 1999;92(5):529–31.

31. Williams SE, Wardman AG, Taylor GA, Peacock M, Cooke NJ. Long term study of the effect of rifampicin and isoniazid on vitamin D metabolism. Tubercle 1985;66(1):49–54.

32. Toppet M, Vainsel M, Cantraine F, Franckson M. Evolution de la phosphatase alcaline sérique sous traitement d'isoniazide et de rifampicine. [Course of serum alkaline phosphatase during treatment with isoniazid and rifampicin.] Arch Fr Pediatr 1985;42(2):79–80.

33. Millar JW. Rifampicin-induced porphyria cutanea tarda. Br J Dis Chest 1980;74(4):405–8.

34. Conen D, Blumberg A, Weber S, Schubothe H. Hämolytische Krise und akutes Nierenversagen unter Rifampicin. [Hemolytic crisis and acute kidney failure from rifampicin.] Schweiz Med Wochenschr 1979;109(15):558–62.

35. De Vriese AS, Robbrecht DL, Vanholder RC, Vogelaers DP, Lameire NH. Rifampicin-associated acute renal failure: pathophysiologic, immunologic, and clinical features. Am J Kidney Dis 1998;31(1):108–15.

36. Shishido Y, Nagayama N, Masuda K, Baba M, Tamura A, Nagai H, Akagawa S, Kawabe Y, Machida K, Kurashima A, Komatsu H, Yotsumoto H. [Agranulocytosis due to anti-tuberculosis drugs including isoniazid (INH) and rifampicin (RFP)—a report of four cases and review of the literature.] Kekkaku 2003;78(11):683–9.

37. van Assendelft AH. Leucopenia caused by two rifampicin preparations. Eur J Respir Dis 1984;65(4):251–8.

38. Pereira J, Hidalgo P, Ocqueteau M, Blacutt M, Marchesse M, Nien Y, Letelier L, Mezzano D. Glycoprotein Ib/IX complex is the target in rifampicin-induced immune thrombocytopenia. Br J Haematol 2000;110(4):907–10.

39. Chouraqui JP, Bessard G, Favier M, Kolodie L, Rambaud P. Hémorragie par avitaminose K chez la femme enceinte et le nouveau-né. [Haemorrhage associated with vitamin K deficiency in pregnant women and newborns. Relationship with rifampicin therapy in two cases.] Therapie 1982;37(4):447–50.

40. Ip M, Cheng KP, Cheung WC. Disseminated intravascular coagulopathy associated with rifampicin. Tubercle 1991;72(4):291–3.

41. Souza CS, Alberto FL, Foss NT. Disseminated intravascular coagulopathy as an adverse reaction to intermittent rifampin schedule in the treatment of leprosy. Int J Lepr Other Mycobact Dis 1997;65(3):366–71.

42. van Assendelft AH. Leucopenia in rifampicin chemotherapy. J Antimicrob Chemother 1985;16(3):407–8.

43. Diamond JR, Tahan SR. IgG-mediated intravascular hemolysis and nonoliguric acute renal failure complicating discontinuous rifampicin administration. Nephron 1984;38(1):62–4.

44. Tahan SR, Diamond JR, Blank JM, Horan RF. Acute hemolysis and renal failure with rifampicin-dependent antibodies after discontinuous administration. Transfusion 1985;25(2):124–7.

45. Criel A, Verwilghen RL. Intravascular haemolysis and renal failure caused by intermittent rifampicin treatment. Blut 1980;40(2):147–50.

46. Hoigne R, Biedermann HP, Naegeli HR. INH-induzierter systemischer Lupus Erythematodes: 2 Beobachtungen mit Reexposition. Schweiz Med Wochenschr 1975;105(50):1726.

47. Rothfield NF, Bierer WF, Garfield JW. Isoniazid induction of antinuclear antibodies. A prospective study. Ann Intern Med 1978;88(5):650–2.

48. George JN, Raskob GE, Shah SR, Rizvi MA, Hamilton SA, Osborne S, Vondracek T. Drug-induced thrombocytopenia: a systematic review of published case reports. Ann Intern Med 1998;129(11):886–90.

49. Zargar SA, Thapa BR, Sahni A, Mehta S. Rifampicin-induced upper gastrointestinal bleeding. Postgrad Med J 1990;66(774):310–11.

50. Smith SJ, Lee AJ, Maddix DS, Chow AW. Pill-induced esophagitis caused by oral rifampin. Ann Pharmacother 1999;33(1):27–31.

51. Moriarty HJ, Scobie BA. Pseudomembranous colitis in a patient on rifampicin and ethambutol. NZ Med J 1980;91(658):294–5.

52. Pessayre D. Present views on isoniazid and isoniazid-rifampicin hepatitis. Agressologie 1982;23(A):13–5.

53. Ji BH, Chen JK, Wang CM, Xia GA. Hepatotoxicity of combined therapy with rifampicin and daily prothionamide for leprosy. Lepr Rev 1984;55(3):283–9.

54. Mandell GL, Sande MA. Antimicrobial agents: drugs used in the chemotherapy of tuberculosis and leprosy. In: Goodman LS, Gilman A. The Pharmacological Basis of Therapeutics. 6th ed. New York: Macmillan Publishing Co Inc, 1980:1200.

55. Mitchell I, Wendon J, Fitt S, Williams R. Anti-tuberculous therapy and acute liver failure. Lancet 1995;345(8949):555–6.

56. Linna O, Uhari M. Hepatotoxicity of rifampicin and isoniazid in children treated for tuberculosis. Eur J Pediatr 1980;134(3):227–9.

57. Prince MI, Burt AD, Jones DE. Hepatitis and liver dysfunction with rifampicin therapy for pruritus in primary biliary cirrhosis. Gut 2002;50(3):436–9.

58. Berg JD, Pandov HI, Sammons HG. Serum total bile acid levels in patients receiving rifampicin and isoniazid. Ann Clin Biochem 1984;21(Pt 3):218–22.

59. Kar HK, Roy RG. Reversible acute renal failure due to monthly administration of rifampicin in a leprosy patient. Indian J Lepr 1984;56(4):835–9.

60. Mauri JM, Fort J, Bartolome J, Camps J, Capdevila L, Morlans M, Martin-Vega C, Piera L. Antirifampicin antibodies in acute rifampicin-associated renal failure. Nephron 1982;31(2):177–9.

61. Warrington RJ, Hogg GR, Paraskevas F, Tse KS. Insidious rifampin-associated renal failure with light-chain proteinuria. Arch Intern Med 1977;137(7):927–30.

62. Winter RJ, Banks RA, Collins CM, Hoffbrand BI. Rifampicin induced light chain proteinuria and renal failure. Thorax 1984;39(12):952–3.

63. Cohn JR, Fye DL, Sills JM, Francos GC. Rifampicin-induced renal failure. Tubercle 1985;66(4):289–93.

64. Covic A, Goldsmith DJ, Segall L, Stoicescu C, Lungu S, Volovat C, Covic M. Rifampicin-induced acute renal failure: a series of 60 patients. Nephrol Dial Transplant 1998;13(4):924–9.

65. Covic A, Gusbeth-Tatomir P, Tarevici Z, Mihaescu T, Covic M. Insuficientă renală acută post-rifampicină—complicatie redutabilă însă putin cunoscută a tratamentulvi tuberculostatic. [Post-rifampicin acute renal failure—serious, but seldom recognized complication of the anti-tuberculosis treatment.] Pneumologia 2001;50(4):225–31.

66. Munteanu L, Golea O, Nicolicioiu M, Tudorache V. Particularitatile insuficientei renale acute (IRA) la bolnavii tratati cu rifampicină. [Specific features of acute renal failure in patients treated with rifampicin.] Pneumologia 2002;51(1):15–20.

67. Prakash J, Kumar NS, Saxena RK, Verma U. Acute renal failure complicating rifampicin therapy. J Assoc Physicians India 2001;49:877–80.

68. Muthukumar T, Jayakumar M, Fernando EM, Muthusethupathi MA. Acute renal failure due to rifampicin: a study of 25 patients. Am J Kidney Dis 2002;40(4):690–6.

69. Bassilios N, Vantelon C, Baumelou A, Deray G. Continuous rifampicin administration inducing acute renal failure. Nephrol Dial Transplant 2001;16(1):190–1.

70. Ogata H, Kubo M, Tamaki K, Hirakata H, Okuda S, Fujishima M. Crescentic glomerulonephritis due to rifampin treatment in a patient with pulmonary atypical mycobacteriosis. Nephron 1998;78(3):319–22.

71. Yoshioka K, Satake N, Kasamatsu Y, Nakamura Y, Shikata N. Rapidly progressive glomerulonephritis due to rifampicin therapy. Nephron 2002;90(1):116–18.

72. Lee CW, Lim JH, Kang HJ. Pemphigus foliaceus induced by rifampicin. Br J Dermatol 1984;111(5):619–22.

73. Miyagawa S, Yamashina Y, Okuchi T, Konoike Y, Kano T, Sakamoto K. Exacerbation of pemphigus by rifampicin. Br J Dermatol 1986;114(6):729–32.

74. Prazuck T, Fisch A, Simonnet F, Noat G. Lyell's syndrome associated with rifampicin therapy of tuberculosis in an AIDS patient. Scand J Infect Dis 1990;22(5):629.

75. Nahata MC, Fan-Havard P, Barson WJ, Bartkowski HM, Kosnik EJ. Pharmacokinetics, cerebrospinal fluid concentration, and safety of intravenous rifampin in pediatric patients undergoing shunt placements. Eur J Clin Pharmacol 1990;38(5):515–17.

76. John SS. Fixed drug eruption due to rifampin. Lepr Rev 1998;69(4):397–9.

77. Griffith DE, Brown BA, Girard WM, Wallace RJ Jr. Adverse events associated with high-dose rifabutin in macrolide-containing regimens for the treatment of Mycobacterium avium complex lung disease Clin Infect Dis 1995;21(3):594–8.

78. Farr B, Mandell GL. Rifampin. Med Clin North Am 1982;66(1):157–68.

79. Bassi L, Di Berardino L, Arioli V, Silvestri LG, Ligniere EL. Conditions for immunosuppression by rifampicin. J Infect Dis 1973;128(6):736–44.

80. Dickinson JM, Aber VR, Mitchison DA. Bactericidal activity of streptomycin, isoniazid, rifampin, ethambutol, and pyrazinamide alone and in combination against Mycobacterium tuberculosis: Am Rev Respir Dis 1977;116(4):627–35.

81. Rook GA. Absence from sera from normal individuals or from rifampin-treated leprosy patients (THELEP trials) of antibody to rifamycin-protein or rifamycin-membrane conjugates. Int J Lepr Other Mycobact Dis 1985;53(1):22–7.

82. Baciewicz AM, Self TH, Bekemeyer WB. Update on rifampin drug interactions. Arch Intern Med 1987;147(3):565–8.

83. Garcia F, Blanco J, Carretero P, Herrero D, Juste S, Garces M, Perez R, Fuentes M. Anaphylactic reactions to topical rifamycin. Allergy 1999;54(5):527–8.

84. Berning SE, Iseman MD. Rifamycin-induced lupus syndrome. Lancet 1997;349(9064):1521–2.

85. Arrizabalaga J, Casas A, Camino X, Iribarren JA, Rodriguez Arrondo F, Von Wichmann MA. Utilidad de la desensibilizacion a rifampicina en el tratamiento de enfermedades producidas por micobacterias en pacientes con SIDA. [The usefulness of the desensitization to rifampin in the treatment of mycobacterial disease in patients with AIDS.] Med Clin (Barc) 1998;111(3):103–4.

86. Morris H, Muckerjee J, Akhtar S, Abdullahi L, Harrison M, Scott G. Use of corticosteroids to suppress drug toxicity in complicated tuberculosis. J Infect 1999;39(3):237–40.

87. Siskind MS, Thienemann D, Kirlin L. Isoniazid-induced neurotoxicity in chronic dialysis patients: report of three cases and a review of the literature. Nephron 1993;64(2):303–6.

88. Paumgartner G. Medikamente in der Muttermilch. Pharma-Kritik (Switzerland) 1979;1:53.

89. Acocella G. Clinical pharmacokinetics of rifampicin. Clin Pharmacokinet 1978;3(2):108–27.

90. Bergamini N, Fowst G, Rifamycin SV. A review. Arzneimittelforschung 1965;15(Suppl 8):951–1002.

91. Thompson JE. The effect of rifampicin on liver morphology in tuberculous alcoholics. Aust NZ J Med 1976;6(2):111–6.

92. Cross FS, Long MW, Banner AS, Snider DE Jr. Rifampin-isoniazid therapy of alcoholic and nonalcoholic tuberculous patients in a U.S. Public Health Service Cooperative Therapy Trial. Am Rev Respir Dis 1980;122(2):349–53.

93. Bolan G, Laurie RE, Broome CV. Red man syndrome: inadvertent administration of an excessive dose of rifampin to children in a day-care center. Pediatrics 1986;77(5):633–5.

94. Broadwell RO, Broadwell SD, Comer PB. Suicide by rifampin overdose. JAMA 1978;240(21):2283–4.

95. Meisel S, Brower R. Rifampin: a suicidal dose. Ann Intern Med 1980;92(2 Pt 1):262–3.

96. Zarembski DG, Fischer SA, Santucci PA, Porter MT, Costanzo MR, Trohman RG. Impact of rifampin on serum amiodarone concentrations in a patient with congenital heart disease. Pharmacotherapy 1999;19(2):249–51.

97. Khalil SAH, El-Khordagui LK, El-Gholmy ZA. Effect of antacids on oral absorption of rifampicin. Int J Pharm 1984;20:99.

98. Centers for Disease Control and Prevention (CDC). Updated guidelines for the use of rifabutin or rifampin for the treatment and prevention of tuberculosis among HIV-infected patients taking protease inhibitors or nonnucleoside reverse transcriptase inhibitors. MMWR Morb Mortal Wkly Rep 2000;49(9):185–9.

99. Duroux P. Surveillance et accidents de la chimiothérapie antituberculeuse. [Surveillance and complications of antituberculosis chemotherapy.] Rev Prat 1979;29(33):2681–90.

100. Greiner B, Eichelbaum M, Fritz P, Kreichgauer HP, von Richter O, Zundler J, Kroemer HK. The role of intestinal P-glycoprotein in the interaction of digoxin and rifampin. J Clin Invest 1999;104(2):147–53.

101. Capone D, Aiello C, Santoro GA, Gentile A, Stanziale P, D'Alessandro R, Imperatore P, Basile V. Drug interaction between cyclosporine and two antimicrobial agents, josamycin and rifampicin, in organ-transplanted patients. Int J Clin Pharmacol Res 1996;16(2–3):73–6.

102. Offermann G, Keller F, Molzahn M. Low cyclosporin A blood levels and acute graft rejection in a renal transplant recipient during rifampin treatment. Am J Nephrol 1985;5(5):385–7.

103. Rubinstein E. Comparative safety of the different macrolides. Int J Antimicrob Agents 2001;18(Suppl 1):S71–6.

104. Jordan MK, Polis MA, Kelly G, Narang PK, Masur H, Piscitelli SC. Effects of fluconazole and clarithromycin on rifabutin and 25-O-desacetylrifabutin pharmacokinetics. Antimicrob Agents Chemother 2000;44(8):2170–2.

105. Baciewicz AM, Self TH. Rifampin drug interactions. Arch Intern Med 1984;144(8):1667–71.

106. Houin G, Tillement JP. Clofibrate and enzymatic induction in man. Int J Clin Pharmacol Biopharm 1978;16(4):150–4.

107. Affrime MB, Lowenthal DT, Rufo M. Failure of rifampin to induce the metabolism of clonidine in normal volunteers. Drug Intell Clin Pharm 1981;15(12):964–6.

108. Joos AA, Frank UG, Kaschka WP. Pharmacokinetic interaction of clozapine and rifampicin in a forensic patient with an atypical mycobacterial infection. J Clin Psychopharmacol 1998;18(1):83–5.

109. Pallardo L, Moreno R, Garcia Martinez J, et al. Rechado agudo tardio del injerto renal inducido por rifampicina. Nefrologia 1987;7:93.

110. Ribera E, Pou L, Fernandez-Sola A, Campos F, Lopez RM, Ocana I, Ruiz I, Pahissa A. Rifampin reduces concentrations of trimethoprim and sulfamethoxazole in serum in human immunodeficiency virus-infected patients. Antimicrob Agents Chemother 2001;45(11):3238–41.

111. Ribera E, Fernandez-Sola A, Juste C, Rovira A, Romero FJ, Armadans-Gil L, Ruiz I, Ocana I, Pahissa A. Comparison of high and low doses of trimethoprim-sulfamethoxazole for primary prevention of toxoplasmic encephalitis in human immunodeficiency virus-infected patients. Clin Infect Dis 1999;29(6):1461–6.

112. Held H. Interaktion von Rifampicin mit Phenprocoumon: Beobachtungen bei tuberkulosekranken Patienten. [Interaction of rifampicin with phenprocoumon.] Dtsch Med Wochenschr 1979;104(37):1311–14.

113. Lee CR, Thrasher KA. Difficulties in anticoagulation management during coadministration of warfarin and rifampin. Pharmacotherapy 2001;21(10):1240–6.

114. Casner PR. Inability to attain oral anticoagulation: warfarin-rifampin interaction revisited. South Med J 1996;89(12):1200–3.

115. Cropp JS, Bussey HI. A review of enzyme induction of warfarin metabolism with recommendations for patient management. Pharmacotherapy 1997;17(5):917–28.

116. Krishna DR, Appa Rao AVN, Ramanakar TV, Prabhakar MC. Pharmacokinetic interaction between dapsone and rifampicin (rifampin) in leprosy patients. Drug Dev Ind Pharm 1986;12:443–9.

117. Ochs HR, Greenblatt DJ, Roberts GM, Dengler HJ. Diazepam interaction with antituberculosis drugs. Clin Pharmacol Ther 1981;29(5):671–8.

118. Takeda M, Nishinuma K, Yamashita S, Matsubayashi T, Tanino S, Nishimura T. Serum haloperidol levels of schizophrenics receiving treatment for tuberculosis. Clin Neuropharmacol 1986;9(4):386–97.

119. Pentikainen PJ, Koivula IH, Hiltunen HA. Effect of rifampicin treatment on the kinetics of mexiletine. Eur J Clin Pharmacol 1982;23(3):261–6.

120. Skolnick JL, Stoler BS, Katz DB, Anderson WH. Rifampin, oral contraceptives, and pregnancy. JAMA 1976;236(12):1382.

121. Barditch-Crovo P, Trapnell CB, Ette E, Zacur HA, Coresh J, Rocco LE, Hendrix CW, Flexner C. The effects of rifampin and rifabutin on the pharmacokinetics and pharmacodynamics of a combination oral contraceptive. Clin Pharmacol Ther 1999;65(4):428–38.

122. Niemi M, Kivisto KT, Backman JT, Neuvonen PJ. Effect of rifampicin on the pharmacokinetics and pharmacodynamics of glimepiride. Br J Clin Pharmacol 2000;50(6):591–5.

123. Teunissen MW, Bakker W, Meerburg-Van der Torren JE, Breimer DD. Influence of rifampicin treatment on antipyrine clearance and metabolite formation in patients with tuberculosis. Br J Clin Pharmacol 1984;18(5):701–6.

124. Pankaj R, Lal S, Rao RS. Effect of probenecid on serum rifampicin levels. Indian J Lepr 1985;57(2):329–33.

125. Damkier P, Hansen LL, Brosen K. Rifampicin treatment greatly increases the apparent oral clearance of quinidine. Pharmacol Toxicol 1999;85(6):257–62.

126. Niemi M, Backman JT, Neuvonen M, Neuvonen PJ, Kivisto KT. Rifampin decreases the plasma concentrations and effects of repaglinide. Clin Pharmacol Ther 2000;68(5):495–500.

127. Kyrklund C, Backman JT, Kivisto KT, Neuvonen M, Laitila J, Neuvonen PJ. Rifampin greatly reduces plasma simvastatin and simvastatin acid concentrations. Clin Pharmacol Ther 2000;68(6):592–7.

128. Chenhsu RY, Loong CC, Chou MH, Lin MF, Yang WC. Renal allograft dysfunction associated with rifampin–tacrolimus interaction. Ann Pharmacother 2000;34(1):27–31.

129. Hartmann A, Halvorsen CE, Jenssen T, Bjorneklett A, Brekke IB, Bakke SJ, Hirschberg H, Tonjum T, Gaustad P. Intracerebral abscess caused by *Nocardia otitidiscaviarum* in a renal transplant patient—cured by evacuation plus antibiotic therapy Nephron 2000;86(1):79–83.

130. Powell-Jackson PR, Jamieson AP, Gray BJ, Moxham J, Williams R. Effect of rifampicin administration on theophylline pharmacokinetics in humans. Am Rev Respir Dis 1985;131(6):939–40.

131. Ahn HC, Yang JH, Lee HB, Rhee YK, Lee YC. Effect of combined therapy of oral anti-tubercular agents on theophylline pharmacokinetics. Int J Tuberc Lung Dis 2000;4(8):784–7.

132. Buniva G, Palminteri R, Berti M. Kinetics of a rifampicin–trimethoprim combination. Int J Clin Pharmacol Biopharm 1979;17(6):256–9.

133. Emmerson AM, Gruneberg RN, Johnson ES. The pharmacokinetics in man of a combination of rifampicin and trimethoprim. J Antimicrob Chemother 1978;4(6):523–31.

134. Altundag MK, Barista I. False-positive urine melanin pigment reaction caused by rifampin. Ann Pharmacother 1998;32(5):610.

Organs and Systems

Skin

A photosensitivity reaction has been attributed to rilmenidine (6).

- A 51-year-old woman developed erythema and swelling on sun-exposed areas and complained of a local burning sensation and pruritus 10 days after she started to take rilmenidine 1 mg/day for mild hypertension. She recovered fully 1 week after rilmenidine withdrawal and treatment with prednisolone. The chronology and the results of patch and photopatch tests suggested a phototoxic reaction to rilmenidine.

The authors suggested that this may have been related to the double bond in the oxazoline ring of the drug.

References

1. Reid JL. Update on rilmenidine: clinical benefits. Am J Hypertens 2001;14(11 Pt 2):S322–4.

2. Ostermann G, Brisgand B, Schmitt J, Fillastre JP. Efficacy and acceptability of rilmenidine for mild to moderate systemic hypertension. Am J Cardiol 1988;61(7):D76–80.

3. Beau B, Mahieux F, Paraire M, Laurin S, Brisgand B, Vitou P. Efficacy and safety of rilmenidine for arterial hypertension. Am J Cardiol 1988;61(7):D95–D102.

4. Fillastre JP, Letac B, Galinier F, Le Bihan G, Schwartz J. A multicenter double-blind comparative study of rilmenidine and clonidine in 333 hypertensive patients. Am J Cardiol 1988;61(7):D81–5.

5. Mahieux F. Rilmenidine and vigilance. Review of clinical studies. Am J Med 1989;87(3C):S67–72.

6. Mota AV, Vasconcelos C, Correia TM, Barros MA, Mesquita-Guimaraes J. Rilmenidine-induced photosensitivity reaction. Photodermatol Photoimmunol Photomed 1998;14(3–4):132–3.

Rilmenidine

General Information

Rilmenidine is an imidazoline derivative that lowers blood pressure by an interaction with imidazoline (II) receptors in the brainstem and kidneys (1).

In a number of trials in hypertension the adverse effects profile of rilmenidine was qualitatively similar to that of clonidine, although the overall incidence of adverse events appeared to be lower. The main complaints were of dry mouth, drowsiness, and constipation (2–4). In one of these reviews, in which the impact on vigilance was particularly examined, it was concluded that although there were dose-related effects there was no statistically significant difference between rilmenidine and placebo in relation to sedation and drowsiness. However, these results consistently showed a rank order among placebo, rilmenidine, and clonidine, leading to progressively greater degrees of sedation (5).

Rimantadine

General Information

Rimantadine hydrochloride, an alpha-methyl derivative of amantadine (alpha-methyl-1-adamantane methylamine hydrochloride), is more active than amantadine against influenza A viruses in vitro and in laboratory animals. It is an alternative to amantadine for the prevention and treatment of influenza A virus infections in adults and for the prevention of influenza in children. Adverse effects have been considered to be less common with rimantadine (SEDA-8, 143), and it is generally tolerated better than amantadine, because it causes fewer nervous system adverse effects (1). Unfortunately, rimantadine is more costly, which has led many institutions to develop influenza treatment guidelines. Both drugs work by blocking the M2 ion channel, which is needed to affect a pH change that helps to initiate viral uncoating.

In a systematic review of seven trials of amantadine versus placebo ($n = 1797$), three of rimantadine versus placebo ($n = 688$), and two of amantadine versus rimantadine ($n = 455$) in the prevention of influenza A illness, there was a relative odds reduction of illness of 64% with amantadine compared with placebo, a 75% reduction with rimantadine compared with placebo, and no significant difference between the two drugs (2). There was a significantly higher risk of central nervous system adverse reactions and premature withdrawal with amantadine compared with placebo, but not with rimantadine compared with placebo. However, there was a significant increase in the risk of gastrointestinal adverse events with rimantadine compared with placebo (OR = 3.34, 95% CI = 1.17, 9.55).

Organs and Systems

Nervous system

The major advantage of rimantadine is a lower risk of central nervous system effects, such as light-headedness, difficulty in concentrating, nervousness, and insomnia, which can be a significant problem with amantadine, particularly in older patients. The English-language literature from 1966 to 1994 has been reviewed (3). In 598 elderly patients, nervous system adverse effects were more common with higher dosages (4.9% at 100 mg/day to 12.5% at 200 mg/day).

Gastrointestinal

The English-language literature from 1966 to 1994 has been reviewed (3). Gastrointestinal effects, including nausea, loss of appetite, diarrhea, and dry mouth, occurred in 8.4% of children under 10 years of age, in 3.1% of adults, and in 2.9% of elderly patients taking 100 mg/day and 17.0% taking 200 mg/day.

Long-Term Effects

Drug tolerance

Emergence of resistance of influenza A virus to rimantadine in vivo has been reported (4), but the incidence of resistance in field isolates appears to be extremely low (5).

References

1. Fleming DM. Managing influenza: amantadine, rimantadine and beyond. Int J Clin Pract 2001;55(3):189–95.
2. Marra F, Marra CA, Stiver HG. A case for rimantadine to be marketed in Canada for prophylaxis of influenza A virus infection. Can Respir J 2003;10(7):381–8.
3. Wintermeyer SM, Nahata MC. Rimantadine: a clinical perspective. Ann Pharmacother 1995;29(3):299–310.
4. Hayden FG, Belshe RB, Clover RD, Hay AJ, Oakes MG, Soo W. Emergence and apparent transmission of rimantadine-resistant influenza A virus in families. N Engl J Med 1989;321(25):1696–702.
5. Ziegler T, Hemphill ML, Ziegler ML, Perez-Oronoz G, Klimov AI, Hampson AW, Regnery HL, Cox NJ. Low incidence of rimantadine resistance in field isolates of influenza A viruses. J Infect Dis 1999;180(4):935–9.

Rimazolium

General Information

Rimazolium is a non-narcotic analgesic that strongly potentiates the analgesic and antagonizes the respiratory depressant effect of morphine alkaloids in animals and prevents the development of tolerance to morphine in animals and humans (1). Although rimazolium is not a new drug, experience with it is very limited.

Organs and Systems

Nervous system

Vertigo, drowsiness, and nausea have been attributed to rimazolium (SED-10, 172) (SEDA-7, 117) (2).

References

1. Furst S, Gyires K, Knoll J. Analgesic profile of rimazolium as compared to different classes of pain killers. Arzneimittelforschung 1998;38(4):552–7.
2. Anonymous. Rimazolio metilsulfato. [Rimazolium methylsulfate.] Drugs of Today 1981;17:567.

Risperidone

See also Neuroleptic drugs

General Information

Risperidone is an atypical benzisoxazole neuroleptic drug. It is a dopamine D_2 receptor antagonist, with antagonistic actions at $5-HT_2$ receptors, alpha-adrenoceptors, and histamine H_1 receptors.

Placebo-controlled studies

Patients with bipolar disorder may benefit from risperidone, but this conclusion has mostly come from open studies with small sample sizes (SEDA-23, 69). Experience with risperidone has been reviewed with data from Canadian studies (1).

In a 6-week open study of risperidone (mean dosage 4.7 mg/day) in combination with mood-stabilizing treatments (usually lithium, carbamazepine, or valproate) for the treatment of schizoaffective disorder in 102 patients, 95 of whom completed the trial, at week 4 most patients had improved symptom severity and 9.3% were completely symptom-free (2). There were no statistically significant differences between baseline and week 4 in the severity of extrapyramidal symptoms, as measured by the UKU Side-Effect Rating Scale subscale for neurological adverse effects; other adverse effects included depressive symptoms ($n = 13$), exacerbation of mania ($n = 5$), drowsiness ($n = 3$), and impotence ($n = 2$).

The efficacy and safety of risperidone (mean dose 2.9, range 1.5–4 mg/day) have been examined in a double-blind, randomized, parallel-group, 6-week study of the treatment of aggression in 35 adolescents with a primary diagnosis of disruptive behavior disorder and subaverage intelligence (3). Risperidone significantly improved aggression, and extrapyramidal symptoms were absent or very mild; there was transient tiredness in 11 of the 19 drug-treated subjects compared with one of the 16 placebo-treated subjects; other adverse effects were sialorrhea ($n = 4$ for risperidone, $n = 0$ for placebo), nausea ($n = 3$ for risperidone, $n = 0$ for placebo), and weight gain (mean of 3.5% of body weight with risperidone). There were no clinically important changes in laboratory parameters, electrocardiography, heart rate, or blood pressure.

In a double-blind, placebo-controlled study of the addition of low-dose risperidone (mean dosage 2.2 mg/day) to a 5-HT re-uptake inhibitor in refractory obsessive-compulsive disorder in 70 adults, 18 of 20 risperidone-treated patients had at least one adverse effect (4). The adverse effects in both groups included sedation ($n = 17$ for risperidone, $n = 8$ for placebo), increased appetite (6 and 3), restlessness (6 and 6), and dry mouth (5 and 5).

The results of two major controlled clinical trials of risperidone in patients with dementia were not conclusive, but risperidone was more effective than placebo in agitated and demented patients (SEDA-25, 68). The long-term data have been reviewed and they suggest that although in the two pivotal previous comparisons of risperidone with placebo the risk of adverse events was similar in the two groups when risperidone was given in the optimal dosage (1 mg/day), during a 12-month open extension of these studies, the incidence of de novo tardive dyskinesia was very low, and there were no clinically important adverse events or changes in vital signs or laboratory signs (5).

Risperidone has been used in bipolar disorder, dementia, disruptive behavior disorder with subaverage intelligence, Tourette's syndrome, and autism (SEDA-23, 69) (SEDA-25, 67) (SEDA-26, 64). The efficacy and safety of low doses of risperidone in the treatment of autism and serious behavioral problems have been studied in 101 children aged 5–17 years with autistic disorder accompanied by severe tantrums, aggression, or self-injurious behavior, who were randomly assigned to risperidone for 8 weeks ($n = 49$; dosage 0.5–3.5 mg/day) or placebo ($n = 52$) (6). Risperidone produced a 57% reduction in the Irritability Score, compared with a 14% reduction in the placebo group; all other parameters were also significantly improved. Risperidone was associated with an average weight gain of 2.7 kg, compared with 0.8 kg with placebo; increased appetite, fatigue, drowsiness, dizziness, and drooling were more common with risperidone. In two-thirds of the children with a positive response to risperidone at 8 weeks, the benefit was maintained at 6 months.

Risperidone was also effective and well tolerated in 118 children aged 5–12 years with subaverage intelligence and severely disruptive behavior in a 6-week, multicenter, double-blind, randomized trial (7). Risperidone produced significantly greater improvement than placebo on the conduct problem subscale of the Nisonger Child Behavior Rating Form from week 1 (respective reductions in score of 15 and 6). The most common adverse effects of risperidone (mean dose at end-point 1.16 mg/day) were headache and somnolence; the extrapyramidal symptom profile of

Table 1 The results of two 12-week, randomized, double-blind studies of risperidone in elderly patients with behavioral symptoms associated with dementia (28,29)

Mean age (years)	Number	Dose (mg/day)	Response (%)	Extrapyramidal symptoms (%)
81	344	Risperidone (1.1)	54	15
		Haloperidol (1.2)	63	22
		Placebo	47	11
83	625	Risperidone (1)	45	13
		Risperidone (2)	50	21
		Placebo	33	7.4

risperidone was comparable to that of placebo, and there were respective mean weight increases of 2.2 and 0.9 kg.

Adults with autistic disorder ($n = 17$) or pervasive developmental disorder not otherwise specified ($n = 14$) participated in a randomized, 12-week, double-blind, placebo-controlled trial of risperidone (8). Among those who completed the study, risperidone ($n = 14$) was superior to placebo ($n = 16$) in reducing the symptoms of autism, and the most prominent adverse effect was mild transient sedation during the initial phase of drug administration. Abnormal gait was reported in one patient taking risperidone.

According to a thorough review, risperidone is more effective than placebo in patients with dementia (9). Nevertheless, the results of the two major controlled clinical trials have not been conclusive (see Table 1). There was no statistical difference between the treatments in the first study, although there was in the second; extrapyramidal symptoms were notably more common with risperidone. In both studies, there was a high rate of placebo response, which implies that these patients responded favorably to the increased care that is given during a clinical trial. Long-term data in patients with dementia are lacking, but they are crucial in identifying tardive dyskinesia.

Observational studies

In a Prescription Event Monitoring study of the safety of risperidone in 7684 patients treated in general practice, information on risperidone prescriptions issued to patients in England was gathered between July 1993 and April 1996 (10). After 6 months, 76% of the patients for whom data were available were still taking risperidone. Drowsiness/sedation was the most frequent reason for stopping risperidone and the most frequently reported event (4.6 cases per 1000 patient-months). Extrapyramidal symptoms were rarely reported, the incidence being 3.2 per 1000 patient-months; they were more frequent in elderly patients (7.8 per 1000 patient-months). There were only four reports of dyskinesias and one report of tardive dyskinesia, which resulted in withdrawal of risperidone. Eight overdoses of risperidone alone were reported, with no serious clinical sequelae. Nine patients took risperidone during ten pregnancies, with seven live births and three early therapeutic terminations. There were no abnormalities among the live births.

Long-term data on the efficacy and tolerability of risperidone are scant, as most of the clinical trials have been of short duration (no longer than 12 weeks). However, some additional data from open studies have emerged. In one study, 386 patients with chronic schizophrenia took risperidone 2–16 mg/day for up to 57 weeks; 247 patients were treated for at least 1 year (11). All but 48 patients (88%) had been treated with antipsychotic drugs before entering the study. At the end of the study, 64% of the patients were rated as having improved on the Clinical Global Impression change scale, and extrapyramidal symptoms (scored on the Extrapyramidal Symptom Rating Scale, ESRS) tended to be lower in severity or remained unchanged over the course of risperidone treatment; 27% of the patients required antiparkinsonian medication during the study, and 6.5% discontinued treatment prematurely because of adverse events. One or more adverse events were reported by 221 patients (57%) during risperidone treatment. Extrapyramidal symptoms occurred in 23%. Insomnia and anxiety were reported by 13% and 12% of patients. Two patients died during the 1-year study: one patient drowned and another committed suicide by hanging after 3.5 months. At the end of the study the mean increase in body weight was 1.8 kg.

In a retrospective study of 97 patients taking risperidone, under 30% of the patients were still taking risperidone after a mean period of follow-up of 102 (range 13–163) weeks (12). Reasons for discontinuation included not achieving the desired therapeutic effect ($n = 39$), non-compliance ($n = 22$), adverse effects ($n = 26$), the patient's not liking the drug and requesting a change to a different medication ($n = 17$), and symptom remission ($n = 6$). The authors stated that in routine clinical practice, the use of risperidone is plagued by many of the same problems of older antipsychotic drugs.

The efficacy and safety of risperidone have been examined in special groups of patients, such as those with psychotic depression (13), autistic disorders (8), bipolar disorder (14), mental retardation (15), and children and adolescents (16).

Patients with bipolar disorders may benefit from risperidone. This has been observed in an open trial of ten patients with rapid cycling bipolar disorder who were refractory to lithium carbonate, carbamazepine, and valproate; eight improved after 6 months of treatment. One patient dropped out through non-adherence to therapy and one because of adverse effects (agitation, anxiety, insomnia, and headache) (14). There was a similar beneficial effect in eight adults with moderate to profound mental retardation (15). Risperidone was associated with a significant reduction in aggression and self-injurious behavior, whereas adverse effects were primarily those of sedation and restlessness.

Eight of a heterogeneous group of eleven children and adolescents (mean age 9.8, range 5.5–16 years) with mood disorders and aggressive behavior, improved with a low dose of risperidone (0.75–2.5 mg/day) (16). Treatment was stopped in two children because of drowsiness; the most bothersome adverse effect of risperidone was weight gain in two cases (mean increase 4 kg).

The medical records of 151 hospitalized elderly psychiatric patients (mean age 71 years) have been analysed (17).

Of 114 patients treated with risperidone (mean duration of treatment 17 days; mean dose 3 mg/day), 78% responded. Adverse events were reported in 20 patients, including new-onset extrapyramidal effects in four; tremor in four; sedation in three; hypotension in three; diarrhea in two; tardive dyskinesia in two; and chest pain, anxiety, restlessness, itching, insomnia, and falls in one each.

A review of both core information and new findings concerning risperidone concluded that it can be associated with transient drowsiness (probably no greater than that observed with haloperidol), postural hypotension (which is avoided by dose titration), weight gain, reduced sexual interest, and erectile dysfunction. Risperidone can also cause dose-dependent hyperprolactinemia (which can cause amenorrhea, sexual dysfunction, and galactorrhea). Risperidone tends not to cause extrapyramidal signs at therapeutic doses (the optimal dose being 6 mg/day) but they do occur dose-dependently (18).

In an 8-week open prospective study of risperidone in 20 patients, mean age 34 (range 19–53) years, adverse effects included giddiness ($n = 3$), headache ($n = 2$), and agitation ($n = 2$); one woman reported galactorrhea and another developed obsessive-compulsive symptoms; 16 of 20 patients were taking antiparkinsonian drugs before the study, compared with 12 patients at the end (19).

Objections have been raised on the ways in which some clinical trials are interpreted (20). Furthermore, it has been stated that a major problem with the risperidone literature is that the original data can be very difficult to decipher or even obtain. Huston and Moher have described their frustration in trying to perform a meta-analysis of the effects of risperidone; they found "obvious redundancy in the results of a single-center trial being published twice," as well as problems with "changing authorship, lack of transparency in reporting, and frequent citation of abstracts and unpublished reports" (21). These concerns were reiterated in an editorial (22).

In a prospective, 6-week open trial in 31 Chinese patients with acute exacerbation of schizophrenia, risperidone doses were titrated to 6 mg/day (if tolerated) over 3 days, but were reduced thereafter if adverse effects occurred (23). Efficacy and adverse effects were assessed on days 0, 4, 14, 28, and 42. End-point steady-state plasma concentrations of risperidone and 9-hydroxyrisperidone were analysed. Of the 30 patients who completed the trial, 17 tolerated the 6 mg dose well, while the other 13 received lower final doses (mean 3.6 mg) for curtailing adverse effects. At end-point, 92% of the 13 low-dose patients had responded to treatment (a 20% or more reduction in the total score on the Positive and Negative Syndrome Scale), compared with 53% of the 17 high-dose subjects. There were no significant between-group differences in other minor efficacy measures. End-point plasma concentrations of the active moieties (risperidone plus 9-hydroxyrisperidone) were 40 ng/ml in the low-dose group and 50 ng/ml in the high-dose group; this difference was not significant, suggesting that the different responses were pharmacokinetic in origin. The results of this preliminary trial suggest that up to 6 mg/day of risperidone is efficacious in treating patients with an acute exacerbation of schizophrenia. Nearly 60% of the patients tolerated 6 mg/day; in the others, reducing the dosage to relieve adverse effects still yielded efficacy.

The efficacy and safety of long-term risperidone have been assessed in children and adolescents ($n = 11$) in a prospective study (24). Subjects with autism or pervasive developmental disorder not otherwise specified took risperidone for 6 months, after which their parents were given the option of continuing for a further 6 months. Weight gain was common, although the rate of increase abated with time. After 6 months two patients developed facial dystonias, which disappeared after reducing the dosage in one case and after withdrawal in the other. Amenorrhea was also observed, but there were no changes in liver function, blood tests, or electroencephalography. The authors concluded that risperidone may be effective and relatively safe in the long-term treatment of behavioral disruption in autistic children and adolescents.

Youths with behavioral disorders (25,26), and patients with disturbing neuroleptic drug-induced extrapyramidal symptoms (27) have been studied. Ten youths (aged 6–14 years) were randomly assigned to receive placebo and 10 to receive risperidone (0.75–1.50 mg/day) for conduct disorder in a preliminary study lasting 10 weeks (25). Of those assigned to risperidone, six completed the course; three completed placebo. Those who took risperidone were significantly less aggressive during the last weeks of the study than those who did not. Eight youths who took risperidone and four who took placebo had at least one adverse effect, including increased appetite ($n = 3$ for risperidone), sedation ($n = 3$ for risperidone; $n = 2$ for placebo), headache ($n = 1$ for risperidone; $n = 1$ for placebo), insomnia ($n = 1$ for risperidone), restlessness ($n = 1$ for risperidone), irritability ($n = 1$ for risperidone), enuresis ($n = 1$ for placebo), and nausea/vomiting ($n = 1$ for risperidone; $n = 1$ for placebo). These adverse effects were mild and transient.

There was marked reduction in aggression in 14 of 26 subjects (10–18 years old) in an open study of risperidone (0.5–4 mg/day) for 2–12 months (26). Two subjects had marked weight gain (8 and 10 kg) in the first 8 weeks; another participant who took lithium (1400 mg/day, serum concentration 0.9 mmol/l) presented with moderate akathisia and hand tremor; in seven, tiredness and sedation occurred after week 8.

Organs and Systems

Cardiovascular

Cardiac arrest was attributed to risperidone in a patient with no history of cardiac disease (30).

One of two children aged 29 and 23 months with autistic disorder developed a persistent tachycardia and dose-related QT_c interval prolongation while taking risperidone (31).

Cardiotoxicity of risperidone has recently been discussed (32) in the light of a death in a patient taking a therapeutic dose (SEDA-22, 68).

Nervous system

Seizures

Stuttering, a rare adverse effect of neuroleptic drugs, is thought to be a harbinger of seizures. Stuttering without seizures has been attributed to risperidone (33).

- A 32-year-old Korean man with delusions took oral risperidone 1.0 mg/day and lorazepam 0.5 mg bd. The dose of risperidone was increased to 4 mg/day over 4 days. On day 5, he began to stutter and could not articulate what he wanted to say without stuttering. The dose of risperidone was increased to 8 mg/day and the stuttering became more pronounced. However, after 1 year of continuous treatment, he did not stutter any more.

The authors suggested that since the patient had a history of stuttering risperidone had reactivated the speech pattern.

Extrapyramidal effects

Risperidone produces dose-related extrapyramidal adverse effects, but at concentrations lower than those of conventional antipsychotic drugs (SEDA-21, 58); at equieffective doses it has fewer such effects than haloperidol (SEDA-21, 57) (SEDA-22, 67) (SEDA-23, 68). The relation between the degree of receptor occupancy and the presence of extrapyramidal symptoms is not clear, as observed in a SPECT study in 20 patients (34). The frequency of risperidone-induced extrapyramidal signs, on the other hand, is intermediate between clozapine and conventional antipsychotic drugs, according to an open study in patients treated for at least 3 months with clozapine ($n = 41$; mean dose 426 mg/day), risperidone ($n = 23$; 4.7 mg/day), or conventional antipsychotic drugs ($n = 42$; 477 mg/day chlorpromazine equivalents) (35). The point prevalence of akathisia was 7.3% in those who took clozapine, 13% in those who took risperidone, and 24% in those who took conventional antipsychotic drugs; the point prevalences of rigidity and cogwheeling were 4.9% and 2.4% respectively with clozapine, 17% and 17% with risperidone, and 36% and 26% with conventional antipsychotic drugs.

A combined analysis of 12 double-blind studies in schizophrenic patients comparing the use of risperidone ($n = 2074$) with placebo ($n = 140$) or haloperidol ($n = 517$) has further stressed the dose-related extrapyramidal effects associated with risperidone (36). After covariance analysis to adjust for baseline ESRS (Extrapyramidal Symptom Rating Scale) scores, sex, race, age, height, duration of symptoms, age at first hospitalization, hospitalization status, and diagnosis, the effects of the maximum dose of risperidone on the mean shift to worse ESRS total scores were 1.4 (CI = 0.73, 2.03) at 1–4 mg/day ($n = 319$); 2.1 (CI = 1.65, 2.50) at 4–8 mg/day ($n = 932$); 3.3 (CI = 2.61, 3.89) at 8–12.5 mg/day ($n = 439$); and 3.8 (CI = 2.99, 4.55) at 13 mg/day or more ($n = 361$). The results also showed a significant dose-dependent increase in the use of antiparkinsonian drugs; the percentages of those requiring antiparkinsonian drugs were 14% at 1–4 mg/day ($n = 319$); 25% at 4–8 mg/day ($n = 900$); 27% at 8–12.5 mg/day ($n = 407$); and 31% at 13 mg/day or more ($n = 335$). Of 882 patients who took risperidone for at least 12 weeks, based on unsolicited reports, two developed tardive dyskinesia.

In an international, multicenter, double-blind study in 183 patients with a first psychotic episode treated with flexible doses of risperidone or haloperidol for 6 weeks, the severity of extrapyramidal symptoms and the use of antiparkinsonian drugs were significantly lower in patients taking low doses (up to 6 mg/day) than high doses (over

6 mg/day) of risperidone or haloperidol (37). These findings are consistent with the suggestion that patients with a first psychotic episode may require low doses of antipsychotic drugs. Furthermore, the severity of extrapyramidal symptoms was significantly lower in the risperidone-treated patients. Also, risperidone-treated subjects were significantly less likely than haloperidol-treated subjects to require concomitant anticholinergic drugs after 4 weeks (20 versus 63%); they had significantly less observable akathisia (24 versus 53%) and significantly less severe tardive dyskinesia. This was observed in a randomized double-blind comparison of risperidone 6 mg/day ($n = 34$) and haloperidol 15 mg/day ($n = 33$) (38).

In a 9-week open study of risperidone for agitated behavior in 15 patients with dementia (modal dose 0.5 mg/day), extrapyramidal symptoms developed at some point during the trial in 8 patients, and cognitive skills were impaired in 3 patients (39). Similarly, in 22 patients with dementia and behavioral disturbances, treated with risperidone 1.5 mg/day (range 0.5 mg qds to 3 mg bd), 50% had significant improvement, but 50% had some extrapyramidal symptoms (40). A further case of a severe extrapyramidal reaction in an old patient with dementia further illustrated these susceptibility factors (41).

Although several cases of sensitivity to risperidone with extrapyramidal signs in Lewy body dementia have been published (SEDA-20, 52), a case of successful treatment without extrapyramidal adverse effects has also been reported (42).

- A 74-year-old man with Lewy body dementia treated with a combination of donepezil (5 mg in the evening) and risperidone (0.25 mg/day) had significant improvement, objectively and subjectively, within 2 weeks.

Akathisia
Restless legs syndrome has been reported in association with risperidone (43).

- A 31-year-old woman with schizoaffective disorder taking risperidone 6 mg/day complained of uncomfortable tingling and tearing sensations deep inside the calves and less severe sensations in her arms after 5 days; the symptoms vanished after replacement by quetiapine 400 mg/day.

Parkinsonism
Intolerable exacerbation of parkinsonism with risperidone has been reported (SEDA-20, 52), and even a 12-year-old boy reportedly developed parkinsonian tremor while taking risperidone (44). However, in contrast, eight patients (five women, three men) with advanced Parkinson's disease, motor fluctuations, and levodopa-induced dyskinesia took part in an open study with a low dosage of risperidone (mean 0.187 mg/day); after an average of 11 months all the patients had moderate to pronounced reductions in levodopa-induced dyskinesias (45).

Whether risperidone should be used in patients with Parkinson's disease is a subject of debate (46,47).

The efficacy and safety of risperidone have been evaluated in 44 patients (25 women and 19 men) with Parkinson's disease (48). There was either complete or near-complete resolution of hallucinations in 23, but an

unsatisfactory response ($n = 6$) or worsening of parkinsonism ($n = 6$) in 12. Excluding patients with diffuse Lewy body disease, there was no significant worsening of scores on the Unified Parkinson's Disease Rating Scale after either 3 or 6 months of treatment, and the presence of dementia did not predict the response to treatment.

The long-term effect of risperidone on basal ganglia volume, measured by MRI scanning, has been studied in 30 patients with a first episode of schizophrenia who took risperidone, 12 patients taking long-term typical neuroleptic drugs, and 23 healthy controls (49). Treatment with risperidone for 1 year (mean dosage 2.7, range 1–6 mg/day) did not alter basal ganglia volume, although there were movement disorders in both groups of treated patients, suggesting effects of both illness and medications.

Tardive dyskinesia
Tardive dyskinesia has occasionally been reported with risperidone (SEDA-20, 53) (SEDA-21, 59) (SEDA-22, 68) (50–55).

The incidence of tardive dyskinesia in patients with chronic schizophrenia taking risperidone is said to be 0.34% per year. Advanced age and dementia may be contributing factors (SEDA-21, 59) (SEDA-22, 68) (SEDA-23, 70).

Tardive dyskinesia/dystonia developed in four patients treated with risperidone at an early intervention facility for young people with psychosis (56). Other cases that have emerged were in:

- a 13-year-old young girl treated with risperidone 6 mg/day (57);
- a 21-year-old woman without previous exposure to other neuroleptic drugs or systemic illnesses that affected the central nervous system (58);
- a 58-year-old man with chronic alcoholism who developed tardive dyskinesia after exposure to risperidone that was aggravated by olanzapine (59).
- a 16-year-old girl who developed buccolingual masticatory tardive dyskinesia after taking risperidone 6 mg/day (60); when she restarted risperidone 2 mg/day, increasing to 6 mg/day later on, the dyskinesia improved.
- a 74-year-old woman who developed persistent tardive dyskinesia following a short trial (3 weeks) of a low dose (0.5 mg bd) of risperidone (61).

Tardive dyskinesia was studied in 330 elderly patients with dementia (mean age 83 years) (62). They were enrolled in a 1-year open study, in which the modal risperidone dose was 0.96 mg/day and the median duration of use was 273 days. The 1-year cumulative incidence of persistent tardive dyskinesia among the 225 patients without dyskinesia at baseline was 2.6%, and patients with dyskinesia at baseline had significant reductions in severity.

Attention deficit hyperactivity disorder (ADHD) may be a susceptibility factor for risperidone-induced tardive dyskinesia and withdrawal dyskinesia. Both conditions have occurred in patients with a past or recent history of attention deficit hyperactivity disorder.

- A 34-year-old woman developed dyskinesia after starting risperidone, with a marked increase in prolactin concentrations (63).

- A 13-year-old boy developed mild mouth movements, neck twisting, and intermittent upward gaze approximately 2 weeks after withdrawal of risperidone (1.5 mg and then 0.5 mg) (64).

Tardive dystonia

Dystonia and tardive dystonia have been attributed to risperidone.

- A 23-year-old man taking risperidone 8 mg/day developed blepharospasm (65).
- A 25-year-old man, who had never taken any other psychotropic medication, developed tardive dyskinesia with severe blepharospasm and tardive dystonia 2 months after withdrawal of risperidone (66).
- Possible risperidone-induced tardive dystonia has been reported in a 47-year-old man (67).

Marked improvement of tardive dystonia after replacing haloperidol with risperidone in a schizophrenic patient has been reported (68).

Pisa syndrome, a tardive axial dystonia with flexion of the trunk towards one side, is a rare reaction that occurs during treatment with neuroleptic drugs (SED-14, 146) (SEDA-24, 57). Two cases related to risperidone have been published.

- A 24-year-old woman with mental retardation and an unspecified psychosis took risperidone 2 mg/day and trihexyphenidyl 2 mg/day and after 2 weeks developed symptoms that included tilting of her body backwards and to the left and tremors and cogwheel rigidity of the limbs (69). Risperidone was withdrawn and olanzapine 5 mg/day started; after 4 weeks there was no improvement and she was then lost to follow-up.
- A 25-year-old man with auditory hallucinations took risperidone 7 mg/day for 15 months plus biperiden 6 mg/day (70). He then complained of leaning to the right and being unable to straighten up. He had tonic flexion of the trunk to the right with slight backward axial rotation. After 5 months of risperidone withdrawal, the condition had not resolved; it later improved with co-beneldopa 400/100 mg/day and then after the addition of cabergoline 0.75 mg/day.

Rabbit syndrome

Rabbit syndrome has been reported in patients taking risperidone.

- A 27-year-old man took risperidone 6 mg/day and after 4 months the dosage was reduced to 4 mg/day; 7 months after the start of treatment he developed fine rapid pouting and puckering of the lips (71). These movements were accompanied by a strange, irritating, involuntary popping sound. The dosage of risperidone was reduced to 2 mg/day and an anticholinergic drug was added. Within days, there was symptomatic improvement, but a trial withdrawal of the anticholinergic drug resulted in worsening of the symptoms and treatment was renewed.
- A 38-year-old man with major depressive disorder and psychotic features developed rabbit syndrome after taking risperidone 4 mg/day and paroxetine 40 mg/day for

4 months; he was also taking simvastatin 10 mg/day, thiamine 100 mg/day, and folic acid 1 mg/day (72).

Neuroleptic malignant syndrome

Neuroleptic malignant syndrome has been reported in patients taking risperidone (73,74); most cases occurred within the first months, and even as early as 12 hours (SEDA-22, 68) (SEDA-23, 70).

Delayed risperidone-induced neuroleptic malignant syndrome has been reported in a 27-year-old man after 21 months (75), and in a 17-year-old girl who took risperidone 0.5 mg bd (76). Risperidone-induced neuroleptic malignant syndrome has also been reported in a 63-year-old woman with probable Lewy body dementia, who had previously had an episode of neuroleptic malignant syndrome with trifluoperazine (77).

A patient with schizoaffective disorder, who developed risperidone-related neuroleptic malignant syndrome, responded satisfactorily to supportive management and vitamin E plus vitamin B6 (78).

Catatonia

Catatonia has been reported in relation to risperidone (SEDA-23, 72) (79,80).

- Catatonia occurred in a 61-year-old woman who was taking risperidone 5 mg/day for prominent paranoid delusions after a post-frontal lobotomy some 35 years ago. The catatonic disorder was dose-dependent and resolved immediately after changing to clozapine.

Pseudotumor cerebri

Two patients with hydrocephalus and learning difficulties developed headache, nausea, vomiting, drowsiness, lethargy, and episodes of collapse after starting to take risperidone for aggressive outbursts; the condition mimicked increased intracranial pressure (81). Withdrawal of the drug resulted in complete resolution of all the symptoms within 72 hours. The authors pointed out the striking degree of overlap between the adverse effects profile of risperidone and the symptoms of raised intracranial pressure due to shunt malfunction, which has not been previously highlighted.

Psychological, psychiatric

Anxiety and behavioral stimulation, characterized by anxiety, insomnia, and restlessness, during risperidone treatment have been reported (SEDA-20, 53) (SEDA-21, 59) (SEDA-23, 71) (82). Six of thirteen outpatients who took part in a 10-week open trial of risperidone had a good initial response, followed by intolerable effects, including feelings of agitation and depression and periods of crying and insomnia (83). The patients who developed this syndrome had a significantly higher mean baseline rating on the Brief Psychiatric Rating Scale anxiety subscale.

Visual distortion with generalized anxiety and panic attacks has been attributed to risperidone (SEDA-22, 69). Visual disturbance resembling hallucinogen persistent perception disorder occurred after each of three consecutive risperidone dosage increases in a 55-year-old woman; there was absence of substance abuse (84).

It has been speculated that the antiserotonergic properties of risperidone could lead to obsessive and depressive symptoms, since a patient taking risperidone 4 mg/day developed major depression and obsessions, which resolved with fluoxetine 29 mg/day, relapsing when fluoxetine was withdrawn (85).

Mania

Mania has rarely been associated with typical neuroleptic drugs, but has been described in patients treated with new antipsychotic drugs, especially risperidone (SEDA-22, 69) (SEDA-23, 71) (86). Risperidone-induced mania occurred in a 23-year-old man and a 21-year-old woman, who developed acute mania with euphoria, psychomotor agitation, and hypersexuality, at dosages of 4–8 mg/day (87).

Nevertheless, risperidone has been used in the treatment of mania in combination with mood stabilizers (SEDA-23, 69) (SEDA-26, 64).

Obsessive-compulsive disorder

Obsessive-compulsive symptoms associated with risperidone have been reported (SEDA-22, 69).

- Obsessive-compulsive symptoms developed in a 26-year-old Chinese woman taking risperidone for a chronic schizophrenic illness (88). She had no history of obsessive-compulsive symptoms. Risperidone 2 mg/day, benzhexol 2 mg/day, and diazepam 10 mg at night had been prescribed after she had had adverse effects with other antipsychotic drugs.
- A man who had taken risperidone 4 mg/day for 18 months developed an obsessional image of a person's face that repeatedly appeared in his mind as he went about his activities; the recurrent images disappeared after the dosage of risperidone was reduced to 3 mg/day (89).

In one case, reintroduction of risperidone did not cause obsessive-compulsive symptoms to re-emerge in a 29-year-old man who had previously developed obsessive-compulsive features when first treated with risperidone (90).

Endocrine

Prolactin

There was a significant rise in baseline serum prolactin concentration in 10 patients after they had taken risperidone for a mean of 12 weeks compared with 10 patients who were tested after a neuroleptic drug-free wash-out period of at least 2 weeks (91). A non-significant increase in serum prolactin has also been observed in an open comparison of risperidone with other neuroleptic drugs in 28 patients (92). However, in a meta-analysis of two independent studies ($n = 404$), prolactin was greatly increased by risperidone (mean change 45–80 ng/ml), a larger effect than with olanzapine and haloperidol (93).

Five patients (four women and one man, aged 30–45 years), who were evaluated for risperidone-induced hyperprolactinemia, had significant hyperprolactinemia, with prolactin concentrations of 66–209 μg/l (94). All but one had manifestations of hypogonadism, and in these four patients, risperidone was continued and a dopamine receptor agonist (bromocriptine or cabergoline) was added; in three patients this reduced the prolactin concentration and alleviated the hypogonadism.

The relation of prolactin concentrations and certain adverse events has been explored by using data from two large randomized, double-blind studies ($n = 2725$; 813 women, 1912 men) (95). Both risperidone and haloperidol produced dose-related increases in plasma prolactin concentrations in men and women, but they were not correlated with adverse events such as amenorrhea, galactorrhea, or reduced libido in women or with erectile dysfunction, ejaculatory dysfunction, gynecomastia, or reduced libido in men. Nevertheless, in five patients risperidone (1–8 mg/day) caused amenorrhea in association with raised serum prolactin concentrations (mean 122 ng/ml, range 61–230 ng/ml; reference range 2.7–20 ng/ml) (96).

Furthermore, risperidone-induced galactorrhea associated with a raised prolactin has been reported (97,98), as have amenorrhea and sexual dysfunction (18).

- Galactorrhea associated with a rise in prolactin occurred after a few weeks of treatment with risperidone in two women aged 24 and 39 (97). One of them was switched to thioridazine, with an improvement in the galactorrhea, and the other continued to take risperidone owing to a robust response; her galactorrhea was partially treated with bromocriptine.
- A 34-year-old woman, who developed amenorrhea while taking risperidone, regained her normal menstrual pattern along with a marked fall in serum prolactin concentration 8 weeks after being switched to olanzapine, whereas amantadine had failed to normalize the menses and had apparently reactivated the psychotic symptoms (99).

The authors suggested that olanzapine may offer advantages for selected patients in whom hyperprolactinemia occurs during treatment with other antipsychotic drugs.

- Galactorrhea and gynecomastia occurred in a 38-year-old hypothyroid man who took risperidone for 14 days (100).

The authors suggested that men with primary hypothyroidism may be particularly sensitive to neuroleptic drug-induced increases in prolactin concentrations.

- A 17-year-old man developed galactorrhea and breast tenderness within weeks of starting to take risperidone.

The authors suggested that patients who have galactorrhea, amenorrhea, or both while taking risperidone should be gradually switched to olanzapine, quetiapine, or clozapine (101). Indeed, when 20 women with schizophrenia who were taking risperidone and had menstrual disturbances, galactorrhea, and sexual dysfunction (SEDA-24, 72) (SEDA-26, 65) were switched from risperidone to olanzapine over 2 weeks and then took olanzapine 5–20 mg/day for 8 further weeks, serum prolactin concentrations fell significantly (102). Scores on the Positive and Negative Syndrome Scale, Abnormal Involuntary Movement Scale, and Simpson–Angus Scale for extrapyramidal symptoms at the end-point were also significantly reduced. There were improvements in menstrual functioning and patients' perceptions of sexual adverse effects.

Amenorrhea presumed to have been induced by risperidone has been successfully treated with

Shakuyaku-kanzo-to, a Japanese herbal medicine that contains *Peoniae radix* and *Glycyrrhizae radix* (103).

Metabolism

Diabetes mellitus

There has been a report of diabetic ketoacidosis in a 42-year-old man, without a prior history of diabetes mellitus, who took risperidone (2 mg bd) (104). The authors pointed out that in premarketing studies of risperidone, diabetes mellitus occurred in 0.01–1% of patients.

Weight gain

Pathological weight gain has been increasingly identified as a problem when atypical neuroleptic drugs are given to children (SEDA-21, 57) (SEDA-22, 69). In one case, unremitting weight gain, triggered by risperidone, was eventually curbed through the use of a diet containing slowly absorbed carbohydrates and a careful balance of carbohydrates, proteins, and fats (105).

- A 9-year-old boy with autism and overactivity was unresponsive to several drugs. Risperidone 0.5 mg bd was effective, reducing his Aberrant Behavior Checklist score from 103 to 57 by the end of the first week. Four weeks later his weight had risen from 34.6 to 37 kg. This rate of weight gain (0.6 kg/week) continued over the next 12 weeks. His weight was then contained by the use of the "Zone" diet, with an emphasis on slowly absorbed carbohydrates (examples include apples, oatmeal, kidney beans, whole-grain pasta, and sweet potatoes) in a calorie-reduced diet containing 30% proteins and 30% fats.

In 37 children and adolescent inpatients treated with risperidone for 6 months, compared with 33 psychiatric inpatients who had not taken atypical neuroleptic drugs, risperidone was associated with significant weight gain in 78% of the treated children and adolescents compared with 24% of those in the comparison group (106). Risperidone dosage, concomitant medicaments, and other demographic characteristics (such as age, sex, pubertal status, and baseline weight and body mass index) were not associated with an increased risk of morbid weight gain.

In contrast, in a multicenter, open study in 127 elderly psychotic patients (median age 72, range 54–89 years) taking risperidone (mean dose 3.7 mg/day) there was no significant weight gain after 12 months (107).

Risperidone-induced obesity can cause sleep apnea (108).

- A 50-year-old man with schizophrenia gained 29 kg over 31 months and developed diabetes while taking risperidone 6 mg/day. He reported difficulty in sleeping and frequent daytime napping that left him unsatisfied, and his wife reported prominent snoring and apnea at night.

Nasal continuous positive airway pressure produced improvement.

Electrolyte balance

Polydipsia with hyponatremia has been reported in patients taking risperidone (109,110).

- A 28-year-old man complained of unbearable thirst 2 weeks after starting risperidone 8 mg/day, and would drink 4–5 liters of water within a variable period of a few minutes to 8 hours; he did not develop hyponatremia (111). The condition lasted about 2 years and remitted after withdrawal of risperidone. After a drug-free interval of 2 weeks, clozapine was started and the condition had not recurred after 6 months.

The mechanism of this effect was unclear. The authors thought that SIADH was unlikely, considering the features of polyuria, a low urine osmolality (172 mosmol/kg), and absence of hyponatremia during polydipsia.

Hematologic

Agranulocytosis, leukopenia, neutropenia, lymphopenia, and thrombocytopenia have been reported in patients taking risperidone (112–115).

- A 40-year-old woman developed agranulocytosis after taking risperidone for 2 weeks (114). She had also developed agranulocytosis after treatment with several other antipsychotic drugs (chlorpromazine, haloperidol, and zuclopenthixol).

Mouth and teeth

Hypersalivation or sialorrhea has been reported with all neuroleptic drugs, and has been associated with risperidone as one of the most frequently mentioned adverse effects in patients with disturbing extrapyramidal symptoms during previous neuroleptic drug treatment (SEDA-25, 68). Hypersalivation is a troublesome adverse effect that can contribute to non-adherence to therapy, but it can be treated with clonidine.

- Hypersalivation in a 22-year-old man was rapidly and markedly reduced by clonidine 0.1 mg bd over 3 days (116).

Liver

Several cases of hepatotoxicity have been reported in adults (117) and boys (SEDA-22, 69) taking long-term risperidone.

- Hepatotoxicity occurred in an 81-year-old man who took only two doses of risperidone 0.5 mg (118).
- In a 25-year-old woman, liver function tests were 2.6–7.4 times higher than the upper limit of the reference range during risperidone therapy (119).
- A 13-year-old girl developed liver enzyme rises and fatty liver infiltration in the context of pre-existing obesity after taking risperidone 0.5 mg/day for 3 days (120).
- Transient increases in liver enzymes induced by risperidone occurred in two men aged 19 and 22 (121).
- Cholestatic jaundice occurred in a 37-year-old man taking risperidone (122).

Urinary tract

Hemorrhagic cystitis has been associated with risperidone (123).

- An 11-year-old boy developed acute dysuria and increased frequency accompanied by gross hematuria. He was taking fluoxetine, valproic acid, benzatropine, haloperidol, clonidine, trazodone, and nasal desmopressin. One week before presentation, risperidone had been introduced instead of haloperidol to improve behavioral control. The risperidone was discontinued and haloperidol resumed, and his symptoms resolved during the following week.

Several cases of urinary incontinence have been associated with risperidone, and the manufacturers report that this adverse effect occurs in up to 1% of patients (SEDA-22, 70). The authors of a report of two patients, in both of whom the adverse effect was clearly temporally related to the drug, stated that at least 28% of patients developed transient urinary incontinence after starting risperidone (124).

Skin

Photosensitivity has been attributed to risperidone.

- A 69-year-old woman taking risperidone developed an erythematous rash with areas of blistering and early desquamation. It was most pronounced in exposed areas, although there was some spread beyond (125).

Sexual function

Prolonged erection has been reported with risperidone (126) (SEDA-24, 71).

- Priapism associated with risperidone occurred in a 19-year-old man who had taken 2 mg/day for 4 days (127).

In one case priapism followed the use of first risperidone and then ziprasidone (128). In two other cases, presumed to be due to risperidone (129,130), penile irrigation with isotonic saline and phenylephrine injection resulted in detumescence. Risperidone has a high affinity for alpha-1 adrenoceptors, and alpha-1 blockade leads to direct arteriolar dilatation, which results in increased blood inflow and reduced outflow secondary to effacement and subsequent obstruction of emissary veins.

Ejaculatory dysfunction has also been associated with risperidone in two cases.

- A 21-year-old patient with bipolar schizoaffective disorder developed absent ejaculation with normal orgasm 3 weeks after starting to take risperidone (131).
- A 37-year-old man with paranoid schizophrenia had ejaculatory difficulty during sexual intercourse with his wife, compatible with retrograde ejaculation, 1–2 weeks after starting to take risperidone (132). He reported complete failure to emit semen but a normal desire, erection, and sense of orgasm. Semen was seen in postcoital urine. The dosage of risperidone was reduced to 3 mg/day and anterograde ejaculation was partially restored.

Immunologic

Risperidone has been rarely associated with allergic reactions (SEDA-22, 70).

Long-Term Effects

Drug withdrawal

Serious withdrawal effects have occasionally been reported with risperidone (SEDA-21, 60) (SEDA-22, 70). Both manic and psychotic symptoms have been described in a patient with chronic schizophrenia after risperidone withdrawal (133).

- A 38-year-old Chinese man responded to risperidone monotherapy for 2 weeks after 19 years of resistance to typical neuroleptic drugs. Three days later he lost his medicine and 2 days later his auditory hallucinations and persecutory delusions recurred. Meanwhile, vivid manic symptoms (such as heightened mood, irritability, reduced need for sleep, hyperactivity, pressured speech, flight of ideas, and grandiosity) emerged for the first time throughout the history of his illness.
- Dyskinesia occurred for 5 days in an 82-year-old woman after withdrawal of risperidone and citalopram, which she had taken for about 3 months (134).

It is not clear whether this was a withdrawal effect or a tardive dyskinesia in response to risperidone.

Second-Generation Effects

Teratogenicity

All neuroleptic drugs cross the placenta and reach the fetus in potentially significant amounts; the best recommendation is to avoid any drug during the first trimester and only to use drugs thereafter if the benefits to the mother and fetus outweigh any possibility of risk (SED-14, 152) (SEDA-22, 54). Risperidone has been used in two women before and throughout pregnancy without developmental abnormalities in the children after 9 months and 1 year; the dosages started at 2 mg/day and were increased to 4–6 mg/day (135). In a large postmarketing study of 7684 patients who took risperidone, nine women took it during ten pregnancies; there were seven live births and three therapeutic terminations of pregnancy (SEDA-23, 69) (136).

Lactation

The distribution and excretion of risperidone and 9-hydroxyrisperidone into the breast milk of a young woman with puerperal psychosis, who was treated with risperidone, has been reported (137).

- A 21-year-old woman with a 2-year history of bipolar disorder stopped all of her medication when she discovered that she was pregnant; she was given risperidone 2.5 months after childbirth, gradually increasing to a steady-state dosage of 6 mg/day. Risperidone and 9-hydroxyrisperidone concentrations in plasma and breast milk were measured, and calculations indicated that a suckling infant would receive only 0.84% of the maternal dose as risperidone and 3.46% as 9-hydroxyrisperidone.

Susceptibility Factors

Genetic factors

Impaired metabolism of risperidone can increase the risk of adverse effects.

- A homozygous non-functional genotype, CYP2D6*4, was found in a 17-year-old patient with schizophrenia who developed severe akathisia, parkinsonism, and drowsiness after taking risperidone 6 mg/day for 3 months; he had high plasma concentrations of risperidone and an active metabolite (138).

Age

Elderly people

Elderly patients with dementia have been said to be at particular risk of developing extrapyramidal adverse effects, even with very low doses.

Delirium occurs in 1.6% of elderly patients newly treated with risperidone (SEDA-22, 70), and cases have been reported in patients of advanced age (139,140). It is suggested that in these patients, treatment should begin with low dosages (0.25–0.5 mg/day) and that the dosage be gradually increased over several days, with close monitoring.

The safety, tolerability, and efficacy of risperidone have been assessed in 103 patients with schizophrenia (52 men and 51 women) aged 65 years or older in an open, multicenter, 12-week study (141). The mean risperidone dose at end-point was 2.4 mg/day. Adverse events occurred in 91 patients and included dizziness ($n = 23$), insomnia ($n = 17$), agitation ($n = 15$), somnolence ($n = 15$), injury ($n = 12$), constipation ($n = 11$), and extrapyramidal disorders ($n = 10$); 11 patients withdrew because of adverse events. Among the 91 patients with normal baseline QT_c intervals (below 450 ms), 9 had a prolonged QT_c interval during the study (range 450–516 ms).

Adverse effects leading to dosage reduction or discontinuation were also observed in a retrospective study in 57 patients mean age 84 (range 66–97) years, who took risperidone (doses 0.5–4 mg/day) for more than 1 year (average 2 years) for dementia-related behavioral disturbances (142). Adverse effects included hypotension ($n = 4$), agitation ($n = 6$), and sedation ($n = 5$), and six patients developed a new movement disorder.

In a retrospective study, a substantial proportion of patients who needed antiparkinsonian medication while taking risperidone (mean daily dose 4.4 mg) were identified. Twelve of fifty-five elderly inpatients (aged over 65 years) taking risperidone received antiparkinsonian drugs (143).

A large proportion of new or worsened extrapyramidal adverse effects (32%) was observed in a review of the charts of 41 patients with dementia (mean age 75 years) treated with risperidone (mean 1.8 mg/day) (144).

Children

There was a high incidence (44%) of new movement disorders in 36 children and adolescents who were treated with risperidone (the highest dose of risperidone was 6 mg/day and the average maintenance dose was 4 mg/day) (145). The higher incidence reported in the latter series has been countered by a contrasting report that the most common adverse effect was excessive weight gain ($n = 10$) in a series of 30 children and adolescents (aged 6–21 years) taking risperidone (0.5–6 mg/day) for attention-deficit disorder (146). Vomiting and drowsiness each occurred in one patient; one patient had withdrawal dyskinesia, but the reintroduction of risperidone and slower withdrawal produced no recurrence.

Other features of the patient

Hypothermia associated with hypothalamic and thermoregulatory dysfunction has been reported in a patient with Prader–Willi syndrome taking risperidone and olanzapine (147). Hypothermia in response to these drugs is said to result from $5-HT_2$ receptor blockade, and it is recommended that patients with hypothalamic dysfunction should be carefully monitored if risperidone or olanzapine are used.

Drug Administration

Drug dosage regimens

The safety and tolerability of a rapid oral loading regimen for risperidone, developed to achieve therapeutic doses within 24 hours, have been evaluated (148). Risperidone was begun in a dose of 1 mg, increasing by 1 mg every 6–8 hours up to 3 mg. Dose increases were contingent on the tolerance of the last administered dose. Of 11 consecutive inpatients who were treated with this protocol, seven tolerated the most rapid titration, achieving a dose of 3 mg bd in 16 hours; three required slightly slower titration and achieved the target dose in 24 hours; one could not tolerate the 3 mg dose but tolerated 2 mg tds; no patient had serious extrapyramidal adverse effects, sedation, or any other adverse event during the rapid titration, and in no case did risperidone have to be withdrawn. The authors concluded that aggressive dosing with risperidone is well tolerated in most psychiatric inpatients.

A randomized double-blind comparison of two dosage regimens of risperidone, 8 mg od and 4 mg bd for 6 weeks, in 211 patients has provided further information (149). Neither efficacy nor ESRS scores differed significantly. At least one adverse event was reported in 72 of the patients taking once-daily therapy and 87 of the patients taking twice-daily therapy. The most frequently reported were insomnia, anxiety, extrapyramidal symptoms, agitation, and headache. The only statistically significant difference between the groups was in the incidence of anxiety, which was reported by 31% of those taking twice-daily therapy and 17% of those taking once-daily therapy.

The optimal dose of risperidone in first-episode schizophrenia has been studied in 17 drug-naive patients (12 women, 5 men; mean age 29 years) (150). The mean optimal dosage of risperidone was 2.70 mg/day. All the patients reached the optimal dose before developing extrapyramidal adverse effects; four developed parkinsonism and one developed akathisia at a mean dosage of 5.20 mg/day. In contrast, acute exacerbations of schizophrenia may require a higher dose.

Drug overdose

During 13 months, a regional poisons center gathered information by telephone on 31 patients with reported risperidone overdose (151). Risperidone was the sole ingestant in 15 cases (1–180 mg). The major effects in this group included lethargy ($n = 7$), spasm/dystonia ($n = 3$), hypotension ($n = 2$), tachycardia ($n = 6$), and dysrhythmias ($n = 1$). One patient who co-ingested imipramine died of medical complications, but symptoms resolved within 24 hours in most of the others; all the patients were asymptomatic at 72 hours after ingestion.

- A 41-year-old man who took risperidone 270 mg developed a prolonged QT_c interval (480 ms) and sinus bradycardia (44/minute), without hemodynamic compromise. After 9 hours, he had episodes of asymptomatic supraventricular tachycardia with a maximum frequency of 150/minute. After 30 hours he was in sinus rhythm with a normal QT_c interval (360 ms). He was discharged 72 hours after admission, asymptomatic and with a normal electrocardiogram.
- A 15-year-old who took 110 mg of risperidone in a suicide attempt developed only transient lethargy, hypotension, and tachycardia without any other significant effects (152).

Drug–Drug Interactions

Carbamazepine

Carbamazepine induces CYP3A, and the metabolism of risperidone, which mainly involves CYP2D6, may also involve CYP3A. Carbamazepine can therefore reduce risperidone plasma concentrations (SEDA-22, 71). However, since carbamazepine alters the biotransformation of many agents, non-specific enzyme induction has been suggested for the risperidone and carbamazepine interaction (153).

Plasma concentrations of risperidone and 9-hydroxyrisperidone were measured in 44 patients (aged 26–63 years) treated with risperidone alone ($n = 23$) or co-medicated with carbamazepine ($n = 11$) (154). Carbamazepine markedly reduced the plasma concentrations of risperidone and 9-hydroxyrisperidone.

Mean plasma concentrations of risperidone and 9-hydroxyrisperidone (5 ng/ml and 35 ng/ml) fell significantly during carbamazepine co-administration (2.5 ng/ml and 19 ng/ml) in 11 schizophrenic patients taking risperidone 6 mg/day and then carbamazepine 400 mg/day for 1 week; the changes in risperidone concentrations correlated positively with the concentration ratio of risperidone/9-hydroxyrisperidone, which was closely associated with CYP2D6 genotype (155).

Conversely, carbamazepine concentrations can increase when risperidone is added; when risperidone 1 mg/day was added in eight patients taking carbamazepine (mean dose 625 mg/day) carbamazepine plasma concentrations increased from 6.7 μg/ml at baseline to 8.0 μg/ml 2 weeks later (156).

- A 23-year-old man had raised 9-hydroxyrisperidone concentrations in association with carbamazepine

dosage reduction and concomitant fluvoxamine therapy (157).
- In a 50-year-old man with deficient CYP2D6 activity, the addition of carbamazepine to pre-existing risperidone therapy resulted in a marked reduction in the plasma concentrations of risperidone and 9-hydroxyrisperidone and an acute exacerbation of his psychosis (158).

Clozapine

Risperidone increases plasma clozapine concentrations (159). The effects of risperidone 3.25 mg/day on cytochrome P450 isozymes have therefore been assessed in eight patients by determination of the metabolism of caffeine (for CYP1A2), dextromethorphan (for CYP2D6), and mephenytoin (for CYP2C19) (159). The results suggested that risperidone is a weak in vivo inhibitor of CYP2D6, CYP2C19, and CYP1A2. The authors concluded that inhibition by risperidone of those isozymes is an unlikely mechanism to explain increased clozapine concentrations.

HIV protease inhibitors

An interaction of risperidone with ritonavir and indinavir has been reported (160).

- A 34-year-old man with AIDS took risperidone 4 mg/day for a Tourette-like tic disorder. Ritonavir and indinavir were added, and 1 week later he developed significantly impaired swallowing, speaking, and breathing, and worsening of his existing tremors.

The authors hypothesized that inhibition of CYP2D6 and CYP3A4 by ritonavir and indinavir may have resulted in accumulation of the active moiety of risperidone.

Lithium

Dystonia occurred in an 81-year-old man who took lithium in addition to risperidone 1 mg/day, valproic acid 2250 mg/day, and benzatropine 4 mg/day (161).

Maprotiline

In three patients, maprotiline plasma concentrations increased when risperidone was added (162). The rise was explained by inhibition of CYP2D6, by which maprotiline is mainly metabolized.

Opioids

Two patients who were hospitalized with a diagnosis of opioid dependence received concomitant treatment with methadone 50 mg/day in one case, and levorphanol 14 mg/day in the other, each in association with risperidone. After several days, both had symptoms of opioid withdrawal despite having no change in their opioid doses (163). The withdrawal symptoms resolved soon after risperidone was withdrawn. According to the authors, this finding suggests that risperidone may precipitate opioid withdrawal in opioid-dependent patients.

Phenytoin

An interaction between risperidone and phenytoin resulted in extrapyramidal symptoms (164).

SSRIs

The possibility of a pharmacodynamic interaction between risperidone and serotonin re-uptake inhibitors has been discussed (165–167). Published cases of amelioration and deterioration have perpetuated the debate. Amelioration was observed in four patients with depression that had responded inadequately to selective serotonin re-uptake inhibitors by the addition of risperidone 1 mg bd (n = 2) or 0.5 mg at night (n = 2) (168).

Fluoxetine

A pharmacokinetic interaction of risperidone with fluoxetine has been reported (SEDA-22, 71). When 10 schizophrenic patients stabilized on risperidone 4–6 mg/day took fluoxetine 20 mg/day for concomitant depression the mean plasma risperidone concentration increased from 12 to 56 ng/ml at week 4; the concentration of 9-hydroxyrisperidone was not significantly affected (169). One patient dropped out after 1 week because of akathisia associated with a markedly increased plasma risperidone concentration.

In an open, 30-day trial, the pharmacokinetics, safety, and tolerability of a combination of risperidone 4 or 6 mg/day with fluoxetine 20 mg/day were evaluated in 11 psychotic inpatients (170). CYP2D6 genotyping showed that three were poor metabolizers and eight were extensive metabolizers. The mean AUC of risperidone increased from 83 and 398 h.ng/ml to 341 and 514 h.ng/ml when risperidone was co-administered with fluoxetine in extensive and poor metabolizers respectively. However, despite this pharmacokinetic interaction, the severity and incidence of extrapyramidal symptoms and adverse events did not increase significantly when fluoxetine was added; 10 of the 11 patients improved clinically.

- Catastrophic deterioration, with the severity of obsessive-compulsive symptoms returning to pretreatment levels, was observed in a 21-year-old man when risperidone was added to fluoxetine in a dosage that was stepped up to 3 mg/day (171).

Fluvoxamine

- A 24-year-old woman with auditory hallucinations taking risperidone 6 mg/day developed neuroleptic malignant syndrome after adding fluvoxamine 50 mg/day (172).

Paroxetine

The serotonin syndrome has been reported during treatment with paroxetine and risperidone (173). A case of edema in a patient taking risperidone and paroxetine has also been reported (174).

The effects of paroxetine 20 mg/day for 4 weeks on steady-state plasma concentrations of risperidone and its active metabolite 9-hydroxyrisperidone have been studied in 10 patients taking risperidone 4–8 mg/day (175). During paroxetine administration, mean plasma risperidone concentrations increased significantly, while 9-hydroxyrisperidone concentrations fell slightly but not significantly; after 4 weeks, the sum of the risperidone and 9-hydroxyrisperidone concentrations increased significantly by 45% over baseline, and the mean plasma risperidone/9-hydroxyrisperidone concentration ratio was also significantly changed. However, the drug combination was generally well tolerated, with the exception of one patient who developed parkinsonian symptoms during the second week, and whose total plasma risperidone and 9-hydroxyrisperidone concentrations increased by 62%.

Venlafaxine

In eight patients with major depressive disorder without psychotic features, who did not respond to serotonin re-uptake inhibitors therapy when risperidone was added, all improved within 1 week. Furthermore, risperidone also seemed to have beneficial effects on sleep disturbance and sexual dysfunction (176). In an open study in 30 healthy subjects who took risperidone 1 mg orally before and after venlafaxine dosing to steady state, the oral clearance of risperidone fell by 38% and the volume of distribution by 17%, resulting in a 32% increase in AUC; renal clearance of 9-hydroxyrisperidone also fell by 20% (177). The authors concluded that these small effects were consistent with the fact that venlafaxine is unlikely to alter the clearance of risperidone, which is mainly by CYP2D6.

Tetracycline

- A possible interaction of risperidone with tetracycline has been reported in a 15-year-old adolescent with Asperger's syndrome, Tourette's syndrome, and obsessive-compulsive disorder (178). Acute exacerbation of motor and vocal tics occurred when tetracycline 250 mg bd was introduced for acne; withdrawal of tetracycline resulted in an improvement in the tics.

Thioridazine

A 23-year-old man had high risperidone plasma concentrations secondary to concurrent thioridazine use (157).

Valproate

Plasma concentrations of risperidone and 9-hydroxyrisperidone were measured in 44 patients (aged 26–63 years) taking risperidone alone (n = 23) or co-medicated with sodium valproate (n = 10) (154). Valproate had no major effect on plasma risperidone concentrations.

However, an anecdotal report has suggested that some individuals may be susceptible to an interaction.

- Catatonia occurred in a 42-year-old woman taking valproic acid, sertraline, and risperidone (79). The catatonic features evolved for the first time after a single dose of valproate and were alleviated by lorazepam; the same catatonic signs recurred after a second dose of valproate and again remitted after lorazepam.

The authors considered that this was a possible interaction, since catatonia has not been reported with valproate alone.

The addition of risperidone 10 mg/day over 2 months to valproate and clonazepam in a 40-year-old woman provoked marked edema in the legs and moderate edema in the arms (179). The authors considered that this was a possible interaction, since edema has not been reported with either of these drugs separately.

In contrast, a beneficial interaction has been observed when valproic acid was added to risperidone; the previous addition of valproic acid to treatment with chlorpromazine had no effect on psychotic symptoms (180).

Diagnosis of Adverse Drug Reactions

A therapeutic target range for serum risperidone concentrations has not been established, but in 20 of 22 patients taking 6 mg/day, which is considered the optimum dosage for most patients, risperidone serum concentrations were 50–150 nmol/l (181). Steady-state serum concentrations of risperidone and 9-hydroxyrisperidone, the active moiety, were also measured in 42 patients; there was no correlation between the serum concentration of the active moiety and adverse effects.

References

1. Iskedjian M, Hux M, Remington GJ. The Canadian experience with risperidone for the treatment of schizophrenia: an overview. J Psychiatry Neurosci 1998;23(4):229–39.
2. Vieta E, Herraiz M, Fernandez A, Gasto C, Benabarre A, Colom F, Martinez-Aran A, Reinares M. Efficacy and safety of risperidone in the treatment of schizoaffective disorder: initial results from a large, multicenter surveillance study. Group for the Study of Risperidone in Affective Disorders (GSRAD). J Clin Psychiatry 2001;62(8):623–30.
3. Buitelaar JK, van der Gaag RJ, Cohen-Kettenis P, Melman CT. A randomized controlled trial of risperidone in the treatment of aggression in hospitalized adolescents with subaverage cognitive abilities. J Clin Psychiatry 2001;62(4):239–48.
4. McDougle CJ, Epperson CN, Pelton GH, Wasylink S, Price LH. A double-blind, placebo-controlled study of risperidone addition in serotonin reuptake inhibitor-refractory obsessive-compulsive disorder. Arch Gen Psychiatry 2000;57(8):794–801.
5. Davidson M. Long-term safety of risperidone. J Clin Psychiatry 2001;62(Suppl. 21):26–8.
6. McCracken JT, McGough J, Shah B, Cronin P, Hong D, Aman MG, Arnold LE, Lindsay R, Nash P, Hollway J, McDougle CJ, Posey D, Swiezy N, Kohn A, Scahill L, Martin A, Koenig K, Volkmar F, Carroll D, Lancor A, Tierney E, Ghuman J, Gonzalez NM, Grados M, Vitiello B, Ritz L, Davies M, Robinson J, McMahon D. Research Units on Pediatric Psychopharmacology Autism Network. Risperidone in children with autism and serious behavioral problems. N Engl J Med 2002;347(5):314–21.
7. Aman MG, De Smedt G, Derivan A, Lyons B, Findling RL. Risperidone Disruptive Behavior Study Group. Double-blind, placebo-controlled study of risperidone for the treatment of disruptive behaviors in children with subaverage intelligence. Am J Psychiatry 2002;159(8):1337–46.
8. McDougle CJ, Holmes JP, Carlson DC, Pelton GH, Cohen DJ, Price LH. A double-blind, placebo-controlled study of risperidone in adults with autistic disorder and other pervasive developmental disorders. Arch Gen Psychiatry 1998;55(7):633–41.
9. Bhana N, Spencer CM. Risperidone: a review of its use in the management of the behavioural and psychological symptoms of dementia. Drugs Aging 2000;16(6):451–71.
10. Mackay FJ, Wilton LV, Pearce GL, Freemantle SN, Mann RD. The safety of risperidone: a post-marketing study on 7684 patients. Hum Psychopharmacol 1998;13:413–18.
11. Moller HJ, Gagiano CA, Addington DE, Von Knorring L, Torres-Plank JF, Gaussares C. Long-term treatment of chronic schizophrenia with risperidone: an open-label, multicenter study of 386 patients. Int Clin Psychopharmacol 1998;13(3):99–106.
12. Binder RL, McNiel DE, Sandberg DA. A naturalistic study of clinical use of risperidone. Psychiatr Serv 1998;49(4):524–6.
13. Muller-Siecheneder F, Muller MJ, Hillert A, Szegedi A, Wetzel H, Benkert O. Risperidone versus haloperidol and amitriptyline in the treatment of patients with a combined psychotic and depressive syndrome. J Clin Psychopharmacol 1998;18(2):111–20.
14. Vieta E, Gasto C, Colom F, Martinez A, Otero A, Vallejo J. Treatment of refractory rapid cycling bipolar disorder with risperidone. J Clin Psychopharmacol 1998;18(2):172–4.
15. Cohen SA, Ihrig K, Lott RS, Kerrick JM. Risperidone for aggression and self-injurious behavior in adults with mental retardation. J Autism Dev Disord 1998;28(3):229–33.
16. Schreier HA. Risperidone for young children with mood disorders and aggressive behavior. J Child Adolesc Psychopharmacol 1998;8(1):49–59.
17. Madhusoodanan S, Suresh P, Brenner R, Pillai R. Experience with the atypical antipsychotics—risperidone and olanzapine in the elderly. Ann Clin Psychiatry 1999;11(3):113–18.
18. Keks NA, Culhane C. Risperidone (Risperdal): clinical experience with a new antipsychosis drug. Expert Opin Investig Drugs 1999;8(4):443–52.
19. Chong SA, Yap HL, Low BL, Choo CH, Chan AO, Wong KE, Mahendran R, Chee KT. Clinical evaluation of risperidone in Asian patients with schizophrenia in Singapore. Singapore Med J 1999;40(1):41–3.
20. Meibach RC, Mazurek MF, Rosebush P. Neurologic side effects in neuroleptic-naive patients treated with haloperidol or risperidone. Neurology 2000;55(7):1069.
21. Huston P, Moher D. Redundancy, disaggregation, and the integrity of medical research. Lancet 1996;347(9007):1024–6.
22. Rennie D. Fair conduct and fair reporting of clinical trials. JAMA 1999;282(18):1766–8.
23. Lane HY, Chiu WC, Chou JC, Wu ST, Su MH, Chang WH. Risperidone in acutely exacerbated schizophrenia: dosing strategies and plasma levels. J Clin Psychiatry 2000;61(3):209–14.
24. Zuddas A, Di Martino A, Muglia P, Cianchetti C. Long-term risperidone for pervasive developmental disorder: efficacy, tolerability, and discontinuation. J Child Adolesc Psychopharmacol 2000;10(2):79–90.
25. Findling RL, McNamara NK, Branicky LA, Schluchter MD, Lemon E, Blumer JL. A double-blind pilot study of risperidone in the treatment of conduct disorder. J Am Acad Child Adolesc Psychiatry 2000;39(4):509–16.
26. Buitelaar JK. Open-label treatment with risperidone of 26 psychiatrically-hospitalized children and adolescents with mixed diagnoses and aggressive behavior. J Child Adolesc Psychopharmacol 2000;10(1):19–26.
27. Heck AH, Haffmans PM, de Groot IW, Hoencamp E. Risperidone versus haloperidol in psychotic patients with disturbing neuroleptic-induced extrapyramidal symptoms: a double-blind, multi-center trial. Schizophr Res 2000;46(2–3):97–105.

28. De Deyn PP, Rabheru K, Rasmussen A, Bocksberger JP, Dautzenberg PL, Eriksson S, Lawlor BA. A randomized trial of risperidone, placebo, and haloperidol for behavioral symptoms of dementia. Neurology 1999;53(5):946–55.

29. Katz IR, Jeste DV, Mintzer JE, Clyde C, Napolitano J, Brecher M. Comparison of risperidone and placebo for psychosis and behavioral disturbances associated with dementia: a randomized, double-blind trial. Risperidone Study Group. J Clin Psychiatry 1999;60(2):107–15.

30. Ravin DS, Levenson JW. Fatal cardiac event following initiation of risperidone therapy. Ann Pharmacother 1997;31(7–8):867–70.

31. Posey DJ, Walsh KH, Wilson GA, McDougle CJ. Risperidone in the treatment of two very young children with autism. J Child Adolesc Psychopharmacol 1999;9(4):273–6.

32. Henretig FM. Risperidone toxicity acknowledged. J Toxicol Clin Toxicol 1999;37:893–4.

33. Lee HJ, Lee HS, Kim L, Lee MS, Suh KY, Kwak DI. A case of risperidone-induced stuttering. J Clin Psychopharmacol 2001;21(1):115–16.

34. Dresel S, Tatsch K, Dahne I, Mager T, Scherer J, Hahn K. Iodine-123-iodobenzamide SPECT assessment of dopamine D_2 receptor occupancy in risperidone-treated schizophrenic patients. J Nucl Med 1998;39(7):1138–42.

35. Miller CH, Mohr F, Umbricht D, Woerner M, Fleischhacker WW, Lieberman JA. The prevalence of acute extrapyramidal signs and symptoms in patients treated with clozapine, risperidone, and conventional antipsychotics. J Clin Psychiatry 1998;59(2):69–75.

36. Lemmens P, Brecher M, Van Baelen B. A combined analysis of double-blind studies with risperidone vs. placebo and other antipsychotic agents: factors associated with extrapyramidal symptoms. Acta Psychiatr Scand 1999;99(3):160–70.

37. Emsley RA. Risperidone in the treatment of first-episode psychotic patients: a double-blind multicenter study. Risperidone Working Group. Schizophr Bull 1999;25(4):721–9.

38. Wirshing DA, Marshall BD Jr, Green MF, Mintz J, Marder SR, Wirshing WC. Risperidone in treatment-refractory schizophrenia. Am J Psychiatry 1999;156(9):1374–9.

39. Lavretsky H, Sultzer D. A structured trial of risperidone for the treatment of agitation in dementia. Am J Geriatr Psychiatry 1998;6(2):127–35.

40. Herrmann N, Rivard MF, Flynn M, Ward C, Rabheru K, Campbell B. Risperidone for the treatment of behavioral disturbances in dementia: a case series. J Neuropsychiatry Clin Neurosci 1998;10(2):220–3.

41. Hong R, Matsuyama E, Nur K. Cardiomyopathy associated with the smoking of crystal methamphetamine. JAMA 1991;265(9):1152–4.

42. Geizer M, Ancill RJ. Combination of risperidone and donepezil in Lewy body dementia. Can J Psychiatry 1998;43(4):421–2.

43. Wetter TC, Brunner J, Bronisch T. Restless legs syndrome probably induced by risperidone treatment. Pharmacopsychiatry 2002;35(3):109–11.

44. Roberts MD. Risperdal and parkinsonian tremor. J Am Acad Child Adolesc Psychiatry 1999;38(3):230.

45. Meco G, Fabrizio E, Alessandri A, Vanacore N, Bonifati V. Risperidone in levodopa induced dyskinesiae. J Neurol Neurosurg Psychiatry 1998;64(1):135.

46. Friedman JH, Ott BR. Should risperidone be used in Parkinson's disease? J Neuropsychiatry Clin Neurosci 1998;10(4):473–5.

47. Workman RH. In reply. J Neuropsychiatry Clin Neurosci 1998;10:474–5.

48. Leopold NA. Risperidone treatment of drug-related psychosis in patients with parkinsonism. Mov Disord 2000;15(2):301–4.

49. Lang DJ, Kopala LC, Vandorpe RA, Rui Q, Smith GN, Goghari VM, Honer WG. An MRI study of basal ganglia volumes in first-episode schizophrenia patients treated with risperidone. Am J Psychiatry 2001;158(4):625–31.

50. Haberfellner EM. Tardive dyskinesia during treatment with risperidone. Pharmacopsychiatry 1997;30(6):271.

51. Saran BM. Risperidone-induced tardive dyskinesia. J Clin Psychiatry 1998;59(1):29–30.

52. Silberbauer C. Risperidone-induced tardive dyskinesia. Pharmacopsychiatry 1998;31(2):68–9.

53. Friedman JH. Rapid onset tardive dyskinesia ("fly catcher tongue") in a neuroleptically naive patient induced by risperidone. Med Health R I 1998;81(8):271–2.

54. Sakkas P, Liappas J, Christodoulou GN. Tardive dyskinesia due to risperidone. Eur Psychiatry 1998;13:107–8.

55. Fischer P, Tauscher J, Kufferle B. Risperidone and tardive dyskinesia in organic psychosis. Pharmacopsychiatry 1998;31(2):70–1.

56. Campbell M. Risperidone-induced tardive dyskinesia in first-episode psychotic patients. J Clin Psychopharmacol 1999;19(3):276–7.

57. Carroll NB, Boehm KE, Strickland RT. Chorea and tardive dyskinesia in a patient taking risperidone. J Clin Psychiatry 1999;60(7):485–7.

58. Hong KS, Cheong SS, Woo JM, Kim E. Risperidone-induced tardive dyskinesia. Am J Psychiatry 1999;156(8):1290.

59. Snoddgrass PL, Labbate LA. Tardive dyskinesia from risperidone and olanzapine in an alcoholic man. Can J Psychiatry 1999;44(9):921.

60. Kumar S, Malone DM. Risperidone implicated in the onset of tardive dyskinesia in a young woman. Postgrad Med J 2000;76(895):316–17.

61. Spivak M, Smart M. Tardive dyskinesia from low-dose risperidone. Can J Psychiatry 2000;45(2):202.

62. Jeste DV, Okamoto A, Napolitano J, Kane JM, Martinez RA. Low incidence of persistent tardive dyskinesia in elderly patients with dementia treated with risperidone. Am J Psychiatry 2000;157(7):1150–5.

63. Silver H, Aharon N, Schwartz M. Attention deficit-hyperactivity disorder may be a risk factor for treatment-emergent tardive dyskinesia induced by risperidone. J Clin Psychopharmacol 2000;20(1):112–14.

64. Lore C. Risperidone and withdrawal dyskinesia. J Am Acad Child Adolesc Psychiatry 2000;39(8):941.

65. Mullen A, Cullen M. Risperidone and tardive dyskinesia: a case of blepharospasm. Aust NZ J Psychiatry 2000;34(5):879–80.

66. Bassitt DP, de Souza Lobo Garcia L. Risperidone-induced tardive dyskinesia. Pharmacopsychiatry 2000;33(4):155–6.

67. Narendran R, Young CM, Pato MT. Possible risperidone-induced tardive dystonia. Ann Pharmacother 2000;34(12):1487–8.

68. Yoshida K, Higuchi H, Hishikawa Y. Marked improvement of tardive dystonia after replacing haloperidol with risperidone in a schizophrenic patient. Clin Neuropharmacol 1998;21(1):68–9.

69. Jagadheesan K, Nizamie SH. Risperidone-induced Pisa syndrome. Aust N Z J Psychiatry 2002;36(1):144.

70. Harada K, Sasaki N, Ikeda H, Nakano N, Ozawa H, Saito T. Risperidone-induced Pisa syndrome. J Clin Psychiatry 2002;63(2):166.

71. Levin T, Heresco-Levy U. Risperidone-induced rabbit syndrome: an unusual movement disorder caused by an atypical antipsychotic. Eur Neuropsychopharmacol 1999;9(1–2):137–9.

72. Hoy JS, Alexander B. Rabbit syndrome secondary to risperidone. Pharmacotherapy 2002;22(4):513–15.

73. Rohrbach P, Collinot JP, Vallet G. Syndrome malin des neuroleptiques induit par la rispéridone. [Neuroleptic malignant syndrome induced by risperidone.] Ann Fr Anesth Reanim 1998;17(1):85–6.

74. Aguirre C, Garcia Monco JC, Mendibil B. Síndrome neuroléptico maligno asociado a risperidona. [Neuroleptic malignant syndrome associated with risperidone.] Med Clin 1998;110:239.

75. Lee MS, Lee HJ, Kim L. A case of delayed NMS induced by risperidone. Psychiatr Serv 2000;51(2):254–5.

76. Robb AS, Chang W, Lee HK, Cook MS. Case study. Risperidone-induced neuroleptic malignant syndrome in an adolescent. J Child Adolesc Psychopharmacol 2000;10(4):327–30.

77. Sechi G, Agnetti V, Masuri R, Deiana GA, Pugliatti M, Paulus KS, Rosati G. Risperidone, neuroleptic malignant syndrome and probable dementia with Lewy bodies. Prog Neuropsychopharmacol Biol Psychiatry 2000;24(6):1043–51.

78. Dursun SM, Oluboka OJ, Devarajan S, Kutcher SP. High-dose vitamin E plus vitamin B6 treatment of risperidone-related neuroleptic malignant syndrome. J Psychopharmacol 1998;12(2):220–1.

79. Lauterbach EC. Catatonia-like events after valproic acid with risperidone and sertraline. Neuropsychiatry Neuropsychol Behav Neurol 1998;11(3):157–63.

80. Bahro M, Kampf C, Strnad J. Catatonia under medication with risperidone in a 61-year-old patient. Acta Psychiatr Scand 1999;99(3):223–6.

81. Edwards RJ, Pople IK. Side-effects of risperidone therapy mimicking cerebrospinal fluid shunt malfunction: implications for clinical monitoring and management. J Psychopharmacol 2002;16(2):177–9.

82. Hori M, Shiraishi H. Risperidone-induced anxiety might also develop "awakening" phenomenon. Psychiatry Clin Neurosci 1999;53(6):682.

83. Ashleigh EA, Larsen PD. A syndrome of increased affect in response to risperidone among patients with schizophrenia. Psychiatr Serv 1998;49(4):526–8.

84. Lauterbach EC, Abdelhamid A, Annandale JB. Posthallucinogen-like visual illusions (palinopsia) with risperidone in a patient without previous hallucinogen exposure: possible relation to serotonin 5HT$_{2a}$ receptor blockade. Pharmacopsychiatry 2000;33(1):38–41.

85. Bakaras P, Georgoussi M, Liakos A. Development of obsessive and depressive symptoms during risperidone treatment. Br J Psychiatry 1999;174:559.

86. Zolezzi M, Badr MG. Risperidone-induced mania. Ann Pharmacother 1999;33(3):380–1.

87. Guzelcan Y, de Haan L, Scholte WF. Risperidone may induce mania. Psychopharmacology (Berl) 2002;162(1):85–6.

88. Mahendran R. Obsessional symptoms associated with risperidone treatment. Aust NZ J Psychiatry 1998;32(2):299–301.

89. Mahendran R, Andrade C, Saxena S. Obsessive-compulsive symptoms with risperidone. J Clin Psychiatry 1999;60(4):261–3.

90. Sinha BN, Duggal HS, Nizamie SH. Risperidone-induced obsessive-compulsive symptoms: a reappraisal. Can J Psychiatry 2000;45(4):397–8.

91. Jones H, Curtis VA, Wright PA, Lucey JV. Risperidone is associated with blunting of D-fenfluramine evoked serotonergic responses in schizophrenia. Int Clin Psychopharmacol 1998;13(5):199–203.

92. Shiwach RS, Carmody TJ. Prolactogenic effects of risperidone in male patients—a preliminary study. Acta Psychiatr Scand 1998;98(1):81–3.

93. David SR, Taylor CC, Kinon BJ, Breier A. The effects of olanzapine, risperidone, and haloperidol on plasma prolactin levels in patients with schizophrenia. Clin Ther 2000;22(9):1085–96.

94. Tollin SR. Use of the dopamine agonists bromocriptine and cabergoline in the management of risperidone-induced hyperprolactinemia in patients with psychotic disorders. J Endocrinol Invest 2000;23(11):765–70.

95. Kleinberg DL, Davis JM, de Coster R, Van Baelen B, Brecher M. Prolactin levels and adverse events in patients treated with risperidone. J Clin Psychopharmacol 1999;19(1):57–61.

96. Kim YK, Kim L, Lee MS. Risperidone and associated amenorrhea: a report of 5 cases. J Clin Psychiatry 1999;60(5):315–17.

97. Popli A, Gupta S, Rangwani SR. Risperidone-induced galactorrhea associated with a prolactin elevation. Ann Clin Psychiatry 1998;10(1):31–3.

98. Schreiber S, Segman RH. Risperidone-induced galactorrhea. Psychopharmacology (Berl) 1997;130(3):300–1.

99. Gazzola LR, Opler LA. Return of menstruation after switching from risperidone to olanzapine. J Clin Psychopharmacol 1998;18(6):486–7.

100. Mabini R, Wergowske G, Baker FM. Galactorrhea and gynecomastia in a hypothyroid male being treated with risperidone. Psychiatr Serv 2000;51(8):983–5.

101. Gupta S, Frank B, Madhusoodanan S. Risperidone-associated galactorrhea in a male teenager. J Am Acad Child Adolesc Psychiatry 2001;40(5):504–5.

102. Kim KS, Pae CU, Chae JH, Bahk WM, Jun TY, Kim DJ, Dickson RA. Effects of olanzapine on prolactin levels of female patients with schizophrenia treated with risperidone. J Clin Psychiatry 2002;63(5):408–13.

103. Yamada K, Kanba S, Yagi G, Asai M. Herbal medicine (Shakuyaku-kanzo-to) in the treatment of risperidone-induced amenorrhea. J Clin Psychopharmacol 1999;19(4):380–1.

104. Croarkin PE, Jacobs KM, Bain BK. Diabetic ketoacidosis associated with risperidone treatment? Psychosomatics 2000;41(4):369–70.

105. Horrigan JP, Sikich L. Diet and the atypical neuroleptics. J Am Acad Child Adolesc Psychiatry 1998;37(11):1126–7.

106. Martin A, Landau J, Leebens P, Ulizio K, Cicchetti D, Scahill L, Leckman JF. Risperidone-associated weight gain in children and adolescents: a retrospective chart review. J Child Adolesc Psychopharmacol 2000;10(4):259–68.

107. Barak Y. No weight gain among elderly schizophrenia patients after 1 year of risperidone treatment. J Clin Psychiatry 2002;63(2):117–19.

108. Wirshing DA, Pierre JM, Wirshing WC. Sleep apnea associated with antipsychotic-induced obesity. J Clin Psychiatry 2002;63(4):369–70.

109. Whitten JR, Ruehter VL. Risperidone and hyponatremia: a case report. Ann Clin Psychiatry 1997;9(3):181–3.

110. Kern RS, Marshall BD, Kuehnel TG, Mintz J, Hayden JL, Robertson MJ, Green MF. Effects of risperidone on polydipsia in chronic schizophrenia patients. J Clin Psychopharmacol 1997;17(5):432–5.

111. Kar N, Sharma PS, Tolar P, Pai K, Balasubramanian R. Polydipsia and risperidone. Aust NZ J Psychiatry 2002;36(2):268–70.

112. Edleman RJ. Risperidone side effects. J Am Acad Child Adolesc Psychiatry 1996;35(1):4–5.

113. Dernovsek Z, Tavcar R. Risperidone-induced leucopenia and neutropenia. Br J Psychiatry 1997;171:393–4.

114. Finkel B, Lerner AG, Oyffe I, Sigal M. Risperidone-associated agranulocytosis. Am J Psychiatry 1998;155(6):855–6.

115. Assion HJ, Kolbinger HM, Rao ML, Laux G. Lymphocytopenia and thrombocytopenia during treatment with risperidone or clozapine. Pharmacopsychiatry 1996;29(6):227–8.

116. Gajwani P, Franco-Bronson K, Tesar GE. Risperidone-induced sialorrhea. Psychosomatics 2001;42(3):276.

117. Fuller MA, Simon MR, Freedman L. Risperidone-associated hepatotoxicity. J Clin Psychopharmacol 1996;16(1):84–5.

118. Phillips EJ, Liu BA, Knowles SR. Rapid onset of risperidone-induced hepatotoxicity. Ann Pharmacother 1998;32(7–8):843.

119. Benazzi F. Risperidone-induced hepatotoxicity. Pharmacopsychiatry 1998;31(6):241.

120. Landau J, Martin A. Is liver function monitoring warranted during risperidone treatment? J Am Acad Child Adolesc Psychiatry 1998;37(10):1007–8.

121. Whitworth AB, Liensberger D, Fleischhacker WW. Transient increase of liver enzymes induced by risperidone: two case reports. J Clin Psychopharmacol 1999;19(5):475–6.

122. Krebs S, Dormann H, Muth-Selbach U, Hahn EG, Brune K, Schneider HT. Risperidone-induced cholestatic hepatitis. Eur J Gastroenterol Hepatol 2001;13(1):67–9.

123. Hudson RG, Cain MP. Risperidone associated hemorrhagic cystitis. J Urol 1998;160(1):159.

124. Agarwal V. Urinary incontinence with risperidone. J Clin Psychiatry 2000;61(3):219.

125. Almond DS, Rhodes LE, Pirmohamed M. Risperidone-induced photosensitivity. Postgrad Med J 1998;74(870):252–3.

126. Tekell JL, Smith EA, Silva JA. Prolonged erection associated with risperidone treatment. Am J Psychiatry 1995;152(7):1097.

127. Sirota P, Bogdanov I. Priapism associated with risperidone treatment. Int J Psychiatry Clin Pract 2000;4:237–9.

128. Reeves RR, Mack JE. Priapism associated with two atypical antipsychotic agents. Pharmacotherapy 2002;22(8):1070–3.

129. Ankem MK, Ferlise VJ, Han KR, Gazi MA, Koppisch AR, Weiss RE. Risperidone-induced priapism. Scand J Urol Nephrol 2002;36(1):91–2.

130. Freudenreich O. Exacerbation of idiopathic priapism with risperidone–citalopram combination. J Clin Psychiatry 2002;63(3):249–50.

131. Kaneda Y. Risperidone-induced ejaculatory dysfunction: a case report. Eur Psychiatry 2001;16(2):134–5.

132. Shiloh R, Weizman A, Weizer N, Dorfman-Etrog P, Munitz H. Risperidone-induced retrograde ejaculation. Am J Psychiatry 2001;158(4):650.

133. Lane HY, Chang WH. Manic and psychotic symptoms following risperidone withdrawal in a schizophrenic patient. J Clin Psychiatry 1998;59(11):620–1.

134. Miller LJ. Withdrawal-emergent dyskinesia in a patient taking risperidone/citalopram. Ann Pharmacother 2000;34(2):269.

135. Ratnayake T, Libretto SE. No complications with risperidone treatment before and throughout pregnancy and during the nursing period. J Clin Psychiatry 2002;63(1):76–7.

136. Mackay FJ, Wilton GL, Pearce SN, Freemantle SN, Mann RD. The safety of risperidone a postmarketing study on 7684 patients. Hum Psychopharmacol 1998;13:413–18.

137. Hill RC, McIvor RJ, Wojnar-Horton R, Hackett LP, Ilett KF. Risperidone distribution and excretion into human milk: report and estimated infant exposure during breast-feeding. J Clin Psychopharmocol 2000;20:285–6.

138. Kohnke MD, Griese EU, Stosser D, Gaertner I, Barth G. Cytochrome P450 2D6 deficiency and its clinical relevance in a patient treated with risperidone. Pharmacopsychiatry 2002;35(3):116–18.

139. Ravona-Springer R, Dolberg OT, Hirschmann S, Grunhaus L. Delirium in elderly patients treated with risperidone: a report of three cases. J Clin Psychopharmacol 1998;18(2):171–2.

140. Tavcar R, Dernovsek MZ. Risperidone-induced delirium. Can J Psychiatry 1998;43(2):194.

141. Madhusoodanan S, Brecher M, Brenner R, Kasckow J, Kunik M, Negron AE, Pomara N. Risperidone in the treatment of elderly patients with psychotic disorders. Am J Geriatr Psychiatry 1999;7(2):132–8.

142. Goldberg RJ. Long-term use of risperidone for the treatment of dementia-related behavioral disturbances in a nursing home population. Int J Geriatr Psychopharmacol 1999;2:1–4.

143. Cates M, Collins R, Woolley T. Antiparkinsonian drug prescribing in elderly inpatients receiving risperidone therapy. Am J Health Syst Pharm 1999;56(20):2139–40.

144. Irizarry MC, Ghaemi SN, Lee-Cherry ER, Gomez-Isla T, Binetti G, Hyman BT, Growdon JH. Risperidone treatment of behavioral disturbances in outpatients with dementia. J Neuropsychiatry Clin Neurosci 1999;11(3):336–42.

145. Demb HB, Nguyen KT. Movement disorders in children with developmental disabilities taking risperidone. J Am Acad Child Adolesc Psychiatry 1999;38(1):5–6.

146. Kewley GD. Risperidone in comorbid ADHD and ODD/CD. J Am Acad Child Adolesc Psychiatry 1999;38(11):1327–8.

147. Phan TG, Yu RY, Hersch MI. Hypothermia induced by risperidone and olanzapine in a patient with Prader–Willi syndrome. Med J Aust 1998;169(4):230–1.

148. Feifel D, Moutier CY, Perry W. Safety and tolerability of a rapidly escalating dose-loading regimen for risperidone. J Clin Psychiatry 2000;61(12):909–11.

149. Nair NP, Reiter-Schmitt B, Ronovsky K, Vyssoki D, Baeke J, Desseilles M, Kindts P, Mesotten F, Peuskens J, Addington D, et al. Therapeutic equivalence of risperidone given once daily and twice daily in patients with schizophrenia. The Risperidone Study Group. J Clin Psychopharmacol 1998;18(2):103–10.

150. Kontaxakis VP, Havaki-Kontaxaki BJ, Stamouli SS, Christodoulou GN. Optimal risperidone dose in drug-naive, first-episode schizophrenia. Am J Psychiatry 2000;157(7):1178–9.

151. Acri AA, Henretig FM. Effects of risperidone in overdose. Am J Emerg Med 1998;16(5):498–501.

152. Catalano G, Catalano MC, Nunez CY, Walker SC. Atypical antipsychotic overdose in the pediatric population. J Child Adolesc Psychopharmacol 2001;11(4):425–34.

153. Lane HY, Chang WH. Risperidone–carbamazepine interactions: is cytochrome P450 3A involved? J Clin Psychiatry 1998;59(8):430–1.

154. Spina E, Avenoso A, Facciola G, Salemi M, Scordo MG, Giacobello T, Madia AG, Perucca E. Plasma concentrations of risperidone and 9-hydroxyrisperidone: effect of comedication with carbamazepine or valproate. Ther Drug Monit 2000;22(4):481–5.

155. Ono S, Mihara K, Suzuki A, Kondo T, Yasui-Furukori N, Furukori H, de Vries R, Kaneko S. Significant pharmacokinetic interaction between risperidone and carbamazepine: its relationship with CYP2D6 genotypes. Psychopharmacology (Berl) 2002;162(1):50–4.

156. Mula M, Monaco F. Carbamazepine–risperidone interactions in patients with epilepsy. Clin Neuropharmacol 2002;25(2):97–100.

157. Alfaro CL, Nicolson R, Lenane M, Rapoport JL. Carbamazepine and/or fluvoxamine drug interaction with risperidone in a patient on multiple psychotropic medications. Ann Pharmacother 2000;34(1):122–3.

158. Spina E, Scordo MG, Avenoso A, Perucca E. Adverse drug interaction between risperidone and carbamazepine in a patient with chronic schizophrenia and deficient

CYP2D6 activity. J Clin Psychopharmacol 2001;21(1):108–9.

159. Eap CB, Bondolfi G, Zullino D, Bryois C, Fuciec M, Savary L, Jonzier-Perey M, Baumann P. Pharmacokinetic drug interaction potential of risperidone with cytochrome P450 isozymes as assessed by the dextromethorphan, the caffeine, and the mephenytoin test. Ther Drug Monit 2001;23(3):228–31.

160. Kelly DV, Beique LC, Bowmer MI. Extrapyramidal symptoms with ritonavir/indinavir plus risperidone. Ann Pharmacother 2002;36(5):827–30.

161. Durrenberger S, de Leon J. Acute dystonic reaction to lithium and risperidone. J Neuropsychiatry Clin Neurosci 1999;11(4):518–19.

162. Normann C, Lieb K, Walden J. Increased plasma concentration of maprotiline by coadministration of risperidone. J Clin Psychopharmacol 2002;22(1):92–4.

163. Wines JD Jr, Weiss RD. Opioid withdrawal during risperidone treatment. J Clin Psychopharmacol 1999;19(3):265–7.

164. Sanderson DR. Drug interaction between risperidone and phenytoin resulting in extrapyramidal symptoms. J Clin Psychiatry 1996;57(4):177.

165. Caley CF. Extrapyramidal reactions from concurrent SSRI and atypical antipsychotic use. Can J Psychiatry 1998;43(3):307–8.

166. Baker RW. Possible dose–response relationship for risperidone in obsessive-compulsive disorder. J Clin Psychiatry 1998;59(3):134.

167. Stein DJ, Hawkridge S, Bouwer C, Emsley RA. Dr Stein and colleagues reply. J Clin Psychiatry 1998;59:134.

168. O'Connor M, Silver H. Adding risperidone to selective serotonin reuptake inhibitor improves chronic depression. J Clin Psychopharmacol 1998;18(1):89–91.

169. Spina E, Avenoso A, Scordo MG, Ancione M, Madia A, Gatti G, Perucca E. Inhibition of risperidone metabolism by fluoxetine in patients with schizophrenia: a clinically relevant pharmacokinetic drug interaction. J Clin Psychopharmacol 2002;22(4):419–23.

170. Bondolfi G, Eap CB, Bertschy G, Zullino D, Vermeulen A, Baumann P. The effect of fluoxetine on the pharmacokinetics and safety of risperidone in psychiatric patients. Pharmacopsychiatry 2002;35(2):50–6.

171. Andrade C. Risperidone may worsen fluoxetine-treated OCD. J Clin Psychiatry 1998;59(5):255–6.

172. Reeves RR, Mack JE, Beddingfield JJ. Neurotoxic syndrome associated with risperidone and fluvoxamine. Ann Pharmacother 2002;36(3):440–3.

173. Hamilton S, Malone K. Serotonin syndrome during treatment with paroxetine and risperidone. J Clin Psychopharmacol 2000;20(1):103–5.

174. Masson M, Elayli R, Verdoux H. Rispéridone et edème: à propos d'un cas. [Risperidone and edema: apropos of a case.] Encephale 2000;26(3):91–2.

175. Spina E, Avenoso A, Facciola G, Scordo MG, Ancione M, Madia A. Plasma concentrations of risperidone and 9-hydroxyrisperidone during combined treatment with paroxetine. Ther Drug Monit 2001;23(3):223–7.

176. Ostroff RB, Nelson JC. Risperidone augmentation of selective serotonin reuptake inhibitors in major depression. J Clin Psychiatry 1999;60(4):256–9.

177. Amchin J, Zarycranski W, Taylor KP, Albano D, Klockowski PM. Effect of venlafaxine on the pharmacokinetics of risperidone. J Clin Pharmacol 1999;39(3):297–309.

178. Steele M, Couturier J. A possible tetracycline–risperidone–sertraline interaction in an adolescent. Can J Clin Pharmacol 1999;6(1):15–17.

179. Sanders RD, Lehrer DS. Edema associated with addition of risperidone to valproate treatment. J Clin Psychiatry 1998;59(12):689–90.

180. Chong SA, Tan CH, Lee EL, Liow PH. Augmentation of risperidone with valproic acid. J Clin Psychiatry 1998;59(8):430.

181. Olesen OV, Licht RW, Thomsen E, Bruun T, Viftrup JE, Linnet K. Serum concentrations and side effects in psychiatric patients during risperidone therapy. Ther Drug Monit 1998;20(4):380–4.

Ritanserin

General Information

Ritanserin, a selective 5-HT$_2$ receptor antagonist, increases slow-wave sleep in healthy volunteers [1]. It improved sleep in middle-aged poor sleepers [2], but on withdrawal after 20 days treatment there was rebound sleep impairment, which was at its worst 3 nights after withdrawal, consistent with its long half-life (40 hours). Ritanserin is thus not a useful hypnotic, but analogues with more appropriate kinetics will be of interest.

References

1. Idzikowski C, Mills FJ, James RJ. A dose-response study examining the effects of ritanserin on human slow wave sleep. Br J Clin Pharmacol 1991;31(2):193–6.

2. Adam K, Oswald I. Effects of repeated ritanserin on middle-aged poor sleepers. Psychopharmacology (Berl) 1989;99(2):219–21.

Ritodrine

See also Beta$_2$-adrenoceptor agonists

General Information

Ritodrine is a beta$_2$-adrenoceptor agonist used in the treatment of premature labor.

The hemodynamic effects of ritodrine have been assessed in 12 fetuses by cardiac and extracardiac Doppler sonography [1]. Ritodrine significantly increased maternal and fetal heart rates, left cardiac stroke volume, and cardiac output. There was also an increase in the pulsatility index of the middle cerebral artery and a fall in the pulsatility index of the umbilical artery during ritodrine infusion. The authors suggested that ritodrine vasodilates fetal vessels in the placenta.

Organs and Systems

Cardiovascular

Ritodrine can cause bradycardia instead of the expected tachycardia (SEDA-8, 145); an unexpected hypertensive crisis has also been reported (SEDA-8, 145). ST segment depression is a consistent finding in patients during ritodrine infusion, and should therefore not always be interpreted as an indication of myocardial ischemia. The electrocardiographic changes are unrelated to the more generally accepted changes in heart rate, glucose, and potassium concentrations and are probably an intrinsic effect of the drug.

Endocrine

Brief infusions of ritodrine (0.15 mg/minute for 4 hours) rapidly increased plasma melatonin concentrations in healthy women (2).

Metabolism

There are two well-documented independent reports of severe ketoacidosis in non-diabetic pregnant subjects; both the beta-agonist therapy and inadequate dietary intake could have played a role (3).

Hematologic

Agranulocytosis has been documented in a pregnant woman given ritodrine (SEDA-17, 165).

Skin

Palmar erythema was observed in 12 of 209 patients who were treated with ritodrine for more than 7 days (SEDA-12, 123).

Immunologic

A petechial rash due to vasculitis has been documented in a pregnant woman given ritodrine (SEDA-17, 165).

Second-Generation Effects

Fetotoxicity

Neonatal jaundice is more frequent in the babies of mothers who received ritodrine during the second or third trimesters of pregnancy (4).

Magnetocardiography has been used to detect fetal cardiac dysrhythmias in 84 pregnant women with normal pregnancies and in 68 women receiving ritodrine for pre-term labor (5). There were dysrhythmias in 3.5% of the fetuses in the normal pregnancy group and in 16% in the ritodrine-treated group.

Drug–Drug Interactions

Atropine

When ritodrine is used to alleviate fetal distress and surgical intervention (cesarean section), atropine premedication must be avoided. The vagolytic action of atropine is synergistic with the action of ritodrine, resulting in severe maternal tachycardia and systolic hypertension (6).

References

1. Gokay Z, Ozcan T, Copel JA. Changes in fetal hemodynamics with ritodrine tocolysis. Ultrasound Obstet gynecol 2001;18(1):44–6.

2. Desir D, Kirkpatrick C, Fevre-Montange M, Tourniaire J. Ritodrine increases plasma melatonin in woman. Lancet 1983;1(8317):184–5.

3. Land JM, A'Court CH, Gillmer MD, Ledingham JG. Severe non-diabetic keto-acidosis causing intrauterine death. Br J Obstet Gynaecol 1992;99(1):77–9.

4. Rugolo S, Russo S, Di Stefano F, Marino I, Baiamonte P, Garraffo S. Influenza di alcuni farmaci sull'ittero fisiologico del neonato. [Effect of some drugs on physiological icterus in the newborn.] Minerva Ginecol 1991;43(12):569–72.

5. Wong CA, Walsh LJ, Smith CJ, Wisniewski AF, Lewis SA, Hubbard R, Cawte S, Green DJ, Pringle M, Tattersfield AE. Inhaled corticosteroid use and bone-mineral density in patients with asthma. Lancet 2000;355(9213):1399–403.

6. Sheybany S, Murphy JF, Evans D, Newcombe RG, Pearson JF. Ritodrine in the management of fetal distress. Br J Obstet Gynaecol 1982;89(9):723–6.

Rituximab

See also Monoclonal antibodies

General Information

Rituximab, a chimeric monoclonal antibody directed against the CD20 antigen of normal and malignant B lymphocytes, produces prolonged depletion of B lymphocytes. It has been used to treat refractory or relapsing follicular non-Hodgkin's lymphoma and has been tried in other B cell malignancies, including low-grade non-Hodgkin's lymphoma and diffuse large B cell lymphoma. There has also been interest in its use to treat autoimmune diseases (1–3) and in reducing anti-HLA antibodies in patients awaiting renal transplantation (4).

A wide range of adverse events has been reported in most patients (5). A transient flu-like syndrome is very common (50–90%), particularly after the first infusion of rituximab, and is often associated with various hypersensitivity-like symptoms (5–20%). In the most severe cases, patients had life-threatening cytokine release syndrome with dyspnea, bronchospasm, hypoxia, hypotension, urticaria, and angioedema. Deaths have been reported in eight of 12 000–14 000 patients after drug launch.

Severe reactions to rituximab are rare, but are seen in patients with bulky tumors or with leukemic involvement with high numbers of CD20 positive cells (6,7) and were ascribed to a rapid tumor lysis syndrome (6,8,9). In 11 patients with malignant B cell leukemia, first-dose reactions were significantly more severe in patients whose baseline lymphocyte count was higher than 50×10^6/l and were also associated with raised peak serum concentrations of tumor necrosis factor alfa and interleukin-6 (10).

Organs and Systems

Cardiovascular

Cardiac dysrhythmias have been reported in 8% of patients treated with rituximab in patients with lymphomas (11).

Respiratory

Desquamative alveolitis has been reported in a 55-year-old woman with mantle-cell lymphoma given rituximab (12).

Sensory systems

A variety of ocular adverse effects, including conjunctivitis, transient ocular edema, and visual changes, occurred in 7% of patients receiving rituximab (11).

Hematologic

The factors associated with toxicity in patients with B cell lymphoma receiving rituximab have been studied in Japan (13). By univariate analysis overall non-hematological toxic effects (grade 2 or greater) were more frequent in patients with extranodal disease and especially in those with bone marrow involvement. Fever was more frequent in patients with raised LDH activity, whereas chills/rigors and vomiting were more frequent in patients with extranodal disease. Patients with raised LDH activity or extranodal disease may therefore require closer monitoring. Hematological toxic effects of grade 3 or worse were more common in women.

- A 26-year-old woman with a diffuse large B cell lymphoma received CHOP (cyclophosphamide, hydroxydaunomycin, Oncovin, and prednisone), rituximab, and radiotherapy (14). She developed a transfusion-dependent anemia. Bone marrow biopsy confirmed pure red cell aplasia and parvovirus infection. She had no antibodies to parvovirus, suggesting that she never had a previous exposure. Intravenous immunoglobulin resulted in a reticulocytosis and recovery of her hemoglobin.

The authors suggested that rituximab had depleted her primary B cells, resulting in an inability to mount a primary immune response to parvovirus infection. Parvovirus is pathogenic to red cell precursors, causing their destruction before release from the bone marrow.

Depletion of B lymphocytes by rituximab was suggested as a likely explanation for the occurrence of chronic parvovirus B19 infection complicated by pure red cell aplasia in a 45-year-old patient (15).

Thrombocytopenia leading to gastrointestinal bleeding has been attributed to rituximab (16).

Skin

Stevens–Johnson syndrome has been attributed to rituximab (17).

- A 33-year-old man with a follicular non-Hodgkin lymphoma entered a phase II trial of rituximab. The first two cycles were given without infusion-related toxicity, but during the second cycle mucositis was noticed. Before the third cycle he developed a pruritic rash on the trunk, grade 2 mucositis, and weight loss. He was given oral fluconazole, aciclovir, and antihistamines, which led to improvement. One week after the third infusion of rituximab he had grade 3 orogenital mucositis and the maculopapular rash on the trunk worsened, with areas of ulceration. Rituximab was withdrawn. Stevens–Johnson syndrome was confirmed by biopsy.

Immunologic

Infusion reactions with rituximab are generally well tolerated, as with most monoclonal antibodies. Most reactions are limited to the first infusion, including nausea, chills, and fever. They occur in over 90% of patients. More serious is the cytokine-release syndrome, which occurs within 60–90 minutes and is characterized by fever, chills, rigors, bronchospasm, hypoxia, hypotension, urticaria, and angioedema. Infusion must be discontinued, and the patient carefully monitored with chest radiography and fluid and electrolyte assessment and treated with oxygen and bronchodilators.

A rapid tumor clearance syndrome can occur within 30–60 minutes, with similar symptoms. Lymphocytes rapidly disappear from the peripheral blood and uric acid and lactate dehydrogenase increase markedly. Treatment includes interruption of the infusion, hydration, allopurinol, oxygen, and bronchodilators. It mainly occurs in patients with high white blood cell counts, such as those with chronic lymphatic leukemia.

Severe viral infections/reactivation that have been reported in patients given rituximab have included fulminant hepatitis B (18), parvovirus-induced red cell aplasia (15), and fatal *Varicella zoster* infection (19). There was a high incidence of reactivation of cytomegalovirus and *V. zoster* virus when rituximab was combined with high-dose chemotherapy in high-risk patients with non-Hodgkin's lymphoma (20).

Long-Term Effects

Tumorigenicity

A second cancer is possible when treating a tumor by mutagenicity or immunosuppression. There may be a link between the therapy given and the development of Merkel cell carcinoma (21).

- A 54-year-old man with stage I follicular lymphocytic lymphoma with cervical lymph nodes underwent splenectomy followed by chemotherapy with chlorambucil and had a partial response. Five months later, when he developed generalized lymphadenopathy and bone marrow involvement, he received fludarabine, cyclophosphamide, and rituximab, with complete remission. Ten months later he developed a Merkel cell carcinoma involving the liver and lymph nodes. The disseminated tumor was chemoresistant and he died. His lymphoma remained in complete clinical remission throughout this time.

Two patients developed a peripheral T cell non-Hodgkin's lymphoma after rituximab therapy, one after 15 months and the other after 18 months (22).

Rituximab was suggested as a possible cause of aggressive peripheral T cell lymphoma in two patients 15 and 18 months after the use of rituximab for low-grade B cell non-Hodgkin's lymphoma (23,24).

Second-Generation Effects

Pregnancy

There are few data on the use of rituximab in pregnancy, but one case has been reported.

- A pregnant woman with relapsed follicular non-Hodgkin's lymphoma took rituximab unintentionally during the first trimester (25). The disease stabilized and following an uncomplicated pregnancy a healthy child was born at full term. Careful hematological and immunological monitoring showed no adverse effects from exposure to rituximab.

References

1. Levine TD. Rituximab in the treatment of dermatomyositis: an open-label pilot study. Arthritis Rheum 2005;52(2):601–7.
2. Keogh KA, Wylam ME, Stone JH, Specks U. Induction of remission by B lymphocyte depletion in eleven patients with refractory antineutrophil cytoplasmic antibody-associated vasculitis. Arthritis Rheum 2005;52(1):262–8.
3. Gottenberg JE, Guillevin L, Lambotte O, Combe B, Allanore Y, Cantagrel A, Larroche C, Soubrier M, Bouillet L, Dougados M, Fain O, Farge D, Kyndt X, Lortholary O, Masson C, Moura B, Remy P, Thomas T, Wendling D, Anaya JM, Sibilia J, Mariette X; Club Rheumatismes et Inflammation (CRI). Tolerance and short term efficacy of rituximab in 43 patients with systemic autoimmune diseases. Ann Rheum Dis 2005;64(6):913–20.
4. Vieira CA, Agarwal A, Book BK, Sidner RA, Bearden CM, Gebel HM, Roggero AL, Fineberg NS, Taber T, Kraus MA, Pescovitz MD. Rituximab for reduction of anti-HLA antibodies in patients awaiting renal transplantation: 1. Safety, pharmacodynamics, and pharmacokinetics. Transplantation 2004;77(4):542–8.
5. Onrust SV, Lamb HM, Balfour JA. Rituximab. Drugs 1999;58(1):79–88.
6. Byrd JC, Waselenko JK, Maneatis TJ, Murphy T, Ward FT, Monahan BP, Sipe MA, Donegan S, White CA. Rituximab therapy in hematologic malignancy patients with circulating blood tumor cells: association with increased infusion-related side effects and rapid blood tumor clearance. J Clin Oncol 1999;17(3):791–5.
7. Davis TA, White CA, Grillo-Lopez AJ, Velasquez WS, Link B, Maloney DG, Dillman RO, Williams ME, Mohrbacher A, Weaver R, Dowden S, Levy R. Single-agent monoclonal antibody efficacy in bulky non-Hodgkin's lymphoma: results of a phase II trial of rituximab. J Clin Oncol 1999;17(6):1851–7.
8. Yang H, Rosove MH, Figlin RA. Tumor lysis syndrome occurring after the administration of rituximab in lymphoproliferative disorders: high-grade non-Hodgkin's lymphoma and chronic lymphocytic leukemia. Am J Hematol 1999;62(4):247–50.
9. van der Kolk LE, Grillo-Lopez AJ, Baars JW, Hack CE, van Oers MH. Complement activation plays a key role in the side-effects of rituximab treatment. Br J Haematol 2001;115(4):807–11.
10. Winkler U, Jensen M, Manzke O, Schulz H, Diehl V, Engert A. Cytokine-release syndrome in patients with B-cell chronic lymphocytic leukemia and high lymphocyte counts after treatment with an anti-CD20 monoclonal antibody (rituximab, IDEC-C2B8). Blood 1999;94(7):2217–24.
11. Foran JM, Rohatiner AZ, Cunningham D, Popescu RA, Solal-Celigny P, Ghielmini M, Coiffier B, Johnson PW, Gisselbrecht C, Reyes F, Radford JA, Bessell EM, Souleau B, Benzohra A, Lister TA. European phase II study of rituximab (chimeric anti-CD20 monoclonal antibody) for patients with newly diagnosed mantle-cell lymphoma and previously treated mantle-cell lymphoma, immunocytoma, and small B cell lymphocytic lymphoma. J Clin Oncol 2000;18(2):317–24.
12. Zerga M, Cerchetti L, Cicco J, Constantini P, De Riz M. Desquamative alveolitis: an unusual complication of treatment with Mabthera. Blood 1999;94(Suppl 1):271.
13. Igarashi T, Kobayashi Y, Ogura M, Kinoshita T, Ohtsu T, Sasaki Y, Morishima Y, Murate T, Kasai M, Uike N, Taniwaki M, Kano Y, Ohnishi K, Matsuno Y, Nakamura S, Mori S, Ohashi Y, Tobinai K; IDEC-C2B8 Study Group in Japan. Factors affecting toxicity, response and progression-free survival in relapsed patients with indolent B-cell lymphoma and mantle cell lymphoma treated with rituximab: a Japanese phase II study. Ann Oncol 2002;13(6):928–43.
14. Song KW, Mollee P, Patterson B, Brien W, Crump M. Pure red cell aplasia due to parvovirus following treatment with CHOP and rituximab for B-cell lymphoma. Br J Haematol 2002;119(1):125–7.
15. Sharma VR, Fleming DR, Slone SP. Pure red cell aplasia due to parvovirus B19 in a patient treated with rituximab. Blood 2000;96(3):1184–6.
16. Hagberg H, Lundholm L. Rituximab, a chimaeric anti-CD20 monoclonal antibody, in the treatment of hairy cell leukaemia. Br J Haematol 2001;115(3):609–11.
17. Lowndes S, Darby A, Mead G, Lister A. Stevens–Johnson syndrome after treatment with rituximab. Ann Oncol 2002;13(12):1948–50.
18. Dervite I, Hober D, Morel P. Acute hepatitis B in a patient with antibodies to hepatitis B surface antigen who was receiving rituximab. N Engl J Med 2001;344(1):68–9.
19. Bermudez A, Marco F, Conde E, Mazo E, Recio M, Zubizarreta A. Fatal visceral varicella-zoster infection following rituximab and chemotherapy treatment in a patient with follicular lymphoma. Haematologica 2000;85(8):894–5.
20. Ladetto M, Zallio F, Vallet S, Ricca I, Cuttica A, Caracciolo D, Corradini P, Astolfi M, Sametti S, Volpato F, Bondesan P, Vitolo U, Boccadoro M, Pileri A, Gianni AM, Tarella C. Concurrent administration of high-dose chemotherapy and rituximab is a feasible and effective chemo/immunotherapy for patients with high-risk non-Hodgkin's lymphoma. Leukemia 2001;15(12):1941–9.
21. Cohen Y, Amir G, Polliack A. Development and rapid dissemination of Merkel-cell carcinomatosis following therapy with fludarabine and rituximab for relapsing follicular lymphoma. Eur J Haematol 2002;68(2):117–19.
22. Cheson BD. Rituximab: clinical development and future directions. Expert Opin Biol Ther 2002;2(1):97–110.
23. Micallef IN, Kirk A, Norton A, Foran JM, Rohatiner AZ, Lister TA. Peripheral T-cell lymphoma following rituximab therapy for B-cell lymphoma. Blood 1999;93(7):2427–8.
24. Tetreault S, Abler SL, Robbins B, Saven A. Peripheral T-cell lymphoma after anti-CD20 antibody therapy. J Clin Oncol 1998;16(4):1635–7.
25. Kimby E, Sverrisdottir A, Elinder G. Safety of rituximab therapy during the first trimester of pregnancy: a case history. Eur J Haematol 2004;72(4):292–5.

Rivastigmine

General Information

Rivastigmine (1) was the second drug after donepezil in a class of second-generation acetylcholinesterase inhibitors to become commercially available. It is now marketed in over 60 countries worldwide, including those in Europe and South America and the United Kingdom. It has central selectivity, suggesting fewer peripheral adverse effects. These include nausea, vomiting, abdominal pain, and anorexia (2,3). Daily doses up to 12 mg were tolerated and produced improvement in patients with Alzheimer's disease (4).

Although therapy with newer as well as older cholinesterase inhibitors can prevent cognitive decline, psychiatric and behavioral disturbances, and impaired ability to perform basic activities of daily living, and improve global state of patients with mild-to-moderately-severe Alzheimer's disease, more potent therapies are needed, particularly for modifying the rate of disease progression. Future research efforts need to focus on identifying predictors and better measures of response, timing of treatment, optimum dosage regimens, longer-term follow-up, and establishing how and when acetylcholinesterase inhibitors should be stopped (5,6).

A meta-analysis of various drugs approved for the treatment of Alzheimer's disease in the USA and Canada has suggested that rivastigmine can delay cognitive impairment and deterioration in global health for at least 6 months in patients with mild-to-moderate Alzheimer's disease (7). Patients taking active treatment will have more favorable ADAS-Cog (Alzheimer's Disease Assessment Scale-Cognitive) scores for at least 6 months, after which their scores will begin to converge with those who are taking placebo. The cost-effectiveness data were inconclusive.

In two studies of rivastigmine, 38% of users suffered from nausea, 23% from vomiting, and 24% from vertigo (8). Over 6 months there was a dropout rate of 25%. The gastrointestinal effects led to significant loss of weight. The positive response rate was only 10%, compared with a 6% response to placebo.

The efficacy and safety of rivastigmine have been investigated in several subsequent studies (9–12). Neurologists generally titrated this drug more slowly than recommended in the prescribing information (9). In daily practice, over 50% of the patients were unable to tolerate rivastigmine, mainly because of cholinergic gastrointestinal adverse effects (10), whereas others have found that the adverse events were most frequently mild and transient (11,12). It has been suggested that early treatment with rivastigmine (6–12 mg/day) is associated with sustained long-term (up to 52 weeks) cognitive benefit in patients with Alzheimer's disease (12).

Organs and Systems

Cardiovascular

Based on an electrocardiographic analysis of pooled data from four 26-week, phase III, multicenter, double-blind, placebo-controlled trials of rivastigmine ($n = 2791$), there were no adverse effects on cardiac function (13). Rivastigmine can therefore be safely given to patients with Alzheimer's disease, without the need for cardiac monitoring.

Psychological, psychiatric

Three patients with dementia, with no prior psychiatric history, deteriorated while taking rivastigmine (14). The time course suggested an association with rivastigmine, and each improved after withdrawal.

Gastrointestinal

Potentially fatal rupture of the esophagus has been associated with untitrated use of rivastigmine tablets in a patient with Alzheimer's disease (15).

- A 67-year-old Caucasian woman had a 2-year history of progressive memory loss. She had arterial hypertension successfully controlled with lisinopril and no history of ethanol abuse. A diagnosis of probable Alzheimer's disease was made, and she was given rivastigmine 1.5 mg/day, increasing to 9 mg/day by weekly increments of 1.5 mg. During the titration period, there were no significant adverse effects. After 13 weeks, weight loss was observed and rivastigmine was withdrawn. After 8 weeks she developed marked cognitive deterioration, and she and her carer were advised to restart rivastigmine 1.5 mg/day. However, she mistakenly took one tablet of 4.5 mg. About 30 minutes later she started to vomit several times. Nearly 2 hours later, she complained of severe chest pain, followed by high-grade fever. A chest X-ray showed mediastinal and soft-tissue emphysema, and a contrast X-ray showed rupture of the distal part of the esophagus. Emergency surgery was performed and she recovered.

Rivastigmine and other acetylcholinesterase inhibitors can produce chest pain because of increased esophageal contractions, although consequent rupture of the esophagus has not previously been reported. In this case, the failure to titrate the dosage of rivastigmine could have resulted in rupture secondary to severe vomiting. This confirms the need for careful titration of the dose of rivastigmine, even when restarting treatment.

The transient use of centrally acting antiemetics during rivastigmine titration may be useful in combination with dose-withholding and titration strategies to allow more patients to reach higher doses, resulting in a rapid and robust therapeutic effect. Patients who were treated with trihexyphenidyl and trimethobenzamide were more likely to be able to maintain or to increase their dose of rivastigmine than patients who were treated with glycopyrrolate or ondansetron (16).

Drug–Drug Interactions

General

Rivastigmine did not interact significantly with a wide range of concomitant medications prescribed for elderly patients with Alzheimer's disease, based on an analysis of 2459 patients (rivastigmine 1696, placebo 763) from four randomized placebo-controlled studies (17). However, the Breslow–Day analysis used in this study detected only differences in the odds ratios of rivastigmine versus placebo among patients taking concomitant medications. Thus, these results have to be cautiously interpreted.

References

1. Gottwald MD, Rozanski RI. Rivastigmine, a brain-region selective acetylcholinesterase inhibitor for treating Alzheimer's disease: review and current status. Expert Opin Invest Drugs 1999;8(10):1673–82.

2. Corey-Bloom J, Anand R, Veach J, for the ENA 713 B352 Study Group. A randomized trial evaluating efficacy and safety of ENA-713 (rivastigmine tartrate), a new acetylcholinesterase inhibitor, in patients with mild to moderately severe Alzheimer's disease. Int J Geriatr Psychopharmacol 1998;1:55–65.

3. Rosler M, Anand R, Cicin-Sain A, Gauthier S, Agid Y, Dal-Bianco P, Stahelin HB, Hartman R, Gharabawi M. Efficacy and safety of rivastigmine in patients with Alzheimer's disease: international randomised controlled trial. BMJ 1999;318(7184):633–8.

4. Forette F, Anand R, Gharabawi G. A phase II study in patients with Alzheimer's disease to assess the preliminary efficacy and maximum tolerated dose of rivastigmine (Exelon). Eur J Neurol 1999;6(4):423–9.

5. Knopman DS. Metrifonate for Alzheimer's disease: is the next cholinesterase inhibitor better? Neurology 1998;50(5):1203–5.

6. Bayer T. Another piece of the Alzheimer's jigsaw. BMJ 1999;318(7184):639.

7. Wolfson C, Oremus M, Shukla V, Momoli F, Demers L, Perrault A, Moride Y. Donepezil and rivastigmine in the treatment of Alzheimer's disease: a best-evidence synthesis of the published data on their efficacy and cost-effectiveness. Clin Ther 2002;24(6):862–86.

8. Van Gool WA. Het effect van rivastigmine bij de ziekte van Alzheimer. Geneesmiddelenbulletin 2000;34:17–22.

9. Schmidt R, Lechner A, Petrovic K. Rivastigmine in outpatient services: experience of 114 neurologists in Austria. Int Clin Psychopharmacol 2002;17(2):81–5.

10. Richard E, Walstra GJ, van Campen J, Vissers E, van Gool WA. [Rivastigmine for Alzheimer disease; evaluation of preliminary results and of structured assessment of efficacy.] Ned Tijdschr Geneeskd 2002;146(1):24–7.

11. Bilikiewicz A, Opala G, Podemski R, Puzynski S, Lapin J, Soltys K, Ochudlo S, Barcikowska M, Pfeffer A, Bilinska M, Paradowski B, Parnowski T, Gabryelewicz T. An open-label study to evaluate the safety, tolerability and efficacy of rivastigmine in patients with mild to moderate probable Alzheimer's disease in the community setting. Med Sci Monit 2002;8(2):PI9–15.

12. Doraiswamy PM, Krishnan KR, Anand R, Sohn H, Danyluk J, Hartman RD, Veach J. Long-term effects of rivastigmine in moderately severe Alzheimer's disease: does early initiation of therapy offer sustained benefits? Prog Neuropsychopharmacol Biol Psychiatry 2002;26(4):705–12.

13. Weber JE, Chudnofsky CR, Boczar M, Boyer EW, Wilkerson MD, Hollander JE. Cocaine-associated chest pain: how common is myocardial infarction? Acad Emerg Med 2000;7(8):873–7.

14. Smith DJ, Yukhnevich S. Adverse reactions to rivastigmine in three cases of dementia. Aust N Z J Psychiatry 2001;35(5):694–5.

15. Simon T, Becquemont L, Mary-Krause M, de Waziers I, Beaune P, Funck-Brentano C, Jaillon P. Combined glutathione-S-transferase M1 and T1 genetic polymorphism and tacrine hepatotoxicity. Clin Pharmacol Ther 2000;67(4):432–7.

16. Jhee SS, Shiovitz T, Hartman RD, Messina J, Anand R, Sramek J, Cutler NR. Centrally acting antiemetics mitigate nausea and vomiting in patients with Alzheimer's disease who receive rivastigmine. Clin Neuropharmacol 2002;25(2):122–3.

17. Grossberg GT, Stahelin HB, Messina JC, Anand R, Veach J. Lack of adverse pharmacodynamic drug interactions with rivastigmine and twenty-two classes of medications. Int J Geriatr Psychiatry 2000;15(3):242–7.

Rocuronium bromide

See also Neuromuscular blocking drugs

General Information

Rocuronium is a steroidal agent related chemically to vecuronium. It is less potent than vecuronium and has a quicker onset of action. The plasma clearance of rocuronium is primarily due to liver uptake and biliary excretion (1). About one-third of an injected dose is excreted unchanged in the urine (1). Good intubating conditions may be expected 90–120 seconds after the injection of 0.6 mg/kg rocuronium. Increasing the dose to 1 mg/kg will give acceptable intubating conditions at 60 seconds. There were no increases in plasma histamine concentrations with doses up to 1.2 mg/kg (2).

Organs and Systems

Cardiovascular

Rocuronium has virtually no cardiovascular adverse effects (2–4). Minor increases in heart rate can occur with higher doses owing to its mild vagolytic properties.

There are several reports of pain during injection of rocuronium (5,6). Eight of 10 patients complained of severe pain, one complained of moderate pain, and another reported an unpleasant sensation (5). This suggests that rocuronium will almost invariably cause pain. The mechanism of this phenomenon is not clear, but there appear to be some similarities to propofol injection pain. Several authors have suggested that rocuronium should not be given to awake patients (5,6). On the other hand, small doses of rocuronium have been used, with some success, to prevent fasciculations and myalgia after suxamethonium (7–10). With regard to the severity of injection pain, rocuronium pretreatment in awake patients does not seem advisable.

Immunologic

Several allergic reactions to rocuronium have been reported (11–20). Based on data from the UK, Australia, and France, it had been suggested that the incidence of such reactions after rocuronium administration parallels its frequency of use, as assessed by its market share, implying that rocuronium does not have unusual allergenic properties (15,21,22). In one hospital, the incidence of such reactions was 1 in 3000 (15) and in another 1 in 6000 (11). Also, the incidence of hypotension, tachycardia, or reduced oxygen saturation (which might suggest an anaphylactoid reaction) was relatively low after rocuronium administration compared with other muscle relaxants in a computerized analysis of 47 295 anesthetic records in one hospital (23).

However, the French Group on the Study of Perianesthetic Anaphylactoid Reactions (GERAP) has reported that the proportion of anaphylactoid reactions to rocuronium was similar to suxamethonium in relation to the individual market shares of these agents (22). There were 41 cases among 452 reported cases of anaphylaxis due to neuromuscular blocking agents that were attributed to rocuronium (24). This would make rocuronium look unfavorable, taking into account the fact that suxamethonium is believed to trigger anaphylactoid reactions more often than any non-depolarizing neuromuscular blocker. The authors assumed that their figures might have been partly due to anesthetists' paying more attention to the effects of drugs that had become available more recently, especially in cases of mild reactions. Reporting bias has also been offered as one possible explanation of 29 reports of anaphylaxis to rocuronium among 150 000 patients in Norway, in contrast to 8 cases among 800 000 patients in the other Scandinavian countries (25). This observation has prompted the Norwegian Medicines Agency to recommend that rocuronium be temporarily withdrawn from routine practice and that it be used for rapid-sequence induction only.

It is difficult to understand why such an increase in the number of reported cases should only be observed in France and Norway and not in other countries in which rocuronium is widely used. For the time being, it is not possible to decide whether anaphylactoid reactions are more common with rocuronium than with other non-depolarizing muscle relaxants. To get a clearer picture, a large longitudinal survey would be needed (26), which is unlikely to be performed, owing to the large number of cases that would be required. We shall probably have to rely on national surveys, like the French one cited above. International networking and pooling of data might be the way forward. All of this will depend on clinicians chasing every case of a suspected anaphylactoid reaction by immunological testing and reporting all confirmed cases to appropriate bodies.

The Norwegian Medicines Agency has recommended that rocuronium bromide should be withdrawn from routine practice, referring to 29 reported cases of anaphylaxis or anaphylactoid reactions among 150 000 administrations over 2.5 years. In response, and with regard to the paucity of reported cases of anaphylaxis to rocuronium in other Nordic countries, the statistical problems of surveying such rare adverse drug reactions have been highlighted (25).

One patient died after developing multiorgan failure due to a reaction to rocuronium (27).

- A 64-year-old obese man, scheduled for a hernia repair, had had previous episodes of venous thromboembolism, for which he was still taking an oral anticoagulant. Previous general anesthesia had been uneventful. General anesthesia was induced with sufentanil 15 µg and propofol 400 mg. He was given rocuronium 50 mg to facilitate endotracheal intubation, and shortly after

developed bronchospasm, severe hypotension, tachycardia, and generalized erythema. He was resuscitated with adrenaline, hydrocortisone, and colloid infusion. However, his further course after admission to the intensive care unit was complicated by persistent hypotension, acute respiratory distress syndrome, acute renal insufficiency, disseminated intravascular coagulation, and pancreatitis, and he died 7 days after the incident. Blood samples drawn at 30 and 60 minutes after the initial presentation showed increased concentrations of histamine and tryptase. Specific IgE antibodies against quaternary ammonium groups were detected, with a positive radioimmunoassay inhibition by rocuronium.

Death caused by an anaphylactic reaction to a muscle relaxant seems to be rare, although mortality rates from intraoperative anaphylaxis in the range of 3.4–6% have been reported (28–31). The incidence of cardiac arrest was 4.9% among patients with anaphylactic reactions to muscle relaxants referred to the French GERAP centers for further testing, but these patients all survived (22).

Second-Generation Effects

Fetotoxicity

The maternofetal transfer or rocuronium, as indicated by a fetal/maternal plasma concentration ratio of 0.16, is between that of vecuronium and pancuronium (32). When rocuronium was used for cesarean section, no adverse effects on the fetus were observed (32). With regard to the duration of rocuronium-induced paralysis and the relatively high incidence of failed intubations in obstetric patients, however, it was agreed that rocuronium should be considered for rapid-sequence intubation for cesarean section only if suxamethonium is contraindicated (33–35).

Susceptibility Factors

Age

In elderly patients, because of reduced hepatic elimination, the duration of action of rocuronium can be prolonged (36,37).

Renal disease

Despite the predominantly biliary elimination of rocuronium, reduced clearance and a prolonged half-life have been reported in patients with chronic renal insufficiency requiring hemodialysis (38,39); however, the duration of action was not longer than in healthy controls (38).

Hepatic disease

The duration of action of rocuronium was significantly prolonged in patients with liver cirrhosis, which might be explained either by a larger central volume of distribution or by a lower plasma clearance (40,41).

Drug–Drug Interactions

Anticonvulsant drugs

The duration of action of rocuronium can be reduced during long-term therapy with anticonvulsants (42). In one study the mean times to recovery of twitch height to 25% of baseline after rocuronium 0.6 mg/kg were 21 minutes in patients taking either carbamazepine or phenytoin versus 45 minutes in controls (43). It was suggested that the dose of rocuronium should be increased in patients taking antiepileptic drugs.

General anesthetics

The neuromuscular blocking effects of rocuronium are potentiated by halothane, enflurane, and isoflurane (44–46).

References

1. Wierda JM, Kleef UW, Lambalk LM, Kloppenburg WD, Agoston S. The pharmacodynamics and pharmacokinetics of Org 9426, a new non-depolarizing neuromuscular blocking agent, in patients anaesthetized with nitrous oxide, halothane and fentanyl. Can J Anaesth 1991;38(4 Pt 1):430–5.
2. Levy JH, Davis GK, Duggan J, Szlam F. Determination of the hemodynamics and histamine release of rocuronium (Org 9426) when administered in increased doses under N_2O/O_2–sufentanil anesthesia. Anesth Analg 1994;78(2):318–21.
3. McCoy EP, Maddineni VR, Elliott P, Mirakhur RK, Carson IW, Cooper RA. Haemodynamic effects of rocuronium during fentanyl anaesthesia: comparison with vecuronium. Can J Anaesth 1993;40(8):703–8.
4. Hudson ME, Rothfield KP, Tullock WC, Firestone LL. Haemodynamic effects of rocuronium bromide in adult cardiac surgical patients. Can J Anaesth 1998;45(2):139–43.
5. Borgeat A, Kwiatkowski D. Spontaneous movements associated with rocuronium: is pain on injection the cause? Br J Anaesth 1997;79(3):382–3.
6. Steegers MA, Robertson EN. Pain on injection of rocuronium bromide. Anesth Analg 1996;83(1):203.
7. Demers-Pelletier J, Drolet P, Girard M, Donati F. Comparison of rocuronium and d-tubocurarine for prevention of succinylcholine-induced fasciculations and myalgia. Can J Anaesth 1997;44(11):1144–7.
8. Findlay GP, Spittal MJ. Rocuronium pretreatment reduces suxamethonium-induced myalgia: comparison with vecuronium. Br J Anaesth 1996;76(4):526–9.
9. Motamed C, Choquette R, Donati F. Rocuronium prevents succinylcholine-induced fasciculations. Can J Anaesth 1997;44(12):1262–8.
10. Tsui BC, Reid S, Gupta S, Kearney R, Mayson T, Finucane B. A rapid precurarization technique using rocuronium Can J Anaesth 1998;45(5 Pt 1):397–401.
11. Allen SJ, Gallagher A, Paxton LD. Anaphylaxis to rocuronium. Anaesthesia 2000;55(12):1223–4.
12. Barthelet Y, Ryckwaert Y, Plasse C, Bonnet-Boyer MC, d'Athis F. Accidents anaphylactiques graves après administration de rocuronium. [Severe anaphylactic reactions after administration of rocuronium.] Ann Fr Anesth Reanim 1999;18(8):896–900.
13. Donnelly T. Anaphylaxis to rocuronium. Br J Anaesth 2000;84(5):696.
14. Heier T, Guttormsen AB. Anaphylactic reactions during induction of anaesthesia using rocuronium for muscle relaxation: a report including 3 cases. Acta Anaesthesiol Scand 2000;44(7):775–81.
15. Neal SM, Manthri PR, Gadiyar V, Wildsmith JA. Histaminoid reactions associated with rocuronium. Br J Anaesth 2000;84(1):108–11.
16. Matthey P, Wang P, Finegan BA, Donnelly M. Rocuronium anaphylaxis and multiple neuromuscular blocking drug sensitivities. Can J Anaesth 2000;47(9):890–3.
17. Yee R, Fernandez JA. Anaphylactic reaction to rocuronium bromide. Anaesth Intensive Care 1996;24(5):601–4.
18. Kierzek G, Audibert J, Pourriat JL. Anaphylaxis after rocuronium. Eur J Anaesthesiol 2003;20(2):169–70.
19. Thomas R, Wood M. Anaphylaxis to rocuronium. Anaesthesia 2003;58(2):196.
20. Joseph P, Benoit Y, Gressier M, Blanc P, Lehot JJ. Accident anaphylactique après administration de rocuronium: intérêt du bilan primaire pour le diagnostic précoce. [Anaphylaxis after rocuronium: advantage of blood tests for early diagnosis.] Ann Fr Anesth Reanim 2002;21(3):221–3.
21. Rose M, Fisher M. Rocuronium: high risk for anaphylaxis? Br J Anaesth 2001;86(5):678–82.
22. Laxenaire MC, Mertes PM. Groupe d'Etudes des Réactions Anaphylactoides Peranesthésiques. Anaphylaxis during anaesthesia. Results of a two-year survey in France. Br J Anaesth 2001;87(4):549–58.
23. Booij LH, Houweling PJ. Rocuronium: high risk for anaphylaxis? Br J Anaesth 2001;87(5):805–6.
24. Laxenaire MC. Epidemiologie des réactions anaphylactoides peranesthesiques. Quatrieme enquete multicentrique (juillet 1994–decembre 1996). Le Groupe d'Etudes des Réactions Anaphylactoides Peranésthesiques. [Epidemiology of anesthetic anaphylactoid reactions. Fourth multicenter survey (July 1994–December 1996).] Ann Fr Anesth Reanim 1999;18(7):796–809.
25. Laake JH, Rottingen JA. Rocuronium and anaphylaxis — a statistical challenge. Acta Anaesthesiol Scand 2001;45(10):1196–203.
26. Fisher M, Baldo BA. Anaphylaxis during anaesthesia: current aspects of diagnosis and prevention. Eur J Anaesthesiol 1994;11(4):263–84.
27. Baillard C, Korinek AM, Galanton V, Le Manach Y, Larmignat P, Cupa M, Samama CM. Anaphylaxis to rocuronium. Br J Anaesth 2002;88(4):600–2.
28. Fisher MM, More DG. The epidemiology and clinical features of anaphylactic reactions in anaesthesia. Anaesth Intensive Care 1981;9(3):226–34.
29. Hatton F, Tiret L, Maujol L, N'Doye P, Vourc'h G, Desmonts JM, Otteni JC, Scherpereel P. Enquête épidémiologique sur les anesthesies. [INSERM. Epidemiological survey of anesthesia. Initial results.] Ann Fr Anesth Reanim 1983;2(5):331–86.
30. Currie M, Webb RK, Williamson JA, Russell WJ, Mackay P. The Australian Incident Monitoring Study. Clinical anaphylaxis: an analysis of 2000 incident reports. Anaesth Intensive Care 1993;21(5):621–5.
31. Mitsuhata H, Matsumoto S, Hasegawa J. [The epidemiology and clinical features of anaphylactic and anaphylactoid reactions in the perioperative period in Japan.] Masui 1992;41(10):1664–9.
32. Abouleish E, Abboud T, Lechevalier T, Zhu J, Chalian A, Alford K. Rocuronium (Org 9426) for caesarean section. Br J Anaesth 1994;73(3):336–41.
33. Abouleish E, Abboud T. Rocuronium for caesarean section. Br J Anaesth 1995;74:347–8.
34. McSwiney M, Edwards C, Wilkins A. Rocuronium for caesarean section. Br J Anaesth 1995;74(3):348.
35. Priestley GS, Swales HA, Gaylard DG. Rocuronium for caesarean section. Br J Anaesth 1995;74(3):348.

36. Bevan DR, Fiset P, Balendran P, Law-Min JC, Ratcliffe A, Donati F. Pharmacodynamic behaviour of rocuronium in the elderly. Can J Anaesth 1993;40(2):127–32.

37. Matteo RS, Ornstein E, Schwartz AE, Ostapkovich N, Stone JG. Pharmacokinetics and pharmacodynamics of rocuronium (Org 9426) in elderly surgical patients. Anesth Analg 1993;77(6):1193–7.

38. Cooper RA, Maddineni VR, Mirakhur RK, Wierda JM, Brady M, Fitzpatrick KT. Time course of neuromuscular effects and pharmacokinetics of rocuronium bromide (Org 9426) during isoflurane anaesthesia in patients with and without renal failure. Br J Anaesth 1993;71(2):222–6.

39. Szenohradszky J, Fisher DM, Segredo V, Caldwell JE, Bragg P, Sharma ML, Gruenke LD, Miller RD. Pharmacokinetics of rocuronium bromide (ORG 9426) in patients with normal renal function or patients undergoing cadaver renal transplantation. Anesthesiology 1992;77(5):899–904.

40. Khalil M, D'Honneur G, Duvaldestin P, Slavov V, De Hys C, Gomeni R. Pharmacokinetics and pharmacodynamics of rocuronium in patients with cirrhosis. Anesthesiology 1994;80(6):1241–7.

41. van Miert MM, Eastwood NB, Boyd AH, Parker CJ, Hunter JM. The pharmacokinetics and pharmacodynamics of rocuronium in patients with hepatic cirrhosis. Br J Clin Pharmacol 1997;44(2):139–44.

42. Loan PB, Connolly FM, Mirakhur RK, Kumar N, Farling P. Neuromuscular effects of rocuronium in patients receiving beta-adrenoreceptor blocking, calcium entry blocking and anticonvulsant drugs. Br J Anaesth 1997;78(1):90–1.

43. Koenig HM, Hoffman WE. The effect of anticonvulsant therapy on two doses of rocuronium-induced neuromuscular blockade. J Neurosurg Anesthesiol 1999;11(2):86–9.

44. Oris B, Crul JF, Vandermeersch E, Van Aken H, Van Egmond J, Sabbe MB. Muscle paralysis by rocuronium during halothane, enflurane, isoflurane, and total intravenous anesthesia. Anesth Analg 1993;77(3):570–3.

45. Olkkola KT, Tammisto T. Quantifying the interaction of rocuronium (Org 9426) with etomidate, fentanyl, midazolam, propofol, thiopental, and isoflurane using closed-loop feedback control of rocuronium infusion. Anesth Analg 1994;78(4):691–6.

46. Shanks CA, Fragen RJ, Ling D. Continuous intravenous infusion of rocuronium (ORG 9426) in patients receiving balanced, enflurane, or isoflurane anesthesia. Anesthesiology 1993;78(4):649–51.

Rofecoxib

See also COX-2 inhibitors

General Information

Rofecoxib is a selective inhibitor of COX-2. Although it was originally introduced with the expectation that it would be safer than conventional NSAIDs, because of less gastrointestinal bleeding, the benefit to harm balance is now considered to be unfavorable during long-term treatment, mainly because of an increased risk of cardiovascular disease (heart attacks and strokes; see the monograph on COX-2 inhibitors), and it has been voluntarily withdrawn by its manufacturers.

Organs and Systems

Nervous system

Aseptic meningitis is a rare adverse effect of non-selective NSAIDs in patients with or without connective tissue disease or rheumatological disease. Rofecoxib has been implicated in five patients (four women and one man), in each case occurring within 12 days of the start of rofecoxib therapy (1). The clinical presentations and cerebrospinal fluid findings were typical of aseptic meningitis. One patient had rheumatoid arthritis. After drug withdrawal and recovery, two consecutive rechallenges in one patient led to relapses.

Urinary tract

Acute renal insufficiency has been reported after the use of rofecoxib in patients with predisposing conditions, such as chronic renal insufficiency, renal transplantation, heart disease, liver cirrhosis, and dehydration (2–5). COX-2 inhibitors should be used with great caution, if at all, in patients with medical problems that are associated with prostaglandin-dependent renal function. From this point of view they do not differ from traditional NSAIDs (6).

- Rofecoxib 12.5 mg bd for arthritic pain was associated with biopsy-proven acute tubulointerstitial nephritis in a 67-year-old woman.

Drug–Drug Interactions

Methotrexate

Methotrexate is often prescribed for the management of rheumatoid arthritis, and some NSAIDs have been reported to interact with it, causing increased plasma methotrexate concentrations, associated with impaired renal function. The safety of concurrent rofecoxib and oral methotrexate has been studied for 3 weeks in 25 patients with rheumatoid arthritis (7). Rofecoxib 12.5–50 mg/day had no effect on the plasma concentrations or renal clearance of methotrexate, but supratherapeutic doses of rofecoxib (75 and 250 mg) caused a significant increase in the plasma methotrexate AUC and reduced its renal clearance.

Warfarin

Significant increases in International Normalized Ratio (INR) have been reported in patients who took rofecoxib and warfarin; in some, the increase in INR was accompanied by a bleeding event (8,9). Careful monitoring of the INR in patients taking warfarin and concomitant rofecoxib is mandatory.

References

1. Bonnel RA, Villalba ML, Karwoski CB, Beitz J. Aseptic meningitis associated with rofecoxib. Arch Intern Med 2002;162(6):713–15.
2. Woywodt A, Schwarz A, Mengel M, Haller H, Zeidler H, Kohler L. Nephrotoxicity of selective COX-2 inhibitors. J Rheumatol 2001;28(9):2133–5.
3. Ofran Y, Bursztyn M, Ackerman Z. Rofecoxib-induced renal dysfunction in a patient with compensated cirrhosis and heart failure. Am J Gastroenterol 2001;96(6):1941.
4. Wahba AL, Soper C. Acute, anuric renal failure associated with two doses of a cyclooxygenase-2 inhibitor. Nephron 2001;89(2):239.
5. Meador R, Kolasinski S. Acute renal failure can occur with inappropriate use of a coxib. J Clin Rheumatol 2001;7:413–14.
6. Rocha JL, Fernandez-Alonso J. Acute tubulointerstitial nephritis associated with the selective COX-2 enzyme inhibitor, rofecoxib. Lancet 2001;357(9272):1946–7.
7. Schwartz JI, Agrawal NG, Wong PH, Bachmann KA, Porras AG, Miller JL, Ebel DL, Sack MR, Holmes GB, Redfern JS, Gertz BJ. Lack of pharmacokinetic interaction between rofecoxib and methotrexate in rheumatoid arthritis patients. J Clin Pharmacol 2001;41(10):1120–30.
8. Anonymous. Interaction of rofecoxib with warfarin. Aust Adv Drug React Bull 2002;21:3.
9. Stading JA, Skrabal MZ, Faulkner MA. Seven cases of interaction between warfarin and cyclooxygenase-2 inhibitors. Am J Health Syst Pharm 2001;58(21):2076–80.

Rokitamycin

See also Macrolide antibiotics

General Information

Rokitamycin is a semisynthetic 16-membered ring macrolide. It is more hydrophobic, and has better bacterial uptake and slower release, more cohesive ribosomal binding, and a longer post-antibiotic effect than other 14-, 15- and 16-membered ring macrolides (1).

Organs and Systems

Immunologic

- Churg–Strauss syndrome has been reported in an 18-year-old woman taking cysteinyl leukotriene receptor antagonists and oral rokitamicin 400 mg bd for 10 days (2).

References

1. Braga PC. Rokitamycin: bacterial resistance to a 16-membered ring macrolide differs from that to 14- and 15-membered ring macrolides. J Chemother 2002;14(2):115–31.
2. Richeldi L, Rossi G, Ruggieri MP, Corbetta L, Fabbri LM. Churg–Strauss syndrome in a case of asthma. Allergy 2002;57(7):647–8.

Romazarit

See also Non-steroidal anti-inflammatory drugs

General Information

Romazarit, a slow-acting drug for use in rheumatoid arthritis, was well tolerated in pharmacokinetic studies. It is structurally similar to clobuzarit, which was withdrawn because of four possible cases of Stevens–Johnson syndrome (SEDA-17, 114).

In a double-blind placebo-controlled study in 224 patients with rheumatoid arthritis romazarit 200 mg or 450 mg bd for up to 24 weeks reduced the rate of progress of the disease. Adverse effects were not reported (1). In a double-blind placebo-controlled in 24 patients with rheumatoid arthritis romazarit 100 mg tds, 350 mg bd, or 350 mg tds was associated with adverse events that were mainly trival and similar in incidence to placebo (2).

References

1. Holford NH, Williams PE, Muirhead GJ, Mitchell A, York A. Population pharmacodynamics of romazarit. Br J Clin Pharmacol 1995;39(3):313–20.
2. Williams PE, Bird HA, Minty S, Helliwell PS, Muirhead GJ, Bentley J, York A. A pharmacokinetic and tolerance study of romazarit in patients with rheumatoid arthritis. Biopharm Drug Dispos 1992;13(2):119–29.

Ropinirole

General Information

Ropinirole is a dopamine receptor agonist.

Organs and Systems

Cardiovascular

Supraventricular extra beats have rarely been reported after low doses of ropinirole and have also been reported after pergolide and levodopa (1). Symptomatic postural hypotension has occurred after even low oral doses of ropinirole (2–5), related to peripheral dopaminergic activity. Hypotensive effects occur within 3 minutes of standing, usually between 2 and 4 hours after an oral dose, associated with non-specific malaise (2). Dizziness occurred in up to 40% of patients in clinical trials. Related symptoms include faintness, malaise, and yawning (2). Bradycardia has occasionally accompanied postural hypotension (4). Syncope has been reported.

Nervous system

Somnolence occurred in 20–40% of patients in clinical trials. Drowsiness or euphoria has occurred in some patients taking oral ropinirole (3,4,6). Dyskinesia occurred in 34% of patients with advanced Parkinson's disease in clinical trials.

Gastrointestinal

Nausea, usually mild and not associated with vomiting, has been reported after oral doses of ropinirole, in both supine and standing positions (1–5). Nausea is related to peripheral dopaminergic activity and has been controlled by pretreatment with domperidone (20 mg) (2,3). In one study in healthy subjects, nausea was not reported in the supine position after oral ropinirole; however, nausea with malaise was common on standing (orthostatic symptoms) (2).

Sexual function

Penile erections have been described with ropinirole (7).

- A 49-year-old man with Parkinson's disease was treated with ropinirole, and the dosage eventually reaching 3 mg tds. He had penile erections 20–30 minutes after each dose, lasting for 10–15 minutes. They were not associated with arousal and were very uncomfortable: he had no history of sexual dysfunction. Their frequency diminished with a reduction in drug dosage, but they stopped completely only on drug withdrawal.

Drug–Drug Interactions

Ciprofloxacin

Ciprofloxacin, an inhibitor of CYP1A2, the major enzyme whereby ropinirole is metabolized, increased the risk of ropinirole-induced adverse effects (nausea, somnolence, dizziness) (8).

Warfarin

Ropinirole has been reported to enhance the effects of warfarin (9).

- A 63-year-old man taking co-careldopa and warfarin 4 mg/day (it is not entirely clear why) was also given ropinirole 0.75 mg/day to allow levodopa sparing. After 9 days of ropinirole his INR had increased to 4.6 from a previously stable value of 1.8–2.1, little changed in 2 years. There was no clinical evidence of bleeding. Warfarin was withheld for 4 days and then restarted at 25% of its previous dose. The ropinirole was then withdrawn because of gastrointestinal adverse effects and the warfarin dosage was restored to its previous level.

The mechanism of this interaction has not been elucidated. Ropinirole is metabolized by CYP1A2, but that is not the major isoform involved in warfarin metabolism.

References

1. Acton G, Broom C. A dose rising study of the safety and effects on serum prolactin of SK&F 101468, a novel dopamine D$_2$-receptor agonist. Br J Clin Pharmacol 1989;28(4):435–41.

2. de Mey C, Enterling D, Meineke I, Yeulet S. Interactions between domperidone and ropinirole, a novel dopamine D$_2$-receptor agonist. Br J Clin Pharmacol 1991;32(4):483–8.
3. Kleedorfer B, Stern GM, Lees AJ, Bottomley JM, Sree-Haran N. Ropinirole (SK and F 101468) in the treatment of Parkinson's disease. J Neurol Neurosurg Psychiatry 1991;54(10):938.
4. Vidailhet MJ, Bonnet AM, Belal S, Dubois B, Marle C, Agid Y. Ropinirole without levodopa in Parkinson's disease. Lancet 1990;336(8710):316–17.
5. Kapoon R, Pirtosek Z, Frankel JP, Stern GM, Lees AJ, Bottomley JM, Haran NS. Treatment of Parkinson's disease with novel dopamine D$_2$ agonist SK&F 101468. Lancet 1989;1(8652):1445–6.
6. Frucht S, Rogers JD, Greene PE, Gordon MF, Fahn S. Falling asleep at the wheel: motor vehicle mishaps in persons taking pramipexole and ropinirole. Neurology 1999;52(9):1908–10.
7. Fine J, Lang AE. Dose-induced penile erections in response to ropinirole therapy for Parkinson's disease. Mov Disord 1999;14(4):701–2.
8. Kaye CM, Nicholls B. Clinical pharmacokinetics of ropinirole. Clin Pharmacokinet 2000;39(4):243–54.
9. Bair JD, Oppelt TF. Warfarin and ropinirole interaction. Ann Pharmacother 2001;35(10):1202–4.

Ropivacaine

See also Local anesthetics

General Information

Ropivacaine is an enantiomeric aminoamide local anesthetic, structurally related to bupivacaine but with a wider margin of safety between concentrations that cause nervous system and cardiovascular effects (1). It is mainly metabolized by CYP1A2.

The safety, pharmacokinetics and efficacy of two doses of ropivacaine (300 and 375 mg) for wound infiltration after surgical incision have been studied in an open non-randomized study of 20 men undergoing elective hernia repair (2). Efficacy was similar. There were wide variations in mean plasma concentrations of ropivacaine, the highest individual plasma concentration of total drug being 3.0 µg/ml for the 375 mg dose. One patient in the low-dose group had two episodes of bradycardia at 2 and 12 hours after drug administration. The first episode corresponded to a total plasma drug concentration of 1.3 mg/ml. Three patients in the high-dose group had several recorded episodes of sinus bradycardia. Two of these were within the first hour of ropivacaine administration and corresponded to plasma concentrations of 2.5 and 2.9 µg/ml. One patient in the 300 mg group complained of dizziness at 12 and 21 hours and of nausea at 12 hours. Another patient in the same group vomited 4 hours after the injection of ropivacaine. Two patients had transient hypesthesia in the leg on the operated side, thought to be due to partial block of the femoral nerve. The authors felt that systemic toxicity due to ropivacaine was unlikely to be a cause of any of these adverse effects and they concluded that high-dose ropivacaine is safe for wound infiltration.

Organs and Systems

Cardiovascular

The effects on the cardiovascular system of ropivacaine are similar to those of bupivacaine, although direct cardiotoxicity is less severe with ropivacaine than bupivacaine in both man and animals (SEDA-22, 143). Hypotension and bradycardia are prominent adverse effects when ropivacaine is used epidurally, particularly with concentrations of ropivacaine over 0.5% (SEDA-20, 129) (SEDA-22, 143); in one series, hypotension was observed in 30% of patients who received ropivacaine, but in only 13% of those given an equivalent dose of bupivacaine (3).

Nervous system

Convulsions have occurred after inadvertent intravenous injection of ropivacaine during regional anesthesia (4,5). CNS adverse effects from ropivacaine occur before or without severe cardiovascular toxicity, as there have been several similar reports of CNS toxicity, but not yet one with severe or fatal cardiotoxicity. This reinforces the claim of increased safety from cardiovascular toxicity with this enantiomeric local anesthetic compared with racemic bupivacaine.

Two episodes of central nervous system toxicity without significant cardiovascular toxicity have been described in a patient who had brachial plexus blocks with excessively high doses of ropivacaine 6 weeks apart (6).

- A 45-year-old woman with rheumatoid arthritis asked for regional anesthesia for arthrodesis of her wrist. An interscalene block was performed with ropivacaine 300 mg (6 mg/kg). After 3 minutes she complained of circumoral numbness and twitching in her throat. She developed irrational speech and perioral twitching and 15 minutes after injection developed involuntary clonic twitching in her left upper arm. She was anesthetized with thiopental and ventilated with 100% oxygen via a bag and mask. She regained consciousness within 20 minutes and at 135 minutes was fully conscious, with complete sensorimotor block of her left upper limb. Six weeks later she had an axillary nerve block with ropivacaine 225 mg (4.5 mg/kg) and lidocaine 200 mg (4 mg/kg) with adrenaline. After 25 minutes she complained of a strange feeling in her tongue and became dysarthric and unresponsive to voice. She was anesthetized with propofol and the arthrodesis was performed under general anesthetic. Postoperatively she had a complete brachial plexus block, which resolved after 6 hours. In both instances the only cardiovascular effect noted was sinus tachycardia (150–170/minute).

A single seizure after epidural ropivacaine has been reported (7).

- A 26-year-old primigravid woman in labor had an epidural anesthetic with ropivacaine (a background infusion of 18 mg/hour and three bolus doses totalling 44 mg, followed by an infusion of 24 mg/hour). She failed to progress and another three boluses totalling 150 mg were given. She received a total of 279 mg of ropivacaine over 5 hours. Immediately after the final bolus she developed oculogyric movements and slurred speech and then twitching of her face and arms. The seizure ceased with thiopental and the operation was carried out uneventfully under general anesthesia. Her serum ropivacaine concentration 1 hour later was 3.5 mg/l check units; in previous studies, symptoms of toxicity during intravenous infusions occurred at plasma concentrations of 1–2 µg/ml.

This shows that it is important to leave adequate time between bolus doses to detect adverse effects.

Inadvertent intravenous injection of ropivacaine resulted in systemic toxicity in two cases (5–8).

- A 13-year-old boy weighing 44 kg was given a bolus of 20 mg of ropivacaine through an 18 G Tuohy needle. No cerebrospinal fluid or blood had been aspirated. However, he immediately complained that his face "felt different," and within 1 minute developed a tonic-clonic seizure and a tachycardia of 160/minute. In a blood sample taken about 35 minutes later the plasma concentration of ropivacaine was 1.4 mg/ml, consistent with intravascular injection. In humans, symptoms of toxicity occur at plasma concentrations of 1–2 mg/ml. The authors thought that the rate of injection of epidural local anesthetic should be slower, which would give a greater safety margin between the onset of facial numbness and seizures.
- A ropivacaine-induced seizure occurred in a 23-year-old woman undergoing postpartum tubal ligation. An epidural that had been inserted for labor the evening before the procedure was used to give ropivacaine 120 mg in increments over 11 minutes. She complained of nervousness and within a few seconds had a generalized tonic-clonic seizure and a sinus tachycardia of 120/minute.

In both of these cases reasonable precautions had been taken to ensure correct catheter placement, but nevertheless systemic toxicity occurred. However, neither patient had any serious cardiotoxicity. However, it is worth emphasizing that large doses of local anesthetics should be given slowly and in divided doses and that lidocaine, one of the least toxic of the commonly used local anesthetics, has more obvious prodromal symptoms than ropivacaine, and could be a useful marker for intravenous injection (9).

Three patients suffered convulsions as a result of inadvertent intravascular injection of ropivacaine during placement of local blocks.

- A 75-year-old woman received ropivacaine 160 mg intravenously through an epidural catheter (10). After completion of the injection, she suddenly became unresponsive and had a generalized tonic-clonic convulsion accompanied by a sinus tachycardia of 120/minute but no other cardiac dysrhythmias.
- A 56-year-old 70 kg woman with a Colles fracture received a brachial plexus block at the humeral canal with 0.75% ropivacaine 40 ml using a nerve stimulator (11). The local anesthetic was administered slowly with negative intermittent aspiration. However, 15 minutes later she had two generalized convulsions, which were treated with diazepam. The total venous ropivacaine concentration measured 2 hours after the block was 2.3 µg/ml.
- A 25-year-old man received ropivacaine 75 mg intravenously during sciatic nerve block (12). The nerve was

located using a nerve stimulator and the injection was performed after elicitation of a distal extensor response. Numerous aspirations were performed during the procedure, but 1 minute after injection he suddenly became unresponsive and developed a tonic-clonic seizure, which resolved after treatment with midazolam and propofol. The only cardiovascular effect was a sinus tachycardia of 130/minute.

In the last case, the authors noted that the motor response to stimulation was maintained throughout the injection; it is generally felt that the motor response to stimulation should disappear after the injection of the first milliliters of local anesthetic; if the response does not disappear the injection should be stopped. In all three cases nervous system toxicity occurred with minimal or no cardiovascular toxicity, which is in keeping with previous reports, confirming the relative safety of ropivacaine; there has still not been one single fatal outcome reported with this agent.

References

1. Markham A, Faulds D. Ropivacaine. A review of its pharmacology and therapeutic use in regional anaesthesia. Drugs 1996;52(3):429–49.
2. Pettersson N, Emanuelsson BM, Reventlid H, Hahn RG. High-dose ropivacaine wound infiltration for pain relief after inguinal hernia repair: a clinical and pharmacokinetic evaluation. Reg Anesth Pain Med 1998;23(2):189–96.
3. Morrison LM, Emanuelsson BM, McClure JH, Pollok AJ, McKeown DW, Brockway M, Jozwiak H, Wildsmith JA. Efficacy and kinetics of extradural ropivacaine: comparison with bupivacaine. Br J Anaesth 1994;72(2):164–9.
4. Korman B, Riley RH. Convulsions induced by ropivacaine during interscalene brachial plexus block. Anesth Analg 1997;85(5):1128–9.
5. Abouleish EI, Elias M, Nelson C. Ropivacaine-induced seizure after extradural anaesthesia. Br J Anaesth 1998;80(6):843–4.
6. Ala-Kokko TI, Lopponen A, Alahuhta S. Two instances of central nervous system toxicity in the same patient following repeated ropivacaine-induced brachial plexus block. Acta Anaesthesiol Scand 2000;44(5):623–6.
7. Bisschop DY, Alardo JP, Razgallah B, Just BY, Germain ML, Millart HG, Trenque TC. Seizure induced by ropivacaine. Ann Pharmacother 2001;35(3):311–13.
8. Plowman AN, Bolsin S, Mather LE. Central nervous system toxicity attributable to epidural ropivacaine hydrochloride. Anaesth Intensive Care 1998;26(2):204–6.
9. Checketts MR, Wildsmith JA. Accidental i.v. injection of local anaesthetics: an avoidable event? Br J Anaesth 1998;80(6):710–11.
10. Cherng CH, Wong CS, Ho ST. Ropivacaine-induced convulsion immediately after epidural administration—a case report. Acta Anaesthesiol Sin 2002;40(1):43–5.
11. Ould-Ahmed M, Drouillard I, Fourel D, Roussaly P, Almanza L, Segalen F. Convulsions induites par 1a ropivacaine lors d'un bloc au canal humeral. [Convulsions induced by ropivacaine after midhumeral block.] Ann Fr Anesth Réanim 2002;21(8):681–4.
12. Petitjeans F, Mion G, Puidupin M, Tourtier JP, Hutson C, Saissy JM. Tachycardia and convulsions induced by accidental intravascular ropivacaine injection during sciatic block. Acta Anaesthesiol Scand 2002;46(5):616–17.

Rosaceae

See also Herbal medicines

General Information

The genera in the family of Rosaceae (Table 1) include avens, cotoneasters, hawthorn, and roses, and a variety of fruits such as apples, loquats, pears, plums, quince, and strawberries.

Table 1 The genera of Rosaceae

Acaena (acaena)
Adenostoma (chamise)
Agrimonia (agrimony)
Alchemilla (lady's mantle)
Amelanchier (serviceberry)
Amelasorbus (amelasorbus)
Aphanes (parsley piert)
Argentina (silverweed)
Aruncus (aruncus)
Cercocarus (mountain mahogany)
Chaenmeles (flowering quince)
Chamebatia (mountain misery)
Chamaebatiaria (fernbush)
Chamaerhodos (little rose)
Coleogyne (coleogyne)
Comarum (comarum)
Cotoneaster (cotoneaster)
Crataegus (hawthorn)
Cydonia (cydonia)
Dalibarda (dalibarda)
Dasiphora (shrubby cinquefoil)
Dryas (mountain avens)
Duchesnea (duchesnea)
Eriobotrya (loquat)
Exochorda (pearlbrush)
Fallugia (Apache plume)
Filipendula (queen)
Fragaria (strawberry)
Geum (avens)
Heteromeles (toyon)
Holodiscus (ocean spray)
Horkelia (horkelia)
Horkeliella (false horkelia)
Ivesia (mousetail)
Kelseya (kelseya)
Kerria (kerria)
Luetkea (luetkea)
Lyonothamnus (lyononthmnus)
Malacomeles (false serviceberry)
Malus (apple)
Mespilus (mespilus)
Neviusia (snow wreath)
Oemleria (oemleria)
Osteomeles (osteomeles)
Peraphyllum (peraphyllum)
Petrophyton (rock spiraea)
Photinia (chokeberry)
Physocarpus (ninebark)
Porteranthus (porteranthus)
Potentilla (cinquefoil)
Prunus (plum)
Pseudocydonia (Chinese-quince)

Purshia (bitterbrush)
Pyracantha (firethorn)
Pyrus (pear)
Quillaja (quillaja)
Rhodotypos (rhodotypos)
Rosa (rose)
Rubus (blackberry)
Sanguisorba (burnet)
Sibbaldia (sibbaldia)
Sibbaldiopsis (sibbaldiopsis)
Sorbaria (false spiraea)
Sorbus (mountain ash)
Spiraea (spiraea)
Stephanandra (stephanandra)
Vauquelinia (rosewood)
Waldsteinia (barren strawberry)

Crataegus species

Crataegus species (hawthorn, maybush, whitethorn) contain a variety of flavonoids, including rhamnosides, schaftosides, and spiraeosides. They have a positive inotropic effect on the heart by a mechanism different from that of cardiac glycosides, catecholamines, and the phosphodiesterase type III inhibitors (1) and are effective in mild heart failure (2).

Adverse effects

The main adverse effects of *Crataegus* are dizziness and vertigo (3).

It has been suggested that the flavonoids in *Crataegus* inhibit P glycoprotein function and might therefore interact with drugs that are substrates of P glycoprotein, such as digoxin. However, in a randomized, crossover trial in eight healthy volunteers *Crataegus* special extract WS 1442 (hawthorn leaves with flowers) had no effect on the pharmacokinetics of digoxin 0.25 mg/day for 10 days (4).

Prunus species

The raw pits or kernels of various *Prunus* species (such as apricot, bitter almond, choke cherry and peach) are promoted as health foods. However, they contain the cyanogenic glycoside, amygdalin, which yields hydrogen cyanide after ingestion.

During the late 1950s, and for about 20 years afterwards, laetrile (l-mandelonitrile-beta-glucuronoside), which is related to amygdalin, was touted as a cure for cancer (http://www.quackwatch.org/01QuackeryRelatedTopics/Cancer/laetrile.html). However, in 1982 Arnold Relman, then Editor of the New England Journal of Medicine, pronounced that "Laetrile has had its day in court. The evidence, beyond reasonable doubt, is that it doesn't benefit patients with advanced cancer, and there is no reason to believe that it would be any more effective in the earlier stages of the disease. . . . The time has come to close the books." (5). Nevertheless, it is being so touted again today.

Adverse effects

When ingested in sufficient quantities *Prunus* species cause cyanide poisoning. For instance, a total consumption of about 48 apricot kernels produced forceful vomiting, headache, flushing, heavy sweating, dizziness, and faintness before vomiting was induced in the emergency room, whereafter the symptoms rapidly subsided. In another case accidental poisoning was fatal (6).

- A 67-year-old woman with lymphoma presented with a neuromyopathy following treatment with laetrile. She had high blood and urinary thiocyanate and cyanide concentrations (7). Sural nerve biopsy specimen showed a mixed pattern of demyelination and axonal degeneration, the latter being prominent. Gastrocnemius muscle biopsy specimen showed a mixed pattern of denervation and myopathy with type II atrophy.

Besides the risk that a large dose can lead to acute cyanide poisoning, there is also the question whether continued ingestion of cyanogenic pits or kernels can cause chronic intoxication.

An outbreak of congenital malformations in swine has been retrospectively associated with the eating of the fruit, leaves, and bark of *Prunus serotina* (wild black cherry) (8). Prospective experimental evidence of teratogenicity was not available at that time, but amygdalin was later reported to be teratogenic in hamsters (9).

References

1. Joseph G, Zhao Y, Klaus W. Pharmakologisches Wirkprofil von Crataegus-Extrakt im Vergleich zu Epinephrin, Amrinon, Milrinon und Digoxin am isoliert perfundierten Meerschweinchenherzen. [Pharmacologic action profile of *Crataegus* extract in comparison to epinephrine, amirinone, milrinone and digoxin in the isolated perfused guinea pig heart.] Arzneimittelforschung 1995;45(12):1261–5.
2. Weihmayr T, Ernst E. Die therapeutische Wirksamkeit von *Crataegus*. [Therapeutic effectiveness of *Crataegus*.] Fortschr Med 1996;114(1–2):27–9.
3. Tauchert M. Efficacy and safety of crataegus extract WS 1442 in comparison with placebo in patients with chronic stable New York Heart Association class-III heart failure. Am Heart J 2002;143(5):910–15.
4. Tankanow R, Tamer HR, Streetman DS, Smith SG, Welton JL, Annesley T, Aaronson KD, Bleske BE. Interaction study between digoxin and a preparation of hawthorn (*Crataegus oxyacantha*). J Clin Pharmacol 2003;43(6):637–42.
5. Relman AS. Closing the books on Laetrile. N Engl J Med 1982;306(4):236.
6. Humbert JR, Tress JH, Braico KT. Fatal cyanide poisoning: accidental ingestion of amygdalin. JAMA 1977;238(6):482.
7. Kalyanaraman UP, Kalyanaraman K, Cullinan SA, McLean JM. Neuromyopathy of cyanide intoxication due to "laetrile" (amygdalin). A clinicopathologic study. Cancer 1983;51(11):2126–33.
8. Selby LA, Menges RW, Houser EC, Flatt RE, Case AA. Outbreak of swine malformations associated with the wild black cherry, *Prunus serotina*. Arch Environ Health 1971;22(4):496–501.
9. Willhite CC. Congenital malformations induced by laetrile. Science 1982;215(4539):1513–15.

Rotavirus vaccine

See also Vaccines

General Information

Rotavirus is the most common cause of severe gastroenteritis in infants and young children aged under 5 years in the USA, resulting in approximately 500 000 physician visits, 50 000 hospitalizations, and 20 deaths each year. Worldwide, rotavirus is a major cause of childhood death, accounting for an estimated 600 000 deaths annually among children aged under 5 years. Rotavirus vaccines offer the opportunity to reduce substantially the occurrence of this disease.

Various oral rotavirus vaccines (live attenuated rotavirus vaccines, including rhesus rotavirus and bovine rotavirus strains; serotype 1 bovine-human rotavirus reassortant vaccine; and both rhesus rotavirus monovalent and tetravalent reassortant vaccines) have been evaluated in clinical trials (SEDA-21, 292).

On August 31, 1998, a tetravalent rhesus-based rotavirus vaccine (RRV-TV) (Rotashield) was licensed in the USA. The Advisory Committee on Immunization Practices (ACIP), the American Academy of Pediatrics, and the American Academy of Family Physicians all recommended routine use of the vaccine in healthy infants. Rotashield was the first rotavirus vaccine to be licensed.

Observational studies

The safety and immunogenicity of two human-bovine reassortant rotavirus candidate vaccines have been evaluated in infants, children, and adults (1). One candidate vaccine contained a single human rotavirus gene, while the other candidate vaccine contained two human rotavirus genes. The remaining genes for both vaccines were derived from bovine rotavirus strain UK. Each of these vaccines was well tolerated and immunogenic. This was also the case in the important group of infants under 6 months of age after a single dose of vaccine.

Placebo-controlled studies

The safety, immunogenicity, and efficacy of a live oral human rotavirus vaccine 89–12 has been assessed in 213 US infants in a randomized, placebo-controlled, double-blind, multicenter trial (2). The infants received two doses of vaccine or placebo and were followed up through one rotavirus season. There was an immune response to vaccine in 94.4% of vaccinees, and vaccine efficacy was 89%. Adverse reactions were mild. Low-grade fever after the first dose was the only adverse effect that was significantly more common with the vaccine than with placebo.

Organs and Systems

Gastrointestinal

Natural rotavirus itself is a causative agent for intussusception (3). In rotavirus disease in Japan, hyperplasia of the intestinal lymphoid tissue is a common pathological finding in necropsy cases, and is identical with that observed in patients who receive the tetravalent rhesus-based rotavirus vaccine.

During the period from 1 September 1998 to 7 July 1999, 15 cases of intussusception among infants who had received rotavirus vaccine were reported to the Vaccine Adverse Event Reporting System (VAERS). Of the 15 infants, 13 (87%) had developed intussusception after the first dose of the three-dose RRV-TV series, and 12 had developed symptoms within 1 week of receiving any dose of RRV-TV. Thirteen of the 15 had received other vaccines concurrently. Intussusception was confirmed radiographically in all 15 patients. Eight infants required surgical reduction, and one required resection of 18 cm of distal ileum and proximal colon. Histopathological examination of the distal ileum showed lymphoid hyperplasia and ischemic necrosis. All the infants recovered. The dates of onset ranged from 21 November 1998 to 24 June 1999. The median age of patients was 3 (range: 2–11) months. Ten were boys. Topographically the cases were scattered, being reported from seven states. Of the 15 cases reported to VAERS, 14 were spontaneous reports and one was identified through active postlicensing surveillance.

The rate of hospitalization for intussusception among infants aged less than 12 months during 1991–97 (before RRV-TV licensure) was 51 per 100 000 infant-years in New York. The manufacturer had distributed about 1.8 million doses of RRV-TV as of June 1 1999, and estimated that 1.5 million doses (83%) had been administered. Given this information, 14–16 intussusception cases among infants would be expected by chance alone during the week after the administration of any dose of RRV-TV. Fourteen of the 15 case-patients were vaccinated before June 1 1999, and of those, 11 developed intussusception within 1 week of receiving RRV-TV.

In prelicensure studies of Rotashield, five cases of intussusception had occurred among 10 054 vaccine recipients and one of 4633 controls, a difference that was not statistically significant. Three of the five cases among vaccinated children occurred within 6–7 days of receiving rotavirus vaccine. On the basis of these data, intussusception was included in the package insert as a potential adverse reaction, and the ACIP recommended postlicensure surveillance for this adverse event following vaccination. In addition, because of concerns about the findings in prelicensing trials, VAERS data were analysed early in the postlicensure period (4).

Although the number of reported intussusception cases occurring within 1 week of receiving any dose of vaccine is in the expected range, it must be borne in mind that reporting of suspected adverse events to VAERS is far from complete, and the actual number of intussusception cases occurring among RRV-TV recipients may be substantially greater than that reported. The data available to date suggest but do not establish a causal association between receipt of rotavirus vaccine and intussusception. However, based on these results, use of the vaccine was suspended in July 1999, pending a review of the data by the Advisory Committee on Immunization Practice (ACIP) (5). In further studies more cases of intussusception (including two deaths) were associated with the administration of Rotashield. Based on the results of an expedited review of the scientific data (indicating a strong association between Rotashield and intussusception) presented to the ACIP, it was recommended in 22 October 1999 that Rotashield should no longer be used. The recommendation was made in cooperation with the FDA, NIH, and Public Health Service officials, along with the manufacturer, Wyeth-Lederle (6). In late 1999 the CDC recommended postponing administration of RRV-TV to children scheduled to receive the vaccine before November 1999, including those who had already have begun the RRV-TV series (4).

The epidemiology of hospitalizations and deaths associated with intussusception among US infants has been described (7). Such data could be useful for further clinical trials with newly developed rotavirus vaccines.

Further studies have confirmed that there is an increased risk of intussusception associated with the use of rhesus rotavirus tetravalent vaccine (RRV-TV). The association has been assessed in infants in 19 states of the USA (8). Each infant hospitalized with intussusception between 1 November 1998 and 30 June 1999 was matched according to age with four healthy controls who had been born at the same hospital. The authors estimated that one case of intussusception would occur for every 4670–9474 infants immunized.

In a retrospective cohort study in 10 managed care organizations there was an increased risk of intussusception in immunized children (9). The risk was greatest at 3–7 days after the first dose of RRV-TV.

In an editorial in the journal Emergency and Office Pediatrics the critical role of physicians in the early detection of adverse events was stressed. Despite the demands of busy clinical practice, all physicians are obliged to be alert to unusual circumstances and to seek answers when unexpected findings—especially related to new drugs, vaccines, or procedures—seem to be more than just coincidence. It is incumbent on them to report these findings and to learn if their experience can be confirmed by colleagues (10).

Current prelicensure trials of newly developed rotavirus vaccines are taking into consideration the experiences gained during the licensure process of Rotashield. Phase 3 clinical trials have included over 10 000 volunteers in order to exclude the potential risk of intussusception.

References

1. Eichelberger MC, Sperber E, Wagner M, Hoshino Y, Dudas R, Hodgins V, Marron J, Nehring P, Casey R, Burns R, Karron R, Clements-Mann ML, Kapikian AZ. Clinical evaluation of a single oral dose of human-bovine (UK) reassortant rotavirus vaccines Wa × UK (P1A[8], G6) and Wa × (DS-1 × UK) (P1A[8], G2). J Med Virol 2002;66(3):407–16.
2. Bernstein DI, Sack DA, Rothstein E, Reisinger K, Smith VE, O'Sullivan D, Spriggs DR, Ward RL. Efficacy of live, attenuated, human rotavirus vaccine 89-12 in infants: a randomised placebo-controlled trial. Lancet 1999;354(9175):287–90.
3. Suzuki H, Katsushima N, Konno T. Rotavirus vaccine put on hold. Lancet 1999;354(9187):1390.
4. Centers for Disease Control and Prevention (CDC). Intussusception among recipients of rotavirus vaccine—United States, 1998–99. MMWR Morb Mortal Wkly Rep 1999;48(27):577–81.
5. Salisbury DM. Association between oral poliovaccine and Guillain-Barré syndrome? Lancet 1998;351(9096):79–80.
6. Recommendations of the Advisory Committee on Immunization Practices (ACIP). US Rotavirus Vaccine. CDC Media Relations, 22 October 1999.
7. Parashar UD, Holman RC, Cummings KC, Staggs NW, Curns AT, Zimmerman CM, Kaufman SF, Lewis JE, Vugia DJ, Powell KE, Glass RI. Trends in intussusception-associated hospitalizations and deaths among US infants. Pediatrics 2000;106(6):1413–21.
8. Murphy TV, Gargiullo PM, Massoudi MS, Nelson DB, Jumaan AO, Okoro CA, Zanardi LR, Setia S, Fair E, LeBaron CW, Wharton M, Livengood JR; Rotavirus Intussusception Investigation Team. Intussusception among infants given an oral rotavirus vaccine. N Engl J Med 2001;344(8):564–72.
9. Kramarz P, France EK, Destefano F, Black SB, Shinefield H, Ward JI, Chang EJ, Chen RT, Shatin D, Hill J, Lieu T, Ogren JM. Population-based study of rotavirus vaccination and intussusception. Pediatr Infect Dis J 2001;20(4):410–16.
10. Liebert PS. Reporting vaccine complications. Emerg Off Pediatr 1999;12:125.

Roxithromycin

See also Macrolide antibiotics

General Information

Roxithromycin is a macrolide antibiotic with actions and uses similar to those of erythromycin.

Observational studies

In 2917 adults, adverse effects of roxithromycin occurred in 4.1% at a dosage of 150 mg/day (1). Nausea (1.3%), abdominal pain (1.2%), and diarrhea (0.8%) were the most frequently reported events, whereas rash, vomiting, headache, dizziness, pruritus, urticaria, and constipation were reported only rarely. Treatment had to be withdrawn in 0.9% of the patients because of adverse effects.

In an uncontrolled study in 24 HIV-infected patients, roxithromycin (300 mg bd for 4 weeks) was effective against cryptosporidial diarrhea (2). The most limiting adverse effects were abdominal pain (two patients), raised hepatic enzymes (two patients), and abdominal pain with raised hepatic enzymes (one patient). Minor symptoms occurred in nine patients.

In 304 infants and children under 14 years adverse effects occurred in 6.9% (3). Treatment was withdrawn in 10 children (two with vomiting, two diarrhea, and six rashes).

In 480 elderly patients (over 65 years), there were adverse events in 3.1% and treatment was withdrawn in 1.9%. The gastrointestinal tract was most often affected, whereas laboratory changes (increases in bilirubin, aspartate transaminase, alanine transaminase, and alkaline phosphatase) were seen in under 0.7%.

Organs and Systems

Cardiovascular

- Torsade de pointes has been reported in an 83-year-old man who developed severe prolongation of the QT interval after taking roxithromycin 300 mg/day for 4 days (4).

Respiratory

Eosinophilic pneumonia of acute onset has been attributed to roxithromycin (5).

- A 21-year-old woman developed a fever of 39°C, a generalized pruritic macular rash, odynophagia, and intense weakness, in conjunction with respiratory difficulties 8 days after starting to take roxithromycin 150 mg bd. Her leukocyte count was 15.4×10^9/l with 9.8% eosinophils and an erythrocyte sedimentation rate of 32 mm/hour. Peripheral infiltrates were evident on the chest X-ray and CT scan, with multiple areas of consolidation and an air bronchogram, mainly peripherally distributed. Bronchoalveolar lavage showed 50% eosinophils. She improved with glucocorticoids and 6 months later was free of respiratory symptoms; a chest X-ray was normal.

Hematologic

In one study lymphopenia or eosinophilia were observed in two of 37 patients (6). However, this finding could not be confirmed in other studies.

Gastrointestinal

During long-term use of roxithromycin 300 mg/day for 2–66 months in nine patients with chronic diffuse sclerosing osteomyelitis of the mandible, diarrhea and stomach discomfort occurred in one case and liver dysfunction in another (7).

Liver

- Cholestatic and hepatocellular liver damage occurred in a previously healthy 20-year-old woman after she took roxithromycin 150 mg bd for 4 days (8).
- Hepatic failure occurred in a previously healthy 5-year-old boy after he was given roxithromycin 50 mg bd for 5 days (9). He developed a non-pruritic, non-urticarial, erythematous, maculopapular, generalized rash, and occasional vomiting. Three days later he became jaundiced, and after 8 days underwent liver transplantation.

Skin

Allergic dermatitis with characteristic distribution pattern called "baboon syndrome" has been reported (10).

- A 58-year-old man developed a pruritic skin eruption after he had taken roxithromycin 300 mg/day for 3 days. Large erythematous plaques covered his buttocks. Roxithromycin was immediately withdrawn and following treatment with oral antihistamines and topical corticosteroids the rash resolved within a few days.

Urticarial rashes have been attributed to roxithromycin.

- Roxithromycin-induced generalized urticaria and tachycardia with a positive prick test and a cross-reaction to erythromycin and clarithromycin has been reported in a 31-year-old woman (11).
- Angioedema and urticaria occurred in a 22-year-old woman a few hours after a second dose of roxithromycin 150 mg for a sore throat (12). The lesions subsided within 12 hours of drug withdrawal and there was no relapse after 3 months of follow-up. A skin prick test was positive for roxithromycin (1 mg/ml) and negative for erythromycin and clarithromycin in the same concentrations.

Immunologic

Roxithromycin had an immunomodulatory action on peripheral blood mononuclear cells in patients with psoriasis (13). The anti-inflammatory activity of roxithromycin is due to reduced production of proinflammatory mediators, cytokines, and co-stimulatory molecules, as has been shown in animal studies (14).

Drug–Drug Interactions

Antacids

Roxithromycin did not interact with antacids containing hydroxides of aluminium and magnesium (1).

Carbamazepine

Roxithromycin did not alter the pharmacokinetics of carbamazepine (15) or interact with warfarin, ranitidine, or antacids containing hydroxides of aluminium and magnesium (1).

Oral contraceptives

Plasma concentrations of oral contraceptive steroids were unchanged when roxithromycin was co-administered (16).

Ranitidine

Roxithromycin did not interact with ranitidine (1).

Statins

In an open, randomized, crossover study in 12 healthy volunteers, roxithromycin did not alter the pharmacokinetics of lovastatin in such a way that dosage adjustment of lovastatin should be necessary during co-administration (17).

- Myopathy occurred in a 73-year-old woman taking simvastatin 80 mg/day and gemfibrozil 600 mg bd 4 days after she started to take roxithromycin 300 mg/day (18).

Theophylline

Roxithromycin altered the pharmacokinetics of theophylline, mainly increasing the C_{max}, prolonging the half-life, and increasing the renal clearance (15). However, while these changes were statistically significant, they were considered clinically irrelevant. There was no effect of roxithromycin on trough concentrations of theophylline.

Warfarin

Roxithromycin did not interact with warfarin (1).

References

1. Young RA, Gonzalez JP, Sorkin EM. Roxithromycin. A review of its antibacterial activity, pharmacokinetic properties and clinical efficacy. Drugs 1989;37(1):8–41.
2. Sprinz E, Mallman R, Barcellos S, Silbert S, Schestatsky G, Bem David D. AIDS-related cryptosporidial diarrhoea: an open study with roxithromycin. J Antimicrob Chemother 1998;41(Suppl B):85–91.
3. Kafetzis DA, Blanc F. Efficacy and safety of roxithromycin in treating paediatric patients. A European multicentre study. J Antimicrob Chemother 1987;20(Suppl B):171–7.
4. Haffner S, Lapp H, Thurmann PA. Unerwunschi te Arzneimittel wirkungen Der konkrete Fall. [Adverse drug reactions—case report.] Dtsch Med Wochenschr 200210;127(19):1021.
5. Perez-Castrillon JL, Jimenez-Garcia R, Martin-Escudero JC, Velasco C. Roxithromycin-induced eosinophilic pneumonia. Ann Pharmacother 2002;36(11):1808–9.
6. Agache P, Amblard P, Moulin G, Barriere H, Texier L, Beylot C, Bergoend H. Roxithromycin in skin and soft tissue infections. J Antimicrob Chemother 1987;20(Suppl B):153–6.
7. Yoshii T, Nishimura H, Yoshikawa T, Furudoi S, Yoshioka A, Takenono I, Ohtsuka Y, Komori T. Therapeutic possibilities of long-term roxithromycin treatment for chronic diffuse sclerosing osteomyelitis of the mandible. J Antimicrob Chemother 2001;47(5):631–7.
8. Hartleb M; Biernat L, Kochel A. Drug-induced liver damage—a three-year study of patients from one gastroenterological department. Med Sci Monit 2002;8(4):CR292–6.
9. Easton-Carter KL, Hardikar W, Smith AL. Possible roxithromycin-induced fulminant hepatic failure in a child. Pharmacotherapy 2001;21(7):867–70.
10. Amichai B, Grunwald MH. Baboon syndrome following oral roxithromycin. Clin Exp Dermatol 2002;27(6):523.
11. Kruppa A, Scharffetter-Kochanek K, Krieg T, Hunzelmann N. Immediate reaction to roxithromycin and prick test cross-sensitization to erythromycin and clarithromycin. Dermatology 1998;196(3):335–6.
12. Gurvinder SK, Tham P, Kanwar AJ. Roxithromycin induced acute urticaria. Allergy 2002;57(3):262.
13. Ohshima A, Takigawa M, Tokura Y. CD8+ cell changes in psoriasis associated with roxithromycin-induced clinical improvement. Eur J Dermatol 2001;11(5):410–15.
14. Shimane T, Asano K, Suzuki M, Hisamitsu T, Suzaki H. Influence of a macrolide antibiotic, roxithromycin, on mast cell growth and activation in vitro. Mediators Inflamm 2001;10(6):323–32.
15. Saint-Salvi B, Tremblay D, Surjus A, Lefebvre MA. A study of the interaction of roxithromycin with theophylline and carbamazepine. J Antimicrob Chemother 1987;20(Suppl B):121–9.
16. Archer JS, Archer DF. Oral contraceptive efficacy and antibiotic interaction: a myth debunked. J Am Acad Dermatol 2002;46(6):917–23.
17. Bucher M, Mair G, Kees F. Effect of roxithromycin on the pharmacokinetics of lovastatin in volunteers. Eur J Clin Pharmacol 2002;57(11):787–91.
18. Huynh T, Cordato D, Yang F, Choy T, Johnstone K, Bagnall F, Hitchens N, Dunn R. HMG CoA reductase-inhibitor-related myopathy and the influence of drug interactions. Intern Med J 2002;32(9–10):486–90.

Rubiaceae

See also Herbal medicines

General Information

The genera in the family of Rubiaceae (Table 1) include cinchona and coffee.

Table 1   The genera of Rubiaceae

Anthocephalus (anthocephalus)
Antirhea (quina)
Asperula (woodruff)
Bobea (ahakea)
Bouvardia (bouvardia)
Calycophyllum (calycophyllum)
Canthium (canthium)
Casasia (casasia)
Catesbaea (lilythorn)
Cephaelis (cephaelis)
Cephalanthus (buttonbush)
Chiococca (milkberry)
Chione (chione)
Cinchona (cinchona)
Coccocypselum (coccocypselum)
Coffea (coffee)
Coprosma (mirrorplant)
Crucianella (crucianella)
Cruciata (bedstraw)
Crusea (mountain saucerflower)
Diodia (buttonweed)
Erithalis (blacktorch)
Ernodea (ernodea)
Exostema (exostema)
Faramea (false coffee)
Galium (bedstraw)
Gardenia (gardenia)
Genipa (genipa)
Geophila (geophila)
Gonzalagunia (gonzalagunia)
Guettarda (guettarda)
Hamelia (hamelia)
Hedyotis (starviolet)
Hillia (hillia)
Hintonina
Houstonia (bluet)
Ixora (ixora)
Kelloggia (kelloggia)
Lasianthus (lasianthus)
Lucya (lucya)
Machaonia (machaonia)
Mitchella (mitchella)
Mitracarpus (girdlepod)
Morinda (morinda)
Neolaugeria (neolaugeria)
Neolamarckia (neolamarckia)
Neonauclea
Nertera (nertera)
Oldenlandia (oldenlandia)
Oldenlandiopsis (creeping-bluet)
Paederia (sewer vine)
Palicourea (cappel)
Pentas (pentas)

Continued

Table 1 Continued

Pentodon (pentodon)
Phialanthus (phialanthus)
Pinckneya (pinckneya)
Psychotria (wild coffee)
Randia (indigoberry)
Richardia (Mexican clover)
Rondeletia (cordobancillo)
Rubia (rubia)
Sabicea (woodvine)
Schradera (schradera)
Scolosanthus (scolosanthus)
Serissa (snowrose)
Sherardia (sherardia)
Spermacoce (false buttonweed)
Strumpfia (strumpfia)
Timonius
Uncaria (uncaria)
Vangueria (vangueria)

Asperula odorata

Asperula odorata (sweet woodruff) is rich in coumarins.

Cephaelis ipecacuanha

The root of *Cephaelis ipecacuanha*, also known as *Psychotria ipecacuanha*, is the source of ipecacuanha, which contains the emetic alkaloids emetine and cephaeline. Ipecacuanha is covered in a separate monograph.

Hintonia latiflora

Hintonia latiflora (copalchi bark) has been advocated as a hypoglycemic agent, an effect that has been attributed to the neoflavonoid coutareagenin (1). Its use has been associated with liver toxicity but a causal relation could not be established (2).

Morinda citrifolia

Morinda citrifolia (noni) is one of the most important traditional Polynesian medicinal plants, which has a large range of therapeutic claims, including antibacterial, antiviral, antifungal, antihelminthic, antitumor, analgesic, hypotensive, anti-inflammatory, and immune enhancing effects (3,4).

Adverse effects
The juice of *M. citrifolia* has been reported to cause hyperkalemia (5).

- A man with chronic renal insufficiency who followed dietary restriction of potassium developed a raised serum potassium concentration (5.8 mmol/l). He insisted that he had followed his dietary regimen as usual, except for taking noni juice, purchased from a health food store. He was treated with sodium polystyrene sulfonate and told to stop taking noni juice. At the next check-up his potassium was still raised; he said that he would never stop taking noni juice and

that his physicians did not understand its healing power.

The potassium concentration in noni juice samples was 56 mmol/l.

Rubia tinctorum

The use of herbal medicines prepared from the root of *Rubia tinctorum* (madder) is no longer permitted in Germany. Root extracts have shown genotoxic effects in several test systems, which are attributed to the presence of the anthraquinone derivative lucidin. One of the other main components, alizarin primeveroside, is transformed into 1-hydroxyanthraquinone when given orally to the rat, in which this metabolite has carcinogenic activity (6).

Uncaria tomentosa

Uncaria tomentosa (cat's claw), an herb from the highlands of the Peruvian Amazon, contains the spiroindole alkaloids isopteropodine and rynchophylline; it has immunomodulatory properties and has been used to treat arthritis and inflammatory bowel disease (7).

Adverse effects

- A 59-year-old woman with mantle-cell lymphoma and no hepatic involvement took a range of unconventional medicines (8). During a routine check-up she had raised liver enzymes, and self-medication with cat's claw was deemed the most likely cause. Cat's claw was withdrawn and her liver tests normalized within 60 days.

References

1. Korec R, Heinz Sensch K, Zoukas T. Effects of the neoflavonoid coutareagenin, one of the antidiabetic active substances of *Hintonia latiflora*, on streptozotocin-induced diabetes mellitus in rats. Arzneimittelforschung 2000;50(2):122–8.
2. In: Hansel R, Keller K, Rimpler H, Schneider G, editors. Hagers Handbuch der Pharmazeutischen Praxis. 5th ed. Berlin: Springer-Verlag, 1993.
3. McClatchey W. From Polynesian healers to health food stores: changing perspectives of *Morinda citrifolia* (Rubiaceae). Integr Cancer Ther 2002;1(2):110–20.
4. Wang MY, West BJ, Jensen CJ, Nowicki D, Su C, Palu AK, Anderson G. *Morinda citrifolia* (noni): a literature review and recent advances in noni research. Acta Pharmacol Sin 2002;23(12):1127–41.
5. Mueller BA, Scott MK, Sowinski KM, Prag KA. Noni juice (*Morinda citrifolia*): hidden potential for hyperkalemia? Am J Kidney Dis 2000;35(2):310–12.
6. De Smet PAGM, Stricker BHC. Meekrapwortel in Duitsland niet langer toegestaan. Pharm Weekbl 1993;128:503.
7. Steinberg PN. Una de gato: una hierba prodigiosa de la selva humeda Peruana. [Cat's claw: an herb from the Peruvian Amazon.] Sidahora 1995:35–6.
8. Gertz MA, Bauer BA. Caring (really) for patients who use alternative therapies for cancer. J Clin Oncol 2001;19(23):4346–9.

Rutaceae

See also Herbal medicines

General Information

The genera in the family of Rutaceae (Table 1) include citrus fruits (citrons, oranges, grapefruit, lemons, limes, tangerines, etc.), angostura, kumquat, pilocarpus, and rue.

Agathosma betulina

Agathosma betulina (buchu) contains diosmin (venosmine), and a synthetic form of diosmin is also available. It has been used to treat the pain and bleeding of hemorrhoids (1).

Adverse effects

Diosmin can rarely cause nausea and epigastric discomfort (SEDA-3, 181) and somnolence (2).

In 12 volunteers, diosmin 500 mg/day for 9 days significantly increased the AUC and C_{max} of metronidazole 800 mg without a change in t_{max}; this effect was attributed to inhibition of CYP3A4 (3).

Table 1 The genera of Rutaceae

Acronychia (acronychia)
Aegle (aegle)
Agathosma (agathosma)
Amyris (torchwood)
Boronia (boronia)
Casimiroa (sapote)
Choisya (Mexican orange)
Citrofortunella (citrofortunella)
Citroncirus (citroncirus)
Citrus (citrus)
Clausena (clausena)
Cneoridium (cneoridium)
Correa (Australian fuschia)
Cusparia (cusparia)
Dictamnus (dictamnus)
Eremocitrus (eremocitrus)
Esenbeckia (jopoy)
Flindersia (flindersia)
Fortunella (kumquat)
Galipea (galipea)
Glycosmis (glycosmis)
Helietta (helietta)
Limonia (limonia)
Melicope (melicope)
Microcitrus (microcitrus)
Murraya (murraya)
Phellodendron (cork tree)
Pilocarpus (pilocarpus)
Platydesma (platydesma)
Poncirus (poncirus)
Ptelea (hoptree)
Ravenia (ravenia)
Ruta (rue)
Severinia (severinia)
Thamnosma (desert rue)
Triphasia (triphasia)
Zanthoxylum (prickly ash)

Citrus auranticum

Volatile plant oils (often incorrectly termed "essential oils") are used in aromatherapy and are usually applied by gentle massage. The oil of *C. auranticum* (bergamot) is often used in this way. It has photosensitive and melanogenic properties and is potentially phototoxic and photomutagenic.

Adverse effects

- Two patients had localized and disseminated bullous phototoxic skin reactions 48–72 hours after exposure to bergamot aromatherapy and ultraviolet light (4). One developed bullous skin lesions after exposure to aerosolized aromatherapy oil in a sauna.

Citrus paradisi (grapefruit)

Grapefruit juice is unusual in that it is not used therapeutically but can cause many drug interactions, since an unidentified constituent of grapefruit inhibits CYP3A4. The drugs most commonly involved are dihydropyridine calcium channel blockers and HMG-CoA reductase inhibitors (5).

Both whole grapefruit and grapefruit juice have been implicated, and the wording used on a warning label in New Zealand to alert patients to potential drug interactions with grapefruit is "Do not take grapefruit or grapefruit juice while being treated with this medicine" (6). Health Canada has advised the public not to take grapefruit or its juice (fresh or frozen) with certain drugs (7). Health Canada has also issued several communication documents to remind health professionals of possible interactions of grapefruit with therapeutic drugs and has worked with drug manufacturers whose products are adversely affected by grapefruit to ensure that the relevant information is printed on the product label.

Of the several hundred chemical entities in grapefruit juice (8), psoralens, mainly 6,7-dihydroxybergamottin, are thought to be the components in grapefruit that are responsible for these interactions, although the flavonoid naringenin, which was originally suspected, cannot be excluded and may have a minor role (9).

The ability of grapefruit to increase the plasma concentrations of some drugs was accidentally discovered when grapefruit juice was used as a blinding agent in a drug interaction study of felodipine and alcohol (10). It was noticed that plasma concentrations of felodipine were much higher when the drug was taken with grapefruit juice than those previously reported for the dose of drug administered. In another study, (11) concurrent administration of grapefruit juice and felodipine increased the AUC, causing increased heart rate, and reduced diastolic blood pressure. Similarly, parallel administration of the juice with midazolam altered psychometric performance tests, while with nisoldipine or nitrendipine there was an increase in heart rate.

Table 2 lists some drugs whose effects are altered by grapefruit juice.

Table 2 Drug–grapefruit juice interactions

Drug	Effect of grapefruit	Reference
Benzodiazepines	Pronounced nervous system effects	(12)
Ciclosporin	Inhibits metabolism and increases blood concentration	(13,14)
Coumarins	Interferes with the analysis of coumarins	(15)
Diazepam	Increases concentration	(16)
Felodipine	Enhances the effects and can cause increased blood pressure and heart rate, headache, flushing, and light-headedness	(17)
Lovastatin	Greatly increases serum concentration	(18)
Nifedipine	Increases plasma concentration	(19)
Nisoldipine	Increases plasma concentration	(20)
Quinidine	Delays absorption and maximal effect on QT interval	(21)
Saquinavir	Increases AUC and C_{max}	(9)
Terfenadine	Increases systemic availability, with cardiotoxicity at higher doses of grapefruit juice concentration	(22)
Triazolam	Increases plasma concentrations	(23)

Dictamnus dasycarpus

Dictamnus dasycarpus (densefruit pittany) contains rutaevin, terpene glycosides (dasycarpusides), sesquiterpene glycosides (dictamnosides), and phenolic glycosides. *D. dasycarpus* is a common ingredient of the complex traditional Chinese herbal medicines that have been associated with liver damage; however, a causative role remains to be established (24–27).

Adverse effects
The UK hepatologists have described two cases of severe liver damage, one fatal, attributed to Chinese herbal mixtures for minor complaints (28). *D. dasycarpus* was implicated in one. There have been other reports of hepatotoxicity due to *D. dasycarpus* (28).

Dermatitis has been attributed to *D. dasycarpus* (29).

The root bark of *D. dasycarpus* is mutagenic in bacteria, due not to dietary flavonoids, but to the furoquinoline alkaloids dictamnine and gamma-fagarine. The clinical relevance of this finding remains to be established.

Pilocarpus species

The leaves of *Pilocarpus* species, including *Pilocarpus jaborandi* (jaborandi) and *Pilocarpus racemosus* (aceitillo), contain pilocarpine or isopilocarpine as major alkaloids as well as a variety of minor alkaloids. Pilocarpine (see separate monograph) is an agonist at acetylcholine receptors, which enhances salivary flow, sweating, and gastrointestinal motility. It can interfere with asthma therapy and the effect of anticholinergic drugs.

Ruta graveolens

Ruta graveolens (rue) contains acridone alkaloids, such as furacridone and gravacridone, quinoline alkaloids, such as graveoline and graveolinine, the furanoquinoline dictamnine, coumarins, such as gravelliferone, isorutarin, rutacultin, rutaretin, and suberenone, and the furanocoumarins 5-methoxypsoralen (bergapten) and 8-methoxypsoralen (xanthotoxine). It has been used as an abortifacient and emmenagogue (30).

Adverse effects
The essential oil of rue can cause contact dermatitis and phototoxic reactions (31,32) and severe hepatic and renal

toxicity. Therapeutic doses can lead to depression, sleep disorders, fatigue, dizziness, and cramps. The sap from fresh leaves can produce painful gastrointestinal irritation, fainting, sleepiness, a weak pulse, abortion, a swollen tongue, and a cool skin.

References

1. Diana G, Catanzaro M, Ferrara A, Ferrari P. Attivita della diosmina pura nel trattamento della malattia emorroidaria. [Activity of purified diosmin in the treatment of hemorrhoids.] Clin Ter 2000;151(5):341–4.
2. Jimenez Gomez R, Saldana Garrido D, Martin Arias LH, Carvajal Garcia Pando A. Somnolencia en el curso de un tratamiento con diosmina. [Somnolence during diosmin treatment.] Med Clin (Barc) 1991;97(5):198–9.
3. Rajnarayana K, Reddy MS, Krishna DR. Diosmin pretreatment affects bioavailability of metronidazole. Eur J Clin Pharmacol 2003;58(12):803–7.
4. Kaddu S, Kerl H, Wolf P. Accidental bullous phototoxic reactions to bergamot aromatherapy oil. J Am Acad Dermatol 2001;45(3):458–61.
5. Anonymous. Grapefruit juice. Specific report of drug interactions. WHO Pharmaceuticals Newslett 2003;1:5.
6. Anonymous. Grapefruit warning label: now official in some countries. Drugs Ther Perspect 1998;12:12–13.
7. Anonymous. Grapefruit juice. Potential for drug interactions. WHO Pharmaceuticals Newslett 2002;3:10–11.
8. Ranganna S, Govindarajan VS, Ramana KV. Citrus fruits—varieties, chemistry, technology, and quality evaluation. Part II. Chemistry, technology, and quality evaluation. A. Chemistry. Crit Rev Food Sci Nutr 1983;18(4):313–86.
9. Fuhr U. Drug interactions with grapefruit juice. Extent, probable mechanism and clinical relevance. Drug Saf 1998;18(4):251–72.
10. Bailey DG, Spence JD, Edgar B, Bayliff CD, Arnold JM. Ethanol enhances the hemodynamic effects of felodipine. Clin Invest Med 1989;12(6):357–62.
11. Rodvold KA, Meyer J. Drug-food interactions with grapefruit juice. Infect Med 1996;13:868–912.
12. Kupferschmidt HH, Ha HR, Ziegler WH, Meier PJ, Krahenbuhl S. Interaction between grapefruit juice and midazolam in humans. Clin Pharmacol Ther 1995;58(1):20–8.
13. Hollander AA, van Rooij J, Lentjes GW, Arbouw F, van Bree JB, Schoemaker RC, van Es LA, van der Woude FJ, Cohen AF. The effect of grapefruit juice on cyclosporine and prednisone metabolism in transplant patients. Clin Pharmacol Ther 1995;57(3):318–24.

14. Brunner LJ, Munar MY, Vallian J, Wolfson M, Stennett DJ, Meyer MM, Bennett WM. Interaction between cyclosporine and grapefruit juice requires long-term ingestion in stable renal transplant recipients. Pharmacotherapy 1998;18(1):23–9.

15. Runkel M, Tegtmeier M, Legrum W. Metabolic and analytical interactions of grapefruit juice and 1,2-benzopyrone (coumarin) in man. Eur J Clin Pharmacol 1996;50(3):225–30.

16. Ozdemir M, Aktan Y, Boydag BS, Cingi MI, Musmul A. Interaction between grapefruit juice and diazepam in humans. Eur J Drug Metab Pharmacokinet 1998;23(1):55–9.

17. Feldman EB. How grapefruit juice potentiates drug bioavailability. Nutr Rev 1997;55(11 Pt 1):398–400.

18. Kantola T, Kivisto KT, Neuvonen PJ. Grapefruit juice greatly increases serum concentrations of lovastatin and lovastatin acid. Clin Pharmacol Ther 1998;63(4):397–402.

19. Hashimoto Y, Kuroda T, Shimizu A, Hayakava M, Fukuzaki H, Morimoto S. Influence of grapefruit juice on plasma concentration of nifedipine. Jpn J Clin Pharmacol Ther 1996;27:599–606.

20. Azuma J, Yamamoto I, Wafase T, Orii Y, Tinigawa T, Terashima S, Yoshikawa K, Tanaka T, Kawano K. Effects of grapefruit juice on the pharmacokinetics of the calcium channel blockers nifedipine and nisoldipine. Curr Ther Res Clin Exp 1998;59:619–34.

21. Min DI, Ku YM, Geraets DR, Lee H. Effect of grapefruit juice on the pharmacokinetics and pharmacodynamics of quinidine in healthy volunteers. J Clin Pharmacol 1996;36(5):469–76.

22. Clifford CP, Adams DA, Murray S, Taylor GW, Wilkins MR, Boobis AR, Davies DS. The cardiac effects of terfenadine after inhibition of its metabolism by grapefruit juice. Eur J Clin Pharmacol 1997;52(4):311–15.

23. Hukkinen SK, Varhe A, Olkkola KT, Neuvonen PJ. Plasma concentrations of triazolam are increased by concomitant ingestion of grapefruit juice. Clin Pharmacol Ther 1995;58(2):127–31.

24. Pillans PI, Eade MN, Massey RJ. Herbal medicine and toxic hepatitis. NZ Med J 1994;107(988):432–3.

25. Kane JA, Kane SP, Jain S. Hepatitis induced by traditional Chinese herbs; possible toxic components. Gut 1995;36(1):146–7.

26. Vautier G, Spiller RC. Safety of complementary medicines should be monitored. BMJ 1995;311(7005):633.

27. Perharic L, Shaw D, Leon C, De Smet PAGM, Murray VSG. Liver damage associated with certain types of traditional Chinese medicines used for skin diseases. Hum Exp Toxicol, in press.

28. McRae CA, Agarwal K, Mutimer D, Bassendine MF. Hepatitis associated with Chinese herbs. Eur J Gastroenterol Hepatol 2002;14(5):559–62.

29. Stekhun FI, Kyrnakov BA. [Dermatitis caused by *Dictamnus dasycarpus*.] Vestn Dermatol Venerol 1962;36:67–70.

30. Conway GA, Slocumb JC. Plants used as abortifacients and emmenagogues by Spanish New Mexicans. J Ethnopharmacol 1979;1(3):241–61.

31. Wessner D, Hofmann H, Ring J. Phytophotodermatitis due to *Ruta graveolens* applied as protection against evil spells. Contact Dermatitis 1999;41(4):232.

32. Schempp CM, Schopf E, Simon JC. Dermatitis bullosa striata pratensis durch *Ruta graveolens* L. (Gartenraute). [Bullous phototoxic contact dermatitis caused by *Ruta graveolens* L. (garden rue), Rutaceae. Case report and review of literature.] Hautarzt 1999;50(6):432–4.

S

Salbutamol

See also Beta$_2$-adrenoceptor agonists

General Information

Salbutamol (albuterol) is a beta$_2$-adrenoceptor agonist used to treat asthma. It is available in various formulations:

- oral formulations (tablets of 2 and 4 mg, a modified-release tablet of 4 or 8 mg, and a syrup 5 mg/ml);
- a multidose pressurized aerosol, which delivers 100 micrograms per puff;
- dry powder form ("Rotacaps" 200 micrograms per capsule, "Accuhaler" 200 micrograms, "Turbuhaler" 100 or 200 micrograms, "Ventodisk" 200 or 400 micrograms per delivered dose);
- individual doses for nebulization ("nebulas") containing 2.5 ml of either 1 or 2 mg/ml salbutamol;
- a multidose vial of respirator solution containing 30 ml (concentration 5 mg/ml);
- formulations for injection, 50 micrograms/ml (5 ml) and 50 micrograms/ml (1 ml), and an intravenous infusion formulation of 1 mg/ml (5 ml).

All of these formulations are used in the treatment of asthma and the intravenous infusion is also used to manage premature labor.

Since salbutamol and its congeners are not entirely selective in their beta$_2$-stimulating action, they retain some stimulant effects on the heart, central nervous system, and carbohydrate and fat metabolism; these only become troublesome with relative overdosage or in particularly susceptible subjects. Adverse effects occur through stimulation of extra-pulmonary beta$_2$-adrenoceptors; they consist of:

- vasodilatation with reflex tachycardia;
- at high doses: direct cardiac stimulation;
- tremor;
- increased blood glucose concentration;
- a fall in serum potassium concentration.

The adverse effects of salbutamol have been reviewed (1).

Organs and Systems

Cardiovascular

Peripheral vasodilatation and palpitation have been reported in patients using salbutamol. These effects usually appear with rapid administration of high doses. Inhalation of 0.4 mg did not affect the heart rate, whereas inhalation of 5 mg raised it by 15/minute (2). Infusion of salbutamol at 0.025 mg/minute had a similar effect. Slight tachycardia can result in a mild rise in blood pressure, whereas at higher doses vasodilatation was more marked and the blood pressure fell. Infusion at 0.125 mg/minute reduced blood pressure by 30 mmHg. Salbutamol 10 puffs, administered from a pressurized aerosol using a spacer, produced significant bronchodilatation without adverse effects in mechanically ventilated patients. Heart rate rose significantly after 28 puffs (SEDA-21, 182).

Patients with severe hypoxemia and low serum potassium have an increased risk of developing extra beats and cardiac dysrhythmias (SEDA-2, 121).

Salbutamol causes an increase in the activity of the MB isoenzyme of creatine kinase, which has been interpreted as meaning that it might be cardiotoxic (3).

The systemic vascular changes produced by the combination of hypoxia and inhaled salbutamol in eight healthy men with mild asthma in a randomized, double-blind, placebo-controlled, crossover trial have been briefly reported (4). Forearm blood flow was measured non-invasively to obtain a measure of forearm vascular resistance (equating with systemic vascular resistance) after inhalation of placebo or salbutamol 800 micrograms under normoxic or hypoxic conditions. Both salbutamol alone and hypoxia alone produced small non-significant falls in forearm vascular resistance, but the combination of salbutamol and hypoxia resulted in a dramatic fall (30%). The authors pointed out that this fall in forearm vascular resistance was equivalent to the effects of glyceryl trinitrate 0.6–0.9 mg sublingually or felodipine 10 mg orally. This study emphasizes the marked cardiovascular changes that can occur with even small doses of salbutamol in people with mild asthma when hypoxia is present and confirms the importance of supplementary oxygen in these patients.

Intravenous and intracoronary salbutamol (10–30 and 1–10 micrograms/minute respectively) and intravenous isoprenaline (1–5 micrograms/minute), a mixed beta$_1$/beta$_2$-adrenoceptor agonist, were infused in 85 patients with coronary artery disease and 22 healthy controls during fixed atrial pacing (5). Both salbutamol and isoprenaline produced large increases in QT dispersion (QT_{onset}, QT_{peak}, and QT_{end}), more pronouncedly in patients with coronary artery disease. Dispersion of the QT interval is thought to be a surrogate marker for cardiac dysrhythmia (6). The authors concluded that beta$_2$-adrenoceptors mediate important electrophysiological effects in human ventricular myocardium and can trigger dysrhythmias in susceptible patients.

In a blind, randomized study, 29 children aged under 2 years, with moderate to severe acute exacerbations of hyper-reactive airways disease, were treated with either a standard dose of nebulized salbutamol (0.15 mg/kg) or a low dose of nebulized salbutamol (0.075 mg/kg) plus nebulized ipratropium bromide 250 micrograms (7). Standard and low-dose nebulized salbutamol was given three times at intervals of 20 minutes and nebulized ipratropium bromide was given once. Clinical improvement, measured as oxygen saturation and respiratory distress, was similar in both groups. QT dispersion was measured at baseline and after treatment and was significantly increased only by the standard dose of nebulized salbutamol.

Respiratory

Although salbutamol generally improves respiratory activity in asthma, arterial hypoxemia can be aggravated if it is used in excess or if parenchymal lung infection is present (8). In patients with bronchiectasis, salbutamol may aggravate hemoptysis (SEDA-9, 125). A feeling of "thick neck," chest heaviness, erythema, and edema of the face experienced in one reported case after the third dose could be reproduced by re-administration of the drug (SEDA-10, 116). Pulmonary edema can occur, even hours after discontinuation of beta$_2$-adrenoceptor stimulants (SEDA-13, 110).

Paradoxical bronchoconstriction has rarely been reported in patients with asthma after the inhalation of beta$_2$-agonists (9).

- A 22-year-old woman with mild asthma developed severe laryngospasm and bronchoconstriction after a fourth and subsequent doses of nebulized salbutamol, given during an acute episode of asthma. Her symptoms responded to adrenaline, but recurred after supervised rechallenge with nebulized orciprenaline (metaproterenol) sulfate. Indirect laryngoscopy excluded vocal cord dysfunction, suggesting that her symptoms of severe wheeze, respiratory distress, and hypoxia were due to bronchoconstriction.

Nervous system

Fine muscle tremor is common, especially when salbutamol is given orally or by injection. With nebulized salbutamol (2.5 or 7.5 mg) tremor was experienced by 14% of patients, and occurred more commonly with the higher doses (SEDA-21, 182). Shaking and nervousness were pronounced enough for 84% of patients taking oral salbutamol 5 mg tds to guess their treatment status correctly (SEDA-21, 180). At high doses agitation has been reported (SED-13, 362); in susceptible persons, hallucinations can develop, particularly in children, but also very occasionally in adults (10). A few patients experience headache.

The often reported observation by parents of asthmatic children that salbutamol causes hyperactivity has been investigated in 19 children before and after the inhalation of 5 ml of a nebulized solution (isotonic saline or salbutamol 5 mg); there was no statistically significant difference in activity (11). The authors hypothesized that the supposed effect on the children's activity might be dose-related or might reflect a propellant effect rather than being a consequence of salbutamol itself.

Sensory systems

Salbutamol has been applied to the eye for glaucoma, but often produces local irritation (12).

Metabolism

With inhaled salbutamol there is as a rule no significant effect on carbohydrate metabolism, but there were significant rises in blood glucose and insulin when intravenous salbutamol infusions were given to healthy pregnant women at term. The rise in blood glucose was significantly greater in pregnant women who were diabetic (SED-13, 363). Oral salbutamol 8 mg bd given for 14 days had no effect on glucose tolerance, but total cholesterol fell significantly by 9%; low-density lipoprotein cholesterol fell by 15%, and HDL increased by 10% (SEDA-21, 182).

Transient lactic acidosis/lactatemia has been reported as an adverse effect of inhaled salbutamol. In five patients who received 5 mg salbutamol by inhalation serum lactate concentrations were 3.2–8.0 mmol/l and arterial blood pH values 7.34–7.43; after 24 hours serum lactate concentrations returned to normal without specific treatment (13). In two other cases, high-dose salbutamol caused lactic acidosis, contributing to respiratory failure in one patient and complicating the assessment and management of acute severe asthma in the other (14). Respiratory compensation for this primary metabolic acidosis, characterized by increased respiratory rate and effort, may be mistaken for increased respiratory distress due to asthma. Lactic acidosis in acute asthma can therefore lead to problems in asthma management, including unwarranted intensification of beta$_2$-adrenoceptor agonist therapy and the initiation of premature or unnecessary mechanical ventilation.

Electrolyte balance

High doses of salbutamol, both intravenously and by nebulizer, can cause hypokalemia (15–17). This occurs by at least two mechanisms. First, beta$_2$-adrenoceptor agonists stimulate the Na/K pump in cell membranes, increasing the influx of potassium (18). Secondly, plasma renin activity and angiotensin II concentrations rise; angiotensin causes release of aldosterone, which is potassium-wasting in the kidney. In eight patients with mild asthma, nebulized salbutamol caused falls in serum potassium concentration from 4.4 mmol/l by a maximum of 0.85 mmol/l 45 minutes after 5 mg and by 1.16 mmol/l after 10 mg (SEDA-22, 189).

When three doses of nebulized salbutamol (0.15–0.3 mg/kg) were given at 30-minute intervals to 46 children with acute severe asthma, aged 10 months to 12 years, the mean potassium concentration fell marginally from 3.9 to 3.7 mmol/l. There was a fall in potassium concentration in 57% of the children and hypokalemia (potassium below 3.5 mmol/l) occurred in 39%. Hypokalemia was more likely to occur in children who had received oral salbutamol in the preceding 7 days. It was concluded that hypokalemia can occur in up to 33% of patients treated with three doses of nebulized salbutamol, particularly if they had previously taken oral salbutamol (SEDA-21, 182). Plasma concentrations of salbutamol correlate with changes in plasma potassium (19).

Musculoskeletal

The question of whether salbutamol can cause a myopathy has been discussed (20).

- A 76-year-old asthmatic woman developed increasing weakness, proximal muscle cramps, and fatigue. She had been using salbutamol spray (600 micrograms/day) and tablets (10 mg/day) for 2 years, and for 6 months had also used inhaled formoterol 24 micrograms/day. There were increases in creatine kinase (494 IU/l; reference range 0–130 IU/l), lactate dehydrogenase (350 IU/l; 0–300 IU/l), and aldolase (10 IU/l; 0–7.5 IU/l). Myopathy was confirmed electrophysiologically and histologically. The three medications were withdrawn and 2 days later her condition began to improve; the muscle pain and weakness disappeared within 3 weeks.

The authors concluded that beta$_2$-adrenoceptor agonist activity had been responsible for the deleterious muscle effects and they proposed that beta$_2$-adrenoceptor agonists should be added to the list of drugs that can cause myopathies. However, the exact effects of beta$_2$-adrenoceptor agonists on human skeletal muscle are not clear. They have also been reported to increase muscle strength and have been used in patients with muscle weakness, including spinal muscular atrophy (21).

- A 47-year-old man presented with severe myalgia and a raised creatine kinase MM isoenzyme (from skeletal muscle) while taking salbutamol from a multidose pressurized inhaler (SEDA-21, 182). The MM creatine kinase activity returned to normal when he stopped salbutamol and rested. When salbutamol was taken by inhaler or orally, the enzyme activity rose. When salbutamol was combined with exercise, even higher concentrations of creatine kinase resulted. A muscle biopsy specimen was consistent with a myopathy.

Immunologic

Hypersusceptibility reactions to salbutamol are extremely rare, but one well-documented allergic reaction has been described (SEDA-13, 109).

Long-Term Effects

Tumorigenicity

Tumor-inducing effects have not been reported in man. Chronic administration to rats produces mesovarian leiomyomas, a form of tumor not known in human subjects. The findings might reflect a species-specific consequence of prolonged beta$_2$-adrenoceptor stimulation of the rat estrous cycle; no tumors developed in mice similarly treated (SEDA-3, 118).

Second-Generation Effects

Pregnancy

Should an abortion occur in pregnant asthmatic patients taking salbutamol, the relaxant effect on the uterine wall is likely to result in marked bleeding (22).

Fetotoxicity

When salbutamol is used to arrest premature labor, effective doses are likely to produce mild fetal tachycardia (for example an increase of 20/minute) (23). In one case, supraventricular tachycardia occurred in the fetus in the 34th week of pregnancy after the mother had been treated with salbutamol; digoxin with and without propranolol was ineffective, but amiodarone controlled the tachycardia (24).

Susceptibility Factors

Age

A modified-release formulation of salbutamol (Proventil Repitabs) 12 mg bd was well tolerated in children. There were no serious adverse events and no changes in vital signs or the electrocardiogram (SEDA-21, 182).

Continuous salbutamol nebulization is relatively safe in children with severe asthma and impending respiratory failure. No chest pain, dysrhythmias, or signs of deterioration occurred (SEDA-21, 183). In one center, children presenting to an emergency department with severe asthma were initially given nebulized salbutamol 2.5–5 mg and intravenous corticosteroids. Children who did not improve continued to receive nebulized salbutamol and in addition 0.015 mg/kg of intravenous salbutamol. There were no clinically important adverse effects, although the children who were given intravenous salbutamol developed more tremor (SEDA-22, 190).

Renal disease

In patients with renal insufficiency (creatinine clearances 7–53, average 24 ml/minute) the clearance of an intravenous dose of salbutamol was more than halved (25). The dosage of salbutamol should be reduced in patients with impaired renal function.

Other features of the patient

Because of the cardiac and metabolic effects of salbutamol, it should be given cautiously with appropriate monitoring in patients with cardiovascular disease, diabetes, and hyperthyroidism.

Drug Administration

Drug formulations

Adverse effects are generally more likely when salbutamol is given by injection. At therapeutic doses, the pressurized aerosol and dry powder inhalers produce equivalent bronchodilatation without significant adverse effects (SEDA-22, 191). Patients with severe asthma tolerate large doses of nebulized salbutamol. In severe asthma there is a reduction in early lung absorption of salbutamol after inhalation, which does not occur in mild asthma. This results in lower plasma concentrations of salbutamol and less tremor (SEDA-22, 191). This is consistent with the findings in 323 patients who attended emergency departments because of severe asthma. Initial treatment with nebulized salbutamol 7.5–10 mg or up to 3.5 mg by pressurized aerosol in 1 hour caused no serious adverse effects. Tremor was noted in about 15% of the patients. About one-third of these patients failed to achieve an adequate therapeutic response to salbutamol. The most serious adverse effect of high-dose salbutamol would be failure to intensify treatment in the non-responders, that is an error of omission (SEDA-22, 190).

The efficacy and safety of salbutamol inhaled using a dry powder inhaler has been compared with salbutamol inhaled using a pressurized metered-dose inhaler (pMDI) in a randomized, open, crossover study in 12 patients with moderate to severe asthma. A total of 1600 micrograms of salbutamol was given on two separate days in a cumulative dose fashion in increments of 100, 100, 200, 400, and 800 micrograms at 3-minute intervals. FEV$_1$ rose progressively with each increment. The dose–response curves showed that powdered salbutamol was 3.0 times as potent (CI = 1.8, 5.8) as salbutamol from the pMDI. Systolic and diastolic blood pressures did not change. Powdered salbutamol caused a greater rise in heart rate. The maximum heart rate was seen at 25–30 minutes after the last dose on each study day. The average maximum heart rate was 95/minute (range 78–109) for the powder and 89/minute (range 76–106) for the pMDI. The relative dose potency of the powder versus the pMDI was 2.0 (CI = 1.3, 3.6) for lowering the serum potassium concentration. The lowest serum potassium concentration in an individual patient was 3.7 mmol/l after 1600 micrograms of the powder. No adverse events were reported on either study day. Four patients reported tremor. In one patient tremor was reported after each dose of powder as well as after 1600 micrograms inhaled from the pMDI. Cumulative doses of 800 and 1600 micrograms of powder caused tremor in the other three patients and two noted tremor after 1600 micrograms inhaled from the pMDI. Tremor was objectively measured and the dose–response curves showed a relative dose potency for the powder versus pMDI of 2.3 (CI = 1.5, 4.4). Thus, salbutamol powder was more potent than salbutamol pMDI for extrapulmonary effects and even more potent as a bronchodilator. It was concluded that use of the dry powder inhaler resulted in greater lung deposition of salbutamol, causing a higher concentration not only in the airways but also in the systemic circulation.

Drug additives

Additives to drug for inhalation, such as disodium edetate or benzalkonium chloride, can cause bronchoconstriction (26). This can lead to reduced therapeutic effectiveness of bronchodilators, for example salbutamol (or ipratropium). Some products do and others do not contain these additives, and an unexpected reduction in response to a bronchodilator may be the result of a change of product.

Drug overdose

After the ingestion of doses of salbutamol averaging 10 times the therapeutic oral dose, tachycardia, widened pulse pressure, agitation, nausea, and vomiting can occur (27–29).

A dose of 200 mg taken by mouth resulted in agitation, tachycardia, and peripheral vasodilatation; these effects were successfully treated with beta-blockers and benzodiazepines (SED-13, 362).

- A 28-year-old woman took an overdose of oral salbutamol (100 mg of salbutamol BP solution) (30). She developed diabetic ketoacidosis, with a serum glucose concentration of 17 mmol/l (308 mg/dl). Diabetic ketoacidosis induced by salbutamol overdose is uncommon in patients without diabetes; however, this patient had a family history of diabetes.

- A 4-year-old girl with accidental salbutamol intoxication (2.3 mg/kg) developed fever (38°C) besides the classical signs of salbutamol intoxication (31). Since she had no identifiable focus of infection the possibility of a thermogenic effect induced by increased adrenergic stimulation due to salbutamol intoxication was considered.

Drug–Drug Interactions

Beta blockers

The effects of salbutamol are antagonized by beta-blockers (32).

Corticosteroids

The risk of hyperglycemia or hypokalemia is increased if corticosteroids are given simultaneously (for example for asthma). In 24 healthy subjects randomized to salbutamol 5 mg, fenoterol 5 mg, or isotonic saline before and after a course of prednisone 30 mg/day for 1 week, changes in plasma potassium and glucose after the nebulized beta-agonist were significantly greater after treatment with prednisone (33). Baseline potassium concentration fell from 3.75 to 3.50 mmol/l. The lowest mean plasma potassium occurred 90 minutes after fenoterol with prednisone pretreatment (2.78 mmol/l).

Diuretics

Treatment with bendroflumethiazide, and presumably other diuretics, augments the hypokalemic and electrocardiographic effects of high-dose inhaled salbutamol; the dysrhythmogenic potential of this interaction can be important in patients with acute exacerbations of chronic airflow obstruction, who have concomitant hypoxemia and ischemic heart disease (SEDA-15, 134).

Formoterol and salmeterol

The interaction of formoterol and salmeterol with salbutamol has been studied in a randomized, double-blind, crossover study in 16 asthmatic patients (34). The patients were taking regular inhaled corticosteroids and were responsive to methacholine challenge, with a PD20 (that is the dose of methacholine that produced a fall in FEV_1 of 20%) of less than 500 micrograms. The patients had methacholine challenges performed 12 hours after a single dose of formoterol 12 micrograms, salmeterol 50 micrograms, placebo, and either a low dose (400 micrograms) or a high dose (1600 micrograms) of salbutamol. With placebo, challenge after high-dose salbutamol resulted in a higher PD20 than after low-dose salbutamol (as expected). However, after both formoterol and salmeterol, the higher dose of salbutamol did not give as great an increase in PD20 over the lower dose of salbutamol. This suggests that prior treatment with formoterol and salmeterol can antagonize the protective effect of salbutamol against bronchoconstriction. This effect may be important in patients with acute asthma.

Theophylline

Salbutamol has additive effects with theophylline, which can potentiate the hypokalemic effect (SEDA-17, 164). In 14 healthy volunteers, theophylline increased salbutamol-induced hypokalemia and in some individuals there was profound hypokalemia (less than 2.5 mmol/l) (35). Combining theophylline with salbutamol increased the tachycardia resulting from the salbutamol infusion. Salbutamol infusion caused a fall in diastolic and a rise in systolic blood pressure, which was not altered by theophylline.

References

1. Sears MR. Adverse effects of beta-agonists. J Allergy Clin Immunol 2002;110(Suppl 6):S322–8.

2. Scherrer M, Bachofen H. Vergleich der Wirkung einer 4.5 Minuten dauernden Aerosolinhalation von Salbutamol und von Trimetoquinol mit derjenigen einer 10–15 Minuten dauernden Tacholoquin-Orciprenalin-Inhalation bei Bronchialasthma. [Comparison of the effect of aerosol inhalation with salbutamol and trimetolquinol of four and a half minutes duration with that of tacholiquin–orciprenalin of fifteen minutes duration in bronchial asthma.] Schweiz Med Wochenschr 1972;102(26):909–14.

3. Chazan R, Tadeusiak W, Jaworski A, Droszcz W. Creatine kinase (CK) and creatine kinase isoenzyme (CK-MB) activity in serum before and after intravenous salbutamol administration of patients with bronchial asthma. Int J Clin Pharmacol Ther Toxicol 1992;30(10):371–3.

4. Burggraaf J, Westendorp RG, in't Veen JC, Schoemaker RC, Sterk PJ, Cohen AF, Blauw GJ. Cardiovascular side effects of inhaled salbutamol in hypoxic asthmatic patients. Thorax 2001;56(7):567–9.

5. Lowe MD, Rowland E, Brown MJ, Grace AA. Beta$_2$-adrenergic receptors mediate important electrophysiological effects in human ventricular myocardium. Heart 2001;86:45–51.

6. Pye M, Quinn AC, Cobbe SM. QT interval dispersion: a non-invasive marker of susceptibility to arrhythmia in patients with sugtained ventricular arrhythmias? Br Heart J 1994;71:511–14.

7. Yuksel H, Coskun S, Polat M, Onag A. Lower arrythmogenic risk of low dose albuterol plus ipratropium. Indian J Pediatr 2001;68(10):945–9.

8. Connett G, Lenney W. Prolonged hypoxaemia after nebulised salbutamol. Thorax 1993;48(5):574–5.

9. Mutlu GM, Moonjelly E, Chan L, Olopade CO. Laryngospasm and paradoxical bronchoconstriction after repeated doses of beta 2-agonists containing edetate disodium. Mayo Clin Proc 2000;75(3):285–7.

10. Khanna PB, Davies R. Hallucinations associated with administration of salbutamol via a nebulizer. BMJ (Clin Res Ed) 1986;292:1430.

11. Hadjikoumi I, Loader P, Bracken M, Milner AD. Bronchodilator therapy and hyperactivity in preschool children. Arch Dis Child 2002;86(3):202–3.

12. Paterson GD, Paterson G. Drug therapy of glaucoma. Br J Ophthalmol 1972;56(3):288–94.

13. Stratakos G, Kalomenidis J, Routsi C, Papiris S, Roussos C. Transient lactic acidosis as a side effect of inhaled salbutamol. Chest 2002;122(1):385–6.

14. Prakash S, Mehta S. Lactic acidosis in asthma: report of two cases and review of the literature. Can Respir J 2002;9(3):203–8.

15. Hung CH, Chu DM, Wang CL, Yang KD. Hypokalemia and salbutamol therapy in asthma. Pediatr Pulmonol 1999;27(1):27–31.

16. Chua S, Razvi K, Wong MT, Tay R, Arulkumaran S. Is there a need to treat hypokalaemia associated with intravenous salbutamol infusion? J Obstet Gynaecol Res 1997;23(4):381–7.

17. Udezue E, D'Souza L, Mahajan M. Hypokalemia after normal doses of neubulized albuterol (salbutamol). Am J Emerg Med 1995;13(2):168–71.

18. Brown MJ, Brown DC, Murphy MB. Hypokalemia from beta$_2$-receptor stimulation by circulating epinephrine. N Engl J Med 1983;309(23):1414–19.

19. Fowler SJ, Lipworth BJ. Pharmacokinetics and systemic beta$_2$-adrenoceptor-mediated responses to inhaled salbutamol. Br J Clin Pharmacol 2001;51(4):359–62.

20. Hellier JP, Baudrimont M, Dussaule JC, Berenbaum F. Reversible selective beta(2)-adrenoceptor agonist-induced myopathy. Rheumatology (Oxford) 2002;41(1):111–13.

21. Kinali M, Mercuri E, Main M, De Biasia F, Karatza A, Higgins R, Banks LM, Manzur AY, Muntoni F. Pilot trial of albuterol in spinal muscular atrophy. Neurology 2002;59(4):609–10.

22. Vinall PS, Jenkins DM. Salbutamol and haemorrhage at spontaneous abortion. Lancet 1977;2(8052–8053):1355.

23. Pincus R. Salbutamol infusion for premature labour—the Australian trials experience. Aust NZ J Obstet Gynaecol 1981;21(1):1–4.

24. Belhassen A, Vaksmann G, Francart C, Vinatier D, Patey P, Monnier JC. Intérêt de l'amiodarone dans le traitement des tachycardies supraventriculaires foetales. A propos d'une observation. [Value of amiodarone in the treatment of fetal supraventricular tachycardia. Apropos of a case.] J Gynecol Obstet Biol Reprod (Paris) 1987;16(6):795–800.

25. Rey E, Luquel L, Richard MO, Mory B, Offenstadt G, Olive G. Pharmacokinetics of intravenous salbutamol in renal insufficiency and its biological effects. Eur J Clin Pharmacol 1989;37(4):387–9.

26. Asmus MJ, Sherman J, Hendeles L. Bronchoconstrictor additives in bronchodilator solutions. J Allergy Clin Immunol 1999;104(2 Pt 2):S53–60.

27. Wiley JF 2nd, Spiller HA, Krenzelok EP, Borys DJ. Unintentional albuterol ingestion in children. Pediatr Emerg Care 1994;10(4):193–6.

28. Lewis LD, Essex E, Volans GN, Cochrane GM. A study of self poisoning with oral salbutamol—laboratory and clinical features. Hum Exp Toxicol 1993;12(5):397–401.

29. Spiller HA, Ramoska EA, Henretig FM, Joffe M. A two-year retrospective study of accidental pediatric albuterol ingestions. Pediatr Emerg Care 1993;9(6):338–40.

30. Habib GS, Saliba WR, Cohen L. Diabetic ketoacidosis associated with oral salbutamol overdose. Am J Med 2002;113(8):701–2.

31. Yilmaz HL, Kucukosmanoglu O, Hennes H, Celik T. Salbutamol intoxication: is salbutamol a drug-inducing fever? A case report and treatment strategy. Eur J Emerg Med 2002;9(2):179–82.

32. Desche P, Cournot A, Duchier J, Prost JF. Airway response to salbutamol and to ipratropium bromide after non-selective and cardioselective beta-blocker. Eur J Clin Pharmacol 1987;32(4):343–6.

33. Taylor DR, Wilkins GT, Herbison GP, Flannery EM. Interaction between corticosteroid and beta-agonist drugs. Biochemical and cardiovascular effects in normal subjects. Chest 1992;102(2):519–24.

34. Aziz I, Lipworth BJ. In vivo effect of albuterol on methacholine-contracted bronchi in conjunction with salmeterol and formoterol. J Allergy Clin Immunol 1999;103(5 Pt 1):816–22.

35. Whyte KF, Reid C, Addis GJ, Whitesmith R, Reid JL. Salbutamol induced hypokalaemia: the effect of theophylline alone and in combination with adrenaline. Br J Clin Pharmacol 1988;25(5):571–8.

Salicaceae

See also Herbal medicines

General Information

The family of Salicaceae contains two genera:

1. *Populus* (cottonwood)
2. *Salix* (willow).

Table 1 Some plant sources of salicylates

Salicylate	Plant species	Common name	Family
Methyl salicylate	*Gaultheria procumbens*	Wintergreen, Eastern teaberry	Ericaceae
	Spiraea alba	White meadowsweet	Rosaceae
Salicin	*Salix songorica*		Salicaceae
Salicylic acid	*Salix alba*	White willow	Salicaceae
	Burchardia multiflora	Milk maids	Colchicaceae
	Callicarpa integerrima		Verbenaceae
	Falcaria vulgaris	Sickleweed	Apiaceae
	Flemingia laevicarpa		Fabaceae
	Genista lucida		Fabaceae
	Populus pseudosimonii		Salicaceae
Saligenin	*Populus pseudosimonii*		Salicaceae

Salix species and salicylates

The barks of various species of *Salix* contain glycosides of saligenin (salicylalcohol), namely the simple O-glycoside salicin and more complex glycosides such as salicortin (1). When taken orally, these glycosides undergo intestinal transformation to saligenin, which is rapidly absorbed and converted by the liver to salicylic acid. When willow bark preparations are used according to current dosage recommendations, they will not provide sufficient salicylic acid to produce acute salicylate poisoning. However, the risk of hypersusceptibility reactions, such as skin reactions and bronchospasm, in sensitive individuals cannot be excluded.

Other natural sources of salicylates are listed in Table 1. There are separate monographs on acetylsalicylic acid (aspirin), benorilate, diflunisal, lysine acetylsalicylate, and salsalate. Methyl salicylate is covered under *Gaultheria procumbens* in the monograph on the Ericaceae.

Reference

1. Kammerer B, Kahlich R, Biegert C, Gleiter CH, Heide L. HPLC–MS/MS analysis of willow bark extracts contained in pharmaceutical preparations. Phytochem Anal 2005;16(6):470–8.

Salicylanilides

See also Disinfectants and antiseptics

General Information

The halogenated salicylanilides, which include closantel, niclosamide, oxyclozanide, rafoxanide, and resorantel, have antiparasitic activity in animals (1). Closantel and rafoxanide are widely used for the control of infestation with *Hemonchus* species and *Fasciola* species in sheep and cattle and *Estrus ovis* in sheep. Niclosamide is used as an anticestode in a wide range

of animals. Other parasites that are susceptible include hematophagous helminths and external parasites such as ticks and mites. Many halogenated salicylanilides, including dibromosalicylanilide, tribromosalicylanilide, and tetrachlorosalicylanilide, have been used in disinfectants.

Organs and Systems

Skin

Photocontact dermatitis can occur after the use of halogenated salicylanilides, such as tribromosalicylanilide in soaps (2) and bithionol in first-aid creams (3). Tetrachlorosalicylanilide caused many cases in the 1960s and was withdrawn, after which there was a striking reduction in the numbers of patients with positive photopatch tests (4). The authors concluded that these results were most likely to have been due to removal from the market of the more potent photosensitizing chemicals and increased familiarity of physicians with this effect. Photosensitivity has also been reported to other analogues in widespread use, such as the dibromo and tribromo derivatives. The photoallergy is localized, but transient generalized reactions can occur.

References

1. Swan GE. The pharmacology of halogenated salicylanilides and their anthelmintic use in animals. J S Afr Vet Assoc 1999;70(2):61–70.
2. Osmundsen PE. Fotokontaktdermatitis forarsaget af tribromsalicylanilid i toiletsaebe. [Photocontact dermatitis caused by tribromosalicylanilide in toilet soap.] Ugeskr Laeger 1967;129(48):1607–10.
3. O'Quinn SE, Kennedy CB, Isbell KH. Contact photodermatitis due to bithionol and related compounds. JAMA 1967;199(2):89–92.
4. Smith SZ, Epstein JH. Photocontact dermatitis to halogenated salicylanilides and related compounds. Our experience between 1967 and 1975. Arch Dermatol 1977;113(10):1372–4.

Salicylates, topical

General Information

Salicylic acid is widely used in dermatology because of its keratolytic properties. Methylsalicylate (the main constituent of oil of wintergreen) is a topical analgesic that is also a constituent of Red Flower Oil and White Flower Oil formulations, popular herbal analgesics used topically in Southeast Asia (1). Some users take small amounts of the oil orally to enhance its analgesic effects. It has been responsible for rare cases of allergic skin reactions.

Salicylism

Many reports have described "salicylism," intoxication due to percutaneous absorption of salicylates, such as methyl salicylate (2). The first symptoms of salicylism are pallor, fatigue and drowsiness, and altered respiration, which becomes more frequent and at the same time deeper, and which can be heard from a distance. Other early signs of intoxication with salicylic acid are nausea, vomiting, changes in the ability to hear, and mental confusion. Several deaths have been recorded, mainly in children.

Other signs and symptoms of salicylism (3–5) include:

fatigue, changes in hearing ability, nuchal rigidity, fever, profuse sweating, and pallor (6);
frequent deep respiration, Cheyne-Stokes respiration, dyspnea, hyperpnea;
drowsiness, mental confusion, stupor, hallucinations, headache, dizziness, tinnitus, slurred speech, agitation, disorientation, lethargy, delusions, aggression, retrograde amnesia, depression, coma, somnolence;
hypoglycemia (SEDA-16, 158) and metabolic acidosis (6); nausea, vomiting, thirst, anorexia, diarrhea.

Accidental ingestion of methylsalicylate in young children has resulted in severe salicylate poisoning, in one case with laryngeal edema (7). A suicide attempt by deliberate ingestion of about 100 ml resulted in severe salicylate poisoning (8).

References

1. Chan TY. Ingestion of medicated oils by adults: the risk of severe salicylate poisoning is related to the packaging of these products. Hum Exp Toxicol 2002;21(4):171–4.
2. Morra P, Bartle WR, Walker SE, Lee SN, Bowles SK, Reeves RA. Serum concentrations of salicylic acid following topically applied salicylate derivatives. Ann Pharmacother 1996;30(9):935–40.
3. Chiaretti A, Schembri Wismayer D, Tortorolo L, Piastra M, Polidori G. Salicylate intoxication using a skin ointment. Acta Paediatr 1997;86(3):330–1.
4. Brubacher JR, Hoffman RS. Salicylism from topical salicylates: review of the literature. J Toxicol Clin Toxicol 1996;34(4):431–6.
5. Treguer H, Le Bihan G, Coloignier M, Le Roux P, Bernard JP. Intoxication salicylée par application locale de vaseline salicylée à 20% chez un psoriasique. [Salicylate poisoning by local application of 20% salicylic acid petrolatum to a psoriatic patient.] Nouv Presse Med 1980;9(3):192–3.
6. Smith WO, Lyons D. Metabolic acidosis associated with percutaneous absorption of salicylic acid. J Okla State Med Assoc 1980;73(1):7–8.
7. Botma M, Colquhoun-Flannery W, Leighton S. Laryngeal oedema caused by accidental ingestion of Oil of Wintergreen. Int J Pediatr Otorhinolaryngol 2001;58(3):229–32.
8. Chan TH, Wong KC, Chan JC. Severe salicylate poisoning associated with the intake of Chinese medicinal oil ("red flower oil"). Aust N Z J Med 1995;25(1):57.

Salmeterol

See also Beta$_2$-adrenoceptor agonists

General Information

Salmeterol is a selective beta$_2$-adrenoceptor agonist that is more potent and has a significantly longer duration of action than salbutamol (SEDA-21, 184). It is used as a supplement to inhaled glucocorticoids for sustained bronchodilatation. It has a much slower onset of effect than salbutamol and is not effective in acute attacks of asthma. It is available as a multidose-pressurized aerosol 0.025 mg/puff, and as a dry powder, Diskhaler or Accuhaler 0.05 mg per dose. The adverse effects profile of salmeterol is the same as that of salbutamol and other beta$_2$-agonists (SEDA-21, 185).

Observational studies

There has been a systematic review of the literature and of unpublished trials with single and chronic doses of inhaled salmeterol 100 micrograms from the GlaxoSmithKline databases (1). The analysis covered data available until early 1999. Of 44 trials that included salmeterol 100 micrograms, data on systemic effects were available from 19 trials that were subsequently included in a pooled weighted analysis. In the chronic dose studies in 1504 patients who took salmeterol for more than 7 days, tremor was reported in 5.6%, palpitation in 1.7%, reduced serum potassium in 0.9%, electrocardiographic events in 0.6%, and increased serum glucose in 0.3%. The smaller systemic effects after chronic administration compared with single salmeterol dosing possibly reflected tachyphylaxis to the systemic cardiovascular and metabolic effects of the drug. The mean systemic effects of salmeterol 100 micrograms are small and of doubtful clinical relevance; unintended use of twice the dose of salmeterol is unlikely to affect patients adversely.

Placebo-controlled studies

In a randomized, double-blind, placebo-controlled, multicenter evaluation of the clinical efficacy and safety of salmeterol 42 micrograms bd in 538 asthmatic patients, mean peak flow rate improved significantly in the patients who used salmeterol (2). The use of supplementary salbutamol, asthma symptom scores, and FEV$_1$ were significantly improved by salmeterol. There were no clinically significant adverse events.

In a double-blind study in 49 stable asthmatic patients who were taking inhaled glucocorticoids, randomized to either salmeterol 50 micrograms or placebo bd for 4 weeks, the bronchodilator response to cumulative doses of inhaled salbutamol was measured before and 12 and 36 hours after the last dose (3). There were no significant differences between salmeterol and placebo in maximal FEV_1 or peak expiratory flow rate responses to inhaled salbutamol at 12 and 36 hours. Asthma control, as judged by lung function and diary card parameters, was significantly better in the patients who took regular salmeterol. There were no serious adverse events. The incidence of non-serious adverse events was similar in the two groups, 56% with salmeterol and 50% with placebo. The most commonly reported adverse events were headache and rhinitis.

Salmeterol 50 micrograms bd and salbutamol 400 micrograms qds have been compared in 165 patients with mild to moderate bronchial asthma in a double-dummy, placebo-controlled, crossover study (4). Relative to placebo, mean morning peak expiratory flow rate increased by 30 l/minute with salmeterol but did not change with salbutamol; evening peak expiratory flow rate increased by 25 l/minute. Salmeterol improved the asthma score compared with placebo, but salbutamol produced no overall difference. Only daytime symptoms were improved by salbutamol. The asthma score fell over time with salbutamol. Both minor and major exacerbation rates were significantly less when patients used salmeterol. Major exacerbations lasted for significantly longer in patients taking salbutamol compared with those taking placebo. Tolerance did not develop to either drug; after withdrawal there was no rebound worsening of asthma control, fall in lung function, or increase in bronchial reactivity to inhaled methacholine. Although salbutamol improved daytime symptoms, there was deterioration in asthma control over time.

The effect of salmeterol on asthma control in 506 patients requiring inhaled corticosteroids has been evaluated in a randomized, double-blind, placebo-controlled study (5). The patients received either salmeterol 42 micrograms bd via a metered-dose inhaler or placebo for 12 weeks. Salmeterol was superior to placebo when assessed by asthma quality-of-life score, global score, asthma symptoms, and improvement in FEV_1, peak expiratory flow rate, and use of supplementary salbutamol to treat exacerbations. Adverse events were reported in 53% of patients taking salmeterol and 51% of patients taking placebo. Most adverse events were not related to treatment. Treatment-related adverse events occurred in 13 patients (5%) taking placebo and 11 patients (4%) taking salmeterol. Twelve patients (2%) did not complete the study because of adverse events, five taking placebo and seven taking salmeterol. In only three patients were the adverse effects considered to be potentially related to the treatment: salmeterol—chest tightness; placebo—shortness of breath and chest pains. Respiratory failure occurred in one patient taking salmeterol and was judged to be possibly related to the drug. Exacerbation of asthma occurred in 59 patients (22%) taking placebo and 53 patients (20%) taking salmeterol. The most common

reason cited for exacerbation of the asthma was respiratory infection.

In a double-blind, multicenter trial in primary care, 911 patients with asthma, who were already receiving maintenance anti-inflammatory therapy, were randomized to treatment with salmeterol (50 micrograms bd) or placebo for six months (6). As expected, the patients treated with salmeterol had higher mean peak expiratory flows, used less rescue salbutamol, and had less disturbed sleep than the patients treated with placebo. The most important result from this study was that the number of severe exacerbations was the same in both groups; in other words, salmeterol did not increase the frequency of severe exacerbations.

Salmeterol 42 micrograms bd has been compared with inhaled ipratropium bromide 36 micrograms/day and inhaled placebo in a randomized, double-blind study for 12 weeks in 405 patients with chronic obstructive pulmonary disease (6). Both salmeterol and ipratropium bromide significantly increased the peak expiratory flow rate compared with placebo. Non-specific ear, nose, and throat symptoms (for example sore throat and upper respiratory tract infections) were more common with salmeterol and ipratropium than placebo. There were no significant differences between the groups in the total number of ventricular and supraventricular extra beats. There was no tolerance to the bronchodilating effects of salmeterol.

In a randomized, double-blind, parallel-group study, 911 asthmatic patients in primary care were randomly assigned to inhaled salmeterol 50 micrograms bd or placebo bd for 24 weeks (7). They continued to use their anti-inflammatory maintenance therapy throughout. Salmeterol produced a significant improvement in peak expiratory flow rate and a reduction in the use of short-acting beta$_2$-agonists. Salmeterol did not increase the number of severe exacerbations of asthma.

Comparative studies

Salmeterol has been compared with several other bronchodilators.

Formoterol

Salmeterol dry powder 50 micrograms bd and formoterol dry powder 12 micrograms bd have been compared in 425 asthmatic patients treated for 6 months in a randomized, open, parallel-group study. Improvements were similar in the two groups, although evening predose peak expiratory flow rate showed a trend in favor of formoterol, statistically significant at 2, 3, and 4 months (8). Both treatments were well tolerated: 193 patients taking salmeterol and 190 taking formoterol reported adverse events. This was not unexpected in a 6-month trial. The most frequent adverse events included viral infections, asthma exacerbation, headache, rhinitis, and chest infections. Exacerbation of asthma was reported as an adverse event by 54 (22%) taking salmeterol and 41 patients (17%) taking formoterol. Adverse events, assessed as possibly/probably drug-related, were reported in 21 (9%) taking salmeterol and 32 (13%) patients taking formoterol. The most frequent drug-related adverse event was headache, reported by 11 patients taking salmeterol and seven taking formoterol. Other adverse events included tremor in two taking salmeterol and five patients taking formoterol, exacerbation of asthma in four patients in each group, and palpitation in four patients taking formoterol.

The relative efficacy of the long-acting beta$_2$-adrenoceptor agonists formoterol and salmeterol has been studied in a randomized, double-blind, crossover trial in 15 patients with asthma taking regular corticosteroids and salbutamol (9). The patients had methacholine challenges performed after varying single doses of formoterol (12, 60, and 120 micrograms) and salmeterol (50, 250, and 500 micrograms). The maximal protective effect of salmeterol against methacholine challenge was reached at 250 micrograms, whereas formoterol showed a dose–response relation, with maximum protection at the highest dose. This confirmed the authors' hypothesis that salmeterol is a partial agonist at beta-adrenoceptors compared with formoterol. The higher affinity of formoterol for beta-adrenoceptors also produced more adverse effects. There was a significant fall in serum potassium concentration after 60 micrograms of formoterol but not after 250 micrograms of salmeterol. The serum potassium concentration was also significantly lower with the highest dose of formoterol compared with the highest dose of salmeterol (minimum concentration 3.1 mmol/l). The highest dose of formoterol also resulted in more tremor than the highest dose of salmeterol. The increases in heart rate and QT$_c$ interval were similar with the two drugs. It should be noted that the doses used in this study were higher than recommended. It remains unclear whether the partial agonist activity of salmeterol is clinically important, but this seems unlikely.

Salbutamol

The effects of single inhaled doses of salmeterol 0.1, 0.2, and 0.4 mg and salbutamol 0.4 mg from a multidose pressurized inhaler have been compared in healthy volunteers (10). At all doses tested, salmeterol produced statistically significant changes in pulse rate, tremor, blood glucose, and plasma potassium concentrations. Tremor, awareness of heartbeat, and headache were reported by the subjects after salmeterol administration.

Theophylline

Inhaled salmeterol 50 micrograms bd has been compared with oral modified-release theophylline in 178 patients with mild to moderate chronic obstructive pulmonary disease (8). Salmeterol caused a significant improvement in mean morning peak expiratory flow rate compared with theophylline and significantly increased the percentage of symptom-free days and nights with no additional requirement for salbutamol. Adverse events occurred in 50% of the patients who took salmeterol, and 49% of those who used theophylline. Adverse events due to the pharmacological properties of the drug were less frequent with salmeterol (4%) than with theophylline (15%).

In a randomized, double-blind study, 943 patients with chronic obstructive pulmonary disease were treated over 12 weeks with either inhaled salmeterol 42 micrograms bd via a metered-dose inhaler or oral modified-release theophylline bd, titrated to serum concentrations of 10–20 micrograms/ml, or with a combination of the two drugs (11). Adverse events potentially related to the study drug were significantly more common in those who took theophylline compared with salmeterol alone. This was most evident for adverse gastrointestinal events (nausea, gastric upset, vomiting, diarrhea). Adverse cardiovascular events occurred in 1–4% and were comparable among the groups. Theophylline-related toxicity was considerable, as nearly 16% of the patients withdrew during the theophylline titration period owing to adverse events.

Organs and Systems

Cardiovascular

No cardiovascular effects are seen at the recommended daily dose. At a dose of 0.1 mg of salmeterol twice a day no change in heart rate or rhythm was seen on a 24-hour electrocardiogram (Holter). No change in blood pressure was seen and no electrocardiographic abnormality related to myocardial ischemia was recorded during 24-hour monitoring (12).

Skin

A single case of a pruritic burning maculopapular rash has been documented and confirmed by patch-testing with the active component (SEDA-17, 165).

Death

When salmeterol was given for one year to 15 407 patients there were no unexpected major adverse events. There were 1022 (6.6%) deaths; 73 patients died of asthma and 39 used salmeterol during the last month of life. Analysis showed that the majority of deaths were due to natural causes. In four of the 39 subjects who died of asthma and who had taken salmeterol the authors thought it possible that death had been related to the use of salmeterol (13).

Long-Term Effects

Drug tolerance

Current guidelines recommend the use of formoterol and salmeterol in addition to inhaled corticosteroids for optimal management of asthma. Both drugs are highly selective beta$_2$-adrenoceptor agonists, with minor pharmacological differences. Several studies have shown that regular use of both formoterol and salmeterol results in the development of tolerance to their bronchoprotective effects, even with treatment periods as short as 1 week. The significance of this tolerance is unclear, but it is potentially important clinically.

Previous studies over periods of up to 8 weeks have established that the bronchoprotective effect of salmeterol abates with regular use, even after only 1 week of regular treatment. The effects of longer-term use of salmeterol on airway hyper-responsiveness have been examined in a randomized, double-blind, placebo-controlled trial in 408 patients with mild asthma (14). These patients were not using inhaled corticosteroids and took salmeterol (42 micrograms bd) or placebo for 24 weeks. Methacholine challenges were performed at 4, 12, and 24 weeks. At 4 weeks salmeterol provided protection against methacholine of about one doubling dose and there was no further change in this protection over the study period. As expected, regular salmeterol produced significant improvements in asthma symptoms. Adverse events were similar in the two groups, apart from headache, which was reported in 14 of 202 patients treated with salmeterol and seven of 206 patients taking placebo. The loss of bronchoprotection that develops with regular salmeterol did not appear to worsen over a 24-week period.

The effect of inhaled budesonide on the loss of bronchoprotection with regular salmeterol has been studied in a randomized, double-blind trial in 18 patients with mild asthma, taking no regular medications (15). After 1 week of regular salmeterol (50 micrograms bd) 12 patients developed tolerance to its protective effect against airway allergen. After another week of salmeterol combined with either inhaled budesonide (500 micrograms bd) or placebo, the patients who took budesonide showed some recovery of the protective effect of salmeterol against airway allergen compared with placebo. The authors suggested upregulation of beta-adrenoceptors as a potential mechanism.

The effect of a bolus of inhaled budesonide on formoterol-induced subsensitivity in airway beta-adrenoceptors has been studied in a randomized, double-blind, crossover study in 10 asthmatic patients taking regular inhaled glucocorticoids (16). Challenge testing with AMP was performed at baseline and after one week of regular formoterol (24 micrograms bd). Before the second challenge the patients were given either a dose of inhaled budesonide (1600 micrograms) or placebo via a dry powder inhaler. After one week of formoterol, the PC_{20} for the second challenge fell significantly (by a factor of 3.9). However, when the second challenge was performed after a bolus of budesonide, there was no fall in the PC_{20}, suggesting protection against formoterol-induced tolerance. Lymphocyte beta-adrenoceptor density fell with regular formoterol, but not after a bolus of budesonide. These results have implications for the treatment of acute severe asthma in patients taking regular long-acting beta$_2$-adrenoceptor agonists. It may be appropriate to give a bolus dose of inhaled glucocorticoids to these patients early in an acute asthma attack, particularly if they are poorly responsive to initial therapy with short-acting bronchodilators.

Drug Administration

Drug formulations

Combination formulations of fluticasone with salmeterol delivered through a dry powder inhaler are intended to provide a combination of an inhaled glucocorticoid and a long-acting beta$_2$-adrenoceptor agonist in one dose, simplifying the treatment regimen and so possibly improving compliance.

Salmeterol 50 micrograms plus fluticasone 500 micrograms bd delivered via a combination inhaler (plus a placebo inhaler) have been compared with the same drug regimen delivered by separate inhalers in a randomized, double-blind trial over 28 weeks in 503 asthmatic patients already taking inhaled glucocorticoids (17).

There was also an arm treated with inhaled fluticasone alone. Outcome variables were peak flow and asthma symptoms. Both combination and concurrent therapy with fluticasone plus salmeterol resulted in significantly better symptom control and higher peak flows than fluticasone alone. There were no significant differences in the effects of fluticasone plus salmeterol delivered in a combination inhaler versus separate inhalers. Drug-related adverse effects were similar in all three treatment groups: most were asthma-related, but hoarseness, dysphonia, and throat irritation were the commonest adverse effects attributed to therapy (1–4%).

The effects of salmeterol 50 micrograms plus fluticasone 250 micrograms delivered via a combination inhaler and via separate inhalers have been compared in 371 asthmatic patients (18). There were equivalent improvements in peak flows and asthma symptoms. Candidiasis, dysphonia, and throat irritation were the commonest adverse effects attributed to treatment and occurred equally in the two groups (35%). Palpitation and tremor, which may have been related to salmeterol, occurred in 2% (for each symptom) of the combination group and in 1% and under 1% of the separate inhaler group. In both of these studies compliance was measured by dose counters on the inhalers and was equivalent in the two groups.

It appears that treatment with fluticasone plus salmeterol delivered via a combination inhaler is as effective as the same drugs given in separate inhalers and has a similar adverse effects profile. Whether treatment with a combination inhaler improves compliance is not yet proven.

Drug–Drug Interactions

Salbutamol

Experimental studies continue to show that regular treatment with either formoterol or salmeterol in patients with asthma can produce subsensitivity to the bronchodilator effects of salbutamol (19,20). This bronchodilator subsensitivity can be partly reversed by a bolus dose of inhaled or systemic corticosteroids. The clinical relevance of these experimental findings is unclear.

References

1. Shrewsbury S, Hallett C. Salmeterol 100 microg: an analysis of its tolerability in single and chronic-dose studies. Ann Allergy Asthma Immunol 2001;87(6):465–73.
2. Busse WW, Casale TB, Murray JJ, Petrocella V, Cox F, Rickard K. Efficacy, safety, and impact on quality of life of salmeterol in patients with moderate persistent asthma. Am J Manag Care 1998;4(11):1579–87.
3. Langley SJ, Masterson CM, Batty EP, Woodcock A. Bronchodilator response to salbutamol after chronic dosing with salmeterol or placebo. Eur Respir J 1998;11(5):1081–5.
4. Taylor DR, Town GI, Herbison GP, Boothman-Burrell D, Flannery EM, Hancox B, Harre E, Laubscher K, Linscott V, Ramsay CM, Richards G, Cowan J, Holbrook N, McLachlan C, Rigby S. Asthma control during long-term treatment with regular inhaled salbutamol and salmeterol. Thorax 1998;53(9):744–52.

5. Kemp JP, Cook DA, Incaudo GA, Corren J, Kalberg C, Emmett A, Cox FM, Rickard K. Salmeterol improves quality of life in patients with asthma requiring inhaled corticosteroids. Salmeterol Quality of Life Study Group. J Allergy Clin Immunol 1998;101(2 Pt 1):188–95.

6. Rennard SI, Anderson W, ZuWallack R, Broughton J, Bailey W, Friedman M, Wisniewski M, Rickard K. Use of a long-acting inhaled beta$_2$-adrenergic agonist, salmeterol xinafoate, in patients with chronic obstructive pulmonary disease. Am J Respir Crit Care Med 2001;163(5):1087–92.

7. D'Urzo AD, Chapman KR, Cartier A, Hargreave FE, Fitzgerald M, Tesarowski D. Effectiveness and safety of salmeterol in nonspecialist practice settings. Chest 2001;119(3):714–9.

8. Vervloet D, Ekstrom T, Pela R, Duce Gracia F, Kopp C, Silvert BD, Quebe-Fehling E, Della Cioppa G, Di Benedetto G. A 6-month comparison between formoterol and salmeterol in patients with reversible obstructive airways disease. Respir Med 1998;92(6):836–42.

9. Palmqvist M, Ibsen T, Mellen A, Lotvall J. Comparison of the relative efficacy of formoterol and salmeterol in asthmatic patients. Am J Respir Crit Care Med 1999;160(1):244–9.

10. Maconochie JG, Forster JK. Dose-response study with high-dose inhaled salmeterol in healthy subjects. Br J Clin Pharmacol 1992;33(3):342–5.

11. ZuWallack RL, Mahler DA, Reilly D, Church N, Emmett A, Rickard K, Knobil K. Salmeterol plus theophylline combination therapy in the treatment of COPD. Chest 2001;119(6):1661–70.

12. Tranfa CM, Pelaia G, Grembiale RD, Naty S, Durante S, Borrello G. Short-term cardiovascular effects of salmeterol. Chest 1998;113(5):1272–6.

13. Mann RD, Kubota K, Pearce G, Wilton L. Salmeterol: a study by prescription-event monitoring in a UK cohort of 15,407 patients. J Clin Epidemiol 1996;49(2):247–50.

14. Rosenthal RR, Busse WW, Kemp JP, Baker JW, Kalberg C, Emmett A, Rickard KA. Effect of long-term salmeterol therapy compared with as-needed albuterol use on airway hyperresponsiveness. Chest 1999;116(3):595–602.

15. Giannini D, Bacci E, Dente FL, Di Franco A, Vagaggini B, Testi R, Paggiaro P. Inhaled beclomethasone dipropionate reverts tolerance to the protective effect of salmeterol on allergen challenge. Chest 1999;115(3):629–34.

16. Aziz I, Lipworth BJ. A bolus of inhaled budesonide rapidly reverses airway subsensitivity and beta2-adrenoceptor down-regulation after regular inhaled formoterol. Chest 1999;115(3):623–8.

17. Aubier M, Pieters WR, Schlosser NJ, Steinmetz KO. Salmeterol/fluticasone propionate (50/500 microg) in combination in a Diskus inhaler (Seretide) is effective and safe in the treatment of steroid-dependent asthma. Respir Med 1999;93(12):876–84.

18. Chapman KR, Ringdal N, Backer V, Palmqvist M, Saarelainen S, Briggs M. Salmeterol and fluticasone propionate (50/250 microg) administered via combination Diskus inhaler: as effective as when given via separate Diskus inhalers. Can Respir J 1999;6(1):45–51.

19. Lipworth BJ, Aziz I. Bronchodilator response to albuterol after regular formoterol and effects of acute corticosteroid administration. Chest 2000;117(1):156–62.

20. van der Woude HJ, Winter TH, Aalbers R. Decreased bronchodilating effect of salbutamol in relieving methacholine induced moderate to severe bronchoconstriction during high dose treatment with long acting beta2 agonists. Thorax 2001;56(7):529–35.

Salsalate

General Information

Salsalate is a compound that contains two salicylate molecules joined by a diazo bond, which is hydrolysed after absorption, yielding two molecules of salicylate.

Organs and Systems

Mouth and teeth

Salicylates can cause ulceration in the mouth from local contact (1).

- A 77-year-old man developed three ulcerated lesions on his tongue because he had difficulty in swallowing salsalate tablets. He was taught how to swallow tablets and instructed to take them with water to avoid prolonged contact of salsalate with the tongue. Three weeks later, his lesions had healed and no new ones had appeared (2).

Gastrointestinal

There is some evidence that salsalate causes less gastric toxicity than aspirin, but salsalate can produce dyspepsia and occult bleeding when used therapeutically in effective doses. In an open study in 66 patients taking salsalate 3 g/day for 6 weeks, three patients were withdrawn because of gastrointestinal upsets; the most common adverse effect was dyspepsia (3).

References

1. Sapir S, Bimstein E. Cholinsalicylate gel induced oral lesion: report of case. J Clin Pediatr Dent 2000;24(2):103–6.
2. Ruscin JM, D'Astroth JD. Lingual lesions secondary to prolonged contact with salsalate tablets. Ann Pharmacother 1998;32(11):1248.
3. Regalado RG. The use of salsalate for control of long-term musculo-skeletal pain: an open, non-comparative assessment. Curr Med Res Opin 1978;5(6):454–60.

Saperconazole

See also Antifungal azoles

General Information

Saperconazole is an experimental, water-insoluble, lipophilic, fluorinated triazole. Its structure resembles that of itraconazole and it has a long half-life. It has a broad antifungal spectrum, including *Cryptococcus* Species and *Aspergillus* species. In early studies in cases of compassionate use, only a few adverse effects were described, including hepatotoxicity (1,2), and its adverse effects were expected to resemble those of itraconazole (3). However, the manufacturers stopped developing it because of concerns about toxicity.

References

1. Lin C, Kim H, Radwanski E, Affrime M, Brannan M, Cayen MN. Pharmacokinetics and metabolism of genaconazole, a potent antifungal drug, in men. Antimicrob Agents Chemother 1996;40(1):92–6.
2. Khoo SH, Denning DW. Cure of chronic invasive sinus aspergillosis with oral saperconazole. J Med Vet Mycol 1995;33(1):63–6.
3. Lyman CA, Walsh TJ. Systemically administered antifungal agents. A review of their clinical pharmacology and therapeutic applications. Drugs 1992;44(1):9–35.

Sapindaceae

See also Herbal medicines

General Information

The genera in the family of Sapindaceae (Table 1) include akee and lychee.

Blighia sapida

Blighia sapida (akee) contains a large amount of a potent hypoglycemic amino acid, glycylglycylglycine, known as hypoglycin.

Adverse effects

Akee poisoning (Jamaican winter vomiting sickness or toxic hypoglycemic syndrome) is a potentially fatal illness. During an outbreak in 1991, symptoms included vomiting (77%), coma (25%), and seizures (24%) (1). In 29 African children, all of whom died in 2–48 hours, there

Table 1 The genera of Sapindaceae

Alectryon (alectryon)
Allophylus (allophylus)
Blighia (akee)
Cardiospermum (balloon vine)
Cupania (cupania)
Cupaniopsis (carrot wood)
Dimocarpus (dimocarpus)
Dodonaea (dodonaea)
Exothea (exothea)
Harpullia (harpullia)
Hypelate (hypelate)
Koelreuteria (koelreuteria)
Litchi (lychee)
Matayba (matayba)
Melicoccus (melicoccus)
Nephelium (nephelium)
Paullinia (bread and cheese)
Sapindus (soapberry)
Schleichera (schleichera)
Serjania (serjania)
Thouinia (thouinia)
Ungnadia (ungnadia)
Urvillea (urvillea)
Xanthoceras (xanthoceras)

were intense thirst (38%) and hypotonia (97%) and the effects were more severe in those with malnutrition.

Chronic poisoning can cause cholestatic jaundice (2).

- A 27-year-old Jamaican man developed jaundice, pruritus, intermittent diarrhea, and right upper quadrant abdominal pain after chronic ingestion of akee fruit. Liver biopsy showed centrilobular zonal necrosis and cholestasis. There was no evidence of another cause.

An anaphylactic reaction to akee has been described (3).

Paullinia cupana

Paullinia cupana (*guaraná*) contains the xanthines theobromine and theophylline as well as flavone glycosides. The crushed seeds of *P. cupana* are made into a dried paste called guaraná, from which a beverage is prepared. All of its effects are directly related to its high content of caffeine-like substances.

Adverse effects

US authors have reported two cases of ventricular extra beats associated with the intake of supplements containing guaraná (4). In both cases the supplements also contained multiple other ingredients, and causality was therefore not certain.

References

1. Meda HA, Diallo B, Buchet JP, Lison D, Barennes H, Ouangre A, Sanou M, Cousens S, Tall F, Van de Perre P. Epidemic of fatal encephalopathy in preschool children in Burkina Faso and consumption of unripe ackee (*Blighia sapida*) fruit. Lancet 1999;353(9152):536–40.
2. Larson J, Vender R, Camuto P. Cholestatic jaundice due to ackee fruit poisoning. Am J Gastroenterol 1994;89(9):1577–8.
3. Lebo DB, Ditto AM, Boxer MB, Grammer LC, Bonagura VR, Roberts M. Anaphylaxis to ackee fruit. J Allergy Clin Immunol 1996;98(5 Pt 1):997–8.
4. Baghkhani L, Jafari M. Cardiovascular adverse reactions associated with guaraná: is there a causal effect? J Herb Pharmacother 2002;2(1):57–61.

Saquinavir

See also Protease inhibitors

General Information

Of all protease inhibitors, saquinavir is the most potent in vitro. However, owing to poor systemic availability (less than 4%), it is the least potent of all protease inhibitors in use, although a formulation with increased availability has been marketed. However, when saquinavir is given together with ritonavir, the strong inhibitory effect on CYP3A4 of the latter results in high plasma concentrations of saquinavir. This interaction has been exploited, with favorable results, both in first-line protease therapy and as salvage treatment in patients with virus resistant to a regimen containing a protease inhibitor. Using 400 mg/400 mg and 800 mg/ 200 mg, the saquinavir soft gelatin capsule AUC increased by 17–23 times compared with saquinavir alone (1). Saquinavir had no clinically significant effect on the pharmacokinetics of ritonavir. Ritonavir as a booster allows a much higher saquinavir concentration to be obtained, allowing twice-daily dosing and a reduced capsule burden.

General adverse effects

Hitherto, no particular or frequent adverse effects attributable to saquinavir have been reported from trials in which saquinavir was used at the licensed dosage of 600 mg tds (2). Diarrhea, usually of only moderate severity, occurring in 3–4% of patients, is the most common single adverse effect (SEDA-22, 310).

As with other HIV-1 protease inhibitors, saquinavir may be associated with drug interactions as a result of the effect of saquinavir on the hepatic cytochrome P450 oxidase system. Although compared with other HIV protease inhibitors, saquinavir has less of an inhibitory effect on cytochrome P450 isozymes; clinically relevant interactions can nevertheless occur. Drug interactions with saquinavir have been reviewed (3).

Organs and Systems

Psychological, psychiatric

Saquinavir can occasionally be associated with acute paranoid psychotic reactions (4).

- A 41-year-old woman took zidovudine and didanosine for HIV-1 infection after an acute seroconversion illness. Zidovudine and didanosine had to be withdrawn because of neutropenia and nausea, so she was given stavudine plus lamivudine without any adverse effects. Saquinavir (600 mg tds) was added 12 months later because of weight loss and a falling CD4 cell count. Within 24 hours of starting to take saquinavir she developed agitated depression with paranoid ideation. After drug withdrawal her mental health returned to normal over 5 days. Over the next 6 weeks stavudine and lamivudine were reintroduced without any adverse effects and continued for a further 11 months. Saquinavir was then reintroduced at the previous dosage, and within 2 days she again became extremely mentally agitated with paranoid ideation. Saquinavir was withdrawn and she recovered within 7 days. She was later given indinavir without problems. Her mother had a history of major depressive illness.

Endocrine

Gynecomastia has been reported in a series of men taking saquinavir (5). In these cases the association was clear (particularly since there was positive dechallenge), but this is a rare effect and has not previously been reported with either this or other protease inhibitors, although it has been associated with the nucleoside analogue reverse transcriptase inhibitor stavudine.

Gastrointestinal

Diarrhea, usually of only moderate severity, which occurs in 3–4% of patients, is the most common single adverse effect of saquinavir (6–8).

Urinary tract

A renal stone has been attributed to saquinavir (9).

- A 42-year-old HIV-positive man with a prior history of *Pneumocystis jiroveci* pneumonia who had been treated with zidovudine and dideoxycytidine started to take saquinavir 600 mg tds. His CD4 cell count rose from 28×10^3/l to 101×10^3/l and zidovudine and dideoxycytidine were replaced by stavudine and lamivudine, because of mild peripheral neuropathy. Saquinavir was continued unchanged. A few months later he developed left-sided loin pain and hematuria and a left renal calculus was seen on ultrasound. A month later the same signs and symptoms recurred and a few weeks later he passed a small black stone in the urine. Ultrasonic lithotripsy was performed, with a good result. Saquinavir was discontinued, after which he had no further renal problems.

This case suggests that saquinavir, like indinavir, may be associated with renal calculus formation in some individuals.

Skin

Adverse skin reactions to saquinavir are exceptional, but erythema multiforme has been reported (10).

- A 32-year-old HIV-positive man, who had been treated with didanosine and lamivudine, added saquinavir (600 mg tds) because of a rising plasma HIV-1 RNA viral load. Five days later he presented with a generalized maculopapular skin eruption, the lesions being centered on a bulla, and erosive lesions on the palate. Histological examination was compatible with erythema multiforme. Saquinavir was discontinued and all the mucocutaneous lesions healed within 15 days. Rechallenge was not attempted.

Long-Term Effects

Tumorigenicity

- Eruptive angiolipomata occurred in a 49-year-old woman after she had taken stavudine 30 mg bd, lamivudine 150 mg bd, and saquinavir 600 mg 8-hourly for 3 months (11). This has also been reported with other protease inhibitors (12,13) and the mechanism is not known. In one case lipomata regressed after the introduction of indinavir (14).

Drug Administration

Drug formulations

A soft gelatin capsule formulation of saquinavir with greater systemic availability than the hard gelatin capsule has been developed. Of 442 patients who used the soft gelatin capsule 1200 mg tds, for 48 weeks, 8% withdrew because of adverse events, which were not necessarily related to saquinavir. No new adverse effects or laboratory abnormalities emerged compared with those previously observed with the hard gelatin capsule. The most frequent adverse effects were gastrointestinal, diarrhea being the most common (15).

Drug–Drug Interactions

Ciclosporin

In an HIV-1-positive kidney transplant recipient, saquinavir increased the trough concentration of ciclosporin three-fold, resulting in fatigue, headache, and gastrointestinal discomfort. Ciclosporin, like saquinavir, is metabolized by CYP3A. Saquinavir plasma concentrations were likewise increased by ciclosporin. All the symptoms disappeared after downward adjustment of the doses of both ciclosporin and saquinavir (16).

Cytotoxic drugs

In 37 patients with HIV-associated non-Hodgkin's lymphoma who were treated with a 96-hour continuous intravenous infusion of cyclophosphamide + doxorubicin + etoposide, severe (grade 3 or 4) mucositis occurred in eight of 12 patients who received concomitant saquinavir (600 mg tds) compared with three of 25 who did not receive saquinavir. Although the authors did not measure saquinavir plasma concentrations, they suggested that this finding may have been explained by inhibition of the metabolism of one or more of the cytotoxic drugs by saquinavir (17).

Erythromycin

In 11 healthy men, erythromycin 250 mg qds increased the AUC of saquinavir (given as a soft gel capsule 1200 mg tds) by 69% when both were given for 7 days (18).

Ketoconazole

In 12 healthy men, ketoconazole 400 mg/day increased the AUC of saquinavir (given as a soft gel capsule 1200 mg tds) by 190% when both were given for 7 days (18).

Midazolam

Saquinavir substantially potentiates the effects of midazolam by raising its blood concentrations (19).

Rifamycins

In 14 healthy men, rifampicin 600 mg/day reduced the AUC of saquinavir (given as a soft gel capsule 1200 mg tds) by 46% when both were given for 14 days; this reduction can be counteracted by the addition of ritonavir (18).

References

1. Buss N, Snell P, Bock J, Hsu A, Jorga K. Saquinavir and ritonavir pharmacokinetics following combined ritonavir and saquinavir (soft gelatin capsules) administration. Br J Clin Pharmacol 2001;52(3):255–64.
2. Pollard RB. Use of proteinase inhibitors in clinical practice. Pharmacotherapy 1994;14(6 Pt 2):S21–9.
3. Vella S, Floridia M. Saquinavir. Clinical pharmacology and efficacy. Clin Pharmacokinet 1998;34(3):189–201.
4. Finlayson JA, Laing RB. Acute paranoid reaction to saquinavir. Am J Health Syst Pharm 1998;55(19):2016–17.
5. Donovan B, Bodsworth NJ, Mulhall BP, Allen D. Gynaecomastia associated with saquinavir therapy. Int J STD AIDS 1999;10(1):49–50.
6. Kitchen VS, Skinner C, Ariyoshi K, Lane EA, Duncan IB, Burckhardt J, Burger HU, Bragman K, Pinching AJ, Weber JN. Safety and activity of saquinavir in HIV infection. Lancet 1995;345(8955):952–5.
7. Collier AC, Coombs RW, Schoenfeld DA, Bassett RL, Timpone J, Baruch A, Jones M, Facey K, Whitacre C, McAuliffe VJ, Friedman HM, Merigan TC, Reichman RC, Hooper C, Corey L. Treatment of human immunodeficiency virus infection with saquinavir, zidovudine, and zalcitabine. AIDS Clinical Trials Group. N Engl J Med 1996;334(16):1011–17.
8. Noble S, Faulds D. Saquinavir. A review of its pharmacology and clinical potential in the management of HIV infection. Drugs 1996;52(1):93–112.
9. Green ST, McKendrick MW, Schmid ML, Mohsen AH, Prakasam SF. Renal calculi developing de novo in a patient taking saquinavir. Int J STD AIDS 1998;9(9):555.
10. Garat H, el Sayed F, Obadia M, Bazex J. Erythème polymorphe au saquinavir. [Erythema multiforme caused by saquinavir.] Ann Dermatol Venereol 1998;125(1):42–3.
11. Dauden E, Alvarez S, Garcia-Diez A. Eruptive angiolipomas associated with antiretroviral therapy. AIDS 2002;16(5):805–6.
12. Dank JP, Colven R. Protease inhibitor-associated angiolipomatosis. J Am Acad Dermatol 2000;42(1 Pt 1):129–31.
13. Bornhovd E, Sakrauski AK, Bruhl H, Walli R, Plewig G, Rocken M. Multiple circumscribed subcutaneous lipomas associated with use of human immunodeficiency virus protease inhibitors? Br J Dermatol 2000;143(5):1113–14.
14. Bates D. Valacyclovir neurotoxicity: two case reports and a review of the literature. Can J Hosp Pharm 2002;55:123–7.
15. Gill MJ. Safety profile of soft gelatin formulation of saquinavir in combination with nucleosides in a broad patient population. NV15182 Study Team. AIDS 1998;12(11):1400–2.
16. Brinkman K, Huysmans F, Burger DM. Pharmacokinetic interaction between saquinavir and cyclosporine. Ann Intern Med 1998;129(11):914–15.
17. Sparano JA, Wiernik PH, Hu X, Sarta C, Henry DH, Ratech H. Saquinavir enhances the mucosal toxicity of infusional cyclophosphamide, doxorubicin, and etoposide in patients with HIV-associated non-Hodgkin's lymphoma. Med Oncol 1998;15(1):50–7.
18. Grub S, Bryson H, Goggin T, Ludin E, Jorga K. The interaction of saquinavir (soft gelatin capsule) with ketoconazole, erythromycin and rifampicin: comparison of the effect in healthy volunteers and in HIV-infected patients. Eur J Clin Pharmacol 2001;57(2):115–21.
19. Palkama VJ, Ahonen J, Neuvonen PJ, Olkkola KT. Effect of saquinavir on the pharmacokinetics and pharmacodynamics of oral and intravenous midazolam. Clin Pharmacol Ther 1999;66(1):33–9.

Satranidazole

General Information

Satranidazole is a highly active amebicidal agent with a slightly wider spectrum than metronidazole against micro-aerophilic and anaerobic bacteria; it is also effective against *Giardia* and *Trichomonas*. It is less toxic than metronidazole, nimorazole, secnidazole, and ornidazole. Gastrointestinal tolerability was good in early studies. Therapeutic doses did not cause an adverse interaction with alcohol (SEDA-12, 707) (1,2).

References

1. Edlind TD, Hang TL, Chakraborty PR. Activity of the anthelmintic benzimidazoles against *Giardia lamblia* in vitro. J Infect Dis 1990;162(6):1408–11.
2. Arya VP. Satranidazole. Drugs Future 1983;8:797.

Sclerosants

General Information

In sclerotherapy an irritant is introduced into varicose veins and esophageal varices, causing a local inflammatory reaction and obliteration of the veins concerned. Sclerosing agents include lauromacrogol 400, monoethanolamine oleate, sodium morrhuate, and sodium tetradecylsulfate.

Lauromacrogol 400 (polidocanol)

Lauromacrogol 400 is a solvent and non-ionic emulsifier. In medicaments it is used as topical anesthetic, an antipruritic, and a sclerosing agent (1).

Monoethanolamine oleate

Monoethanolamine oleate is an alkaline viscous liquid that is irritant and is used as a sclerosant.

Sodium morrhuate

Sodium morrhuate is a fatty acid extract of cod liver oil; its sclerosant effect was discovered with the use of the agent in treating leprosy (2). Sodium morrhuate is cytotoxic, as demonstrated by autopsy studies in 10 patients (3).

Sodium tetradecylsulfate

Sodium tetradecylsulfate is an anionic surfactant used as a sclerosant.

Treatment of esophageal varices

Bleeding esophageal varices are treated by inserting a needle-tipped catheter through an endoscope to the site of the varices, and injecting a sclerosing agent directly into the bleeding varix. The common mechanism of action of all sclerosing agents is destruction of endothelial surfaces, with subsequent thrombosis, leading to intimal fibrosis and obliteration of the vessel lumen (4).

Adverse effects occur in 10–15% of patients. These include severe local edema and necrosis at the site of sclerosis (5), bacterial peritonitis (6), and pneumococcal bacteremia (7). Fever, chest pain, and odynophagia are common after esophageal sclerotherapy, but they tend to be of short duration (8).

In one review (9) complications of endoscopic variceal sclerotherapy were studied retrospectively in 267 patients who had been treated with endoscopic variceal injection for esophageal variceal hemorrhage in the period 1988–94. Local complications were: transient dysphagia (73%), chest pain (65%), esophageal ulceration (63%), ulcerogenic bleeding (14%), post-therapeutic hemorrhage (13%), esophageal strictures (10%), pleural effusions (9%), subfebrile temperatures (6.4%), pericarditis (0.4%), and esophageal perforation (0.4%). No patient died from sclerotherapy-induced adverse effects.

Sclerotherapy has also been used in the extremities for treating varicose and telangiectatic leg veins (10,11). Telangiectatic matting can develop bluish areas due to post-treatment neovascularization, in which new blood vessels, less than 0.2 mm in diameter, appear distally to the treated site, most commonly on the thigh. The incidence of this has been reported to be between 5 and 35%. Resolution often occurs spontaneously over 3–12 months, although in some patients it may be permanent or require further sclerotherapy to which it can be resistant (12).

Organs and Systems

Cardiovascular

Vascular thrombosis due to sclerosants is due to direct damage to vascular endothelium and red cells, aggregation of platelets, and aggregation of granulocytes at the venous wall endothelium. Where sodium morrhuate is concerned, these effects probably derive from its surfactant properties and its high arachidonate content (13). Other sclerosant agents in current use (lauromacrogol 400, monoethanolamine oleate, and sodium tetradecylsulfate) cause effects similar to sodium morrhuate.

Cardiac arrest has been reported in a child who received lauromacrogol 400 to sclerose a symptomatic peripheral venous malformation (14).

- A 5-year-old child with Klippel–Trenaunay syndrome, a cutaneous capillary malformation in the right leg, and a venous malformation of the lateral and posterior aspects of the right thigh and buttock had an injection of 4 ml of 1% lauromacrogol 400 into the malformation in the leg after oral premedication with midazolam 5 mg and atropine 0.5 mg and anesthesia with thiopental 80 mg and vecuronium bromide 2 mg for tracheal intubation. Shortly after the injection the patient developed rapidly progressive sinus bradycardia with eventual asystolic cardiac arrest. Anesthesia was discontinued and cardiopulmonary resuscitation, with 100% oxygen, external cardiac message, and intravenous orciprenaline 0.05 mg, was successful.

Respiratory

Fever and pneumonia have been reported after the use of sodium morrhuate sclerosant solution (SEDA-14, 456).

Gastrointestinal

Following the use of sclerosants, such as monoethanolamine oleate 5%, to treat esophageal varices, patients commonly experience early dysphagia and retrosternal pain, as might be expected. More serious complications can arise later if the fibrosis that is a natural consequence of the treatment extends too far, or if the sclerosant escapes from the veins that are being treated. Complications can include fibrosis (leading, for example, to esophageal stricture) as well as perforation, sepsis, and respiratory problems. Mediastinal pain can be precipitated by excessively deep or large injections. Mesenteric thrombosis has been claimed to occur as a complication and would not be unexpected; chylothorax and cerebral embolism have also been described.

Immunologic

Contact allergic reactions to lauromacrogol 400 have been reported (15). Patch testing with lauromacrogol 400 may yield irritant reactions. In a retrospective study of 8739 patients tested with a topical drug patch test series, 3186 patients were tested with 0.5% lauromacrogol 400 in water (16). There was slight irritation in 0.88%, weakly positive reactions in 0.97%, and strongly positive reactions in 0.25%. In 6202 patients tested with lauromacrogol 400 3% in petrolatum, there was slight skin irritation in 0.48%, weakly positive reactions in 1.77%, and strongly positive reactions in 0.34%. Among the 649 patients tested with both formulations, concurrence was moderate.

Long-Term Effects

Tumorigenicity

A number of case reports have suggested that sclerosant therapy could be carcinogenic (SEDA-15, 401).

References

1. Feied CF, Jackson JJ, Bren TS, Bond OB, Fernando CE, Young VC, Hashemiyoon RB. Allergic reactions to polidocanol for vein sclerosis. Two case reports. J Dermatol Surg Oncol 1994;20(7):466–8.
2. Rogers L. Intravenous sclerosing solutions. BMJ 1930;1:59.
3. Hammerschmidt DE, Craddock PR, McCullough F, Kronenberg RS, Dalmasso AP, Jacob HS. Complement activation and pulmonary leukotasis during nylon fiber filtration leukapheresis. Blood 1978;51(4):721–30.
4. Yamaki T, Nozaki M, Sasaki K. Color duplex-guided sclerotherapy for the treatment of venous malformations. Dermatol Surg 2000;26(4):323–8.
5. Chait S, Adler OB, Rosenberger A. Intramural dissection of the oesophagus after sclerotherapy. Value of CT. Rofo 1990;152(1):107–8.
6. Tam F, Chow H, Prindiville T, Cornish D, Haulk T, Trudeau W, Hoeprich P. Bacterial peritonitis following esophageal injection sclerotherapy for variceal hemorrhage. Gastrointest Endosc 1990;36(2):131–3.
7. Low DE, Shoenut JP, Kennedy JK, Harding GK, Den Boer B, Micflikier AB. Infectious complications of endoscopic injection sclerotherapy. Arch Intern Med 1986;146(3):569–71.
8. Zeller FA, Cannan CR, Prakash UB. Thoracic manifestations after esophageal variceal sclerotherapy. Mayo Clin Proc 1991;66(7):727–32.
9. Jaspersen D, Schwacha H, Sauer B, Wzatek J, Schorr W, Graf zu Dohna P, Hammar CH. Komplikationen der endoskopischen Sklerotherapie von Ösophagusvarizen. [Complications of endoscopic sclerotherapy of esophageal varices.] Leber Magen Darm 1995;25(4):171–4.
10. Davis LT, Duffy DM. Determination of incidence and risk factors for postsclerotherapy telangiectatic matting of the lower extremity: a retrospective analysis. J Dermatol Surg Oncol 1990;16(4):327–30.
11. Weiss RA, Weiss MA. Resolution of pain associated with varicose and telangiectatic leg veins after compression sclerotherapy. J Dermatol Surg Oncol 1990;16(4):333–6.
12. Duffy DM. Small vessel sclerotherapy: an overview. Adv Dermatol 1988;3:221–42.
13. Stroncek DF, Hutton SW, Silvis SE, Vercellotti GM, Jacob HS, Hammerschmidt DE. Sodium morrhuate stimulates granulocytes and damages erythrocytes and endothelial cells: probable mechanism of an adverse reaction during sclerotherapy. J Lab Clin Med 1985;106(5):498–504.
14. Marrocco-Trischitta MM, Guerrini P, Abeni D, Stillo F. Reversible cardiac arrest after polidocanol sclerotherapy of peripheral venous malformation. Dermatol Surg 2002;28(2):153–5.
15. Frosch PJ, Schulze-Dirks A. Kontaktallergie durch Polidocanol (Thesis). [Contact allergy caused by polidocanol (thesis).] Hautarzt 1989;40(3):146–9.
16. Uter W, Geier J, Fuchs T; IVDK Study Group. Contact allergy to polidocanol, 1992 to 1999. J Allergy Clin Immunol 2000;106(6):1203–4.

Secnidazole

General Information

Secnidazole is more active and gives more prolonged blood concentrations than metronidazole; it is effective in hepatic amebiasis. Gastrointestinal adverse effects are less common (SEDA-11, 597) (1).

Reference

1. Andre LJ. Traitement de l'amibiase par le secnidazole. Ann Gastroenterol Hepatol 1979;15:221.

Secretin

General Information

Secretin is a peptide hormone that stimulates pancreatic secretion. It has been used to treat autism, without success (1–3).

Synthetic porcine secretin and biologically derived porcine secretin have been compared in a double-blind, randomized, crossover study in 12 volunteers (4). The two formulations had identical effects and were safe and well tolerated. One subject reported transient mild flushing with both formulations. Otherwise, physical examination, clinical laboratory assessments, and electrocardiograms were normal.

In 10 healthy volunteers secretin suppressed peptone-stimulated gastric acid secretion and serum gastrin and inhibited acid output (5). There was a significant correlation between percentage inhibition of acid secretion and plasma secretin concentrations, which were greatly above those seen physiologically. Serum lipase and trypsin activities increased significantly. Most of the subjects lost fluid from diuresis and diarrhea, and serum sodium and total protein concentrations increased significantly.

Organs and Systems

Mineral balance

In seven healthy controls, seven patients with duodenal ulcer, seven with primary hyperparathyroidism, and one with an excluded gastric antrum, intravenous secretin 3 U/kg/hour for 90 minutes increased total protein and the protein-bound calcium fraction but did not alter the ionized calcium fraction (6).

References

1. Sandler AD, Sutton KA, DeWeese J, Girardi MA, Sheppard V, Bodfish JW. Lack of benefit of a single dose of synthetic human secretin in the treatment of autism and pervasive developmental disorder. N Engl J Med 1999;341(24):1801–6.
2. Carey T, Ratliff-Schaub K, Funk J, Weinle C, Myers M, Jenks J. Double-blind placebo-controlled trial of secretin: effects on aberrant behavior in children with autism. J Autism Dev Disord 2002;32(3):161–7.
3. Coplan J, Souders MC, Mulberg AE, Belchic JK, Wray J, Jawad AF, Gallagher PR, Mitchell R, Gerdes M, Levy SE. Children with autistic spectrum disorders. II: parents are unable to distinguish secretin from placebo under double-blind conditions. Arch Dis Child 2003;88(8):737–9.
4. Jowell PS, Robuck-Mangum G, Mergener K, Branch MS, Purich ED, Fein SH. A double-blind, randomized, dose response study testing the pharmacological efficacy of synthetic porcine secretin. Aliment Pharmacol Ther 2000;14(12):1679–84.
5. Londong W, Londong V, Hanssen LE, Schwanner A. Gastric effects and side effects of synthetic secretin in man. Regul Pept 1981;2(4):231–44.
6. Schwille PO, Scholz D, Samberger NM, Kayser PE. Studies on the calcemic effect of intravenous secretin in humans. Acta Hepatogastroenterol (Stuttg) 1975;22(3):192–200.

Selaginellaceae

See also Herbal medicines

General Information

The family of Selaginellaceae contains the single genus *Selaginella*.

Selaginella doederleinii

Selaginella doederleinii (spike moss) has been used as an alternative anticancer treatment.

Adverse effects

- A 52-year-old woman with cholangiocarcinoma developed severe bone marrow suppression after taking *S. doederleinii* daily for 2 weeks (1). She developed severe pancytopenia with skin ecchymoses and gum bleeding. A bone marrow smear and biopsy showed severe hypocellularity without malignant cell infiltration. One week after withdrawal her blood count became normal.

Reference

1. Pan KY, Lin JL, Chen JS. Severe reversible bone marrow suppression induced by *Selaginella doederleinii*. J Toxicol Clin Toxicol 2001;39(6):637–9.

Selective serotonin re-uptake inhibitors (SSRIs)

See also Individual agents

General Information

The selective serotonin re-uptake inhibitors (SSRIs) that are currently available are fluoxetine, fluvoxamine, paroxetine, sertraline, citalopram, and escitalopram. They are widely marketed and are in many countries a major alternative to tricyclic antidepressants in the treatment of depression. The SSRIs are structurally diverse, but they are all inhibitors of serotonin uptake, with much less effect on noradrenaline. They have slight or no inhibitory effect on histaminergic, adrenergic, serotonergic, dopaminergic, and cholinergic receptors (1).

The SSRIs are eliminated mainly through hepatic metabolism. Their half-lives are about 1 day for fluvoxamine, paroxetine, and sertraline (2–5), 1.5 days for citalopram (6), and 2–3 days for fluoxetine (7). Norfluoxetine, the main metabolite of fluoxetine, is a potent and selective serotonin re-uptake inhibitor, and since this metabolite also has a very long half-life (7–15 days) it contributes significantly to the clinical effect. Norsertraline, the desmethylated metabolite of sertraline, is also an inhibitor of serotonin re-uptake, but with much lower potency than sertraline; although its half-life is about 2.5 times longer than that of sertraline, it is not considered to contribute to the clinical effect (3). The main metabolite of citalopram, desmethylcitalopram, is pharmacologically active but has much lower potency than the parent compound (1). The metabolites of fluvoxamine and paroxetine are inactive with respect to monoamine uptake (2). Escitalopram oxalate is the S-enantiomer of citalopram (8). The therapeutic activity of citalopram resides in the S-isomer and escitalopram binds with high affinity to the human serotonin transporter; R-citalopram is about 30-fold less potent. The half-life of escitalopram is 27–32 hours. Escitalopram and citalopram have negligible effects on CYP isozymes.

The major advantages of SSRIs over the tricyclic antidepressants are their less pronounced anticholinergic adverse effects and lack of severe cardiotoxicity. However, some studies have shown some degree of nervousness or agitation, sleep disturbances, gastrointestinal symptoms, and perhaps sexual adverse effects more commonly in patients treated with SSRIs than in those treated with tricyclic antidepressants. SSRIs may also be associated with an increased risk of suicide, particularly in children under 16 (9).

There seems to be little difference between SSRIs with respect to frequency and severity of adverse effects. The most common adverse effects are gastrointestinal disturbances (nausea, diarrhea/loose stools, constipation; incidence 6–37%), nervous system effects (insomnia, somnolence, tremor, dizziness and headache; 11–26%), and effects on the autonomic nervous system (dryness of the mouth and sweating; 9–30%) (2,10). Weight gain or weight loss have been documented relatively infrequently (2). A high frequency of sexual disturbances has been reported. SSRIs may selectively inhibit hepatic enzymes, causing pharmacokinetic interactions with other drugs that are metabolized by these enzymes; a pharmacodynamic interaction can also occur when SSRIs are given in combination with other serotonergic drugs, which may give rise to serotonergic hyperstimulation, the "serotonin syndrome." The SSRIs are safer than the tricyclic antidepressants in overdose.

A meta-analysis of 20 short-term studies of five SSRIs (citalopram, fluoxetine, fluvoxamine, paroxetine, and sertraline) has been published (11). There were no overall differences in efficacy, but fluoxetine had a slower onset of action. Analysis of tolerability showed the expected adverse effects profile, the most common adverse event being nausea, followed by headache, dizziness, and tremor. The rate of withdrawal from treatment because of adverse effects was significantly greater with fluvoxamine (RR = 1.9; CI = 1.2, 3.0). Data available from the UK Committee on Safety of Medicines suggested that withdrawal reactions were most common with paroxetine and least common with fluoxetine (presumably because of the long half-life of its active metabolite norfluoxetine). There were more gastrointestinal reactions to fluvoxamine and paroxetine. This pattern was reflected in prescription-event monitoring data. Citalopram and sertraline were least likely to cause drug interactions, but citalopram was implicated more often in fatal overdoses.

Organs and Systems

Nervous system

Movement disorders

Extrapyramidal symptoms (including akathisia, dystonia, dyskinesia, tardive dyskinesia, parkinsonism, and bruxism) have been reported in association with SSRIs, especially in the presence of predisposing factors (SEDA-14, 14) (12). Current data suggest that SSRIs should be used with caution in patients with parkinsonism (see the monograph on fluoxetine). Concomitant treatment with neuroleptic drugs and high concentrations of SSRIs seems to predispose to extrapyramidal symptoms. Elderly patients and women are also at increased risk.

It is believed that SSRIs produce movement disorders by facilitating inhibitory serotonin interactions with dopamine pathways. While all SSRIs are potent inhibitors of serotonin re-uptake, they have other pharmacological actions that might contribute to their clinical profile. Sertraline has an appreciable affinity for the dopamine re-uptake site, and for this reason might be presumed less likely to cause movement disorders than other SSRIs. However, there is little clinical evidence to support this suggestion and a case of sertraline-induced parkinsonism has been reported (13).

SSRI-induced movement disorders have been comprehensively reviewed (14). The use of SSRIs was associated with a range of movement disorders, the most frequent of which was akathisia. However, clinician-based reports of adverse events solicited from SSRI manufacturers suggested that parkinsonism might occur with an equal frequency but with a later onset during treatment. As suggested before (SEDA-22, 12), concomitant treatment with antipsychotic drugs and lithium, as well as pre-existing brain damage, predisposes to the development of movement disorders with SSRIs. Case reports have suggested that akathisia can be associated with suicidal impulses.

Spontaneous reports received by the Netherlands Pharmacovigilance Foundation between 1985 and 1999 have been analysed in a case-control study (15). Relative to other antidepressants, SSRIs were about twice as likely to be implicated in spontaneous reports of extrapyramidal reactions (OR = 2.2; 95% CI = 1.2, 3.9). The risk was greater in patients who were also taking neuroleptic drugs. This result suggests that SSRIs have a modestly increased risk of producing extrapyramidal reactions compared with other antidepressants. However, increased reporting can be influenced by increased awareness. In addition, no account was apparently taken in this study of relative prescription rates of different antidepressants.

Withdrawal of SSRIs usually results in remission of symptoms of extrapyramidal movement disorders. However, occasionally, SSRIs can unmask a vulnerability to Parkinson's disease, and can also worsen established Parkinson's disease (SEDA-22, 23) (see monographs on citalopram and sertraline) (16).

Serotonin syndrome

The serotonin syndrome is a well-established complication of SSRI treatment. It is usually associated with high doses of SSRIs or the use of SSRIs in combination with other serotonin-potentiating agents, such as monoamine oxidase inhibitors (SEDA-22, 24).

- A 45-year-old man had definite symptoms of serotonin toxicity (hypomania, myoclonus, sweating, and shivering), first when taking a low therapeutic dose of citalopram (20 mg/day) and then with low-dose sertraline (25 mg/day); he was also taking zolpidem (17).

The authors speculated that the combination of zolpidem with an SSRI might have predisposed to the serotonin syndrome. It is also possible that some people (for example poor metabolizers) are idiosyncratically vulnerable to serotonin toxicity at low doses of SSRIs.

Sleep

SSRIs can cause insomnia and daytime somnolence; however, the symptoms seem to reflect a sleep–wake cycle disorder. It is conceivable that disruptions in the normal pattern of melatonin secretion, particularly a delay in the normal early morning fall in plasma concentrations could be involved in the pathophysiology of these symptoms. The fact that fluvoxamine is the SSRI that is most likely to cause sleep disorders supports a role of melatonin, which is increased by fluvoxamine but not by other SSRIs (18).

Sensory systems

Tricyclic antidepressants can precipitate acute glaucoma through their anticholinergic effects. There are also reports that SSRIs can cause acute glaucoma, presumably by pupillary dilatation (see the monograph on paroxetine and fluoxetine).

Psychological, psychiatric

Like other antidepressants, SSRIs are occasionally associated with manic episodes, even in patients with no history of bipolar disorder. Some argue that the affected patients may have had an underlying predisposition to bipolar illness.

In a retrospective chart review of 167 patients with a variety of anxiety disorders, excluding patients with evidence of current or previous mood disorder, manic episodes were recorded in five patients, a rate of 3% (19). While this might suggest a clear effect of SSRIs to induce mania, two of the patients were taking clomipramine, a tricyclic antidepressant, albeit a potent serotonin re-uptake inhibitor. In addition, all the affected patients had additional diagnoses of histrionic or borderline personality disorder, known to be associated with mood instability. It is still therefore plausible that SSRIs cause mania only in patients with an underlying predisposition, although this may be more subtle than a personal or family history of bipolar illness.

Visual hallucinations are rare during antidepressant drug treatment, except after overdosage.

- A 38-year-old man with a history of chronic depression developed on waking visual hallucinations of different geometric shapes after treatment with both sertraline and fluoxetine. Eventually he responded to treatment

with nefazodone, which did not cause hallucinations (20).

Many drugs that cause visual hallucinations (for example lysergic acid diethylamide) have agonist activity at $5\text{-}HT_2$ receptors, and it is conceivable that in these patients both sertraline and fluoxetine caused sufficient activation of post-synaptic $5\text{-}HT_2$ receptors to produce this visual disturbance. Although nefazodone can increase 5-HT neurotransmission, it is also a $5\text{-}HT_2$-receptor antagonist, so presumably does not activate $5\text{-}HT_2$ receptors.

Endocrine

Serotonin pathways are involved in the regulation of prolactin secretion. Amenorrhea, galactorrhea, and hyperprolactinemia have been reported in patients taking SSRIs (see the monographs on fluoxetine, fluvoxamine, paroxetine, and sertraline).

Electrolyte balance

SSRIs can reportedly cause hyponatremia (SEDA-18, 20) (SEDA-26, 13). In a case-control study of hyponatremia in 39 071 psychiatric inpatients and outpatients, the incidence of antidepressant-induced hyponatremia was 2.1% (21). SSRI users had a three times higher risk of developing hyponatremia relative to users of other antidepressant drugs (OR = 3.1; 95% CI = 1.3, 8.6). Additional risk factors included older age and concomitant treatment with diuretics.

SSRIs can cause hyponatremia in elderly patients (SEDA-18, 20, 21).

- A 45-year-old woman developed hyponatremia complicated by rhabdomyolysis while taking citalopram and the antipsychotic drug chlorprothixene for depressive psychosis (22). The hyponatremia became apparent 2 weeks after the dose of citalopram was increased to 40 mg/day, when she complained of weakness and lethargy.

SSRI-induced hyponatremia is unusual in non-geriatric populations, but the chlorprothixene may have played a role in this case.

There have been other reports of hyponatremia with SSRIs (23,24). Hyponatremia is probably more common with SSRIs than with tricyclic antidepressants and predominantly but not exclusively affects older patients. Most reports involve fluoxetine, but this might represent greater patient exposure. All SSRIs and venlafaxine can produce this adverse effect (SEDA-23, 21) (SEDA-25, 14). According to published reports, the median time to the onset of hyponatremia is 13 days (range 3–120) and the presentation is of inappropriate secretion of antidiuretic hormone (23). Symptoms, such as lethargy and confusion, can be non-specific, so awareness of the possibility of SSRI-induced hyponatremia, particularly in elderly people, is needed.

Fluid balance

The syndrome of inappropriate secretion of antidiuretic hormone (SIADH) is a possible adverse effect of the SSRIs (SEDA-14, 14) (SEDA-18, 20) (SEDA 21, 11) (25). The mechanism is not known. Several of the affected patients have been elderly, and old people may be at greater risk.

Hematologic

SSRIs have in rare cases been reported to produce bruising, bleeding, prolonged bleeding time, increased prothrombin time, and other hematological disturbances (SEDA-24, 15) (see the monographs on fluoxetine, fluvoxamine, paroxetine, and sertraline). The suggested mechanism of these adverse effects is reduced granular storage of serotonin in platelets, leading to disturbances of platelet function, especially in predisposed patients with mild underlying platelet disorders (26,27). An alternative mechanism is increased capillary fragility. Some patients appear to have a pre-existing susceptibility, for example, by virtue of treatment with other medications that might predispose to bleeding.

Five children, aged 8–15 years, developed bruising or epistaxis 1–12 weeks after starting SSRI treatment (28). In all cases the bleeding problem resolved when the SSRI was withdrawn or the dose lowered. In a review of 30 cases of SSRI-induced bleeding disorders the most common events were bruising, petechiae, purpura, and epistaxis, though gastrointestinal hemorrhage was also reported (29). The mean age of the affected patients was 42 years and the female:male ratio was 3:4. Symptoms were sometimes associated with prolonged bleeding time or platelet aggregation disorders, but often these indices were normal.

Gastrointestinal

Gastrointestinal adverse effects are one of the major disadvantages of SSRIs. The most common is nausea, and the incidence is said to be 20% or more for paroxetine (30,31), sertraline (32), fluvoxamine (5), fluoxetine (33), and citalopram (10,34). Although nausea can lead to drug withdrawal, it usually disappears after a few weeks. Other gastrointestinal symptoms that occur commonly with fluoxetine and sertraline are loose stools and diarrhea (32,33,35), while constipation has been more often reported with fluvoxamine (5) and paroxetine (30,31).

In a case-control study, current exposure to SSRIs was associated with an increased risk of upper gastrointestinal bleeding (RR = 3.0; CI = 2.1, 4.4) (36). The risk was substantially greater in subjects taking both SSRIs and non-steroidal anti-inflammatory drugs (NSAIDs) (RR = 16; CI = 6.6, 37). However, there was also an increased risk of bleeding with trazodone (RR = 8.6; CI = 2.1, 35), which does not block the uptake of 5-HT in therapeutic doses. Thus, the association between certain kinds of antidepressant drugs and upper gastrointestinal bleeding appears to be real.

Liver

SSRIs are rarely hepatotoxic and have only occasionally been reported (see the monographs on fluoxetine, paroxetine, and sertraline).

Skin

Skin reactions to SSRIs have been reported (SEDA-17, 20) (SEDA-18, 20), including Stevens–Johnson syndrome

(37), and rash due to fluoxetine occurs in a few percent of patients (38) (see also the monographs on fluoxetine, fluvoxamine, and sertraline).

Sexual function

Impaired sexual function

The adverse sexual effects of SSRIs have been reviewed (39). The use of SSRIs is most often associated with delayed ejaculation and absent or delayed orgasm, but reduced desire and arousal have also been reported. Estimates of the prevalence of sexual dysfunction with SSRIs vary from a small percentage to over 80%. Prospective studies that enquire specifically about sexual function have reported the highest figures. Similar sexual disturbances are seen in patients taking SSRIs for the treatment of anxiety disorders (40), showing that SSRI-induced sexual dysfunction is not limited to patients with depression. It is not clear whether the relative incidence of sexual dysfunction differs between the SSRIs, but it is possible that paroxetine carries the highest risk (39).

The ability of SSRIs to cause delayed ejaculation has been used in controlled trials of men with premature ejaculation (41,42). Of the SSRIs, paroxetine and sertraline produced the most benefit in terms of increase in time to ejaculation, but fluvoxamine did not differ from placebo. Clomipramine was more effective than the SSRIs but caused most adverse effects. From a practical point of view many patients might prefer to take medication for sexual dysfunction when needed rather than on a regular daily basis, and it would be of interest to study the beneficial effects of SSRIs on premature ejaculation when used in this way.

Laboratory studies have shown that fluvoxamine differs from paroxetine, sertraline, and fluoxetine in not delaying the time to ejaculation. The effect of citalopram to delay ejaculation is also relatively modest (43). There are, however, many other ways in which SSRIs can interfere with sexual function, for example by causing loss of sexual interest and erectile difficulties. In an open, prospective study of 1000 Spanish patients taking a variety of antidepressants, there was an overall incidence of sexual dysfunction of 59% (44). The highest rates, 60–70%, were found with SSRIs (including fluvoxamine) and venlafaxine. The lowest rates were found with mirtazapine (24%), nefazodone (8%), and moclobemide (4%). Spontaneous resolution of this adverse effect was uncommon—80% of subjects had no improvement in sexual function over 6 months of treatment. This study suggests very high rates of sexual dysfunction in patients taking SSRIs and venlafaxine. However, in investigations of this nature, it can be difficult to tease out the effect of the drug from that of the underlying disorder. Nevertheless, while depressive symptoms should improve in most patients over 6 months of treatment, the sexual dysfunction in these subjects tended not to remit, suggesting that the antidepressant was the main culprit.

Increased sexual function

Occasionally, SSRIs are associated with increased sexual desire and behavior.

- A 27-year-old married woman with a borderline personality disorder was admitted to hospital with depression and suicidal ideation (45). Over 3 weeks she was given fluvoxamine in doses up to 150 mg/day, but because of lack of response the dosage was increased to 200 mg/day; 3 days later she reported that her sex drive was greater than it had ever been before and that she felt she could not control it. There was no evidence of mania. Within a week of withdrawal of fluvoxamine her sexual desire had returned to its previous level.

Patients with borderline personality disorder may behave in a sexually disinhibited manner and have mood swings. In this patient, however, it did not appear as though the hypersexuality was part of a manic syndrome, and she was clear that the sexual feelings were unusually great for her. Support for a role of the SSRI in this adverse effect comes from a series of five patients (four taking citalopram and one paroxetine) who had an unusual increase in sexual interest, with preoccupation with sexual thoughts, promiscuity, and excessive interest in pornography (46). In some of the cases symptoms such as diminished need for sleep suggested the possibility of a manic syndrome.

These reports suggest that occasionally SSRIs can be associated with increased sexual desire and behavior. This might be associated with mood instability, for example in a manic or mixed affective state, but in some people personality factors are likely to be important.

Treatment of sexual dysfunction due to SSRIs

Various treatments have been advocated to ameliorate sexual dysfunction in SSRI-treated patients, including 5-HT$_2$-receptor antagonists (cyproheptadine, mianserin, nefazodone) and 5-HT$_3$-receptor antagonists such as granisetron (39). One of the most popular remedies is the use of dopaminergic agents, such as amfebutamone.

In a prospective study, 47 patients who complained of SSRI-induced sexual dysfunction took amfebutamone (bupropion) 75–150 mg 1–2 hours before sexual activity (47). If this was unsuccessful they were titrated to a dosage of 75 mg tds on a regular basis. Amfebutamone improved sexual function in 31 patients (66%). Anxiety and tremor were the most frequently reported adverse events, and seven patients discontinued for this reason. However, it should be noted that more serious adverse events (panic attacks, delirium, and seizures) have been reported when amfebutamone (bupropion) and SSRIs are combined (39).

In a placebo-controlled, parallel-group study of buspirone and amantadine in 57 patients with fluoxetine-induced sexual dysfunction, there was an overall improvement in all three treatment groups and no significant differences between them (48). These data suggest that anecdotal reports of treatment benefit in SSRI-induced sexual dysfunction should be regarded with caution.

Reproductive system

Vaginal bleeding and menorrhagia have been rarely reported with SSRI treatment and the mechanism is uncertain. SSRIs have been associated with bleeding diatheses, which might explain these observations (SEDA-24, 15) (SEDA-25, 14). Another possibility is an action of serotonin pathways on the neural

regulation of gonadotropin release. More cases have been reported.

- A 67-year-old woman developed vaginal bleeding after taking sertraline 25 mg/day for 3 days (49). The sertraline was withdrawn and the bleeding stopped 48 hours later.
- A 41-year-old woman developed vaginal bleeding after taking venlafaxine 75 mg/day, a dose at which selective serotonin blockade is the predominant pharmacological action (50). The vaginal bleeding stopped 24 hours after venlafaxine withdrawal and occurred again on rechallenge.

Immunologic

Infection risk: three cases of *Herpes simplex* reactivation associated with fluoxetine have been described (SEDA-16, 10).

Death

Severe adverse reactions to SSRIs that were reported to Health Canada's database in 1986–1996 have been reviewed (51). There were 295 severe adverse reactions with 87 deaths. Of the fatal cases, 65 were due to intentional overdose. The other 22 deaths were due chiefly to other forms of suicide or were accidental or indeterminate (12 cases). Of the rest there were three cases of neuroleptic malignant syndrome and individual cases of cardiac or respiratory disease in which the role of SSRIs was less clear.

This report shows that the major causes of death in patients taking SSRIs are related to the risks of depression itself, particularly self-harm. SSRIs themselves appear to be relatively safe. It is possible, however, that the cases of neuroleptic malignant syndrome could have been misdiagnosed forms of the serotonin syndrome, which, like the neuroleptic malignant syndrome, can present with hyperthermia and changes in consciousness and is usually produced by pharmacodynamic interactions between SSRIs and other serotonin-potentiating compounds (SEDA-25, 24). In general, the risks of SSRIs are increased by co-prescription, and fatal overdose with SSRIs usually involves a mixture of psychotropic drugs and/or alcohol.

Sudden death has been reported in three elderly women with pulmonary disease and atrial fibrillation who had recently started taking fluoxetine. The authors recommended caution in such patients, although no causal link with fluoxetine was established (SEDA-17, 19).

Long-Term Effects

Drug withdrawal

Reports of withdrawal reactions after abrupt withdrawal of SSRIs continue to accumulate, and several reviews have summarized case reports of withdrawal symptoms (52,53).

SSRIs with shorter half-lives, such as fluvoxamine and paroxetine (qv), have a higher incidence of withdrawal symptoms than long-acting ones, but withdrawal effects have been reported, albeit rarely, after withdrawal of fluoxetine (qv) (SEDA-20, 8) (54) and citalopram (55). Patients taking high doses, long-term treatment, or both are at increased risk of developing withdrawal symptoms (54,56).

In a randomized, placebo-controlled trial, sudden withdrawal of paroxetine produced significant withdrawal symptoms by as early as the second day, while patients taking fluoxetine remained asymptomatic for the five-day withdrawal period (57). Patients taking sertraline had an intermediate level of abstinence symptoms. Both paroxetine- and sertraline-treated patients reported impaired functioning during the withdrawal period, while those taking fluoxetine did not. These findings are consistent with earlier reports that suggested that acute withdrawal symptoms after fluoxetine withdrawal are unusual, presumably because of the long half-life of its active metabolite, norfluoxetine.

Second-Generation Effects

Teratogenicity

Tricyclic antidepressants appear to be generally free of teratogenic effects, but the status of newer antidepressants is unclear. Since 1993 four controlled prospective studies of antidepressant exposure during pregnancy have been published, involving about 400 women, most of whom took fluoxetine at various stages during pregnancy (58). There was no evidence that fluoxetine or other SSRIs caused an increase in intrauterine death, significant birth defects, or growth impairment. Follow-up behavioral studies of infants exposed to SSRIs during pregnancy also showed no difference from controls.

Fetotoxicity

An increasing number of women are being exposed to SSRIs during pregnancy. It is therefore important to establish as carefully as possible whether SSRIs have teratogenic effects (SEDA-24, 15). In a retrospective study of the impact on birth outcome of the timing of fluoxetine exposure in 64 pregnant women there were no major differences between infants exposed to fluoxetine early in pregnancy (the first or second trimesters only) and those exposed to fluoxetine throughout the third trimester and delivery (59). However, the infants in the late-exposed group were about twice as likely to be admitted to a special-care nursery. No specific pattern of neonatal difficulties could be found to account for this difference, and it is possible that the excess of neonatal problems in the late-onset treatment group was due to worse depression in the women who took antidepressants at around the time of delivery.

Withdrawal effects of SSRI treatment may be apparent in neonates shortly after delivery. These include jitteriness, hypoglycemia, hypothermia, and respiratory distress (60).

Lactation

The benefit : harm balance of breast-feeding during antidepressant treatment is difficult to compute and must be done on an individual basis. In general, breast-feeding with SSRIs is regarded as safe, as the amount of drug ingested by the infant is very low. However, adverse effects in the child are reported occasionally (SEDA-25, 15) and it is difficult to exclude completely the possibility of long-term effects on brain development in the infant. Clearly, the lower the concentration of SSRI in the infant the less likely are problems of acute and longer-term toxicity. In two cases treatment of breast-feeding mothers with fluvoxamine (300 mg/day) was associated with undetectable concentrations of fluvoxamine (below 2.5 ng/ml) in the plasma of both infants (61). These results are encouraging, but further data will be needed before it can be concluded that fluvoxamine has an advantage over other SSRIs in this respect. Because fluoxetine has a long half-life it may be advisable not to use it in breast-feeding women.

Drug Administration

Drug overdose

The SSRIs are in general considered to be less toxic in overdose than tricyclic antidepressants. From a review of cases of overdose with SSRI during 10 years it was concluded that SSRIs are rarely fatal in overdose when taken alone (62). In moderate overdoses of up to 30 times the daily dose, symptoms were either minor or absent. In higher doses, typical symptoms included drowsiness, tremor, nausea, and vomiting. At extremely high doses (over 75 times the usual daily dose), there were more serious toxic effects, including seizures, electrocardiographic changes, and disturbances of consciousness. When an SSRI overdose was taken in combination with alcohol or other drugs, toxicity increased, and almost all deaths involving SSRIs were in combination with other drugs.

Drug–Drug Interactions

General

For the SSRIs there are two types of interaction of major concern: SSRIs can selectively inhibit hepatic drug metabolizing enzymes, giving rise to pharmacokinetic interactions (SEDA-22, 13), and pharmacodynamic interactions can occur when SSRIs are given in combination with other serotonergic drugs, which can cause serotonergic hyperstimulation: the "serotonin syndrome." Fluoxetine gives rise to special concern, since reactions can occur weeks after withdrawal, owing to the long half-life of both parent compound and metabolite. Of the various SSRIs, citalopram seems the least likely to produce this effect. Paroxetine and fluoxetine can cause interactions with tricyclic antidepressants, neuroleptic drugs, and some antidysrhythmic drugs that are metabolized by CYP2D6.

In 31 healthy men and women (mean age 28 years) the ability of four SSRIs (fluoxetine, fluvoxamine, paroxetine, and sertraline) to inhibit CYP2D6 activity was assessed in vivo, as judged by the dextromethorphan test (63). All were extensive metabolizers of dextromethorphan. After 8 days treatment at therapeutic doses, four of eight paroxetine-treated and five of eight fluoxetine-treated subjects had become poor metabolizers, presumably because of the inhibitory effect of the two SSRIs on CYP2D6 activity. In contrast, none of the eight fluvoxamine-treated or seven sertraline-treated subjects showed this effect. This in vivo study has confirmed the potent inhibitory effect of fluoxetine and paroxetine on CYP2D6 and the relative sparing by fluvoxamine and sertraline. However, fluvoxamine is a potent inhibitor of CYP1A2 and CYP3A3/4 (SEDA-22, 13). In addition, at higher doses (over 100 mg/day at steady state) sertraline can inhibit CYP2D6.

The drugs that can cause a serotonin syndrome when they are combined with SSRIs include monoamine oxidase inhibitors (including reversible inhibitors of monoamine oxidase types A and B), dextromethorphan, tryptophan, lithium, pentazocine, and carbamazepine (SEDA-17, 23) (SEDA-18, 22) (64).

Buspirone

The serotonin syndrome can occur with therapeutic doses of SSRIs (see above), but it occurs most commonly when SSRIs are co-administered with other drugs that also potentiate serotonin function. Recent case reports have suggested that there is a risk of the serotonin syndrome when SSRIs are combined with buspirone (65).

Dextromethorphan

SSRIs inhibit hepatic CYP isozymes and can thereby increase the activity of co-administered drugs that are metabolized by this route (SEDA-22, 13) (SEDA-24, 15). In healthy volunteers randomly allocated to fluoxetine (20 mg/day), sertraline (100 mg/day), or paroxetine (20 mg/day) the activity of CYP2D6 was measured by dextromethorphan testing once steady state had been achieved and the medication was withdrawn (66). Extrapolated calculations showed that the mean time for full CYP2D6 recovery after fluoxetine (63 days) was significantly longer than that for sertraline (25 days) or paroxetine (20 days). Accordingly, even after SSRIs have been withdrawn, the potential for drug interactions persists for substantial periods of time, particularly in the case of fluoxetine.

Monoamine oxidase inhibitors

Monoamine oxidase inhibitors, including reversible inhibitors of monoamine oxidase types A and B, can cause a serotonin syndrome when they are combined with SSRIs (SEDA-17, 23) (SEDA-18, 22) (64).

Nefazodone

The serotonin syndrome can occur with therapeutic doses of SSRIs (see above), but it occurs most commonly when SSRIs are co-administered with other drugs that also potentiate serotonin function. Recent case reports have suggested that there is a risk of the serotonin syndrome when SSRIs are combined with nefazodone (67).

Neuroleptic drugs

Interactions of SSRIs with neuroleptic drugs have been reported (68–70).

Sibutramine

The serotonin syndrome has been attributed to a combination of citalopram and sibutramine.

- A 43-year-old woman who had taken citalopram 40 mg/day for 2 years was given sibutramine for obesity and a few hours after the first dose of 10 mg had irritability, racing thoughts, pressure of speech, agitation, shivering, and sweating (71). These symptoms persisted for 3 days, during which time she continued to take sibutramine. The day after sibutramine was withdrawn the symptoms resolved.

The serotonin syndrome can present with hypomanic features, and the clinical picture and rapid onset in this case suggested that the addition of sibutramine to citalopram provoked serotonin toxicity. Sibutramine blocks the re-uptake of serotonin, dopamine, and noradrenaline. Whether the serotonin toxicity seen here resulted purely from the combined effects of both citalopram and sibutramine in blocking serotonin re-uptake is unclear. It is possible, for example, that potentiation of dopamine and noradrenaline activity by sibutramine might also have been involved.

Tricyclic antidepressants

Interactions of SSRIs with tricyclic antidepressants have been reported. For example, plasma concentrations of tricyclic antidepressants rise after the addition of fluoxetine (72,73), fluvoxamine (74,75), and sertraline (76).

Triptans

Drugs used in the treatment of acute migraine, such as sumatriptan and rizatriptan, are 5-HT$_{1B/1D}$-receptor agonists and could theoretically interact pharmacodynamically with SSRIs to cause serotonin toxicity. Triptans are metabolized mainly by monoamine oxidase, which makes pharmacokinetic interactions with SSRIs unlikely. Although case series have suggested that sumatriptan can be safely combined with SSRIs (SEDA-22, 14), there are occasional reports of toxicity.

References

1. Hyttel J. Pharmacological characterization of selective serotonin reuptake inhibitors (SSRIs). Int Clin Psychopharmacol 1994;9(Suppl. 1):19–26.
2. Leonard BE. The comparative pharmacology of new antidepressants. J Clin Psychiatry 1993;54(Suppl.):3–15.
3. Doogan DP, Caillard V. Sertraline: a new antidepressant. J Clin Psychiatry 1988;49(Suppl.):46–51.
4. Kaye CM, Haddock RE, Langley PF, Mellows G, Tasker TC, Zussman BD, Greb WH. A review of the metabolism and pharmacokinetics of paroxetine in man. Acta Psychiatr Scand Suppl 1989;350:60–75.
5. Benfield P, Ward A. Fluvoxamine: a review of its pharmacodynamic and pharmacokinetic properties, and therapeutic efficacy in depressive illness. Drugs 1986;32(4):313–34.
6. Kragh-Sorensen P, Overo KF, Petersen OL, Jensen K, Parnas W. The kinetics of citalopram: single and multiple dose studies in man. Acta Pharmacol Toxicol (Copenh) 1981;48(1):53–60.

7. Bergstrom RF, Lemberger L, Farid NA, Wolen RL. Clinical pharmacology and pharmacokinetics of fluoxetine: a review. Br J Psychiatry Suppl 1988;3:47–50.

8. Burke WJ. Escitalopram. Expert Opin Investig Drugs 2002;11(10):1477–86.

9. Whittington CJ, Kendall T, Fonagy P, Cottrell D, Cotgrove A, Boddington E. Selective serotonin reuptake inhibitors in childhood depression: systematic review of published versus unpublished data. Lancet 2004;363(9418):1341–5.

10. Dencker SJ, Hopfner Petersen HE. Side effect profile of citalopram and reference antidepressants in depression. In: Montgomery SA, editor. Citalopram—The New Antidepressant from Lundbeck Research. Amsterdam: Excerpta Medica, 1989:31.

11. Edwards JG, Anderson I. Systematic review and guide to selection of selective serotonin reuptake inhibitors. Drugs 1999;57(4):507–33.

12. Gill HS, DeVane CL, Risch SC. Extrapyramidal symptoms associated with cyclic antidepressant treatment: a review of the literature and consolidating hypotheses. J Clin Psychopharmacol 1997;17(5):377–89.

13. Di Rocco A, Brannan T, Prikhojan A, Yahr MD. Sertraline induced parkinsonism: a case report and an in-vivo study of the effect of sertraline on dopamine metabolism. J Neural Transm 1998;105(2–3):247–51.

14. Gerber PE, Lynd LD, Leo RJ. Selective serotonin-reuptake inhibitor-induced movement disorders. Ann Pharmacother 1998;32(6):692–8.

15. Gray NA, Zhou R, Du J, Moore GJ, Manji HK. The use of mood stabilizers as plasticity enhancers in the treatment of neuropsychiatric disorders. J Clin Psychiatry 2003;64(Suppl. 5):3–17.

16. Stadtland C, Erfurth A, Arolt V. De novo onset of Parkinson's disease after antidepressant treatment with citalopram. Pharmacopsychiatry 2000;33(5):194–5.

17. Voirol P, Hodel PF, Zullino D, Baumann P. Serotonin syndrome after small doses of citalopram or sertraline. J Clin Psychopharmacol 2000;20(6):713–14.

18. Hartter S, Wang X, Weigmann H, Friedberg T, Arand M, Oesch F, Hiemke C. Differential effects of fluvoxamine other antidepressants on the biotransformation of melatonin. J Clin Psychopharmacol 2001;21(2):167–74.

19. Levy D, Kimhi R, Barak Y, Aviv A, Elizur A. Antidepressant-associated mania: a study of anxiety disorders patients. Psychopharmacology (Berl) 1998;136(3):243–6.

20. Bourgeois JA, Thomas D, Johansen T, Walker DM. Visual hallucinations associated with fluoxetine and sertraline. J Clin Psychopharmacol 1998;18(6):482–3.

21. Movig KLL, Leufkens HGM, Lenderink AW, van den Akker VGA, Hodiamont PPG, Goldschmidt HMJ, Egberts ACG. Association between antidepressant drug use and hyponatremia: a case–control study. Br J Clin Pharmacol 2002;53(4):363–9.

22. Zullino D, Brauchli S, Horvath A, Baumann P. Inappropriate antidiuretic hormone secretion and rhabdomyolysis associated with citalopram. Thérapie 2000;55(5):651–2.

23. Odeh M, Beny A, Oliven A. Severe symptomatic hyponatremia during citalopram therapy. Am J Med Sci 2001;321(2):159–60.

24. Movig KLL, Egberts ACG, Van den Akker VGA, Goldschmidt HMJ, Leufkens HGM, Lenderink AW. SSRIs are different than other antidepressant agents: a larger risk of hyponatremia. Pharm Weekbl 2001;136:461–3.

25. Staab JP, Yerkes SA, Cheney EM, Clayton AH. Transient SIADH associated with fluoxetine. Am J Psychiatry 1990;147(11):1569–70.

26. Skop BP, Brown TM. Potential vascular and bleeding complications of treatment with selective serotonin reuptake inhibitors. Psychosomatics 1996;37(1):12–16.

27. Pai VB, Kelly MW. Bruising associated with the use of fluoxetine. Ann Pharmacother 1996;30(7–8):786–8.

28. Lake MB, Birmaher B, Wassick S, Mathos K, Yelovich AK. Bleeding and selective serotonin reuptake inhibitors in childhood and adolescence. J Child Adolesc Psychopharmacol 2000;10(1):35–8.

29. Nelva A, Guy C, Tardy-Poncet B, Beyens MN, Ratrema M, Benedetti C, Ollagnier M. Syndromes hemorragiques sons antidepresseurs inhibiteurs selectifs de la recapture de la serotonine (ISRS). A propos de sept cas et revue de la literature. [Hemorrhagic syndromes related to selective serotonin reuptake inhibitor (SSRI) antidepressants Seven case reports and review of the literature.] Rev Méd Interne 2000;21(2):152–60.

30. Dunbar GC. An interim overview of the safety and tolerability of paroxetine. Acta Psychiatr Scand Suppl 1989;350:135–7.

31. Boyer WF, Blumhardt CL. The safety profile of paroxetine. J Clin Psychiatry 1992;53(Suppl.):61–6.

32. Murdoch D, McTavish D. Sertraline: a review of its pharmacodynamic and pharmacokinetic properties, and therapeutic potential in depression and obsessive-compulsive disorder. Drugs 1992;44(4):604–24.

33. Stokes PE. Fluoxetine: a five-year review. Clin Ther 1993;15(2):216–43.

34. Shaw DM, Crimmins R. A multicenter trial of citalopram and amitriptyline in major depressive illness. In: Montgomery SA, editor. Citalopram—The New Antidepressant from Lundbeck Research. Amsterdam: Excerpta Medica, 1989:43.

35. Nemeroff CB. Evolutionary trends in the pharmacotherapeutic management of depression. J Clin Psychiatry 1994;55(Suppl.):3–15.

36. de Abajo FJ, Rodriguez LA, Montero D. Association between selective serotonin reuptake inhibitors and upper gastrointestinal bleeding: population based case-control study. BMJ 1999;319(7217):1106–9.

37. Jan V, Toledano C, Machet L, Machet MC, Vaillant L, Lorette G. Stevens–Johnson syndrome after sertraline. Acta Dermatol Venereol 1999;79(5):401.

38. Cooper GL. The safety of fluoxetine—an update. Br J Psychiatry Suppl 1988;3:77–86.

39. Rosen RC, Lane RM, Menza M. Effects of SSRIs on sexual function: a critical review. J Clin Psychopharmacol 1999;19(1):67–85.

40. Labbate LA, Grimes JB, Arana GW. Serotonin reuptake antidepressant effects on sexual function in patients with anxiety disorders. Biol Psychiatry 1998;43(12):904–7.

41. Kim SC, Seo KK. Efficacy and safety of fluoxetine, sertraline and clomipramine in patients with premature ejaculation: a double-blind, placebo controlled study. J Urol 1998;159(2):425–7.

42. Waldinger MD, Hengeveld MW, Zwinderman AH, Olivier B. Effect of SSRI antidepressants on ejaculation: a double-blind, randomized, placebo-controlled study with fluoxetine, fluvoxamine, paroxetine, and sertraline. J Clin Psychopharmacol 1998;18(4):274–81.

43. Waldinger MD, Olivier B. Sexual dysfunction and fluvoxamine therapy. J Clin Psychiatry 2001;62(2):126–7.

44. Montejo AL, Llorca G, Izquierdo JA, Rico-Villademoros F. Incidence of sexual dysfunction associated with antidepressant agents: a prospective multicenter study of 1022 outpatients. Spanish Working Group for the Study of Psychotropic-Related Sexual Dysfunction. J Clin Psychiatry 2001;62(Suppl. 3):10–21.

45. Hori H, Yoshimura R, Nakamura J. Increased libido in a woman treated with fluvoxamine: a case report. Acta Psychiatr Scand 2001;103(4):312–14.

46. Greil W, Horvath A, Sassim N, Erazo N, Grohmann R. Disinhibition of libido: an adverse effect of SSRI? J Affect Disord 2001;62(3):225–8.

47. Ashton AK, Rosen RC. Bupropion as an antidote for serotonin reuptake inhibitor-induced sexual dysfunction. J Clin Psychiatry 1998;59(3):112–15.

48. Michelson D, Bancroft J, Targum S, Kim Y, Tepner R. Female sexual dysfunction associated with antidepressant administration: a randomized, placebo-controlled study of pharmacologic intervention. Am J Psychiatry 2000; 157(2):239–43.

49. Smith M, Robinson D. Sertraline and vaginal bleeding—a possible association. J Am Geriatr Soc 2002;50(1):200–1.

50. Linnebur SA, Saseen JJ, Pace WD. Venlafaxine-associated vaginal bleeding. Pharmacotherapy 2002;22(5):652–5.

51. Dalfen AK, Stewart DE. Who develops severe or fatal adverse drug reactions to selective serotonin reuptake inhibitors? Can J Psychiatry 2001;46(3):258–63.

52. Haddad P. Newer antidepressants and the discontinuation syndrome. J Clin Psychiatry 1997;58(Suppl. 7):17–21; discussion 22.

53. Coupland NJ, Bell CJ, Potokar JP. Serotonin reuptake inhibitor withdrawal. J Clin Psychopharmacol 1996;16(5):356–62.

54. Zajecka J, Tracy KA, Mitchell S. Discontinuation symptoms after treatment with serotonin reuptake inhibitors: a literature review. J Clin Psychiatry 1997;58(7):291–7.

55. Fernando AT 3rd, Schwader P. A case of citalopram withdrawal. J Clin Psychopharmacol 2000;20(5):581–2.

56. Lejoyeux M, Ades J. Antidepressant discontinuation: a review of the literature. J Clin Psychiatry 1997;58(Suppl. 7):11–5.

57. Michelson D, Fava M, Amsterdam J, Apter J, Londborg P, Tamura R, Tepner RG. Interruption of selective serotonin reuptake inhibitor treatment. Double-blind, placebo-controlled trial. Br J Psychiatry 2000;176:363–8.

58. Wisner KL, Gelenberg AJ, Leonard H, Zarin D, Frank E. Pharmacologic treatment of depression during pregnancy. JAMA 1999;282(13):1264–9.

59. Cohen LS, Heller VL, Bailey JW, Grush L, Ablon JS, Bouffard SM. Birth outcomes following prenatal exposure to fluoxetine. Biol Psychiatry 2000;48(10):996–1000.

60. Gerola O, Fiocchi S, Rondini G. Rischi da farmaci antidepressivi in gravidanza: revisione della letteratura e presentazione di un caso di sospetta sindrome da astinenza da paroxetina in neonato. [Risk of antidepressant drugs in pregnancy: review of the literature and presentation of a case of suspected sevotonin syndrome caused by abstinence of paroxetine in neonate.] Riv Ital Pediatr 1999;25:216–18.

61. Piontek CM, Wisner KL, Perel JM, Peindl KS. Serum fluvoxamine levels in breastfed infants. J Clin Psychiatry 2001;62(2):111–13.

62. Barbey JT, Roose SP. SSRI safety in overdose. J Clin Psychiatry 1998;59(Suppl. 15):42–8.

63. Alfaro CL, Lam YW, Simpson J, Ereshefsky L. CYP2D6 status of extensive metabolizers after multiple-dose fluoxetine, fluvoxamine, paroxetine, or sertraline. J Clin Psychopharmacol 1999;19(2):155–63.

64. Sporer KA. The serotonin syndrome. Implicated drugs, pathophysiology and management. Drug Saf 1995;13(2):94–104.

65. Manos GH. Possible serotonin syndrome associated with buspirone added to fluoxetine. Ann Pharmacother 2000;34(7–8):871–4.

66. Liston HL, DeVane CL, Boulton DW, Risch SC, Markowitz JS, Goldman J. Differential time course of cytochrome P450 2D6 enzyme inhibition by fluoxetine, sertraline, and paroxetine in healthy volunteers. J Clin Psychopharmacol 2002;22(2):169–73.

67. Smith DL, Wenegrat BG. A case report of serotonin syndrome associated with combined nefazodone and fluoxetine. J Clin Psychiatry 2000;61(2):146.

68. Hamilton S, Malone K. Serotonin syndrome during treatment with paroxetine and risperidone. J Clin Psychopharmacol 2000;20(1):103–5.

69. Spina E, Avenoso A, Facciola G, Scordo MG, Ancione M, Madia A. Plasma concentrations of risperidone and 9-hydroxyrisperidone during combined treatment with paroxetine. Ther Drug Monit 2001;23(3):223–7.

70. de Jong J, Hoogenboom B, van Troostwijk LD, de Haan L. Interaction of olanzapine with fluvoxamine. Psychopharmacology (Berl) 2001;155(2):219–20.

71. Benazzi F. Organic hypomania secondary to sibutramine–citalopram interaction. J Clin Psychiatry 2002;63(2):165.

72. Aranow AB, Hudson JI, Pope HG Jr, Grady TA, Laage TA, Bell IR, Cole JO. Elevated antidepressant plasma levels after addition of fluoxetine. Am J Psychiatry 1989;146(7):911–13.

73. Preskorn SH, Beber JH, Faul JC, Hirschfeld RM. Serious adverse effects of combining fluoxetine and tricyclic antidepressants. Am J Psychiatry 1990;147(4):532.

74. Spina E, Campo GM, Avenoso A, Pollicino MA, Caputi AP. Interaction between Fluvoxamine and imipramine/desipramine in four patients. Ther Drug Monit 1992;14(3):194–6.

75. Härtter S, Wetzel H, Hammes E, Hiemke C. Inhibition of antidepressant demethylation and hydroxylation by fluvoxamine in depressed patients. Psychopharmacology (Berl) 1993;110(3):302–8.

76. Lydiard RB, Anton RF, Cunningham I. Interaction between sertraline and tricyclic antidepressants. Am J Psychiatry 1993;150(7):1125–6.

Selegiline

See also Monoamine oxidase inhibitors

General Information

Selegiline is a relatively selective and irreversible inhibitor of monoamine oxidase type B, which has been used in the treatment of Parkinson's disease. It was originally suggested that selegiline may be neuroprotective. However, in a prospective double-blind study no such action was seen (1). On the other hand, selegiline does delay the start of disability, determined by the need for levodopa and progression of parkinsonian signs and symptoms (2).

However, the Parkinson's Disease Research Group in the UK reported that after a mean follow-up period of 5.6 years, mortality was increased in randomized patients with Parkinson's disease who took levodopa together with selegiline compared with patients who took levodopa alone (2). This unexpected conclusion was interpreted as a result of methodological failures. In a meta-analysis of five long-term, prospective, randomized trials of selegiline, the treated group did not have an increase in mortality (3).

Organs and Systems

Cardiovascular

Unwanted effects of selegiline on cardiovascular regulation have been investigated as a potential cause for the unexpected mortality in the UK Parkinson's Disease Research Group trial (4). Head-up tilt caused selective and often severe orthostatic hypotension in nine of 16 patients taking selegiline and levodopa, but had no effect on nine patients taking levodopa alone. Two patients taking selegiline lost consciousness with unrecordable blood pressures and another four had severe symptomatic hypotension. The normal protective rises in heart rate and plasma noradrenaline were impaired. The abnormal response to head up tilt was reversed by withdrawal of selegiline. The authors proposed that these findings might be due to either non-selective inhibition of monoamine oxidase or effects of amfetamine and metamfetamine.

Nervous system

Selegiline is metabolized to amfetamine and metamfetamine, and can therefore cause insomnia (SEDA-17, 167).

Gastrointestinal

Selegiline has rarely re-activated pre-existing peptic ulcer disease (5).

Sexual function

Hypersexuality has been attributed to selegiline (6).

- A 72-year-old man who had taken levodopa for over 20 years started to take selegiline 10 mg/day. He developed a strong impulse for cross-dressing, which he had never experienced before. The behavior ceased when the selegiline was withdrawn.

It is not clear whether this effect was due to an interaction of levodopa with selegiline or due to a direct effect of selegiline itself.

Drug–Drug Interactions

Dopamine

An interaction of selegiline with dopamine has been described (7).

- A 75-year-old critically ill man taking selegiline 10 mg/day was given intravenous dopamine 3.5 micrograms/kg/minute. Within 50 minutes his systolic pressure had risen from 105 to 228 mmHg. Within 30 minutes of stopping the infusion his systolic blood pressure fell to 121 mmHg. Rather surprisingly, two rechallenges were attempted on that day and the next, at doses of 1.03 and 0.9 micrograms/kg/minute. Severe hypertension occurred on both occasions, with return to normal pressures very soon after the dopamine was discontinued.

As the authors pointed out, the selectivity of selegiline for monoamine oxidase type B may be less than was once thought, and co-administration of the drug with dopamine may be risky.

Fluoxetine and paroxetine

When given alongside fluoxetine selegiline can produce a sudden increase in blood pressure. The combined use of selective serotonin re-uptake inhibitors, such as fluoxetine or paroxetine, with selegiline has reportedly caused muscle rigidity, autonomic instability, and agitation or delirium. However, these possibilities are rare, and the serotonin syndrome is even rarer.

Levodopa

The Parkinson's Disease Research Group in the UK have reviewed an earlier report that there was excess mortality in patients with early disease treated with a combination of levodopa and selegiline (8). They have confirmed that there was about a 35% greater mortality in those on combined treatment compared with patients treated with levodopa alone. The excess deaths were all attributed to Parkinson's disease. The authors did not present any explanation for these findings, but they very reasonably suggested that the combination is inappropriate in early disease and should be used only with caution if at all in the later stages of the disease.

Tricyclic antidepressants

The combined use of tricyclic antidepressants and selegiline has been associated with hyperpyrexia, tremors, agitation, restlessness, reduced level of consciousness, and in rare instances death (9).

References

1. Tetrud JW, Langston JW. The effect of Deprenyl (selegiline) on the natural history of Parkinson's disease. Science 1989;245(4917):519–22.
2. The Parkinson Study Group. Effects of tocopherol and deprenyl on the progression of disability in early Parkinson's disease. N Engl J Med 1993;328(3):176–83.
3. Olanow CW, Myllyla VV, Sotaniemi KA, Larsen JP, Palhagen S, Przuntek H, Heinonen EH, Kilkku O, Lammintausta R, Maki-Ikola O, Rinne UK. Effect of selegiline on mortality in patients with Parkinson's disease: a meta-analysis. Neurology 1998;51(3):825–30.
4. Churchyard A, Mathias CJ, Boonkongchuen P, Lees AJ. Autonomic effects of selegiline: possible cardiovascular toxicity in Parkinson's disease. J Neurol Neurosurg Psychiatry 1997;63(2):228–34.
5. Robin DW. Selegiline in the treatment of Parkinson's disease. Am J Med Sci 1991;302(6):392–5.
6. Riley DE. Reversible transvestic fetishism in a man with Parkinson's disease treated with selegiline. Clin Neuropharmacol 2002;25(4):234–7.
7. Rose LM, Ohlinger MJ, Mauro VF. A hypertensive reaction induced by concurrent use of selegiline and dopamine. Ann Pharmacother 2000;34(9):1020–4.
8. Ben-Shlomo Y, Churchyard A, Head J, Hurwitz B, Overstall P, Ockelford J, Lees AJ. Investigation by Parkinson's Disease Research Group of United Kingdom into excess mortality seen with combined levodopa and selegiline treatment in patients with early, mild Parkinson's disease: further results of randomised trial and confidential inquiry. BMJ 1998;316(7139):1191–6.
9. Anonymous. Eldepryl and antidepressant interaction. FDA Med Bull 1995;25:6.

Selenium

General Information

Selenium is a non-metallic element (symbol Se; atomic no. 34) that was discovered by Berzelius in 1817.

The major functions of selenium can be attributed to its antioxidative properties and its role in the regulation of thyroid hormone metabolism. Selenium is important as a nutritional factor, and the US Food and Nutrition Board's Committee on Dietary Allowances has, perhaps somewhat arbitrarily, proposed a recommended daily intake of 50–200 micrograms/day.

Selenium has functions in many selenoproteins and also in relation to the immune response. There is an association between low plasma selenium concentrations and oral cancer (1). Selenium compounds inhibit tumorigenesis in a variety of animal models, and added selenium in human diets might reduce the risk of cancer (SEDA-21, 240).

Uses

Selenium-based drugs show some promise in several diseases, as orally active antihypertensive, anticancer, antiviral, antimicrobial, and immunosuppressive drugs, and organoselenium compounds reduce oxidative tissue damage and edema (2).

Selenium sulfide is used as an antiseborrheic agent and as a shampoo in the treatment of *Tinea versicolor*. Selenite is also found in mineral supplements and is used in parenteral nutrition. However, selenium has gained undeserved popularity as a constituent of health foods and alternative tonics, perhaps because selenium deficiency has been implicated in the pathogenesis of some forms of malnutrition in children. However, even in children with selenium deficiency the benefit to harm balance has not been established. Indeed, in protein deficiency it seems to be particularly toxic. Nor is there any serious basis for its reputation as a remedy for cystic fibrosis, to prevent aging, or as a sexual stimulant.

General adverse effects

As is evident from veterinary practice and animal studies, selenium has both acute and chronic toxic effects on many organs. Endemic selenium poisoning of populations in an area of China produced a picture resembling arsenic poisoning (3). It is not possible to say what effects have gone unrecorded, or perhaps what effects irregular use in alternative medicines might have at various ages. In countries where selenium is in vogue, physicians should be aware of its potential risks and should enquire about the possible use of selenium products in the home, either in adults or children.

An FDA overview has described 12 cases of selenium intoxication in the USA due to ingestion of "superpotent" selenium tablets, the estimated total ingested doses ranging from 27 to 2310 mg (4). Nausea, vomiting, nail changes, fatigue, and irritability were the most common symptoms; some subjects had watery diarrhea, abdominal cramps, dry hair, paresthesia, and a garlic-like odor on the breath. Many of these symptoms resembled the pattern of endemic poisoning seen in China (3). In one case,

selenium poisoning resulted from a gross underestimation of the selenium content of a nutritional supplement.

Various aspects of selenium have been reviewed, including its toxicology and selenium deficiency (5–7) and its protective effects against cancer (8).

Organs and Systems

Neuromuscular function

The incidence of amyotrophic lateral sclerosis has been studied in some 5000 residents in an area of Italy in which they had accidentally been exposed to drinking water with a high selenium content for 9 years (9). The findings pointed to a possible association between overexposure to environmental selenium and amyotrophic lateral sclerosis.

Endocrine

One report suggests that therapeutic use of selenium in the form of selenite could precipitate hypothyroidism, but the circumstances were complex and iodine deficiency seems to have played a major role (10).

Urinary tract

Selenium 400 micrograms/day for 2 weeks in a boy of 17 and 25 micrograms/day for 2 weeks in an 11-month-old infant were thought to have caused renal damage, manifested primarily by sodium loss (11). However, there is little evidence that selenium is nephrotoxic, and the patients in question had cystic fibrosis, which could have caused sodium depletion.

Skin

Selenium sulfide can cause local irritation (SED-12, 685). Photosensitive dermatitis (pityriasis versicolor) occurred in an adult man after a second application of 2.5% selenium sulfide (12).

Reproductive system

Suppression of lactation has been ascribed to the use of selenium sulfide shampoo, but the causal relation was not proven (SEDA-16, 158).

Immunologic

Selenium can cause allergic reactions (12–14).

Drug Administration

Drug overdose

Fatal suicidal selenium poisoning has been described (15), although the patient had ingested not only selenious acid 90 mg/kg but also cupric sulfate 60 mg/kg. At autopsy, pulmonary edema, congestion of the kidneys, and hemorrhagic and erosive gastric mucosa were found.

Drug–Drug Interactions

Cisplatin

Selenium appears to accentuate the nephrotoxic effects of cisplatin and its vascular toxicity (SEDA-21, 241).

References

1. Carinci F, Felisatti P. Selenio e carcinoma orale. Revisione della letteratura. [Selenium and oral cancer. Review of the literature.] Minerva Stomatol 1996;45(7–8):345–8.
2. May SW. Selenium-based pharmacological agents: an update. Expert Opin Investig Drugs 2002;11(9):1261–9.
3. Yang GQ, Wang SZ, Zhou RH, Sun SZ. Endemic selenium intoxication of humans in China. Am J Clin Nutr 1983;37(5): 872–81.
4. Anonymous. Toxicity with superpotent selenium. FDA Drug Bull 1984;14(2):19.
5. Barceloux DG. Selenium. J Toxicol Clin Toxicol 1999;37(2):145–72.
6. Rayman MP. The importance of selenium to human health. Lancet 2000;356(9225):233–41.
7. Combs GF Jr. Chemopreventive mechanisms of selenium. Med Klin (Munich) 1999;94(Suppl 3):18–24.
8. Combs GF Jr, Clark LC, Turnbull BW. An analysis of cancer prevention by selenium. Biofactors 2001;14(1–4): 153–9.
9. Vinceti M, Guidetti D, Pinotti M, Rovesti S, Merlin M, Vescovi L, Bergomi M, Vivoli G. Amyotrophic lateral sclerosis after long-term exposure to drinking water with high selenium content. Epidemiology 1996;7(5):529–32.
10. Hofbauer LC, Spitzweg C, Magerstadt RA, Heufelder AE. Selenium-induced thyroid dysfunction. Postgrad Med J 1997;73(856):103–4.
11. Snodgrass W, Rumack BH, Sullivan JB Jr, Peterson RG, Chase HP, Cotton EK, Sokol R. Selenium: childhood poisoning and cystic fibrosis. Clin Toxicol 1981;18(2):211–20.
12. Mani MZ. Photosensitivity to Selsun shampoo. Indian J Dermatol Venereol Leprol 1994;60:49–50.
13. Jirasek L, Kalensky J. Precitlivelost na platinu, rhodium, zlato, med', antimom a jine vzacne kovy a profesionalni dermatitidy zpusobene selenem. [Hypersensitivity to platinum, rhodium, gold, copper, antimony and other precious metals and occupational dermatitis caused by selenium.] Cesk Dermatol 1975;50(6):361–8.
14. Diskin CJ, Tomasso CL, Alper JC, Glaser ML, Fliegel SE. Long-term selenium exposure. Arch Intern Med 1979;139(7):824–6.
15. Matoba R, Kimura H, Uchima E, Abe T, Yamada T, Mitsukuni Y, Shikata I. An autopsy case of acute selenium (selenious acid) poisoning and selenium levels in human tissues. Forensic Sci Int 1986;31(2):87–92.

Sertindole

See also Neuroleptic drugs

General Information

Sertindole is an antipsychotic drug that was approved in several countries in 1997, but was suspended in January 2000, following concerns about reports of cardiac dysrhythmias and sudden death (SEDA-22, 71) (SEDA-25,

71) (1). To gather further information, data collected for prescription-event-monitoring (PEM) studies have been analysed (2). Patients taking sertindole ($n = 462$; 5482 months of observation) were compared with patients taking risperidone or olanzapine ($n = 16\ 542$; 139 987 months of observation). There were seven deaths in the sertindole group and 415 in the other, and the death rates were not significantly different, although the confidence intervals were wide because of the relatively small number of patients in the sertindole group. There were six cases of prolonged QT_c interval in the patients taking sertindole and one in the controls. The authors concluded that the sertindole group was too small to rule out an association between sertindole and cardiovascular deaths.

On 28 June 2001 an ad hoc expert committee was convened to review the available clinical and preclinical data related to the cardiovascular activity of sertindole and to consider whether such data supported the then current marketing authorization status of sertindole (3). Based on a re-evaluation of all the available data, including additional data submitted by the Marketing Authorization Holder, it was concluded that the re-introduction of sertindole could be supported by further clinical safety data, strong safeguards (including extensive contraindications and warnings for patients at risk of cardiac dysrhythmias), a reduction in the recommended maximum dose from 24 mg to 20 mg in all but exceptional cases, and extensive electrocardiographic monitoring before and during treatment. The Committee for Proprietary Medicinal Products (CPMP) of The European Agency for the Evaluation of Medicinal Products later recommended lifting the ban on sertindole-containing medicinal products on the basis of additional data provided by the marketing authorization holders (see monthly report from October, 2001: www. emea.eu.int).

Organs and Systems

Cardiovascular

Sertindole was associated with 27 deaths (16 cardiac) in 2194 patients who were enrolled in premarketing studies; further fatal cases have been collected, and the Committee on Safety of Medicines has described reports of 36 deaths (including some sudden cardiac deaths) and 13 serious but non-fatal dysrhythmias also associated with sertindole (4).

References

1. Rawlins M. Suspension of availability of Serdolect (sertindole). Media Release 1998;2:3–7.
2. Wilton LV, Heeley EL, Pickering RM, Shakir SA. Comparative study of mortality rates and cardiac dysrhythmias in post-marketing surveillance studies of sertindole and two other atypical antipsychotic drugs, risperidone and olanzapine. J Psychopharmacol 2001;15(2):120–6.
3. EMEA. The European Agency for the Evaluation of Medicinal Products. http://www.emea.eu.int/pdfs/human/referral/Sertindole/285202en.pdf.
4. Committee on Safety of Medicines-Medicines Control Agency. Cardiac arrhythmias with pomizode (Orap). Curr Probl Pharmacovigilance 1995;21:1.

Sertraline

See also Selective serotonin re-uptake inhibitors (SSRIs)

General Information

Sertraline hydrochloride has an average half-life of about 26 hours, and mean peak plasma concentrations occur at 4.5–8.4 hours. The dosage is 50–200 mg/day orally. Its major metabolite, *N*-desmethylsertraline, is less active than sertraline. Adverse effects are as for the SSRIs in general.

Organs and Systems

Cardiovascular

Angina occurred in an elderly woman shortly after she started to take sertraline and on rechallenge (1).

Nervous system

Parkinsonism
Sertraline has an appreciable affinity for the dopamine re-uptake site, and for this reason might be presumed less likely to cause movement disorders than other SSRIs. However, there is little clinical evidence to support this suggestion and cases of sertraline-induced parkinsonism have been reported (2).

- A 70-year-old woman, who had been taking sertraline 100 mg/day for 7 months, gave a 6-month history of resting tremor and loss of dexterity in the right hand. She had mild bradykinesia and cogwheel rigidity in the right arm and leg. She had not taken any other medications. A brain MRI scan was normal. The sertraline was withdrawn and within 1 month all the neurological symptoms and signs had remitted.
- An 81-year-old woman took sertraline 100 mg/day for depression and 6 months later presented with tremor and difficulty in moving her right arm and leg (3). A diagnosis of right hemiparkinsonism was made and the sertraline was withdrawn. Her extrapyramidal symptoms resolved within 3 months, but 14 months later she developed parkinsonism and was treated with levodopa and carbidopa.
- A 70-year-old man developed parkinsonian symptoms 1 month after starting to take sertraline 100 mg/day (4). Withdrawal of sertraline resulted in amelioration but not complete remission of his symptoms which then required treatment with carbidopa and levodopa.

In these cases presumably the sertraline prematurely precipitated Parkinson's disease. Two cases of sertraline-induced akathisia have been reported (SEDA-18, 19).

Serotonin syndrome
Treatment with serotonin-potentiating drugs in usual therapeutic doses can sometimes produce the serotonin syndrome. There are also case reports of this reaction with single doses of SSRIs (see also the monograph on fluvoxamine) (5).

Serotonin syndrome after a single dose of sertraline 100 mg has been reported in a 16-year-old girl (6). It responded to a single 4 mg dose of the serotonin antagonist cyproheptadine.

There was therapeutic benefit from cyproheptadine in a case of serotonin syndrome in a 2-year-old girl who accidentally swallowed ten 50 mg tablets of sertraline (7).

Endocrine

Serotonin pathways are involved in the regulation of prolactin secretion. Galactorrhea has also been reported in a patient taking sertraline, in whom lactation ceased after withdrawal (SEDA-18, 20) and in another case (8).

Hematologic

Prolonged bleeding time has been reported with sertraline (9).

Sertraline has been associated with agranulocytosis (10).

Liver

Hepatitis has been associated with sertraline (11).

Hepatitis has also been reported with paroxetine (SEDA-21, 12).

Skin

Stevens–Johnson syndrome has been reported in a 96-year-old woman who had taken sertraline (dosage not stated) for 3 weeks (12). The lesions involved the skin, oral mucosa, and conjunctiva. The eruption disappeared within 7 days of sertraline withdrawal.

Hair

Hair loss has been associated with sertraline (13).

Sexual function

Sexual disturbance has also been associated with sertraline (14), and a high frequency of such adverse effects has been reported in studies in which high doses were used. In a double-blind, placebo-controlled study of sertraline and amitriptyline in patients with major depression, male sexual dysfunction, mainly ejaculatory disturbance, was reported significantly more often with sertraline (in 21% of the patients) (15). Male sexual dysfunction in 15% of sertraline-treated patients has also been reported (16).

Priapism is occasionally associated with the use of psychotropic drugs, such as trazodone, that are α_1-adrenoceptor antagonists. It has also been reported in a man taking sertraline (17).

- A 47-year-old man presented with a 4-day history of priapism and moderate pain. Several brief but otherwise similar episodes had occurred during the previous month. He had a history of depression and had been taking sertraline 200 mg/day and dexamfetamine 10 mg/day. He received intracorporeal methoxamine, but when this proved ineffective he was treated with intracorporeal adrenaline and a shunt procedure. However, detumescence was incomplete. At follow-up after several weeks the priapism had resolved and he had not become impotent (a significant risk in cases of prolonged priapism). He was given nefazodone with no recurrence of erectile dysfunction.

The dosage of sertraline used in this case was high and the combined use of dexamfetamine may also have been relevant.

Long-Term Effects

Drug withdrawal

Withdrawal symptoms have been reported with sertraline (18). All the symptoms, including gastrointestinal discomfort, insomnia, and influenza-like symptoms, remitted when sertraline was reinstituted.

Drug Administration

Drug overdose

In 40 patients who took up to 8 g of sertraline there were no serious sequelae (19).

One of the largest overdoses of sertraline has been reported (20).

- A 51-year-old woman took about 8 g of sertraline, about 80 times the usual daily dose. On admission to hospital she was somnolent but rousable. Her electrocardiogram showed a transiently prolonged QT_c interval (510 ms falling to 470 ms). On the third day she developed agitation, disorientation, myoclonus, and pyrexia (38.5 °C), was treated with supportive measures, and recovered over the next 3 days.

While cardiac toxicity was not prominent in this case, the patient developed clear evidence of the serotonin syndrome, which proved self-limiting.

Drug–Drug Interactions

Carbamazepine

Sertraline is a substrate for a number of CYP450 isozymes, including CYP2C9, CYP2C19, and CYP3A4. Several case reports have shown loss of antidepressant activity of sertraline at usual therapeutic doses when depressed patients have also taken drugs that induce CYP3A4, including carbamazepine (21).

Erythromycin

Drug interactions leading to the serotonin syndrome usually result from pharmacodynamic mechanisms. However, the antibiotic erythromycin may have precipitated the serotonin syndrome in a patient taking sertraline by a pharmacokinetic mechanism (22).

- A 12-year-old boy, who had taken sertraline 37.5 mg/day for 5 weeks for obsessive-compulsive disorder, started to take erythromycin 200 mg bd. Within 4 days he began to feel anxious; this was followed over the next 10 days by panic, restlessness, irritability, tremulousness, and confusion. These symptoms resolved within 72 hours of withdrawal of sertraline and erythromycin.

The authors proposed that in this case erythromycin had inhibited sertraline metabolism by inhibiting CYP3A. This could have led to increased concentrations of sertraline and signs of serotonin toxicity. Unfortunately sertraline concentrations were not measured to confirm this suggestion.

Rifampicin

Sertraline is a substrate for a number of CYP450 isozymes, including CYP2C9, CYP2C19, and CYP3A4. Several case reports have shown loss of antidepressant activity of sertraline at usual therapeutic doses when depressed patients have also taken drugs that induce CYP3A4, including rifampicin (23).

References

1. Sunderji R, Press N, Amin H, Gin K. Unstable angina associated with sertraline. Can J Cardiol 1997;13(9):849–51.
2. Di Rocco A, Brannan T, Prikhojan A, Yahr MD. Sertraline induced parkinsonism. A case report and an in-vivo study of the effect of sertraline on dopamine metabolism. J Neural Transm 1998;105(2–3):247–51.
3. Pina Latorre MA, Modrego PJ, Rodilla F, Catalan C, Calvo M. Parkinsonism and Parkinson's disease associated with long-term administration of sertraline. J Clin Pharm Ther 2001;26(2):111–12.
4. Gregory RJ, White JF. Can sertraline induce parkinson's disease? Psychosomatics 2001;42(2):163–4.
5. Gill M, LoVecchio F, Selden B. Serotonin syndrome in a child after a single dose of fluvoxamine. Ann Emerg Med 1999;33(4):457–9.
6. Mullins ME, Horowitz BZ. Serotonin syndrome after a single dose of fluvoxamine. Ann Emerg Med 1999;34(6):806–7.
7. Horowitz BZ, Mullins ME. Cyproheptadine for serotonin syndrome in an accidental pediatric sertraline ingestion. Pediatr Emerg Care 1999;15(5):325–7.
8. Lesaca TG. Sertraline and galactorrhea. J Clin Psychopharmacol 1996;16(4):333–4.
9. Calhoun JW, Calhoun DD. Prolonged bleeding time in a patient treated with sertraline. Am J Psychiatry 1996;153(3):443.
10. Trescoli-Serrano C, Smith NK. Sertraline-induced agranulocytosis. Postgrad Med J 1996;72(849):446.
11. Hautekeete ML, Colle I, van Vlierberghe H, Elewaut A. Symptomatic liver injury probably related to sertraline. Gastroenterol Clin Biol 1998;22(3):364–5.
12. Jan V, Toledano C, Machet L, Machet MC, Vaillant L, Lorette G. Stevens-Johnson syndrome after sertraline. Acta Derm Venereol 1999;79(5):401.
13. Bourgeois JA. Two cases of hair loss after sertraline use. J Clin Psychopharmacol 1996;16(1):91–2.
14. Cooper GL. The safety of fluoxetine – an update. Br J Psychiatry Suppl 1988;3:77–86.
15. Reimherr FW, Chouinard G, Cohn CK, Cole JO, Itil TM, LaPierre YD, Masco HL, Mendels J. Antidepressant efficacy of sertraline: a double-blind, placebo- and amitriptyline-controlled, multicenter comparison study in outpatients with major depression. J Clin Psychiatry 1990;51(Suppl. B):18–27.
16. Doogan DP. Toleration and safety of sertraline: experience worldwide. Int Clin Psychopharmacol 1991;6(Suppl. 2):47–56.
17. Rand EH. Priapism in a patient taking sertraline. J Clin Psychiatry 1998;59(10):538.

18. Louie AK, Lannon RA, Ajari LJ. Withdrawal reaction after sertraline discontinuation. Am J Psychiatry 1994;151(3):450–1.
19. Lau GT, Horowitz BZ. Sertraline overdose. Acad Emerg Med 1996;3(2):132–6.
20. Brendel DH, Bodkin JA, Yang JM. Massive sertraline overdose. Ann Emerg Med 2000;36(5):524–6.
21. Khan A, Shad MU, Preskorn SH. Lack of sertraline efficacy probably due to an interaction with carbamazepine. J Clin Psychiatry 2000;61(7):526–7.
22. Lee DO, Lee CD. Serotonin syndrome in a child associated with erythromycin and sertraline. Pharmacotherapy 1999;19(7):894–6.
23. Markowitz JS, DeVane CL. Rifampin-induced selective serotonin reuptake inhibitor withdrawal syndrome in a patient treated with sertraline. J Clin Psychopharmacol 2000; 20(1):109–10.

Sevoflurane

See also General anesthetics

General Information

Sevoflurane is an isoflurane-related anesthetic, which is pleasant to breathe and has a rapid onset and offset of action. It can be used for both the induction and maintenance of anesthesia.

It has become popular in day surgery, despite little evidence of clear advantages over current alternatives.

Inhalational induction of anesthesia is common in children, and sevoflurane is challenging the tradition of halothane induction in children. Deep anesthesia with sevoflurane can be obtained rapidly, and recovery is also faster than with halothane.

Compound A

Compound A is a haloalkene degradation product of sevoflurane metabolism by carbon dioxide absorbers, and it has been suggested that prolonged low-flow closed-circuit anesthesia with sevoflurane may maximize exposure to the degradation product. Compound A can cause convulsions and neural damage in rats (1). It also causes nephrotoxicity and hepatotoxicity in rats, particularly if barium hydroxide lime is used (2).

Organs and Systems

Cardiovascular

In 28 subjects given either sevoflurane + nitrous oxide or enflurane + nitrous oxide anesthesia, sevoflurane caused fewer cardiodepressant effects than enflurane (3). Nevertheless, in 10 healthy subjects atrial contraction and left ventricular diastolic function, including active relaxation, passive compliance, and elastic recoil were impaired by sevoflurane (1 MAC) (4).

Sevoflurane has a similar effect on regional blood flow to other halogenated anesthetics, although it is perhaps slightly less of a coronary artery vasodilator than isoflurane. It reduces myocardial contractility and does not potentiate adrenaline-induced cardiac dysrhythmias (5).

It also reduces baroreflex function, and in that respect is similar to other halogenated anesthetics. Coronary artery disease is not a risk factor for the use of these agents (6).

In contrast to isoflurane and desflurane, sevoflurane tends not to increase the heart rate, and is usually well tolerated for induction of anesthesia in young children. However, profound bradycardia was reported in four unpremedicated children aged 6 months to 2 years during anesthesia induction with sevoflurane 8% and nitrous oxide 66% (7). The episodes were not associated with loss of airway or ventilation. In three of the children there was spontaneous recovery of heart rate when the sevoflurane concentration was reduced; the other child received atropine because of evidence of significantly reduced cardiac output. In a previous study of sevoflurane induction of anesthesia in children with atropine premedication there was also a low incidence of this complication (8), which is probably due to excessive sevoflurane concentrations.

The effects of sevoflurane on cardiac conduction have been studied in 60 healthy unpremedicated infants (9). They received sevoflurane either as a continuous concentration of 8% from a primed circuit or in incrementally increasing doses. Nodal rhythm occurred in 12 cases. The mean duration of the nodal rhythm was 62 seconds in the incremental group and 90 seconds in the 8% group. All of the dysrhythmias were self-limiting and there were no ventricular or supraventricular dysrhythmias. No adverse events occurred as a result of the dysrhythmias. This study highlights the importance of using electrocardiographic monitoring when inducing anesthesia with volatile agents.

- Complete atrioventricular block occurred in a 10-year-old child with a history of hypertension, severe renal dysfunction, incomplete right bundle branch block, and a ventricular septal defect that had been repaired at birth (10). After slow induction with sevoflurane and nitrous oxide 66%, complete atrioventricular block occurred when the inspired sevoflurane concentration was 3% and reverted to sinus rhythm after withdrawal of the sevoflurane. The dysrhythmia recurred at the end of the procedure, possibly caused by lidocaine, which had infiltrated into the abdominal wound, and again at 24 hours in association with congestive cardiac failure following absorption of peritoneal dialysis fluid.

Congenital or acquired forms of the long QT syndrome can result in polymorphous ventricular tachycardia (torsade de pointes). Many drugs, including inhalational anesthetics, alter the QT interval, and sevoflurane prolongs the rate-corrected QT interval (QT_c). In a randomized study of whether sevoflurane-associated QT_c prolongation was rapidly reversed when propofol was used instead, 32 patients were randomly allocated to one of two groups (11). All received sevoflurane induction and maintenance for the first 15 minutes. In one group, sevoflurane was then withdrawn, and anesthesia was maintained with propofol for another 15 minutes; the other group continued to receive sevoflurane for 30 minutes. Sevoflurane-associated QT_c prolongation was fully reversed within 15 minutes when propofol was substituted.

A case of torsade de pointes has been attributed to sevoflurane anesthesia (12).

- A 65-year-old woman, who had had normal preoperative serum electrolytes and a normal QT interval with sinus rhythm, received hydroxyzine and atropine premedication followed by thiopental and vecuronium for anesthetic induction. Endotracheal intubation was difficult and precipitated atrial fibrillation, which was refractory to disopyramide 100 mg. Anesthesia was then maintained with sevoflurane 2% and nitrous oxide 50%. Ten minutes later ventricular tachycardia ensued, refractory to intravenous lidocaine, disopyramide, and magnesium. DC cardioversion resulted in a change to a supraventricular tachycardia, which then deteriorated to torsade de pointes. External cardiac massage and further DC cardioversion were initially unsuccessful, but the cardiac rhythm reverted to atrial fibrillation 10 minutes after the sevoflurane was switched off. Two weeks later she had her operation under combined epidural and general anesthesia, with no changes in cardiac rhythm.

In this case the role of excessive sympathetic drive as a result of the difficult intubation and the lack of opioid use during induction must be considered, even if sevoflurane played a role in precipitating the dysrhythmia.

Respiratory

In a randomized study of the respiratory effects of high concentrations of halothane and sevoflurane in 21 healthy boys undergoing inguinal or penile surgery, there was similar respiratory depression with each agent (13). Minute ventilation fell by about 50% as a result of a reduction in tidal volume, despite an increase in respiratory rate.

Nervous system

Despite a fall in mean arterial pressure, with a consequent reduction in cerebral perfusion pressure, sevoflurane should be a suitable agent for neuroanesthesia (14). Even in patients with ischemic cerebrovascular diseases, both the CO_2 response and cerebral autoregulation were well maintained during sevoflurane anesthesia (0.88 MAC) (15).

A case of acute dystonia has been reported during induction of anesthesia with sevoflurane (16).

- A 19-year-old man with schizophrenia, who was taking cyamemazine (a phenothiazine) 75 mg/day, and dihydroergotamine 180 mg/day to avoid neuroleptic drug-induced hypotension, had no history of involuntary movements, and neurological examination was normal preoperatively. Anesthesia was induced with midazolam 5 mg oral premedication and an inhalational induction using 4–5 maximum breaths of sevoflurane 8% and nitrous oxide 50% in oxygen. One minute after loss of consciousness, he developed a torticollic posture and stiffness, rapidly extending to the left trapezius and scalene muscles. There was severe rotation of the head accompanied by trismus and opisthotonos. An intravenous injection of the muscle relaxant atracurium 30 mg resolved the muscle spasms. Subsequent anesthesia was uneventful.

Dystonia after inhalational anesthesia is rare and is presumably due to an alteration in the dynamic relation between dopaminergic and other receptors in the brain.

Sevoflurane can cause epileptiform activity on the electroencephalogram, especially during emergence from anesthesia. It has also been associated with epileptiform discharges in volunteer studies, but clinical convulsions appear to very be rare. Two cases of epileptiform activity during sevoflurane anesthesia have been reported in healthy volunteers (17). They were taking part in a study of the effects of sevoflurane on regional cerebral blood flow and received twice the minimum alveolar concentration (MAC) of sevoflurane (4.4%). The only other drug administered was rocuronium, a muscle relaxant. Sevoflurane was used at up to twice its MAC, to induce burst suppression of the electroencephalogram. One of the subjects had partial motor seizure activity in the form of slight clonic movements in the right and then later in the left leg. There was an associated increase in heart rate (from 65 to 79 beats/minute) and systolic blood pressure (from 85 to 106 mmHg) and rhythmic epileptiform discharges on the electroencephalogram. The second subject had epileptiform activity on his electroencephalogram, consisting of partial and secondarily generalized discharges lasting for 2 and 3 minutes respectively. There were no clinical signs of an epileptic seizure. Burst suppression appeared on the electroencephalogram in both subjects before the seizure activity, and the Bispectral Index increased dramatically during the epileptiform discharge to maximum values of 44 and 73 respectively. As expected, regional cerebral blood flow and regional metabolism of the epileptic focus fell interictally and increased ictally. Although the concentrations of sevoflurane used in this study were high compared with usual anesthetic practice, further human studies are warranted, because prolonged epileptiform discharge is known to be harmful.

In another case, epileptiform activity was reported during sevoflurane anesthesia, but not with propofol in the same individual (18).

- A 62-year-old woman with no personal or family history of seizures had general relaxant anesthesia for plastic surgery using a total intravenous anesthetic technique with propofol, remifentanil, and cisatracurium, after benzodiazepine premedication. Routine electroencephalographic monitoring showed continuous slowing followed by burst suppression (consistent with very deep anesthesia), but no epileptiform activity. At a second procedure, and following identical benzodiazepine premedication and induction with propofol, anesthesia was maintained with sevoflurane (plus remifentanil for analgesia and cisatracurium for neuromuscular blockade). During the procedure, sevoflurane was increased from 2% to 8%. After 5 minutes, at an end-tidal concentration of 5.9%, there was epileptiform activity on the electroencephalogram. There were no hemodynamic changes.

Epileptiform activity on the electroencephalogram in association with sevoflurane induction has also been reported in a prospective study of 20 non-premedicated healthy children in whom electroencephalographic monitoring was started before sevoflurane induction (19). At 2

MAC there was epileptiform activity in two boys, with spontaneously resolving myoclonic movements.

Epileptiform activity on the electroencephalogram in association with sevoflurane has also been reported in two children aged 3 and 5 years in a center in which electroencephalographic monitoring is routine (20). In both cases the activity occurred after several minutes of anesthesia, when the sevoflurane concentrations were increased to 7–8%. The epileptiform activity resolved after a reduction in sevoflurane concentrations. No seizure activity was noted.

In a prospective, observational study in 30 children undergoing adenoidectomy anesthesia was induced with midazolam and thiopental (both potent anticonvulsants) and maintained with sevoflurane; no electroencephalographic epileptiform activity was observed (21).

Generalized tonic–clonic seizures have been reported in association with the use of sevoflurane.

- Generalized tonic–clonic seizure-like movements lasting 40 seconds occurred in a healthy 32-year-old man after emergence from sevoflurane-based anesthesia (22).
- A 19-year-old man with a history of metamfetamine abuse 3 weeks earlier, but no personal or family history of seizure activity had anesthesia induced with midazolam 1 mg, nitrous oxide 50%, and sevoflurane 8% (23). The sevoflurane was subsequently reduced to 2%. After radical orchidectomy the sevoflurane and nitrous oxide were withdrawn and oxygen 100% was given and 2 minutes later rhythmic jerking movements began in the legs and quickly spread to the rest of the body. The movements were accompanied by an arched back and a stiff neck. Arterial oxygen saturation dropped to 50% and ventilation was controlled, again using sevoflurane 8%. The duration of the seizure was about 4 minutes. The sevoflurane was again withdrawn 3 minutes later, and a similar seizure occurred. This time it was controlled with midazolam 1 mg and propofol 30 mg. Recovery was marked only by mild disorientation. Postoperative computerized tomography showed a ganglioneuroma in the posterior cortex. The electroencephalogram was normal.

These reports show that clinicians need to be aware of the possibility of generalized seizures, especially in patients who are predisposed to seizures.

Peripheral neuropathy has been reported in two healthy men anesthetized with 1.25 MAC sevoflurane at 2 l/minute fresh gas flow for 8 hours. Their average concentrations of compound A were 45 and 28 ppm. Both had had previous minor injuries in the regions in which the neuropathies were reported. The authors suggested that compound A, or other factors associated with sevoflurane anesthesia, may predispose patients to peripheral neuropathy. Both men were volunteers for earlier published studies comparing the nephrotoxic properties of sevoflurane and desflurane, sponsored by Baxter PPD, New Jersey, the manufacturer of desflurane, a rival inhalational anesthetic agent; these reports need to be regarded with caution.

Neuromuscular function

Prolongation of rapacuronium-induced neuromuscular blockade by sevoflurane has been studied in a randomized, placebo-controlled comparison with suxamethonium in 40 children (24). Patients received sevoflurane and nitrous oxide anesthesia followed by rapacuronium 2 mg/kg. The study was stopped after only seven patients had been recruited, because the mean time to return of twitch height to 25% of baseline was 26 minutes. This time represents a stage at which neuromuscular blockade can be reversed and in this case it was twice as long as predicted from experience in adult patients. The authors suggested that the prolonged neuromuscular relaxation was due to the interaction of sevoflurane with rapacuronium, because such prolongation has not been observed using other inhalation agents.

Psychological, psychiatric

Delirium during emergence from sevoflurane anesthesia has often been documented. Four patients, an adult and three children aged 3–8 years, who were able to recount the experience, have been reported (25). They had full recall of postoperative events, were terrified, agitated, and distressed, and hence presented with acute organic mental state dysfunction which was short-lived. Two were disoriented and had paranoid ideation. They were not in any pain or were not distressed by pain if it was present. The authors hypothesized that misperception of environmental stimuli associated with sevoflurane's particular mode of action may have been the underlying cause of this phenomenon. Anxiolytic premedication and effective analgesia did not necessarily prevent the problem.

The effect of intravenous clonidine 2 micrograms/kg on the incidence and severity of postoperative agitation has been assessed in a double-blind, randomized, placebo-controlled trial in 40 boys who had anesthetic induction with sevoflurane after oral midazolam premedication (26). There was agitation in 16 of those who received placebo and two of those who received clonidine; the agitation was severe in six of those given placebo and none of those given clonidine.

The effects of intravenous and caudal epidural clonidine on the incidence and severity of postoperative agitation have been assessed in a randomized, double-blind study in 80 children, all of whom received sevoflurane as the sole general anesthetic for induction and maintenance (27). A caudal epidural block was performed before surgery for analgesia with 0.175% bupivacaine 1 ml/kg. The children were assigned randomly to four groups: (I) clonidine 1 microgram/kg added to the caudal bupivacaine; (II) clonidine 3 micrograms/kg added to the caudal bupivacaine; (III) clonidine 3 micrograms/kg intravenously; and (IV) no clonidine. The incidences of agitation were 22, 0, 5, and 39% in the four groups respectively. Thus, clonidine 3 micrograms/kg effectively prevented agitation after sevoflurane anesthesia independent of the route of administration.

The effect of a single preoperative dose of the opioid oxycodone on emergence behavior has been studied in a randomized trial in 130 children (28). Oxycodone prophylaxis had no effect on post-sevoflurane delirium.

The effect of a single bolus dose of midazolam before the end of sevoflurane anesthesia has been investigated in a double-blind, randomized, placebo-controlled trial in 40 children aged 2–7 years (29). Midazolam significantly reduced the incidence of delirium after anesthesia. However, when it was used for severe agitation midazolam only reduced the severity without abolishing agitation. The authors concluded that midazolam attenuates, but does not abolish, agitation after sevoflurane anesthesia.

Liver

Sevoflurane can be used to induce hypotension during neurosurgery. Hypotensive anesthesia has little effect on postoperative liver function (30).

- A 3-day-old boy underwent inguinal herniorrhaphy under sevoflurane anesthesia, and 2 days later developed vomiting, anorexia, and fever (31). His aspartate transaminase, alanine transaminase, and lactate dehydrogenase activities were increased and peaked 12–16 days after the operation. Viral markers were negative, as was a lymphocyte stimulation test with sevoflurane. Toxic (not allergic) liver damage due to exposure to sevoflurane was considered to be the most probable diagnosis.

In a randomized study of the renal and hepatic effects of prolonged low-flow anesthesia with sevoflurane or isoflurane in patients undergoing prolonged operations (over 8 hours), using a technique that maximized compound A production, there were no differences in markers of hepatocellular injury at 24 or 72 hours (32).

The effect of minimal-flow (as opposed to low-flow) anesthesia with sevoflurane and isoflurane has been examined in a randomized trial in 76 patients (33). There were no significant differences between the groups in blood chemistry markers of hepatic function, despite high exposure to Compound A in the patients who received sevoflurane.

Plasma activity of alpha-glutathione S-transferase activity (αGT) is a more sensitive and specific marker of hepatocellular injury than transaminase activity and it correlates better with hepatic histology. Anesthesia with halothane leads to transiently raised αGT activity, but propofol and isoflurane do not. In a randomized study of plasma αGT activity during and after low-flow anesthesia with sevoflurane or isoflurane, there were no significant differences in αGT activities between the two groups during or after anesthesia (34).

Thus, the evidence suggests that sevoflurane is as safe as isoflurane in low-flow anesthesia with respect to liver dysfunction.

Urinary tract

The effects of sevoflurane, isoflurane, and desflurane on macroscopic renal structure have been studied in 24 patients undergoing nephrectomy (35). All anesthetics were administered using a fresh gas flow of 1 l/minute and a sodium hydroxide absorber and had an average duration of 3 hours. No injury to nephrons was observed by pathologists blinded to which anesthetic agent had been used. Postoperative creatinine concentrations and urine volumes did not differ significantly between the groups.

- Transient renal tubular dysfunction has been reported in a patient with asthma requiring mechanical ventilation who received sevoflurane for 9 days (36). Soda lime was not used, and the cumulative dose was 298 MAC-hours. Serum and urinary inorganic fluoride concentrations reached maximum concentrations of 71 and 2047 µmol/l respectively. Markers of renal tubular injury were also greatly raised (urinary N-acetyl-beta-D-glucosaminidase and beta$_2$-microglobulin). However, urine volume, creatinine clearance, and serum creatinine and urea concentrations were unaffected.

There has been a meta-analysis of 22 controlled trials in 3436 patients (82% ASA I or II, 16% ASA III, and 2% ASA IV) (37). The trials had compared sevoflurane for anesthesia maintenance with isoflurane, propofol, or enflurane. Serum creatinine and blood urea nitrogen were used to assess preoperative and postoperative renal function. The duration of anesthesia was 0.5–11 hours. Most patients (97%) were exposed to less than 4 MAC-hours of volatile agent. Falls in the serum creatinine and blood urea nitrogen were significantly smaller with isoflurane than with sevoflurane. In patients who received concurrent aminoglycosides, sevoflurane was associated with a small increase in serum creatinine. The following factors had no effect on renal function: the type of anesthetic circuit, the choice of carbon dioxide absorber, the inorganic fluoride ion concentration, the duration of anesthesia, the use of nitrous oxide, or how sick patients were. When all patients were considered, the incidences of clinically significant increases in serum creatinine were the same between agents. In patients with baseline creatinine values greater than 132 µmol/l (1.5 mg/dl), the incidence of clinically important increases in serum creatinine was significantly higher in both treatment groups compared with baseline. This meta-analysis has provided strong evidence that sevoflurane does not contribute to clinically significant renal insufficiency.

Renal impairment often follows cardiac surgery, but in a randomized trial in elective coronary artery surgery in 354 patients, sevoflurane did not produce greater increases in serum creatinine concentrations than isoflurane or propofol (38).

The role of compound A

Sevoflurane is metabolized to compound A by carbon dioxide absorbers. It is nephrotoxic in rats, but nephrotoxicity in humans has not been proven. The accumulation of compound A is greatest with low fresh gas flows and barium hydroxide absorbers, both of which cause higher temperatures in the absorber. Current anesthetic practice is to use sodium hydroxide for carbon dioxide absorption, because it produces less compound A than barium hydroxide.

There has been controversy over whether compound A causes significant renal damage in humans. The potential for renal damage using sevoflurane was investigated in 42 patients without renal disease scheduled for surgery lasting more than 4 hours (39). The patients were given low-flow sevoflurane or isoflurane (fresh gas flow 1 l/minute/m^2) or high-flow sevoflurane (6 l/minute/m^2). None of these increased blood urea nitrogen concentrations, creatinine concentrations, or creatinine clearance.

There were no significant differences in beta$_2$-microglobulin, a marker of tubular function, or urinary glucose concentrations. However, there was an increase in the 24-hour urinary excretion of N-acetyl-beta-glucosaminidase, a marker of proximal tubular necrosis, with both doses of sevoflurane but not with isoflurane. There were no significant differences in the serum and urinary fluoride concentrations between the two sevoflurane groups, despite the higher concentration of compound A (29 versus 3.9 ppm) in the expired gases of those who received low-flow sevoflurane. The maximum 24-hour protein excretion was higher with low-flow sevoflurane compared with the other two groups.

The effect of the nephrotoxic aminoglycoside antibiotic amikacin on renal function during low-flow sevoflurane anesthesia has been studied in a randomized study in 37 men undergoing orthopedic surgery (40). Markers of renal tubular injury (urinary N-acetyl-beta-D-glucosaminidase and beta$_2$-microglobulin) were not abnormally raised, and urine volume, creatinine clearance, and serum creatinine and urea concentrations were unaffected. The duration of anesthesia and compound A concentrations were similar in the two groups.

In a randomized study of the renal and hepatic effects of prolonged low-flow anesthesia with sevoflurane or isoflurane in patients undergoing prolonged operations (over 8 hours), using a technique that maximized compound A production, there were no significant differences between the groups in serum creatinine or urea concentrations, creatinine clearance, or urinary protein or glucose excretion at 24 or 72 hours (32). Proteinuria and glycosuria were common in both groups. There was no correlation between exposure to compound A and any measure of renal function. There were no differences in markers of hepatocellular injury. There was no evidence of nephrotoxicity of sevoflurane even at high degrees of exposure to compound A for as long as 17 hours.

The effect on renal function of minimal-flow (as opposed to low-flow) anesthesia with sevoflurane and isoflurane has been examined in a randomized trial in 76 patients (33). There were no significant differences between the groups in blood chemistry markers of renal or hepatic function or in urinary markers of tubular injury, despite high exposure to compound A in the patients who received sevoflurane.

These studies have confirmed earlier findings that although there is biochemical evidence of renal damage after sevoflurane anesthesia, there are no clinically significant effects.

The role of fluoride

Serum and urinary inorganic fluoride concentrations can rise after inhalation of sevoflurane, because of hepatic metabolism (41). The authors concluded that lengthy sevoflurane anesthesia could alter renal function, although there was no other evidence of nephrotoxicity. Although patients with normal renal function are probably not at risk during normal anesthesia with sevoflurane, those with pre-existing renal impairment may be at risk.

A randomized, open study in 26 patients with renal dysfunction who received either isoflurane or sevoflurane for operations lasting up to 6 hours showed no significant differences in postoperative creatinine clearances. However, there was a significant increase in the plasma fluoride ion concentration with sevoflurane (42). In 10 adults who were given repeat high-flow sevoflurane anesthesia there was no evidence of renal or hepatic injury and no increases in serum or urine fluoride concentrations that would indicate an increase in sevoflurane metabolism with repeated use (43).

Renal function has been assessed after low fresh gas flow anesthesia (1 l/minute or less) with either sevoflurane or isoflurane in a multicenter study of 254 patients (44). The mean duration of anesthesia was 3.0 MAC-hours in both groups. Peak serum fluoride concentrations were significantly higher (40 µmol/l) after sevoflurane compared with isoflurane (3 µmol/l), and 26 patients had peak fluoride concentrations over 50 µmol/l, a concentration that is associated with renal dysfunction after methoxyflurane anesthesia. There were no significant differences in the renal function of the two groups, as measured by serum creatinine, urea, glycosuria, proteinuria, urine pH, or specific gravity. Absence of renal dysfunction, despite high serum fluoride concentrations after sevoflurane anesthesia, was consistent with previous reports. It appears that low fresh gas flow anesthesia with sevoflurane is not associated with clinically significant renal damage.

The role of aquaporins

Aquaporin-2 is a protein involved in regulation of water permeability in the kidneys. The effects of sevoflurane- and propofol-based anesthesia on urine concentrating ability and aquaporin-2 concentrations have been compared in 30 patients undergoing major surgical procedures given sevoflurane + nitrous oxide or propofol + nitrous oxide (45). Sevoflurane caused a transient 25% fall in aquaporin-2 concentrations 90 minutes after surgery, rather than the usual 40% increase, which occurred in the propofol group. By 3 hours after surgery the aquaporin concentrations in the sevoflurane group had increased and were similar to those in the propofol group. There was a 40% fall in urine osmolarity in the sevoflurane group, but recovery occurred by 3 hours postoperatively. This effect is the likely cause of the occasional cases of polyuria reported in association with sevoflurane anesthesia, rather than nephrotoxicity caused by fluoride ion or compound A.

Musculoskeletal

There have been reports of rhabdomyolysis after anesthesia with halothane, enflurane, and isoflurane in patients with muscular dystrophy, in whom suxamethonium was not used. Rhabdomyolysis has also been reported after sevoflurane anesthesia (46).

- An 11-year-old boy with Duchenne's muscular dystrophy underwent strabismus repair. He also had asthma, for which he was taking prednisone 25 mg/day and theophylline. He underwent inhalational induction with sevoflurane 4% and nitrous oxide 64%; tracheal intubation was then performed without the use of a muscle relaxant. Anesthesia was maintained using sevoflurane 1.5–3.0% and nitrous oxide 64%. He also received hydrocortisone 100 mg and diclofenac 25 mg. The operation lasted 51 minutes and anesthesia was uneventful. He suffered heel pain during the first few hours postoperatively, and 3 hours postoperatively passed 300 ml of dark red urine, containing large amounts of myoglobin. His serum enzymes increased from preoperative values, serum aspartate transaminase from 76 to 458 IU/l, alanine transaminase from 136 to 254 IU/l, and creatine kinase from 4430 to 55 700 IU/l. He was treated with dantrolene 1 mg/kg and recovered over the next day.

The history and finding in this case are strongly diagnostic of rhabdomyolysis. The most likely cause of rhabdomyolysis in this patient was thought to be inhalation of sevoflurane.

Rhabdomyolysis triggered by sevoflurane in a child with Duchenne muscular dystrophy has been reported in one case (47).

Body temperature

Malignant hyperthermia has occurred in people treated with sevoflurane.

- In the case of a 4-year-old girl, dantrolene was effective; susceptibility to malignant hyperthermia was later confirmed by muscle biopsy (48).
- A 28-year-old man, who developed malignant hyperthermia after anesthesia induced with isoflurane and maintained with sevoflurane, died 4 days later, despite cooling and intravenous dantrolene (49).

Other cases of malignant hyperthermia have been reported in patients who received sevoflurane (50,51). Although it is highly likely that sevoflurane caused malignant hyperpyrexia in these cases, suxamethonium was also given and was also a suspect.

Of two other cases (52,53), the second was remarkable, in that the specific-treatment dantrolene was not available, and yet the patient survived with aggressive active cooling and general supportive measures, including sodium bicarbonate.

In more than 3000 cases in Japan, there were two cases of malignant hyperthermia, one fatal (49). In this case isoflurane had been used early in anesthesia, and could have been at least in part responsible. There was some reason to consider that the patient, a 12-year-old girl, had a family propensity to malignant hyperthermia, as indicated by higher resting Pi/Pcr values. However, sevoflurane itself can trigger malignant hyperthermia in swine (54).

Susceptibility Factors

Renal disease

It has been thought that patients with chronically impaired renal function might be at increased risk of nephrotoxicity due to sevoflurane, because of an increased fluoride load due to reduced excretion. However, this was not confirmed in 41 patients undergoing elective surgery, with a stable increased preoperative serum creatinine concentration, who were randomly allocated to receive sevoflurane ($n = 21$) or enflurane ($n = 20$) at a fresh gas inflow rate of 4 l/minute for

maintenance of anesthesia (55). Peak serum inorganic fluoride concentrations were significantly higher after sevoflurane than after enflurane anesthesia. Laboratory measures of renal function remained stable throughout the postoperative period in both groups. No patient had permanent deterioration of pre-existing renal insufficiency and none required dialysis.

Other features of the patient

Insulinoma

- A 56-year-old woman with insulinoma, operated under sevoflurane anesthesia, had an uneventful perioperative course, and the authors suggested that sevoflurane suppressed the spontaneous release of insulin (56).

Sevoflurane may therefore be useful for anesthesia in patients with insulinoma.

Transplantation

- A 29-year-old man was anesthetized after renal transplantation with sevoflurane + nitrous oxide + oxygen for replacement of the head of the left femur (57). His serum fluoride concentration was always below 40 μmol/l and sevoflurane had little effect on the transplanted kidney.

It seems therefore that sevoflurane might be suitable for patients with renal transplants.

Drug–Drug Interactions

Dexmedetomidine

In 45 adult patients undergoing elective surgery, the α_2-adrenoceptor agonist dexmedetomidine in a concentration of 0.7 ng/ml reduced the minimum alveolar concentration of sevoflurane required to suppress movement to skin incision by 17%, but a plasma concentration of 0.39 ng/ml had no effect (58). The larger reductions in isoflurane requirements found in earlier studies of dexmedetomidine were probably due to the use of potent opioids and intravenous induction as part of the anesthetic.

Fentanyl

The minimum alveolar concentrations of sevoflurane required to suppress movements and adrenergic responses to surgery in the presence of the potent opioid fentanyl have been quantified in 226 adults (59). Fentanyl 3 ng/ml and 6 ng/ml reduced sevoflurane requirements to suppress movement to pain by 61% and 74%, respectively, and requirements to suppress the adrenergic responses to pain by 83% and 91%, respectively. There was no further reduction in sevoflurane requirements at concentrations of fentanyl above 6 ng/ml. The degree of interaction was similar to that seen in previous studies of other volatile anesthetic + opioid combinations.

Ketorolac

Ketorolac, which can cause renal vasoconstriction by inhibiting cyclo-oxygenase, is often given to patients anesthetized with sevoflurane, which is also potentially nephrotoxic. The effect of ketorolac has been assessed in a placebo-controlled, randomized study in 30 women undergoing breast surgery with sevoflurane anesthesia (60). There were no differences in several markers of renal injury in those who did or did not receive ketorolac.

Probenecid

The effect of the uricosuric agent probenecid in prolonged sevoflurane anesthesia has been examined in 64 patients randomized to receive high-flow or low-flow anesthesia with sevoflurane with or without preoperative oral probenecid (61). There were no differences in urea, creatinine, or creatinine clearance among the treatments. However, patients who received low-flow sevoflurane had some evidence of renal tubular injury (raised urinary markers) compared with those who received either high-flow anesthesia or probenecid.

References

1. Goldberg ME, Larijani GE, Eger EI 2nd. Peripheral neuropathy in healthy men volunteers anesthetized with 1.25 MAC sevoflurane for 8 hours Pharmacotherapy 1999;19(10):1173–6.
2. Kharasch ED. Compound A: Toxikologie und klinische Relevanz. [Compound A: toxicology and clinical relevance.] Anaesthesist 1998;47(Suppl 1):S7–S10.
3. Kikura M, Ikeda K. Comparison of effects of sevoflurane/nitrous oxide and enflurane/nitrous oxide on myocardial contractility in humans. Load-independent and noninvasive assessment with transesophageal echocardiography. Anesthesiology 1993;79(2):235–43.
4. Kitahata H, Tanaka K, Kimura H, Saito T. [Effects of sevoflurane on left ventricular diastolic function using transesophageal echocardiography.] Masui 1993;42(3):358–64.
5. Ebert TJ, Harkin CP, Muzi M. Cardiovascular responses to sevoflurane: a review. Anesth Analg 1995;81(Suppl 6):S11–22.
6. Malan TP Jr, DiNardo JA, Isner RJ, Frink EJ Jr, Goldberg M, Fenster PE, Brown EA, Depa R, Hammond LC, Mata H. Cardiovascular effects of sevoflurane compared with those of isoflurane in volunteers. Anesthesiology 1995;83(5):918–28.
7. Townsend P, Stokes MA. Bradycardia during rapid inhalation induction with sevoflurane in children. Br J Anaesth 1998;80(3):410.
8. Sigston PE, Jenkins AM, Jackson EA, Sury MR, Mackersie AM, Hatch DJ. Rapid inhalation induction in children: 8% sevoflurane compared with 5% halothane. Br J Anaesth 1997;78(4):362–5.
9. Green DH, Townsend P, Bagshaw O, Stokes MA. Nodal rhythm and bradycardia during inhalation induction with sevoflurane in infants: a comparison of incremental and high-concentration techniques. Br J Anaesth 2000;85(3):368–70.
10. Maruyama K, Agata H, Ono K, Hiroki K, Fujihara T. Slow induction with sevoflurane was associated with complete atrioventricular block in a child with hypertension, renal dysfunction, and impaired cardiac conduction. Paediatr Anaesth 1998;8(1):73–8.
11. Kleinsasser A, Loeckinger A, Lindner KH, Keller C, Boehler M, Puehringer F. Reversing sevoflurane-associated Q-Tc prolongation by changing to propofol. Anaesthesia 2001;56(3):248–50.
12. Abe K, Takada K, Yoshiya I. Intraoperative torsade de pointes ventricular tachycardia and ventricular fibrillation during sevoflurane anesthesia. Anesth Analg 1998;86(4):701–2.
13. Walpole R, Olday J, Haetzman M, Drummond GB, Doyle E. A comparison of the respiratory effects of high concentrations of halothane and sevoflurane. Paediatr Anaesth 2001;11(2):157–60.
14. Takahashi H, Murata K, Ikeda K. Sevoflurane does not increase intracranial pressure in hyperventilated dogs. Br J Anaesth 1993;71(4):551–5.
15. Kitaguchi K, Ohsumi H, Kuro M, Nakajima T, Hayashi Y. Effects of sevoflurane on cerebral circulation and metabolism in patients with ischemic cerebrovascular disease. Anesthesiology 1993;79(4):704–9.
16. Bernard JM, Le Roux D, Pereon Y. Acute dystonia during sevoflurane induction. Anesthesiology 1999;90(4):1215–16.
17. Kaisti KK, Jaaskelainen SK, Rinne JO, Metsahonkala L, Scheinin H. Epileptiform discharges during 2 MAC sevoflurane anesthesia in two healthy volunteers. Anesthesiology 1999;91(6):1952–5.
18. Schultz B, Schultz A, Grouven U, Korsch G. Epilepsietypische EEG-Aktivitat: Auftreten bei Sevofluran-anflutung und nicht unter Propofolapplikation. [Epileptoform EEG activity: occurrence under sevoflurane and not during propofol application.] Anaesthesist 2001;50(1):43–5.
19. Conreux F, Best O, Preckel MP, Lhopitault C, Beydon L, Pouplard F, Granry JC. Effects electroencephalograhiques du sevoflurane a l'induction chez le jeune enfant: etude prospective sur 20 cas. [Electroencephalographic effects of sevoflurane in pediatric anesthesia: a prospective study of 20 cases.] Ann Fr Anesth Reanim 2001;20(5):438–45.
20. Schultz A, Schultz B, Grouven U, Korsch G. Epileptiform activity in the EEGs of two nonepileptic children under sevoflurane anaesthesia. Anaesth Intensive Care 2000;28(2):205–7.
21. Ohkoshi N, Shoji S. Reversible ageusia induced by losartan: a case report. Eur J Neurol 2002;9(3):315.
22. Terasako K, Ishii S. Postoperative seizure-like activity following sevoflurane anesthesia. Acta Anaesthesiol Scand 1996;40(8 Pt 1):953–4.
23. Hilty CA, Drummond JC. Seizure-like activity on emergence from sevoflurane anesthesia. Anesthesiology 2000;93(5):1357–9.
24. Cara DM, Armory P, Mahajan RP. Prolonged duration of neuromuscular block with rapacuronium in the presence of sevoflurane. Anesth Analg 2000;91(6):1392–3.
25. Wells LT, Rasch DK. Emergence "delirium" after sevoflurane anesthesia: a paranoid delusion? Anesth Analg 1999;88(6):1308–10.
26. Kulka PJ, Bressem M, Tryba M. Clonidine prevents sevoflurane-induced agitation in children. Anesth Analg 2001;93(2):335–8.
27. Tabak F, Mert A, Ozaras R, Biyikli M, Ozturk R, Ozbay G, Senturk H, Aktuglu Y. Losartan-induced hepatic injury. J Clin Gastroenterol 2002;34(5):585–6.
28. Neunteufl T, Berger R, Pacher R. Endothelin receptor antagonists in cardiology clinical trials. Expert Opin Investig Drugs 2002;11(3):431–43.
29. Kulka PJ, Bressem M, Wiebalck A, Tryba M. Prophylaxe des "Postsevoflurandelirs" mit Midazolam. [Prevention of "post-sevoflurane delirium" with midazolam.] Anaesthesist 2001;50(6):401–5.
30. Hasegawa J, Mitsuhata H, Matsumoto S, Komatsu H, Mizunuma T. [The effects of induced hypotension with sevoflurane and PGE_1 on liver functions during neurosurgery.] Masui 1992;41(5):772–8.
31. Watanabe K, Hatakenaka S, Ikemune K, Chigyo Y, Kubozono T, Arai T. [A case of suspected liver dysfunction induced by sevoflurane anesthesia.] Masui 1993;42(6):902–5.
32. Kharasch ED, Frink EJ Jr, Artru A, Michalowski P, Rooke GA, Nogami W. Long-duration low-flow

sevoflurane and isoflurane effects on postoperative renal and hepatic function. Anesth Analg 2001;93(6):1511–20.

33. Goeters C, Reinhardt C, Gronau E, Wusten R, Prien T, Baum J, Vrana S, Van Aken H. Minimal flow sevoflurane and isoflurane anaesthesia and impact on renal function. Eur J Anaesthesiol 2001;18(1):43–50.

34. Higuchi H, Adachi Y, Wada H, Kanno M, Satoh T. Comparison of plasma alpha glutathione S-transferase concentrations during and after low-flow sevoflurane or isoflurane anaesthesia. Acta Anaesthesiol Scand 2001;45(10):1226–9.

35. Pertek JP, Le Chaffotec L, Cormier L, Champigneulle J, Omar-Amrani M, Meistelman C. Effects of sevoflurane and isoflurane or desflurane on kidney structure and function in patients undergoing nephrectomy. Cah Anesthesiol 1999;47:365–70.

36. Ishikawa M, Miyazaki M, Ohta Y. Transient renal tubular dysfunction in a patient with severe asthmatic attack treated with sevoflurane. J Anesth 2001;15(1):49–52.

37. Mazze RI, Callan CM, Galvez ST, Delgado-Herrera L, Mayer DB. The effects of sevoflurane on serum creatinine and blood urea nitrogen concentrations: a retrospective, twenty-two-center, comparative evaluation of renal function in adult surgical patients. Anesth Analg 2000;90(3):683–8.

38. Story DA, Poustie S, Liu G, McNicol PL. Changes in plasma creatinine concentration after cardiac anesthesia with isoflurane, propofol, or sevoflurane: a randomized clinical trial. Anesthesiology 2001;95(4):842–8.

39. Higuchi H, Sumita S, Wada H, Ura T, Ikemoto T, Nakai T, Kanno M, Satoh T. Effects of sevoflurane and isoflurane on renal function and on possible markers of nephrotoxicity. Anesthesiology 1998;89(2):307–22.

40. Higuchi H, Adachi Y. Renal function in surgical patients after administration of low-flow sevoflurane and amikacin. J Anesth 2002;16(1):17–22.

41. Kobayashi Y, Ochiai R, Takeda J, Sekiguchi H, Fukushima K. Serum and urinary inorganic fluoride concentrations after prolonged inhalation of sevoflurane in humans. Anesth Analg 1992;74(5):753–7.

42. McGrath BJ, Hodgins LR, DeBree A, Frink EJ Jr, Nossaman BD, Bikhazi GB. A multicenter study evaluating the effects of sevoflurane on renal function in patients with renal insufficiency. J Cardiovasc Pharmacol Ther 1998;3(3):229–34.

43. Nishiyama T, Hanaoka K. Inorganic fluoride kinetics and renal and hepatic function after repeated sevoflurane anesthesia. Anesth Analg 1998;87(2):468–73.

44. Groudine SB, Fragen RJ, Kharasch ED, Eisenman TS, Frink EJ, McConnell S, Ebert TJ, Muzi M, Hannon V, Jellish WS, Johnson JO, Jones RM, Sebel PS, Vinik HR, Boyd G. Comparison of renal function following anesthesia with low-flow sevoflurane and isoflurane. J Clin Anesth 1999;11(3):201–7.

45. Morita K, Otsuka F, Ogura T, Takeuchi M, Mizobuchi S, Yamauchi T, Makino H, Hirakawa M. Sevoflurane anaesthesia causes a transient decrease in aquaporin-2 and impairment of urine concentration. Br J Anaesth 1999;83(5):734–9.

46. Obata R, Yasumi Y, Suzuki A, Nakajima Y, Sato S. Rhabdomyolysis in association with Duchenne's muscular dystrophy. Can J Anaesth 1999;46(6):564–6.

47. Takahashi H, Shimokawa M, Sha K, Sakamoto T, Kawaguchi M, Kitaguchi K, Furuya H. [Sevoflurane can induce rhabdomyolysis in Duchenne's muscular dystrophy.] Masui 2002;51(2):190–2.

48. Otsuka H, Komura Y, Mayumi T, Yamamura T, Kemmotsu O, Mukaida K. Malignant hyperthermia during sevoflurane anesthesia in a child with central core disease. Anesthesiology 1991;75(4):699–701.

49. Ochiai R, Toyoda Y, Nishio I, Takeda J, Sekiguchi H, Fukushima K, Kohda E. Possible association of malignant

hyperthermia with sevoflurane anesthesia. Anesth Analg 1992;74(4):616–18.

50. Hoshino K, Yamashiro Y, Nitta K, Kawaguchi H, Fukui H, Ikeda M, Ooshima Y. A case of postoperative malignant hyperthermia after 15 hours induced anesthesia. Hiroshima J Anesth 1996;32:15–18.

51. Yamamoto Y, Tanaka H, Ikeda K. A case in which it was difficult to differentiate between malignant hyperthermia and thyroid storm. Anesth Resusc 1996;32S:85–9.

52. Massaro F, De Klerk DYJ, Snoeck MMJ. A case of malignant hyperthermia during use of sevoflurane. Ned Tijdschr Anesthesiol 2001;14:71–3.

53. Baris S, Karakaya D, Guldogus F, Sarihasan B, Tekat A. A case of malignant hyperthermia during sevoflurane anesthesia. Turk J Med Sci 2001;31:171–3.

54. Shulman M, Braverman B, Ivankovich AD, Gronert G. Sevoflurane triggers malignant hyperthermia in swine. Anesthesiology 1981;54(3):259–60.

55. Conzen PF, Nuscheler M, Melotte A, Verhaegen M, Leupolt T, Van Aken H, Peter K. Renal function and serum fluoride concentrations in patients with stable renal insufficiency after anesthesia with sevoflurane or enflurane. Anesth Analg 1995;81(3):569–75.

56. Matsumoto M, Sakai H. [Sevoflurane anesthesia for a patient with insulinoma.] Masui 1992;41(3):446–9.

57. Saitoh K, Hirabayashi Y, Fukuda H, Shimizu R. [Sevoflurane anesthesia in a patient following renal transplantation.] Masui 1993;42(5):746–9.

58. Fragen RJ, Fitzgerald PC. Effect of dexmedetomidine on the minimum alveolar concentration (MAC) of sevoflurane in adults age 55 to 70 years. J Clin Anesth 1999;11(6):466–70.

59. Katoh T, Kobayashi S, Suzuki A, Iwamoto T, Bito H, Ikeda K. The effect of fentanyl on sevoflurane requirements for somatic and sympathetic responses to surgical incision. Anesthesiology 1999;90(2):398–405.

60. Laisalmi M, Eriksson H, Koivusalo AM, Pere P, Rosenberg P, Lindgren L. Ketorolac is not nephrotoxic in connection with sevoflurane anesthesia in patients undergoing breast surgery. Anesth Analg 2001;92(4):1058–63.

61. Higuchi H, Wada H, Usui Y, Goto K, Kanno M, Satoh T. Effects of probenecid on renal function in surgical patients anesthetized with low-flow sevoflurane. Anesthesiology 2001;94(1):21–31.

Sfericase

General Information

Sfericase is a crystallized alkaline protease that breaks down various protein bases. It is given in enterolytic tablets containing 10 000 units of sfericase. It is prescribed in a dose of two tablets to be taken three times a day. In 73 patients with chronic respiratory diseases there were no significant adverse effects (1).

Reference

1. Itoh K, Kounou O, Morise M, Iwakura M, Misutani N, Katayama T, Senda Y, Hirano Y, Torii Y, Ogura Y, et al. Clinical effects of proteinase, sfericase (AI-794), on chronic bronchitis and similar diseases. Int J Clin Pharmacol Ther Toxicol 1984;22(1):32–8.

Sibutramine

See also Anorectic drugs

General Information

Sibutramine is an appetite suppressant that inhibits the re-uptake of noradrenaline and serotonin. It is used in the adjunctive management of obesity in individuals with a body mass index (BMI) of $30\,kg/m^2$ or more (and no associated co-morbidity) or in individuals with a BMI of $27\,kg/m^2$ or more in the presence of other risk factors such as type 2 diabetes or hypercholesterolemia.

The safety and efficacy of sibutramine 10 mg/day in 109 obese patients (BMI over $30\,kg/m^2$, ages 16–65 years) has been evaluated in a double-blind, placebo-controlled, parallel-group, prospective study over a period of 6 months (1). There was a significant loss of body weight and significantly reduced BMI and waist measurement. There were 45 adverse events in 32 patients taking sibutramine; the most frequent were dry mouth ($n = 19$), increased blood pressure ($n = 5$), constipation ($n = 5$), and tachycardia ($n = 5$); two patients withdrew owing to adverse events. There were 29 adverse events in 23 patients taking placebo, mainly increased blood pressure ($n = 11$) and dry mouth ($n = 10$). In contrast, in an earlier study (2) there was no significant increase in systolic or diastolic blood pressures or heart rate.

Although serious adverse events have not been reported, there is no evidence of the long-term safety of sibutramine (3). Several new randomized clinical trials have assessed long-term weight reduction efficacy, tolerability, and safety of sibutramine. In a 1-year placebo-controlled study in primary care, sibutramine 10 mg/day ($n = 122$) or 15 mg/day ($n = 123$) with dietary advice produced and maintained more weight loss than dietary advice alone (4). None of the patients taking sibutramine or placebo ($n = 114$) was withdrawn because of a raised blood pressure.

There were comparable results in 44 patients who took sibutramine 10 mg/day for 12 months in a double-blind, placebo-controlled, crossover design (5). After sibutramine withdrawal, the patients gained weight but did not reach baseline body weight. There were no significant adverse events of sibutramine withdrawal. Early sibutramine administration produced better effects than administration after a period of dieting.

Further trials have confirmed the efficacy of sibutramine as a weight-loss agent in doses of 10–20 mg/day. The benefit of sibutramine is not only in its ability to induce weight loss, but also in its ability to maintain the weight loss effect for up to 2 years. However, once sibutramine is withdrawn, weight gain commonly occurs. Thus, sibutramine is considered effective in the management of obese patients who require pharmacotherapy as part of a multimodal approach to weight reduction (6).

In a multicenter, double-blind, randomized, parallel-group, placebo-controlled trial in 22 European centers for specialist diabetes care over 6 months, sibutramine, in conjunction with moderate caloric restriction, enabled obese patients with type 2 diabetes taking sulfonylureas to achieve clinically significant weight loss (7). This was associated with additional improvement in glycemic control in a limited number of patients who lost at least 10% of their baseline body weight.

Sibutramine was approved in Italy in April 2001 but was taken off the market there on 6 March 2002, after 50 reported adverse reactions (mainly tachycardia, hypertension, and dysrhythmias, in seven cases serious), and two deaths from cardiac arrest (8). Subsequently, the Secretariat of the European Medicines Evaluation Agency began a comprehensive benefit : harm balance assessment of sibutramine, which remains on the market in several European countries; these include the UK (where there were 215 reports of 411 adverse events, 95 serious and 2 deaths) and France (where there were 99 reports of adverse events, 10 serious but no deaths). From February 1998 to September 2001, the Food and Drug Administration (FDA) in the USA received reports of 397 adverse events (143 cardiac dysrhythmias and 29 deaths, 19 due to cardiovascular causes, 10 involving people under 50 years of age, and 3 involving women under 30 years of age) (9). In Canada, 28 adverse reactions (mainly hypertension and dysrhythmias, but no deaths) were reported from December 2000 to February 2002, including one case of chest pain, one of stroke, and two of eye hemorrhage; in three of these cases, the patients were concurrently taking a contraindicated antidepressant (10). The safety of sibutramine needs further postmarketing surveillance.

In a placebo-controlled study, sibutramine 10 mg/day for 6 months caused weight loss and a reduction in left ventricular mass in 86 obese hypertensive patients, with no changes in blood pressure or antihypertensive therapy (11). Baseline investigations included echocardiography, 24-hour ambulatory blood pressure monitoring, and hepatic enzyme measurements. Compared with placebo, sibutramine produced a greater weight loss, an increase in heart rate, and a reduction in left ventricular mass/height index. The two groups had comparable increases in alkaline phosphatase activity and comparable adjustments in antihypertensive therapy. The most frequent adverse effects associated with sibutramine were dry mouth and arthralgia; higher frequencies of insomnia and irritability, as suggested in other studies, were not found. The alterations reported in alkaline phosphatase may be associated with mobilization of visceral adipose tissue (12) and cannot be attributed to the use of sibutramine.

Organs and Systems

Cardiovascular

Cardiovascular risk factors associated with obesity, including dyslipidemia, particularly raised triglyceride concentrations and reduced high-density lipoprotein concentrations, can be improved with weight loss during sibutramine treatment (4,5,13). In general, improvements in serum lipids are proportional to the degree of body weight loss, whether that weight loss occurs with sibutramine or with placebo (13,14).

In a study of the efficacy and safety of sibutramine in obese white and African Americans with hypertension, the most common adverse event resulting in withdrawal among those taking sibutramine was hypertension (5.3 versus 1.4% of patients taking placebo) (15).

The observation that sibutramine, which blocks the re-uptake of noradrenaline and serotonin and to a lesser extent dopamine (6), causes a raised blood pressure has been a cause of concern (1,16). Some insight into this problem and its magnitude comes from two recent studies (17,18). Most studies have shown a positive relation between blood pressure and weight (19). The failure of the blood pressure to fall with weight loss in normotensive and hypertensive patients treated with sibutramine differs from the fall seen with orlistat (20–22) or weight loss induced by life-style modifications (23,24). In the case of sibutramine, the potentially detrimental effect due to the failure of the blood pressure to fall with weight loss may be offset by the reductions in lipids, insulin, and uric acid that occur with weight loss (25).

Intermittent use of sibutramine has been proposed to reduce potential concerns about its effect on blood pressure. An alternative strategy would be to identify those patients who respond to sibutramine with weight loss but who have minimal changes in blood pressure (25).

The effects of sibutramine on weight loss, blood pressure, and pulse rate in hypertensive obese patients, whose blood pressure was well controlled with a beta-blocker either alone or with a thiazide diuretic, have been evaluated in a 12-week, double-blind, placebo-controlled, parallel-group, randomized study in 69 patients (17). Sibutramine was effective and well tolerated and did not exacerbate pre-existing hypertension controlled with beta-blockers. Despite the presence of apparently effective beta-blockade, there were modest increases in pulse rate in those who took sibutramine, suggesting that mechanisms other than increased sympathetic tone may, at least in part, mediate this effect. Based on the potential for increased blood pressure and pulse rate, obese patients with well-controlled hypertension who are taking sibutramine should be monitored periodically (17).

In a 52-week, multicenter, randomized, double-blind, placebo-controlled, parallel-group study in 220 hypertensive patients with obesity (BMI 27–40 kg/m^2), whose hypertension was well controlled with an angiotensin converting enzyme (ACE) inhibitor with or without a thiazide diuretic, sibutramine 20 mg/day safely and effectively achieved weight loss without compromising blood pressure control (18). Blood pressure remained in the target range in patients who took sibutramine or placebo, although sibutramine was associated with a small mean increase in blood pressure and a modest increase in pulse rate.

Drug–Drug Interactions

Citalopram

Hypomania in a unipolar depressed woman has been attributed to concomitant use of sibutramine and citalopram (26). The close temporal relation between the onset and the disappearance of hypomania with the introduction and withdrawal of sibutramine suggested a causal link. This report suggests that combining sibutramine with a serotonin re-uptake inhibitor could cause hypomania in people with unipolar major depressive disorder with a family history of bipolar disorder.

Finasteride

Soon after the introduction of finasteride to treat alopecia, a 30-year-old man taking sibutramine developed paranoid psychotic behavior (27). This drug interaction was demonstrated by careful clinical follow-up and the use of Naranjo's algorithm.

References

1. Fanghanel G, Cortinas L, Sanchez-Reyes L, Berber A. A clinical trial of the use of sibutramine for the treatment of patients suffering essential obesity. Int J Obes Relat Metab Disord 2000;24(2):144–50.
2. Lean ME. Sibutramine—a review of clinical efficacy. Int J Obes Relat Metab Disord 1997;21(Suppl. 1):S30–6.
3. Arterburn D, Noel PH. Extracts from "Clinical Evidence". Obesity BMJ 2001;322(7299):1406–9.
4. Smith IG, Goulder MA. On Behalf of the Members of the Sibutramine Clinical Study 1047 Team. Randomized placebo-controlled trial of long-term treatment with sibutramine in mild to moderate obesity. J Fam Pract 2001;50(6):505–12.
5. Fanghanel G, Cortinas L, Sanchez-Reyes L, Berber A. Second phase of a double-blind study clinical trial on sibutramine for the treatment of patients suffering essential obesity: 6 months after treatment cross-over. Int J Obes Relat Metab Disord 2001;25(5):741–7.
6. Luque CA, Rey JA. The discovery and status of sibutramine as an anti-obesity drug. Eur J Pharmacol 2002;440(2–3):119–28.
7. Serrano-Rios M, Melchionda N, Moreno-Carretero E. Spanish Investigators. Role of sibutramine in the treatment of obese Type 2 diabetic patients receiving sulphonylurea therapy. Diabet Med 2002;19(2):119–24.
8. Health Canada. Ottawa. Advisory: Health Canada investigates safety of Meridia (sibutramine). www.hc-sc.gc.ca/english/protection/warnings/2002/2002-21e.htm, 27/03/2002.
9. Wooltorton E. Obesity drug sibutramine (Meridia): hypertension and cardiac arrhythmias. CMAJ 2002;166(10):1307–8.
10. Deitel M. Sibutramine warning: hypertension and cardiac arrhythmias reported. Obes Surg 2002;12(3):422.
11. Faria AN, Ribeiro Filho FF, Lerario DD, Kohlmann N, Ferreira SR, Zanella MT. Effects of sibutramine on the treatment of obesity in patients with arterial hypertension. Arq Bras Cardiol 2002;78(2):172–80.
12. Luyckx FH, Desaive C, Thiry A, Dewe W, Scheen AJ, Gielen JE, Lefebvre PJ. Liver abnormalities in severely obese subjects: effect of drastic weight loss after gastroplasty. Int J Obes Relat Metab Disord 1998;22(3):222–6.
13. Dujovne CA, Zavoral JH, Rowe E, Mendel CM. Sibutramine Study Group. Effects of sibutramine on body weight and serum lipids: a double-blind, randomized, placebo-controlled study in 322 overweight and obese patients with dyslipidemia. Am Heart J 2001;142(3):489–97.
14. Toubro S, Hansen DL, Hilsted JC, Porsborg PA, Astrup AV. STORM Study Group. Effekt af sibutramin til vaegttabsvedligeholdelse: en randomiseret klinisk kontrolleret undersogelse. [The effect of sibutramine for the maintenance of weight loss: a randomized controlled clinical trial.] Ugeskr Laeger 2001;163(21):2935–40.
15. McMahon FG, Fujioka K, Singh BN, Mendel CM, Rowe E, Rolston K, Johnson F, Mooradian AD. Efficacy and safety of sibutramine in obese white and African American patients with hypertension: a 1-year, double-blind,

placebo-controlled, multicenter trial. Arch Intern Med 2000;160(14):2185–91.

16. James WP, Astrup A, Finer N, Hilsted J, Kopelman P, Rossner S, Saris WH, Van Gaal LF. STORM Study Group. Effect of sibutramine on weight maintenance after weight loss: a randomised trial. Sibutramine Trial of Obesity Reduction and Maintenance. Lancet 2000;356(9248):2119–25.

17. Sramek JJ, Leibowitz MT, Weinstein SP, Rowe ED, Mendel CM, Levy B, McMahon FG, Mullican WS, Toth PD, Cutler NR. Efficacy and safety of sibutramine for weight loss in obese patients with hypertension well controlled by beta-adrenergic blocking agents: a placebo-controlled, double-blind, randomised trial J Hum Hypertens 2002;16(1):13–19.

18. McMahon FG, Weinstein SP, Rowe E, Ernst KR, Johnson F, Fujioka K. Sibutramine in Hypertensives Clinical Study Group. Sibutramine is safe and effective for weight loss in obese patients whose hypertension is well controlled with angiotensin-converting enzyme inhibitors. J Hum Hypertens 2002;16(1):5–11.

19. Cutler JA. Randomized clinical trials of weight reduction in nonhypertensive persons. Ann Epidemiol 1991;1(4):363–70.

20. Rossner S, Sjostrom L, Noack R, Meinders AE, Noseda G. European Orlistat Obesity Study Group. Weight loss, weight maintenance, and improved cardiovascular risk factors after 2 years treatment with orlistat for obesity. Obes Res 2000;8(1):49–61.

21. Davidson MH, Hauptman J, DiGirolamo M, Foreyt JP, Halsted CH, Heber D, Heimburger DC, Lucas CP, Robbins DC, Chung J, Heymsfield SB. Weight control and risk factor reduction in obese subjects treated for 2 years with orlistat: a randomized controlled trial. JAMA 1999;281(3):235–42.

22. Hauptman J, Lucas C, Boldrin MN, Collins H, Segal KR. Orlistat in the long-term treatment of obesity in primary care settings. Arch Fam Med 2000;9(2):160–7.

23. Stamler R, Stamler J, Grimm R, Gosch FC, Elmer P, Dyer A, Berman R, Fishman J, Van Heel N, Civinelli J, Mc Donald A. Nutritional therapy for high blood pressure. Final report of a four-year randomized controlled trial—the Hypertension Control Program. JAMA 1987;257(11):1484–91.

24. Anonymous. The Hypertension Prevention Trial: three-year effects of dietary changes on blood pressure. Hypertension Prevention Trial Research Group. Arch Intern Med 1990;150(1):153–62.

25. Bray GA. Sibutramine and blood pressure: a therapeutic dilemma. J Hum Hypertens 2002;16(1):1–3.

26. Benazzi F. Organic hypomania secondary to sibutramine–citalopram interaction. J Clin Psychiatry 2002;63(2):165.

27. Sucar DD, Sougey EB, Neto JB. Psychotic episode induced by potential drug interaction of sibutramine and finasteride. Rev Bras Psiquiatr 2002;24:30–3.

Sildenafil

General Information

Sildenafil is a potent inhibitor of phosphodiesterase type V, and therefore of the breakdown of cyclic guanosine monophosphate (cGMP) in the corpora cavernosa. The increased concentration of cGMP leads to nitric oxide-mediated relaxation of the smooth muscle cells and vasodilatation in the corpus cavernosum, which is essential for normal erection. Thus, sildenafil increases the penile response to sexual stimulation and is effective in erectile dysfunction (1,2).

The main adverse effects reported in clinical studies were flushing, headache, dyspepsia, visual disturbances, and rhinitis, some of which show that vasodilatation is not confined to the corpora cavernosa. They were mild, and only 1–2% of the patients discontinued sildenafil because of adverse effects.

The adverse effects of a single dose of sildenafil 50 mg have been evaluated in a placebo-controlled study in 40 young healthy volunteers (3). The most commonly reported adverse effects with sildenafil and placebo respectively were flushing (75 and 0%), headache (50 and 5%), and dyspepsia (15 and 5%). This adverse effects profile was similar to that observed in clinical trials. Heart rate changed significantly, but blood pressure did not.

There have been several case reports of the use of sildenafil to ameliorate rebound pulmonary hypertension (4).

- A six-week-old 3.1 kg girl developed severe pulmonary hypertension and systemic hypotension after the removal of a bilateral pulmonary vein obstruction due to a left atrial membrane. Nitric oxide 20 ppm reduced the pulmonary arterial pressure from 57 to 33 mmHg, and plasma cGMP concentrations increased from 12 nmol/l at baseline to 28 nmol/l with nitric oxide. After three unsuccessful weaning attempts, due to rebound, sildenafil 1 mg was given via a nasogastric tube and nitric oxide was withdrawn 90 minutes later, with minimal increase in pulmonary artery pressure and a rise in cGMP concentration to 45 nmol/l.

- A 3.5 kg newborn girl, who underwent corrective surgery for an infradiaphragmatic totally anomalous pulmonary venous connection, had postoperative systemic hypotension, low cardiac output, and pulmonary hypertension. Inhaled nitric oxide 20 ppm improved her pulmonary hemodynamics but could not be withdrawn by the third postoperative day, owing to reflex pulmonary hypertension. Sildenafil 1 mg via nasogastric tube again allowed withdrawal of nitric oxide, with preservation of plasma cGMP concentrations above baseline.

- A 4-month-old 4.1 kg boy with severe bilateral pulmonary vein stenosis developed moderate pulmonary hypertension after surgical revision. Sildenafil 1.1 mg via nasogastric tube did not increase the plasma cGMP concentration or reduce the rebound effect.

The authors suggested that in this case the effect of sildenafil may have been reduced by impaired gastrointestinal absorption. They speculated that exogenous nitric oxide inhibits nitric oxide synthase activity, with a consequent reduction in pulmonary vascular smooth muscle cGMP concentration. Phosphodiesterase type V inhibitors, such as sildenafil, increase cGMP concentration and ameliorate the rebound effect.

Organs and Systems

Cardiovascular

In several reviews, in which the same data have been analysed, sildenafil has been rated as being well tolerated

(5,6) and extremely safe (7). Concerns about its cardio-vascular safety profile have stemmed primarily from sporadic reports of myocardial infarction and stroke.

- One patient without a history of previous chest pain or risk factors for cardiovascular disease, developed a well-documented myocardial infarction 30 minutes after he took sildenafil 50 mg and before any attempt at sexual intercourse (8).

The interpretation of these sporadic cases is controversial, although some have argued that the reported cardiovascular adverse effects occur more often with sildenafil than with other pharmacological treatments of erectile dysfunction. It is at present unclear whether there is an increased risk with sildenafil. For example, in placebo-controlled trials there have been no differences in the incidences of myocardial infarction, angina, or coronary artery disorders between sildenafil and placebo (9). Exclusion criteria in clinical trials may have prevented the inclusion of patients who are at increased risk of adverse events. On the other hand, sexual activity itself increases cardiac workload and the risk of myocardial infarction. Patients with cardiovascular disease should be cautious in their use of sildenafil.

Cardiac dysrhythmias have been reported in patients who have taken sildenafil.

- A 54-year-old man with hypertrophic cardiomyopathy, for which he took verapamil, felt unwell after a single tablet of sildenafil (10). Holter monitoring after repeat sildenafil showed an increase in ventricular extra beats and episodes of non-sustained ventricular tachycardia. On echocardiography, left ventricular dimensions were reduced and the subaortic gradient was markedly increased.
- Two other patients with severely depressed left ventricular function developed ventricular tachycardia (11).

Ear, nose, throat

Two men developed prolonged epistaxis a few hours after taking sildenafil 50 mg to enhance their sexual performance (before the nose bleeding started); both had well-controlled hypertension (12). Epistaxis is not an unusual problem in elderly people with hypertension, and venous engorgement is thought to be the main causative factor. Whether this is amplified by sildenafil (and/or by sexual activity) is an open question.

Nervous system

Clinical trials of sildenafil have not shown increased risks of stroke or myocardial infarction. However, postmarketing drug surveillance programs have mentioned strokes associated with sildenafil, and case reports have been published.

- A 50-year-old man took sildenafil 50 mg, and 2 hours later developed a right-sided hemiparesis and altered hemibody sensation, a right-facial paresis, and slurred speech (13). The symptoms gradually disappeared 4 hours later, but recurred the next week when he took sildenafil 100 mg. On the second occasion the symptoms did not resolve, and an MRI scan showed a recent infarct in the left internal capsule and lateral

thalamus. No other cause of the stroke was found by evaluation of the heart and extracranial vessels. The symptoms gradually improved over 6 months.
- A 44-year-old man developed a severe headache and vomiting after taking four tablets of sildenafil (of unknown strength) followed by sexual intercourse (14). A CT scan showed a left-sided temporal intracranial hemorrhage. He died of cerebral edema and pneumonia a few days later. Autopsy showed no vascular abnormality.
- A 67-year-old man took two tablets of sildenafil 25 mg 1 hour apart (15). He complained of headache, confusion, and nervousness after the first tablet, his symptoms increased, and he developed language difficulty after the second tablet. He did not have sexual intercourse. A few days later, an MRI scan showed a large left temporal subcortical hemorrhage. The symptoms resolved partially over a few days.

Whereas the suspected mechanism for ischemic stroke is analogous to that leading to myocardial infarction (hypoperfusion distal to a critical lesion), intracerebral bleeding (14,15) may be more difficult to explain. The authors considered the likelihood of sildenafil-induced spontaneous intracerebral hemorrhage due to the vasodilatory effects of the drug on the cerebral vasculature (as evidenced by headache, flushing, and nasal congestion).

- A third-nerve palsy occurred 36 hours after a second dose of sildenafil in a 56-year-old man.

The authors suggested that sildenafil had caused systemic hypotension sufficient to cause neurological dysfunction, but 36 hours is a long lag time for a drug with a half-life of only a few hours (16).

Unexpected functional disturbances, which occur shortly after the use of sildenafil, are likely to be attributed to the drug.

- A 51-year-old man had transient global amnesia 30 minutes after taking sildenafil 25 mg (17).
- A 79-year-old man had acute vertigo, vomiting, and tinnitus resembling vestibular neuronitis 2 hours after first taking 50 mg; the symptoms lasted for 24 hours (18).
- Generalized tonic-clonic seizures have been reported after a first 50 mg tablet in two men aged 54 and 63, neither of whom had organic brain lesions on imaging; one had tonic-clonic seizures again on rechallenge with the drug 3 months later (19).

Sensory systems

Sildenafil has weak inhibitory effects on phosphodiesterase type V in the retina, leading to temporary changes in the perception of color hue and brightness. The importance of reversible changes in the electroretinogram observed in volunteers after sildenafil 100 mg, ascribed to inhibition of phosphodiesterase type 5 in the retina, is unclear (20–22).

There have been reports of a temporal association between vascular events in the eye and sildenafil administration.

- A fit, healthy, 69-year-old man presented with sudden painless loss of vision in the left eye a few hours after taking sildenafil 100 mg (23). Fundus examination showed occlusion of a branch of the retinal artery. No cardiovascular abnormality was detected.

- A 52-year-old man developed sweating, headache, and blurred vision in his left eye 1 hour after a first dose of sildenafil 50 mg (24). The same symptoms recurred on the next night, after a second dose of sildenafil. Fundoscopy a few days later showed an ischemic optic neuropathy.
- A 42-year-old man presented with anterior ischemic optic neuropathy, leading to a visual field defect in that eye within 24 hours of having taken sildenafil (25).

Anterior ischemic optic neuropathy is a disorder whose pathophysiology is poorly understood. The difference between the intraocular pressure and the perfusion pressure in the posterior ciliary arteries determines the circulation in the optic disc, and a reduction in this difference may contribute to ischemia.

Several other cases of non-arteritic ischemic optic neuropathy have been reported in men taking sildenafil (26,27).

Liver

- A 68-year-old man with alcoholic cirrhosis and small esophageal varices (degree of severity classified as Child I) started bleeding after taking sildenafil 25 mg for the first time (28).

Sudden overload of the portal venous system related to splanchnic vasodilatation was a possible provoking factor in this case. Gastroesophageal reflux secondary to a lower esophageal sphincter tone and causing mucosal erosion was an alternative explanation.

Sexual function

Whereas priapism has not been reported with sildenafil in controlled clinical trials, it is being mentioned in postmarketing drug surveillance programs, and two case reports have appeared in a healthy young man and a patient with sickle cell trait (29,30).

Death

There has been debate on the risk of death after sildenafil: can it be entirely attributed to co-existing cardiovascular disease with an inherent high risk of mortality, particularly during sexual activity, or does the drug contribute (31,32).

- A 44-year-old man developed an acute myocardial infarction after taking sildenafil but before sexual intercourse (33).

This case appears to point to the drug as a potential trigger in people with unknown critical coronary lesions

A postmarketing survey over the first 6 months of sales of sildenafil in the USA (April to the middle of November 1998) has reported details on 130 patients who died after having been given sildenafil (over 3.5 million having received a prescription for it). As expected, deaths were mostly cardiovascular. There was a close time relation to the administration of sildenafil (within 4–5 hours) in 44 patients, 27 of whom died during or immediately after sexual intercourse. The disturbing finding was that 16 men also either took or were given

glyceryl trinitrate, contrary to product labeling and to several warnings (34). A survey conducted in the UK on recreational use of sildenafil among night-club customers detected combined use of sildenafil with amyl nitrate. As both drugs are vasodilators, combined use may expose users to the same risk as the combination with glyceryl trinitrate (35).

Long-Term Effects

Drug tolerance

Potential tachyphylaxis with long-term use of sildenafil has been discussed following a survey in which 200 patients were questioned twice, 2 years apart, about the effects of sildenafil; on the second occasion 20% of them reported needing an increased dose, and 17% had discontinued therapy because of lack of effect (36). However, others have commented that more likely reasons for the loss of effect over time included worsening of the disease (37–41), reducing testosterone concentrations with age (38,39), or lack of proper arousal (42). Although the mRNA for phosphodiesterase type 5 is down-regulated in the retina by long-term administration of sildenafil in rats (43), it is not known whether that happens in human corpus cavernosum, nor whether long-term sildenafil use is associated with tachyphylaxis.

Drug Administration

Drug overdose

A case of suspected overdose of sildenafil has been reported (44).

- A 56-year-old man with a history of diabetes mellitus and hypertension was found dead at home, with an empty package of sildenafil (12 tablets of 50 mg) near the body. The concentration of sildenafil in postmortem blood was high. Autopsy showed a dilated cardiomyopathy and diffuse coronary atherosclerosis, but an overdose of sildenafil was suspected to have provoked a fatal ventricular dysrhythmia.

Drug–Drug Interactions

Calcium channel blockers

Retrospective analysis of clinical trials has suggested that the concomitant use of antihypertensive drugs did not lead to an increase in adverse events in patients also taking sildenafil (45).

Hypertensive patients taking amlodipine, in contrast to glyceryl trinitrate, had only a minor supplementary fall in blood pressure when challenged with a single dose of sildenafil, and a few had a mild to moderate headache (46).

Diltiazem is metabolized by CYP3A4 and was held responsible for unanticipated prolonged hypotension after sublingual glyceryl trinitrate in a patient who underwent coronary angiography 2 days after last using sildenafil (47).

Indinavir

A drug interaction between sildenafil and HIV antiretroviral drugs is suspected, since both are metabolized by and act as inhibitors of the same cytochrome P450 isoforms (48). A pharmacokinetic study of sildenafil in HIV-positive patients taking indinavir has shown that the AUC of sildenafil was 4.4 times higher than data from historical controls (49). The magnitude of the interaction suggested that a lower starting dose of sildenafil may be more appropriate in patients taking indinavir.

Nitrates

The concomitant use of nitrates and sildenafil can precipitate a hypotensive reaction, and this combination should therefore be avoided (50,51). More than 3.6 million prescriptions for sildenafil were issued as of August 1998; of 69 deaths, 12 were attributable to the interaction with nitrates, as reported to the FDA.

Potentiation by sildenafil of the hypotensive effects of glyceryl trinitrate and amlodipine has been investigated. The fall in systolic blood pressure with glyceryl trinitrate was amplified four-fold by sildenafil in healthy subjects.

The pressure-lowering effect of a step-wise intravenous infusion of glyceryl trinitrate was significantly increased in 12 healthy volunteers treated for 4 days with sildenafil 25 mg tds; episodes of symptomatic hypotension were also more frequent with sildenafil (52). When sublingual glyceryl trinitrate was used, the reduction in systolic blood pressure was fourfold greater in association with sildenafil.

Tacrolimus

The effects of sildenafil can be potentiated by drugs that are metabolized by CYP3A4. Tacrolimus is an example. When sildenafil was given to patients with kidney transplants taking regular tacrolimus, peak concentrations were much higher and the half-life much longer than expected from data in healthy volunteers (53). However, an effect of the underlying disease and other concomitant drugs obviously could not be excluded.

References

1. Boolell M, Gepi-Attee S, Gingell JC, Allen MJ. Sildenafil, a novel effective oral therapy for male erectile dysfunction. Br J Urol 1996;78(2):257–61.
2. Goldstein I, Lue TF, Padma-Nathan H, Rosen RC, Steers WD, Wicker PA. Oral sildenafil in the treatment of erectile dysfunction. Sildenafil Study Group. N Engl J Med 1998;338(20):1397–404.
3. Dundar M, Kocak I, Dundar SO, Erol H. Evaluation of side effects of sildenafil in group of young healthy volunteers. Int Urol Nephrol 2001;32(4):705–8.
4. Atz AM, Wessel DL. Sildenafil ameliorates effects of inhaled nitric oxide withdrawal. Anesthesiology 1999;91(1):307–10.
5. Padma-nathan H, Eardley I, Kloner RA, Laties AM, Montorsi F. A 4-year update on the safety of sildenafil citrate (Viagra). Urology 2002;60(2 Suppl 2):67–90.
6. Fink HA, Mac Donald R, Rutks IR, Nelson DB, Wilt TJ. Sildenafil for male erectile dysfunction: a systematic review and meta-analysis. Arch Intern Med 2002;162(12):1349–60.
7. Lim PH, Moorthy P, Benton KG. The clinical safety of Viagra. Ann NY Acad Sci 2002;962:378–88.
8. Feenstra J, van Drie-Pierik RJ, Lacle CF, Stricker BH. Acute myocardial infarction associated with sildenafil. Lancet 1998;352(9132):957–8.
9. Morales A, Gingell C, Collins M, Wicker PA, Osterloh IH. Clinical safety of oral sildenafil citrate (Viagra) in the treatment of erectile dysfunction. Int J Impot Res 1998;10(2):69–73.
10. Stauffer JC, Ruiz V, Morard JD. subaortic obstruction after sildenafil in a patient with hypertrophic cardiomyopathy. N Engl J Med 1999;341(9):700–1.
11. Shah PK. Sildenafil in the treatment of erectile dysfunction. N Engl J Med 1998;339(10):699.
12. Hicklin LA, Ryan C, Wong DK, Hinton AE. Nose-bleeds after sildenafil (Viagra). J R Soc Med 2002;95(8):402–3.
13. Morgan JC, Alhatou M, Oberlies J, Johnston KC. Transient ischemic attack and stroke associated with sildenafil (Viagra) use. Neurology 2001;57(9):1730–1.
14. Buxton N, Flannery T, Wild D, Bassi S. Sildenafil (Viagra)-induced spontaneous intracerebral haemorrhage. Br J Neurosurg 2001;15(4):347–9.
15. Monastero R, Pipia C, Camarda LK, Camarda R. Intracerebral haemorrhage associated with sildenafil citrate. J Neurol 2001;248(2):141–2.
16. Wigley FM, Korn JH, Csuka ME, Medsger TA Jr, Rothfield NF, Ellman M, Martin R, Collier DH, Weinstein A, Furst DE, Jimenez SA, Mayes MD, Merkel PA, Gruber B, Kaufman L, Varga J, Bell P, Kern J, Marrott P, White B, Simms RW, Phillips AC, Seibold JR. Oral iloprost treatment in patients with Raynaud's phenomenon secondary to systemic sclerosis: a multicenter, placebo-controlled, double-blind study. Arthritis Rheum 1998;41(4):670–7.
17. Savitz SA, Caplan LR. Transient global amnesia after sildenafil (Viagra) use. Neurology 2002;59(5):778.
18. Hamzavi J, Schmetterer L, Formanek M. Vestibular symptoms as a complication of sildenafil: a case report. Wien Klin Wochenschr 2002;114(1–2):54–5.
19. Gilad R, Lampl Y, Eshel Y, Sadeh M. Tonic–clonic seizures in patients taking sildenafil. BMJ 2002;325(7369):869.
20. Vobig MA, Klotz T, Staak M, Bartz-Schmidt KU, Engelmann U, Walter P. Retinal side-effects of sildenafil. Lancet 1999;353(9150):375.
21. Zrenner E. No cause for alarm over retinal side-effects of sildenafil. Lancet 1999;353(9150):340–1.
22. Vobig MA. Retinal side-effects of sildenafil. Lancet 1999;353(9162):1442.
23. Tripathi A, O'Donnell NP. Branch retinal artery occlusion; another complication of sildenafil. Br J Ophthalmol 2000;84(8):934–5.
24. Egan R, Pomeranz H. Sildenafil (Viagra) associated anterior ischemic optic neuropathy. Arch Ophthalmol 2000;118(2):291–2.
25. Payne B, Sasse B, Franzen D, Hailemariam S, Gemsenjager E. Manifold manifestations of ergotism. Schweiz Med Wochenschr 2000;130(33):1152–6.
26. Pomeranz HD, Smith KH, Hart WM Jr, Egan RA. Sildenafil-associated nonarteritic anterior ischemic optic neuropathy. Ophthalmology 2002;109(3):584–7.
27. Boshier A, Pambakian N, Shakir SA. A case of nonarteritic ischemic optic neuropathy (NAION) in a male patient taking sildenafil. Int J Clin Pharmacol Ther 2002;40(9):422–3.
28. Tzathas C, Christidou A, Ladas SD. Sildenafil (Viagra) is a risk factor for acute variceal bleeding. Am J Gastroenterol 2002;97(7):1856.
29. Sur RL, Kane CJ. Sildenafil citrate-associated priapism. Urology 2000;55(6):950.
30. Kassim AA, Fabry ME, Nagel RL. Acute priapism associated with the use of sildenafil in a patient with sickle cell trait. Blood 2000;95(5):1878–9.

31. Kloner RA. Cardiovascular risk and sildenafil. Am J Cardiol 2000;86(2A):F57–61.

32. Mitka M. Some men who take Viagra die—why? JAMA 2000;283(5):590, 593.

33. Muniz AE, Holstege CP. Acute myocardial infarction associated with sildenafil (Viagra) ingestion. Am J Emerg Med 2000;18(3):353–5.

34. Jackson G, Sweeney M, Osterloh IH. Sildenafil citrate (Viagra): a cardiovascular overview. Br J Cardiol 1999;6:325–33.

35. Aldridge J, Measham F. Sildenafil (Viagra) is used as a recreational drug in England. BMJ 1999;318(7184):669.

36. El-Galley R, Rutland H, Talic R, Keane T, Clark H. Long-term efficacy of sildenafil and tachyphylaxis effect. J Urol 2001;166(3):927–31.

37. Billups KL. Re: Long-term efficacy of sildenafil and tachyphylaxis effect. J Urol 2002;168(1):204–5.

38. Carson CC. Re: Long-term efficacy of sildenafil and tachyphylaxis effect. J Urol 2002;168(1):205.

39. Guay AT. Re: Long-term efficacy of sildenafil and tachyphylaxis effect. J Urol 2002;168(1):205–6.

40. Mumtaz FH, Khan MA, Mikhailidis DP, Morgan RJ. Long-term efficacy of sildenafil and tachyphylaxis effect. J Urol 2002;168(1):206.

41. Tomera K. Re: Long-term efficacy of sildenafil and tachyphylaxis effect. J Urol 2002;168(1):206.

42. Basson R, Robinow O. Re: Long-term efficacy of sildenafil and tachyphylaxis effect. J Urol 2002;168(1):204.

43. Steers WD. Tachyphylaxis and phosphodiesterase type 5 inhibitors. J Urol 2002;168(1):207.

44. Tracqui A, Miras A, Tabib A, Raul JS, Ludes B, Malicier D. Fatal overdosage with sildenafil citrate (Viagra): first report and review of the literature. Hum Exp Toxicol 2002;21(11):623–9.

45. Stauffer JC, Ruiz V, Morard JD. Subaortic obstruction after sildenafil in a patient with hypertrophic cardiomyopathy. N Engl J Med 1999;341(9):700–1.

46. Spencer CM, Gunasekara NS, Hills C. Zolmitriptan: a review of its use in migraine. Drugs 1999;58(2):347–74.

47. Khoury V, Kritharides L. Diltiazem-mediated inhibition of sildenafil metabolism may promote nitrate-induced hypotension. Aust NZ J Med 2000;30(5):641–2.

48. Granier I, Garcia E, Geissler A, Boespflug MD, Durand-Gasselin J. Postpartum cerebral angiopathy associated with the administration of sumatriptan and dihydroergotamine—a case report. Intensive Care Med 1999;25(5):532–4.

49. Liston H, Bennett L, Usher B Jr, Nappi J. The association of the combination of sumatriptan and methysergide in myocardial infarction in a premenopausal woman. Arch Intern Med 1999;159(5):511–13.

50. Kloner RA, Jarow JP. Erectile dysfunction and sildenafil citrate and cardiologists. Am J Cardiol 1999;83(4):576–82.

51. Cheitlin MD, Hutter AM Jr, Brindis RG, Ganz P, Kaul S, Russell RO Jr, Zusman RM. Use of sildenafil (Viagra) in patients with cardiovascular disease. Technology and Practice Executive Committee. Circulation 1999;99(1):168–77.

52. Webb DJ, Freestone S, Allen MJ, Muirhead GJ. Sildenafil citrate and blood-pressure-lowering drugs: results of drug interaction studies with an organic nitrate and a calcium antagonist. Am J Cardiol 1999;83(5A):C21–8.

53. Christ B, Brockmeier D, Hauck EW, Friemann S. Interactions of sildenafil and tacrolimus in men with erectile dysfunction after kidney transplantation. Urology 2001;58(4):589–93.

Silicone

General Information

Silicones are polymers of alternating atoms of silicon and oxygen, whose viscosity depends on the molecular weight: the longer the molecule the more viscous.

When silicones were used for the first time, more than 35 years ago, they were proposed as excellent, inert, seemingly harmless compounds (1) and they have been used in various medical applications, including the construction of joint prostheses and breast implants and in tissue augmentation procedures. However, reports of silicone-induced granulomatous reactions in man and animals subsequently appeared (2,3) and silicones were prohibited in many countries as cosmetic materials. However, silicones are nevertheless still used (4). The FDA has issued a ruling requiring the filing of a premarket approval application or a notice of completion of a product development protocol for silicone inflatable breast prostheses, a generic type of medical device intended to or reconstruct the female breast. This device is made of a silicone shell that is inflated with sterile isotonic saline (5). The agency has taken this action because the requirement of premarket approval will provide an opportunity to assess more fully the risks and benefits of these devices, in order to determine whether there is reasonable assurance of their safety and effectiveness, or what regulatory course should be taken in the absence of such assurance. Silicone gel-filled breast prostheses have already been subjected to this requirement.

Local complications have been associated with both types of breast prostheses, including rupture, pain, capsular contracture, disfigurement, and serious infection, which may lead to medical interventions and repeated surgery. The practice of injecting liquid silicone has largely been abandoned by plastic surgeons (6), but unfortunately there are still people who perform these injections injudiciously (7).

- A 26-year-old male-to-female transsexual received an injection of 100 ml of liquid silicone of unknown grade into her upper lateral thighs to gain female contours (8). Four years later she developed pain and a massively swollen right ankle with signs of inflammation. An MRI scan showed massive diffuse and localized silicone infiltration throughout the soft tissues of the legs.

This case provides further evidence that severe morbidity can be associated with the subcutaneous injection of large volumes of liquid silicone.

Silicone implants sometimes provoke systemic adverse effects. More than 20 women developed muscle pain, joint pain and swelling, pulmonary disease including pleural effusions, pulmonary infiltrates, and reduced pulmonary diffusing capacity, dry eyes, dysphagia, bladder dysfunction, neurological abnormalities, and skin disease (including localized and diffuse scleroderma-like changes) (9).

Organs and Systems

Sensory systems

Silicone oil injection has been used to treat retinal detachment. Six patients who had had previous silicone oil injection had the oil extracted, partial introduction of perfluorocarbon liquids, extraction of epiretinal membranes, endodiathermy, retinotomy, retinectomy, complete filling of the intraocular cavity with perfluorocarbon, endophotocoagulation, and silicone oil injection (10). All maintained the reattached retina. One developed a macular epiretinal membrane. Another developed a macular epiretinal membrane with subfoveal perfluorocarbon and a relapse of the retinal re-detachment when the silicone oil was extracted and it had to be re-introduced. Four of the patients developed different degrees of cataracts; the other two were aphakic.

Other reported complications include pupillary block glaucoma, secondary glaucoma, and corneal complications, including band-shaped keratopathy (11). Pupillary block in aphakic eyes can be prevented by placing peripheral iridectomy at the 6 o'clock position, since silicone is lighter than water.

After silicone injection, glaucoma is more common in diabetic aphakic eyes than in phakic or non-diabetic eyes; on the other hand, corneal complications are less frequent in diabetic than in non-diabetic eyes; in non-diabetic eyes the complications are more frequent in aphakic than in phakic eyes (11). In a 2-year-follow up study of 105 eyes (including 27 aphakic eyes), operated on for retinal detachment by silicone oil injection after pars plana vitrectomy, cataract was a constant complication in all phakic eyes (12). Intraocular hypertension was common in both phakic and aphakic eyes (30 and 33% of cases respectively) and responded poorly to medical or surgical treatment. Other complications occurred less often; they were corneal edema, conjunctival hyperemia, and uveitis. Pain required evisceration of 2 eyes.

A heavier-than-water fluorinated silicone oil was used in the treatment of 30 selected cases of complicated retinal detachment due to proliferative vitreoretinopathy ($n = 19$), proliferative diabetic retinopathy with traction detachment ($n = 2$), giant retinal tears ($n = 5$), ruptured globe with retinal detachment ($n = 2$), massive choroidal effusion with retinal detachment ($n = 1$), and acute retinal necrosis with retinal detachment ($n = 1$) (13). Initial retinal reattachment was achieved in all cases. Complications included redetachment ($n = 7$), cataract ($n = 6$), raised intraocular pressure ($n = 4$), hypotony ($n = 4$), keratopathy ($n = 3$), uveitis synechia formation ($n = 3$), phthisis ($n = 2$), choroidal hemorrhage ($n = 1$), and vitreous hemorrhage ($n = 1$).

Skin

Foreign body giant cell granulomas were first reported after liquid silicone injection in 1965 (14) and are usually observed near silicone-injected areas (15). There have been many reports of cysts and granulomatous reactions to silicone at application sites and distal sites after hematogenous or lymphatic migration (15–17).

- An otherwise healthy 59-year-old woman had received acupuncture for a sprained ankle several times over the previous year (18). She had numerous 2–5 mm waxy orange-brown papules on the dorsal aspects of both feet and ankles. A punch biopsy of one of these showed a mixed lichenoid, spongiotic, and granulomatous dermatitis. Macrophages, including many foreign body-type giant cells, were arranged in a granuloma annulare-like pattern around dermal collagen with focal mucinous alteration. Ultrastructural examination showed macrophages containing amorphous foreign material consistent with silicone. The acupuncturist had switched to silicone-plated acupuncture needles over the recent months, and she was believed to have cutaneous granulomas secondary to silicone deposition (18). She was treated with potent topical steroids and continued acupuncture with non-coated needles. The lesions slowly resolved over the ensuing months.

This case raises the possibility of silicone deposition from cutaneous manipulation with silicone-coated instruments over a relatively short duration of time. In addition, the case is remarkable in that the latency from exposure to the foreign material to the onset of lesions was relatively short (6–12 months).

Facial granulomatous lesions and a connective tissue-like disorder have been attributed to silicone deposition following injection of silicone into the breasts (19).

- A 56-year-old Japanese woman developed eyelid edema and erythema on her face and arms and 2 weeks later annular erythema on both arms, sicca syndrome, and progressive loss of sweating on her forehead. Laboratory studies, including muscle enzymes, antinuclear antibodies, and serum immunoelectrophoresis, were unremarkable. One month later, she developed skin lesions around the eyelids that resembled lupus miliaris disseminatus faciei. A biopsy showed non-caseating epithelioid granulomas in the mid-dermis, especially around the sweat glands. A CT scan of the chest showed fibrous implant capsules in each breast, due to silicone injections 30 years before. Electron microscopy of a nodule from the lower eyelid showed particles of silicone within the granulomas. The silicone was thought to have been derived from the material that had been injected into her breasts. After subcutaneous mastectomy and axial lymphadenectomy the facial edema disappeared rapidly, but the nodules remained.

Silicone gel breast prostheses are associated with a mild foreign body response resulting in the formation of a collagenous capsule around the prosthesis (20,21). Although many such patients may have evidence of a microscopic granulomatous foreign body reaction on examination of the capsular material at explantation of a prosthesis, it is unusual to have large palpable granulomas, even in the presence of rupture or leakage (22). Nevertheless, rare patients have had severe local inflammation and complications resulting from silicone migration to the axilla, arm, or abdominal wall (23,24). Three patients had significant problems with deforming granulomas after implant rupture (25). More importantly, they suffered the consequences of silicone gel migrating down the arm. Once silicone gel leaves the implant it is not biologically inert and in some people it can elicit profound pathological responses.

Silicone granulomas are usually observed near silicone-injected areas (15).

Siliconized dressings can cause pigmentation abnormalities (26).

Musculoskeletal

Foreign-body reactions to silicone can complicate silicone elastomer joint prostheses, manifesting as synovitis and/or lymphadenopathy, sometimes at remote locations (27).

Silicone can cause fibromyalgia (SEDA-22, 526).

Immunologic

There is a possible association between silicone breast implants and underlying connective tissue diseases (9,28–30).

In patients with symptoms of connective tissue diseases it has been assumed that rupture of the gel-filled prosthesis was the most likely cause of the symptoms. Although the prosthesis was intact in some patients, amorphous silicone-like material was identified by light microscopy in surgically removed fibrous tissue. In one study (31), granulomatous inflammatory reactions developed when silicone elastomers were used as skin expanders. This was attributed to leakage of particles of the plastic material through the expander wall. Lymphadenitis and destructive synovitis following silicone implants (especially joint prostheses) have been described before (32,33), while use of silicone in dialysis tubing also led to dissemination of silicone causing splenomegaly and deposits in liver, bone marrow, skin and visceral lymph nodes. Exposure for less than 53 months did not elicit these complications (34,35).

Immunological abnormalities in the form of increased autoantibodies, specifically antinuclear antibodies, anti-thyroid antibodies, rheumatoid factor, and increased immune complexes, have been evaluated and documented (36). In addition, abnormalities in lymphocyte subsets have been reported, with reduced lymphocytic mitogenic response, as well as abnormalities in the ratios of T-helper to T-suppressor cells (37). Several mechanisms have been suggested, among them that silicone oozes through the intact capsule of the implants, enters the lymphatic system, and causes an immunological reaction (38); this reaction causes further development of autoimmune disease through an adjuvant effect, with possible immune dysregulation (39).

More evidence for the antigenicity of silicone has been provided in studies that have shown specific silicone antibodies directed against silanized albumin in the sera of two patients exposed to silastic tubing (40). In 520 patients, aged 28–65 years, who had had silicone breast implants for 3–22 years, the most common symptoms were fatigue (96%), myalgia (86%), morning stiffness (86%), insomnia (77%), attention deficit (74%), night sweats (43%), cervical lymphadenopathy (78%), and axillary lymphadenopathy (55%).

Clinical, histopathological, and fibroblast studies have been carried out in 30 patients given subcutaneous injections of silicone (41). The mean time between the injection and the onset of symptoms was 6 years. All the patients had sclerodermatous skin changes, subcutaneous nodules, edema, and/or hyperpigmentation at the site(s) of injection(s); five individuals also had skin changes at sites far from the injection; 13 patients had clinical features of an autoimmune disease; 11 patients gave a history of arthralgias, including four who had symmetrical non-erosive polyarthritis; 20 of 28 patients had positive antinuclear antibodies. This report confirms the association between the injection of silicon and the development of autoimmune disease (human adjuvant disease). Pneumonitis and pulmonary edema following subcutaneous injection of silicone have been reported earlier (42–44).

In an evaluation of the frequency and clinical characteristics of the underlying connective tissue disorders associated with silicone breast implants, 300 women with silicone breast implants were studied (45). In addition to a history and physical examination, C reactive protein, rheumatoid factor, and autoantibodies were determined. Criteria for fibromyalgia and/or chronic fatigue syndrome were met by 54%; connective tissue diseases were detected in 11%; and undifferentiated connective tissue disease or human adjuvant disease in 10.6%. A variety of disorders, such as angioedema, frozen shoulder, and a multiple sclerosis-like syndrome, were also found. Several other miscellaneous conditions, including recurrent and unexplained low grade fever, hair loss, skin rash, symptoms of the sicca syndrome, Raynaud's phenomenon, carpal tunnel syndrome, memory loss, headaches, chest pain, and shortness of breath were also seen. Of 93 patients who underwent explantation, 70% reported improvement in their systemic symptoms.

References

1. Symmers WS. Silicone mastitis in "topless" waitresses and some other varieties of foreign-body mastitis. BMJ 1968;3(609):19–22.
2. Okano Y, Nishikai M, Sato A. Scleroderma, primary biliary cirrhosis, and Sjögren's syndrome after cosmetic breast augmentation with silicone injection: a case report of possible human adjuvant disease. Ann Rheum Dis 1984;43(3):520–2.
3. Bridges AJ, Conley C, Wang G, Burns DE, Vasey FB. A clinical and immunologic evaluation of women with silicone breast implants and symptoms of rheumatic disease. Ann Intern Med 1993;118(12):929–36.
4. Silver RM, Sahn EE, Allen JA, Sahn S, Greene W, Maize JC, Garen PD. Demonstration of silicon in sites of connective-tissue disease in patients with silicone-gel breast implants. Arch Dermatol 1993;129(1):63–8.
5. Anonymous. Silicone inflatable breast prosthesis-requirement for premarket approval. WHO Pharm Newslett 1999;9/12:22.
6. Behar TA, Anderson EE, Barwick WJ, Mohler JL. Sclerosing lipogranulomatosis: a case report of scrotal injection of automobile transmission fluid and literature review of subcutaneous injection of oils. Plast Reconstr Surg 1993;91(2):352–61.
7. Chen TH. Silicone injection granulomas of the breast: treatment by subcutaneous mastectomy and immediate subpectoral breast implant. Br J Plast Surg 1995;48(2):71–6.
8. Hofer SOP, Damen A, Nicolai CPA. Large volume liquid silicone injection in the upper thighs: a never ending story. Eur J Plast Surg 2000;23:241–4.
9. Vasey FB, Espinoza LR, Martinez-Osuna P, Seleznick MJ, Brozena SJ, Penske NA. Silicone and rheumatic disease: replace implants or not? Arch Dermatol 1991;127(6):907.

10. Vilaplana Blanch D, Escoto Gonzalez R, Guinot Saera A. Tratamiento del redesprendimiento de la retina en ojos con aceite de silicona intraocular. [Treatment of retinal re-detachment in eyes with intraocular silicone oil.] Arch Soc Esp Oftalmol 2001;76(4):241–8.

11. Ando F. Usefulness and limit of silicone in management of complicated retinal detachment. Jpn J Ophthalmol 1987;31(1):138–46.

12. Roussat B, Ruellan YM. Traitement du decollement de réine par vitrectomie et injection d'huile de silicone. Résultats a long terme et complications dans 105 cas. [Treatment of retinal detachment by vitrectomy and injection of silicone oil. Long-term results and complications in 105 cases.] J Fr Ophthalmol 1984;7(1):11–18.

13. Gremillion CM Jr, Peyman GA, Liu KR, Naguib KS. Fluorosilicone oil in the treatment of retinal detachment. Br J Ophthalmol 1990;74(11):643–6.

14. Ballantyne DL Jr, Rees TD, Seidman I. Silicone fluid: response to massive subcutaneous injections of dimethyl-polysiloxane fluid in animals. Plast Reconstr Surg 1965;36(3):330–8.

15. Travis WD, Balogh K, Abraham JL. Silicone granulomas: report of three cases and review of the literature. Hum Pathol 1985;16(1):19–27.

16. Ellenbogen R, Rubin L. Injectable fluid silicone therapy. Human morbidity and mortality. JAMA 1975;234(3):308–9.

17. Savrin RA, Martin EW Jr, Ruberg RL. Mass lesion of the breast after augmentation mammoplasty. Arch Surg 1979;114(12):1423–4.

18. Alani RM, Busam K. Acupuncture granulomas. J Am Acad Dermatol 2001;45(Suppl 6):S225–6.

19. Suzuki K, Aoki M, Kawana S, Hyakusoku H, Miyazawa S. Metastatic silicone granuloma: lupus miliaris disseminatus faciei-like facial nodules and sicca complex in a silicone breast implant recipient. Arch Dermatol 2002;138(4):537–8.

20. Barker DE, Retsky MI, Schultz S. "Bleeding" of silicone from bag-gel breast implants, and its clinical relation to fibrous capsule reaction. Plast Reconstr Surg 1978;61(6):836–41.

21. van Diest PJ, Beekman WH, Hage JJ. Pathology of silicone leakage from breast implants. J Clin Pathol 1998;51(7):493–7.

22. Brown SL, Silverman BG, Berg WA. Rupture of silicone-gel breast implants: causes, sequelae, and diagnosis. Lancet 1997;350(9090):1531–7.

23. Teuber SS, Ito LK, Anderson M, Gershwin ME. Silicone breast implant-associated scarring dystrophy of the arm. Arch Dermatol 1995;131(1):54–6.

24. Sanger JR, Matloub HS, Yousif NJ, Komorowski R. Silicone gel infiltration of a peripheral nerve and constrictive neuropathy following rupture of a breast prosthesis. Plast Reconstr Surg 1992;89(5):949–52.

25. Teuber SS, Reilly DA, Howell L, Oide C, Gershwin ME. Severe migratory granulomatous reactions to silicone gel in 3 patients. J Rheumatol 1999;26(3):699–704.

26. Williams G, Withey S, Walker CC. Longstanding pigmentary changes in paediatric scalds dressed with a non-adherent siliconised dressing. Burns 2001;27(2):200–2.

27. Kircher T. Silicone lymphadenopathy: a complication of silicone elastomer finger joint prostheses. Hum Pathol 1980;11(3):240–4.

28. Spiera H, Kerr LD. Scleroderma following silicone implantation: a cumulative experience of 11 cases. J Rheumatol 1993;20(6):958–61.

29. Gutierrez FJ, Espinoza LR. Progressive systemic sclerosis complicated by severe hypertension: reversal after silicone implant removal. Am J Med 1990;89(3):390–2.

30. Endo LP, Edwards NL, Longley S, Corman LC, Panush RS. Silicone and rheumatic diseases. Semin Arthritis Rheum 1987;17(2):112–18.

31. Maturri L, Azzolini A, Campiglio GL, Tardito E. Are synthetic prostheses really inert? Preliminary results of a study on the biocompatibility of Dacron vascular prostheses and silicone skin expanders. Int Surg 1991;76(2):115–18.

32. Atkinson RE, Smith RJ. Silicone synovitis following silicone implant arthroplasty. Hand Clin 1986;2(2):291–9.

33. Nalbandian RM, Swanson AB, Maupin BK. Long-term silicone implant arthroplasty. Implications of animal and human autopsy findings. JAMA 1983;250(9):1195–8.

34. Bommer J, Ritz E, Waldherr R. Silicone-induced splenomegaly: treatment of pancytopenia by splenectomy in a patient on hemodialysis. N Engl J Med 1981;305(18):1077–9.

35. Bommer J, Waldherr R, Gastner M, Lemmes R, Ritz E. Iatrogenic multiorgan silicone inclusions in dialysis patients. Klin Wochenschr 1981;59(20):1149–57.

36. Vojdani A, Brautbar N, Campbell AW. Antibody to silicone and native macromolecules in women with silicone breast implants. Immunopharmacol Immunotoxicol 1994;16(4):497–523.

37. Vojdani A, Brautbar N, Campbell AW. Antibody to silicone and native macromolecules in women with silicone breast implants. Immunopharmacol Immunotoxicol 1994;16(4):497–523.

38. McGrath MH, Burkhardt BR. The safety and efficacy of breast implants for augmentation mammaplasty. Plast Reconstr Surg 1984;74(4):550–60.

39. Vojdani A, Campbell A, Brautbar N. Immune functional impairment in patients with clinical abnormalities and silicone breast implants. Toxicol Ind Health 1992;8(6):415–29.

40. Goldblum RM, Pelley RP, O'Donell AA, Pyron D, Heggers JP. Antibodies to silicone elastomers and reactions to ventriculoperitoneal shunts. Lancet 1992;340(8818):510–13.

41. Cabral AR, Alcocer-Varela J, Orozco-Topete R, Reyes E, Fernandez-Dominguez L, Alarcon-Segovia D. Clinical, histopathological, immunological and fibroblast studies in 30 patients with subcutaneous injections of modelants including silicone and mineral oils. Rev Invest Clin 1994;46(4):257–66.

42. Chastre J, Basset F, Viau F, Dournovo P, Bouchama A, Akesbi A, Gibert C. Acute pneumonitis after subcutaneous injections of silicone in transsexual men. N Engl J Med 1983;308(13):764–7.

43. Celli BR, Kovnat DM. Acute pneumonitis after subcutaneous injections of silicone. N Engl J Med 1983;309(14):856–7.

44. Manresa JM, Manresa F. Silicone pneumonitis. Lancet 1983;2(8363):1373.

45. Cuellar ML, Gluck O, Molina JF, Gutierrez S, Garcia C, Espinoza R. Silicone breast implant—associated musculoskeletal manifestations. Clin Rheumatol 1995;14(6):667–72.

Silver salts and derivatives

General Information

Silver is a white precious metal (symbol Ag; atomic no. 47). The symbol derives from the Latin word argentum. It is found in various minerals, including argyrodite, cerargyrite, chlorargyrite, dyscrasite, iodyrite, and sylvanite.

Silver compounds are still used in medicine to a limited extent, notably in dermatological formulations, nose-drops, and eye-drops, the essential effect being to precipitate protein. If sufficient silver is absorbed, for example from long use or application to extensive burns, there can be accumulation in many tissues (1). Although silver is well tolerated, the frequency of exposure results in frequent reports of complications (SEDA-22, 250).

Silver nitrate

Silver nitrate is used as a caustic, antiseptic, and astringent agent. The silver ion is precipitated by the chloride in tissue fluids, so that it does not readily penetrate.

Silver nitrate is effective in vitro against *Neisseria gonorrheae* and *Staphylococcus aureus* in a concentration of about 0.1% and against *Escherichia coli* in a concentration of about 0.01%. It is effective in vivo against most strains of *Staphylococcus aureus* and *Staphylococcus epidermidis* and also has activity against *Pseudomonas aeruginosa*, but is less active against other gram-negative species, such as *Enterobacter* and *Klebsiella* (2). It does not penetrate eschar to any significant degree. The non-histotoxic concentrations of 0.5% used in burns are bacteriostatic. Thick cotton dressings saturated with the solution are applied to thoroughly debrided areas. The dressings must be re-wetted every 23 hours with fresh solution to prevent development of histotoxic concentrations over 2% at the wound surface. In the treatment of burns, silver nitrate has been largely replaced by silver sulfadiazine.

Silver sulfadiazine

Silver sulfadiazine (3) is a white, highly insoluble compound synthesized from silver nitrate and the sulfonamide sodium sulfadiazine. It is used in burns as a 1% formulation in a water-soluble cream base. It has in vitro activity against a wide range of burn wound microbial pathogens, including *S. aureus*, *E. coli*, *Klebsiella* species, *P. aeruginosa*, *Proteus* species, other Enterobacteriaceae, and *Candida albicans*. Its penetration into eschar is considered to be better than that of silver nitrate. Silver from silver sulfadiazine cream is rapidly absorbed and deposited in large amounts throughout the body (4).

Uses of silver compounds

Silver nitrate and silver sulfadiazine are used to treat burns (5,6).

Ophthalmic use of silver nitrate solution for prophylaxis of ophthalmia neonatorum due to gonorrhea should be considered as obsolete; silver nitrate is highly irritant and antibiotics provide better alternatives.

Silver is used in various medical devices. There is concern about the use of silver-containing formulations of uncontrolled composition (for example colloidal silver) with supposed activity in a host of microbial diseases. Despite the supposed anti-infective efficacy of silver-coated medical prostheses, in the majority of studies these prostheses have not been proven to be infection-resistant (7).

Silver fluoride has been used in dental care for the treatment of deep caries. However, application of 40% silver fluoride to deep carious lesions or its use as a spot application agent can cause 3–4 mg of fluoride to reach the systemic circulation (8). It has therefore been suggested that solutions of lower strength (1–4%), which may be as effective as a 40% solution, should be used. Similarly, the high concentration is contraindicated in children because of systemic access of fluoride (9).

Silver has been used in anti-smoking formulations designed to alter taste sensation. In 21 adults who use silver acetate chewing gum for 12 weeks as a smoking deterrent, serum concentrations of silver rose and quickly returned to normal after withdrawal (10). In most cases the number of silver granules in skin biopsies, observed by autometallography, increased after the gum had been used for 12 weeks. However, no-one developed clinical signs of argyria.

Over-the-counter products containing colloidal silver or silver salts have been marketed for use in adults and children for a wide variety of diseases, including AIDS, cancer, tuberculosis, malaria, systemic lupus erythematosus, syphilis, scarlet fever, herpesvirus infections, pneumonia, typhoid, tetanus, and many others. The US Food and Drug Administration has issued a ruling that a colloidal silver product for any medical use will first have to be approved by the FDA under drug application procedures (11).

Argyria

Argyria is a characteristic smoke-gray discoloration of the skin and a bluish discoloration of the mucous membranes reminiscent of cyanosis (12,13). The discoloration is permanent. The deposited pigment may be partly silver sulfide and partly metallic silver, formed by photoactivated reduction.

Accumulation in the deeper tissues occurs at the same time, but as a rule has no clinical consequences (14). One disputed report dating from 1984 (15) concerned two patients with what was regarded as systemic argyria following the uncontrolled use for several years of nose-drops containing silver salts; they had dyspnea, palpitation, weakness, a slightly reduced CO_2 diffusion capacity and in one case "functional adrenal hypofunction."

Delayed wound healing has been suggested as one adverse effect of presence of silver in the system.

Argyria has followed the use of dietary supplements containing colloidal silver protein (16).

- A 56-year-old man developed blue color changes of his fingernails. His face had a dusky appearance, and there was no scleral or conjunctival discoloration or hyperpigmentation of the gums. His fingernails had a blue-gray proximal band of discoloration, as did the lunulae of both thumbnails. His toenails were not involved and the rest of his skin showed no discoloration. His serum silver concentration was 85 (reference range below 5) ng/ml. He had taken colloidal silver for the previous 3 years as an allergy and cold medication, following the recommended regimen of 1 teaspoon of a 200 ppm silver solution tds.

Generalized argyria has occurred in patients treated with eye-drops containing silver nitrate. In one case the diagnosis was confirmed by a skin biopsy showing deposits of metallic silver in the dermis (17). Argyria should be considered in the differential diagnosis of focal pigmented conjunctival lesions (18).

- An 82-year-old woman with strabismus amblyopia, for which she had had surgery as a child, developed an asymptomatic pigmented conjunctival lesion in the right eye, mainly involving the underlying subconjunctival connective tissue and the insertion of the lateral rectus muscle; there was no scleral thinning. Biopsy of the conjunctiva and lateral rectus muscle showed numerous extracellular black pigment granules, many of which were aligned in a linear array along the muscle fibers. Energy dispersive X-ray microanalysis showed the pigmentation to be due to silver deposits. During strabismus surgery a silver clip had probably been used to shorten the lateral rectus muscle.

Vaginal argyria has been attributed to a combination of silver sulfadiazine and Aci-Jel (a buffered acid jelly containing acetic acid) (19).

- A 67-year-old woman with a sore vulva applied Flamazine cream (containing 1% silver sulfadiazine) topically for nearly 10 years and then Aci-Jel. She developed widespread black deposits in the vagina consistent with argyria. There were dark pigmented areas around the urethral meatus, Skene's ducts, and hymeneal remnants, and a circumferential deposit around the upper third of the vagina. Biopsies showed mild acanthosis and a mild chronic inflammatory infiltrate in the upper dermis, with black pigment granules 0.5–2 μm in size in the superficial dermis. Electron probe analysis confirmed the presence of silver. The creams were withdrawn and 6 months later the vagina showed no signs of argyria.

It is likely that reducing agents in the gel base of Aci-Jel interacted with the silver sulfadiazine, causing deposition of silver and discoloration of the vagina.

- A patient with schizophrenia developed systemic argyria from chronic and excessive ingestion of an anti-smoking formulation that contained silver (20). Seizures developed after he had taken the pills for 40 years. There was an extremely high concentration of silver in the serum.

The authors suggested that systemic silver can cause seizures.

Argyria and hepatotoxicity has been reported after the use of a silver-coated wound dressing, Acticoat, in the treatment of 30% mixed depth burns in a 17-year-old boy (21). Silver concentrations were high in the plasma (107 μg/kg) and urine (28 μg/kg).

Organs and Systems

Cardiovascular

A chronic inflammatory reaction in a prosthetic valve has been attributed to silver (22).

- A prosthetic mitral valve (St Jude Medical Silzone) that had been implanted in a 72-year-old woman became partially detached 4 months later, causing acute cardiac failure. The mitral annulus was ulcerated and there were multiple erosions in the tissues in contact with the valve. Histology showed chronic inflammation,

with hemosiderin deposits and giant cells. She was not allergic to silver.

The silver-coated sewing cuff had caused a chronic inflammatory reaction because of a toxic reaction to silver. The Silzone valve was withdrawn from the market in January 2000.

Nervous system

Peripheral neuropathy from long-term treatment of venous leg ulcers with silver sulfadiazine cream has been observed in one patient (13).

Sensory systems

The use of 1% silver nitrate eye-drops in prophylaxis of ophthalmia neonatorum has been periodically reviewed and compared with other prophylactic measures. There seems to be no case in which permanent damage to the eye was actually proven to have been caused by a single application of a correctly used 1% silver nitrate solution (23). However, silver nitrate has largely been replaced by antimicrobial drugs.

The reaction of the tissues in the front of the eye during the first 5 days after delivery has been examined in a double-blind study in 40 neonates with and without prophylaxis with silver nitrate solution (24). There was no significant difference in the frequency of pathological changes in the palpebrae, conjunctiva bulbi et tarsi, or cornea between the two groups and the same frequency of palpebral edema and conjunctival hyperemia. Repeated application of silver nitrate solutions in low concentrations can cause discoloration of the conjunctiva due to argyria (25).

Several cases of chemical burns of the eyes in newborn babies have been reported (26) but most of these complications followed incorrect administration of the formulation.

The clinical significance and incidence of chemical conjunctivitis due to silver nitrate has been investigated in 1000 newborn infants (27). Rinsing after instillation does not reduce the conjunctival irritation. Although 90% of the infants had conjunctivitis in the first 6 hours of life, in most cases it cleared within 24 hours. Chemical conjunctivitis did not increase the incidence of secondary infections. In 1980 the American Academy of Pediatrics pointed out the need for continued prophylaxis for all newborn infants, and proposed a 1% silver nitrate solution in single dose ampules or single-use tubes of an ophthalmic ointment with 1% tetracycline or 0.5% erythromycin. However, in infants of mothers with clinically apparent gonorrhea aqueous crystalline penicillin G should be injected.

In a double-blind, controlled study of a possible causal relation between 1% silver nitrate solution and 1% tetracycline solution in prophylaxis of ophthalmia neonatorum there was no statistically significant difference in the incidence of nasolacrimal duct obstruction between the two groups at either 2 weeks or 2 months of age (28).

Concentrations of silver nitrate of 5–50% applied accidentally to the eye have caused severe injuries with permanent corneal opacification and cataract in some cases (25).

Psychological, psychiatric

In one case there was a rapid decline in mental function at silver concentrations of 191 ng/ml, but the patient was seriously ill in other respects and although high concentrations of silver were found in the brain postmortem, it is not at all clear that the silver was responsible for the mental state (29).

Nutrition

Failure to thrive in a child has been attributed to silver toxicity (30).

- A 12-month-old girl with failure to thrive had been treated with various supplements and alternative therapies (including a blend of kelp, *Lactobacillus acidophilus*, wheat, rye, and barley) or colloidal silver. The silver was given in the form of a suspension and was thought to be effective in boosting immunity. The serum silver concentration was 3.4 (reference range below 0.02) µmol/l. Silver was withdrawn and her serum silver concentrations normalized some months later.

Electrolyte balance

Electrolyte disturbances are the major adverse effect of the use of silver nitrate in burns, since the distilled water vehicle used to carry the silver nitrate is hypotonic, and since the silver salts that are formed in the tissues, primarily silver chloride and silver sulfide, are insoluble (31). The hypotonicity produces absorption of large amounts of water into the body, with a dilutional effect and the leaking of significant quantities of body minerals, including sodium, potassium, magnesium, calcium, and chloride. Deficiency of chloride is caused by the formation of silver chloride on the treated surface. Up to 350 mmol/day of sodium can be lost per square meter of treated body surface area. Problems occur particularly in patients with burns that exceed 20% of the body surface and in infants, unless a regular replacement schedule is established. Maximum deficiency can occur within a matter of 6–8 hours after the start of therapy. Continuous oral or intravenous electrolyte supplementation and careful monitoring of electrolyte balance are necessary.

Hematologic

Methemoglobinemia due to silver nitrate occurs via bacterial reduction of nitrate to nitrite, which is subsequently absorbed (32). The diagnosis should be suspected if the skin or blood appears cyanotic or gray in the presence of normal arterial PO_2. The diagnosis should always be confirmed with measurement of blood methemoglobin concentration. In the treatment of burns with silver nitrate solutions, the possible occurrence of methemoglobinemia must be considered, especially when organisms are cultured from the wounds. The silver nitrate should be withdrawn if this complication occurs. Treatment of the methemoglobinemia with reducing agents is rarely required.

- Fatal methemoglobinemia occurred in a 3-year-old Caucasian girl who had burns involving 82% of the body surface and had been treated by painting the burns with silver nitrate solution (33). By the fourth

day, low-grade fever was evident and *Aerobacter cloacae*, which was resistant to silver nitrate 0.5%, was cultured from the scar tissue. The child became cyanotic and died after 27 days. Methemoglobin constituted 70% of her hemoglobin; there was no other evident cause of death. The *A. cloacae* cultured from the skin was tested and reduced nitrate to nitrite.

- A 12-month-old girl, with necrotizing fasciitis at the site of a cutaneous infection on her left trunk, became unresponsive, lethargic, and in shock, and underwent immediate aggressive tissue debridement (34). Later wound irrigation was carried out with a solution of silver nitrate 0.5% and 20 days later she became cyanotic and dyspneic. Her methemoglobin concentration was 38%. Intravenous methylene blue restored her oxygen saturation and reduced the dyspnea and cyanosis. Her methemoglobin concentration fell to 0.8%.

Transient leukopenia with a disproportionate reduction in neutrophilic leukocytes has been reported during treatment with sulfadiazine silver (35). This adverse effect appears to run a typical course: sulfadiazine-induced leukopenia reaches a nadir within 2–4 days of starting therapy, with a characteristic fall in the neutrophil count and a relative increase in the number of band forms. The erythrocyte count is not affected. By 2–3 days after the onset of leukopenia, the leukocyte count returns to normal. The leukocyte count tends to recover whether or not the silver sulfadiazine is withdrawn and may also be an intrinsic response to burn injury and unrelated to the use of silver sulfadiazine.

The use of silver sulfadiazine has been associated with acute hemolytic anemia (22).

Fatal pancytopenia has been reported from the extensive use of topical silver sulfadiazine.

- An 11-month-old infant with second- and third-degree burns over 30% of the body was treated topically with silver sulfadiazine (36). From day 2 there was significant neutropenia, maximal at day 3. The silver sulfadiazine was withdrawn. The neutropenia was followed by anemia, which was maximal on day 5. Finally, thrombocytopenia developed. In spite of blood transfusions and recovery of the neutropenia and thrombocytopenia, infection occurred and the patient died from respiratory failure.

Mouth and teeth

In one case severe ulceration of the anterior ventral surface of the tongue was caused by ill-advised cautery of a small ulcer with a silver nitrate stick (37). Only silver nitrate solutions of 5–10% should be used to cauterize mucous membranes or when a strong germicidal action is desired.

Urinary tract

Intrapelvic instillation of silver nitrate is sometimes still used in the treatment of essential hematuria. In one case ureteric stenosis developed as a consequence (38).

Nephrotic syndrome following topical therapy with silver sulfadiazine has been reported once (39).

Anuria has occurred after silver nitrate irrigation for intractable bladder hemorrhage caused by cyclophosphamide chemotherapy (40). The level of obstruction was the ureterovesical junction on the one hand, and the collecting ducts of the renal papillae on the other. Therapy consisted of rigorous endoscopic evacuation of deposited coagulate from the bladder, after which the urinary output rapidly returned to normal.

Skin

Three infants treated for umbilical granuloma with silver nitrate suffered chemical burns to the periumbilical area; conservative treatment led to good outcomes (41).

- A 29-year-old woman complained of increasing black discoloration of the tip of her left middle finger, resembling gangrene (42). She had been applying silver nitrate to her finger for the treatment of a small granuloma and had developed localized tissue necrosis, secondary to application of the silver nitrate, on withdrawal of which she recovered completely.

In consequence, it is recommended that the practice of unsupervised local application of silver nitrate to the fingers should be discontinued.

Höllensteinstift 10 (Pharma Winter, Leipzig, Germany) is a stick that contains 90% silver nitrate and 10% potassium nitrate, and has corrosive, germicidal, and astringent characteristics; it is used in the treatment of hypergranulation and common warts.

- A 28-year-old woman used Höllensteinstift 10 inappropriately (43). Intending to treat her periorbital folds, she removed the outside layer of paraffin, moistened the tip, and applied the stick to the lower parts of the lids, accidentally transferring parts of the corrosive agent to the skin in the periorbicular region. After some time, she felt a burning sensation, rinsed her face with water, and so distributed the agent widely to both cheeks and increased the pain. Self-treatment with several ointments did not bring relief. On the next day she developed brown discoloration of the facial skin, particularly in the periorbital region, pain, and torsion of the skin in the affected area. Initial treatment consisted of soap solution (to wash out the silver particles) and panthenol ointment (to support the process of healing). The lesions disappeared completely.

Cutaneous sensitivity reactions, typically maculopapular rashes, occur in under 5% of patients who use silver sulfadiazine and rarely require withdrawal (44).

Immunologic

A meta-analysis of the clinical and economic effects of chlorhexidine and silver sulfadiazine antiseptic-impregnated catheters has been undertaken (45). The costs of hypersensitivity reactions were considered as part of the analysis, and the use of catheters impregnated with antiseptics resulted in reduced costs. The analysis used the higher estimated incidence of hypersensitivity reactions occurring in Japan, where the use of chlorhexidine impregnated catheters is still banned (46).

Susceptibility Factors

Renal disease

If silver sulfadiazine is used in a patient with impaired renal function, accumulation of silver can occur.

- In a patient with end-stage renal disease, there was a marked increase in serum silver concentration during treatment with silver sulfadiazine cream 200 g/day for 2 weeks (29). The serum concentration of silver reached a maximum of 291 ng/ml and there was rapid deterioration of mental status. Silver sulfadiazine was withdrawn, but the patient died after 4 months. At autopsy, there were very high concentrations of silver in the brain tissues (617 and 824 ng/g in the cerebrum and cerebellum respectively).

In this patient both plasma exchange and hemofiltration were effective in reducing the serum silver concentration, and their effects were additive, but hemodialysis was ineffective. However, none of these maneuvers affected brain silver concentrations.

Drug Administration

Drug formulations

A modification of silver sulfadiazine by the incorporation of cerium nitrate is believed to enhance its efficacy. In 60 patients with moderate and severe burns randomly assigned to topical silver sulfadiazine either alone ($n = 30$) or in combination with cerium nitrate ($n = 30$), there were four deaths in those who were given sulfadiazine alone and only one in those who were given the combination (47). Wound infection did not differ significantly between the groups. The rate of re-epithelialization of partial thickness burns was faster by 8 days in those given the combination, and the relatively dry shell-like eschar allowed planned excisions with immediate autologous grafting and the tissue underneath was ready to accept grafting 11 days earlier. There was a higher incidence of transient stinging pain with the combination, but this was effectively managed with analgesics when necessary.

References

1. Hollinger MA. Toxicological aspects of topical silver pharmaceuticals. Crit Rev Toxicol 1996;26(3):255–60.
2. Chataigner D, Garnier R, Sans S, Efthymiou ML. Intoxication aiguë accidentelle par un désinfectant hospitalier. 45 cas dont 13 d'évolution mortelle. [Acute accidental poisoning with hospital disinfectant. 45 cases of which 13 with fatal outcome.] Presse Méd 1991;20(16):741–3.
3. Monafo WW, West MA. Current treatment recommendations for topical burn therapy. Drugs 1990;40(3):364–73.
4. Coombs CJ, Wan AT, Masterton JP, Conyers RA, Pedersen J, Chia YT. Do burn patients have a silver lining? Burns 1992;18(3):179–84.
5. Klasen HJ. Historical review of the use of silver in the treatment of burns. I. Early uses. Burns 2000;26(2):117–30.
6. Klasen HJ. A historical review of the use of silver in the treatment of burns. II. Renewed interest for silver. Burns 2000;26(2):131–8.
7. Darouiche RO. Anti-infective efficacy of silver-coated medical prostheses. Clin Infect Dis 1999;29(6):1371–7.
8. Gotjamanos T. Safety issues related to the use of silver fluoride in paediatric dentistry. Aust Dent J 1997;42(3):166–8.
9. Gotjamanos T, Orton V. Abnormally high fluoride levels in commercial preparations of 40 per cent silver fluoride

solution: contraindications for use in children. Aust Dent J 1998;43(6):422–7.

10. Jensen EJ, Rungby J, Hansen JC, Schmidt E, Pedersen B, Dahl R. Serum concentrations and accumulation of silver in skin during three months treatment with an anti-smoking chewing gum containing silver acetate. Hum Toxicol 1988;7(6):535–40.

11. Anonymous. Colloidal silver or silver salts—final rule: no longer acceptable in over the counter products. WHO Pharm Newslett 1999;9/12:1.

12. Tanner LS, Gross DJ. Generalized argyria. Cutis 1990;45(4):237–9.

13. Payne CM, Bladin C, Colchester AC, Bland J, Lapworth R, Lane D. Argyria from excessive use of topical silver sulpha-diazine. Lancet 1992;340(8811):126.

14. Lee SM, Lee SH. Generalized argyria after habitual use of AgNO₃. J Dermatol 1994;21(1):50–3.

15. Dupont T, Gomez J, Cuvillier P, Beaujot S, Haguenoer J, Lefrancois H. Argyrie généralisée médicamenteuse: intérêt des dosages sériques et urinaires. A propos de 2 cas. [Drug-induced generalized argyria. Value of blood and urine ana-lysis. Apropos of 2 cases.] LARC Med 1984;4(2):103–5.

16. Gulbranson SH, Hud JA, Hansen RC. Argyria following the use of dietary supplements containing colloidal silver protein. Cutis 2000;66(5):373–4.

17. Nielsen IO, Kjaerbo E. Generaliseret argyri sekundaert til brug af solvnitratholdige ojendraber. [Generalized argyria due to the use of eyedrops containing silver nitrate.] Ugeskr Laeger 1989;151(1):33–4.

18. Holck DE, Klintworth GK, Dutton JJ, Foulks GN, Manning FJ. Localized conjunctival argyrosis: a late sequela of strabismus surgery. Ophthalmic Surg Lasers 2000;31(6):495–8.

19. Thomas K, Sproston AR, Kingsland CR. A case of vaginal argyrosis: all that glistens isn't gold. BJOG 2001;108(8):890–1.

20. Ohbo Y, Fukuzako H, Takeuchi K, Takigawa M. Argyria and convulsive seizures caused by ingestion of silver in a patient with schizophrenia. Psychiatry Clin Neurosci 1996;50(2):89–90.

21. Trop M, Novak M, Rodl S, Hellbom B, Kroell W, Goessler W. Silver-coated dressing acticoat caused raised liver enzymes and argyria-like symptoms in burn patient. J Trauma 2006;60(3):648–52.

22. Tozzi P, Al-Darweesh A, Vogt P, Stumpe F. Silver-coated prosthetic heart valve: a double-bladed weapon. Eur J Cardiothorac Surg 2001;19(5):729–31.

23. Barsam PC. Specific prophylaxis of gonorrheal ophthalmia neonatorum. A review. N Engl J Med 1966;274(13):731–4.

24. Graf H, Retzke U, Schilling C, Schmidt M. Die Reaktion des vorderen Augenabschnittes auf die Crede-Prophylaxe. [Reaction of the anterior eye segment to preventive Crede treatment.] Zentralbl Gynakol 1994;116(11):639–42.

25. Grant WM. Toxicology of the Eye. 2nd ed. Springfield, IL: Charles C Thomas, 1974:917.

26. Huber-Spitzy V, Arocker W, Schmidt C. Ophthalmia neo-natorum. Klin Monatsbl Augenheilkd 1987;191(5):341–3.

27. Nishida H, Risemberg HM. Silver nitrate ophthalmic solution and chemical conjunctivitis. Pediatrics 1975;56(3):368–73.

28. Hick JF, Block DJ, Ilstrup DM. A controlled study of silver nitrate prophylaxis and the incidence of nasolacrimal duct obstruction. J Pediatr Ophthalmol Strabismus 1985;22(3):92–3.

29. Iwasaki S, Yoshimura A, Ideura T, Koshikawa S, Sudo M. Elimination study of silver in a hemodialyzed burn patient treated with silver sulfadiazine cream. Am J Kidney Dis 1997;30(2):287–90.

30. McIntyre E, Wilcox J, McGill J, Lewindon PJ. Silver toxi-city in an infant of strict vegan parents. J Pediatr Gastroenterol Nutr 2001;33(4):501–2.

31. Connelly DM. Silver nitrate. Ideal burn wound therapy? NY State J Med 1970;70(12):1642–4.

32. Strauch B, Buch W, Grey W, Laub D. Methemoglobinemia: a complication of silver nitrite therapy used in burns. AORN J 1969;10(4):54–6.

33. Ternberg JL, Luce E. Methemoglobinemia: complication of the silver nitrate treatment of burns. Surgery 1968;63:328.

34. Chou TD, Gibran NS, Urdahl K, Lin EY, Heimbach DM, Engrav LH. Methemoglobinemia secondary to topical silver nitrate therapy—a case report. Burns 1999;25(6):549–52.

35. Caffee HH, Bingham HG. Leukopenia and silver sulfadia-zine. J Trauma 1982;22(7):586–7.

36. Blangy H, Simon D, Levy-Cloez A, Feillet F, Fyad JP, Trechot P, Gillet P, Lascombes P. Sulfadiazine argentique topique et bicytopénie: 1er cas. [Topic silver sulfadiazine bicytopenia: first case.] Therapie 2002;57(3):307–9.

37. Frost DE, Barkmeier WW, Abrams H. Aphthous ulcer—a treatment complication. Report of a case. Oral Surg Oral Med Oral Pathol 1978;45(6):863–9.

38. Vijan SR, Keating MA, Althausen AF. Ureteral stenosis after silver nitrate instillation in the treatment of essential hematuria. J Urol 1988;139(5):1015–16.

39. Owens CJ, Yarbrough DR 3rd., Brackett NC Jr. Nephrotic syndrome following topically applied sulfadiazine silver therapy. Arch Intern Med 1974;134(2):332–5.

40. Raghavaiah NV, Soloway MS. Anuria following silver nitrate irrigation for intractable bladder hemorrhage. J Urol 1977;118(4):681–2.

41. Chamberlain JM, Gorman RL, Young GM. Silver nitrate burns following treatment for umbilical granuloma. Pediatr Emerg Care 1992;8(1):29–30.

42. Sankar NS, Donaldson D. Lessons to be learned: a case study approach. Finger discoloration due to silver nitrate exposure: review of uses and toxicity of silver in clinical practice. J R Soc Health 1998;118(6):371–4.

43. Schepler H, Kessler J, Hartmann B. Abuse of silver-nitrate solution for planing periorbital folds. Burns 2002;28(1):90–1.

44. Hoffmann S. Silver sulfadiazine: an antibacterial agent for topical use in burns. A review of the literature. Scand J Plast Reconstr Surg 1984;18(1):119–26.

45. Veenstra DL, Saint S, Sullivan SD. Cost-effectiveness of antiseptic-impregnated central venous catheters for the pre-vention of catheter-related bloodstream infection. JAMA 1999;282(6):554–60.

46. Raad I, Hanna H. Intravascular catheters impregnated with antimicrobial agents: a milestone in the prevention of bloodstream infections. Support Care Cancer 1999;7(6):386–90.

47. de Gracia CG. An open study comparing topical silver sulfadiazine and topical silver sulfadiazine–cerium nitrate in the treatment of moderate and severe burns. Burns 2001;27(1):67–74.

Simvastatin

See also HMG Co-A reductase inhibitors

General Information

Simvastatin is an HMG Co-A reductase inhibitor. Its most serious adverse effect is rhabdomyolysis, which is enhanced by other drugs that inhibit CYP3A4 (1).

Organs and Systems

Cardiovascular

Transient hypotension attributable to simvastatin may have been related to reduced production of corticosteroids (2).

Respiratory

Hypersensitivity reactions can occur with statins (SEDA-13, 1328) (3), and an otherwise unexplained case of interstitial lung disease and pleural effusion developed during treatment with simvastatin for 6 months; the number of eosinophils in the bronchoalveolar lavage fluid normalized a few days after withdrawal (4).

Psychological, psychiatric

In the 4S study there were five suicides in the simvastatin group and four in controls (5).

Endocrine

In 521 patients taking simvastatin 40–80 mg/day, serum cortisol concentrations were on average reduced by 3–7% (6). In the men there was a 10% fall in serum testosterone. However, there were no reports of sexual dysfunction.

Simvastatin up to 40 mg/day was given to 98 boys and 75 girls, aged 10–17 years, for 48 weeks without any adverse effects beyond a small fall in dehydroepiandrosterone (7). Of special note was the observation that simvastatin had no adverse effects on growth or pubertal development.

Metabolism

- A 53-year-old man taking simvastatin 40 mg/day developed rhabdomyolysis and hepatitis and had a raised serum lactate concentration (8.3 mmol/l; reference range 0.5–2.2) (8). Everything resolved 7 days after drug withdrawal.

Lactic acidosis in this patient supports the view that interference with the mitochondrial respiratory chain may play a role in the toxicity of the statins.

Hematologic

Thrombocytopenia is a rare adverse effect of simvastatin (9).

- Severe thrombocytopenia occurred in a 75-year-old woman taking simvastatin 5 mg/day and was resistant to therapy until she developed pneumonia. Recovery from the thrombocytopenia coincided with an increased interleukin concentration in the blood (10).
- There was a close temporal association with thrombotic thrombocytopenic purpura in a 43-year-old man after his second dose of simvastatin (11).

Other cases have been reported (12–15).

Liver

Cholestatic hepatitis occurred in a man with cirrhosis of the liver given simvastatin 20 mg/day (16).

Pancreas

Pancreatitis has been reported with simvastatin (17–22).

Urinary tract

It has been claimed that physicians should bear in mind the nephrotoxic potential of this drug (23), but there is no definite evidence that simvastatin is associated with the development of proteinuria (24).

Skin

- A 66-year-old man had persistent photosensitivity after using simvastatin intermittently (25). The clinical, histopathological, and photobiological features met the criteria for chronic actinic dermatitis.

Musculoskeletal

Rhabdomyolysis has been reported in patients taking simvastatin (26,27). Of 66 patients who took simvastatin for 1 year, two had myalgia and weakness with creatine kinase activity above 3000 (normally less than 100) (28).

- Simvastatin 5 mg/day caused rhabdomyolysis in a 61-year-old man not taking interacting drugs (29).

In a meta-analysis of megatrials with simvastatin, the overall incidence of myopathy was 0.025% (30). The authors suggested that potent inhibitors of CYP3A4 greatly increase the risk, but that weak inhibitors do not. Episodes of gout occurred in three of nine patients with chronic renal insufficiency who took simvastatin (31).

Immunologic

Lupus-like syndrome has been associated with simvastatin, with antibodies to double-stranded DNA in the serum (32).

- Simvastatin-induced lupus erythematosus was suspected in a 79-year-old white man after 3 months (33). He had signs of pleuropericarditis that resolved within 2 weeks of withdrawal.

Second-Generation Effects

Teratogenicity

Of 169 women exposed to simvastatin during pregnancy, three delivered babies with malformations and there were two fetal deaths (34). These results are comparable to what would be expected in the general population. However, based on a general consideration of risk, statins should not be used during pregnancy and only in exceptional circumstances should they be given to any woman of childbearing age.

Drug–Drug Interactions

Calcium channel blockers

In a meta-analysis of megatrials of simvastatin, the overall incidence of myopathy was 0.025%; the same proportion of those with myositis had used calcium channel blockers as the proportion overall, suggesting that there is no important interaction between these two groups of drugs (30).

However, diltiazem interacts with lovastatin although not with pravastatin (SEDA-24, 511), and an interaction has also been observed with simvastatin in a 75-year-old man who developed impaired renal function (35). He had extreme weakness and muscle pain.

Ciclosporin

In a patient with glucocorticoid-resistant nephrotic syndrome taking simvastatin and ciclosporin, there was an increase in lactic dehydrogenase activity, suggesting tissue injury, in the absence of an increase in creatine kinase (36).

Clarithromycin

Lovastatin has been reported to interact with clarithromycin (SEDA-14, 1531) (37), and a similar reaction has been observed with simvastatin (38).

- A 64-year-old African-American man developed worsening renal insufficiency, raised creatine kinase activity, diffuse muscle pain, and severe muscle weakness. He had been taking simvastatin for about 6 months and clarithromycin for sinusitis for about 3 weeks. He was treated aggressively with intravenous hydration, sodium bicarbonate, and hemodialysis. A muscle biopsy showed necrotizing myopathy secondary to a toxin. He continued to receive intermittent hemodialysis until he died from infectious complications 3 months after admission.

Gemfibrozil

- Severe rhabdomyolysis occurred in a 52-year-old woman taking a combination of gemfibrozil and simvastatin (39).

Grapefruit juice

Simvastatin should be avoided in patients using grapefruit juice (40).

Itraconazole

Itraconazole probably inhibits simvastatin metabolism (SEDA 21, 459).

Rifamycins

Rifampicin greatly reduced the plasma concentrations of simvastatin and simvastatin acid in 10 healthy volunteers in a randomized, crossover study (41). Because the half-life of simvastatin was not affected by rifampicin, induction of CYP3A4-mediated first-pass metabolism of simvastatin in the intestine and liver probably explains this interaction.

Warfarin

An interaction with warfarin with resulting acute rhabdomyolysis has been observed in a patient taking simvastatin (42). This has not been observed with other statins.

References

1. Kivisto KT, Kantola T, Neuvonen PJ. Different effects of itraconazole on the pharmacokinetics of fluvastatin and lovastatin. Br J Clin Pharmacol 1998;46(1):49–53.
2. French J, White H. Transient symptomatic hypotension in patients on simvastatin. Lancet 1989;2(8666):807–8.
3. Tobert JA, Shear CL, Chremos AN, Mantell GE. Clinical experience with lovastatin. Am J Cardiol 1990;65(12):F23–6.
4. De Groot RE, Willems LN, Dijkman JH. Interstitial lung disease with pleural effusion caused by simvastatin. J Intern Med 1996;239(4):361–3.
5. Pedersen TR, Tobert JA. Benefits and risks of HMG-CoA reductase inhibitors in the prevention of coronary heart disease: a reappraisal. Drug Saf 1996;14(1):11–24.
6. Stein EA, Davidson MH, Dobs AS, Schrott H, Dujovne CA, Bays H, Weiss SR, Melino MR, Stepanavage ME, Mitchel YB. Efficacy and safety of simvastatin 80 mg/day in hypercholesterolemic patients. The Expanded Dose Simvastatin U.S. Study Group. Am J Cardiol 1998;82(3):311–16.
7. de Jongh S, Ose L, Szamosi T, Gagne C, Lambert M, Scott R, Perron P, Dobbelaere D, Saborio M, Tuohy MB, Stepanavage M, Sapre A, Gumbiner B, Mercuri M, van Trotsenburg AS, Bakker HD, Kastelein JJ; Simvastatin in Children Study Group. Efficacy and safety of statin therapy in children with familial hypercholesterolemia: a randomized, double-blind, placebo-controlled trial with simvastatin. Circulation 2002;106(17):2231–7.
8. Goli AK, Goli SA, Byrd RP Jr, Roy TM. Simvastatin-induced lactic acidosis: a rare adverse reaction? Clin Pharmacol Ther 2002;72(4):461–4.
9. McCarthy LJ, Dlott JS, Orazi A, Waxman D, Miraglia CC, Danielson CF. Thrombotic thrombocytopenic purpura: yesterday, today, tomorrow. Ther Apher Dial 2004;8(2):80–6.
10. Yamada T, Shinohara K, Katsuki K. Severe thrombocytopenia caused by simvastatin in which thrombocyte recovery was initiated after severe bacterial infection. Clin Drug Invest 1998;16:172–4.
11. McCarthy LJ, Porcu P, Fausel CA, Sweeney CJ, Danielson CF. Thrombotic thrombocytopenic purpura and simvastatin. Lancet 1998;352(9136):1284–5.
12. Possamai G, Bovo P, Santonastaso M. Thrombocytopenic purpura during therapy with simvastatin. Haematologica 1992;77(4):357–8.
13. Koduri PR. Simvastatin and thrombotic thrombocytopenic purpura. Lancet 1998;352(9145):2020.
14. Groneberg DA, Barkhuizen A, Jeha T. Simvastatin-induced thrombocytopenia. Am J Hematol 2001;67(4):277.
15. Sundram F, Roberts P, Kennedy B, Pavord S. Thrombotic thrombocytopenic purpura associated with statin treatment. Postgrad Med J 2004;80(947):551–2.
16. Horiuchi Y, Maruoka H. Petechial eruptions due to simvastatin in a patient with diabetes mellitus and liver cirrhosis. J Dermatol 1997;24(8):549–51.
17. Ramdani M, Schmitt AM, Liautard J, Duhamel O, Legroux P, Gislon J, Pariente EA, Agay D, Faure D. Pancreatite aiguë a la simvastatine: deux cas. [Simvastatin-induced acute pancreatitis: two cases.] Gastroenterol Clin Biol 1991;15(12):986.
18. Couderc M, Blanc P, Rouillon JM, Bauret P, Larrey D, Michel H. Un nouveau cas de pancréatite aiguë après la prise de simvastatine. [A new case of simvastatin-induced acute pancreatitis.] Gastroenterol Clin Biol 1991;15(12):986–7.
19. Andersen V, Sonne J, Andersen M. Spontaneous reports on drug-induced pancreatitis in Denmark from 1968 to 1999. Eur J Clin Pharmacol 2001;57(6–7):517–21.
20. McDonald KB, Garber BG, Perreault MM. Pancreatitis associated with simvastatin plus fenofibrate. Ann Pharmacother 2002;36(2):275–9.
21. Pezzilli R, Ceciliato R, Corinaldesi R, Barakat B. Acute pancreatitis due to simvastatin therapy: increased severity after rechallenge. Dig Liver Dis 2004;36(9):639–40.
22. Lons T, Chousterman M. La simvastatine: une nouvelle molécule responsable de pancréatite aiguë? [Simvastatin: a new drug responsible for acute pancreatitis?] Gastroenterol Clin Biol 1991;15(1):93–4.
23. Gorrie MJ, MacGregor MS, Rodger RS. Acute on chronic renal failure induced by simvastatin. Nephrol Dial Transplant 1996;11(11):2328–9.

24. La Belle P, Mantel G. Simvastatin and proteinuria. Lancet 1991;337(8745):864.

25. Granados MT, de la Torre C, Cruces MJ, Pineiro G. Chronic actinic dermatitis due to simvastatin. Contact Dermatitis 1998;38(5):294–5.

26. Berland Y, Vacher Coponat H, Durand C, Baz M, Laugier R, Musso JL. Rhabdomyolysis with simvastatin use. Nephron 1991;57(3):365–6.

27. Deslypere JP, Vermeulen A. Rhabdomyolysis and simvastatin. Ann Intern Med 1991;114(4):342.

28. Emmerich J, Aubert I, Bauduceau B, Dachet C, Chanu B, Erlich D, Gautier D, Jacotot B, Rouffy J. Efficacy and safety of simvastatin (alone or in association with cholestyramine). A 1-year study in 66 patients with type II hyperlipoproteinaemia. Eur Heart J 1990;11(2):149–55.

29. Pershad A, Cardello FP. Simvastatin and rhabdomyolysis—a case report and brief review. J Pharm Technol 1999;15:88–9.

30. Gruer PJ, Vega JM, Mercuri MF, Dobrinska MR, Tobert JA. Concomitant use of cytochrome P450 3A4 inhibitors and simvastatin. Am J Cardiol 1999;84(7):811–15.

31. Harris DC, Simons LA, Mitchell P, Stewart JH. Management of non-nephrotic hyperlipidaemia of chronic renal failure with simvastatin. Med J Aust 1991;155(8):573.

32. Noel B, Panizzon RG. Lupus-like syndrome associated with statin therapy. Dermatology 2004;208(3):276–7.

33. Khosla R, Butman AN, Hammer DF. Simvastatin-induced lupus erythematosus. South Med J 1998;91(9):873–4.

34. Freyssinges C, Ducrocq MB. Simvastatine et grossesse. [Simvastatin and pregnancy.] Therapie 1996;51(5):537–42.

35. Peces R, Pobes A. Rhabdomyolysis associated with concurrent use of simvastatin and diltiazem. Nephron 2001;89(1):117–18.

36. Ogawa D, Maruyama K, Miyatake N, Kashihara N, Makino H. Concomitant use of simvastatin and cyclosporin A increases LDH in nephrotic syndrome. Nephron 1998;80(3):351–2.

37. Grunden JW, Fisher KA. Lovastatin-induced rhabdomyolysis possibly associated with clarithromycin and azithromycin. Ann Pharmacother 1997;31(7–8):859–63.

38. Lee AJ, Maddix DS. Rhabdomyolysis secondary to a drug interaction between simvastatin and clarithromycin. Ann Pharmacother 2001;35(1):26–31.

39. Tal A, Rajeshawari M, Isley W. Rhabdomyolysis associated with simvastatin–gemfibrozil therapy. South Med J 1997;90(5):546–7.

40. Lilja JJ, Kivisto KT, Neuvonen PJ. Grapefruit juice–simvastatin interaction: effect on serum concentrations of simvastatin, simvastatin acid, and HMG-CoA reductase inhibitors. Clin Pharmacol Ther 1998;64(5):477–83.

41. Kyrklund C, Backman JT, Kivisto KT, Neuvonen M, Laitila J, Neuvonen PJ. Rifampin greatly reduces plasma simvastatin and simvastatin acid concentrations. Clin Pharmacol Ther 2000;68(6):592–7.

42. Mogyorosi A, Bradley B, Showalter A, Schubert ML. Rhabdomyolysis and acute renal failure due to combination therapy with simvastatin and warfarin. J Intern Med 1999;246(6):599–602.

Sirolimus

General Information

Sirolimus is a macrocyclic lactone immunosuppressant that has anti-rejection activity through inhibition of T cell activation. In contrast to tacrolimus and ciclosporin, sirolimus has no effect on calcineurin activity.

Sirolimus is being investigated for the prophylaxis of renal rejection in combination with ciclosporin and glucocorticoids (1).

Comparative studies

In a 12-month study in 719 patients with renal transplants, the combination of sirolimus, ciclosporin, and prednisone in 558 patients (284 taking sirolimus 2 mg/day and 274 taking 5 mg/day) produced significantly more acne, diarrhea, dyslipidemia, headache, hirsutism, hyperkalemia, hypertension, lymphocele formation, and thrombocytopenia compared with 161 patients who took azathioprine, ciclosporin, and prednisone (2). Serum creatinine concentrations were significantly higher at 6 and 12 months in those who took sirolimus. Most of these adverse effects were thought to represent exacerbations of ciclosporin adverse effects, except for diarrhea (8–32%), dyslipidemia (30–42%), lymphocele formation (12–15%), and thrombocytopenia (9–18%), which were more probably related to sirolimus.

That the adverse events profile of sirolimus is different from that of ciclosporin has been further suggested in 83 patients taking primary immunosuppressant regimens containing sirolimus (41 patients) or ciclosporin (42 patients) (3). Arthralgia (20%), hypercholesterolemia (44%), hypertriglyceridemia (51%), leukopenia (39%), thrombocytopenia (37%), and pneumonia (17%) were significantly more frequent in patients taking sirolimus, particularly during the first 2 months of treatment, that is until sirolimus trough concentrations were carefully monitored. Serum creatinine concentrations were lower in the sirolimus group, confirming that sirolimus probably has no direct nephrotoxic effect.

Organs and Systems

Respiratory

Progressive diffuse interstitial pneumonitis has been reported as a possible adverse effect of sirolimus (4), and by 2000 the FDA was aware of at least 34 cases (5). Although the reports were insufficient to conclude that sirolimus was responsible in most cases, eight patients recovered after sirolimus withdrawal.

Bronchiolitis obliterans with organizing pneumonia has been attributed to sirolimus in two renal transplant patients (6). Both improved rapidly after sirolimus withdrawal or dosage reduction.

Metabolism

The most striking consequence of treatment with sirolimus is dose-dependent hyperlipidemia with significant increases in both cholesterol and triglyceride serum concentrations, which resolve after dosage reduction or sirolimus withdrawal (7).

In a 1-year follow-up of 40 renal transplant patients treated with various dosages of sirolimus (0.5–$7\,\text{mg/m}^2$/day) in addition to a ciclosporin-based regimen, there were significant increases in serum cholesterol and triglycerides, and significant falls in white blood cell and platelet counts, compared with historical controls (1). These effects correlated with sirolimus trough concentrations but not dosages. One patient had to discontinue sirolimus because of hyperlipidemia refractory to treatment.

In six patients with renal transplants treated with sirolimus, mean total plasma cholesterol, triglyceride, and apolipoprotein concentrations increased (8). The authors suggested that sirolimus increases lipase activity in adipose tissue and reduces lipoprotein lipase activity, resulting in increased hepatic synthesis of triglycerides, increased secretion of VLDL, and increased hypertriglyceridemia.

Hematologic

Thrombocytopenia, probably related to sirolimus, as well as significant reversible reductions in platelet and white blood cell counts have been found (SEDA-20, 346).

In 119 patients taking sirolimus, thrombocytopenia (defined as a platelet count below $150 \times 10^9/l$) and leukopenia (white blood cell count below $5.0 \times 10^9/l$) occurred in 78 and 63% respectively (9). The incidence, but not the severity, of these effects correlated with sirolimus whole-blood trough concentrations. Most cases occurred within the first 4 weeks of treatment and the severity was usually limited. There was spontaneous resolution in 89% of the patients and sirolimus dosage reduction or temporary withdrawal was necessary in only 7% and 4% of the patients respectively. None of the patients required permanent withdrawal.

Immunologic

Two reports have recently suggested that sirolimus can produce features of the capillary leak syndrome in patients with psoriasis (10).

- A 53-year-old woman with severe psoriasis for 3 years, who had previously taken ciclosporin, sulfasalazine, and topical glucocorticoids, was given sirolimus $8\,mg/m^2/day$, and 3 days later had fever, leg edema, dyspnea, weight gain, anemia, and hypotension. A chest X-ray showed pulmonary congestion and cardiomegaly. Empirical antibiotics were unsuccessful, and all symptoms progressively disappeared after sirolimus withdrawal.
- A 58-year-old man took sirolimus $8\,mg/m^2/day$ for severe psoriasis with arthritis. He also took ibuprofen, co-trimoxazole, and paracetamol. Within 1 month he developed nocturnal fever, dizziness, orthostatic hypotension, leg edema, and anemia. All his symptoms subsided after sirolimus withdrawal, furosemide treatment, and erythrocyte transfusion.

No other causes were found, and the authors noted that of 34 psoriatic patients given sirolimus, three had leg edema and a reduced hematocrit. Based on limited in vitro findings, they suggested that sirolimus might enhance apoptosis of activated lymphocytes and thereby cytokine release.

Drug–Drug Interactions

Ciclosporin

Combination of sirolimus with ciclosporin virtually eliminates acute rejection. However, the adverse effects of both drugs are potentiated, increasing the nephrotoxicity of ciclosporin (11).

In a single-dose, open, crossover study in 15 men and six women, the systemic availability of sirolimus 10 mg was markedly increased by concomitant ciclosporin 300 mg, C_{max}, t_{max}, and AUC being increased by 116, 92, and 230% respectively (12,13). However, when sirolimus was given 4 hours after ciclosporin, the increases were only 37, 58, and 80%. Ciclosporin did not affect the half-life or mean residence time of sirolimus. Sirolimus did not significantly affect the systemic availability of ciclosporin.

Diltiazem

In 18 healthy subjects, in a randomized, crossover study of the pharmacokinetics of a single oral dose of sirolimus 10 mg, a single dose of diltiazem 120 mg, and the combination, diltiazem increased exposure to sirolimus, presumably by inhibiting its first-pass metabolism (13).

Tacrolimus

Combination of sirolimus with tacrolimus virtually eliminates acute rejection. However, the adverse effects of both drugs are potentiated, increasing the nephrotoxicity of tacrolimus (11).

References

1. Kahan BD, Podbielski J, Napoli KL, Katz SM, Meier-Kriesche HU, Van Buren CT. Immunosuppressive effects and safety of a sirolimus/cyclosporine combination regimen for renal transplantation. Transplantation 1998;66(8):1040–6.
2. Kahan BD. Efficacy of sirolimus compared with azathioprine for reduction of acute renal allograft rejection: a randomised multicentre study. The Rapamune US Study Group. Lancet 2000;356(9225):194–202.
3. Groth CG, Backman L, Morales JM, Calne R, Kreis H, Lang P, Touraine JL, Claesson K, Campistol JM, Durand D, Wramner L, Brattstrom C, Charpentier B. Sirolimus (rapamycin)-based therapy in human renal transplantation: similar efficacy and different toxicity compared with cyclosporine. Sirolimus European Renal Transplant Study Group. Transplantation 1999;67(7):1036–42.
4. Morelon E, Stern M, Kreis H. Interstitial pneumonitis associated with sirolimus therapy in renal-transplant recipients. N Engl J Med 2000;343(3):225–6.
5. Singer SJ, Tiernan R, Sullivan EJ. Interstitial pneumonitis associated with sirolimus therapy in renal-transplant recipients. N Engl J Med 2000;343(24):1815–16.
6. Mahalati K, Murphy DM, West ML. Bronchiolitis obliterans and organizing pneumonia in renal transplant recipients. Transplantation 2000;69:1531–2.
7. Brattstrom C, Wilczek H, Tyden G, Bottiger Y, Sawe J, Groth CG. Hyperlipidemia in renal transplant recipients treated with sirolimus (rapamycin). Transplantation 1998;65(9):1272–4.
8. Morrisett JD, Abdel-Fattah G, Hoogeveen R, Mitchell E, Ballantyne CM, Pownall HJ, Opekun AR, Jaffe JS, Oppermann S, Kahan BD. Effects of sirolimus on plasma lipids, lipoprotein levels, and fatty acid metabolism in renal transplant patients. J Lipid Res 2002;43(8):1170–80.
9. Hong JC, Kahan BD. Sirolimus-induced thrombocytopenia and leukopenia in renal transplant recipients: risk factors, incidence, progression, and management. Transplantation 2000;69(10):2085–90.

10. Kaplan MJ, Ellis CN, Bata-Csorgo Z, Kaplan RS, Endres JL, Fox DA. Systemic toxicity following administration of sirolimus (formerly rapamycin) for psoriasis: association of capillary leak syndrome with apoptosis of lesional lymphocytes. Arch Dermatol 1999;135(5):553–7.

11. Johnson RW. Sirolimus (Rapamune) in renal transplantation. Curr Opin Nephrol Hypertens 2002;11(6):603–7.

12. Zimmerman JJ, Harper D, Getsy J, Jusko WJ. Pharmacokinetic interactions between sirolimus and microemulsion cyclosporine when orally administered jointly and 4 hours apart in healthy volunteers. J Clin Pharmacol 2003;43(10):1168–76.

13. Bottiger Y, Sawe J, Brattstrom C, Tollemar J, Burke JT, Hass G, Zimmerman JJ. Pharmacokinetic interaction between single oral doses of diltiazem and sirolimus in healthy volunteers. Clin Pharmacol Ther 2001;69(1):32–40.

Sitafloxacin

See also Fluoroquinolones

General Information

Sitafloxacin is a quinolone antibiotic that is effective against methicillin-resistant *Staphylococcus aureus*.

Organs and Systems

Liver

In a phase II, open, multicenter, randomized study sitafloxacin 400 mg/day caused mild transient increases in alanine transaminase and alkaline phosphatase in 69 patients but no effects on other enzymes (1).

Skin

Data obtained in albino mice have suggested that the phototoxic potential of sitafloxacin is milder than that of lomefloxacin or sparfloxacin (2).

Drug Administration

Drug formulations

After oral administration sitafloxacin 500 mg is rapidly absorbed, with a systemic availability of 89% (3). By 48 hours, about 61% is excreted unchanged in the urine after oral administration and about 75% after intravenous administration. For both routes, the high renal clearance of sitafloxacin implies active tubular secretion.

References

1. Feldman C, White H, O'Grady J, Flitcroft A, Briggs A, Richards G. An open, randomised, multi-centre study comparing the safety and efficacy of sitafloxacin and imipenem/cilastatin in the intravenous treatment of hospitalised patients with pneumonia. Int J Antimicrob Agents 2001;17(3):177–88.

2. Shimoda K, Ikeda T, Okawara S, Kato M. Possible relationship between phototoxicity and photodegradation of sitafloxacin, a quinolone antibacterial agent, in the auricular skin of albino mice. Toxicol Sci 2000;56(2):290–6.

3. O'Grady J, Briggs A, Atarashi S, Kobayashi H, Smith RL, Ward J, Ward C, Milatovic D. Pharmacokinetics and absolute bioavailability of sitafloxacin, a new fluoroquinolone antibiotic, in healthy male and female Caucasian subjects. Xenobiotica 2001;31(11):811–22.

Sitamaquine

General Information

Sitamaquine (1) is an 8-aminoquinoline that has been used to treat kala-azar (visceral leishmaniasis) (2) and is being tested for activity against *Pneumocystis jiroveci* (1).

In a phase-II, open, dose-escalating safety and efficacy study in 22 Brazilian patients with kala-azar, five groups were given different oral regimens, containing 1.0–3.25 mg of sitamaquine, for 28 days (3). There was nephrotoxicity with 2.5 mg/kg/day in two patients and in the single patient who took 3.25 mg/kg/day. Interstitial nephritis with acute tubular necrosis was proven by biopsy in two patients. Headache and gastrointestinal adverse effects occurred in under 5%. Methemoglobinemia of less than 6% after 7 days was common.

References

1. Yeates C. Sitamaquine (GlaxoSmithKline/Walter Reed Army Institute). Curr Opin Investig Drugs 2002;3(10):1446–52.

2. Sangraula H, Sharma KK, Rijal S, Dwivedi S, Koirala S. Orally effective drugs for kala-azar (visceral leishmaniasis): focus on miltefosine and sitamaquine. J Assoc Physicians India 2003;51:686–90.

3. Dietze R, Carvalho SF, Valli LC, Berman J, Brewer T, Milhous W, Sanchez J, Schuster B, Grogl M. Phase 2 trial of WR6026, an orally administered 8-aminoquinoline, in the treatment of visceral leishmaniasis caused by *Leishmania chagasi*. Am J Trop Med Hyg 2001;65(6):685–9.

Smallpox vaccine

See also Vaccines

General Information

The last case of smallpox occurred in 1977, and the eradication of smallpox was declared complete by the World Health Assembly in 1980. Since then, routine smallpox vaccination has ceased in all countries, because it is no longer required and because serious adverse reactions sometimes occur after both primary vaccination and revaccination (SED-8, 709) (SED-11, 685) (SEDA-1, 247) (SEDA-3, 262) (SEDA-4, 227) (SEDA-6, 289) (SEDA-13, 289) (SEDA-15, 357) (1–5). However, the threat of bioterrorism has made it necessary to consider prevention and control

Table 1 Frequencies of some complications per 1 000 000 smallpox vaccinations

Complication	Primarily vaccinated	Revaccinated
Vaccinia gangrenosa	0.9	0.7
Eczema vaccinatum	10.0	0.9
Generalized vaccinia	23.4	1.2
Accidental infections	25.3	0.8

strategies through vaccination and the potential hazards associated with the administration of smallpox vaccine.

Adverse reactions to smallpox vaccination vary from what may be called a "normal" reaction via anomalous reactions to real complications. These can be divided into two categories (6):

1. complications in which sequelae or a fatal outcome are rare (sensitivity, rashes, generalized vaccinia, and autoinoculation vaccinia);
2. complications that may well be fatal or have permanent sequelae (postvaccinial encephalomyelitis, vaccinia necrosum, eczema vaccinatum).

Both categories of complications are much less common after revaccination than after primary vaccination. *Vaccinia* virus can also spread by contact to other subjects and cause adverse effects (7,8).

In an Australian survey of 5 000 000 vaccinations carried out between 1960 and 1976, the frequency of all complications was 188 per million and the death rate 1.5 per million. The ratio of reactions in women to reactions in men was 1.6, increasing with age. Paradoxically, of eight reports of cardiac complications seven concerned men (9).

The frequencies of some complications in 1968 in the USA per 1 000 000 smallpox vaccinations in primarily vaccinated and revaccinated subjects are shown in Table 1 (7).

Recombinant DNA technology using *Vaccinia* virus

Because of its great genetic potential, *Vaccinia* virus is an ideal medium for recombined genes originating from different organisms. In order to use *Vaccinia* virus, efforts have been made to attenuate it further, either by inactivating the genes responsible for virulence (SEDA-15, 357) or by introducing human lymphokine genes into its genome.

Vaccinia DNA can tolerate large insertions into nonessential regions of the genome, and this opens the door to the making of polyvalent live *Vaccinia* recombinations. A major obstacle to their use as vaccines is that severe complications can occur after vaccination, especially in immunodeficient individuals. On the other hand, there is evidence that recombinant *Vaccinia* viruses have reduced pathogenicity. A genetically engineered *Vaccinia* virus expressing murine interleukin-2 has been described (10), and it has been shown that athymic nude mice infected with the *Vaccinia* virus recover from the virus infection rapidly, whereas mice infected with a control virus develop progressive vaccinia.

One attempt to develop safe and efficacious live recombinant vaccines is the use of low neurovirulent strains of vaccinia virus: LC 16 m O (m O) or LC 16 m 8 (m 8). A recombinant *Vaccinia* virus vaccine (RVV) expressing hepatitis B surface antigen likely to form the basis of a safe live RV vaccine against hepatitis B has been constructed (11).

Little is known of the ways in which orthopoxviruses are maintained in nature (12). There is a possibility that strains of *Vaccinia* used as vaccines may become established in nature, as *Vaccinia* may have become established in Indian buffaloes, and/or undergo genetic hybridization with existing orthopoxviruses (12). Enthusiasm for these new prospects should not be allowed to compromise the requirement for obtaining additional scientific information essential to ensure safety, efficacy, and the exercise of all reasonable caution in mounting field investigations (13).

There have already been accusations that two patients with AIDS, treated with an experimental vaccine prepared using a *Vaccinia* virus that had apparently been inactivated and genetically engineered to express HIV proteins, may have died from vaccinia gangrenosa (14,15). On the other hand, there is evidence that recombinant *Vaccinia* viruses have reduced pathogenicity (SEDA-13, 289).

Protection of laboratory workers exposed to orthopoxviruses

In 1980, the US Public Health Service first recommended the use of *Vaccinia* (smallpox) vaccine to protect laboratory workers occupationally exposed to orthopoxviruses. In 1991, the Centers for Disease Control, Atlanta, Georgia, published recommendations on *Vaccinia* vaccine. From 1983 to 1991, 4649 doses of smallpox vaccine were administered, of which 57% were given in 1989–91. The proportion of primary vaccinations increased from 4% in 1983–88 to 14% in 1989–91. Of vaccinees 93% reported no signs or symptoms after vaccination. Reported adverse reactions were mild: lymphadenopathy, fever or chills, and tenderness at the site of vaccination. No severe adverse effects were reported. However, one vaccinee reported a spontaneous abortion 5 months after primary vaccination (16).

A somewhat different note has been sounded from the Committee on Occupational Medical Practice of the American College of Occupational and Environmental Medicine. The committee pointed out that risks to laboratory workers resulting from spontaneous infection are presumably similar to those involved in vaccination. The positive aspect of immunization is that it renders possible control over the time and initial site of entry of the virus. In the Committee's opinion, it is important for scientists and technicians to understand the US Public Health Service recommendations and to have the opportunity to receive *Vaccinia* immunization. They should also understand the possible drawbacks and have the opportunity to refuse vaccination (17). These different recommendations in the USA are also reflected in different national recommendations in other countries.

Accidental needle-stick inoculation of *Vaccinia* virus has been reported (18).

- A 26-year-old laboratory worker, who had been vaccinated against smallpox in childhood, developed a pustule and erythema on his left thumb 3 days after an accidental needle-stick while working with *Vaccinia* virus. Further pustules occurred on the fourth and fifth fingers of the same hand, accompanied by a large erythematous lesion on the left forearm, secondary bacterial infection, and axillary lymphadenopathy. After surgical excision of the necrotic tissue, he improved slowly and the lesions healed in about 3 weeks.

Smallpox and bioterrorism

The threat of bioterrorism has made it necessary to consider again prevention and control strategies through vaccination and the potential hazards associated with the administration of smallpox vaccine. Guidelines for prevention and control of smallpox have been elaborated in many countries. The guidelines distinguish between pre-event vaccination programs (worldwide no re-emergence of smallpox) and postevent vaccination programs (re-emergence of smallpox confirmed). Taking into account the risk of smallpox vaccination, most countries have elaborated plans for postevent vaccination programs. During the US pre-event vaccination program, in 1 per 20 000 members of the military who received primary smallpox vaccination, cardiac inflammation (myocarditis and/or pericarditis), including one death (myocardial infarction), has been reported. Compared with the rate reported in an unvaccinated military population during 1998–2000, the rate of myocarditis/pericarditis was substantially increased. However, there were no cases after revaccination. In 2003, among 38 257 civilian health-care and public health workers vaccinated against smallpox, 17 suspected and 5 probable cases of myocarditis/pericarditis were reported. The other adverse events include one case of suspected encephalitis, three of generalized *Vaccinia*, three of ocular *Vaccinia*, and 21 of inadvertent inoculation.

During the US pre-event smallpox vaccination program, there were no reports of eczema vaccinatum, progressive *Vaccinia*, or fetal *Vaccinia* (19,20).

During a meeting in June 2003, the Global Advisory Committee on Vaccine Safety considered two expert reports on the safety of smallpox vaccination in detail. They concluded that there is a real risk of serious adverse events, including safety issues that have not previously been recognized. Therefore, if the vaccine is being used in mass campaigns, it would be very important to include adverse events monitoring. The committee found that the available data were insufficient to define the risk after primary vaccination compared with the risk of revaccination after a long interval (21).

Organs and Systems

Cardiovascular

Acute myocarditis after vaccination against smallpox has been reported (22). Fatal myocarditis is rare, but electrocardiographic evidence of myocarditis has been found more frequently; this adverse effect is probably not always noticed (23–25). Pericarditis after smallpox vaccination has also been described (26).

All case reports of myocarditis/pericarditis after smallpox vaccination have been carefully evaluated. It was concluded that the data are consistent with a causal relation between myocarditis/pericarditis and smallpox vaccination; however, no causal association between ischemic cardiac events and smallpox has been identified (19,20).

- A 57-year-old woman with a history of hypertension, a transient ischemic attack, and carotid endarterectomy died 22 days after smallpox vaccination. Histopathological evaluation showed no evidence of cardiac inflammation.

Pericarditis after smallpox vaccination has been described (26).

The Advisory Committee on Immunization Practices (ACIP) has recommended that people who have underlying heart disease, with or without symptoms, or who have three or more known major cardiac risk factors (that is hypertension, diabetes, hypercholesterolemia, heart disease at age 50 years in a first-degree relative, and smoking) should be excluded from the pre-event smallpox vaccination program (27).

During the period of routine smallpox vaccination, only rare reports of cardiac inflammation (pericarditis, fatal myocarditis, and electrocardiographic evidence of myocarditis) were published in the world literature (SED-8, 709). To determine the risk of cardiac death after smallpox vaccination, death certificates were analysed from a period in 1947 when 6 million New York City residents were vaccinated after a smallpox outbreak; the incidence of cardiac deaths did not increase after the vaccination campaign (28).

Respiratory

Pneumonia has been observed after smallpox vaccination (2).

Nervous system

Neurological complications of smallpox vaccination can cause paralysis; of 26 patients with such symptoms, most were children under 2 years (29).

The most dreaded complication of smallpox vaccination is postvaccinial encephalitis or encephalomyelitis, which is said to occur even without a cutaneous vaccination reaction (30), although this occurs rarely, if at all (2,31). It is mainly a complication of primary vaccination. There is increased morbidity with increasing age, especially around puberty. It is rare after revaccination.

Two conditions must be distinguished: a histopathological picture characterized by diffuse perivenous focal encephalitis and a condition based on a disturbance of the blood–brain barrier, that is an encephalopathy that characteristically occurs in infants. The incubation period of postvaccinial encephalomyelitis is 9–13 days. Its onset is mostly sudden. The clinical picture varies. Mortality is high (30–50%). Recovery may be complete, but there are often neurological sequelae, such as paresis and extrapyramidal disturbances.

The frequency of postvaccinial encephalomyelitis in different countries has varied considerably. Per million primary vaccinations 68 cases were recorded in Bavaria, 48 in the Netherlands, 15 in the UK, and 1.8 in the USA. The frequency increases with age beyond the first year (5). In 53 034 primarily vaccinated army recruits in the Netherlands there were 11 cases (1:5000) (32). In 1968 the frequency in the USA was 2.8 per million primarily vaccinated. There were no cases among 8.5 million revaccinations (8). In very young infants sudden death can occur (33), but information about frequency is difficult to assess, because of the occurrence of sudden unexplained deaths ("cot" deaths).

The risk of postvaccinial encephalomyelitis is reduced by simultaneous administration of hyperimmune *Vaccinia* gamma globulin (32) or by pre-immunization with an antigen from formol-inactivated *Vaccinia* virus (34,35). However, cases of postvaccinial encephalomyelitis have been described even after these procedures (32,36).

- A 13-year-old girl died of neuromyelitis optica. By inoculation of rabbits it was shown that the brain tissue contained *Vaccinia* antigen. Moreover, there were high titres against *Vaccinia* virus in both sera and spinal fluid. In infancy this patient had been vaccinated against smallpox (37).
- Accidental administration of 10 doses of smallpox vaccine to an already vaccinated girl resulted in a clinical picture characterized by neuraxitis with general tonic-clonic convulsions. Complete cure was attained after treatment with hyperimmune antivaccinia globulins and methisazone (38).

Polyneuropathy (39) and bacterial meningitis (40) have been described after smallpox vaccination.

Sensory systems

Ears
Disturbances of hearing and balance are described after smallpox vaccination (41).

Eyes
Vaccinial lesions on the eyelids and the conjunctivae are seen after secondary infection with *Vaccinia* virus by scratching (42,43). From these lesions a keratitis can develop, which sometimes extends to deeper layers of the cornea, with concomitant iridocyclitis. Papillitis with myelitis has been described after revaccination (44).

Metabolism

Diabetes mellitus occurred in a 1-year-old child about 4 weeks after smallpox vaccination (45).

Hematologic

Thrombocytopenic purpura is a rare complication of smallpox vaccination (46). Postvaccinial lymphadenitis can occur (47).

Mouth and teeth

Of 2568 people who were given oral vaccination, five bit open the vaccine-containing capsule or tablet, with release of the virus, and developed vaccinia lesions on the tongue, gums, or nares (48).

Urinary tract

Nephritis is a very rare complication of smallpox vaccination (49).

Skin

A 20-year-old man had active eczematous lesions on both wrists. After vaccination widespread *Vaccinia* developed in non-eczematous skin around the eyes and mouth, while the eczematous regions were unaffected. The possible reason was the use of a glucocorticoid ointment (50).

Skin reactions after smallpox vaccination can cause the following complications (2,3):

- Ectopic pocks near the vaccination site (vaccinia serpiginosa).
- Secondary vaccinia, which is caused by spreading of Vaccinia virus from the vaccination site to other body sites by scratching.
- Generalized vaccinia (vaccinia generalisata). Here the *Vaccinia* virus is spread by the blood stream and vaccinial lesions can develop all over the body some 9–10 days after vaccination.
- Eczema vaccinatum. This serious complication occurs most often in infants with active infantile eczema and occasionally in adults who have eczema or some other skin disease. It is seen after vaccination or contact with vaccinated persons with vaccinial lesions. The first symptoms are observed at the eczematous spots 3–4 days after vaccination. In many cases generalization of the vaccinial lesions follows. The estimated mortality is 25–30%.
- Progressive vaccinia (vaccinia gangrenosa). About 7 days after a normal vaccinial reaction the lesion extends, penetrates the underlying tissue, and becomes necrotic. Ulcers are formed, and the process spreads to adjacent areas of the skin. Secondary bacterial infection is common. This rare complication may be due to some abnormality of serum proteins, interfering with immunity, such as agammaglobulinemia or hypogammaglobulinemia. Mortality is high (51–53).
- Keloid from vaccinial scars.

Abnormal hair growth (54), herpes virus infections (55), and malignant changes in smallpox vaccination scars have also been observed (56,57). Allergic skin reactions sometimes occur, for example urticaria and purpura (58) and possibly photosensitivity reactions.

Musculoskeletal

Osteomyelitis and periosteitis are exceedingly rare sequels to smallpox vaccination (59,60).

Acute arthritis has been described after smallpox vaccination (61).

Death

In France 4 113 109 primary vaccinations during 1968–77 have been surveyed. There were 30 deaths that could have been associated with the vaccine, 23 in the first year of life (62). The relation was considered certain in one case, probable in 5, possible in 6, and doubtful in 18. In the certain case there may have been immunodeficiency. In the second group there were three cases of acute encephalitis. Among the doubtful cases were 12 patients who had neurological symptoms.

Second-Generation Effects

Pregnancy

The incidence of abortions is said to be higher in women who have recently received smallpox vaccination; in some cases the aborted fetus showed evidence of *Vaccinia* infection (63).

Fetotoxicity

Although routine smallpox vaccination of infants was discontinued in the UK in 1971, some 20–28 cases of complications of vaccination continue to be reported yearly to the Committee on Safety of Medicines (64), including both cross-infection and fetal infection (64).

Susceptibility Factors

HIV infection is a risk factor for vaccinia generalisata, making it important to have *Vaccinia* immune globulin available for outbreak control (65).

- Vaccinia generalisata developed after smallpox vaccination (co-administrated with other vaccines) of an army recruit with asymptomatic HIV infection (66). After 2–3 weeks he developed cryptococcal meningitis, and a diagnosis of AIDS was made. While being treated for the meningitis he developed generalized vaccinia. He was treated with *Vaccinia* immune globulin and recovered from his vaccinia generalisata.

References

1. Moss B, Fuerst TR, Flexner C, Hugin A. Roles of vaccinia virus in the development of new vaccines. Vaccine 1988;6(2):161–3.
2. Herrlich A, Ehrengut W, Schleussing H. Die Pockenschutzimpfung. Der Impfschaden. Herrlich A, editor. Handbuch der Schutzimpfungen. 1st ed. Berlin: Springer-Verlag, 1965:60.
3. Dixon CW, editor. Treatment and Nursing. Sequelae Complications. Smallpox. 1st ed. London: J and A Churchill Ltd, 1962:143.
4. Copeman PW, Banatvala JE. The skin and vaccination against smallpox. Br J Dermatol 1971;84(2):169–73.
5. Dick G. Routine smallpox vaccination. BMJ 1971;3(767):163–6.
6. WHO Scientific Group. Human viral and rickettsial vaccines. World Health Organ Tech Rep Ser 1966;325:1–79.
7. Lane JM, Ruben FL, Neff JM, Millar JD. Complications of smallpox vaccination, 1968: results of ten statewide surveys. J Infect Dis 1970;122(4):303–9.
8. Lane JM, Ruben FL, Neff JM, Millar JD. Complications of smallpox vaccination, 1968. N Engl J Med 1969;281(22):1201–8.
9. Feery BJ. Adverse reactions after smallpox vaccination. Med J Aust 1977;2(6):180–3.
10. Ramshaw IA, Andrew ME, Phillips SM, Boyle DB, Coupar BE. Recovery of immunodeficient mice from a vaccinia virus/IL-2 recombinant infection. Nature 1987;329(6139):545–6.
11. Watanabe K, Kobayashi H, Kajiyama K, Morita M, Yasuda A, Gotoh H, Saeki S, Sugimoto M, Saito H, Kojima A. Improved recombinant LC16m0 or LC16m8 vaccinia virus successfully expressing hepatitis B surface antigen. Vaccine 1989;7(1):53–9.
12. Baxby D, Gaskell RM, Gaskell CJ, Bennett M. Ecology of orthopoxviruses and use of recombinant vaccinia vaccines. Lancet 1986;2(8511):850–1.
13. Brown F, Schild GC, Ada GL. Recombinant vaccinia viruses as vaccines. Nature 1986;319(6054):549–50.
14. Dorozynski A, Anderson A. Deaths in vaccine trials trigger French inquiry. Science 1991;252(5005):501–2.
15. Guillaume JC, Saiag P, Wechsler J, Lescs MC, Roujeau JC. Vaccinia from recombinant virus expressing HIV genes. Lancet 1991;337(8748):1034–5.
16. Stokes SL, Atkinson WL, Becher JA, Williams WW. Vaccination against orthopoxvirus infection and adverse events among laboratory personnel, United States, 1983–1991. Personal communication, 1992.
17. Perry GF. Occupational Medicine Forum: Pro and cons of vaccinia immunization. J Occup Med 1992;34:757.
18. Moussatche N, Tuyama M, Kato SE, Castro AP, Njaine B, Peralta RH, Peralta JM, Damaso CR, Barroso PF. Accidental infection of laboratory worker with vaccinia virus. Emerg Infect Dis 2003;9(6):724–6.
19. Centers for Disease Control and Prevention (CDC). Update: adverse events following civilian smallpox vaccination—United States, 2003. MMWR Morb Mortal Wkly Rep 2003;52(34):819–20.
20. Centers for Disease Control and Prevention (CDC). Update: adverse events following smallpox vaccination—United States, 2003. MMWR Morb Mortal Wkly Rep 2003;52(13):278–82.
21. Global Advisory Committee on Vaccine Safety, 11–12 June 2003. Wkly Epidemiol Rec 2003;78(32):282–4.
22. Baldini G, Bani E. Sulle complicanze cardiache in corso di vaccinazione jenneriana. (Contributo clinico ed ec-grafie.) [Cardiac complications in Jennerian vaccination (Clinical and electrocardiographic studies).] Minerva Pediatr 1979;31(1):35–9.
23. Finlay-Jones LR. Fatal myocarditis after vaccination against smallpox. Report of a case. N Engl J Med 1964;270:41–2.
24. Mead J. Serum transaminase and electrocardiographic findings after smallpox vaccination: case report. J Am Geriatr Soc 1966;14(7):754–6.
25. Bessard G, Marchal A, Avezou F, Pont J, Rambaud P. Un nouveau cas de myocardite après vaccination anti-variolique. [A new case of myocarditis following smallpox vaccination.] Pediatrie 1974;29(2):179–84.
26. Price MA, Alpers JH. Acute pericarditis following smallpox vaccination. Papua N Guinea Med J 1968;11:30.
27. Centers for Disease Control and Prevention (CDC). Supplemental recommendations on adverse events following smallpox vaccine in the pre-event vaccination program: recommendations of the Advisory Committee on Immunization Practices. MMWR Morb Mortal Wkly Rep 2003;52(13):282–4.
28. Centers for Disease Control and Prevention (CDC). Cardiac deaths after a mass smallpox vaccination campaign—New York City, 1947. MMWR Morb Mortal Wkly Rep 2003;52(39):933–6.
29. Koen M. Paralyses following smallpox vaccination and revaccination. Probl Infect Parasit Dis 1978;6:64.
30. Rockoff A, Spigland I, Lorenstein B, Rose AL. Postvaccinal encephalomyelitis without cutaneous vaccination reaction. Ann Neurol 1979;5(1):99–101.
31. De Vries E, editor. Postvaccinal Perivenous Encephailitis. Amsterdam: Elsevier, 1960.
32. Nanning W. Prophylactic effect of antivaccinia gamma-globulin against post-vaccinal encephalitis. Bull World Health Organ 1962;27:317–24.
33. De Vries E. Plotselinge dood na pokkenvaccinatie bij zeer jonge kinderen. [Sudden death following smallpox

vaccination in very young children.] Ned Tijdschr Geneeskd 1964;108:2061–3.

34. Herrlich A. Welchen Nutzen hat die Prophylaxe der post-vakzinalen Enzephalitis? [What is the advantage of a prevention of postvaccinal encephalitis? A comparative evaluation of present methods.] Dtsch Med Wochenschr 1964;89:968–74.

35. Dietzsch HJ. Kasuistik: Enzephalitis nach Pocken Erstimpfung trotz Vorbehandlung mit Vakzineantigen. [Encephalitis following 1st smallpox vaccination despite pretreatment with vaccine antigens.] Kinderarztl Prax 1966;34(9):425–8.

36. Eggers C. Die postvakzinale Polyneuritis als Komplikation nach Pockenschützimpfung. [The post-vaccinal polyneuritis as complication following smallpox-vaccination.] Monatsschr Kinderheilkd 1974;122(4):169–71.

37. Adams JM, Brown WJ, Eberle ED, Vorlty A. Neuromyelitis optica: severe demyelination occurring years after primary smallpox vaccination. Rev Roum Neurol 1973;10(3):227–31.

38. Bertaggia A. Nevrassite da inoculazione accidentale in dose massiva di vaccino antiaioloso per via sottocutanea in soggetto vaccinato e rivaccinate contro il vaiolo. Trattamento e guarigione con immunoglobuline iperimmuni antivacciniche e methisazone. [Neuraxitis due to accidental inoculation of a massive subcutaneous dose of smallpox vaccine in a subject vaccinated and revaccinated against smallpox. Treatment and recovery with antivaccinal hyperimmune immunoglobulins and methisazone.] Minerva Pediatr 1975;27(29):1586–91.

39. Herrlich A. Über Vakzineantigen: Versuch einer Prophylaxe neuraler Impfschäden. [Vaccine antigen; an experiment in prevention of neural vaccinal complications.] Munch Med Wochenschr 1959;101(1):12–14.

40. Stickl H, Helming M. Eitrige Meningitiden nach der Pockenschutzimpfung. [Purulent meningitides following smallpox vaccination. On the problem of post-vaccinal decrease of resistance.] Dtsch Med Wochenschr 1966;91(29):1307–10.

41. Wirth G. Schädigung des Hör- und Gleichgewichtsorganes nach Wiederimpfung gegen Pocken ohne Impfenzephalitis. [Labyrinthine lesion following smallpox revaccination without vaccinia encephalitis.] Z Laryngol Rhinol Otol 1973;52(7):526–32.

42. Paufique L, Durand L, Magnard G, Dorne PA. Complications oculopalpébrales de la vaccination antivariolique: vaccine palpébrale. [Oculo-palpebral complications of smallpox vaccination: palpebral vaccinia.] Bull Soc Ophtalmol Fr 1968;68(7):673–7.

43. Ross J, Gorin M. Vaccinia infection of the eyelids: two case reports. Eye Ear Nose Throat Mon 1969;48(6):363–5.

44. Mathur SP, Makhija JM, Mehta MC. Papillitis with myelitis after revaccination. Indian J Med Sci 1967;21(7):469–71.

45. Schneider H. Diabetesmanifestation nach Pockenimpfung. [Manifestation of diabetes after smallpox vaccination.] Kinderarztl Prax 1975;43(3):101–7.

46. Burke PJ, Shah NR. Thrombocytopenic purpura after smallpox vaccine. Pa Med 1981;84(9):49–50.

47. Hartsock RJ. Postvaccinial lymphadenitis. Hyperplasia of lymphoid tissue that simulates malignant lymphomas. Cancer 1968;21(4):632–49.

48. Stickl H, Jung EG. Störungen des Impfverlaufes bei der Oral Impfung gegen Pocken. [Abnormal postvaccination course after oral smallpox immunisation.] Dtsch Med Wochenschr 1977;102(31):1118–19.

49. von Vacano D. Akute diffuse Glomerulonephritis nach Pockenschutzimpfung. [Acute diffuse glomerulonephritis following smallpox vaccination.] Monatsschr Kinderheilkd 1968;116(11):596–8.

50. Gundersen SG, Bjorvatn B. Vaccinia and topical steroids: a case report. Acta Derm Venereol 1980;60(5):445–7.

51. Stoop JW. Een patiëntje met vaccinia progressive et generalisata. [A patient with progressive and generalized vaccinia.] Ned Tijdschr Geneeskd 1972;116(44):1981–4.

52. Ziegler HK, Schock V. [Vaccinia generalisata progressiva in a case of alymphocytosis.] Z Kinderheilkd 1969;106(3):206–12.

53. Chandra RK, Kaveramma B, Soothill JF. Generalised non-progressive vaccinia associated with IgM deficiency. Lancet 1969;1(7597):687–9.

54. Kumar LR, Goyal BG. Pigmented hairy scar following smallpox vaccination. Indian J Pediatr 1968;35(245):283–4.

55. Warren WS, Salvatore MA. Herpesvirus hominis infection at a smallpox vaccination site. JAMA 1968;205(13):931–3.

56. Gordon HH. Complications of smallpox vaccination: Basal cell carcinoma, keloids, acute bullons reaction. Cutis 1974;13:444.

57. Haider S. Keratoacanthoma in a smallpox vaccination site. Br J Dermatol 1974;90(6):689–90.

58. Coskey RJ, Bryan HG. Photosensitivity secondary to smallpox vaccination. Cutis (NY) 1970;6:761.

59. Bennett NM, Yung AP, Lehmann NI. Periostitis following smallpox vaccination. Med J Aust 1968;1(24):1052–3.

60. Singhal RK. Osteo-articular complications of smallpox vaccination. J Indian Med Assoc 1970;55(1):20–2.

61. Silby HM, Farber R, O'Connell CJ, Ascher J, Marine EJ. Acute monarticular arthritis after vaccination. Report of a case with isolation of vaccinia virus from synovial fluid. Ann Intern Med 1965;62:347–50.

62. Martin-Bouyer C, Foulon G, de Solan M, Torgal J, N'Guyen K, Martin-Bouyer G. Etude des décès imputés à la vaccination antivariolique en France, de 1968 à 1977. [Deaths due to smallpox vaccination in France 1968–1977.] Arch Fr Pediatr 1980;37(3):199–206.

63. Tondury G, Kistler G. Die Gefährdung des ungeborenen bei Pockenschutzimpfung in graviditate. Prav-Med 1973;18:45.

64. Du Mont GC, Beach RC. Continuing mortality and morbidity from smallpox vaccination. BMJ 1979;1(6175):1398–9.

65. Heymann DL. Smallpox containment updated: considerations for the 21st century. Int J Infect Dis 2004;8(Suppl 2):S15–20.

66. La Force FM. Immunization of children infected with human immunodeficiency virus. WHO/EPI/GEN/86.6 Rev 1, Geneva, 1986.

Snakebite antivenom

See also Vaccines

General Information

Snakebite is an important medical emergency in some parts of the rural tropics. In most tropical countries it is an occupational disease of farmers, plantation workers, herders, and hunters. Every year thousands of people die in Africa, Central America, South Asia, and South-East Asia because of envenomation after snakebite. In India alone, an estimated 15–20 000 people die each year due to snakebite. In Sri Lanka, the overall incidence of snakebite exceeds 400 per 100 000 population per year, one of the highest in the world.

Antivenom (also known as antivenin, antivenene, and antisnakebite serum) is the concentrated enzyme-refined immunoglobulin of animals, usually horses or sheep, that have been exposed to venom. It is the only specific treatment currently available for the management of snakebite envenoming and has proved effective against many of the lethal and damaging effects of venoms. The most widely used antivenoms are F(ab')2-equine polyspecific antivenoms, raised against the venoms of many poisonous snakes. In the management of snakebite, the most important clinical decision is whether or not to give antivenom, because only some snake-bitten patients need it, it can produce severe reactions, and it is expensive and often in short supply.

Antivenom is most effective by intravenous injection. The range of venoms neutralized by an antivenom is usually stated in the package insert. If the biting species of snake is known, the appropriate monospecific antivenom should be used. In countries where several species produce similar signs, snakebite victims are treated with polyspecific antivenom, which contains a lower concentration of specific antibody to each species than the monospecific antivenom.

Organs and Systems

Immunologic

Antivenom treatment can be complicated by early reactions (anaphylaxis), pyrogenic reactions, or late reactions (serum sickness-type). The incidence and severity of early reactions is proportional to the dose of antivenom and the speed with which it enters the blood stream (1,2). These reactions usually develop within 10–180 minutes of starting antivenom therapy. The reported incidence of early reactions after intravenous antivenom in snakebite patients, which ranges from 43% (3) to 81% (4), appears to increase with the dose and decrease when refined antivenom is used and administration is by intramuscular rather than intravenous injection. Unless patients are watched carefully for 3 hours after treatment, mild reactions can be missed and deaths misattributed to the envenoming itself. In most cases symptoms are mild: urticaria, nausea, vomiting, diarrhea, headache, and fever; however, in up to 40% of cases severe systemic anaphylaxis develops, with bronchospasm, hypotension, or angioedema. However, deaths are rare (5).

Early reactions respond well to adrenaline given by intramuscular injection of 0.5–1 ml of a 0.1% solution (1:1000, 1 mg/ml) in adults (children 0.01 ml/kg) at the first sign of trouble. Antihistamines also should be given by intravenous injection to counteract the effects of histamine released during the reaction.

Pyrogenic reactions result from contamination of antivenom by endotoxin-like compounds. High fever develops 1–2 hours after treatment and is associated with rigors, followed by vasodilatation and a fall in blood pressure. Febrile convulsions can occur in children. Patients should be cooled and given antipyretic drugs by mouth, powdered and washed down a nasogastric tube, or by suppository.

Late (serum sickness-type) reactions develop 5–24 days after treatment. Symptoms include fever, itching, urticaria, arthralgia (which can involve the temporomandibular joint), lymphadenopathy, periarticular swellings, mononeuritis multiplex, albuminuria, and rarely encephalopathy. This is an immune complex disease which responds to antihistamines or, in more severe cases, to glucocorticoids.

Early antivenom reactions are not usually Type I IgE-mediated reactions to equine serum proteins and are not predicted by hypersensitivity tests. Several methods have been used to reduce acute adverse reactions to antivenom. A small test dose of antivenom to detect patients who may develop acute adverse reactions to the antivenom has no predictive value, can itself cause anaphylaxis, and is no longer recommended (5). Prophylactic use of hydrocortisone and antihistamines before infusion with antivenom is also practiced widely, although the theoretical basis for their use is unclear. Antihistamines counter only the effects of histamine after its release and do not prevent further release; one small randomized controlled trial showed no benefit from the routine use of antihistamines (6). Hydrocortisone takes time to act and may be ineffective as a prophylactic against acute adverse reactions that can develop almost immediately after antivenom treatment, which is very often administered urgently to snakebite victims. One study has suggested that intravenous hydrocortisone is ineffective in preventing acute adverse reactions to antivenom, but if given together with intravenous chlorphenamine it can reduce these reactions (7). However, this trial recruited only 52 patients and was not designed to study the efficacy of chlorphenamine alone, making it difficult to give a clear interpretation of the results and recommendations on pretreatment with glucocorticoids and antihistamines to prevent acute reactions to antivenom. In one study of 105 patients, low-dose adrenaline given subcutaneously immediately before administration of antivenom to snakebite victims significantly reduced the incidence of acute adverse reactions to the serum (3). However, this trial did not enroll sufficient participants to establish safety adequately, a major concern regarding the use of adrenaline in a prophylactic role, particularly the risk of intra-cerebral haemorrhage. Therefore, further studies on the safety of this treatment are required before it can be recommended routinely. For the present, the only available alternative to prevention is the early detection of adverse reactions to antivenom and the ready availability of drugs such as adrenaline for their prompt treatment.

References

1. Anonymous. Antivenom therapy and reactions. Lancet 1980;1(8176):1009–10.
2. Reid HA. Antivenom reactions and efficacy. Lancet 1980;1(8176):1024–5.
3. Premawardhena AP, de Silva CE, Fonseka MM, Gunatilake SB, de Silva HJ. Low dose subcutaneous adrenaline to prevent acute adverse reactions to antivenom serum in people bitten by snakes: randomised, placebo controlled trial. BMJ 1999;318(7190):1041–3.
4. Ariaratnam CA, Sjostrom L, Raziek Z, Kularatne SA, Arachchi RW, Sheriff MH, Theakston RD, Warrell DA. An open, randomized comparative trial of two antivenoms

for the treatment of envenoming by Sri Lankan Russell's viper *(Daboia russelii russelii)*. Trans R Soc Trop Med Hyg 2001;95(1):74–80.

5. Malasit P, Warrell DA, Chanthavanich P, Viravan C, Mongkolsapaya J, Singhthong B, Supich C. Prediction, prevention, and mechanism of early (anaphylactic) antivenom reactions in victims of snake bites. BMJ (Clin Res Ed) 1986;292(6512):17–20.

6. Fan HW, Marcopito LF, Cardoso JL, Franca FO, Malaque CM, Ferrari RA, Theakston RD, Warrell DA. Sequential randomised and double blind trial of promethazine prophylaxis against early anaphylactic reactions to antivenom for bothrops snake bites. BMJ 1999;318(7196):1451–2.

7. Gawarammana IB, Kularatne SA, Dissanayake WP, Kumarasiri RP, Senanayake N, Ariyasena H. Parallel infusion of hydrocortisone +/− chlorpheniramine bolus injection to prevent acute adverse reactions to antivenom for snakebites. Med J Aust 2004;180(1):20–3.

Sodium hypochlorite

See also Disinfectants and antiseptics

General Information

Sodium hypochlorite is widely used as a cleaning agent and to deal with blood spillages. Chlorine gas is released during the use of hypochlorite. Alkaline hypochlorite solutions with 0.25% "available chlorine" have been used to clean and disinfect wounds.

Accidental injection

Local injection
A patient developed ulceration and paresthesia of the lip with facial swelling after accidental injection of Milton solution (sodium hypochlorite 1%, sodium chloride 16.5%) into the upper lip when a sharp needle was used for irrigation (1). The ulceration healed within 6 weeks, the paresthesia within 3 months. In similar cases hypochlorite solution (25 mg NaClO) was accidentally injected into periapical tissue (2), and into the mandibular branch of the facial nerve (90 mg NaClO) (3).

Intraperitoneal infusion
Accidental intraperitoneal infusion of hypochlorite solution on two occasions (the first time about 10 ml of a 5% solution the second time more diluted) has been reported (4). After the infusion the patient felt severe abdominal pain accompanied by nausea but not by vomiting. Raised peritoneal solute transport rates and reduced ultrafiltration gradually subsided, but they did not return to pre-infusion values.

Intravenous infusion
Accidental intravenous infusion has been reported (5–7).

- A 68-year-old man received an accidental infusion of a 1% sodium hypochlorite solution. After 1 hour and an infusion volume of 150 ml the infusion was stopped. By this time he had a slow heart rate, mild hypotension, and an increased respiratory rate. The blood cell count, hemoglobin, serum electrolyte, creatinine, and urea concentrations, and transaminase activities were normal and hemolysis did not occur. Treatment with NaCl 0.9% and dextrose at an infusion rate of 300 ml/hour was started immediately with the goal of maintaining an adequate diuresis. Furosemide and dopamine hydrochloride were also administered. His blood pressure and respiratory rate promptly returned to normal, but the bradycardia persisted for 3 days despite atropine sulfate (5).

- During dialysis a patient received an accidental infusion of 30 ml of a 5.25% solution of hypochlorite. This led to cardiorespiratory arrest and massive hemolysis with hyperkalemia, although the patient eventually recovered (7).

- In a third case, intravenous infusion of 60 ml of an oral and 0.3 ml of a parenteral 5.25% solution in a suicide attempt did not result in any serious effects (6).

Organs and Systems

Respiratory

Chlorine gas, released during the use of hypochlorite, can cause mucous membrane irritation, bronchospasm, pneumonia, and pulmonary edema. It is believed that when hypochlorite is used as a cleaning substance in low concentrations it does not cause respiratory damage, but in a comparison of pulmonary function tests in 23 cleaning workers and 14 technical personnel, as a control group, even low concentrations of hypochlorite affected pulmonary function, causing irritation in the airways (8).

References

1. Linn JL, Messer HH. Hypochlorite injury to the lip following injection via a labial perforation. Case report. Aust Dent J 1993;38(4):280–2.

2. Becker GL, Cohen S, Borer R. The sequelae of accidentally injecting sodium hypochlorite beyond the root apex. Report of a case. Oral Surg Oral Med Oral Pathol 1974;38(4):633–8.

3. Herrmann JW, Heicht RC. Complications in therapeutic use of sodium hypochlorite. J Endod 1979;5(5):160.

4. Dedhia NM, Schmidt LM, Twardowski ZJ, Khanna R, Nolph KD. Long-term increase in peritoneal membrane transport rates following incidental intraperitoneal sodium hypochlorite infusion. Int J Artif Organs 1989;12(11):711–14.

5. Marroni M, Menichetti F. Accidental intravenous infusion of sodium hypochlorite. DICP 1991;25(9):1008–9.

6. Froner GA, Rutherford GW, Rokeach M. Injection of sodium hypochlorite by intravenous drug users. JAMA 1987;258(3):325.

7. Hoy RH. Accidental systemic exposure to sodium hypochlorite (Chlorox) during hemodialysis. Am J Hosp Pharm 1981;38(10):1512–14.

8. Demiralay R. Effects of the use of hypochlorite as a cleaning substance on pulmonary functions. Turk J Med Sci 2001;31:51–7.

Solanaceae

See also Herbal medicines

General Information

The genera in the family of Solanaceae (Table 1) include deadly nightshade, henbane, jimson weed, peppers, petunia, and tobacco.

Anisodus tanguticus

Anisodus tanguticus (Zangqie), a traditional Chinese herbal medicine, contains hyoscyamine and related toxic tropane alkaloids (1). Its active ingredient anisodamine has been used to treat snakebite (2).

Brugmansia species

Brugmansia candida (*Datura candida*, angel's trumpet) and *Brugmansia suaveolens* (*Datura suaveolens*, angel's tears) are ornamental flowers that have been used for hallucinogenic effects. Both contain tropane alkaloids, such as hyoscine, hyoscyamine, meteloidine, and norhyoscine, which have anticholinergic properties.

Table 1 The genera of Solanaceae

Acnistus (acnistus)
Atropa (belladonna)
Bouchetia (bouchetia)
Browallia (browallia)
Brugmansia (brugmansia)
Brunfelsia (rain tree)
Calibrachoa (calibrachoa)
Capsicum (pepper)
Cestrum (jessamine)
Chamaesaracha (five eyes)
Datura (jimson weed)
Goetzea (goetzea)
Hunzikeria (hunzikeria)
Hyoscyamus (henbane)
Jaborosa (jaborosa)
Jaltomata (false holly)
Leucophysalis (leucophysalis)
Lycianthes (lycianthes)
Lycium (desert thorn)
Mandragora (mandrake)
Margaranthus (margaranthus)
Nectouxia (nectouxia)
Nicandra (nicandra)
Nicotiana (tobacco)
Nierembergia (cupflower)
Nothocestrum (aiea)
Oryctes (oryctes)
Petunia (petunia)
Physalis (ground cherry)
Quincula (quincula)
Salpichroa (salpichroa)
Salpiglossis (salpiglossis)
Schizanthus (schizanthus)
Scopolia
Solanum (nightshade)
Solandra (solandra)
Streptosolen (streptosolen)

Adverse effects

Anticholinergic toxicity can result from the alkaloids that *Brugmansia* species contain (3).

- A 53-year-old woman was admitted to hospital with vertigo, blurred vision, palpitation, mydriasis of the right eye, and tachycardia (120/minute) (4). She reported that she had been cutting leaves from an angel's trumpet when a drop of sap had entered her right eye.
- A 76-year-old man drank 3 teaspoons (15 ml) of a homemade wine made from *B. suaveolens* over 1 hour and about 1.5 hours later developed respiratory distress and weakness (5).

There have been reports of young men who had confusion and other signs of central nervous system involvement after taking angel's trumpet (6).

After ocular exposure to sap from *B. suaveolens*, seven patients developed unilateral mydriasis, at least three also had ipsilateral cycloplegia, and one developed transient tachycardia (7).

Capsicum annuum

Capsicum annuum (chili pepper) contains a variety of carotenoids, including capsanthin, capsorubin, beta-carotene, cryptoxanthin, lutein, phytofluene, and xanthophyll, and steroids, including capsicoside. One of the main constituents is capsaicin, which produces an intense burning sensation when it comes into contact with the skin, eyes, or mucous membranes and which gives peppers their burning taste. A hot shower or bath before topical application to the skin intensifies the burning sensation. Capsaicin is used internally for various conditions, including colic and for improving peripheral circulation, and externally for unbroken chilblains. A cream for topical application has been used to relieve the pain of postherpetic neuralgia and other pain syndromes.

Adverse effects

Sensitization to *C. annuum* has been reported in a patient who was allergic to latex (8).

Taken orally in regular high doses capsaicin can act as a carcinogen and could promote gastric cancer, but in low doses it seems to have anticarcinogenic activity (9).

Datura stramonium

Datura stramonium (Jimson weed) is a naturally occurring plant that is ingested to induce hallucinogenic effects. Toxicity after ingestion is due to an atropine-containing alkaloid that is present in all parts of the plant but is particularly concentrated in the seeds.

Adverse effects

Intoxication with *Datura* species is often reported (10–12). Eleven patients aged 13–21 years ingested large quantities of Jimson weed pods and seeds (13). The signs and symptoms were classical of atropine poisoning. In milder cases there was asymptomatic mydriasis and tachycardia and in the more severely affected agitation, disorientation, and hallucinations. Nine of the 11 were admitted for observation. None died and none required pharmacological intervention with physostigmine to reverse the anticholinergic symptoms.

Lycium barbarum

Lycium barbarum (Chinese wolfberry) contains a variety of steroids. A tea prepared from it is used in China as a general tonic.

Adverse effects

An interaction of *L. barbarum* with warfarin has been described.

- A 61-year-old woman, who had taken warfarin for atrial fibrillation in weekly doses of 18–19 mg for years and had been completely stable, developed a raised INR after she consumed a tea made from Chinese wolfberry (14). Four days after drinking the tea (180 ml/day), she had an INR of 4.1. After withdrawal of the herbal tea her INR returned to within the target range and remained stable.

Although an extract of *L. barbarum* inhibited CYP2C9 in vitro, the effect was weak and the authors thought that another mechanism must have been involved.

Mandragora species

Mandragora (mandrake) species contain toxic tropane alkaloids, such as hyoscyamine and/or scopolamine.

Adverse effects

The tropane alkaloids in *Mandragora* species are powerful anticholinergic agents and can cause peripheral symptoms (for example blurred vision, dry mouth) and central effects (for example drowsiness, delirium) (15). They can potentiate the effects of synthetic drugs with similar pharmacological activity.

In 15 patients anticholinergic effects were due to poisoning by *Mandragora autumnalis* intermingled with leaves of chard (*Beta vulgaris*) and spinach (*Spinacia oleracea*) (16). The latency from the time of ingestion was 1–4 hours. There was no correlation between latency and severity. All had blurred vision and dryness of mouth, nine had difficult in micturition, nine dizziness, nine headache, eight vomiting, two difficulty in swallowing, and two abdominal pain. All had blushing, a reactive mydriasis, and tachycardia. The skin and mucosae were dry in 14. There was hyperactivity/hallucination in 14 and agitation/delirium in nine. One patient developed a florid psychotic episode. Prostigmine (2–6 mg) was given to 11 patients and physostigmine (0.5–2 mg) to six. The time to a definite response was variable (3–36 hours). The patients treated with physostigmine had better reversal of the psychoneurological symptoms.

In some cases of poisoning, formulations of ginseng may have been adulterated with *Mandragora officinarum* (17).

Anaphylaxis has been reported after the administration of a homeopathic preparation of mandragora (18).

Nicotiana tabacum

The leaves of *Nicotiana tabacum* (tobacco) contain the toxic alkaloid, nicotine as a major constituent and several other pyridine alkaloids as minor constituents. Although tobacco enemas have been abandoned in official medicine because of their life-threatening toxicity, unorthodox self-

medication with this agent has not completely died out. A case report in the 1970s described nausea and confusion, followed by hypotension and bradycardia, due to an enema apparently prepared from 5 to 10 cigarettes. Transdermal nicotine is now widely used as an aid to smoking cessation. Nicotine is covered in a separate monograph.

Scopolia species

Scopolia species (scopola) contain tropane alkaloids, such as atropine, hyoscine (scopolamine), hyoscyamine, and tropane. They can cause anticholinergic symptoms (19).

References

1. De Smet PA. Health risks of herbal remedies. Drug Saf 1995;13(2):81–93.
2. Li QB, Pan R, Wang GF, Tang SX. Anisodamine as an effective drug to treat snakebites. J Nat Toxins 1999;8(3):327–30.
3. Finlay P. Anticholinergic poisoning due to *Datura candida*. Trop Doct 1998;28(3):183–4.
4. Roemer HC, von Both H, Foellmann W, Golka K. Angel's trumpet and the eye. J R Soc Med 2000;93(6):319.
5. Smith EA, Meloan CE, Pickell JA, Oehme FW. Scopolamine poisoning from homemade "moon flower" wine. J Anal Toxicol 1991;15(4):216–19.
6. Greene GS, Patterson SG, Warner E. Ingestion of angel's trumpet: an increasingly common source of toxicity. South Med J 1996;89(4):365–9.
7. Havelius U, Asman P. Accidental mydriasis from exposure to angel's trumpet (*Datura suaveolens*). Acta Ophthalmol Scand 2002;80(3):332–5.
8. Gallo R, Cozzani E, Guarrera M. Sensitization to pepper (*Capsicum annuum*) in a latex-allergic patient. Contact Dermatitis 1997;37(1):36–7.
9. Surh YJ, Lee SS. Capsaicin in hot chili pepper: carcinogen, co-carcinogen or anticarcinogen? Food Chem Toxicol 1996;34(3):313–16.
10. Guharoy SR, Barajas M. Atropine intoxication from the ingestion and smoking of jimson weed (*Datura stramonium*). Vet Hum Toxicol 1991;33(6):588–9.
11. Coremans P, Lambrecht G, Schepens P, Vanwelden J, Verhaegen H. Anticholinergic intoxication with commercially available thorn apple tea. J Toxicol Clin Toxicol 1994;32(5):589–92.
12. Centers for Disease Control and Prevention (CDC). Jimson weed poisoning—Texas, New York, and California, 1994. MMWR Morb Mortal Wkly Rep 1995;44(3):41–4.
13. Tiongson J, Salen P. Mass ingestion of jimson weed by eleven teenagers. Del Med J 1998;70(11):471–6.
14. Lam AY, Elmer GW, Mohutsky MA. Possible interaction between warfarin and *Lycium barbarum* L. Ann Pharmacother 2001;35(10):1199–201.
15. Piccillo GA, Mondati EG, Moro PA. Six clinical cases of *Mandragora autumnalis* poisoning: diagnosis and treatment. Eur J Emerg Med 2002;9(4):342–7.
16. Jimenez-Mejias ME, Montano-Diaz M, Lopez Pardo F, Campos Jimenez E, Martin Cordero MC, Ayuso Gonzalez MJ, Gonzalez de la Puente. Intoxicacion atropinica por *Mandragora autumnalis*. Descripcion de quince casos. [Atropine poisoning by *Mandragora autumnalis*. A report of 15 cases.] Med Clin (Barc) 1990;95(18):689–92.
17. Chan TY. Anticholinergic poisoning due to Chinese herbal medicines. Vet Hum Toxicol 1995;37(2):156–7.
18. Helbling A, Brander KA, Pichler WJ, Muller UB. Anaphylactic shock after subcutaneous injection of

mandragora D3, a homeopathic drug. J Allergy Clin Immunol 2000;106(5):989–90.

19. Cuculic M, Kalodera Z, Sindik J, Kvasic D, Petricic J. [Familial poisoning with the root of the plant, *Scopolia carniolica* Jacq.] Arh Hig Rada Toksikol 1988;39(3):345–8.

Somatostatin and analogues

General Information

Somatostatin was first isolated from the hypothalamus, and was shown to inhibit growth hormone release. It has since been found in neuroendocrine tissues throughout the body. It has multiple effects, via five distinct receptors, and acts as a neurotransmitter, in the regulation of growth hormone and thyrotropin release, as a regulator of gastrointestinal and pancreatic function, and as an immune modulator. Synthetic analogues are selective for receptor subtypes 2 and 5, and have different clinical and adverse effects profiles to the native hormone, as well as having longer half-lives. Analogues of somatostatin include depreotide, edotreotide, ilatreotide, lanreotide, octreotide, pasireotide, pentetreotide, and vapreotide (all rINNs).

Octreotide, an octapeptide somatostatin analogue, is usually given subcutaneously in three divided doses per day. Longer-acting analogues with similar efficacy and adverse effects to octreotide, but which can be given every 14–28 days, have been developed (1,2). The therapeutic indications and adverse effects of octreotide have been reviewed (SEDA-13, 1309) (3).

Organs and Systems

Cardiovascular

Both somatostatin and octreotide cause transient increases in mean arterial pressure and mean pulmonary pressure when given intravenously to patients with cirrhosis, more marked with bolus administration than with continuous infusion (4). This may be either direct or mediated by inhibition of gut vasodilatory peptides (SEDA-24, 505) (5) and is not usually associated with significant clinical effects.

Severe hypertension with associated headache, nausea, and vomiting was reported within 2 weeks of administration of octreotide LAR 20 mg in a 26-year-old diabetic woman with autonomic neuropathy (5). Rechallenge with octreotide 75 µg resulted in a transient hypertensive episode lasting 3 hours.

- Exacerbation of pre-existing hypertension was also reported in a 22-month-old boy during octreotide infusion (6).

There has been one report of acute pulmonary edema during octreotide and intravenous fluid therapy for variceal bleeding (7).

Sinus bradycardia (less than 50/minute) is reported in up to 25% of acromegalic patients taking octreotide, and conduction abnormalities are also commonly reported in these patients. This adverse effect is reported only rarely in other recipients of somatostatin or octreotide, probably reflecting the high rate of cardiac abnormalities due to acromegaly (8).

Nervous system

Dizziness occurred in 7.4% of 68 patients randomized to somatostatin and 8.2% of 73 randomized to octreotide, both by rapid infusion, to control variceal bleeding, in which the effectiveness of somatostatin and its analogues is probably via a transient reduction in heart rate and cardiac output (9).

Metabolism

Somatostatin and its analogues inhibit insulin secretion in the short term, before receptor down-regulation. Mild hyperglycemia occurs during octreotide infusion in up to 23% of adults (10,11), and occasionally in children (12). This is not usually clinically significant (3). However, in an open, retrospective comparison of octreotide and lanreotide in 38 patients with acromegaly, one patient in each group stopped therapy because of worsening glycemic control (13).

In a meta-analysis of trials for variceal bleeding, hyperglycemia occurred in 41 of 310 patients who received somatostatin, octreotide, or vapreotide, compared with 26 of 318 patients who received placebo (14).

Reports of the effects of octreotide on glucose metabolism in acromegaly are inconsistent and are complicated by the high prevalence of insulin resistance and overt diabetes in acromegaly. In 10 patients with acromegaly who used modified-release lanreotide for 19 months followed by modified-release octreotide for 21 months after a 3-month washout period, mean fasting glucose, the glucose response to oral glucose tolerance testing, and glycated hemoglobin all increased after octreotide but not lanreotide (15). However, the study was small and the order of the two medications was not randomized.

In patients with insulinoma, octreotide can cause clinically important hypoglycemia, because of suppression of counter-regulatory hormone secretion (16).

Hematologic

- A 42-year-old woman, treated with octreotide infusion 50 mg/hour for cirrhosis-related gastrointestinal bleeding on two occasions 9 months apart, had an immediate fall in platelet count on both occasions, resolving after octreotide withdrawal (17). The thrombocytopenia was not severe (nadir platelet counts 62 and 55×10^9/l) and did not require specific treatment.

The rapid fall in platelet count in this case suggests an immunological mechanism, although this was not directly demonstrated.

Gastrointestinal

Transient gastrointestinal symptoms (nausea, diarrhea, abdominal discomfort, and flatulence) occur in up to 50% of patients during the first few days of treatment, but usually resolve spontaneously after the first 1–2 weeks of treatment (13,18). Nausea and vomiting occur in up to 25% of patients after somatostatin and are also common after octreotide (19). Two of 15 patients in a phase I trial of malignant gastrinoma had to stop using long-acting octreotide because of severe nausea (20).

Diarrhea is common soon after starting octreotide but usually resolves within 2 weeks without specific treatment. In a randomized, double-blind, placebo-controlled trial in 203 mostly postmenopausal women with locally recurrent or metastatic breast carcinoma, all of whom were also taking tamoxifen, and who had estrogen-receptor positive and/or progesterone-receptor positive tumors, octreotide was added to the basic treatment in 99 cases (21). The adverse events experienced by 10% or more of the patients and attributed to octreotide were gastrointestinal: diarrhea (53%), nausea (16%), and abdominal pain (11%); diarrhea occurred in only 11% of the controls.

One of 10 patients with rheumatoid arthritis in an open study stopped using long-acting octreotide because of severe diarrhea and weight loss of 3 kg (22). These effects are dose-related and are similar in healthy volunteers, acromegalic patients, and patients with gastrointestinal tumors (3).

Octreotide 100 µg given subcutaneously to five healthy subjects 30 minutes before meals for 7 days increased fecal fat excretion; however, steatorrhea occurred in only two cases; fecal bile acid excretion fell to about 25% (23)

Biliary tract

Biliary sludge and gallstones are frequent adverse effects of both octreotide (2) and its longer acting analogues, compared with 10–25% of the general population (24). Cholelithiasis develops in up to 20% of patients in the long term, secondary to reduced gall-bladder contractility, but only 1% of patients develop symptoms per year of treatment (25). There is prospective evidence that gallstones develop earlier in patients on higher doses of octreotide (24). Rebound gall-bladder hypermotility can occur on withdrawal of octreotide and can be associated with biliary colic or pancreatitis (SEDA-13, 1309) (26,27).

Patients treated with octreotide have impaired meal-stimulated gall-bladder emptying and altered bile chemical composition, similar to spontaneous cholelithiasis. In 16 patients with acromegaly the serum deoxycholic acid concentration increased in proportion to large bowel transit time (28). In 11 patients gall-bladder emptying was slower in patients given octreotide LAR than lanreotide SR, but was impaired in both groups compared with pretreatment values (29).

Fasting gall-bladder volume increased progressively in seven patients with acromegaly treated with once-monthly long-acting octreotide; gallstones formed de novo in six patients within 8 months and one had symptomatic biliary colic (30). Gallstones have also been reported in children receiving prolonged octreotide therapy (12).

Ursodiol appeared to reverse gall-bladder abnormalities in seven of 10 patients. Data from this study also showed earlier development of sludge in recipients of higher doses of octreotide (24).

Hair

Reversible hair loss has been reported in a few patients after both octreotide (31) and lanreotide (32).

Immunologic

Antibodies to somatostatin analogues have been reported only rarely. However, in one study octreotide antibodies were demonstrated in 63 (27%) of 231 patients treated with subcutaneous octreotide for more than 3 years, rising to 57% after 5 years and 72% after 8 years (33). The antibodies did not reduce clinical efficacy.

- A 64-year-old woman, who had had monthly intramuscular injections of long-acting octreotide in the buttocks for 6 years, had increased uptake of ^{111}In-pentetreotide in both buttocks, thought to represent granuloma formation at the injection sites (34). Localized granulomas have previously been described in isolated cases after intramuscular somatostatin analogues, and somatostatin receptors are expressed in high density in activated lymphocytes.

Allergic reactions to somatostatin are rare. Of 97 cirrhotic patients randomized to subcutaneous octreotide, one stopped therapy because of erythematous itchy skin, which then resolved (11).

Second-Generation Effects

Pregnancy

Octreotide is a small peptide that can pass the placental barrier, and it is not recommended for use in pregnant women.

Placental transfer was significant in the first reported pregnancy with long-acting octreotide (35). The dose of octreotide was reduced after an ultrasound suggested intrauterine growth retardation. The female infant had a low birth weight (11th percentile) but caught up to the 50th percentile by 3 months of age. Her development was normal during 18 months of follow-up.

Of seven women who took somatostatin analogues during pregnancy, five stopped taking it when the pregnancy was diagnosed (36). One had a single injection of modified-release lanreotide before pregnancy was diagnosed, with no apparent adverse effects on the infant (37). No fetal malformations or delay in postnatal development have been reported.

Susceptibility Factors

Age

Children are generally not given long-term octreotide because of concerns about its effect on growth. Although growth was reported as normal in a few case series, "catch-up" growth was also described after octreotide was withdrawn (12).

Drug–Drug Interactions

Erythromycin

Pretreatment with octreotide enhanced the gastric prokinetic effects of erythromycin in eight healthy subjects, suggesting that octreotide may be clinically useful in patients with tachyphylaxis to this effect of erythromycin (38).

Midodrine

In a controlled study of octreotide and midodrine (an alpha-adrenoceptor agonist) in patients with orthostatic hypotension, the pressor effect of the two drugs was synergistic (39).

Morphine

Somatostatin and its analogues have been reported to be OP$_3$ (μ) opioid receptor antagonists (40). Somatostatin infusions significantly reduced the effectiveness of morphine analgesia in a case report of three patients with cancer.

References

1. Caron P, Morange-Ramos I, Cogne M, Jaquet P. Three year follow-up of acromegalic patients treated with intramuscular slow-release lanreotide. J Clin Endocrinol Metab 1997;82(1):18–22.
2. Davies PH, Stewart SE, Lancranjan L, Sheppard MC, Stewart PM. Long-term therapy with long-acting octreotide (Sandostatin-LAR) for the management of acromegaly. Clin Endocrinol (Oxf) 1998;48(3):311–16.
3. Lamberts SW, van der Lely AJ, de Herder WW, Hofland LJ. Octreotide. N Engl J Med 1996;334(4):246–54.
4. Hadengue A. Somatostatin or octreotide in acute variceal bleeding. Digestion 1999;60(Suppl 2):31–41.
5. Pop-Busui R, Chey W, Stevens MJ. Severe hypertension induced by the long-acting somatostatin analogue Sandostatin LAR in a patient with diabetic autonomic neuropathy. J Clin Endocrinol Metab 2000;85(3):943–6.
6. Beckman RA, Siden R, Yanik GA, Levine JE. Continuous octreotide infusion for the treatment of secretory diarrhea caused by acute intestinal graft-versus-host disease in a child. J Pediatr Hematol Oncol 2000;22(4):344–50.
7. Jenkins SA, Shields R, Davies M, Elias E, Turnbull AJ, Bassendine MF, James OF, Iredale JP, Vyas SK, Arthur MJ, Kingsnorth AN, Sutton R. A multicentre randomised trial comparing octreotide and injection sclerotherapy in the management and outcome of acute variceal haemorrhage. Gut 1997;41(4):526–33.
8. Herrington AM, George KW, Moulds CC. Octreotide-induced bradycardia. Pharmacotherapy 1998;18(2):413–16.
9. Zhang HB, Wong BC, Zhou XM, Guo XG, Zhao SJ, Wang JH, Wu KC, Ding J, Lam SK, Fan DM. Effects of somatostatin, octreotide and pitressin plus nitroglycerine on systemic and portal haemodynamics in the control of acute variceal bleeding. Int J Clin Pract 2002;56(6):447–51.
10. Corley DA, Cello JP, Adkisson W, Ko WF, Kerlikowske K. Octreotide for acute esophageal variceal bleeding: a meta-analysis. Gastroenterology 2001;120(4):946–54.
11. Erstad BL. Octreotide for acute variceal bleeding. Ann Pharmacother 2001;35(5):618–26.
12. Lam JC, Aters S, Tobias JD. Initial experience with octreotide in the pediatric population. Am J Ther 2001; 8(6):409–15.
13. Razzore P, Colao A, Baldelli R, Gaia D, Marzullo P, Ferretti E, Ferone D, Jaffrain-Rea ML, Tamburrano G, Lombardi G, Camanni F, Ciccarelli E. Comparison of six months therapy with octreotide versus lanreotide in acromegalic patients: a retrospective study. Clin Endocrinol (Oxf) 1999;51(2):159–64.
14. Banares R, Albillos A, Rincon D, Alonso S, Gonzalez M, Ruiz-del-Arbol L, Salcedo M, Molinero LM. Endoscopic treatment versus endoscopic plus pharmacologic treatment for acute variceal bleeding: a meta-analysis. Hepatology 2002;35(3):609–15.
15. Ronchi C, Epaminonda P, Cappiello V, Beck-Peccoz P, Arosio M. Effects of two different somatostatin analogues on glucose tolerance in acromegaly. J Endocrinol Invest 2002;25(6):502–7.
16. Stehouwer CD, Lems WF, Fischer HR, Hackeng WH, Naafs MA. Aggravation of hypoglycemia in insulinoma patients by the long-acting somatostatin analogue octreotide (Sandostatin). Acta Endocrinol (Copenh) 1989;121(1):34–40.
17. Demirkan K, Fleckenstein JF, Self TH. Thrombocytopenia associated with octreotide. Am J Med Sci 2000;320(4):296–7.
18. Bienvenu B, Timsit J. Sauna-induced diabetic ketoacidosis. Diabetes Care 1999;22(9):1584.
19. Abraldes JG, Bosch J. Somatostatin and analogues in portal hypertension. Hepatology 2002;35(6):1305–12.
20. Shojamanesh H, Gibril F, Louie A, Ojeaburu JV, Bashir S, Abou-Saif A, Jensen RT. Prospective study of the antitumor efficacy of long-term octreotide treatment in patients with progressive metastatic gastrinoma. Cancer 2002;94(2):331–43.
21. Bajetta E, Procopio G, Ferrari L, Martinetti A, Zilembo N, Catena L, Alu M, Della TS, Alberti D, Buzzoni R. A randomized, multicenter prospective trial assessing long-acting release octreotide pamoate plus tamoxifen as a first line therapy for advanced breast carcinoma. Cancer 2002;94(2):299–304.
22. Paran D, Elkayam O, Mayo A, Paran H, Amit M, Yaron M, Caspi D. A pilot study of a long acting somatostatin analogue for the treatment of refractory rheumatoid arthritis. Ann Rheum Dis 2001;60(9):888–91.
23. Nakamura T, Kudoh K, Takebe K, Imamura K, Terada A, Kikuchi H, Yamada N, Arai Y, Tando Y, Machida K, et al. Octreotide decreases biliary and pancreatic exocrine function, and induces steatorrhea in healthy subjects. Intern Med 1994;33(10):593–6.
24. Avila NA, Shawker TH, Roach P, Bradford MH, Skarulis MC, Eastman R. Sonography of gallbladder abnormalities in acromegaly patients following octreotide and ursodiol therapy: incidence and time course. J Clin Ultrasound 1998;26(6):289–94.
25. Hussaini SH, Pereira SP, Veysey MJ, Kennedy C, Jenkins P, Murphy GM, Wass JA, Dowling RH. Roles of gall bladder emptying and intestinal transit in the pathogenesis of octreotide induced gall bladder stones. Gut 1996;38(5):775–83.
26. Rhodes M, James RA, Bird M, Clayton B, Kendall-Taylor P, Lennard TW. Gallbladder function in acromegalic patients taking long-term octreotide: evidence of rebound hypermotility on cessation of treatment. Scand J Gastroenterol 1992;27(2):115–18.
27. Sadoul JL, Benchimol D, Thyss A, Freychet P. Acute pancreatitis following octreotide withdrawal. Am J Med 1991;90(6):763–4.
28. Veysey MJ, Thomas LA, Mallet AI, Jenkins PJ, Besser GM, Wass JA, Murphy GM, Dowling RH. Prolonged large bowel transit increases serum deoxycholic acid: a risk factor for octreotide induced gallstones. Gut 1999;44(5):675–81.
29. Turner HE, Lindsell DR, Vadivale A, Thillainayagam AV, Wass JA. Differing effects on gall-bladder motility of lanreotide SR and octreotide LAR for treatment of acromegaly. Eur J Endocrinol 1999;141(6):590–4.
30. Moschetta A, Stolk MF, Rehfeld JF, Portincasa P, Slee PH, Koppeschaar HP, Van Erpecum KJ, Vanberge-Henegouwen GP. Severe impairment of postprandial

cholecystokinin release and gall-bladder emptying and high risk of gallstone formation in acromegalic patients during Sandostatin LAR. Aliment Pharmacol Ther 2001;15(2):181–5.

31. Vecht J, Lamers CB, Masclee AA. Long-term results of octreotide-therapy in severe dumping syndrome. Clin Endocrinol (Oxf) 1999;51(5):619–24.

32. Suliman M, Jenkins R, Ross R, Powell T, Battersby R, Cullen DR. Long-term treatment of acromegaly with the somatostatin analogue SR-lanreotide. J Endocrinol Invest 1999;22(6):409–18.

33. Kaal A, Orskov H, Nielsen S, Pedroncelli AM, Lancranjan I, Marbach P, Weeke J. Occurrence and effects of octreotide antibodies during nasal, subcutaneous and slow release intramuscular treatment. Eur J Endocrinol 2000;143(3):353–61.

34. Rideout DJ, Graham MM. Buttock granulomas: a consequence of intramuscular injection of Sandostatin detected by In-111 octreoscan. Clin Nucl Med 2001;26(7):650.

35. Fassnacht M, Capeller B, Arlt W, Steck T, Allolio B. Octreotide LAR treatment throughout pregnancy in an acromegalic woman. Clin Endocrinol (Oxf) 2001;55(3):411–15.

36. Herman-Bonert V, Seliverstov M, Melmed S. Pregnancy in acromegaly: successful therapeutic outcome. J Clin Endocrinol Metab 1998;83(3):727–31.

37. de Menis E, Billeci D, Marton E, Gussoni G. Uneventful pregnancy in an acromegalic patient treated with slow-release lanreotide: a case report. J Clin Endocrinol Metab 1999;84(4):1489.

38. Athanasakis E, Chrysos E, Zoras OJ, Tsiaoussis J, Karkavitsas N, Xynos E. Octreotide enhances the accelerating effect of erythromycin on gastric emptying in healthy subjects. Aliment Pharmacol Ther 2002;16(8):1563–70.

39. Hoeldtke RD, Horvath GG, Bryner KD, Hobbs GR. Treatment of orthostatic hypotension with midodrine and octreotide. J Clin Endocrinol Metab 1998;83(2):339–43.

40. Ripamonti C, De Conno F, Boffi R, Ascani L, Bianchi M. Can somatostatin be administered in association with morphine in advanced cancer patients with pain? Ann Oncol 1998;9(8):921–3.

Somatropin

General Information

Established indications for somatropin (growth hormone) include growth hormone deficiency in children, Turner's syndrome, Noonan's syndrome, and renal insufficiency in children. Other well-studied indications include idiopathic short stature, adult growth hormone deficiency, osteoporosis, and catabolic states associated with acute and chronic illness and injury. Body composition, respiratory muscle function, physical strength, and height improved in a 12-month trial of somatropin in 54 children with Prader–Willi syndrome (1).

The adverse effects of somatropin differ between adults and children. In adults, adverse effects are commoner in men, in heavier patients, and in adult-onset growth hormone deficiency. Efficacy is no greater in those who develop adverse effects. The higher rate of adverse effects is due to the higher dose of somatropin when calculated according to body weight, and also to lower sensitivity to somatropin in women than in men (2–4). Rapid dose escalation also increases the rate of adverse effects. To minimize adverse effects, it is recommended that treatment be started at a low dosage, that is 0.4–0.8 U/day, and titrated according to the age-specific concentration of IGF-1 (2,3,5).

Adverse effects are commoner in patients using higher doses. Starting at a low dose, increasing the dose gradually, and titrating individual doses against age-specific IGF-I concentrations may minimize adverse events.

Organs and Systems

Cardiovascular

The effect of somatropin on cardiovascular risk is complex, as growth hormone reduces visceral fat and total cholesterol and increases HDL cholesterol concentrations (6–8).

Edema, both generalized and peripheral, is common in adults given somatropin, as is hypertension. Symptoms are usually mild and resolve in many patients despite continuing treatment (9). Increased left ventricular wall thickness has been reported in both adults and children, although in children this is thought to reflect an increase in overall mass and is not thought to be of clinical significance (10,11).

In an open study in five patients with severe dilated cardiomyopathy given high-dose somatropin 4 IU/day (1.3 mg/day) for 3 months, ventricular dysrhythmias worsened in all patients during treatment, from Lown class 2 or 3 to 4A or 4B, and returned to baseline when treatment was stopped (12).

- A 7-year-old boy developed cardiomegaly and edema within a month of starting somatropin, 0.7 IU/kg/week; when the dose was reduced to 0.35 IU/kg/week his heart size returned to normal (13).

This is a reminder that the adverse effects of somatropin are dose-related within the therapeutic range and that dose escalation should be gradual.

Nervous system

Somatropin extracted from cadaveric human pituitaries was used to treat growth hormone-deficient patients until several cases of the fatal degenerative neurological disorder Creutzfeldt–Jakob disease were reported in the mid-1980s. Of 267 cases of iatrogenic Creutzfeldt–Jakob disease, 139 were caused by human cadaver-derived somatropin (SEDA-25, 479).

This disease develops when an abnormal prion protein present in the cadaveric material induces a cascade of conformational changes in host protein. Creutzfeldt–Jakob disease in recipients of somatropin differs from the sporadic form, in that it usually presents with cerebellar signs rather than cognitive impairment, and also in the prominence of prion protein amyloid plaques in nervous tissue (14). In a review, 139 cases of Creutzfeldt–Jakob disease were identified worldwide in people treated with cadaveric somatropin before recombinant human growth hormone became available in the mid-1980s (15). The prevalence of this fatal neurodegenerative condition in recipients of somatropin ranges from 0.3% in the USA to 4.4% in France. Creutzfeldt–Jakob disease has been reported to start at 4–30 years after therapy with cadaveric somatropin (14), so that further cases are anticipated and continue to be reported (16).

- A case has been reported in Brazil, 28 years after somatropin therapy (17).
- An 18-year-old man from Qatar presented with a 3-month history of unsteadiness, dysarthria, and left-sided weakness, followed by visual, hearing, and memory loss, 13 years after somatropin therapy (18).

This is the first case from Qatar, but it is possible that other cases there have not been reported.

People exposed to a contaminated batch of somatropin have about a 6% chance of developing Creutzfeldt–Jakob disease (19), although there are no reliable predictors of risk in an individual. The risk varies to some extent with the mode of preparation of the product, but it seems unlikely that it can be entirely eliminated. The natural product was therefore withdrawn from the market in most countries, but was rapidly replaced by biosynthetic somatropin preparations

Carpal tunnel syndrome due to somatropin is probably dose-dependent and was reported in 4.8% of subjects in a double-blind trial (9).

Headache is a common adverse effect of somatropin. It often occurs early in treatment and usually responds to temporary dosage reduction followed by gradual re-escalation (1,20). It can be an early indicator of the rare complication pseudotumor cerebri (idiopathic intracranial hypertension), particularly in high-risk groups, such as children with renal insufficiency, and may require further investigation. Headache was reported in 13% of 75 prepubertal children treated with a modified-release formulation of somatropin over 12 months (21).

Somatropin can cause idiopathic intracranial hypertension (pseudotumor cerebri), characterized by headache, papilledema, visual disturbance, and sometimes nausea and vomiting (22). Less common features include extra-ocular palsy, present in up to 48% of affected patients (22), mood changes, and somnolence. There have been 30 cases reported worldwide (23); chronic renal insufficiency, Turner's syndrome, obesity, and biochemical growth hormone deficiency are all associated with an increased risk. About half of the reported cases occurred within the first 8 weeks of treatment, and all responded to dose reduction or withdrawal of human growth hormone. Fundoscopy is recommended before starting somatropin and regularly during the first few months, although the absence of papilledema does not exclude the diagnosis. Up to 48% of children with intracranial hypertension due to somatropin also develop a sixth nerve palsy (23).

- A non-obese 6-year-old girl with Ullrich–Turner syndrome developed headache, vomiting, and blurred vision, with papilledema and increased cerebrospinal fluid pressure 5 months after starting somatropin 0.9 IU/kg/week (24). The cerebrospinal fluid pressure normalized after somatropin was withdrawn, and increased again when therapy was restarted. Her visual acuity was reduced to less than 30% in the right eye.

According to the authors there have been 40 cases of pseudotumor cerebri associated with somatropin therapy

worldwide, owing to stimulation of cerebrospinal fluid production or reduced drainage.

Sensory systems

Retinal changes, clinically indistinguishable from diabetic retinopathy, were reported in two non-diabetic recipients of somatropin (25).

- An obese 31-year-old man developed non-proliferative retinopathy and macular edema with reduced visual acuity after 14 months' therapy, which improved after somatropin was withdrawn.
- An 11-year-old girl with Turner's syndrome developed unilateral neovascularization after receiving somatropin for 22 months.

These patients improved but did not completely resolve after somatropin was withdrawn.

Somatropin concentrations correlate with retinopathy in patients with diabetes. There are no prospective clinical reports of retinal findings in adult recipients of somatropin, and these are awaited to determine the true frequency of this complication.

Endocrine

Thyroid function tests are often altered by somatropin because of increased conversion of T4 to T3, but this is clinically insignificant at low doses (SEDA-21, 453). One child with Prader–Willi syndrome had a fall in serum thyroxine concentration during somatropin therapy and needed thyroxine replacement (26). Hypothyroidism developed in 11 of 46 growth hormone-deficient children treated with somatropin (27). Prior abnormalities in hypothalamic-pituitary function and alterations in thyroid hormone metabolism, probably both, contributed to the high incidence of hypothyroidism, which was similar to that in previous studies.

Three adolescent boys with chronic renal insufficiency, treated with somatropin during the pubertal growth spurt, developed severe hyperparathyroidism (28). It is unclear whether this was coincidental or whether growth hormone and sex steroid hormones had a synergistic effect.

There have been occasional reports of gynecomastia attributed to somatropin (SEDA-21, 453).

Metabolism

Hyperinsulinemia is common in recipients of somatropin, but the long-term effects are controversial. This issue is becoming increasingly important as more adult patients are treated and the duration of therapy is extended. Growth hormone deficiency is itself associated with insulin resistance (29). Plasma concentrations of glucose and hemoglobin A_{1C} increase, especially in the first 6–12 months, indicating relative insulin resistance (30,31); the increases are often within the reference ranges (4,32).

Plasma glucose is inconsistently described as showing a sustained increase within the reference range, a transient increase, or no change. This reflects both the small non-controlled populations reported and possible selection bias, with exclusion of some patients because of hyperglycemia before the start of a cohort study (32). Hyperglycemia has occasionally been reported in patients receiving very high doses of human growth hormone for catabolic conditions, but has usually not required specific treatment (33). In a 6-month randomized study of 74 men and 57 women aged over 65 years, diabetes or glucose intolerance developed in 18 men treated with somatropin compared with seven controls (34).

Diabetes mellitus was previously not thought to be more common in recipients of somatropin than in the general population (SEDA-13, 1308) (35). However, longer-term observations have shown a three-fold incidence compared with predicted rates of type II diabetes, probably representing a younger age of onset rather than an increase in de novo cases (36).

In 78 children treated with somatropin for 7 years the mean fasting glucose concentration increased significantly compared with baseline after both 1 and 6 years of somatropin treatment, but remained the reference range and was not higher at 6 years than at 1 year (30).

In a 5-year study, 67 children treated with somatropin all had a sustained increase in fasting and oral glucose-stimulated insulin concentrations. This was most significant in children on dialysis and with renal transplants (37). In another study, insulin secretion in response to intravenous glucose was increased in 14 children with renal insufficiency, but returned to baseline after 12 months. However, increased insulin concentrations persisted in nine girls with Turner's syndrome (38). Concomitant glucocorticoid and somatropin treatment in children with juvenile arthritis caused a small but significant rise in blood glucose and glycosylated hemoglobin, which returned to pretreatment concentrations after somatropin was withdrawn (39).

Of 21 children, 15 developed hyperglycemia in a study of high-dose somatropin (0.2 mg/kg/day) for burns (40). In another study of 29 children with renal insufficiency (a group known to have insulin resistance), integrated insulin concentrations increased significantly in the first year of somatropin treatment, with no associated change in plasma glucose or glycated hemoglobin (41).

In a retrospective study, the fasting glucose:insulin ratio, a marker of insulin resistance, fell more in girls with Turner syndrome than in children with idiopathic short stature during somatropin therapy. The lower glucose:insulin ratio was due to increased fasting insulin and correlated with increased body mass index (42).

- Diabetes occurred 2 months after somatropin was begun in a 14 year-old girl, with restoration of normoglycemia after it was withdrawn (43).

In a postmarketing review of over 20 000 patients, type II diabetes was three times more common than expected, probably because at-risk individuals became diabetic at an earlier age than predicted (36). In a postmarketing review of 23 333 children and adolescents (52 375 treatment years), the incidence of type I diabetes was not significantly increased. However, type II diabetes occurred in 46 and 28 per 100 000 treatment years in children aged 10–19 and 6–14 years respectively (six times greater in both age groups than published reference values). There was no difference in incidence between boys and girls. A further 42 children developed abnormal glucose tolerance (44). Diabetes and glucose intolerance did not resolve after somatropin was withdrawn. Children who became diabetic were usually pubertal and had received somatropin for a longer period. Obesity, a risk factor for type II diabetes in the general population, was uncommon in these children.

Experience in adults is more limited, and monitoring is essential (45). Studies of somatropin in adults have consistently shown increased plasma concentrations of glucose, glycated hemoglobin, and insulin (46,47). Glucose intolerance and frank diabetes mellitus have been frequently reported in small series (46,48). Hyperglycemia not requiring specific treatment has been reported more often in adult patients (9) and in patients receiving high-dose somatropin to treat wasting associated with burns or HIV infection (33,49), but the overall incidence has not been compared with that in the general population.

In 25 patients a depot formulation of somatropin was associated with a non-sustained increase in glucose and insulin concentrations, more pronounced in men (50).

In a double-blind, placebo-controlled study of 24 growth hormone-deficient adults treated for 4 months with somatropin 2 IU/day, the treated patients had a significant increase in fasting plasma glucose and insulin concentrations, and increased insulin resistance, determined by insulin AUC during oral and intravenous glucose tolerance testing (8). Similarly, a group of 30 adolescents who were not growth hormone-deficient, and who were treated with somatropin for a mean of 7.9 years, had significantly reduced insulin sensitivity and raised plasma glucose concentrations during treatment, returning to control concentrations after somatropin was withdrawn (51). One of these patients developed glucose intolerance.

In a study of high-dose somatropin (0.1 mg/kg/day) in 20 patients with severe burns (a condition that causes insulin resistance), 60% of the treated patients required insulin therapy for hyperglycemia compared with 25% of the controls (52). This study was limited by the fact that the treated patients had more severe burns than the controls.

In a high-dose study in eight HIV-positive men, oral glucose tolerance worsened in the first month of human growth hormone 3 mg/day, then improved toward baseline. Mild glucose intolerance was still present after 6 months, despite a reduction in visceral fat. One man with pre-existing glucose intolerance developed symptomatic diabetes within 2 weeks of starting somatropin (53).

- Acanthosis nigricans, which is characterized by dark velvety thickening of the skin on the nape of the neck and in the groins and axillae, has been described in a non-obese 10-year-old boy with achondroplasia who received somatropin 3–4 IU/week for 7 years (54).

There has been one previous report of acanthosis nigricans in a woman who received human pituitary extract (55). This condition is usually seen in hyperinsulinemic states, including diabetes mellitus and acromegaly; overstimulation at the IGF-I receptor is probably the final common pathway.

Mineral balance

Hypercalcemia, usually mild and not requiring specific treatment, was reported in 43 of 100 patients receiving high-dose somatropin in intensive care (SEDA-13, 1308) (56).

Fluid balance

Edema is three times more frequent with a dose of somatropin of 0.025 mg/kg/day than 0.0125 mg/kg/day (57). In a randomized, controlled study of 33 obese women, three of nine who received somatropin and two of seven who received somatropin plus insulin-like growth factor-1 withdrew from the study, because of intolerable edema, compared with none in the placebo group. Most patients receiving somatropin required diuretic treatment for edema in this study, in which dose was calculated according to body weight (58). In a randomized, placebo-controlled trial of growth hormone replacement in 166 hormone-deficient adults, 48% of the treated group and 30% of the placebo group reported mild to moderate edema, which resolved in 70% of subjects despite continued treatment (9).

Hematologic

Leukemia has been reported in several patients treated with somatropin. However, when other risk factors are accounted for, there is no current evidence that it increases the risk significantly above population levels (SEDA-23, 468) (59).

- Acute myelogenous leukemia was diagnosed in a 25-year-old man with hypopituitarism, 4 months after he started to use somatropin three times a week (60).

The time interval in this case was too short to implicate somatropin as a definite cause.

Gastrointestinal

Nausea, which did not require specific treatment, occurred within 72 hours after an injection of long-acting somatropin in six of 25 patients (50).

Skin

Injection site reactions to somatropin are common and include nodules, pain, and erythema. They usually resolve spontaneously (21,27). In a 2-year study of once- or twice-monthly injections of a modified-release formulation of somatropin in 56 prepubertal children, injection site reactions were common, especially in the first year of treatment. These included skin nodules in 56% of injections, erythema in 49%, and lipoatrophy in 12% (61).

- A 12-year-old boy developed lipohypertrophy at the site of somatropin injection (62). Site rotation gave partial resolution.
- A 51-year-old woman with both panhypopituitarism and liver disease developed localized abdominal lipohypertrophy during somatropin therapy (63).

The authors of the second report speculated that hepatic IGF-1 secretion was compromised and that peripheral somatropin reached supraphysiological concentrations.

Lipoatrophy, a transient loss of subcutaneous fat identifiable as skin dimpling, occurred in 11% of injections in 75 children who were given modified-release somatropin for 12 months (21) and in one of 68 children in another study (27). Site rotation is recommended to prevent lipodystrophy.

Non-neoplastic pigmented nevi may increase in number in patients treated with somatropin (SEDA-21, 453).

Musculoskeletal

Arthralgia and proximal myalgia are common with somatropin, especially with large doses or rapid dose escalation (3,49,57,58).

A slipped capital femoral epiphysis was reported in 26 of 16 500 patients in one study: it is less common in children with idiopathic short stature than those with a known cause of growth failure (64).

Growth acceleration makes scoliosis more apparent in less than 1% of children treated with somatropin, many of whom also receive spinal irradiation. A causative role for somatropin has not been substantiated (65).

There are conflicting reports on a possible increased risk of fractures in children with osteogenesis imperfecta treated with somatropin, many of whom have a qualitative defect in collagen (66,67).

- A boy with osteogenesis imperfecta, with no previous fractures, who received somatropin from age 5 to 14, had four fractures during his pubertal growth spurt, similar to two previous case reports (68).

Immunologic

Patients treated with recombinant somatropin commonly develop antibodies against growth hormone; the incidence is 22–88% (69). There were low titers of antigrowth hormone antibody, with no reduction in growth response, in 44% of children who used modified-release somatropin once a month and in 68% who used it twice a month (21). Antibodies almost never have clinical significance, but the fourth case of reduced growth due to neutralizing antibodies against growth hormone has been reported in a 9-year-old boy; growth resumed after he was changed to a methionyl-free human formulation of somatropin (69).

Systemic allergic reactions to somatropin are very rare, but can be overcome by desensitization (SEDA-13, 1308) (70). Although early studies suggested a higher rate of renal transplant rejection in recipients of somatropin than in controls (SEDA-21, 452), this was not confirmed in a long-term prospective study (71).

- In a 15-year-old boy with previously quiescent lupus nephritis, laboratory markers of disease activity rose during somatropin treatment and returned to baseline concentrations within 3 months after withdrawal (72).

Long-Term Effects

Tumorigenicity

The incidence of malignancy is increased in acromegaly, in which growth hormone is present in excess. Patients treated with growth hormone have therefore been carefully monitored. The first report of leukemia in Japanese children treated with growth hormone (73) prompted a worldwide survey. There have been reports of 44 new cases of leukemia in growth hormone recipients, of which only 20 were acute lymphoblastic leukemia. This is much less than the expected 80–85% of new childhood leukemia (74).

A review of Japanese patients found that of the 15 patients who had developed hematological malignancies since 1975, 6 had other risk factors for leukemia, such as Fanconi's syndrome or prior chemotherapy or radiotherapy. The incidence of leukemia in this study was 3 per 100 000, similar to that in the general population of the same age (59). The National Cooperative Growth Study (NCGS—a postmarketing database that includes 19 846 patient-years since the time of growth hormone exposure) similarly reported no increase in the incidence of new leukemia when patients with other risk factors were excluded from the analysis (75).

The recurrence rate of intracranial tumors has been addressed in a number of large observational studies. Reports from the NCGS database (which includes 1262 children with brain tumors) and from England have shown no increase in intracranial tumor recurrence in patients treated with growth hormone (76,77). For patients with craniopharyngioma, postoperative irradiation reduced the recurrence rate, but growth hormone therapy did not increase the risk (78).

In the NCGS study extracranial non-leukemia malignancy rates were similarly not increased in patients treated with growth hormone compared with those who were not (79).

Despite theoretical concerns, there is no evidence that either intracranial or extracranial malignancy, new or recurrent, is increased in subjects treated with growth hormone (76,78,79). Despite this, certain precautions are still recommended for children who have previously been treated for cancer. The diagnosis of growth hormone deficiency should be clearly established (74) and it is recommended that treatment be delayed for at least 1 year after tumor therapy has been completed (36).

In a cohort study in 1848 British patients who received human pituitary-derived growth hormone from 1959 to 1985 (30 000 patient-years), there were two cases of colorectal cancer (0.25 expected) and two cases of Hodgkin's disease (0.85 expected); the standardized mortality ratios were 10.8 and 11.4 respectively (80). However, the number of cancers was small and the doses used were higher than typically today, and these results should be interpreted with caution.

Second-Generation Effects

Teratogenicity

Only a few pregnancies have been reported in women treated with somatropin. Eight women with hypopituitarism were followed prospectively during 12 pregnancies at a mean daily pregestation dose of 0.5 mg/day. The dose of somatropin was gradually reduced during the second trimester and withdrawn at the start of the third trimester. No congenital abnormalities were observed and weight and length at birth were normal (81).

Susceptibility Factors

Age

Most of the information about the long-term safety of somatropin in children has been derived from databases

voluntarily maintained by two pharmaceutical companies; thus, there may be under-reporting. Other trials have generally been of short duration, with few participants, and may thus have been subject to type II error. The effectiveness and safety of somatropin in children has been the subject of a systematic review (82).

Sex

Somatropin is being increasingly prescribed for growth hormone-deficient adults. Men have more adverse effects than women, probably because of a greater IGF-1 response (83). This was also seen in 74 elderly men and 57 elderly women in a controlled trial, and was not influenced by concomitant sex steroid therapy (34).

Drug Administration

Drug dosage regimens

One recommended regimen is to start somatropin in a dosage of 0.15 mg/day and titrate upward (SEDA-14, 1521). Very high dosages (0.1–0.2 mg/kg/day, 10–20 times higher than replacement dosages given to adults with growth hormone deficiency) were given to 532 critically ill patients in intensive care units in two placebo-controlled trials (84). Mortality was significantly higher in the treated group than in the placebo group (42 versus 18%). Morbidity was also increased in somatropin recipients, who needed longer ventilator times.

Early studies using doses of somatropin that have been derived from pediatric experience had a high rate of adverse effects, and doses have been progressively reduced. In a 6-month, multicenter, randomized study, 302 adults were given somatropin 3 micrograms/kg/day, increasing to 6 micrograms/kg/day after 3 months, and 293 were given 6 micrograms/kg/day, increasing to 12 micrograms/kg/day (85). The lower dose was associated with significantly fewer adverse events (in particular, arthralgia in 12 versus 20%). However, 78% of women or patients with childhood-onset growth hormone deficiency had subnormal IGF-1 concentrations, suggesting that treatment should be titrated to IGF-1 concentrations and adverse effects.

Drug–Drug Interactions

Ciclosporin

Growth hormone increases the activity and regulates the gene expression of hepatic CYP3A4 (86). Mean blood concentrations of ciclosporin were lower during somatropin therapy in an open study in 16 prepubertal kidney transplant recipients, despite stable weight-related doses, suggesting that the metabolism of ciclosporin was increased by somatropin. Two patients had acute episodes of rejection during somatropin therapy; one of these may have been related to the fall in ciclosporin concentration (87).

Estradiol

In eight postmenopausal growth hormone-deficient women randomized to estradiol, either orally 2 mg/day or transdermally 100 micrograms/day, together with incremental doses of somatropin in an 8-week, crossover study, oral but not transdermal estrogen reduced IGF-1 concentrations, protein synthesis, and postprandial lipid oxidation rates (88). This confirms the results of a previous report (89). The mechanism is not known, but high portal estrogen concentrations after oral estrogen administration probably alter hepatic growth hormone metabolism.

References

1. Carrel AL, Myers SE, Whitman BY, Allen DB. Growth hormone improves body composition, fat utilization, physical strength and agility, and growth in Prader–Willi syndrome: A controlled study. J Pediatr 1999;134(2):215–21.
2. Blethen S. Dosing, monitoring, and safety in adults with growth hormone deficiency. Endocrinologist 1998;16:994–9.
3. Drake WM, Coyte D, Camacho-Hubner C, Jivanji NM, Kaltsas G, Wood DF, Trainer PJ, Grossman AB, Besser GM, Monson JP. Optimizing growth hormone replacement therapy by dose titration in hypopituitary adults. J Clin Endocrinol Metab 1998;83(11):3913–19.
4. Hayes FJ, Fiad TM, McKenna TJ. Gender difference in the response of growth hormone (GH)-deficient adults to GH therapy. Metabolism 1999;48(3):308–13.
5. Meling TR. Growth hormone deficiency in adults: the role of replacement therapy. Biodrugs 1998;9:351–62.
6. Weaver JU, Monson JP, Noonan K, John WG, Edwards A, Evans KA, Cunningham J. The effect of low dose recombinant human growth hormone replacement on regional fat distribution, insulin sensitivity, and cardiovascular risk factors in hypopituitary adults. J Clin Endocrinol Metab 1995;80(1):153–9.
7. Attanasio AF, Lamberts SW, Matranga AM, Birkett MA, Bates PC, Valk NK, Hilsted J, Bengtsson BA, Strasburger CJ. Adult growth hormone (GH)-deficient patients demonstrate heterogeneity between childhood onset and adult onset before and during human GH treatment. Adult Growth Hormone Deficiency Study Group. J Clin Endocrinol Metab 1997;82(1):82–8.
8. Rosenfalck AM, Fisker S, Hilsted J, Dinesen B, Volund A, Jorgensen JO, Christiansen JS, Madsbad S. The effect of the deterioration of insulin sensitivity on beta-cell function in growth-hormone-deficient adults following 4-month growth hormone replacement therapy. Growth Horm IGF Res 1999;9(2):96–105.
9. Cuneo RC, Judd S, Wallace JD, Perry-Keene D, Burger H, Lim-Tio S, Strauss B, Stockigt J, Topliss D, Alford F, Hew L, Bode H, Conway A, Handelsman D, Dunn S, Boyages S, Cheung NW, Hurley D. The Australian Multicenter Trial of Growth Hormone (GH) Treatment in GH-Deficient Adults. J Clin Endocrinol Metab 1998;83(1):107–16.
10. Daubeney PE, McCaughey ES, Chase C, Walker JM, Slavik Z, Betts PR, Webber SA. Cardiac effects of growth hormone in short normal children: results after four years of treatment. Arch Dis Child 1995;72(4):337–9.
11. Crepaz R, Pitscheider W, Radetti G, Paganini C, Gentili L, Morini G, Braito E, Mengarda G. Cardiovascular effects of high-dose growth hormone treatment in growth hormone-deficient children. Pediatr Cardiol 1995;16(5):223–7.
12. Frustaci A, Gentiloni N, Russo MA. Growth hormone in the treatment of dilated cardiomyopathy. N Engl J Med 1996;335(9):672–3.
13. Oczkowska U. Przejsciowe powiekszenie sylwetki serca jako nietypowe powiklanie leczenia hormonen wzrostu. [Transient cardiac enlargement: an unusual adverse event associated with growth hormone therapy.] Endokrynol Diabetol Chor Przemiany Materii Wieku Rozw 2001;7(1):53–6.
14. Brown P, Preece MA, Will RG. "Friendly fire" in medicine: hormones, homografts, and Creutzfeldt–Jakob disease. Lancet 1992;340(8810):24–7.
15. Brown P, Preece M, Brandel JP, Sato T, McShane L, Zerr I, Fletcher A, Will RG, Pocchiari M, Cashman NR, d'Aignaux JH, Cervenakova L, Fradkin J, Schonberger LB, Collins SJ. Iatrogenic Creutzfeldt–Jakob disease at the millennium. Neurology 2000;55(8):1075–81.
16. Gibbons RV, Holman RC, Belay ED, Schonberger LB. Creutzfeldt–Jakob disease in the United States: 1979-1998. JAMA 2000;284(18):2322–3.
17. Caboclo LO, Huang N, Lepski GA, Livramento JA, Buchpiguel CA, Porto CS, Nitrini R. Iatrogenic Creutzfeldt–Jakob disease following human growth hormone therapy: case report. Arq Neuropsiquiatr 2002;60(2-B):458–61.
18. Hamad A, Hamad A, Sokrab TE, Momeni S. Iatrogenic Creutzfeldt–Jakob disease at the millennium. Neurology 2001;56(7):987.
19. Huillard d'Aignaux J, Alperovitch A, Maccario J. A statistical model to identify the contaminated lots implicated in iatrogenic transmission of Creutzfeldt–Jakob disease among French human growth hormone recipients. Am J Epidemiol 1998;147(6):597–604.
20. Toogood AA, Shalet SM. Growth hormone replacement therapy in the elderly with hypothalamic–pituitary disease: a dose-finding study. J Clin Endocrinol Metab 1999;84(1):131–6.
21. Reiter EO, Attie KM, Moshang T Jr, Silverman BL, Kemp SF, Neuwirth RB, Ford KM, Saenger P; Genentech, Inc.-Alkermes, Inc. Collaborative Study Group. A multicenter study of the efficacy and safety of sustained release GH in the treatment of naive pediatric patients with GH deficiency. J Clin Endocrinol Metab 2001;86(10):4700–6.
22. Malozowski S, Tanner LA, Wysowski DK, Fleming GA, Stadel BV. Benign intracranial hypertension in children with growth hormone deficiency treated with growth hormone. J Pediatr 1995;126(6):996–9.
23. Crock PA, McKenzie JD, Nicoll AM, Howard NJ, Cutfield W, Shield LK, Byrne G. Benign intracranial hypertension and recombinant growth hormone therapy in Australia and New Zealand. Acta Paediatr 1998;87(4):381–6.
24. Bechtold S, Butenandt O, Meidert A, Boergen KP, Schmidt H. Persistent papilledema in Ullrich–Turner syndrome treated with growth hormone. Clin Pediatr (Phila) 2001;40(11):629–31.
25. Koller EA, Green L, Gertner JM, Bost M, Malozowski SN. Retinal changes mimicking diabetic retinopathy in two non-diabetic, growth hormone-treated patients. J Clin Endocrinol Metab 1998;83(7):2380–3.
26. Lindgren AC. Side effects of growth hormone treatment in Prader–Willi syndrome. Endocrinologist 2000;10(Suppl 1):S63–4.
27. Bercu BB, Murray FT, Frasier SD, Rudlin C, O'Dea LS, Brentzel J, Hanson B, Landy H. Long-term therapy with recombinant human growth hormone (Saizen) in children with idiopathic and organic growth hormone deficiency. Endocrine 2001;15(1):43–9.
28. Picca S, Cappa M, Rizzoni G. Hyperparathyroidism during growth hormone treatment: a role for puberty? Pediatr Nephrol 2000;14(1):56–8.
29. Johansson JO, Fowelin J, Landin K, Lager I, Bengtsson BA. Growth hormone-deficient adults are insulin-resistant. Metabolism 1995;44(9):1126–9.
30. Sas T, Mulder P, Aanstoot HJ, Houdijk M, Jansen M, Reeser M, Hokken-Koelega A. Carbohydrate metabolism during long-term growth hormone treatment in children

with short stature born small for gestational age. Clin Endocrinol (Oxf) 2001;54(2):243–51.

31. Wuhl E, Haffner D, Offner G, Broyer M, van't Hoff W, Mehls O; European Study Group on Growth Hormone Treatment in Children with Nephropathic Cystinosis. Long-term treatment with growth hormone in short children with nephropathic cystinosis. J Pediatr 2001;138(6):880–7.

32. Jeffcoate W. Growth hormone therapy and its relationship to insulin resistance, glucose intolerance and diabetes mellitus: a review of recent evidence. Drug Saf 2002;25(3):199–212.

33. Singh KP, Prasad R, Chari PS, Dash RJ. Effect of growth hormone therapy in burn patients on conservative treatment. Burns 1998;24(8):733–8.

34. Blackman MR, Sorkin JD, Munzer T, Bellantoni MF, Busby-Whitehead J, Stevens TE, Jayme J, O'Connor KG, Christmas C, Tobin JD, Stewart KJ, Cottrell E, St Clair C, Pabst KM, Harman SM. Growth hormone and sex steroid administration in healthy aged women and men: a randomized controlled trial. JAMA 2002;288(18):2282–92.

35. Czernichow P, Albertsson-Wikland K, Tuvemo T, Gunnarsson R. Growth hormone treatment and diabetes: survey of the Kabi Pharmacia International Growth Study. Acta Paediatr Scand Suppl 1991;379:104–7.

36. Frisch H. Pharmacovigilance: the use of KIGS (Pharmacia and Upjohn International Growth Database) to monitor the safety of growth hormone treatment in children. Endocrinol Metabol 1997;4(Suppl B):83–6.

37. Haffner D, Nissel R, Wuhl E, Schaefer F, Bettendorf M, Tonshoff B, Mehls O. Metabolic effects of long-term growth hormone treatment in prepubertal children with chronic renal failure and after kidney transplantation. The German Study Group for Growth Hormone Treatment in Chronic Renal Failure. Pediatr Res 1998;43(2):209–15.

38. Filler G, Amendt P, Kohnert KD, Devaux S, Ehrich JH. Glucose tolerance and insulin secretion in children before and during recombinant growth hormone treatment. Horm Res 1998;50(1):32–7.

39. Touati G, Prieur AM, Ruiz JC, Noel M, Czernichow P. Beneficial effects of one-year growth hormone administration to children with juvenile chronic arthritis on chronic steroid therapy. I. Effects on growth velocity and body composition. J Clin Endocrinol Metab 1998;83(2):403–9.

40. Hart DW, Wolf SE, Chinkes DL, Lal SO, Ramzy PI, Herndon DN. Beta-blockade and growth hormone after burn. Ann Surg 2002;236(4):450–6.

41. Hertel NT, Holmberg C, Ronnholm KA, Jacobsen BB, Olgaard K, Meeuwisse GW, Rix M, Pedersen FB. Recombinant human growth hormone treatment, using two dose regimens in children with chronic renal failure—a report on linear growth and adverse effects. J Pediatr Endocrinol Metab 2002;15(5):577–88.

42. Burgert TS, Vuguin PM, DiMartino-Nardi J, Attie KM, Saenger P. Assessing insulin resistance: application of a fasting glucose to insulin ratio in growth hormone-treated children. Horm Res 2002;57(1-2):37–42.

43. Filler G, Franke D, Amendt P, Ehrich JH. Reversible diabetes mellitus during growth hormone therapy in chronic renal failure. Pediatr Nephrol 1998;12(5):405–7.

44. Cutfield WS, Wilton P, Bennmarker H, Albertsson-Wikland K, Chatelain P, Ranke MB, Price DA. Incidence of diabetes mellitus and impaired glucose tolerance in children and adolescents receiving growth-hormone treatment. Lancet 2000;355(9204):610–13.

45. Jeffcoate W. Can growth hormone therapy cause diabetes? Lancet 2000;355(9204):589–90.

46. Florakis D, Hung V, Kaltsas G, Coyte D, Jenkins PJ, Chew SL, Grossman AB, Besser GM, Monson JP. Sustained reduction in circulating cholesterol in adult hypopituitary patients given low dose titrated growth hormone

replacement therapy: a two year study. Clin Endocrinol (Oxf) 2000;53(4):453–9.

47. Rosenfalck AM, Maghsoudi S, Fisker S, Jorgensen JO, Christiansen JS, Hilsted J, Volund AA, Madsbad S. The effect of 30 months of low-dose replacement therapy with recombinant human growth hormone (rhGH) on insulin and C-peptide kinetics, insulin secretion, insulin sensitivity, glucose effectiveness, and body composition in GH-deficient adults. J Clin Endocrinol Metab 2000;85(11):4173–81.

48. Fernholm R, Bramnert M, Hagg E, Hilding A, Baylink DJ, Mohan S, Thoren M. Growth hormone replacement therapy improves body composition and increases bone metabolism in elderly patients with pituitary disease. J Clin Endocrinol Metab 2000;85(11):4104–12.

49. Nguyen BY, Clerici M, Venzon DJ, Bauza S, Murphy WJ, Longo DL, Baseler M, Gesundheit N, Broder S, Shearer G, Yarchoan R. Pilot study of the immunologic effects of recombinant human growth hormone and recombinant insulin-like growth factor in HIV-infected patients. AIDS 1998;12(8):895–904.

50. Cook DM, Biller BM, Vance ML, Hoffman AR, Phillips LS, Ford KM, Benziger DP, Illeperuma A, Blethen SL, Attie KM, Dao LN, Reimann JD, Fielder PJ. The pharmacokinetic and pharmacodynamic characteristics of a long-acting growth hormone (GH) preparation (Nutropin Depot) in GH-deficient adults. J Clin Endocrinol Metab 2002;87(10):4508–14.

51. Bareille P, Azcona C, Matthews DR, Conway GS, Stanhope R. Lipid profile, glucose tolerance and insulin sensitivity after more than four years of growth hormone therapy in non-growth hormone deficient adolescents. Clin Endocrinol (Oxf) 1999;51(3):347–53.

52. Demling RH. Comparison of the anabolic effects and complications of human growth hormone and the testosterone analogue, oxandrolone, after severe burn injury. Burns 1999;25(3):215–21.

53. Lo JC, Mulligan K, Noor MA, Schwarz JM, Halvorsen RA, Grunfeld C, Schambelan M. The effects of recombinant human growth hormone on body composition and glucose metabolism in HIV-infected patients with fat accumulation. J Clin Endocrinol Metab 2001;86(8):3480–7.

54. Downs AM, Kennedy CT. Somatotrophin-induced acanthosis nigricans. Br J Dermatol 1999;141(2):390–1.

55. Nordlund JJ, Lerner AB. Cause of acanthosis nigricans. N Engl J Med 1975;293(4):200.

56. Knox JB, Demling RH, Wilmore DW, Sarraf P, Santos AA. Hypercalcemia associated with the use of human growth hormone in an adult surgical intensive care unit. Arch Surg 1995;130(4):442–5.

57. Blethen S. Dosing, monitoring, and safety of growth hormone-replacement therapy in adults with growth hormone deficiency. Endocrinologist 1998;8:S36–40.

58. Thompson JL, Butterfield GE, Gylfadottir UK, Yesavage J, Marcus R, Hintz RL, Pearman A, Hoffman AR. Effects of human growth hormone, insulin-like growth factor I, and diet and exercise on body composition of obese postmenopausal women. J Clin Endocrinol Metab 1998;83(5):1477–84.

59. Nishi Y, Tanaka T, Takano K, Fujieda K, Igarashi Y, Hanew K, Hirano T, Yokoya S, Tachibana K, Saito T, Watanabe S. Recent status in the occurrence of leukemia in growth hormone-treated patients in Japan. GH Treatment Study Committee of the Foundation for Growth Science, Japan. J Clin Endocrinol Metab 1999;84(6):1961–5.

60. Aktan M, Tanakol R, Nalcaci M, Dincol G. Leukemia in a patient treated with growth hormone. Endocr J 2000;47(4):471–3.

61. Silverman BL, Blethen SL, Reiter EO, Attie KM, Neuwirth RB, Ford KM. A long-acting human growth hormone (Nutropin Depot): efficacy and safety following two years of treatment in children with growth hormone deficiency. J Pediatr Endocrinol Metab 2002;15(Suppl 2):715–22.

62. Ruvalcaba RH, Kletter GB. Abdominal lipohypertrophy caused by injections of growth hormone: a case report. Pediatrics 1998;102(2 Pt 1):408–10.

63. Mersebach H, Feldt-Rasmussen UF. Lokaliseret lipohypertrophia under behandling med vaeksthormon. [Localized lipohypertrophy during growth hormone therapy.] Ugeskr Laeger 2002;164(14):1930–2.

64. Blethen SL, Rundle AC. Slipped capital femoral epiphysis in children treated with growth hormone. A summary of the National Cooperative Growth Study experience. Horm Res 1996;46(3):113–16.

65. Allen DB. Safety of human growth hormone therapy: current topics. J Pediatr 1996;128(5 Pt 2):S8–13.

66. Antoniazzi F, Bertoldo F, Mottes M, Valli M, Sirpresi S, Zamboni G, Valentini R, Tato L. Growth hormone treatment in osteogenesis imperfecta with quantitative defect of type I collagen synthesis. J Pediatr 1996;129(3):432–9.

67. Kodama H, Kubota K, Abe T. Osteogenesis imperfecta: are fractures and growth hormone treatment linked? J Pediatr 1998;132(3 Pt 1):559–60.

68. Noda H, Onishi H, Saitoh K, Nakajima H. Growth hormone therapy may increase fracture risk in a pubertal patient with osteogenesis imperfecta. J Pediatr Endocrinol Metab 2002;15(2):217–18.

69. Pitukcheewanont P, Schwarzbach L, Kaufman FR. Resumption of growth after methionyl-free human growth hormone therapy in a patient with neutralizing antibodies to methionyl human growth hormone. J Pediatr Endocrinol Metab 2002;15(5):653–7.

70. Walker SB, Weiss ME, Tattoni DS. Systemic reaction to human growth hormone treated with acute desensitization. Pediatrics 1992;90(1 Pt 1):108–9.

71. Guest G, Berard E, Crosnier H, Chevallier T, Rappaport R, Broyer M. Effects of growth hormone in short children after renal transplantation. French Society of Pediatric Nephrology. Pediatr Nephrol 1998;12(6):437–46.

72. Yap HK, Loke KY, Murugasu B, Lee BW. Subclinical activation of lupus nephritis by recombinant human growth hormone. Pediatr Nephrol 1998;12(2):133–5.

73. Anonymous. Leukaemia in patients treated with growth hormone. Lancet 1988;1(8595):1159–60.

74. Moshang T Jr. Use of growth hormone in children surviving cancer. Med Pediatr Oncol 1998;31(3):170–2.

75. Allen DB, Rundle AC, Graves DA, Blethen SL. Risk of leukemia in children treated with human growth hormone: review and reanalysis. J Pediatr 1997;131(1 Pt 2):S32–6.

76. Moshang T Jr, Rundle AC, Graves DA, Nickas J, Johanson A, Meadows A. Brain tumor recurrence in children treated with growth hormone: the National Cooperative Growth Study experience. J Pediatr 1996;128(5 Pt 2):S4–7.

77. Ogilvy-Stuart AL, Ryder WD, Gattamaneni HR, Clayton PE, Shalet SM. Growth hormone and tumour recurrence. BMJ 1992;304(6842):1601–5.

78. Price DA, Wilton P, Jonsson P, Albertsson-Wikland K, Chatelain P, Cutfield W, Ranke MB. Efficacy and safety of growth hormone treatment in children with prior craniopharyngioma: an analysis of the Pharmacia and Upjohn International Growth Database (KIGS) from 1988 to 1996. Horm Res 1998;49(2):91–7.

79. Tuffli GA, Johanson A, Rundle AC, Allen DB. Lack of increased risk for extracranial, nonleukemic neoplasms in recipients of recombinant deoxyribonucleic acid growth hormone. J Clin Endocrinol Metab 1995;80(4):1416–22.

80. Swerdlow AJ, Higgins CD, Adlard P, Preece MA. Risk of cancer in patients treated with human pituitary growth hormone in the UK, 1959–85: a cohort study. Lancet 2002;360(9329):273–7.

81. Wiren L, Boguszewski CL, Johannsson G. Growth hormone (GH) replacement therapy in GH-deficient women during pregnancy. Clin Endocrinol (Oxf) 2002;57(2):235–9.

82. Bryant J, Cave C, Mihaylova B, Chase D, McIntyre L, Gerard K, Milne R. Clinical effectiveness and cost-effectiveness of growth hormone in children: a systematic review and economic evaluation Health Technol Assess 2002;6(18):1–168.

83. Attanasio AF, Bates PC, Ho KK, Webb SM, Ross RJ, Strasburger CJ, Bouillon R, Crowe B, Selander K, Valle D, Lamberts SW; Hypoptiuitary Control and Complications Study International Advisory Board. Human growth hormone replacement in adult hypopituitary patients: long-term effects on body composition and lipid status—3-year results from the HypoCCS Database. J Clin Endocrinol Metab 2002;87(4):1600–6.

84. Takala J, Ruokonen E, Webster NR, Nielsen MS, Zandstra DF, Vundelinckx G, Hinds CJ. Increased mortality associated with growth hormone treatment in critically ill adults. N Engl J Med 1999;341(11):785–92.

85. Kehely A, Bates PC, Frewer P, Birkett M, Blum WF, Mamessier P, Ezzat S, Ho KK, Lombardi G, Luger A, Marek J, Russell-Jones D, Sonksen P, Attanasio AF. Short-term safety and efficacy of human GH replacement therapy in 595 adults with GH deficiency: a comparison of two dosage algorithms. J Clin Endocrinol Metab 2002;87(5):1974–9.

86. Liddle C, Goodwin BJ, George J, Tapner M, Farrell GC. Separate and interactive regulation of cytochrome P450 3A4 by triiodothyronine, dexamethasone, and growth hormone in cultured hepatocytes. J Clin Endocrinol Metab 1998;83(7):2411–16.

87. Sanchez CP, Salem M, Ettenger RB. Changes in cyclosporine A levels in pediatric renal allograft recipients receiving recombinant human growth hormone therapy. Transplant Proc 2000;32(8):2807–10.

88. Wolthers T, Hoffman DM, Nugent AG, Duncan MW, Umpleby M, Ho KK. Oral estrogen antagonizes the metabolic actions of growth hormone in growth hormone-deficient women. Am J Physiol Endocrinol Metab 2001;281(6):E1191–6.

89. Cook DM, Ludlam WH, Cook MB. Route of estrogen administration helps to determine growth hormone (GH) replacement dose in GH-deficient adults. J Clin Endocrinol Metab 1999;84(11):3956–60.

Sotalol

See also Beta-adrenoceptor antagonists

General Information

Sotalol is a non-selective beta-adrenoceptor antagonist with no partial agonist or membrane-stabilizing activity. It is also a class III antidysrhythmic drug. The beta-adrenoceptor antagonist properties of D,L-sotalol reside in the L-isomer, the D-isomer having class III antidysrhythmic activity and no clinically significant beta-blocking action (1).

Quinidine and sotalol have been compared in a prospective multicenter trial of 121 patients after conversion of atrial fibrillation (2). Patients with low left ventricular ejection fractions (below 0.4) or high left atrial diameters (over 5.2 cm) were excluded. After 6 months the percentages of patients remaining in sinus rhythm were similar in the two groups (around 70%), but when the dysrhythmia recurred, it occurred later with sotalol than with quinidine (69 versus 10 days). There was also a difference between patients who had been converted from recent onset atrial fibrillation, in whom sotalol was more effective than quinidine, and in patients who had had chronic atrial fibrillation for more than 3 days, in whom quinidine was more effective. There were significant adverse effects requiring withdrawal of therapy in 17 patients, of whom nine were taking quinidine; three patients had gastrointestinal symptoms, two had central nervous symptoms, two had allergic reactions, one had undefined palpitation, and one had QT interval prolongation. One patient taking quinidine, a 65-year-old man, had frequent episodes of non-sustained ventricular tachycardia.

Organs and Systems

Cardiovascular

Sotalol prolongs the QT interval and can predispose to torsade de pointes (3), sustained ventricular tachycardia, and cardiac arrest, especially in those taking 160 mg/day or more (SEDA-16, 191). Torsade de pointes has been reported in 1.2% of those exposed (data on file, Bristol-Myers Squibb, Princeton, New Jersey). In a review it was concluded that torsade de pointes is also more likely in patients with depressed left ventricular function and a history of sustained ventricular tachydysrhythmias (4).

Several publications involving 962 patients treated with an intravenous infusion of racemic sotalol have been reviewed, with the aim of describing the risk of torsade de pointes (5). Torsade de pointes occurred in only one case (0.1%; 95% CI = 0.003, 0.6), which is less often than with oral sotalol (2–4%). This difference can be explained by the shorter duration of treatment. The other reported complications were hypotension (0.3%), severe bradycardia (0.2%), and atrioventricular block necessitating drug withdrawal (0.03%).

In a survey of 1288 patients taking sotalol, dysrhythmias occurred in 56, in 24 cases torsade de pointes (3). There was no relation between these dysrhythmias and previously associated factors, such as bradycardia, a long QT interval, and hypokalemia, but in patients on hemodialysis even a low dosage (40 mg bd) can be associated with torsade de pointes (6). Similar prodysrhythmic effects have been reported in children (7).

Death

A trial of the efficacy of D-sotalol in patients with left ventricular dysfunction (8) was discontinued early when an interim analysis of 2762 patients showed an overall mortality of 3.9% in the D-sotalol group, compared with 2% in the placebo group (9).

Susceptibility Factors

Some patients with thyrotoxicosis have occult cardiac dysfunction. However, the use of beta-blockers in the treatment of thyrotoxicosis can have severe consequences in terms of severe cardiac dysfunction (10).

- A 52-year-old woman developed atrial fibrillation with a ventricular rate of 220/minute. She had had thyrotoxicosis 20 years before, but was taking no medications. She had an 8-month history of weight loss with a normal appetite. During the previous month she had had excessive sweating, palpitation, and exercise intolerance. The diagnosis was thyroid storm. She was given intravenous sotalol 1 mg/kg over 15 minutes and within 5 minutes sinus rhythm was restored, with improvement of symptoms. However, immediately after the infusion she had an episode of ventricular tachycardia followed by sinus bradycardia, with a resultant fall in blood pressure, followed by an asystolic cardiac arrest. She underwent endotracheal intubation and was treated with inotropes. Right-heart catheterization showed severe cardiac dysfunction (cardiac index 1.2 l/minute). She made an uneventful recovery.

Patients with severe hyperthyroidism can have an occult cardiomyopathy that makes them extremely sensitive to beta-blockers. The long duration of action of sotalol in this case necessitated prolonged inotropic and vasopressor support. A shorter-acting beta-blocker, such as esmolol, could theoretically be safer in such cases.

References

1. Yasuda SU, Barbey JT, Funck-Brentano C, Wellstein A, Woosley RL. d-Sotalol reduces heart rate in vivo through a beta-adrenergic receptor-independent mechanism. Clin Pharmacol Ther 1993;53(4):436–42.
2. de Paola AA, Veloso HH. Efficacy and safety of sotalol versus quinidine for the maintenance of sinus rhythm after conversion of atrial fibrillation. SOCESP Investigators. The Cardiology Society of Sao Paulo. Am J Cardiol 1999;84(9):1033–7.
3. Soyka LF, Wirtz C, Spangenberg RB. Clinical safety profile of sotalol in patients with arrhythmias. Am J Cardiol 1990;65(2):A74–81.
4. Hohnloser SH, Woosley RL. Sotalol. N Engl J Med 1994;331(1):31–8.
5. Marill KA, Runge T. Meta-analysis of the risk of torsades de pointes in patients treated with intravenous racemic sotalol. Acad Emerg Med 2001;8(2):117–24.
6. Huynh-Do U, Wahl C, Sulzer M, Buhler H, Keusch G. Torsades de pointes during low-dosage sotalol therapy in haemodialysis patients. Nephrol Dial Transplant 1996;11(6):1153–4.
7. Pfammatter JP, Paul T, Lehmann C, Kallfelz HC. Efficacy and proarrhythmia of oral sotalol in pediatric patients. J Am Coll Cardiol 1995;26(4):1002–7.
8. Waldo AL, Camm AJ, deRuyter H, Freidman PL, MacNeil DJ, Pitt B, Pratt CM, Rodda BE, Schwartz PJ. Survival with oral d-sotalol in patients with left ventricular dysfunction after myocardial infarction: rationale, design, and methods (the SWORD trial). Am J Cardiol 1995;75(15):1023–7.
9. Choo V. SWORD slashed. Lancet 1994;344:1358.

10.   Fraser T, Green D. Weathering the storm: beta-blockade and the potential for disaster in severe hyperthyroidism. Emerg Med (Fremantle) 2001;13(3):376–80.

Sparfloxacin

See also Fluoroquinolones

General Information

Sparfloxacin is a fluoroquinolone with activity against the major respiratory pathogens and atypical pathogens that cause pneumonia. Photosensitivity, nausea, and diarrhea have been the most common adverse events reported in trials, and sparfloxacin is contraindicated in patients with QT interval prolongation (1).

In an in vivo study in rats, endotoxin reduced the biliary excretion of sparfloxacin and its glucuronide, probably owing to impairment of hepatobiliary transport systems and renal handling (2).

Observational studies

The efficacy and safety of sparfloxacin (400 mg loading dose followed by 200 mg/day for 10 days) in the treatment of acute bacterial maxillary sinusitis have been evaluated in 253 patients (3). The overall success rate was 92%. The majority of adverse events were mild or moderate and the most frequent were photosensitivity reactions, headache, nausea, and diarrhea.

Comparative studies

Analysis of safety data from six multicenter phase III trials in 1585 patients comparing sparfloxacin with standard drugs (cefaclor, ciprofloxacin, clarithromycin, erythromycin, and ofloxacin) showed that 25% of patients treated with sparfloxacin and 28% of patients treated with the other drugs had at least one adverse event considered to be related to the study medication (4). Photosensitivity reactions were seen in 7.4% of treatment episodes with sparfloxacin, compared with 0.5% of episodes with the other drugs. Gastrointestinal reactions, insomnia, and alterations in taste were more common in patients taking the comparator drugs. The mean change from baseline QT interval corrected for heart rate (QT_c) was significantly greater with sparfloxacin, but no ventricular dysrhythmias were detected. Study medication was withdrawn in 8.9% of patients taking the comparator drugs and in 6.6% of those taking sparfloxacin.

Organs and Systems

Cardiovascular

Some quinolones can prolong the QT interval, with a risk of cardiac dysrhythmias.

Sparfloxacin causes greater prolongation of the QT interval than other quinolones (5), as has been shown in in vitro comparisons. Compared with grepafloxacin, moxifloxacin, and ciprofloxacin, sparfloxacin caused the greatest prolongation of the action potential duration (6), and in an in vitro comparison of sparfloxacin, ciprofloxacin, gatifloxacin, gemifloxacin, grepafloxacin, levofloxacin, moxifloxacin, sitafloxacin, tosufloxacin, and trovafloxacin, sparfloxacin caused the largest increase in QT interval (7). In an in vivo study in conscious dogs with stable idioventricular automaticity and chronic complete atrioventricular block, oral sparfloxacin 60 mg/kg caused torsade de pointes, leading to ventricular fibrillation within 24 hours, while 6 mg/kg did not (8). In halothane-anesthetized dogs, intravenous sparfloxacin 0.3 mg/kg prolonged the effective refractory period, and an extra 3.0 mg/kg reduced the heart rate and prolonged the effective refractory period and ventricular repolarization phase to a similar extent, suggesting that a backward shift of the relative repolarization period during the cardiac cycle may be the mechanism responsible for the dysrhythmogenic effect of sparfloxacin. Data from in vitro electrophysiological studies of the effect of sparfloxacin, ofloxacin, and levofloxacin on repolarization of rabbit Purkinje fibers indicate that the prolongation of the action potential is observed only with sparfloxacin (9).

In a double-blind, randomized, placebo-controlled, crossover study of a single oral dose of sparfloxacin in 15 healthy volunteers, prolongation of the QT interval was about 4% greater with sparfloxacin than with placebo (10). An independent Safety Board concluded from the results of various phase I and phase II studies that the increase in the QT_c interval associated with sparfloxacin is moderate, averaging 3%, and that the few serious adverse cardiovascular events that have been reported during postmarketing surveillance all occurred in patients with underlying heart disease (11).

In 25 patients taking sparfloxacin for multiresistant tuberculosis, there were six cases of moderate prolongation of the electrocardiographic QT interval (30–40 ms compared to baseline) without clinical symptoms (12).

- A 37-year-old woman who was taking sparfloxacin as part of modified antituberculosis drug therapy developed torsade de pointes (13).

Sensory systems

Abnormal taste developed in 17 of 175 patients treated with clarithromycin 250 mg bd for 10 days for community-acquired pneumonia, compared with three of 167 patients treated with sparfloxacin (14). Mild to moderate gastrointestinal disturbances were the most common adverse events and were reported in 13 and 11% respectively.

Skin

During the first 9 months of marketing of sparfloxacin, 371 severe phototoxic reactions were reported to the French pharmacovigilance system or the manufacturers, reporting rate of 0.4 per thousand treated patients (about 4–25 times that reported with other fluoroquinolones) (15).

Phototoxicity occurred in four of nine patients with multidrug-resistant tuberculosis treated with a combination of sparfloxacin (400 mg/day), ethionamide, and kanamycin (initially for 3–4 months) (16). It occurred after several months of treatment and was presumably due to the sparfloxacin. Sparfloxacin more commonly causes photosensitivity than ciprofloxacin, levofloxacin, or ofloxacin, which are also effective antituberculosis drugs (15,17). Skin reactions can be severe enough to require withdrawal of sparfloxacin in some patients. In view of this, other fluoroquinolones, particularly ofloxacin, are preferable to sparfloxacin in the management of multi-drug-resistant tuberculosis.

In 25 patients taking sparfloxacin for multidrug-resistant tuberculosis, there were five mild phototoxic reactions (12).

Long-Term Effects

Mutagenicity

DNA damage produced by sparfloxacin and UVA in retinal pigment epithelial cells in vitro was remedied by antioxidants, suggesting a possible in vivo strategy for preventing or minimizing retinal damage in humans (18).

Susceptibility Factors

Patients with a history of cardiac disease and patients taking other medications with effects on cardiac repolarization should not be given sparfloxacin, in order to prevent any cumulative inhibitory effect on cardiac repolarization.

Drug–Drug Interactions

Antacids

The absorption of sparfloxacin is impaired by antacids containing aluminium or magnesium (19). In an open, single-dose (400 mg), randomized, four-way crossover study in 20 male volunteers (aged 18–38 years), Maalox (30 ml) given 4 hours after sparfloxacin did not cause a statistically significant reduction in the rate and extent of sparfloxacin absorption. In contrast, Maalox given 2 hours before or 2 hours after sparfloxacin did reduce its absorption: AUC fell by 23 and 17% respectively and mean C_{max} by 29 and 13% (20).

Cisapride

Concomitant administration of cisapride increased the rate of absorption and increased the peak concentration of sparfloxacin without having a significant effect on systemic availability (21,22).

Sucralfate

Co-administration of sucralfate leads to a 44% reduction in the systemic availability of sparfloxacin (22). In eight healthy Japanese, the absorption of sparfloxacin (300 mg orally) was reduced when sucralfate (1.5 g orally) was administered concurrently or 2 hours after sparfloxacin, but not 4 hours after sparfloxacin (23).

References

1. Schentag JJ. Sparfloxacin: a review. Clin Ther 2000; 22(4):372–87.
2. Nadai M, Zhao YL, Wang L, Nishio Y, Takagi K, Kitaichi K, Takagi K, Yoshizumi H, Hasegawa T. Endotoxin impairs biliary transport of sparfloxacin and its glucuronide in rats. Eur J Pharmacol 2001;432(1):99–105.
3. Garrison N, Spector S, Buffington D, Stafford C, Granito K, Zhang H, Talbot GH. Sparfloxacin for the treatment of acute bacterial maxillary sinusitis documented by sinus puncture. Ann Allergy Asthma Immunol 2000;84(1):63–71.
4. Lipsky BA, Dorr MB, Magner DJ, Talbot GH. Safety profile of sparfloxacin, a new fluoroquinolone antibiotic. Clin Ther 1999;21(1):148–59.
5. Stahlmann R. Clinical toxicological aspects of fluoroquinolones. Toxicol Lett 2002;127(1–3):269–77.
6. Patmore L, Fraser S, Mair D, Templeton A. Effects of sparfloxacin, grepafloxacin, moxifloxacin, and ciprofloxacin on cardiac action potential duration. Eur J Pharmacol 2000;406(3):449–52.
7. Hagiwara T, Satoh S, Kasai Y, Takasuna K. A comparative study of the fluoroquinolone antibacterial agents on the action potential duration in guinea pig ventricular myocardia. Jpn J Pharmacol 2001;87(3):231–4.
8. Chiba K, Sugiyama A, Satoh Y, Shiina H, Hashimoto K. Proarrhythmic effects of fluoroquinolone antibacterial agents: in vivo effects as physiologic substrate for torsades. Toxicol Appl Pharmacol 2000;169(1):8–16.
9. Adamantidis MM, Dumotier BM, Caron JF, Bordet R. Sparfloxacin but not levofloxacin or ofloxacin prolongs cardiac repolarization in rabbit Purkinje fibers. Fundam Clin Pharmacol 1998;12(1):70–6.
10. Demolis JL, Charransol A, Funck-Brentano C, Jaillon P. Effects of a single oral dose of sparfloxacin on ventricular repolarization in healthy volunteers. Br J Clin Pharmacol 1996;41(6):499–503.
11. Jaillon P, Morganroth J, Brumpt I, Talbot G. Overview of electrocardiographic and cardiovascular safety data for sparfloxacin. Sparfloxacin Safety Group. J Antimicrob Chemother 1996;37(Suppl A):161–7.
12. Lubasch A, Erbes R, Mauch H, Lode H. Sparfloxacin in the treatment of drug resistant tuberculosis or intolerance of first line therapy. Eur Respir J 2001;17(4):641–6.
13. Kakar A, Byotra SP. Torsade de pointes probably induced by sparfloxacin. J Assoc Physicians India 2002;50:1077–8.
14. Ramirez J, Unowsky J, Talbot GH, Zhang H, Townsend L. Sparfloxacin versus clarithromycin in the treatment of community-acquired pneumonia. Clin Ther 1999;21(1):103–17.
15. Pierfitte C, Royer RJ, Moore N, Begaud B. The link between sunshine and phototoxicity of sparfloxacin. Br J Clin Pharmacol 2000;49(6):609–12.
16. Singla R, Gupta S, Gupta R, Arora VK. Efficacy and safety of sparfloxacin in combination with kanamycin and ethionamide in multidrug-resistant pulmonary tuberculosis patients: preliminary results. Int J Tuberc Lung Dis 2001;5(6):559–63.
17. Stahlmann R, Lode H. Toxicity of quinolones. Drugs 1999;58(Suppl 2):37–42.
18. Verna LK, Holman SA, Lee VC, Hoh J. UVA-induced oxidative damage in retinal pigment epithelial cells after H_2O_2 or sparfloxacin exposure. Cell Biol Toxicol 2000;16(5):303–12.
19. Shiba K, Hori S, Shimada J. Interaction between oral sparfloxacin and antacid in normal volunteers. Eur J Clin Microbiol Infect Dis 1991;(Special issue):583–5.
20. Johnson RD, Dorr MB, Talbot GH, Caille G. Effect of Maalox on the oral absorption of sparfloxacin. Clin Ther 1998;20(6):1149–58.
21. Goa KL, Bryson HM, Markham A. Sparfloxacin. A review of its antibacterial activity, pharmacokinetic properties, clinical efficacy and tolerability in lower respiratory tract infections. Drugs 1997;53(4):700–25.

22. Zix JA, Geerdes-Fenge HF, Rau M, Vockler J, Borner K, Koeppe P, Lode H. Pharmacokinetics of sparfloxacin and interaction with cisapride and sucralfate. Antimicrob Agents Chemother 1997;41(8):1668–72.
23. Kamberi M, Nakashima H, Ogawa K, Oda N, Nakano S. The effect of staggered dosing of sucralfate on oral bio-availability of sparfloxacin. Br J Clin Pharmacol 2000;49(2):98–103.

Sparteine

General Information

Sparteine is a major quinolizidine alkaloid found in a variety of plants:

- *Ammodendron conollyi*
- *Anagyris fetida*
- *Baptisia australis*
- *Baptisia tinctoria*
- *Chelidonium majus*
- *Cytisus scoparius*
- *Genista lucida*
- *Lupinus argentus*
- *Lupinus laxus*
- *Lupinus luteus*
- *Lupinus niger*
- *Lupinus polyphyllus*
- *Sarothamnus scoparius*
- *Sophora pachycarpa*
- *Sophora secundiflora*
- *Spartium junceum*
- *Spartium scoparium.*

Sparteine has been used as a marker of the metabolic activity of CYP2D6 (1). Pharmacokinetic studies have shown that its metabolic oxidation exhibits genetic polymorphism and that about 6–9% of the Caucasian population are poor metabolizers. Quinidine, haloperidol, and moclobemide are all potent inhibitors of the oxidative metabolism of sparteine (2).

Among the reported effects of sparteine are reduced cardiac conductivity, stimulation of uterine motility, circulatory collapse, and respiratory arrest. Sparteine was contained in a slimming aid ("Herbal Slimming Aid," UK). It was formerly used to induce labor; at the very least it should be considered contraindicated during pregnancy.

References

1. Ozawa S, Soyama A, Saeki M, Fukushima-Uesaka H, Itoda M, Koyano S, Sai K, Ohno Y, Saito Y, Sawada J. Ethnic differences in genetic polymorphisms of CYP2D6, CYP2C19, CYP3As and MDR1/ABCB1. Drug Metab Pharmacokinet 2004;19(2):83–95.
2. De Smet PA. Health risks of herbal remedies. Drug Saf 1995;13(2):81–93.

Spectinomycin

General Information

Spectinomycin is an aminocyclitol antibiotic, distinct from the aminoglycosides. It has been used mainly in single-dose treatment of gonorrhea (2 g intramuscularly), and for treating organisms with multiple antibiotic resistance (1–3). Apart from induration at the site of injection, tolerance in otherwise healthy individuals has been good, even with doses of 8 g/day for 21 days. Allergic reactions have been observed, but are rare. Spectinomycin-resistant gonococci have been found (4,5).

Long-Term Effects

Drug tolerance

Aminoglycoside adenylyltransferase (aadA) genes mediate resistance to streptomycin and spectinomycin. In a pathogenic porcine *Escherichia coli*, the novel aaA5 has now been described integrated with a trimethoprim resistance gene (6). The aadA6 gene has been sequenced from *Pseudomonas aeruginosa* and can confer high-level resistance to spectinomycin in *E. coli* (7). All strains of multidrug resistant *Vibrio cholerae* O1 El Tor isolated in Albania were resistant to spectinomycin, and resistance to this antibiotic was mediated by the aadA1 gene cassette located in the bacterial chromosome within a class 1 integron (8). Another class 1 integron that contained aadA2 was found in pathogenic *Salmonella typhimurium* isolates from France and was also chromosomally located (9). An aadA gene has also been described in *Enterococcus faecalis* (10).

Resistance of *E. coli* isolates from chicken in Saudia Arabia was 96% compared with 71% among human isolates (11). Serotyping showed an overlap between human and chicken strains, suggesting that these animals may serve as a resistance pool for humans.

References

1. Stolz E, Zwart HG, Michel MF. Sensitivity to ampicillin, penicillin, and tetracyline of gonococci in Rotterdam. Br J Vener Dis 1974;50(3):202–7.
2. Levy B, Brown J, Fowler W. Spectinomycin in gonorrhoea. Br J Clin Pract 1974;28(5):174–6.
3. Novak E, Gray JE, Pfeifer RT. Animal and human tolerance of high-dose intramuscular therapy with spectinomycin. J Infect Dis 1974;130(1):50–5.
4. Zenilman JM, Nims LJ, Menegus MA, Nolte F, Knapp JS. Spectinomycin-resistant gonococcal infections in the United States, 1985–1986. J Infect Dis 1987;156(6):1002–4.
5. Boslego JW, Tramont EC, Takafuji ET, Diniega BM, Mitchell BS, Small JW, Khan WN, Stein DC. Effect of spectinomycin use on the prevalence of spectinomycin-resistant and of penicillinase-producing *Neisseria gonorrhoeae*. N Engl J Med 1987;317(5):272–8.
6. Sandvang D. Novel streptomycin and spectinomycin resistance gene as a gene cassette within a class 1 integron

isolated from *Escherichia coli*. Antimicrob Agents Chemother 1999;43(12):3036–8.

7. Naas T, Poirel L, Nordmann P. Molecular characterisation of In51, a class 1 integron containing a novel aminoglycoside adenylyltransferase gene cassette, aadA6, in *Pseudomonas aeruginosa*. Biochim Biophys Acta 1999;1489(2–3):445–51.

8. Falbo V, Carattoli A, Tosini F, Pezzella C, Dionisi AM, Luzzi I. Antibiotic resistance conferred by a conjugative plasmid and a class I integron in *Vibrio cholerae* O1 El Tor strains isolated in Albania and Italy. Antimicrob Agents Chemother 1999;43(3):693–6.

9. Poirel L, Guibert M, Bellais S, Naas T, Nordmann P. Integron- and carbenicillinase-mediated reduced susceptibility to amoxicillin–clavulanic acid in isolates of multidrug-resistant *Salmonella enterica* serotype typhimurium DT104 from French patients. Antimicrob Agents Chemother 1999;43(5):1098–104.

10. Clark NC, Olsvik O, Swenson JM, Spiegel CA, Tenover FC. Detection of a streptomycin/spectinomycin adenylyltransferase gene (aadA) in *Enterococcus faecalis*. Antimicrob Agents Chemother 1999;43(1):157–60.

11. Al-Ghamdi MS, El-Morsy F, Al-Mustafa ZH, Al-Ramadhan M, Hanif M. Antibiotic resistance of *Escherichia coli* isolated from poultry workers, patients and chicken in the eastern province of Saudi Arabia. Trop Med Int Health 1999;4(4):278–83.

Spiramycin

See also Macrolide antibiotics

General Information

Spiramycin is a macrolide antibiotic with activity primarily against *Staphylococcus aureus*, beta-hemolytic streptococci, and viridans streptococci. Since spiramycin is retained in bone and the salivary glands and reaches prolonged high concentrations in the saliva, it is used mainly by dentists and otorhinolaryngologists. Because of high concentration in the tonsillar lymphoid tissue it has been proposed that spiramycin be used in the prevention of meningococcal infections. It does not reach the cerebrospinal fluid. Its toxicity is relatively low. Adverse effects include nausea, vomiting, diarrhea, and skin rashes (1).

Organs and Systems

Cardiovascular

QT interval prolongation (2) and torsade de pointes (3) occur rarely in patients taking spiramycin.

Hematologic

Hematological toxicity, including bone marrow suppression (4) and hemolysis (5), has been observed, especially during combined treatment with spiramycin and pyrimethamine for toxoplasmosis.

Liver

Cholestatic hepatitis occurred in a patient taking spiramycin (6).

Immunologic

A peculiar hypersensitivity reaction was reported in an employee of a pharmaceutical company who developed attacks of sneezing, coughing, and breathlessness while working with spiramycin; he had immediate positive skin prick tests to spiramycin and developed blood eosinophilia during asthma attacks (7).

Henoch–Schönlein purpura occurred in a patient taking spiramycin (8).

Drug–Drug Interactions

Neuroleptic drugs

Acute dystonia was observed during spiramycin therapy in a patient who was being treated with neuroleptic drugs (9).

References

1. Johnson RH, Rozanis J, Schofield ID, Haq MS. The effect of spiramycin on plaque accumulation and gingivitis. Dent J 1978;44(10):456–60.

2. Stramba-Badiale M, Guffanti S, Porta N, Frediani M, Beria G, Colnaghi C. QT interval prolongation and cardiac arrest during antibiotic therapy with spiramycin in a newborn infant. Am Heart J 1993;126(3 Pt 1):740–2.

3. Verdun F, Mansourati J, Jobic Y, Bouquin V, Munier S, Guillo P, Pages Y, Boschat J, Blanc JJ. Torsades de pointes sous traitement par spiramycine et mequitazine. A propos d'un cas. [Torsades de pointe with spiramycine and metiquazine therapy. Apropos of a case.] Arch Mal Coeur Vaiss 1997;90(1):103–6.

4. Switala I, Dufour P, Ducloy AS, Vinatier D, Bernardi C, Monnier JC, Plantier I, Fortier B. Aplasie medullaire au cours du traitement d'une toxoplasmose congenitale lors d'une grossesse gemellaire. [Medullary aplasia during treatment for congenital toxoplasmosis in a twin pregnancy.] J Gynecol Obstet Biol Reprod (Paris) 1993;22(5):513–16.

5. Sarma PS. Oxidative haemolysis after spiramycin. Postgrad Med J 1997;73(864):686–7.

6. Denie C, Henrion J, Schapira M, Schmitz A, Heller FR. Spiramycin-induced cholestatic hepatitis. J Hepatol 1992;16(3):386.

7. Davies RJ, Pepys J. Asthma due to inhaled chemical agents—the macrolide antibiotic spiramycin. Clin Allergy 1975;5(1):99–107.

8. Valero Prieto I, Calvo Catala J, Hortelano Martinez E, Abril L, de Medrano V, Glez-Cruz Cervellera MI, Herrera Ballester A, Orti E. Purpura de schönlein–Henoch asociada a espiramicina y con importantes manifestaciones digestiwas. [Schoenlein–Henoch purpura associated with spiramycin and with important digestive manifestations.] Rev Esp Enferm Dig 1994;85(1):47–9.

9. Benazzi F. Spiramycin-associated acute dystonia during neuroleptic treatment. Can J Psychiatry 1997;42(6):665–6.

Spironolactone

See also Diuretics

General Information

Spironolactone is a competitive antagonist at aldosterone receptors. It acts through its active metabolite, canrenone. Canrenone itself has also been used as a potassium-sparing diuretic for intravenous use and its potassium salt has been used orally, in the hope of avoiding the hormonal adverse effects of spironolactone.

Spironolactone has been used as a potassium-sparing diuretic in cardiac failure and in the management of ascites and edema associated with hepatic cirrhosis with secondary hyperaldosteronism. It is also used to treat hyperaldosteronism due to adrenal tumors or adrenal hyperplasia. It has a weak positive inotropic effect and a modest antihypertensive effect, in keeping with its natriuretic action.

Although spironolactone has been available for more than 30 years, its efficacy and safety in patients with heart failure have only recently been recognized in the Randomized Aldosterone Evaluation Study (RALES), in which it reduced mortality (1). Based on this and numerous smaller trials, the use of spironolactone, in conjunction with ACE inhibitors, other diuretics, and possibly beta-blockers or digoxin, represents a promising strategy for patients with severe heart failure. Its main adverse effects are hyperkalemia and antiadrenergic complications (SED-14, 675).

General adverse effects

The major limitation to the use of spironolactone is its liability to cause (sometimes lethal) hyperkalemia, particularly in the elderly, in patients with reduced renal function, and in patients who simultaneously take potassium supplements or ACE inhibitors. As with other diuretics, hyponatremia and dehydration can occur. Other less frequent adverse effects are gastrointestinal intolerance, neurological symptoms, and skin rashes. Hypersensitivity rashes and a lupus–like syndrome have been reported rarely. A few cases of mammary carcinoma have been reported and potential human metabolic products of spironolactone are carcinogenic in rodents. Second-generation effects have not been reported.

Organs and Systems

Nervous system

Central nervous system effects, such as weakness, drowsiness, and confusion, have been reported in patients taking spironolactone. Because most patients with such adverse effects were taking spironolactone for edema and ascites in hepatic cirrhosis, it is not yet clear whether they were caused by the drug itself or by hepatic encephalopathy. The incidence of these complaints in such patients is quite high (9.8%) (SED-9, 357).

Electrolyte balance

The beneficial effects of spironolactone in congestive cardiac failure and hypertension are additive to those of ACE inhibitors. In the RALES, patients taking an ACE inhibitor who were randomized to spironolactone 25–50 mg/day had only a 0.3 mmol/l increase in median potassium concentration (1). Although the difference between the spironolactone and placebo groups was statistically significant, the mean increase was not clinically important, and the incidence of serious hyperkalemia was minimal in both groups of patients.

However, since the publication of RALES the incidence of hyperkalemia attributable to spironolactone has increased. Trends in the rate of spironolactone prescriptions and the rate of hospitalization for hyperkalemia in ambulatory patients before and after the publication of RALES have been examined in a population time-based series analysis (2). Among patients treated with ACE inhibitors who had recently been hospitalized for heart failure, the spironolactone prescription rate increased immediately after the publication of RALES, from 3.4% in 1994 to 15% in late 2001. The rate of hospitalization for hyperkalemia rose from 0.2% in 1994 to 11% and the associated mortality rose from 0.3 to 2.0 per 1000 patients. These increases were particularly marked in elderly people.

It is essential to identify patients who are likely to develop serious hyperkalemia during combined treatment and to evaluate the associated morbidity and mortality. Spironolactone is used in patients with end-stage renal disease undergoing either peritoneal (3) or maintenance hemodialysis (4), although there is scant experimental evidence to support such use in advanced dialysis-dependent renal disease. Carefully selected dialysis patients exposed to doses of spironolactone ranging from 25 mg three times a week to 25 mg/day appeared not to have an increased frequency of hyperkalemia. However, these studies were preliminary and the results should not be extrapolated to the general dialysis population. If spironolactone is contemplated in patients with end-stage renal disease, periodic surveillance is necessary and other causes of hyperkalemia, such as ACE inhibitor therapy and/or a high potassium intake, should be controlled.

Close laboratory monitoring and judicious use of spironolactone is needed to reduce the risk of hyperkalemia. The excess of hyperkalemia in clinical practice compared with RALES can be explained largely by the use of higher doses of spironolactone and the inclusion of patients with lower glomerular filtration rates and whose aldosterone-mediated compensatory distal tubular potassium excretion is already attenuated (5). Such patients include elderly people, people with diabetes, and those taking beta-blockers, non-steroidal anti-inflammatory drugs, potassium salts, potassium-sparing diuretics, or trimethoprim.

Hematologic

Rare cases of agranulocytosis have been reported in patients taking spironolactone (SEDA-22, 239).

- Agranulocytosis occurred in an 87-year-old man with congestive heart failure who took spironolactone 25 mg/day for 3 weeks (6). The agranulocytosis rapidly reversed after withdrawal of spironolactone and a short course of granulocyte-colony-stimulating-factor.

- A 43-year-old woman with cirrhosis and hepatocellular carcinoma took spironolactone for 7 days before leukopenia was detected (7). The leukocyte count returned to normal 8 days after withdrawal of spironolactone.

In general, the onset of agranulocytosis with spironolactone ranges from 4 days to 5 weeks and it takes 5–7 days to resolve without the aid of a growth factor.

Gastrointestinal

Nausea and vomiting are more common with spironolactone than with other diuretics (SED-9, 358) and were reported in 11% of patients in the Boston Collaborative Drug Surveillance Program (8). These symptoms can be reduced in patients taking high doses by spreading the dose out during the day.

Liver

Two cases of spironolactone-induced parenchymal hepatitis have been reported. The patients recovered uneventfully (SEDA-20, 205).

- A 50-year-old woman taking spironolactone for androgenic alopecia developed hepatitis with minimal cholestasis 6 weeks after starting therapy (9). After withdrawal of spironolactone, her symptoms resolved and liver function tests improved. She was not rechallenged.

Skin

Rashes (sometimes with eosinophilia), lichen planus (SED-9, 358), and a lupus–like syndrome with a positive rechallenge (SEDA-5, 230) have been reported, but on the whole skin reactions seem to be rare.

Cutaneous vasculitis has been attributed to spironolactone (SED-11, 430). It is unclear whether a patient presenting with erythema annulare centrifugum while taking spironolactone (10) had a similar reaction.

Other reported adverse effects of spironolactone include urticaria, alopecia, and chloasma (SEDA-14, 185).

- A 76-year-old patient developed eczema-like lesions and severe pruritus; histological and immunological investigations showed pemphigoid (11). The skin lesions regressed spontaneously within 15 days of spironolactone withdrawal and no relapse was noted over the next 30 months.

Sexual function

Because of its antiandrogenic action, spironolactone causes gynecomastia, reduced libido, and erectile failure in 4–30% of men. These effects seem to be both dose- and time-dependent.

Reproductive system

Spironolactone causes breast tenderness and enlargement, mastodynia, infertility, chloasma, altered vaginal lubrication, and reduced libido in women, probably because of estrogenic effects on target tissue. Menstrual irregularities were experienced by almost all women taking spironolactone 400 mg/day and most developed amenorrhea at doses of 100–200 mg/day. Normal menstruation was resumed within 2 months of withdrawal.

Very high doses of spironolactone (over 450 mg/day) can cause infertility, but such doses are rarely used. As with other diuretics, studies with spironolactone have mostly been small, not placebo-controlled, and often anecdotal (SEDA-18, 235).

In patients with hepatic cirrhosis, gynecomastia was twice as common during treatment with spironolactone than with potassium canrenoate (42 versus 20%) at equiactive doses (12). This difference may be related to structural characteristics unique to metabolites of spironolactone, namely a thiol group at the 7-alpha position (SEDA-11, 200).

Long-Term Effects

Tumorigenicity

Spironolactone is antiandrogenic and increases the peripheral metabolism of testosterone to estradiol (13). It often causes gynecomastia in men and breast enlargement and soreness in women. Five cases of mammary carcinoma have been reported. Potential human metabolic products of spironolactone are carcinogenic in rodents, and the UK Committee on Safety of Medicines in 1988 restricted the approved indications for the drug, removing the indications of essential hypertension and idiopathic edema (14).

Susceptibility Factors

Age

It has been argued that potassium-sparing diuretics present a real risk of renal insufficiency when they are used in elderly people (15). In large-scale studies in elderly hypertensive patients there is indeed some slight increase in the incidence of renal insufficiency when combinations including potassium-sparing diuretics are used. Although the overall incidence of nephrotoxicity is quite low, elderly patients and those with prior renal dysfunction are at particular risk. Special care is necessary in these circumstances.

Renal disease

In patients with renal insufficiency there is an increased risk of hyperkalemia with spironolactone; serum potassium should be monitored regularly.

Hepatic disease

Hepatic failure carries an unwarranted risk unless serum potassium is regularly monitored (16).

Drug–Drug Interactions

ACE inhibitors

Co-administration of potassium-sparing diuretics with ACE inhibitors can cause severe hyperkalemia (SED-14, 674).

The effects of ACE inhibitors plus spironolactone have been evaluated in 25 patients (11 men, 14 women, mean age 74 years, five with diabetes mellitus) with a mean serum potassium concentration of 7.7 mmol/l (17). The mean serum creatinine was 336 µmol/l, the mean arterial pH 7.3, and the mean plasma bicarbonate 18 mmol/l. The main causes of acute renal insufficiency were dehydration ($n = 12$) and worsening heart failure ($n = 9$). The mean dose of spironolactone was 57 mg/day and 12 patients were also taking other drugs that can cause hyperkalemia. Two patients died and two were resuscitated and survived. Hemodialysis was necessary in 17 patients. The mean duration of hospitalization was 12 days. The combination of ACE inhibitors and spironolactone should be used cautiously in patients with chronic renal insufficiency, diabetes, older age, worsening cardiac failure, a risk of dehydration (for example diarrhea), and in those who are taking other drugs that can cause hyperkalemia (18). A dose of spironolactone of 25 mg/day should be exceeded only with caution. In four similar elderly patients with underlying renal insufficiency taking spironolactone there was an increased risk of hyperkalemia associated with diarrhea (19).

In a population-based, nested, case-control study, all patients aged 66 years or over who were taking an ACE inhibitor and who had been hospitalized for hyperkalemia were evaluated for interacting medications (20). Compared with controls taking ACE inhibitors who did not have hyperkalemia, before adjusting for confounding variables, the patients were 27 times more likely to have received a prescription for a potassium-sparing diuretic (type not specified) in the week before hospitalization. There was no such association between hospital admission for hyperkalemia and the use of indapamide in patients taking ACE inhibitors.

Angiotensin receptor antagonists

In eight healthy subjects, treatment with spironolactone and losartan increased mean plasma potassium concentration by 0.8 mmol/l (up to 5.0 mmol/l) and reduced mean urinary potassium excretion from 108 to 87 mmol/l (21). Until more data are available, it is prudent to consider angiotensin II receptor antagonists similar to ACE inhibitors as risk factors for hyperkalemia in patients taking potassium-sparing diuretics.

Antipyrine

Spironolactone has a weak enzyme-inducing effect and enhances the metabolic breakdown of phenazone (antipyrine) (SED-9, 358).

Aspirin

The renal tubular secretion of canrenone, the main metabolite of spironolactone, is blocked by aspirin (22), abolishing the diuretic response, although the antihypertensive effect is apparently not affected (23).

Carbenoxolone

Spironolactone abolishes the ulcer-healing properties of carbenoxolone (24).

Colestyramine

Colestyramine in combination with spironolactone has been reported to cause severe hyperkalemia (25), presumably because it causes exchange of chloride for bicarbonate in the small bowel, predisposing to hyperchloremic acidosis.

Digitoxin

Spironolactone has a weak enzyme-inducing effect and enhances the metabolic breakdown of digitoxin (SED-9, 358) (26). However, this effect may not be significant, because in six healthy subjects spironolactone prolonged the half-life of digitoxin from 142 to 192 hours (27).

Digoxin

Spironolactone increases steady-state digoxin concentrations by about 30%, probably by inhibiting the renal tubular secretion of digoxin by P glycoprotein. There may also be a pharmacodynamic interaction with digoxin. The clinical importance of these observations is uncertain (SEDA-9, 209).

NSAIDs

Some non-steroidal anti-inflammatory drugs, notably indometacin and mefenamic acid, inhibit the excretion of canrenone (28).

Warfarin

It has been suggested that spironolactone may reduce the anticoagulant effect of warfarin (SED-11, 430).

Interference with Diagnostic Tests

Radioimmunoassay of digoxin

Overestimation of the digoxin concentration
Spironolactone can alter the results of some digoxin radioimmunoassays, because it and its metabolites, such as canrenone and 7-alpha-thiomethylspironolactone, are immunoreactive with some forms of antidigoxin antibody (29–31). This results in an overestimate of the true digoxin concentration, because the assay reads the interfering substances as digoxin.

In a study of the use of the TDx II assay in 80 children and adults, there was apparent digoxin immunoreactivity in 3.7% of healthy subjects ($n = 80$), 3.6% of pregnant women ($n = 28$), 10% of patients with renal transplants ($n = 31$), and 23% of immature infants ($n = 40$) (32).

Underestimation of the digoxin concentration
In contrast to this, it has also been reported that spironolactone and its metabolite canrenone caused falsely low readings in a common assay for digoxin (AXSym MEIA) because of negative cross-reactivity (33). Misleading subtarget concentrations were repeatedly reported, and falsely guided increases in drug doses, resulting in digoxin intoxication.

In another study canrenoate interfered with the immunoassay of digoxin (33), reducing the apparent digoxin concentration. The effect was largest with the AxSym MEIA II assay, and there was also some interference with the EMIT assay. However, the TDx assay was not affected. Spironolactone also caused some interference in the AxSym assay but less than canrenoate. In this case the failure to measure high digoxin concentrations resulted in clinical toxicity in a 71-year-old man who was given 3.8 mg over 11 days.

In nine assays (AxSYM, IMx, TDx, Emit, Dimension, aca, TinaQuant, Elecsys, and Vitros) interference by spironolactone, canrenone, and three metabolites was sought in vitro, and all routine digoxin measurements using the AxSYM system over 16.5 months ($n = 3089$) were reviewed (34). There was a reduction in the expected concentrations by canrenone (3125 ng/ml) in the following assays: AxSYM (42% of expected), IMx (51%), and Dimension (78%). There was positive bias in aca (0.7 ng/ml), TDx (0.62 ng/ml), and Elecsys (>0.58 ng/ml). Of 669 routinely monitored patients, 25 had falsely low results and 19 of them actually had potentially toxic digoxin concentrations; this was attributable to concurrent therapy with spironolactone, canrenone, hydrocortisone, or prednisolone. However, standard doses of spironolactone (up to 50 mg/day) in patients with heart failure produced less than 11% inhibition.

Although several modern digoxin assays suffer from potentially negative interference from spironolactone and canrenone (34), there are assays that are less susceptible to interference by spironolactone (35). Laboratories should determine the false negative potential of the analytical method that they use.

References

1. Pitt B, Zannad F, Remme WJ, Cody R, Castaigne A, Perez A, Palensky J, Wittes J. The effect of spironolactone on morbidity and mortality in patients with severe heart failure. Randomized Aldactone Evaluation Study Investigators. N Engl J Med 1999;341(10):709–17.

2. Juurlink DN, Mamdani MM, Lee DS, Kopp A, Austin PC, Laupacis A, Redelmeier DA. Rates of hyperkalemia after publication of the Randomized Aldactone Evaluation Study. N Engl J Med 2004;351(6):543–51.

3. Hausmann MJ, Liel-Cohen N. Aldactone therapy in a peritoneal dialysis patient with decreased left ventricular function. Nephrol Dial Transplant 2002;17(11):2035–6.

4. Hussain S, Dreyfus DE, Marcus RJ, Biederman RW, McGill RL. Is spironolactone safe for dialysis patients? Nephrol Dial Transplant 2003;18(11):2364–8.

5. McMurray JJ, O'Meara E. Treatment of heart failure with spironolactone—trial and tribulations. N Engl J Med 2004;351(6):526–8.

6. Hui CH, Das PK, Horvath N. Spironolactone and agranulocytosis. Aust NZ J Med 2000;30(4):515.

7. Hsiao SH, Lin YJ, Hsu MY, Wu TJ. Spironolactone-induced agranulocytosis: a case report. Kaohsiung J Med Sci 2003;19(11):574–8.

8. Ochs HR, Greenblatt DJ, Bodem G, Smith TW. Spironolactone. Am Heart J 1978;96(3):389–400.

9. Thai KE, Sinclair RD. Spironolactone-induced hepatitis. Australas J Dermatol 2001;42(3):180–2.

10. Carsuzaa F, Pierre C, Dubegny M. Erythème annulaire centrifugé à l'Aldactone. [Erythema annulare centrifugum caused by Aldactone.] Ann Dermatol Venereol 1987;114(3):375–6.

11. Modeste AB, Cordel N, Courville P, Gilbert D, Lauret P, Joly P. Pemphigoide regressive après arrêt d'un diurétique contenant de l'Aldactone. [Bullous pemphigoid induced by spironolactone.] Ann Dermatol Venereol 2002;129(1 Pt 1):56–8.

12. Emili M, Cuppone R, Ricci GL. Comparative clinical study of spironolactone and potassium canrenoate. A randomized

13. evaluation with double cross-over. Arzneimittelforschung 1988;38(10):1492–5.

13. Rose LI, Underwood RH, Newmark SR, Kisch ES, Williams GH. Pathophysiology of spironolactone-induced gynecomastia. Ann Intern Med 1977;87(4):398–403.

14. Committee on Safety of Medicines. Spironolactone. Curr Probl 1988:21.

15. Bailey RR. Adverse renal reactions to non-steroidal anti-inflammatory drugs and potassium-sparing diuretics. Adv Drug React Bull 1988;131:492.

16. Rado JP, Marosi J, Szende L, Tako J. Hyperkalemic changes during spironolactone therapy for cirrhosis and ascites, with special reference to hyperkalemic intermittent paralysis. J Am Geriatr Soc 1968;16(8):874–86.

17. Schepkens H, Vanholder R, Billiouw JM, Lameire N. Life-threatening hyperkalemia during combined therapy with angiotensin-converting enzyme inhibitors and spironolactone: an analysis of 25 cases. Am J Med 2001;110(6):438–41.

18. Vanpee D, Swine CH. Elderly heart failure patients with drug-induced serious hyperkalemia. Aging (Milano) 2000;12(4):315–19.

19. Berry C, McMurray JJ. Serious adverse events experienced by patients with chronic heart failure taking spironolactone. Heart 2001;85(4):E8.

20. Juurlink DN, Mamdani M, Kopp A, Laupacis A, Redelmeier DA. Drug–drug interactions among elderly patients hospitalized for drug toxicity. JAMA 2003;289(13):1652–8.

21. Henger A, Tutt P, Hulter HM, Krapf R. Acid-base effects of inhibition of aldosterone and angiotensin II action in chronic metabolic acidosis in humans. J Am Soc Nephrol 1999;10:121A.

22. McInnes GT, Shelton JR, Ramsay LE. Evaluation of aldosterone antagonists in healthy man. Methods Find Exp Clin Pharmacol 1982;4(1):49–71.

23. Hollifield JW. Failure of aspirin to antagonize the antihypertensive effect of spironolactone in low-renin hypertension. South Med J 1976;69(8):1034–6.

24. Doll R, Langman MJ, Shawdon HH. Treatment of gastric ulcer with carbenoxolone: antagonistic effect of spironolactone. Gut 1968;9(1):42–5.

25. Zapater P, Alba D. Acidosis and extreme hyperkalemia associated with cholestyramine and spironolactone. Ann Pharmacother 1995;29(2):199–200.

26. Taylor SA, Rawlins MD, Smith SE. Spironolactone—a weak enzyme inducer in man. J Pharm Pharmacol 1972;24(7):578–9.

27. Carruthers SG, Dujovne CA. Cholestyramine and spironolactone and their combination in digitoxin elimination. Clin Pharmacol Ther 1980;27(2):184–7.

28. Tweeddale MG. Antagonism between antipyretic analgesic drugs and spironolactone in man. Clin Res 1974;22:727A.

29. Huffman DH. The effect of spironolactone and canrenone on the digoxin radioimmunoassay. Res Commun Chem Pathol Pharmacol 1974;9(4):787–90.

30. Pleasants RA, Williams DM, Porter RS, Gadsden RH Sr. Reassessment of cross-reactivity of spironolactone metabolites with four digoxin immunoassays. Ther Drug Monit 1989;11(2):200–4.

31. Valdes R Jr, Jortani SA. Unexpected suppression of immunoassay results by cross-reactivity: now a demonstrated cause for concern. Clin Chem 2002;48(3):405–6.

32. Capone D, Gentile A, Basile V. Possible interference of digoxin-like immunoreactive substances using the digoxin fluorescence polarization immunoassay. J Appl Ther Res 1999;2:305–8.

33. Steimer W, Muller C, Eber B, Emmanuilidis K. Intoxication due to negative canrenone interference in digoxin drug monitoring. Lancet 1999;354(9185):1176–7.

34. Steimer W, Muller C, Eber B. Digoxin assays: frequent, substantial, and potentially dangerous interference by spironolactone, canrenone, and other steroids. Clin Chem 2002;48(3):507–16.

35. Datta P, Dasgupta A. A new turbidometric digoxin immunoassay on the ADVIA 1650 analyzer is free from interference by spironolactone, potassium canrenoate, and their common metabolite canrenone. Ther Drug Monit 2003;25(4):478–82.

Stavudine

See also Nucleoside analogue reverse transcriptase inhibitors (NRTIs)

General Information

Stavudine is a nucleoside analogue reverse transcriptase inhibitor. Its most important adverse effects are peripheral neuropathy and increases in hepatic transaminases, both of which usually resolve on withdrawal.

Organs and Systems

Nervous system

The principal toxic effect of stavudine is a peripheral neuropathy, with symptoms similar to the neuropathy associated with didanosine and zalcitabine (1,2). The development of this neuropathy depends on the duration of treatment, with an increasing risk after 12 weeks of treatment. A prior history of neuropathy increases the risk of stavudine-induced neuropathy. After withdrawal, the symptoms usually improve within 2 weeks, although they can persist for several months.

Metabolism

Lipodystrophy, a syndrome characterized by fat redistribution, hyperglycemia/insulin resistance, and dyslipidemia, can be associated with long-term HIV infection or with highly active antiretroviral therapy (HAART). In 1035 patients, those who took stavudine were 1.35 times more likely to report lipodystrophy (3). However, the study was retrospective, and other factors unrelated to specific drug therapy may have had a greater effect on the adjusted odds ratio.

Hematologic

A modest dose-related macrocytosis without an associated anemia can occur during treatment with stavudine (1,2).

Liver

Asymptomatic increases in hepatic transaminases, which are not clearly dose-related, can occur during treatment with stavudine, requiring dosage modification because of moderate or severe toxicity in about 10% of patients (1,2).

Urinary tract

Renal tubular dysfunction and hypophosphatemia occurred in a patient who was taking both stavudine and lamivudine (4).

Sexual function

Painful bilateral gynecomastia and hypersexuality, possibly related to the use of stavudine, have been reported (5).

- A 25-year-old HIV-infected man reported hot flushes and headaches during the first days of treatment with stavudine (40 mg bd), followed by swelling and tenderness under both nipples. He also reported increased libido, premature ejaculation, and persistent erections. He denied illicit drug use. He had bilateral gynecomastia. Luteinizing hormone and testosterone concentrations were within the reference ranges, excluding primary causes of gynecomastia. One month after withdrawal of stavudine, the swelling and tenderness had abated and his sexual symptoms had resolved. He was not rechallenged with the drug.

The authors argued that although idiopathic gynecomastia could not be ruled out, the temporal relation between withdrawal of the drug and improvement in his symptoms suggested a causative role of stavudine.

In a Swiss case-control study gynecomastia was associated with stavudine in 47 cases. Blood concentrations of luteinizing hormone were above the reference range in 40% of the cases and 29% had reduced testosterone concentrations (6).

Drug–Drug Interactions

Isoniazid

A distal sensory neuropathy is the commonest neurological complication in HIV-infected individuals, and has been documented in up to 30% of patients with AIDS. There is evidence from a retrospective case-note review in 30 individuals that co-administration of stavudine and isoniazid increases the incidence of distal sensory neuropathy. Of 22 patients taking stavudine in combination with other drugs, all took isoniazid for tuberculosis and 12 developed a distal sensory neuropathy, with a median time to onset of 5 months (7). Those taking stavudine alone had an incidence of 11%.

References

1. Riddler SA, Anderson RE, Mellors JW. Antiretroviral activity of stavudine (2′,3′-didehydro-3′-deoxythymidine, D4T). Antiviral Res 1995;27(3):189–203.

2. Skowron G. Biologic effects and safety of stavudine: overview of phase I and II clinical trials. J Infect Dis 1995;171(Suppl 2):S113–17.

3. Heath KV, Hogg RS, Chan KJ, Harris M, Montessori V, O'Shaughnessy MV, Montanera JS. Lipodystrophy-associated morphological, cholesterol and triglyceride abnormalities in a population-based HIV/AIDS treatment database. AIDS 2001;15(2):231–9.

4. Morris AA, Baudouin SV, Snow MH. Renal tubular acidosis and hypophosphataemia after treatment with nucleoside reverse transcriptase inhibitors. AIDS 2001;15(1):140–1.

5. Melbourne KM, Brown SL, Silverblatt FJ. Gynecomastia with stavudine treatment in an HIV-positive patient. Ann Pharmacother 1998;32(10):1108.

6. Strub C, Kaufmann GR, Flepp M, Egger M, Kahlert C, Cavassini M, Battegay M; Swiss HIV Cohort Study. Gynecomastia and potent antiretroviral therapy. AIDS 2004;18(9):1347–9.

7. Breen RA, Lipman MC, Johnson MA. Increased incidence of peripheral neuropathy with co-administration of stavudine and isoniazid in HIV-infected individuals. AIDS 2000;14(5):615.

Stem cell factor

General Information

Stem cell factor amplifies the proliferation and mobilization of myeloid, erythroid, and megakaryocyte colonies when combined with a lineage-specific hemopoietic growth factor (for example G-CSF, IL-3). Stem cell factor, added to other recombinant hemopoietic cytokines, is used to increase the mobilization of peripheral blood progenitor cells.

In preliminary trials, transient allergic-type reactions, that is urticaria, respiratory symptoms, and injection-site reactions, resulting from dose-dependent mast cell degranulation, were easily prevented by classical premedication (1).

In 102 patients with multiple myeloma, stem cell factor plus G-CSF produced more frequent injection site reactions and more frequent skin reactions (25 versus 2%), namely rash, erythema, urticaria, pruritus, and abnormal pigmentation, compared with G-CSF alone (2). These reactions occurred despite systemic prophylactic antihistamines. Other adverse effects occurred with similar frequency in the two groups of patients.

Organs and Systems

Immunologic

Stem cell factor produces direct mast cell stimulation with subsequent allergic-type reactions. Despite careful premedication with diphenhydramine, ranitidine, inhaled salbutamol, and pseudoephedrine, such reactions were still observed in 3% of patients (3).

References

1. Maslak P, Nimer SD. The efficacy of IL-3, SCF, IL-6, and IL-11 in treating thrombocytopenia. Semin Hematol 1998;35(3):253–60.

2. Facon T, Harousseau JL, Maloisel F, Attal M, Odriozola J, Alegre A, Schroyens W, Hulin C, Schots R, Marin P, Guilhot F, Granena A, De Waele M, Pigneux A, Meresse V, Clark P, Reiffers J. Stem cell factor in combination with filgrastim after chemotherapy improves peripheral blood progenitor cell yield and reduces apheresis requirements in multiple myeloma patients: a randomized, controlled trial. Blood 1999;94(4):1218–25.

3. Shpall EJ, Wheeler CA, Turner SA, Yanovich S, Brown RA, Pecora AL, Shea TC, Mangan KF, Williams SF, LeMaistre CF, Long GD, Jones R, Davis MW, Murphy-Filkins R, Parker WR, Glaspy JA. A randomized phase 3 study of peripheral blood progenitor cell mobilization with stem cell factor and filgrastim in high-risk breast cancer patients. Blood 1999;93(8):2491–501.

Stepronin

General Information

The adverse effects of stepronin, a sulfhydryl compound, which is used in rheumatoid arthritis, are similar to those of penicillamine. In a long-term open study, treatment had to be interrupted in 30% of 36 patients because of severe adverse effects (1). Seven patients had mucocutaneous reactions (dermatitis, pruritus, stomatitis, glossitis, ageusia), three proteinuria, and one thrombocytopenia and leukopenia.

Reference

1. Nervetti A, Salaffi F, Manganelli P, et al. Terapia di fondo dell'artrite reumatoide con stepronina: studio long-term di 3 anni. Reumatismo 1988;40:287.

Sterculiaceae

See also Herbal medicines

General Information

The genera in the family of Sterculiaceae (Table 1) include cola, theobroma, and sterculia.

Table 1 The genera of Sterculiaceae

Ayenia (ayenia)
Brachychiton (brachychiton)
Chiranthodendron (chiranthodendron)
Cola (cola)
Firmiana (parasol tree)
Fremontodendron (flannel bush)
Guazuma (guazuma)
Helicteres (helicteres)
Heritiera
Hermannia (hermannia)
Kleinhovia (kleinhovia)
Melochia (melochia)
Pentapetes (pentapetes)
Sterculia (sterculia)
Theobroma (theobroma)
Waltheria (waltheria)

Sterculia species

The family of *Sterculia* plants (sterculia) yield a fiber that has bulk laxative effects. It is covered in the monograph on Laxatives.

Stiripentol

See also Antiepileptic drugs

General Information

The clinical pharmacology and adverse effects of stiripentol have been reviewed (1).

The effects of stiripentol have been studied in 41 children with severe myoclonic epilepsy in infancy in a randomized, placebo-controlled, add-on trial (2). There were adverse effects in 21 patients taking stiripentol (drowsiness and loss of appetite) compared with five taking placebo, and the adverse effects disappeared when the doses of other antiepileptic drugs were reduced in 12 of the 21 cases.

Drug–Drug Interactions

Clobazam

When stiripentol 50 mg/kg was given to 20 children taking clobazam, mean serum clobazam and norclobazam concentrations increased about two-fold and three-fold respectively; a mean 25% reduction in clobazam dose was required because of adverse effects (3).

Valproic acid

Serum concentrations of concomitantly administered valproic acid rose by about 20% (3). These findings are in agreement with evidence that stiripentol is a potent metabolic inhibitor.

References

1. Willmore LJ. Clinical pharmacology of new antiepileptic drugs. Neurology 2000;55(11 Suppl. 3):S17–24.
2. Chiron C, Marchand MC, Tran A, Rey E, D'Athis P, Vincent J, Dulac O, Pons G. Stiripentol in severe myoclonic epilepsy in infancy: a randomised placebo-controlled syndrome-dedicated trial. STICLO Study Group. Lancet 2000;356(9242):1638–42.
3. Rey E, Tran A, D'Athis P, Chiron C, Dulac O, Vincent J, Pons G. Stiripentol potentiates clobazam in childhood epilepsy: a pharmacological study. Epilepsia 1999;40(Suppl. 7):112–13.

Streptogramins

General Information

Pristinamycin (rINN) is a synergistic combination of streptogramin A (pristinamycin IIA) and streptogramin B (pristinamycin IB). It is active against the main bacteria that cause respiratory tract infections and could be useful in the treatment of acute or recurrent sinusitis, community-acquired pneumonia, or periodontal infection with *Actinobacillus actinomycetemcomitans* (1–5).

Quinupristin (rINN) and dalfopristin (rINN) are two semisynthetic pristinamycin derivatives that are given in combination parenterally. The combination has a broad spectrum of activity against Gram-positive bacteria, including multidrug resistant bacilli. A comprehensive review has been published (6). Quinupristin + dalfopristin can be used to treat macrolide-resistant streptococci, staphylococcal infections after failure of conventional therapy, or vancomycin-resistant *Enterococcus faecium* (and probably *Enterococcus raffinosus*), but not vancomycin-resistant *Enterococcus faecalis*, *Enterococcus avium*, *Enterococcus casseliflavus*, or *Enterococcus gallinarum* (7–19). Adverse effects include arthralgia, myalgia, and pain at the infusion site (20).

Observational studies

In a small, open, phase II pilot study, low-dose quinupristin + dalfopristin (5 mg/kg intravenously every 8 hours; $n = 11$) and high-dose quinupristin + dalfopristin (7.5 mg/kg intravenously every 8 hours; $n = 15$) were compared with vancomycin (1 g intravenously every 12 hours; $n = 13$) in the treatment of catheter-related staphylococcal bacteremia (21). In patients with a baseline pathogen, the outcome was comparable in all groups. Adverse clinical events in the quinupristin + dalfopristin group consisted of arm and chest pain, chills, fever, arthritis, and phlebitis or pain at the injection site; quinupristin + dalfopristin was withdrawn in 12% of patients (compared with 15% of vancomycin-treated patients).

In healthy volunteers receiving quinupristin + dalfopristin, 7.5 mg/kg infused over 1 hour bd, mean fecal antibiotic concentrations were 291 and 42 µg/g of feces for quinupristin and dalfopristin respectively by the fifth day of treatment (22).

Comparative studies

The pooled results of two multicenter, phase III, randomized comparisons of quinupristin + dalfopristin (7.5 mg/kg intravenously every 12 hours; $n = 450$) with established comparators (cefazolin, oxacillin, vancomycin; $n = 443$) for complicated skin and skin structure infections have been reported (23). The success rate was equivalent in the two groups: 63% of patients given quinupristin + dalfopristin (versus 54%) reported at least one adverse event, most commonly nausea, vomiting, rash, pain, or pruritus. Although most of the adverse events were mild to moderate, the drug was withdrawn in 19% of patients treated with quinupristin + dalfopristin (versus 4.7%) owing to an untoward event. Adverse venous events (atrophy, edema, hemorrhage, hypersensitivity, inflammation, thrombophlebitis, pain) were reported by 66% of patients treated with quinupristin + dalfopristin (versus 28%) and required withdrawal of the drug in 12% of these patients (versus 2%).

General adverse effects

The adverse effects of quinupristin + dalfopristin include arthralgia, myalgias, reversible rises in serum alkaline phosphatase, itching, diarrhea, vomiting, and pain at the infusion site; adverse effects occurred in 2.5–4.6% of patients (24–31).

Organs and Systems

Electrolyte balance

The combination of quinupristin + dalfopristin has been associated with hyponatremia, probably secondary to inappropriate secretion of antidiuretic hormone (32).

- A 67-year-old woman with peripheral neuropathy, IgM paraproteinemia, and chronic obstructive pulmonary disease developed dyspnea and hyponatremia, and a small-cell lung cancer was diagnosed. She was given 3 cycles of chemotherapy (etoposide, cyclophosphamide, and doxorubicin). Her serum sodium concentrations normalized. On day 103, she was given quinupristin + dalfopristin (7.5 mg/kg every 8 hours) because of septicemia with vancomycin-resistant E. faecium. The serum sodium concentration thereafter fell (day 110: 117 mmol/l; serum osmolarity: 268 mosm/l; urine osmolarity: 426 mosm/l). Therapy was withdrawn on day 111, and the sodium concentration gradually returned to normal.

Gastrointestinal

In a multicenter, open, randomized trial in 204 patients with erysipelas treated with either oral pristinamycin 1 g tds or intravenous then oral penicillin, adverse events related to treatment were significantly more common with pristinamycin; they were mostly mild or moderate and mainly involved the gastrointestinal tract (33).

Pristinamycin can cause pseudomembranous colitis.

- An 85-year-old woman developed a severe illness (severe diarrhea and vomiting, abdominal tenderness, peritoneal irritation, and systemic toxicity) 8 days after receiving pristinamycin 3 g/day for 10 days (34). An assay for Clostridium difficile was positive. She was treated with metronidazole and her symptoms resolved after 72 hours.

Liver

In 25 liver transplant recipients who received intravenous quinupristin + dalfopristin 7.5 mg/kg 8-hourly for vancomycin-resistant E. faecium infection, hyperbilirubinemia developed, but there was no evidence of drug-specific histological injury (35).

Skin

In a retrospective study of children taking quinupristin + dalfopristin, rash (2%) was the most frequent adverse event, but only one patient with rash discontinued quinupristin + dalfopristin because of it (31).

Patch tests can be used to confirm pristinamycin-induced drug eruptions. In 11 patients with cutaneous drug reactions after oral pristinamycin, patch tests (with pristinamycin diluted to 20% aqueous and 20% petrolatum) were performed 1–3 months after treatment with pristinamycin (36). There were positive patch tests in nine, and there was no relapse of the drug eruption during patch-testing; 30 control patients had negative tests.

Mean antibiotic concentrations of pristinamycin in dermal interstitial fluid (from suction bullae) are low; nevertheless, the concentrations achieved should theoretically inhibit the growth of group A streptococci (37).

Musculoskeletal

Of seven patients with end-stage renal insufficiency who received quinupristin + dalfopristin, two developed myalgias (38).

Of 32 patients who received quinupristin + dalfopristin, at least 15 developed arthralgias and/or myalgias (39).

Immunologic

The combination of quinupristin + dalfopristin reduces cytokine production in stimulated monocytes from healthy volunteers, suggesting significant immunomodulatory activity (40).

Long-Term Effects

Drug resistance

The relative frequency of resistance to macrolides, lincosamides, and streptogramins (MLS resistance) has been assessed in a series of 2091 staphylococcus isolates collected during a 3-week period in 1995 in 32 French hospitals. A total of 294 strains (144 Staphylococcus aureus, 150 coagulase-negative staphylococci) exhibited resistance to at least one of these groups of antibiotics. Resistance to pristinamycin was phenotypically detected in ten S. aureus strains (seven isolates from the same hospital and possibly of the same clone) and three coagulase-negative staphylococcus isolates. It was associated with resistance to type A streptogramins encoded by vat or vatB genes and was associated with the erm genes (41).

A short report demonstrated the absence of a reliable correlation between killing kinetics and normal laboratory tests for pristinamycin susceptibility testing of some pneumococci (42). Eight selected multiresistant clinical isolates and two reference pristinamycin-resistant Streptococcus pneumoniae strains were studied. Disk diffusion susceptibility and MICs were determined by the agar dilution method, and all clinical isolates appeared to be susceptible to pristinamycin, whereas the two reference strains were not. In contrast, time-kill experiments identified a limited bactericidal effect of pristinamycin in three clinical and both reference strains. These three strains had been classified as pristinamycin-resistant by the Vitek-II system, which uses a kinetic turbidimetric measurement of bacterial growth. Epidemiological information is hindered by the use of highly selected strains for the study.

The in vitro activity of pristinamycin has been evaluated in 200 isolates of S. pneumoniae strains with various degrees of susceptibility to penicillin G and erythromycin (43). All the strains were susceptible to pristinamycin, irrespective of their susceptibility to penicillin G or erythromycin.

After 5 days administration of quinupristin + dalfopristin 7.5 mg/kg infused over 1 hour bd, the fecal microflora in 20 healthy volunteers increased significantly during treatment and returned within 12 weeks to baseline concentrations after the end of treatment. There were anerobes and enterococci resistant to erythromycin or to quinupristin + dalfopristin, but glycopeptide-resistant enterococci did not emerge (22).

The relevance of resistance to virginiamycin

Virginiamycin is a streptogramin that has been used in animals as a growth-promoter. Increasing use of virginiamycin has been associated with a high rate of resistance to quinupristin + dalfopristin (44). Acquired resistance to virginiamycin, which is active against Gram-positive lactic acid-producing bacteria, can be detected in *E. faecium* and *E. faecalis* strains isolated from animals and food (45), including strains from poultry, in which high resistance against virginiamycin was found in Belgium (46). Streptogramin resistance is associated with the resistance genes vatA and vatG in *E. faecium* of both animals and man (44). Because virginiamycin has been used in animals and streptogramins have been used infrequently in man, an animal origin of resistance has been suggested, and spread of resistance via the food chain to humans is probable (47).

Susceptibility Factors

Renal disease

The disposition of quinupristin, dalfopristin, and their primary metabolites was similar in eight non-infected patients on peritoneal dialysis compared with eight matched healthy volunteers after the administration of quinupristin + dalfopristin 7.5 mg/kg (48). Since dialysis clearance was insignificant, the combination was thought to be inadequate for the therapy of dialysis-associated peritonitis.

The pharmacokinetics of a single intravenous injection of quinupristin + dalfopristin (7.5 mg/kg over 1 hour) have been assessed in 13 patients with severe chronic renal insufficiency (creatinine clearance 6–28 ml/minute/$1.73 m^2$) (49). Although the mean peak plasma drug concentration and AUC of quinupristin plus its active derivatives and of both unchanged dalfopristin and dalfopristin plus its active derivatives were about 1.3–1.4 times higher than in healthy volunteers, the authors concluded that no formal reduction in the dosage of quinupristin + dalfopristin is necessary in patients with chronic renal insufficiency.

Drug–Drug Interactions

CYP3A4

Quinupristin + dalfopristin can inhibit the metabolism of agents that are metabolized by CYP3A4 (50).

References

1. Leclercq R. Activité in vitro de la pristinamycine sur les germes respiratoires. [In vitro activity of pristinamycin on respiratory bacteria.] Presse Méd 1999;28(Suppl 1):6–9.
2. Klossek JM, Mayaud C. Conclusions: quelle stratégie antibiotique dans les infections respiratoires de l'adulte? [Conclusion: what is the choice of antibiotics in adult respiratory tract infections?] Presse Méd 1999;28(Suppl 1):16–18.
3. Poirier R. La place de la pristinamycine dans les pneumopathies aiguës communautaires de l'adulte. [Pristinamycin in the treatment of acute communicable pneumopathies in adults.] Presse Méd 1999;28(Suppl 1):13–15.
4. Pessey JJ. Place de la pristinamycine dans le traitement des sinusites aiguës de l'adulte en ville. [Pristinamycin in the outpatient treatment of acute sinusitis in adults.] Presse Méd 1999;28(Suppl 1):10–12.
5. Madinier IM, Fosse TB, Hitzig C, Charbit Y, Hannoun LR. Resistance profile survey of 50 periodontal strains of Actinobacillus actinomyectomcomitans. J Periodontol 1999;70(8):888–92.
6. Lamb HM, Figgitt DP, Faulds D. Quinupristin/dalfopristin: a review of its use in the management of serious gram-positive infections. Drugs 1999;58(6):1061–97.
7. Betriu C, Redondo M, Palau ML, Sanchez A, Gomez M, Culebras E, Boloix A, Picazo JJ. Comparative in vitro activities of linezolid, quinupristin–dalfopristin, moxifloxacin, and trovafloxacin against erythromycin-susceptible and -resistant streptococci. Antimicrob Agents Chemother 2000;44(7):1838–41.
8. Elsner HA, Sobottka I, Feucht HH, Harps E, Haun C, Mack D, Ganschow R, Laufs R, Kaulfers PM. Nosocomial outbreak of vancomycin-resistant *Enterococcus faecium* at a German university pediatric hospital. Int J Hyg Environ Health 2000;203(2):147–52.
9. von Eiff C, Reinert RR, Kresken M, Brauers J, Hafner D, Peters G. Nationwide German multicenter study on prevalence of antibiotic resistance in staphylococcal bloodstream isolates and comparative in vitro activities of quinupristin–dalfopristin. J Clin Microbiol 2000;38(8):2819–23.
10. Johnson AP, Warner M, Hallas G, Livermore DM. Susceptibility to quinupristin/dalfopristin and other antibiotics of vancomycin-resistant enterococci from the UK, 1997 to mid-1999. J Antimicrob Chemother 2000;46(1):125–8.
11. McGeer AJ, Low DE. Vancomycin-resistant enterococci. Semin Respir Infect 2000;15(4):314–26.
12. Levison ME, Mallela S. Increasing antimicrobial resistance: therapeutic implications for enterococcal infections. Curr Infect Dis Rep 2000;2(5):417–23.
13. Bergogne-Berezin E. Resistances et nouvelles stratégies antibiotiques. Nouveaux antibiotiques antistaphylococciques. [Resistance and new antibiotic strategies. New antistaphylococcal antibiotics.] Presse Méd 2000;29(37):2023–7.
14. Livermore DM. Antibiotic resistance in staphylococci. Int J Antimicrob Agents 2000;16(Suppl 1):S3–10.
15. Bhavnani SM, Ballow CH. New agents for Gram-positive bacteria. Curr Opin Microbiol 2000;3(5):528–34.
16. Bush K, Macielag M. New approaches in the treatment of bacterial infections. Curr Opin Chem Biol 2000;4(4):433–9.
17. Jones RN. Perspectives on the development of new antimicrobial agents for resistant gram-positive pathogens. Braz J Infect Dis 2000;4(1):1–8.
18. Murray BE. Problems and perils of vancomycin resistant enterococci. Braz J Infect Dis 2000;4(1):9–14.
19. Lundstrom TS, Sobel JD. Antibiotics for Gram-positive bacterial infections. Vancomycin, teicoplanin, quinupristin/dalfopristin, and linezolid. Infect Dis Clin North Am 2000;14(2):463–74.
20. Delgado G Jr, Neuhauser MM, Bearden DT, Danziger LH. Quinupristin–dalfopristin: an overview. Pharmacotherapy 2000;20(12):1469–85.
21. Raad I, Bompart F, Hachem R. Prospective, randomized dose-ranging open phase II pilot study of quinupristin/dalfopristin versus vancomycin in the treatment of catheter-related staphylococcal bacteremia. Eur J Clin Microbiol Infect Dis 1999;18(3):199–202.
22. Scanvic-Hameg A, Chachaty E, Rey J, Pousson C, Ozoux ML, Brunel E, Andremont A. Impact of quinupristin/

dalfopristin (RP59500) on the faecal microflora in healthy volunteers J Antimicrob Chemother 2002;49(1):135–9.

23. Nichols RL, Graham DR, Barriere SL, Rodgers A, Wilson SE, Zervos M, Dunn DL, Kreter B. Treatment of hospitalized patients with complicated Gram-positive skin and skin structure infections: two randomized, multicentre studies of quinupristin/dalfopristin versus cefazolin, oxacillin or vancomycin. Synercid Skin and Skin Structure Infection Group. J Antimicrob Chemother 1999;44(2):263–73.

24. Raad I, Hachem R, Hanna H, Girgawy E, Rolston K, Whimbey E, Husni R, Bodey G. Treatment of vancomycin-resistant enterococcal infections in the immunocompromised host: quinupristin–dalfopristin in combination with minocycline. Antimicrob Agents Chemother 2001;45(11):3202–4.

25. Rehm SJ, Graham DR, Srinath L, Prokocimer P, Richard MP, Talbot GH. Successful administration of quinupristin/dalfopristin in the outpatient setting. J Antimicrob Chemother 2001;47(5):639–45.

26. Linden PK, Moellering RC Jr, Wood CA, Rehm SJ, Flaherty J, Bompart F, Talbot GH; Synercid Emergency-Use Study Group. Treatment of vancomycin-resistant *Enterococcus faecium* infections with quinupristin/dalfopristin. Clin Infect Dis 2001;33(11):1816–23.

27. Verma A, Dhawan A, Philpott-Howard J, Rela M, Heaton N, Vergani GM, Wade J. Glycopeptide-resistant *Enterococcus faecium* infections in paediatric liver transplant recipients: safety and clinical efficacy of quinupristin/dalfopristin. J Antimicrob Chemother 2001;47(1):105–8.

28. Allington DR, Rivey MP. Quinupristin/dalfopristin: a therapeutic review. Clin Ther 2001;23(1):24–44.

29. Bonfiglio G, Furneri PM. Novel streptogramin antibiotics. Expert Opin Investig Drugs 2001;10(2):185–98.

30. Blondeau JM, Sanche SE. Quinupristin/dalfopristin. Expert Opin Pharmacother 2002;3(9):1341–64.

31. Loeffler AM, Drew RH, Perfect JR, Grethe NI, Stephens JW, Gray SL, Talbot GH. Safety and efficacy of quinupristin/dalfopristin for treatment of invasive Gram-positive infections in pediatric patients. Pediatr Infect Dis J 2002;21(10):950–6.

32. Cole RP, Roberts WD, Cheng MD. Hyponatremia associated with quinupristin–dalfopristin. Ann Intern Med 2000;133(6):485.

33. Bernard P, Chosidow O, Vaillant L; French Erysipelas Study Group. Oral pristinamycin versus standard penicillin regimen to treat erysipelas in adults: randomised, non-inferiority, open trial. BMJ 2002;325(7369):864.

34. Gavazzi G, Barnoud R, Lamloum M, Coume M, Fillipi M, Debray M, Couturier P, Franco A. Colite pseudomembraneuse après pristinamycine. [Pseudomembranous colitis after pristinamycin.] Rev Med Interne 2001;22(7):672–3.

35. Linden PK, Bompart F, Gray S, Talbot GH. Hyperbilirubinemia during quinupristin–dalfopristin therapy in liver transplant recipients: correlation with available liver biopsy results. Pharmacotherapy 2001;21(6):661–8.

36. Mayence C, Dompmartin A, Verneuil L, Michel M, Leroy D. Value of patch tests in pristinamycin-induced drug eruptions. Contact Dermatitis 1999;40(3):161–2.

37. Vaillant L, Le Guellec C, Jehl F, Barruet R, Sorensen H, Roiron R, Autret-Leca E, Lorette G. Diffusions comparées de l'acide fusidique, de l'oxacilline et de la pristinamycine dans le liquide interstitiel dermique après administration orale repetée. [Comparative diffusion of fusidic acid, oxacillin, and pristinamycin in dermal interstitial fluid after repeated oral administration.] Ann Dermatol Venereol 2000;127(1):33–9.

38. Olsen KM, Rebuck JA, Rupp ME. Arthralgias and myalgias related to quinupristin–dalfopristin administration. Clin Infect Dis 2001;32(4):e83–6.

39. Khan AA, Slifer TR, Araujo FG, Remington JS. Effect of quinupristin/dalfopristin on production of cytokines by human monocytes. J Infect Dis 2000;182(1):356–8.

40. Schwenger V, Mundlein E, Dagrosa EE, Fahr AM, Zeier M, Mikus G, Andrassy K. Treatment of life-threatening multi-resistant staphylococcal and enterococcal infections in patients with end-stage renal failure with quinupristin/dalfopristin: preliminary report. Infection 2002;30(5):257–61.

41. Lina G, Quaglia A, Reverdy ME, Leclercq R, Vandenesch F, Etienne J. Distribution of genes encoding resistance to macrolides, lincosamides, and streptogramins among staphylococci. Antimicrob Agents Chemother 1999;43(5):1062–6.

42. Schlegel L, Sissia G, Fremaux A, Geslin P. Diminished killing of pneumococci by pristinamycin demonstrated by time-kill studies. Antimicrob Agents Chemother 1999;43(8):2099–100.

43. Lozniewski A, Lion C, Mory F, Weber M. Comparison of the in vitro activity of pristinamycin and quinupristin/dalfopristin against *Streptococcus pneumoniae*. Pathol Biol (Paris) 2000;48(5):463–6.

44. Hayes JR, McIntosh AC, Qaiyumi S, Johnson JA, English LL, Carr LE, Wagner DD, Joseph SW. High-frequency recovery of quinupristin-dalfopristin-resistant *Enterococcus faecium* isolates from the poultry production environment. J Clin Microbiol 2001;39(6):2298–9.

45. Butaye P, Devriese LA, Haesebrouck F. Phenotypic distinction in *Enterococcus faecium* and *Enterococcus faecalis* strains between susceptibility and resistance to growth-enhancing antibiotics. Antimicrob Agents Chemother 1999;43(10):2569–70.

46. Butaye P, Devriese LA, Haesebrouck F. Differences in antibiotic resistance patterns of *Enterococcus faecalis* and *Enterococcus faecium* strains isolated from farm and pet animals. Antimicrob Agents Chemother 2001;45(5):1374–8.

47. Voegel LP. Path of drug resistance from farm to clinic. Science 2002;295(5555):625.

48. Johnson CA, Taylor CA 3rd, Zimmerman SW, Bridson WE, Chevalier P, Pasquier O, Baybutt RI. Pharmacokinetics of quinupristin–dalfopristin in continuous ambulatory peritoneal dialysis patients. Antimicrob Agents Chemother 1999;43(1):152–6.

49. Chevalier P, Rey J, Pasquier O, Leclerc V, Baguet JC, Meyrier A, Harding N, Montay G. Pharmacokinetics of quinupristin/dalfopristin in patients with severe chronic renal insufficiency. Clin Pharmacokinet 2000;39(1):77–84.

50. Fost DA, Leung DY, Martin RJ, Brown EE, Szefler SJ, Spahn JD. Inhibition of methylprednisolone elimination in the presence of clarithromycin therapy. J Allergy Clin Immunol 1999;103(6):1031–5.

Strychnine

General Information

Strychnine is an alkaloid that is found in *Nux vomica*. It causes excitation of all parts of the central nervous system, with a characteristic motor pattern. Strychnine is a competitive antagonist at inhibitory neurotransmitter glycine receptors in the spinal cord, brain stem, and higher centers. It thus increases neuronal activity and excitability, leading to increased muscular activity. Since strychnine convulsions also occur in decerebrate animals, the convulsion is termed a "spinal convulsion," but other parts of the central nervous system are also stimulated by doses that produce motor manifestations in a decerebrate animal. Strychnine does not selectively stimulate the medulla and cannot therefore be regarded as a useful analeptic drug (1).

The features of strychnine poisoning occur at 15–30 minutes after ingestion. They include heightened awareness, muscle twitches and spasms, and hypersensitivity to stimuli. In severe toxicity, painful generalized convulsions can occur without loss of consciousness. Respiratory arrest secondary to respiratory muscle spasm also occurs and is the usual mode of death. Prolonged muscular spasm can lead to hyperthermia, lactic acidosis, rhabdomyolysis, and acute renal insufficiency due to myoglobinuria.

Drug Administration

Drug overdose

Two cases of strychnine poisoning with characteristic signs and symptoms have been described (2,3). Management included gastric lavage, the administration of activated charcoal, sedation with midazolam and phenobarbital, and paralysis with vecuronium, along with respiratory support and forced hydration. In some countries strychnine is available as a pest control agent, resulting in occasional poisoning. Early diagnosis and prompt management can save the patient, despite the consumption of a large dose of strychnine.

- A 33-year-old man attempted suicide by self-injection of strychnine intramuscularly (4). A few seconds after the first injection he developed dizziness and light-headedness. Ten minutes after the second injection he had seizures, opisthotonos, and tetany. He was rescued with a benzodiazepine and ventilatory support.

A case of fatal poisoning due to strychnine has been described, and the concentrations of strychnine in various body fluids and organs have been detailed (5). The half-life of strychnine in a case of poisoning in a 42-year-old man who survived was 12 hours (6).

References

1   Curtis DR. The pharmacology of spinal postsynaptic inhibition. Prog Brain Res 1969;31:171–89.
2   Oberpaur B, Donoso A, Claveria C, Valverde C, Azocar M. Strychnine poisoning: an uncommon intoxication in children. Pediatr Emerg Care 1999;15(4):264–5.
3   Adam JC, Cheize P, Adam F. Strychnine poisoning: about one case. JEUR 1999;12:128–30.
4   Mesquida S, Pumariega H, Ruano O, De los Rios D. Intoxicacion por inyeccion intramuscular de estricnina. [Intoxication caused by intramuscular injection of strychnine.] Rev Toxicol 2001;18:15–16.
5   Rosano TG, Hubbard JD, Meola JM, Swift TA. Fatal strychnine poisoning: application of gas chromatography and tandem mass spectrometry. J Anal Toxicol 2000;24(7):642–7.
6   Wood D, Webster E, Martinez D, Dargan P, Jones A. Survival after deliberate strychnine self-poisoning, with toxicokinetic data. Crit Care 2002;6(5):456–9.

Substances that affect the skin: Contact allergy

General Information

Contact allergy is the most frequently described adverse effect of topical drugs and cosmetics; the diagnosis can be established by patch-testing (1–4) and review articles (5).

In allergic contact dermatitis due to topical medicaments (6), any constituent of the formulation can be responsible for the adverse event—the vehicle, preservative, emulsifier, perfume, or the active drug. Hence, patch tests should be carried out with all active and supposedly inactive ingredients of the incriminated topical drug.

When cosmetic allergy is suspected (SEDA-11, 142) (SEDA-13, 117) (7), the patient should be tested with the suspected products. Skin care products can be tested as the marketed formulation. However, some cosmetics, notably those that contain detergents such as soaps, shampoos, and bath foams, can cause false-negative and false-positive patch test reactions. Their ingredients should therefore preferably be tested separately when contact allergy to such products is strongly suspected (8). Natural botanical extracts are being increasingly used in cosmetics. Consumers tend to regard these natural substances as safe. However, patients with positive patch tests to *Aloe vera*, arnica, *Centella asiatica*, chamomile, cucumber, lavender oil, peppermint, rosemary, sage, St John's wort (photosensitivity), tea tree oil, and witch hazel have been reported (9).

Ingredient labeling, which has been mandatory in the European Union since 1 January, 1997, has greatly facilitated the investigation of patients with suspected cosmetic dermatitis (SEDA-22, 159) (10).

There have been useful review articles on cosmetic allergy (8), preservatives (11), fragrances (SEDA-20, 149) (12), topical drugs (6), glucocorticoids (13), and antihistamines (14).

Table 1 lists alphabetically a large number of ingredients of cosmetics and topical drugs that can act as sensitizers; some drugs are accidental contactants, for example in the pharmaceutical industry or in health personnel. For each compound, the concentration and vehicle for patch-testing, known or generally held to be adequate, are mentioned.

Substances that are not listed in any standard table should be patch-tested with great caution; control tests are mandatory when positive reactions are obtained, so as to exclude false-positive irritant patch test reactions.

We have attempted to estimate the sensitizing potential of each particular drug using the following scale:

1—sensitization is common;
2—sensitization can occur;
3—sensitization is unusual;
4—sensitization is rare.

These estimates are based on literature data and personal experience (4).

Table 1 Patch test concentrations and vehicles for skin testing of ingredients of topical drugs and cosmetics

Chemical	Patch test concentration and vehicle	Frequency of sensitization	References	Comments
Acetarsone	1–5% petrolatum	4	(SEDA-20, 158)	
Acetylsalicylic acid	2% petrolatum	4	(SEDA-18, 164) (36)	
Aciclovir	5% petrolatum	4	(SEDA-14, 125)	
Adrenaline[3]	0.1–1% aqua	4	(3)	
Aescin	2% aqua	4	(SEDA-17, 188)	
Alcohol[1]	10% aqua, pure	4	(SEDA-12, 133) (37)	b, d
Alkylammonium amidobenzoate	0.1 and 0.01% petrolatum	4	(SEDA-17, 188) (38,39)	
Amalgam	5% petrolatum	3	(SEDA-19, 158)	
Ambroxol hydrochloride	0.5% aqua	4	(SEDA-14, 125)	
Amcinonide[2]	1% epi (45% alcohol, 10% propylene glycol, 45% isopropyl alcohol)	3	(SEDA-15, 140)	
Amerchol CAB	Pure	2	(SEDA-17, 188)	
Aminoethanolamine	0.005, 0.1, and 0.5% in aqua		(40)	
ϵ-Aminocaproic acid[3]	1% aqua	4	(SEDA-17, 189)	
3-(Aminomethyl)-pyridyl salicylate	1% aqua	3	(SEDA-14, 125)	
4-Amino-3-nitrophenol	2% petrolatum		(41)	
Amlexanox	0.01–1% aqua or petrolatum	3	(SEDA-16, 155)	
Ammoniated mercury	1% petrolatum	2	(SEDA-19, 159)	d
Ammonium bisulfate[1]	0.1 and 0.5% aqua	4	(SEDA-21, 165)	
Ammonium persulfate	2.5% petrolatum	3	(3)	e, b
Amorolfine	1% petrolatum or aqua	4	(SEDA-21, 165)	
Ampicillin	5% petrolatum	4	(SEDA-9, 136)	b
α-Amylcinnamic alcohol[4]	2% petrolatum	2	(SEDA-8, 158)	
α-Amylcinnamic aldehyde[4]	2% petrolatum	2	(SEDA-8, 158) (42)	
Anethole	5% petrolatum		(43)	
Apomorphine	0.05% aqua	4	(SEDA-17, 188)	
Arnica, tincture of	20% petrolatum	3	(3)	
Atropine sulfate[3]	1% petrolatum	4	(3)	
Auranofin	0.2% petrolatum	2	(SEDA-19, 158)	
Avocado oil	Pure	4	(SEDA-12, 134)	
Azidamfenicol	5% petrolatum	4	(SEDA-12, 132)	
Azulene	1% petrolatum	4	(SEDA-20, 157)	
Bacitracin[3]	20% petrolatum	2	(SEDA-18, 171)	b
Basic blue 99	0.5% petrolatum	4	(3)	b
Basic red 22	1% aqua		(44)	
Beclomethasone dipropionate[2]	5% petrolatum	4	(SEDA-15, 140)	
Beeswax	30% petrolatum	2	(SEDA-21, 165)	
Befunolol	1% aqua	3	(SEDA-17, 188)	
Benzalkonium chloride[1,3]	0.05% aqua	3	(SEDA-7, 161)	
Benzarone	2% petrolatum and pure	4	(SEDA-10, 127)	
Benzocaine[3]	5% petrolatum	1	(3)	a, b, d
Benzoic acid[1]	5% petrolatum	2	(3)	b
Benzoin tincture	10% alcohol or glycerol	3	(SEDA-10, 127)	b
Benzophenone	Not reported		(45)	
Benzophenone-2	2% petrolatum		(46)	
Benzophenone-3 (oxybenzone)	2% petrolatum	3	(SEDA-2, 137)	a
Benzophenone-10 (mexenone)	2% petrolatum	3	(SEDA-18, 171)	a
Benzoxonium chloride[1]	0.05% aqua	3	(SEDA-13, 127)	
Benzoyl peroxide	1% petrolatum	2	(SEDA-9, 152)	b, e
Benzydamine hydrochloride	5% petrolatum	3	(SEDA-17,188) (36)	a
Benzyl alcohol[1]	5%petrolatum	3	(SEDA-8, 154)	b
Benzyl benzoate[4]	5% petrolatum	3	(SEDA-8,154)	
Benzyl salicylate[4]	1% petrolatum	3	(3)	
Betamethasone-17-valerate[2]	5% petrolatum	3	(SEDA-15, 140)	
Betamethasone sodium phosphate[2]	5% petrolatum	4	(SEDA-15, 140)	
Betaxolol hydrochloride	1–5% aqua	4	(SEDA-17, 188)	
Bifonazole	1% alcohol or methylethylketone	4	(SEDA-20, 156)	
Bismuth tribromophenol	Pure	4	(SEDA-9, 136)	
Black iron oxide	5% petrolatum		(47)	
Boric acid	2% aqua	4	(SEDA-19, 162)	
Bornelone	5% petrolatum	4	(SEDA-9, 140)	
2-Bromo-2-nitropropane-1,3-diol[1]	0.25–0.5% petrolatum	2	(SEDA-9, 136)	

Continued

Table 1 Continued

Chemical	Patch test concentration and vehicle	Frequency of sensitization	References	Comments
Bronopol (2-bromo-2-nitropropane-1,3-diol)	Not stated	1	(48)	
Budesonide[2]	1% petrolatum	2	(SEDA-17, 185)	
Bufexamac	5% petrolatum	2	(SEDA-22, 169) (36)	
Buphenine hydrochloride	1% alcohol	4	(SEDA-10, 127)	
Bupivacaine			(SEDA-18, 172)	
Butoxyethyl nicotinate	2.5% petrolatum	4	(SEDA-15, 146)	
tert-Butyl alcohol	70% aqua	4	(SEDA-8, 159) (37)	b
tert-Butyl hydroquinone	1% petrolatum	4	(SEDA-9, 140)	
Butyl aminobenzoate	2% petrolatum	2	(SEDA-16, 155)	
Butylated hydroxyanisole[1]	2–5% petrolatum	3	(3)	
Butylated hydroxytoluene[1]	2–5% petrolatum	3	(3)	
1,3-Butylene glycol	5% aqua	4	(SEDA-22, 171) (49)	
Butylhydroxyanisole	2% petrolatum	2	(50)	
Butylmethoxybenzoylmethane	2% petrolatum	3	(SEDA-18, 171)	
Calcipotriol	0.4–10 µg/ml isopropyl alcohol	4	(SEDA-21, 164) (51)	d, e
Capric/caprylic triglyceride	1% (vehicle not stated)		(52)	
Carboxyvinyl polymer	0.2% aqua	4	(SEDA-20, 158)	
Carmustine	0.1% aqua	1	(53)	
Carprofen	10% petrolatum	4	(SEDA-18, 164) (36)	a
Carvone[4]	1–5% petrolatum	4	(SEDA-20, 157) (54)	
Castor oil	Pure	3	(SEDA-21, 165)	
Centelase	1% powder in petrolatum	3	(SEDA-12, 132)	
Ceramide, hydrophilized	0.25% petrolatum	1	(55)	
Cetrimide	0.1% aqua	1	(56)	
Cetrimonium bromide[1]	0.05% aqua	3	(SEDA-8, 126)	c
Cetyl alcohol	30% petrolatum	3	(3)	b
Cetylpyridinium chloride	0.05% aqua	3	(SEDA-9, 136)	
Cetylstearyl alcohol (Lanette)	30% petrolatum	3	(SEDA-9, 136) (57)	
Chamomile, oil of	25% olive oil	3	(3)	
Chitosan gluconate	10% aqua	4	(SEDA-19, 162)	
Chloral hydrate	1-5 MEK	4	(SEDA-12, 132)	
Chloramphenicol[3]	1% alcohol or 5–10% petrolatum	2	(SEDA-10, 127)	b
Chlordantoin	0.1–1% petrolatum	4	(3)	
Chlorhexidine[1,3]	1% aqua	3	(SEDA-13, 125)	a, b, e
Chlorhexidine digluconate	0.5–1% alcohol	1	(58)	
		1	(59)	
Chloroacetamide[1]	0.2% petrolatum or aqua	3	(SEDA-20, 157)	
p-Chloro-m-cresol[1]	1–2% petrolatum	3	(3)	b
2-Chloro-p-phenylenediamine	1% petrolatum	2	(60)	
Chloro-2-phenylphenol[1]	1% aqua	3	(3)	a
Chloroxylenol[1]	0.5–1% petrolatum	3	(SEDA-15, 148)	
		1	(61)	
Chlorphenesin	1% petrolatum	4	(SEDA-22, 171)	
Chlorphenamine maleate[3,5]	2% petrolatum	4	(SEDA-17, 191)	f
Chlorquinaldol	5% petrolatum	3	(SEDA-9, 136)	
		1	(62)	
CI 12010 (solvent Red 3)	1% petrolatum	4	(SEDA-16, 156)	
CI 12085 (D and C Red No. 36)	2% petrolatum	3	(SEDA-11, 140)	
CI 26100 (D and C Red No. 17)	2% petrolatum	4	(SEDA-7, 164)	
CI 47000 (D and C Yellow No. 11)	0.1% petrolatum	3	(SEDA-14, 129)	
Cicloproxolamine	1% petrolatum	1	(63)	
Cinchocaine	5% petrolatum	4	(SEDA-20, 158)	
Cinnamic alcohol[4]	1% petrolatum	2	(SEDA-2, 140) (42)	
Cinnamic aldehyde[4]	1% petrolatum	2	(SEDA-22, 168) (42)	a, b
Cinoxicam	2% petrolatum	4	(SEDA-18, 164) (36)	
Clindamycin phosphate	1% aqua	3	(SEDA-20, 158)	d
Clobetasol-17-propionate[2]	0.05–10% petrolatum	3	(SEDA-15, 140)	b
Clobetasone butyrate[2]	0.5–1% petrolatum	3	(SEDA-9, 137)	
		1	(64)	
Clonidine	1% petrolatum	1	(SEDA-15, 144) (65,66)	d
Clotrimazole	1% methylethylketone or alcohol	4	(SEDA-20, 158)	

Chemical	Patch test concentration and vehicle	Frequency of sensitization	References	Comments
Cloxyquine (5-chloro-8-hydroxyquinoline)	5% petrolatum	4	(SEDA-20, 158)	
Cocaethylene	10% petrolatum	1	(67)	
Cocamide DEA	0.5% petrolatum	4	(SEDA-12, 134)	
Cocamidopropyl betaine	1% aqua	2	(SEDA-19, 151)	
Cocamidopropyl hydroxysultaine	1% aqua	1	(68)	
Cocamidopropyl PG-dimonium chloride	2.5% aqua	4	(SEDA-21, 165)	
Cocobetaine	2% aqua	4	(SEDA-8, 158)	
Codeine	0.001–0.033% aqua	4	(SEDA-11, 139)	
Colistin sodium methanesulfonate	1–10% petrolatum	4	(SEDA-21, 165)	
Colophony (rosin)	30% petrolatum	1	(SEDA-22, 171)	
Crocein scarlet MOO and solvent yellow 3	1% plastibase	1	(69)	
Croconazole	2% petrolatum	3	(SEDA-21, 166)	
Crotamiton	10% aqua	4	(SEDA-15, 146)	
Cyclomethycaine	1% petrolatum	3	(3)	
Cyclopentolate	0.5–1.0% aqua	4	(SEDA-21, 165)	
Cyclopyroxolamine	10% petrolatum or 1% alcohol	4	(SEDA-20, 158)	
Decyl oleate	1% petrolatum	4	(SEDA-17, 188)	
Desoximetasone[2]	1% epi (45% alcohol, 10% propylene glycol, 45% isopropyl alcohol)	4	(SEDA-15, 140)	a
Dexchlorpheniramine maleate	1% aqua	4	(SEDA-15, 146)	
Dexpanthenol	5% petrolatum	3	(SEDA-22, 171)	f
Diazolidinyl urea[1]	2% aqua or petrolatum	3	(SEDA-19, 158)	
Dibromopropamidine	5% petrolatum	4	(SEDA-13, 125)	
Dibutylphthalate	5% petrolatum	4	(SEDA-17, 188)	
		1	(67)	
Dicaprylyl maleate	10% (vehicle not stated)	2	(52)	
Dichlorodifluoromethane	Pure	4	(SEDA-19, 162)	
Dichlorophene[1]	1% petrolatum	4	(SEDA-20, 157)	a
Diclofenac sodium	2.5–10% petrolatum	3	(SEDA-18, 164) (36)	
		1	(70)	
Diethyl sebacate			(SEDA-22, 171)	
	5% petrolatum	4	(SEDA-24, 173)	
	30% alcohol	1	(71)	
	30% alcohol	3	(SEDA-22, 171)	
Diethylstilbestrol	1% petrolatum	4	(3)	b, d
Diflucortolone 21-valerate[2]	1% petrolatum	4	(SEDA-10, 127)	
2,7-Dihydroxynaphthalene	0.1% aqua	4	(SEDA-22, 171)	
Dihydrostreptomycin	1% petrolatum	3	(3)	
Dihydroxyacetone	10% aqua	4	(SEDA-16, 155)	
Diisopropanolamine	1% petrolatum	4	(SEDA-15, 146)	
Diisopropyl sebacate	3–10% alcohol	4	(SEDA-16, 155)	
Dimethindene maleate[5]	Commercial preparation	4	(SEDA-18, 172)	
Diphenhydramine[5]	1% petrolatum	3	(SEDA-21, 164)	a, d
Dipicolinic acid	0.1% petrolatum	4	(SEDA-14, 125)	
Dipivalyl adrenaline hydrochloride	0.5% aqua	4	(SEDA-17, 188)	
Dipropylene glycol	0.5% petrolatum or aqua	4	(SEDA-20, 158)	
Disodium cocoamphodipropionate	0.3–1% aqua	4	(SEDA-21, 165)	
Disodium ricinoleamido MEA sulfosuccinate	0.1% aqua	4	(SEDA-21, 165)	
Dithranol (cignolin, anthralin)	0.03% acetone	4	(SEDA-7, 161)	e
Dodecyl (=lauryl) gallate	0.25% petrolatum	3	(SEDA-12, 132) (72)	
Dodecyl malamic acid	1% petrolatum	4	(SEDA-8, 154)	
Dorzolamide	0.01–10% aqua and petrolatum		(73)	
Doxepin	0.05–5% petrolatum	1	(SEDA-19, 158)	a, d
			(SEDA-19, 159)	
		1	(74,75)	
Drometrizole	5% petrolatum	4	(SEDA-9, 140)	
Dyclonine hydrochloride	1% petrolatum	4	(SEDA-10, 128)	
Econazole nitrate	1% alcohol or MEK	3	(SEDA-20, 156)	

Continued

Table 1 Continued

Chemical	Patch test concentration and vehicle	Frequency of sensitization	References	Comments
Enilconazole	1% alcohol or MEK	4	(SEDA-20, 156)	
Enoxolone (18-glycyrrhetinic acid)	10% petrolatum	4	(SEDA-17, 188)	
	10% petrolatum	1	(76)	
Eosin (tetrabromofluorescein)	1% petrolatum	4	(SEDA-20, 158)	
Epinephrine, see adrenaline				
Erythromycin	5% petrolatum	3	(SEDA-8, 154)	a
Erythromycin lactobionate	1–10% petrolatum	4	(SEDA-21, 165)	
Esculin	1% petrolatum	4	(SEDA-5, 155)	
Essential oils[4]	2% petrolatum	2	(SEDA-17, 189)	
17-β-Estradiol	1% petrolatum or alcohol 96%	3	(SEDA-21, 165)	d
Estradiol benzoate	0.05% MEK	4	(SEDA-14, 126)	b, d
2-Ethoxyethyl-p-methoxycinnamate	2% petrolatum	3	(SEDA-18, 171)	a
Ethoxyquin	0.5% alcohol or petrolatum	2	(SEDA-9, 137)	
Ethyl chloride	Pure	4	(SEDA-19, 162)	
Ethylenediamine tetraacetate (EDTA)	1% petrolatum	3	(SEDA-12, 132)	
Ethyl diglycol (carbitol) chitosan gluconate	Unknown		(77)	
Ethylhexylglycerine	10% petrolatum	1	(78)	
Ethyl lactate	1% petrolatum	4	(SEDA-13, 125)	
Ethyl mercuric chloride[1]	0.05% petrolatum	2	(SEDA-18, 174) (79)	d
Ethyl sebacate	1% petrolatum	4	(SEDA-15, 146)	
Etofenamate	2% petrolatum	4	(SEDA-18, 164) (36)	b
Eucalyptol (*Malaleuca alternifolia*)	1% petrolatum	1	(80)	
Eucerin	Pure	3	(3)	
Eugenol[4]	5% petrolatum	1	(SEDA-20, 157) (42)	b
Eumulgin L	10% aqua or petrolatum	4	(SEDA-22, 171)	
Eusolez 8021	2% petrolatum	2	(SEDA-7, 164)	
Fenticonazole	5% petrolatum	4	(SEDA-20, 158)	
Fepradinol	5% DMSO or 2% alcohol	3	(SEDA-18, 172)	
Feprazone	5% petrolatum	4	(SEDA-18, 164) (36)	
Flufenamic acid	2–5% petrolatum	4	(SEDA-18, 164) (36)	
Fluocinolone acetonide[2]	1% petrolatum	4	(SEDA-9, 137)	
Fluocortin butyl[2]	1% alcohol	3	(SEDA-15, 140)	
5-Fluorouracil	5% petrolatum	4	(SEDA-10, 128)	a, e
Flurandrenolide	1% petrolatum	3	(SEDA-10, 128)	
Gallate esters	0.1–1% petrolatum	3	(3)	
Gentamicin[3]	20% petrolatum	2	(SEDA-14, 126)	b, d
Gentian violet	0.25% aqua	4	(SEDA-22, 171)	b, d
Geraniol[4]	2% petrolatum	2	(SEDA-7, 164) (42)	
Glucocorticoids[2]	1% alcohol 94%	1	(SEDA-21, 158) (13)(81,82)	d, e
Glutaraldehyde[1]	1% aqua	3	(SEDA-8, 155)	
Glycerol	10% aqua	4	(3)	
Glyceryl diisostearate	2% petrolatum	4	(SEDA-18, 172)	
Glyceryl PABA	5% petrolatum	3	(SEDA-2, 137)	a
Glyceryl stearate	10–30% petrolatum	4	(SEDA-14, 128)	
		1	(83)	
Glyceryl thioglycolate	1% petrolatum	2	(SEDA-10, 128)	
Glyceryl trinitrate	2% petrolatum	3	(SEDA-15, 144)	d
Glyceryl trinitrate (Percutol)	2% petrolatum	1	(65,66)(84)	
Glyceryl trinitrate TTS	0.2% aqua	1	(85)	
	0.5% ethanol			
Guaiazulene	1% petrolatum	4	(SEDA-21, 157)	
Henna	10% petrolatum	4	(SEDA-22, 171)	b, d
Heparin	Commercial preparation	4	(SEDA-14, 126)	
Hexachlorophene[1]	1% petrolatum	4	(3)	a, d, e
Hexamidine	0.15% aqua	3	(SEDA-10, 128)	
cis-3-Hexenyl salicylate[4]	3% petrolatum	4	(SEDA-8, 158)	
Hexetidine	0.1% petrolatum	4	(SEDA-7, 161)	

Chemical	Patch test concentration and vehicle	Frequency of sensitization	References	Comments
Hexyl laurate	30% petrolatum	4	(SEDA-15, 146)	
Hinokitiol	0.1% alcohol	4	(SEDA-8, 158)	
Hirudin	20% alcohol extract	4	(SEDA-21, 165)	
Homomenthyl salicylate (homosalate)	2% petrolatum	4	(SEDA-3, 131a)	
4-Homosulfanilamide (mafenide)	5% petrolatum	2	(SEDA-17, 189)	d
Hydrocortisone acetate[2]	25% petrolatum	3	(3)	a
Hydrocortisone-17-butyrate[2]	1% alcohol	2	(SEDA-17, 185)	
Hydrogen peroxide	3% aqua	4	(SEDA-19, 162)	
Hydroquinone	1% petrolatum	4	(SEDA-22, 171)	
		1	(86)	
Hydroxycitronellal[4]	5% petrolatum	1	(SEDA-2, 140) (42)	
Hydroxyethyl salicylate	1% petrolatum	4	(SEDA-20, 158)	
	5% aqua	1	(87)	
17-α-Hydroxyprogesterone	1% alcohol	3	(SEDA-18, 170)	
Hydroxypropylcellulose	5% aqua	4	(SEDA-13, 125)	
Ibuprofen	5% petrolatum	3	(SEDA-18, 164) (36)	f
Ibuprofen piconol	1–5% petrolatum	3	(SEDA-13, 125)	
Ibuproxam	2.5% petrolatum	3	(SEDA-18, 164) (36)	
Ichthyol (ichthammol)	5% petrolatum	3	(SEDA-9, 136)	
Idoxuridine[3]	1% petrolatum	3	(SEDA-7, 162)	
Indometacin	5% petrolatum	4	(SEDA-18, 164) (36)	
Interferon-β-hydrochloride[3]	Eye drops pure and diluted 1:32	4	(SEDA-16, 155)	
Iodine, tincture of	0.5% aqua (open test)	3	(3)	b, d, e
Iodoform	10% petrolatum	3	(88)	
3-Iodo-2-propynyl-butylcarbamate	0.1% petrolatum	3168	(89)	
Isoconazole	1% alcohol or methylethylketone	3	(SEDA-20, 156)	
Isoeugenol[4]	5% petrolatum	1	(42)	
Isopropyl alcohol[1]	20% aqua	3	(SEDA-7, 162) (37)	b
Isopropyl dibenzoylmethane	2% petrolatum	2	(SEDA-18, 171)	a, b
Isopropyl myristate	20% petrolatum	4	(3)	
Isopropyl palmitate	2% petrolatum	4	(SEDA-8, 155)	
Isostearyl alcohol	5% alcohol and pure	4	(SEDA-12, 135)	b
Isothipendyl hydrochloride	1% petrolatum	4	(SEDA-9, 137)	
Isotretinoin	0.05–0.01% petrolatum	4	(SEDA-21, 165)	
Jasmin synthetic[4]	10% petrolatum	2	(3)	
Jojoba oil	20% olive oil	3	(SEDA-7, 164)	
Kanamycin[3]	20% petrolatum	3	(3)	
Kathon CG[1]	100 ppm aqua	1	See methyl(chloro)-isothiazoline	
Ketoconazole	1% alcohol or methylethylketone	4	(SEDA-20, 156)	
Ketoprofen	5% petrolatum	3	(SEDA-22, 170) (90)	a, f
Kojic acid	1–5% aqua	2	(SEDA-20, 156)	
Krameria triandra (red rhatany)	1% petrolatum 2% ethanol		(91)	
Lactic acid	3% aqua	4	(SEDA-18, 172)	
Lanette wax	30% paraffinum liquidum	3	(SEDA-2, 139)	
Lanoconazole	0.1, 1, and 10% (?)	4	(SEDA-21, 166) (92)	
Lanolin	Pure	3	(3)	
Laurylpyridinium chloride[1]	0.1% aqua	4	(SEDA-13, 127)	
Lawsone(2-hydroxy-1,4-naphthoquinone)	5% petrolatum	4	(SEDA-12, 135)	
Levobunolol hydrochloride[3]	1% aqua	3	(SEDA-17, 189)	
Lidocaine	2% aqua	3	(SEDA-18, 172)	b, d
Lilial[4]	1% petrolatum	4	(SEDA-8, 159)	
Linalool[4]	30% petrolatum	3	(SEDA-9, 140)	
Lincomycin hydrochloride	1% aqua	4	(SEDA-10, 128)	
Mandelic acid	5% petrolatum	4	(SEDA-18, 172)	
Masoprocol (nordihydro-guaiaretic acid)	1% "cream"	2	(SEDA-18, 171)	e
Matricaria chamomilla (German chamomile)	1% (?)		(93)	

Continued

Table 1   Continued

Chemical	Patch test concentration and vehicle	Frequency of sensitization	References	Comments
Mechlorethamine hydrochloride (nitrogen mustard)	0.02% aqua (open test)	1	(SEDA-22, 172) (94)	b
Melia azadirachata (Psorigon)	1–10%, vehicle not stated		(95)	
Mephenesin	5% petrolatum	3	(SEDA-22, 170)	
Mepivacaine	1% aqua	4	(SEDA-16, 155)	
Mercuric chloride[1]	0.05% petrolatum	2	(SEDA-17, 186)	d
Mercuric oxide, yellow	1% petrolatum	3	(SEDA-21, 165)	d
Mesulfen	5% petrolatum	4	(SEDA-8, 155)	e
Metaoxedrine, see phenylephrine				
Methoxypolyethylene glycol/ 17-dodecyl glycol copolymer (Elfacos OW 100)	10% petrolatum		(96)	
8-Methoxypsoralen	0.1% alcohol	4	(SEDA-19, 162)	a
4-Methylbenzylidene camphor	2% petrolatum	3	(SEDA-18, 171)	a
Methylbutetisalicylate	30% petrolatum		(97)	
Methyl(chloro)isothiazolinone (Kathon CG)[1]	100 ppm aqua	1	(98)	a
Methyldibromoglutaronitrile[1]	0.3–0.5% petrolatum	1	(SEDA-19, 152) (99)	
Methylglucose dioleate	5% petrolatum	4	(SEDA-20, 159) (100)	
Methylglucose sesquistearate	5% petrolatum	4	(SEDA-10, 130)	
Methylionone[4]	10% petrolatum	4	(SEDA-14, 128)	
Methyloctine carbonate[4]	1% MEK	4	(SEDA-13, 125)	
6-Methylprednisolone aceponate[2]	1% alcohol	4	(SEDA-22, 171)	
Methylsalicylate[4]	2% petrolatum	4	(3)	b
Metipranolol[3]	2% aqua	4	(SEDA-13, 125)	
Metoprolol[3]	3% aqua	4	(3)	
Metronidazole	1% petrolatum 50% petrolatum	4	(SEDA-22, 171) (101)	
Miconazole nitrate	1% alcohol or MEK	3	(SEDA-20, 156)	
Microcrystalline wax	Pure	4	(SEDA-10, 130)	
Minoxidil	1% alcohol 2% ethanol	3	(SEDA-11, 139) (102)	a, d
Monobenzylether of hydroquinone	1% petrolatum	3	(3)	
Mupirocin	1–10% petrolatum	4	(SEDA-20, 159)	
Musk ambrette[4]	5% petrolatum	3	(SEDA-7, 164)	a
Mycanodin	2% petrolatum	4	(3)	a
Myristyl picolinium chloride	1% petrolatum	4	(SEDA-20, 159)	
Myrrh	Unknown		(103)	
Naftifine	1% petrolatum or 5% alcohol	3	(SEDA-20, 159)	
Neo-ballistol	1% (?)		(104)	
Neomycin[3]	20% petrolatum	2	(3)	b
Neticonazole	1–10% petrolatum	4	(SEDA-22, 171)	
Nicotine	10% aqua	2	(SEDA-18, 170)	a, b
Nifuratel	1% acetone	3	(SEDA-15, 147)	
Nitrocellulose	10% isopropyl alcohol	4	(SEDA-22, 171)	
Nitrofurazone	1% petrolatum	2	(3)	
Nonoxynols	2% aqua	3	(3)	
Noxurol (Clostridiopeptidase A)	(?)		(105) (106)	
Nystatin	100 000 U/g in PEG-400	3	(3)	
Oak moss[4]	2% petrolatum	1	(42)	
Octyl dimethyl PABA	2% petrolatum	3	(SEDA-18, 171)	a
Octyl dodecanol	5–10% paraffinum liquidum	4	(SEDA-22, 171)	
Oleamidopropyl dimethylamine	0.1% petrolatum	2	(SEDA-14, 128)	
Oleth-3-phosphate	1% petrolatum	4	(SEDA-22, 171)	
Oleyl alcohol	10% petrolatum	3	(SEDA-22, 172)	
Olive oil	Pure	4	(SEDA-15, 147) (107)	
Omeprazole	0.25–1% petrolatum	4	(SEDA-12, 133)	
Oxiconazole	1% alcohol or MEK	4	(SEDA-20, 156)	
Oxybenzone			See benzophenone-3	
Oxyphenbutazone	1% petrolatum	3	(SEDA-18, 164) (36)	b, f

Chemical	Patch test concentration and vehicle	Frequency of sensitization	References	Comments
PABA (para-aminobenzoic acid)[3]	2–5% petrolatum	2	(SEDA-18, 171)	a
Palmitoyl hydrolysed milk protein	10% petrolatum	4	(SEDA-13, 126)	
Parabens	Parabens mix European Standard Series		(108)	
Patchouli oil	10% petrolatum	4	(SEDA-17, 189)	
D-Panthenyl ethyl ether[4]	30% petrolatum	4	(SEDA-9, 141)	
Pentaerythritol ester of rosin	10–20% petrolatum	3	(SEDA-19, 162)	
Petrolatum	Pure	4	(SEDA-9, 138)	
Phenobarbital	0.1% aqua or 20% propylene glycol	4	(SEDA-12,133)	
Phenothiazine derivatives[5]	2% petrolatum	1	(3)	a
Phenoxybenzamine	1% aqua	4	(SEDA-1, 136)	c
Phenoxyethanol[1]	1% petrolatum	4	(SEDA-10, 128)	
Phenylbutazone	5% petrolatum	3	(SEDA-22, 170) (36)	
Phenyldimethicone	2% petrolatum	4	(SEDA-10, 130)	
Phenylephrine	0.5–1% petrolatum 5% aqua	4	(SEDA-19, 162) (109) (3)	
Phenylmercuric acetate[1]	0.01% aqua	2	(3)	b, d
Phenylmercuric borate[1]	0.01% aqua	2	(3)	b, d
2-Phenyl-5-methylbenzoxazole	2% petrolatum	4	(SEDA-14, 128)	a
Phenylsalicylate (Salol)	1% petrolatum	4	(SEDA-20, 157)	
Phthalic anhydride/trimellitic anhydride/glycols co-polymer	1% petrolatum	1	(110)	
Picric acid	1% aqua	4	(SEDA-16, 155)	
Pigment red 57:1	1% petrolatum	4	(SEDA-18, 172)	
Piketoprofen	1–5% petrolatum	4	(SEDA-20, 159)	
Pilocarpine[3]	4% petrolatum	4	(SEDA-18, 172)	
Piperazine	1% petrolatum	3	(SEDA-8, 156)	c
Piroxicam	0.5% petrolatum	2	(SEDA-18, 164) (36)	a
Pivampicillin	5% petrolatum	1	(SEDA-17, 189)	c
Polidocanol	5% petrolatum	3	(3)	d
Polyethylene glycol	Pure	3	(SEDA-15, 144)	b
Polymyxin B[3]	3% petrolatum	4	(3)	
Polyoxyethylene oleylether	1% petrolatum		(111)	
Polysorbate 40 (Tween 40)	5% petrolatum	3	(SEDA-2, 139)	
Polysorbate 80 (Tween 80)	10% petrolatum	3	(SEDA-2, 139) (57)	
Polyvinylpyrrolidone/eicosene co-polymer	1% petroleum	1	(112)	
Polyvinylpyrrolidone/1-triacontene co-polymer	10% petrolatum		(113)	
Potassium coco-hydrolysed animal protein	5 and 30% aqua	4	(SEDA-14, 129)	
Povidoneiodine	10% aqua or petrolatum	3	(SEDA-18, 172)	b, d
Pramocaine	2% aqua	4	(SEDA-9, 138)	
Prednicarbate	10% ethanol 1% ethanol		(114)	
Prednisolone (pivalate)[2]	1% epi (45% alcohol, 10% propylene glycol, 45% isopropyl alcohol)	3	(SEDA-13, 126)	
Prilocaine	2% aqua	3	(SEDA-18, 172)	d
Prime yellow carnauba wax	50% mineral oil	1	(67)	
Procaine[3]	1% petrolatum	1	(3)	a
Proflavine dihydrochloride	1% petrolatum	1	(SEDA-13, 126)	
Promethazine hydrochloride[5]	1% petrolatum	1	(3)	a, b, d
Propantheline bromide	55 petrolatum	3	(SEDA-9, 141)	
Propolis	10% petrolatum	2	(SEDA-17, 181)	
Propylene glycol	2% petrolatum	3	(SEDA-9, 159) (115)	b, e
Propyl gallate	1% petrolatum	3	(SEDA-22, 172)	a
PVP/hexadecene co-polymer	5% petrolatum		(116)	
Pyrazinobutazone	1–5% petrolatum	4	(SEDA-17, 191)	f
Pyridoxine 3,4-dioctanoate	1% petrolatum	4	(SEDA-8, 159)	
Pyridoxine hydrochloride	10% petrolatum	4	(SEDA-10, 128)	
Pyrocatechol	2% petrolatum	4	(SEDA-14, 129)	

Continued

Table 1 Continued

Chemical	Patch test concentration and vehicle	Frequency of sensitization	References	Comments
Pyrrolnitrin	1% petrolatum	3	(SEDA-9, 138)	
Quaternium-22	0.1 and 0.01 aqua		(117)	
Quinidine sulfate	1% aqua	3	(SEDA-7, 163)	a, c
Quinine	1% aqua	4	(SEDA-18, 173)	a, c
Resorcinol	2% petrolatum	3	(SEDA-21, 165)	b, d, e
Rhus aculeatus	0.8–1.6% alcohol	4	(SEDA-2, 138)	e
Rifamycin	0.5% petrolatum	4	(SEDA-11, 139)	b
Salbutamol sulfate	5% petrolatum	4	(SEDA-18, 173)	
Salicylic acid	2% petrolatum	4	(SEDA-2, 137)	b, d, e
Scopolamine[3]	1% petrolatum	3	(SEDA-15, 144) (65,66)	d
Sertaconazole	1–5% petrolatum	4	(SEDA-20, 159)	
Sesame oil	Pure	3	(SEDA-13, 127)	
Shellac	20% alcohol and pure	4	(SEDA-12, 135)	
		6	(118)	
Silicic acid	5% petrolatum and pure	4	(SEDA-14, 133)	
Silver nitrate	1% aqua	4	(SEDA-17, 189)	
Silver sulfadiazine cream	Pure	3	(SEDA-10, 129)	
Sisomicin sulfate	1–10% petrolatum	4	(SEDA-21, 165)	
Sodium benzoate[1]	1–2% aqua or petrolatum	3	(SEDA-17, 189)	b
Sodium cromoglicate[3]	2% aqua	4	(SEDA-14, 127)	
Sodium dihydroxyacetyl phosphate	5% petrolatum		(119)	
Sodium fusidate	2% petrolatum	3	(SEDA-8, 156)	
Sodium metabisulfite	2% petrolatum	1	(64)	
Sodium myristoyl sarcosinate	1% aqua	1	(120)	
Sodium ricinoleamido MEA-sulfosuccinate	5% petrolatum	4	(SEDA-15, 148)	
Sodium sulfite	2–5% petrolatum	3	(SEDA-17, 190)	b
Sorbic acid[1]	2% petrolatum	3	(SEDA-17, 190)	b
Sorbitan laurate	5% aqua	4	(SEDA-9, 139)	b
Sorbitan oleate	5% petrolatum	4	(SEDA-8, 156) (57)	
Sorbitan sesquioleate	2% petrolatum	3	(SEDA-18, 173) (57)	
Sorbitan stearate	5% petrolatum	3	(57)	
Soybean extract	1, 10, and 20% petrolatum		(121)	
Spearmint (Mentha spicata)	2% (?)		(105,106)	
Spearmint oil	1–5% petrolatum		(122,123)	
Spiramycin	10% aqua or petrolatum	3	(3)	c
Spironolactone	1% alcohol or petrolatum	3	(SEDA-19, 162)	
Squaric acid dibutyl ester	0.05% acetone	1	(SEDA-9, 138)	b
Stearic acid	5–10% petrolatum	4	(SEDA-14, 129)	
		1	(83)	
Stearyl alcohol	30% petrolatum	3	(3)	b
Stearyl alcohol in Efudix cream	(?)		(124)	
Storax (styrax)	2% petrolatum	2	(3)	
Streptomycin	1% petrolatum	2	(3)	b
Sulconazole	1% alcohol or methylethylketone	4	(SEDA-20, 156)	
Sulfonamides	5% petrolatum	1	(3)	a
Suprofen	0.1% petrolatum	3	(SEDA-18, 164) (36)	a
Tacalcitol	0.0002% alcohol	4	(SEDA-20, 157)	
Tannin	1–10% petrolatum or aqua	4	(SEDA-19, 162)	
TEA-PEG-3 cocamide sulfate	1% aqua	4	(SEDA-10, 130)	
Tea tree oil	15 petrolatum and pure	3	(SEDA-22, 172) (125)	f
Tetracaine	1% petrolatum	2	(SEDA-9, 138)	
Tetrahydroxypropyl ethylenediamine	10% petrolatum		(126)	
Thiabendazole	2% petrolatum	4	(SEDA-17, 190)	a
Thiomersal[1,3]	0.1% petrolatum	1	SEDA-19, 160) (115,127)	b, d
Thioxolone	0.5% alcohol	4	(SEDA-13, 126)	
Thuja essential oil	Pure	4	(SEDA-18, 173)	
Thymol	1% petrolatum	4	(SEDA-20, 157)	
Tiaprofenic acid	1% petrolatum	3	(SEDA-18, 164) (36)	a, f
Timolol maleate	0.5% petrolatum	4	(SEDA-16, 156)	

Chemical	Patch test concentration and vehicle	Frequency of sensitization	References	Comments
Tioconazole[3]	2% petrolatum or alcohol	2	(SEDA-21, 164)	
Tiopronin	6.66 mg/ml solution	4	(SEDA-20, 157)	
Tixocortol pivalate[2]	1% petrolatum	1	(SEDA-17, 185)	
Tobramycin	20% aqua or petrolatum	3	(SEDA-15, 147)	
Tocopherols	10% petrolatum	3	(SEDA-19, 162)	b
Tocopheryl linoleate	10% petrolatum	2	(SEDA-19, 165)	
Tolazoline[3]	<10% aqua	4	(SEDA-11, 139)	
Tolnaftate	1% petrolatum	4	(SEDA-20, 157)	
Tosufloxacin tosilate	20% petrolatum on previously affected site		(128)	
Tosylamide/formaldehyde resin	10% petrolatum	1	(SEDA-17, 186)	
Transdermal therapeutic systems (TTS)		1–4	(65,66)	
Tretinoin	0.005% alcohol	4	(SEDA-21, 165)	d, e
Triamcinolone acetonide[2]	1% alcohol	2	(3)	
Triclosan[1]	2% petrolatum	3	(129)	a
Trideceth-2-carboxamide monoethanolamine	0.5% aqua	1	(130)	
Triethanolamine	1–55% petrolatum	3	(SEDA-15, 143) (131)	
Triethanolamine polypeptide oleate condensate	1% petrolatum	4	(3)	
Triethanolamine stearate	5% petrolatum	4	(SEDA-8, 159)	
Trifluorothymidine	1% petrolatum	4	(SEDA-6, 149)	
Trilaureth-4-phosphate	0.5–1% petrolatum	4	(SEDA-10, 130)	
Trimebutine	0.15–4.8 mg/ml aqua		(132)	
Triphenylmethane dyes	2% aqua	4	(3)	d
Tromantadine hydrochloride	1% petrolatum	2	(SEDA-9, 138)	
Tropicamide	5% aqua	4	(SEDA-18, 173)	
Tylosin	5% petrolatum	3	(SEDA-9, 138)	
Tyrothricin	20% petrolatum	3	(3)	
Undecylenamide DEA	0.1–1% aqua	4	(SEDA-17, 190)	
Undecylenic acid	2% petrolatum	4	(3)	
Usnic acid	1% petrolatum	4	(SEDA-20, 157)	
Virginiamycin	5% petrolatum	3	(3)	b
Vitamin A (retinol palmitate)	0.1% petrolatum	4	(SEDA-21, 165)	
Vitamin B$_1$	10% petrolatum	4	(3)	c
Vitamin E	10% petrolatum	3	(SEDA-21, 165)	c
Vitamin K$_4$	0.1% petrolatum	4	(3)	c
Witch hazel	10% alcohol distillate	4	(SEDA-19, 162)	
Xanthocillin	1–10% petrolatum	3	(3)	
Zinc pyrithione	1% petrolatum	3	(SEDA-10, 130)	a
Zinc ricinoleate	Commercial preparation	4	(SEDA-12, 135) (133)	

[1]For allergy to preservatives, see (11,134,135).

[2]For glucocorticoid allergy, see (13,81,82) and (SEDA-21, 158). For patch-testing glucocorticoids, a 1% concentration in 70% alcohol can be adequate. However, as alcoholic solutions can only be kept in storage for 1–2 months and can cause irritation, petrolatum is the usual choice of vehicle (SEDA-21, 159).

[3]For allergy to ophthalmic drugs, see (136).

[4]For allergy to fragrances, see (12) (SEDA-20, 149).

[5]For allergy to antihistamines, see (14).

In the column "Frequency of sensitization" the following scale for the occurrence of sensitization is used:

1 = common;
2 = can occur;
3 = unusual;
4 = rare.

In the column "Comment" the following symbols are used:

a = photosensitivity reported;
b = immediate contact reactions reported;
c = accidental contactant;
d = see also separate monograph;
e = has also caused irritant dermatitis;
f = systemic contact dermatitis reported.

Contact allergy in the anogenital region

Allergic contact dermatitis is a common anogenital disease. The predominant complaints are itching and burning. Scratching, mainly at night, and lichenification can lead to painful erosions. Topical medicaments, body care products, popular remedies, and sanitary products are the main sources of contact allergens in the anogenital area.

Epidemiology

During 1992–1997, 1008 patients with anogenital complaints (2% of the whole test population of 54 500 patients) were patch-tested in the Departments of Dermatology of the Information Network of Dermatological Clinics (IVDK). The standard series recommended by the German Contact Dermatitis Research Group (DKG) was tested in 978 of these patients. Other specific allergens were tested according to each patient's history. In most cases topical drugs, ointment bases, and preservatives were included, and in 466 cases patients' own products were also patch-tested. In 351 patients (35%), the final diagnosis of allergic contact dermatitis was confirmed (15). Similar numbers were reported from the UK, where anogenital dermatosis was diagnosed in 201 women in a contact dermatitis clinic over 14 years. In 79 cases (39%) the diagnosis of allergic contact dermatitis was confirmed by patch tests with the European standard series, a medicament series, a glucocorticoid series, and the patients' own medicaments, if necessary. In another UK study, 39 of 135 patients tested (29%) with persisting vulval symptoms had contact hypersensitivity (16). There is evidence that the vulval region and the perianal region should be considered separately, since patients with dermatosis that only involves the vulva have positive patch tests less often than patients with dermatosis of the vulva and the perianal area or patients who have only perianal involvement (17).

Allergens and sources

The most frequent allergens in the study of the IVDK are listed in Table 2, and Table 3 gives information about the patch test results obtained with topical drugs, ointment bases, and preservatives.

All allergens that led to positive reactions in at least 1% of the patients tested are listed (15).

Although the spectrum is comparable to that of all patients tested between 1992 and 1997, there are some allergens of pronounced significance for the anogenital region. Cinchocaine HCl ranked fourth among contact allergens

Table 2 The most frequent allergens among patients with anogenital complaints

Allergen	Number tested	Number with a positive reaction (%)[1]	Number with a positive reaction (%)[2]	IVDK total 1992–7 (%)[3]
Nickel sulfate	962	86 (8.9)	12.6	16–17
Balsam of Peru	962	74 (7.7)	6.6	6.5–8
Fragrance mix	960	71 (4.7)	7.2	10–13
Cinchocaine HCl (dibucaine HCl)	592	50 (4.8)	7.4	*
Thiomersal	961	48 (5.0)	5.6	5–7
Methyldibromoglutaronitrile/ 2-phenoxyethanol	958	39 (1.4)	3.1	2–3
Paraphenylenediamine	959	39 (1.4)	3.7	4–5.5
(Chloro)methylisothiazolinone (CMI/MI)	951	32 (3.4)	3.7	~2.5
Benzocaine	962	31 (2.3)	2.7	~1.5
Phenylmercuric acetate	736	28 (3.8)	4.0	4–8
Neomycin sulfate	962	23 (2.4)	2.1	~2.5
Wool wax alcohol	962	22 (2.3)	2.1	2.5–4
Amerchol L-101	561	21 (3.7)	2.9	*
Colophony (rosin)	961	19 (2.0)	2.3	2.5–3.5
Mercury amide chloride (ammoniated mercury)	962	19 (2.0)	1.7	~2.5
Propolis	598	17 (2.8)	2.5	*
Parabens mix	962	17 (1.8)	1.6	~1.5
Benzoylperoxide	218	15 (6.9)	7.6	*
Octylgallate	560	15 (2.7)	2.8	*
Methyldibromoglutaronitrile	508	14 (2.8)	2.1	*
Cobalt chloride	960	13 (1.4)	2.0	4.5–5
Propylene glycol	744	12 (1.6)	1.5	*
Formaldehyde	961	12 (1.2)	1.5	~2
Hexylresorcinol	476	11 (2.3)	2.1	*
Para-*tert*-butylphenol Formaldehyde resin (PTBP-FR)	955	11 (1.2)	1.4	~1
Thiuram mix	961	11 (1.1)	1.1	~2.5

[1]Percentage of positive reactions.
[2]Age- and sex-standardized frequency of sensitization.
[3]Range of the age- and sex-standardized frequency of sensitization in all patients tested ($n = 54\,500$).
*Allergens were tested in selected patients only; so a comparison in this way makes no sense.
 All allergens that led to positive reactions in more than 1% of the total population (that is 10 patients) are listed.
 Source: IVDK 1992–1997 ($n = 1008$) (15).

Table 3 Patch test results obtained with topical drugs, ointment bases, and preservatives

Allergen	Test formulation	Number tested	Number with a positive reaction (%)
Bufexamac	5% petrolatum	534	9 (1.7)
Framycetin sulfate	20% petrolatum	268	7 (2.6)
Lidocaine HCl	15% petrolatum	524	6 (1.1)
Tincture of *Arnica montana*	20% petrolatum	241	5 (1.2)
Clotrimazole	5% petrolatum	272	5 (1.8)
Iodochlorhydroxyquin (clioquinol)	5% petrolatum	303	5 (1.7)
Chamomile extract	2.5% petrolatum	173	5 (2.9)
Tetracaine HCl (amethocaine HCl)	1% petrolatum	306	4 (1.3)
Panthenol	5% petrolatum	323	4 (1.2)
Chloramphenicol	10% petrolatum	244	3 (1.2)
Mafenide	10% petrolatum	299	3 (1.0)
tert-Butyl hydroquinone	1% petrolatum	710	8 (1.1)
Benzalkonium chloride	0.1% petrolatum	740	8 (1.1)
Bronopol	0.5% petrolatum	728	7 (1.0)
Chloroacetamide	0.2% petrolatum	743	7 (0.9)

in this region. Furthermore, there were more positive patch test results to (chloro)methylisothiazolinone (CMI/MI) and to benzocaine among patients with anogenital complaints compared with the whole test population (15).

Topical local anesthetics play an important role in anogenital contact allergy (15–19). Cinchocaine is commonly used in topical antihemorrhoidal formulations and is a well-known sensitizer (20). Although benzocaine is not as widely used in topical anesthetic formulations in Germany, patients with anogenital dermatitis were at higher risk of sensitization. Amide-type local anesthetics, like lidocaine HCl and tetracaine, are less potent sensitizers (21). Contact allergy to local anesthetics is more often observed among patients with perianal complaints than patients with perianal and vulval or only vulval dermatitis (17).

Topical antibiotics are often used in the treatment of dermatitis with bacterial superinfection. However, in Germany sensitization to the aminoglycoside antibiotic neomycin was less frequent in patients with anogenital dermatitis (15) compared with the UK, where 15 of 79 patients with positive patch tests and anogenital complaints were positive to neomycin (17). Framycetin contact sensitivity was frequent in the UK, partly through cross-reactivity with neomycin (16).

Another important substance in hemorrhoidal formulations is bufexamac, a non-steroidal anti-inflammatory drug that is a well-known sensitizer and sometimes elicits severe dermatitis (22). Bufexamac should therefore always be included in patch tests for anogenital dermatitis.

Glucocorticoid contact allergy is well known (SEDA-21, 158) and has to be particularly suspected in chronic conditions affecting the perianal area (17), after long-term topical medication, and in cases of failure to ameliorate dermatitis with corticosteroids. Patch tests should then be performed both with the recommended markers, budesonide (0.1% petrolatum) and tixocortol pivalate (1% petrolatum), and with the patient's own formulations.

Antifungal drugs are comparatively rare contact allergens in the anogenital region in relation to their widespread use. Clotrimazole and nystatin are preferred. In the study of the IVDK, patch tests with clotrimazole were performed in only 272 patients, leading to five positive reactions (15). In the UK study on anogenital dermatosis, five women out of 201 patients tested had positive reactions to antifungal drugs, but was unfortunately not specified in the article (17). If sensitization to nystatin is suspected, polyethylene glycol should be used as a vehicle for patch-testing (23). Imidazoles can cross-react with one another (SEDA-20, 156). Most cases of contact allergy occurred with miconazole, econazole, tioconazole, and isoconazole (24).

Moist toilet paper is a rare source of contact allergens. The most important allergens in moist toilet paper are preservatives, such as CMI/MI and dibromoglutaronitril + 2-phenoxyethanol (Euxyl K 400) (25–27). These substances were also incriminated in the study of the IVDK (15) and are also found in body care products. In Germany, when CMI/MI was replaced by iodopropyl butylcarbamate (IPBC) in moist toilet paper, one case of contact allergy to IPBC was soon described (28).

Other sources of preservatives are topical medicaments and body care products. Parabens, chloracetamide, and formaldehyde-releasing preservatives, like diazolidinyl urea, imidazolidinyl urea, bronopol, and quaternium 15, should also be considered (15).

Ointment bases do not seem to cause contact allergy in the anogenital region too often, despite wide use. Wool wax alcohol and amerchol L-101 are the most important (15,17). Contact sensitivity to balsam of Peru and fragrance mix is not infrequent and reflects the ubiquitous presence of these substances (16).

Topical remedies are very popular in self-treatment and patients will often not report this, since they do not regard them as medicaments. Furthermore, patients often do not suspect that "natural" remedies cause adverse effects. Some substances lead to a considerable number of allergic reactions, for example chamomile extract and tincture of *Arnica montana* (15). Propolis also has pronounced sensitizing capacity (29), and sensitization to aged tea tree oil is being reported with increasing frequency (30).

Contact allergy from rubber additives in condoms is sometimes suspected, and there are anecdotal reports (31). However, in the study of the IVDK, condoms were patch-tested in 17 patients without positive results (15).

Although sensitization to nickel sulfate is common in patients with anogenital contact dermatitis and in patients with dermatitis in other body sites, the relevance to anogenital complaints of sensitization to nickel sulfate should always be doubted (15,16,32). However, direct transmission of nickel from the hands to the anogenital region has to be taken into account, and food can be a rare source of nickel contact in the anogenital area. In these cases relevance can be proved by oral nickel provocation and a nickel-restricted diet for a limited period may be justified (33).

Prediction of contact allergens

Certain chemical substructures, so-called toxophores, can be associated with an increased risk of skin sensitization. These have been codified in a set of 57 rules known as the DEREK (Deductive Estimation of Risk from Existing Knowledge) knowledge-based computer system (34). This rulebase has been subjected to extensive validation and continues to be refined. The predictive ability of the sensitization rule set was assessed by processing the structures of the first 84 chemical substances in the list of contact allergens issued by the German Federal Institute for Health Protection of Consumers (BgVV). The rules identified toxophores for skin sensitization in the structures of 71 of the 84 chemicals. After refinement, by extension of the scope of the existing rules and by generation of new rules with a sound mechanistic rationale for the biological activity, the rules identified toxophores for skin sensitization for 82 of the 84 chemicals.

Conclusions

Contact allergy should always be suspected in patients with anogenital dermatitis, especially if the perianal area is involved. In patients with other chronic inflammatory diseases of the anogenital region, for example lichen sclerosus, contact allergy should also be excluded, since long-term use of topical medicants on compromised skin carries an increased risk of sensitization.

Patch tests in patients with anogenital eczema should include the standard series: cinchocaine HCl, propolis, bufexamac, and other ingredients of topical formulations according to the patient's history. In cases of doubt, the repeated open application test (ROAT) is recommended. Patients should be advised to apply the suspected product three times a day for 3 days to an area of healthy skin on measuring $5\,cm \times 5\,cm$ the flexural site of the forearm (35).

References

1. Rycroft RJG, Frosch PJ, Menné T, editors. Textbook of Contact Dermatitis. 3rd ed. Berlin: Springer-Verlag, 1999.
2. Rietschel RL, Fowler JF Jr, editors. Fisher's Contact Dermatitis. 4th ed. Baltimore: Williams and Wilkins, 1995.
3. De Groot AC. Patch Testing. Test Concentrations and Vehicles for 3700 Allergens. Amsterdam: Elsevier, 1994.
4. De Groot AC, Weyland JW, Nater JP. Unwanted Effects of Cosmetics and Drugs used in Dermatology. 3rd ed. Amsterdam: Elsevier, 1994.
5. Fischer T. Design considerations for patch testing. Am J Contact Dermatitis 1994;5:70–5.
6. Guin JD, Kincannon J. Contact allergens—what's new? Medication-induced contact reactions. Clin Dermatol 1997;15(4):511–25.
7. De Groot AC. Adverse Reactions to Cosmetics. Thesis, University of Groningen, 1988.
8. De Groot AC. Contact allergens—what's new? Cosmetic dermatitis. Clin Dermatol 1997;15(4):485–91.
9. Kiken DA, Cohen DE. Contact dermatitis to botanical extracts. Am J Contact Dermatitis 2002;13(3):148–52.
10. de Groot AC, Weijland JW. Conversion of common names of cosmetic allergens to the INCI nomenclature. Contact Dermatitis 1997;37(4):145–50.
11. Gruvberger B, Bruze M. Contact allergens—what's new? Preservatives. Clin Dermatol 1997;15(4):493–7.
12. de Groot AC, Frosch PJ. Adverse reactions to fragrances. A clinical review. Contact Dermatitis 1997;36(2):57–86.
13. Isaksson M, Dooms-Goossens AN. Contact allergens—what's new? Corticosteroids. Clin Dermatol 1997;15(4):527–31.
14. Szolar-Platzer C, Maibach HI. Allergic contact dermatitis to topically applied antihistamines. Dermatosen 1996;44:205–12.
15. Bauer A, Geier J, Elsner P. Allergic contact dermatitis in patients with anogenital complaints. J Reprod Med 2000;45(8):649–54.
16. Marren P, Wojnarowska F, Powell S. Allergic contact dermatitis and vulvar dermatoses. Br J Dermatol 1992;126(1):52–6.
17. Goldsmith PC, Rycroft RJ, White IR, Ridley CM, Neill SM, McFadden JP. Contact sensitivity in women with anogenital dermatoses. Contact Dermatitis 1997;36(3):174–5.
18. Brenan JA, Dennerstein GJ, Sfameni SF, Drinkwater P, Marin G, Scurry JP. Evaluation of patch testing in patients with chronic vulvar symptoms. Australas J Dermatol 1996;37(1):40–3.
19. Lewis FM, Harrington CI, Gawkrodger DJ. Contact sensitivity in pruritus vulvae: a common and manageable problem. Contact Dermatitis 1994;31(4):264–5.
20. Wilkinson JD, Andersen KE, Lahti A, Rycroft RJ, Shaw S, White IR. Preliminary patch testing with 25% and 15% "caine"-mixes. The EECDRG. Contact Dermatitis 1990;22(4):244–5.
21. Fisher A. Contact dermatitis. 3rd ed. Philadelphia: Lea & Febiger, 1995.
22. Bauer A, Greif C, Gebhardt M, Elsner P. Schwere Epikutantestreaktion auf Bufexamac in einem Hämorrhoidal-Therapeutikum. [A severe epicutaneous test reaction to the bufexamac in a hemorrhoidal therapeutic preparation.] Dtsch Med Wochenschr 1999;124(40):1168–70.
23. de Groot AC, Conemans JM. Nystatin allergy. Petrolatum is not the optimal vehicle for patch testing. Dermatol Clin 1990;8(1):153–5.
24. Dooms-Goossens A, Matura M, Drieghe J, Degreef H. Contact allergy to imidazoles used as antimycotic agents. Contact Dermatitis 1995;33(2):73–7.
25. De Groot AC, van Ginkel CJ, Weijland JW. Methyldibromoglutaronitrile (Euxyl K 400): an important "new" allergen in cosmetics. J Am Acad Dermatol 1996;35(5 Pt 1):743–7.
26. Van Ginkel CJ, Rundervoort GJ. Increasing incidence of contact allergy to the new preservative 1,2-dibromo-2,4-dicyanobutane (methyldibromoglutaronitrile). Br J Dermatol 1995;132(6):918–20.
27. Blecher P, Korting HC. Tolerance to different toilet paper preparations: toxicological and allergological aspects. Dermatology 1995;191(4):299–304.
28. Bryld LE, Agner T, Rastogi SC, Menne T. Iodopropynyl butylcarbamate: a new contact allergen. Contact Dermatitis 1997;36(3):156–8.
29. Hausen BM, Evers P, Stuwe HT, Konig WA, Wollenweber E. Propolis allergy (IV). Studies with further sensitizers from propolis and constituents common to propolis, poplar buds and balsam of Peru. Contact Dermatitis 1992;26(1):34–44.
30. Hausen BM, Reichling J, Harkenthal M. Degradation products of monoterpenes are the sensitizing agents in tea tree oil. Am J Contact Dermatitis 1999;10(2):68–77.

31. Bircher AJ, Hirsbrunner P, Langauer S. Allergic contact dermatitis of the genitals from rubber additives in condoms. Contact Dermatitis 1993;28(2):125–6.

32. Lucke TW, Fleming CJ, McHenry P, Lever R. Patch testing in vulval dermatoses: how relevant is nickel? Contact Dermatitis 1998;38(2):111–12.

33. Bresser H. Orale Nickelprovokation und nickelarme Diät. Indikation und praktische Durchfuhrung. [Oral nickel provocation and a nickel-free diet. Indications and practical implementation.] Hautarzt 1992;43(10):610–15.

34. Langowski J, Barratt M. Validation and development of the DEREK skin sensitisation rulebase by analysis of the BGVV list of contact allergens. ATLA 1999;27:104.

35. Johansen JD, Bruze M, Andersen KE, Frosch PJ, Dreier B, White IR, Rastogi S, Lepoittevin JP, Menne T. The repeated open application test: suggestions for a scale of evaluation. Contact Dermatitis 1998;39(2):95–6.

36. Warin RP, Smith RJ. Chronic urticaria. Investigations with patch and challenge tests. Contact Dermatitis 1982;8(2):117–21.

37. Ophaswongse S, Maibach HI. Alcohol dermatitis: allergic contact dermatitis and contact urticaria syndrome. A review. Contact Dermatitis 1994;30(1):1–6.

38. Schnuch A. Osmaron B is a rare occupational, but a frequent cosmetic, allergen. Contact Dermatitis 2001;44(2):133–4.

39. Haapasaari K, Niinimaki A. Allergic contact dermatitis from alkylammonium amidobenzoate (Osmaron B). Contact Dermatitis 2000;42(4):244–5.

40. Foti C, Bonamonte D, Mascolo G, Tiravanti G, Rigano L, Angelini G. Aminoethylethanolamine: a new allergen in cosmetics? Contact Dermatitis 2001;45(3):129–33.

41. Blanco R, de la Hoz B, Sanchez-Fernandez C, Sanchez-Cano M. Allergy to 4-amino-3-nitrophenol in a hair dye. Contact Dermatitis 1998;39(3):136.

42. Johansen JD, Menne T. The fragrance mix and its constituents: a 14-year material. Contact Dermatitis 1995;32(1):18–23.

43. Franks A. Contact allergy to anethole in toothpaste associated with loss of taste. Contact Dermatitis 1998;38(6):354–5.

44. Salim A, Orton D, Shaw S. Allergic contact dermatitis from Basic Red 22 in a hair-colouring mousse. Contact Dermatitis 2001;45(2):123.

45. Guin JD. Eyelid dermatitis from benzophenone used in nail enhancement. Contact Dermatitis 2000;43(5):308–9.

46. Jacobs MC. Contact allergy to benzophenone-2 in toilet water. Contact Dermatitis 1998;39(1):42.

47. Saxena M, Warshaw E, Ahmed DD. Eyelid allergic contact dermatitis to black iron oxide. Am J Contact Dermatitis 2001;12(1):38–9.

48. Choudry K, Beck MH, Muston HL. Allergic contact dermatitis from 2-bromo-2-nitropropane-1,3-diol in Metrogel. Contact Dermatitis 2002;46(1):60–1.

49. Diegenant C, Constandt L, Goossens A. Allergic contact dermatitis due to 1,3-butylene glycol. Contact Dermatitis 2000;43(4):234–5.

50. Orton DI, Shaw S. Allergic contact dermatitis from pharmaceutical grade BHA in Timodine, with no patch test reaction to analytical grade BHA. Contact Dermatitis 2001;44(3):191–2.

51. Park YK, Lee JH, Chung WG. Allergic contact dermatitis from calcipotriol. Acta Dermatol Venereol 2002;82(1):71–2.

52. Laube S, Davies MG, Prais L, Foulds IS. Allergic contact dermatitis from medium-chain triglycerides in a moisturizing lotion. Contact Dermatitis 2002;47(3):171.

53. Thomson KF, Sheehan-Dare RA, Wilkinson SM. Allergic contact dermatitis from topical carmustine. Contact Dermatitis 2000;42(2):112.

54. Corazza M, Levratti A, Virgili A. Allergic contact cheilitis due to carvone in toothpastes. Contact Dermatitis 2002;46(6):366–7.

55. Yajima J. Allergic contact dermatitis due to hydrophilized ceramide. Contact Dermatitis 2002;47(4):245.

56. Lee JY, Wang BJ. Contact dermatitis caused by cetrimide in antiseptics. Contact Dermatitis 1995;33(3):168–71.

57. Pasche-Koo F, Piletta PA, Hunziker N, Hauser C. High sensitization rate to emulsifiers in patients with chronic leg ulcers. Contact Dermatitis 1994;31(4):226–8.

58. Lauerma AI. Simultaneous immediate and delayed hypersensitivity to chlorhexidine digluconate. Contact Dermatitis 2001;44(1):59.

59. Barrazza V. Connubial allergic contact balanitis due to chlorhexidine. Contact Dermatitis 2001;45(1):42.

60. Hansson C, Thorneby-Andersson K. Allergic contact dermatitis from 2-chloro-*p*-phenylenediamine in a cream dye for eyelashes and eyebrows. Contact Dermatitis 2001;45(4):235–6.

61. Malakar S, Panda S. Post-inflammatory depigmentation following allergic contact dermatitis to chloroxylenol. Br J Dermatol 2001;144(6):1275–6.

62. Rodriguez A, Cabrerizo S, Barranco R, de Frutos C, de Barrio M. Contact cross-sensitization among quinolines. Allergy 2001;56(8):795.

63. Foti C, Diaferio A, Bonamonte D. Allergic contact dermatitis from ciclopirox olamine. Australas J Dermatol 2001;42(2):145.

64. Harrison DA, Smith AG. Concomitant sensitivity to sodium metabisulfite and clobetasone butyrate in Trimovate cream. Contact Dermatitis 2002;46(5):310.

65. Mofenson HC, Caraccio TR, Miller H, Greensher J. Lidocaine toxicity from topical mucosal application. With a review of the clinical pharmacology of lidocaine. Clin Pediatr (Phila) 1983;22(3):190–2.

66. Eldad A, Neuman A, Weinberg A, Benmeir P, Rotem M, Wexler MR. Silver sulphadiazine-induced haemolytic anaemia in a glucose-6-phosphate dehydrogenase-deficient burn patient. Burns 1991;17(5):430–2.

67. Chowdhury MM. Allergic contact dermatitis from prime yellow carnauba wax and coathylene in mascara. Contact Dermatitis 2002;46(4):244.

68. Guin JD. Reaction to cocamidopropyl hydroxysultaine, an amphoteric surfactant and conditioner. Contact Dermatitis 2000;42(5):284.

69. Bajaj AK, Misra A, Misra K, Rastogi S. The azo dye solvent yellow 3 produces depigmentation. Contact Dermatitis 2000;42(4):237–8.

70. Kerr OA, Kavanagh G, Horn H. Allergic contact dermatitis from topical diclofenac in Solaraze gel. Contact Dermatitis 2002;47(3):175.

71. Tanaka M, Kobayashi S, Murata T, Tanikawa A, Nishikawa T. Allergic contact dermatitis from diethyl sebacate in lanoconazole cream. Contact Dermatitis 2000;43(4):233–4.

72. Wong GA, Shear NH. Melkersson-Rosenthal syndrome associated with allergic contact dermatitis from octyl and dodecyl gallates. Contact Dermatitis 2003;49(5):266–7.

73. Aalto-Korte K. Contact allergy to dorzolamide eyedrops. Contact Dermatitis 1998;39(4):206.

74. Buckley DA. Contact allergy to doxepin. Contact Dermatitis 2000;43(4):231–2.

75. Horn HM, Tidman MJ, Aldridge RD. Allergic contact dermatitis due to doxepin cream in a patient with dystrophic epidermolysis bullosa. Contact Dermatitis 2001;45(2):115.

76. Tanaka S, Otsuki T, Matsumoto Y, Hayakawa R, Sugiura M. Allergic contact dermatitis from enoxolone. Contact Dermatitis 2001;44(3):192.

77. Pereira F, Pereira C, Lacerda MH. Contact dermatitis due to a cream containing chitin and a Carbitol. Contact Dermatitis 1998;38(5):290–1.

78. Linsen G, Goossens A. Allergic contact dermatitis from ethylhexylglycerin. Contact Dermatitis 2002;47(3):169.

79. Pirker C, Moslinger T, Wantke F, Gotz M, Jarisch R. Ethylmercuric chloride: the responsible agent in thimerosal hypersensitivity. Contact Dermatitis 1993;29(3):152–4.

80. Vilaplana J, Romaguera C. Allergic contact dermatitis due to eucalyptol in an anti-inflammatory cream. Contact Dermatitis 2000;43(2):118.

81. Dooms-Goossens A. Allergy to inhaled corticosteroids: a review. Am J Contact Dermatitis 1995;6:1–3.

82. Whitmore SE. Delayed systemic allergic reactions to corticosteroids. Contact Dermatitis 1995;32(4):193–8.

83. Kimura M, Kawada A, Ogino M, Murayama Y. Simultaneous contact sensitivity to hydroxystearic acid and C18-36 acid triglyceride in lip glosses. Contact Dermatitis 2002;47(2):115.

84. McKenna KE. Allergic contact dermatitis from glyceryl trinitrate ointment. Contact Dermatitis 2000;42(4):246.

85. Perez-Calderon R, Gonzalo-Garijo MA, Rodriguez-Nevado I. Generalized allergic contact dermatitis from nitroglycerin in a transdermal therapeutic system. Contact Dermatitis 2002;46(5):303.

86. Barrientos N, Ortiz-Frutos J, Gomez E, Iglesias L. Allergic contact dermatitis from a bleaching cream. Am J Contact Dermatitis 2001;12(1):33–4.

87. Horak J, Hemmer W, Focke M, Gotz M, Jarisch R. Contact dermatitis from anti-inflammatory gel containing hydroxyethyl salicylate. Contact Dermatitis 2002;47(2):120–1.

88. Roest MA, Shaw S, Orton DI. Allergic contact otitis externa due to iodoform in BIPP cavity dressings. Contact Dermatitis 2002;46(6):360.

89. Bryld LE, Agner T, Menne T. Allergic contact dermatitis from 3-iodo-2-propynyl-butylcarbamate (IPBC)—an update. Contact Dermatitis 2001;44(5):276–8.

90. Lowe NJ, Chizhevsky V, Gabriel H. Photo(chemo)therapy: general principles. Clin Dermatol 1997;15(5):745–52.

91. Goday Bujan JJ, Oleaga Morante JM, Yanguas Bayona I, Gonzalez Guemes M, Soloeta Arechavala R. Allergic contact dermatitis from krameria triandra extract. Contact Dermatitis 1998;38(2):120–1.

92. Le Coz CJ, Heid E. Allergic contact dermatitis from methoxy PEG-17/dodecyl glycol copolymer (Elfacos OW 100). Contact Dermatitis 2001;44(5):308–9.

93. Rodriguez-Serna M, Sanchez-Motilla JM, Ramon R, Aliaga A. Allergic and systemic contact dermatitis from *Matricaria chamomilla* tea. Contact Dermatitis 1998;39(4):192–3.

94. Goulden V, Layton AM, Cunliffe WJ. Long-term safety of isotretinoin as a treatment for acne vulgaris. Br J Dermatol 1994;131(3):360–3.

95. Ahmed I, Charles-Holmes R. Contact allergy to Psorigon. Contact Dermatitis 2000;42(5):276.

96. Umebayashi Y, Ito S. Allergic contact dermatitis due to both lanoconazole and neticonazole ointments. Contact Dermatitis 2001;44(1):48–9.

97. Valsecchi R, Aiolfi M, Leghissa P, Cologni L, Cortinovis R. Contact dermatitis from methyl butetisalicylate. Contact Dermatitis 1998;38(6):360–1.

98. Gavish D, Katz M, Gottehrer N, Israeli A, Lijovetzky G, Holubar K. Cholestatic jaundice, an unusual side effect of etretinate. J Am Acad Dermatol 1985;13(4):669–70.

99. Erdmann SM, Sachs B, Merk HF. Allergic contact dermatitis due to methyldibromo glutaronitrile in Euxyl K 400 in an ultrasonic gel. Contact Dermatitis 2001;44(1):39–40.

100. Corazza M, Levratti A, Virgili A. Allergic contact dermatitis due to methyl glucose dioleate. Contact Dermatitis 2001;45(5):308.

101. Gastaminza G, Anda M, Audicana MT, Fernandez E, Munoz D. Fixed-drug eruption due to metronidazole with positive topical provocation. Contact Dermatitis 2001;44(1):36.

102. Sanchez-Motilla JM, Pont V, Nagore E, Rodriguez-Serna M, Sanchez JL, Aliaga A. Pustular allergic contact dermatitis from minoxidil. Contact Dermatitis 1998;38(5):283–4.

103. Al-Suwaidan SN, Gad el Rab MO, Al-Fakhiry S, Al Hoqail IA, Al-Maziad A, Sherif AB. Allergic contact dermatitis from myrrh, a topical herbal medicine used to promote healing. Contact Dermatitis 1998;39(3):137.

104. Sigl B. Kontaktallergie auf Neo-Ballistol. Dermatosen 1998;46:170–2.

105. Bonamonte D, Mundo L, Daddabbo M, Foti C. Allergic contact dermatitis from *Mentha spicata* (spearmint). Contact Dermatitis 2001;45(5):298.

106. Lisi P, Brunelli L. Extensive allergic contact dermatitis from a topical enzymatic preparation (Noruxol). Contact Dermatitis 2001;45(3):186–7.

107. Wong GA, King CM. Occupational allergic contact dermatitis from olive oil in pizza making. Contact Dermatitis 2004;50(2):102–3.

108. Shaffer MP, Williford PM, Sherertz EF. An old reaction in a new setting: the paraben paradox. Am J Contact Dermatitis 2000;11(3):189.

109. Rafael M, Pereira F, Faria MA. Allergic contact blepharoconjunctivitis caused by phenylephrine, associated with persistent patch test reaction. Contact Dermatitis 1998;39(3):143–4.

110. Moffitt DL, Sansom JE. Allergic contact dermatitis from phthalic anhydride/trimellitic anhydride/glycols copolymer in nail varnish. Contact Dermatitis 2002;46(4):236.

111. Itoh M, Kantoh H, Fukuzawa M, Kurikawa Y. A case of contact dermatitis due to Restamin ointment. J Med Soc Toho Univ 1998;45:518–22.

112. Le Coz CJ, Lefebvre C, Ludmann F, Grosshans E. Polyvinylpyrrolidone (PVP)/eicosene copolymer: an emerging cosmetic allergen. Contact Dermatitis 2000;43(1):61–2.

113. Stone N, Varma S, Hughes TM, Stone NM. Allergic contact dermatitis from polyvinylpyrrolidone (PVP)/1-triacontene copolymer in a sunscreen. Contact Dermatitis 2002;47(1):49.

114. Kim HJ, Lim YS, Choi HY, K.B. M. A case of allergic contact dermatitis due to Dermatop ointment and Plancollotion. Korean J Dermatol 1998;36:460–3.

115. Funk JO, Maibach HI. Propylene glycol dermatitis: re-evaluation of an old problem. Contact Dermatitis 1994;31(4):236–41.

116. Scheman A, Cummins R. Contact allergy to PVP/hexadecene copolymer. Contact Dermatitis 1998;39(4):201.

117. Scheman AJ. Contact allergy to quaternium-22 and shellac in mascara. Contact Dermatitis 1998;38(6):342–3.

118. Le Coz CJ, Leclere JM, Arnoult E, Raison-Peyron N, Pons-Guiraud A, Vigan M; Members of Revidal-Gerda. Allergic contact dermatitis from shellac in mascara. Contact Dermatitis 2002;46(3):149–52.

119. Lomholt H, Rastogi SC, Andersen KE. Allergic contact dermatitis from sodium dihydroxycetyl phosphate, a new cosmetic allergen? Contact Dermatitis 2001;45(3):143–5.

120. Malanin KE. Allergic contact dermatitis caused by a mixture of sodium myristoyl sarcosinate and sodium myristoate in a cosmetic product. Contact Dermatitis 2002;47(1):50.

121. Shaffrali FC, Gawkrodger DJ. Contact dermatitis from soybean extract in a cosmetic cream. Contact Dermatitis 2001;44(1):51–2.

122. Skrebova N, Brocks K, Karlsmark T. Allergic contact cheilitis from spearmint oil. Contact Dermatitis 1998;39(1):35.

123. Worm M, Jeep S, Sterry W, Zuberbier T. Perioral contact dermatitis caused by L-carvone in toothpaste. Contact Dermatitis 1998;38(6):338.

124. Yesudian PD, King CM. Allergic contact dermatitis from stearyl alcohol in Efudix cream. Contact Dermatitis 2001;45(5):313–14.

125. Khanna M, Qasem K, Sasseville D. Allergic contact dermatitis to tea tree oil with erythema multiforme-like id reaction. Am J Contact Dermatitis 2000;11(4):238–42.

126. Kirkup ME, Sansom JE. Contact sensitivity to tetrahydroxypropyl ethylenediamine in a sunscreen, without cross-sensitivity to ethylenediamine. Contact Dermatitis 2000;43(2):121–2.

127. Moller H. All these positive tests to thimerosal. Contact Dermatitis 1994;31(4):209–13.

128. Sangen Y, Kawada A, Asai M, Aragane Y, Yudate T, Tezuka T. Fixed drug eruption induced by tosufloxacin tosilate. Contact Dermatitis 2000;42(5):285.

129. Wong CS, Beck MH. Allergic contact dermatitis from triclosan in antibacterial handwashes. Contact Dermatitis 2001;45(5):307.

130. Bowling JC, Scarisbrick J, Warin AP, Downs AM. Allergic contact dermatitis from trideceth-2-carboxamide monoethanolamine (MEA) in a hair dye. Contact Dermatitis 2002;47(2):116–17.

131. Chu CY, Sun CC. Allergic contact dermatitis from triethanolamine in a sunscreen. Contact Dermatitis 2001;44(1):41–2.

132. Reyes JJ, Farina MC. Allergic contact dermatitis due to trimebutine. Contact Dermatitis 2001;45(3):164.

133. Magerl A, Heiss R, Frosch PJ. Allergic contact dermatitis from zinc ricinoleate in a deodorant and glyceryl ricinoleate in a lipstick. Contact Dermatitis 2001;44(2):119–21.

134. Fransway AF, Schmitz NA. The problem of preservation in the 1990s. II. Formaldehyde and formaldehyde-releasing biocides: Incidence of cross-reactivity and the significance of the positive response to formaldehyde. Am J Contact Dermatitis 1991;2:78–88.

135. Fransway AF. The problem of preservation in the 1990s. III. Agents with preservation function independent of formaldehyde release. Am J Contact Dermatitis 1991;2:145–74.

136. Herbst RA, Maibach HI. Contact dermatitis caused by allergy to ophthalmic drugs and contact lens solutions. Contact Dermatitis 1991;25(5):305–12.

Substances that affect the skin: Contact urticaria

Contact urticaria (1–4) refers to a wheal-and-flare response to the application of chemicals to the intact skin. Various cutaneous and extracutaneous symptoms and signs have been described, justifying the term "contact urticaria syndrome." The broad spectrum of clinical manifestations is classified in Table 1. The symptoms usually develop within 20–30 minutes after contact with the offending chemical, but later reactions after several hours have also been recorded.

Most cases of contact urticaria are of non-immunological origin, presumably due to the direct release of histamine, slow-reacting substance of anaphylaxis (SRS-A), bradykinin, or other vasoactive substances. Topical drugs and ingredients of cosmetics that have caused non-immunological contact urticaria are listed in Table 2.

Contact urticaria of immunological origin is less common, although many topical drugs have caused it in previously sensitized individuals. In several reports, passive-transfer tests were positive, and specific antibodies have occasionally been demonstrated, indicating an immunological phenomenon. Topical drugs and ingredients of cosmetics that have caused immunological contact urticaria are listed in Table 3; in most of these cases, the contact urticaria was of probable immunological origin.

Some cases of contact urticarial reactions cannot be ascribed with certainty to either immunological or non-immunological mechanisms; the classical example of this category of contact urticaria of uncertain mechanism is that caused by the bleaching agent ammonium persulfate. Also belonging to this category are several topical substances that have caused contact urticaria on patch-testing, the clinical significance of which is uncertain, for example nickel sulfate, butylated hydroxyanisole (BHA),

Table 2 Agents that have caused non-immunological contact urticaria (1,4)

Alcohols	Eugenol
Balsam of Peru	Formaldehyde
Benzaldehyde	Iodine
Benzocaine	Methyl green
Benzoic acid/benzoin tincture	Methyl salicylate
Camphor	Monoethyl fumarate (SEDA-16, 153)
Cantharides	Nicotinic acid esters (SEDA-17, 187)
Capsaicin	Parabens
Chlorocresol	Phenol
Cinnamic acid	Propylene glycol (SEDA-19, 159)
Cinnamic aldehyde (SED-9, 249)	Resorcinol
Cinnamon oil	Sodium benzoate
Diethyl fumarate (SEDA-16, 153)	Sorbic acid
Dimethylsulfoxide (SED-9, 249)	Sulfur

Table 1 Staging and symptoms of the contact urticaria syndrome (3,4)

Cutaneous reactions only			Extracutaneous reactions	
Stage 1	Localized urticaria Dermatitis/dermatosis Non-specific symptoms (itching, tingling, burning, etc.)		Stage 3	Bronchial asthma Rhinoconjunctivitis Otolaryngeal symptoms Gastrointestinal symptoms
Stage 2	Generalized urticaria		Stage 4	Anaphylactoid reactions

Table 3 Agents known or believed to have caused immunological contact urticaria (1–4)

Acetylsalicylic acid	Lanolin alcohol (SEDA-5, 152)
Acrylic acid (SEDA-18, 175)	Latex
Albendazole	Lidocaine (SEDA-15, 149)
Aminophenazone (aminopyrine)	Lindane
Ampicillin	Mechlorethamine hydrochloride (SEDA-22, 172)
Amyl alcohol	Menthol
Bacitracin	Merbromin
Balsam of Peru	Mercurochrome (SEDA-19, 163)
Basic blue 99	Metamizole
Benzocaine	Methotrimeprazine
Benzoic acid	Methylethylketone
Benzophenone	Mexiletine hydrochloride (SEDA-18, 175)
Benzoyl peroxide	Mezlocillin (SEDA-15, 149)
Benzyl alcohol	Monoamylamine
Buserelin acetate	Myrrh
Butyl alcohol	Neomycin
Butylated hydroxyanisole (BHA)	Nickel sulfate
Butylated hydroxytoluene (BHT)	Nicotine
Caraway seed oil	Nicotinyl alcohol
Cefotiam hydrochloride (SEDA-19, 163)	Nifuroxime
Cephalosporins	Orthophenylphenate
Cetyl alcohol	Oxyphenbutazone
Chamomile	Para-aminodiphenylamine (SEDA-5, 152)
Chloramine	Parabens
Chloramphenicol	Parahydroxybenzoic acid
Chlorhexidine (SEDA-21, 166)	Paraphenylenediamine derivatives (SEDA-21, 166)
Chlorocresol (SEDA-12, 137)	Penicillin
Chlorproethazine (SEDA-17, 187)	Pentamidine isethionate
Chlorpromazine (6)	Phenylmercuric salts
Clioquinol (iodochlorhydroxyquinoline) (SEDA-5, 152)	Polyethylene glycol
Clobetasol 17-propionate (SEDA-8, 153)	Polypropylene (Polysorbate 60)
Colophony	Povidone iodine (SEDA-20, 157)
Corn starch	Pristinamycin
Denatonium benzoate	Procaine hydrochloride
Diethyl fumarate	Promethazine hydrochloride
Diethyl toluamide (SEDA-8, 153)	Propipocaine hydrochloride (SEDA-15, 149)
1,3-Diiodo-2-hydroxypropane	Propyl alcohol
Dinitrochlorobenzene	Propylene glycol
Diphenylcyclopropenone (SEDA-14, 132)	Protein hydrolysate (SEDA-15, 149)
Dipyrone	Pyrazolone derivatives (SEDA-9, 139)
Disodium cromoglicate (SEDA-12, 137)	Pyrethrin (SEDA-15, 149)
Emulgade F	Rifamycin (SEDA-17, 191)
Estrogen cream	Salicylic acid
Ethyl alcohol	Sisomycin (SEDA-12, 139)
Ethylenediamine dihydrochloride	Sodium hypochlorite
Etofenamate	Sodium sulfite
Formaldehyde (SEDA-8, 153)	Sorbitan laurate (SEDA-9, 139)
Gelatine	Squaric acid dibutyl ester
Gentamicin (SEDA-12, 139)	Steartrimonium hydrolysed animal protein (SEDA-21, 166)
Gentian violet	Stearyl alcohol
Glyceryl trinitrate	Streptomycin
Hamamelis	Sulfur
Henna	Tetracycline (SEDA-9, 139)
Hexanetriol	Thiomersal
Hydrolysed protein (SEDA-21, 166)	Thuja
Isopropyl alcohol	α-Tocopherol
Isopropyl dibenzoylmethane	Tropicamide
Labetalol	Vanillin
	Virginiamycin

butylated hydroxytoluene (BHT), ethyl vanillin, potassium bichromate, parabens, and ethylenediamine (5).

The diagnosis of contact urticaria can usually be confirmed by an open test. However, such tests should be performed with great caution, since anaphylactoid reactions due to the testing procedure have been described (3,4).

Reports of contact urticaria to ingredients of drugs and cosmetics are listed in Table 4 and Table 5 (7–11).

Table 4 Contact urticaria to ingredients of topical drugs and cosmetics

Allergen	Allergen-containing product	20-minute patch test	Skin prick test	Reference
Cyclopentolate hydrochloride	Eye drops (Colircursi cicloplejico 1%)	Eye drops +	Not performed	(12)
Di(2-ethylhexyl) phthalate (DOP)	PVC grip cotton gloves	Rubbing with PVC grip+	Gas chromatography extracts + DOP + Di-*n*-butylmaleate +	(13)
Glyceryl thioglycolate	Hair permanent fluid	1% in petrolatum +	Not performed	(14)
Panthenol	Hair conditioner	Hair conditioner Panthenol 30% in petrolatum	Hair conditioner + Panthenol +++	(15)
Wheat hydrolysate	Body cream	Body cream ++	Wheat hydrolysate ++	(16)

Table 5 Contact urticaria to relatively rare antigens in drugs and cosmetics

Allergen	Allergen-containing product	Patch tests	Skin prick tests	Reference
Benzophenone 3	Sunscreens	Benzophenone 3 + (concentration not stated)	Not done	(17)
Benzyl alcohol	Bacteriostatic saline	10 cm wheal after 24 hours (concentration not stated)	Not done	(18)
Cyclopentolate hydrochloride	Eye drops	Eye drops 1% +	Not done	(12)
Di-(2-ethylhexyl) phthalate (DOP)	PVC grip cotton gloves	Rubbing with PVC +	Gas chromatography extracts + DOP + Di-*n*-butylmaleate	(13)
Geraniol	Various cosmetics	Geraniol + (concentration not stated)	Not done	(19)
Glyceryl thioglycolate	Hair permanent fluid	1% in petrolatum +	Not done	(14)
Panthenol	Hair conditioner	Panthenol 30% in petrolatum −	Hair conditioner + Panthenol +++	(15)
Phenoxyethanol	Body lotion	Phenoxyethanol 1% pet + Euxyl K 400 1.5% + Own cosmetics + Not done	Phenoxyethanol 1%+ Euxyl K 400 1.5%+ Body lotion +++ Euxyl K 400 ++ Phenoxyethanol 1%+, 5%+,10%++	(20) (21)
Potassium persulfate	Hair dye	Nickel sulfate	Potassium persulfate (dilution not stated) 5 mm wheal	(22)
Wheat hydrolysate	Body cream	Body cream ++	Wheat hydrolysate ++	(16)

+, ++, +++ indicate increasing intensity of reaction.

References

1. De Groot AC, Weyland JW, Nater JP. Unwanted Effects of Cosmetics and Drugs used in Dermatology. 3rd ed. Amsterdam: Elsevier, 1994.
2. Hannuksela M. Mechanisms in contact urticaria. Clin Dermatol 1997;15(4):619–22.
3. Warner MR, Taylor JS, Leow YH. Agents causing contact urticaria. Clin Dermatol 1997;15(4):623–35.
4. Zajonz C, Frosch PJ. Ursachen von Kontakturticaria unter besonderer Berücksichtigung von Arbeitsstoffen. [Etiology of contact urticaria with special reference to occupational substances.] Hautarzt 1994;45(2):65–73.
5. Warin RP, Smith RJ. Chronic urticaria. Investigations with patch and challenge tests. Contact Dermatitis 1982; 8(2):117–21.
6. Leliever WC. Topical gentamicin-induced positional vertigo. Otolaryngol Head Neck Surg 1985;93(4):553–5.
7. Trattner A, Ingber A. Topical treatment with minoxidil 2% and smoking intolerance. Ann Pharmacother 1992;26(2):198–9.
8. Wolff K. Should PUVA be abandoned? N Engl J Med 1997;336(15):1090–1.
9. Ramsay B, Marks JM. Bronchoconstriction due to 8-methoxypsoralen. Br J Dermatol 1988;119(1):83–6.
10. Hughes RA. Arthritis precipitated by isotretinoin treatment for acne vulgaris. J Rheumatol 1993;20(7):1241–2.
11. Barth JH, Macdonald-Hull SP, Mark J, Jones RG, Cunliffe WJ. Isotretinoin therapy for acne vulgaris: a re-evaluation of the need for measurements of plasma lipids and liver function tests. Br J Dermatol 1993;129(6):704–7.
12. Munoz-Bellido FJ, Beltran A, Bellido J. Contact urticaria due to cyclopentolate hydrochloride. Allergy 2000;55(2):198–9.

13. Sugiura K, Sugiura M, Hayakawa R, Sasaki K. Di(2-ethylhexyl) phthalate (DOP) in the dotted polyvinyl-chloride grip of cotton gloves as a cause of contact urticaria syndrome. Contact Dermatitis 2000;43(4):237–8.

14. Engasser P. Type I and type IV immune responses to glyceryl thioglycolate. Contact Dermatitis 2000;42(5):298.

15. Schalock PC, Storrs FJ, Morrison L. Contact urticaria from panthenol in hair conditioner. Contact Dermatitis 2000;43(4):223.

16. Varjonen E, Petman L, Makinen-Kiljunen S. Immediate contact allergy from hydrolyzed wheat in a cosmetic cream. Allergy 2000;55(3):294–6.

17. Yesudian PD, King CM. Severe contact urticaria and ana-phylaxis from benzophenone-3(2-hydroxy 4-methoxy ben-zophenone). Contact Dermatitis 2002;46(1):55–6.

18. Guin JD, Goodman J. Contact urticaria from benzyl alcohol presenting as intolerance to saline soaks. Contact Dermatitis 2001;45(3):182–3.

19. Yamamoto A, Morita A, Tsuji T, Suzuki K, Matsunaga K. Contact urticaria from geraniol. Contact Dermatitis 2002;46(1):52.

20. Hernandez B, Ortiz-Frutos FJ, Garcia M, Palencia S, Garcia MC, Iglesias L. Contact urticaria from 2-phenoxy-ethanol. Contact Dermatitis 2002;47(1):54.

21. Bohn S, Bircher AJ. Phenoxyethanol-induced urticaria. Allergy 2001;56(9):922–3.

22. Estrada Rodriguez JL, Gozalo Reques F, Cechini Fernandez C, Rodriguez Prieto MA. Contact urticaria due to potassium persulfate. Contact Dermatitis 2001; 45(3):177.

Substances that affect the skin: Discoloration, necrosis, and miscellaneous adverse effects

Drugs that cause discoloration of the skin, nails, and mucous membranes are listed in Table 1. Pigmented contact dermatitis has been reviewed (1).

Drugs that cause necrosis of the skin and mucous membranes are listed in Table 2.

Other adverse effects of topical drugs and cosmetics are listed in Table 3.

Table 2 Drugs that have caused necrosis of skin and mucous membranes

Drug	References
Adrenaline	(SEDA-10, 131)
Arsenious oxide	(SED-9, 249)
Cetrimonium bromide	(SED-9, 249)
Dequalinium	(26)
Fluorouracil	(SEDA-5, 155)
Fuchsin–silver nitrate	(27)
Gentian violet (crystal violet)	(SEDA-12, 138)
Glucocorticoids	(SEDA-7, 166)
Phenol	(SED-9, 250)
Povidone iodine	(SEDA-5, 152)

Table 1 Discoloration of the skin and appendages

Drug	Adverse effect	References
Amorolfine nail lacquer	Bluish or yellow-brown discoloration of the nail plate	(SEDA-21, 166)
Benzoyl peroxide	Discoloration of hair and postinflammatory pigmentation; hypopigmentation	(2,3)
Butylated hydroxyanisole	Depigmentation	(4)
Butylated hydroxytoluene	Depigmentation	(5)
Carmustine (BCNU)	Pigmentation	(6)
Chlorhexidine	Discoloration of the teeth and tongue	(SED-9, 249)
Cinnamic aldehyde	Depigmentation	(SEDA-6, 153)
Clioquinol	Red discoloration of white hair	(SEDA-9, 143)
Coal tar dyes	"Pigmented cosmetic dermatitis"	(7)
Diethylstilbestrol	Brown discoloration of nipples and linea alba; systemic effects caused by percutaneous absorption	(SEDA-9, 250)
Dihydroxyacetone	Brown pigmentation ("sunless tanning")	(8)
Dinitrochlorobenzene	Yellow discoloration of grey hair	(SEDA-4, 107)
Diphencyprone	Triggering of vitiligo	(SEDA-14, 132)
Dithranol	Brown-purplish discoloration of skin, nails, and hair	(9,10)
Fluorouracil	Hyperpigmentation of the skin and nails (melanonychia)	(SEDA-5, 155) (11)
Glucocorticoids	Hyperpigmentation and hypopigmentation	(12)
Glutaral (glutaraldehyde)	Brown discoloration	(SED-9, 249)
Hydroquinones	Pigmentation and depigmentation; nail staining	(SEDA-8, 161) (13–15)
Iron salts	Brown discoloration (sometimes permanent)	(16,17)
4-Isopropylcatechol	Depigmentation	(18)
Mechlorethamine hydroquinone	Pigmentation	(19)
Mercury compounds	Depigmentation	(20)
Perfume ingredients	Contact allergy has caused pigmentation of the face	(21)
Petrolatum	Hyperpigmentation	(22)
Phenols	Depigmentation and hyperpigmentation	(SEDA-7, 166)
Resorcinol	Darkens fair hair; orange-brown discoloration of lacquered nails	(23)
Selenium sulfide	Green hair discoloration	(SEDA-22, 173)
Silver nitrate	Slate grey discoloration (argyria)	(24)
Thiotepa	Periorbital leukoderma	(SEDA-5, 155)
Tretinoin	Hypopigmentation	(25)

Table 3 Miscellaneous adverse effects of topical drugs (for additional references see SED-9, 249)

Drug	Common uses	Adverse effects	References
Benzonyl peroxide	Acne treatment	Co-carcinogen (?)	(SEDA-7, 168)
Benzyl benzoate	Antiscabetic drug	Pemphigoid (?)	(28)
Cetrimonium bromide	Antiseptic	Matting of hair	(29)
Clonidine patches	Antihypertensive	Activation of *Herpes simplex*; hyperpigmentation	(SEDA-13, 128)
Coal tar	Psoriasis; eczema	Carcinogen (?)	(30,31)
Dinitrochlorobenzene	Treatment of alopecia areata	Yellow discoloration of grey hair; enhancement of allergy to non-related allergens; mutagen (?); carcinogen (?)	(SEDA-4, 107) (SEDA-6, 149) (32) (SEDA-10, 131) (SEDA-109, 195)
5-Fluorouracil	Topical antimitotic drug	Telangiectasia; bilateral cicatricial ectropion; exacerbation of *Herpes labialis*; pain, edema, livedo reticularis; erosions	(SEDA-7, 166) (SEDA-7, 166) (SEDA-5, 155)
Fusidic acid	Antibacterial agent	Acanthosis nigricans	(SEDA-17, 192)
Idoxuridine	Antiviral drug	Carcinogen (?); mutagen (?); teratogen (?)	(33–35)
Lindane	Antiscabetic drug	Morphea	(SEDA-16, 159)
Mechlorethamine hydrochloride	Nitrogen mustard; topical antimitotic drug	Carcinogen; suppression of immunological defences; Stevens–Johnson syndrome	(SEDA-22, 172) (19)
Nicotinic acid	Treatment of alopecia	Acanthosis nigricans	(SEDA-11, 142)
Petrolatum	Vehicle constituent	Acne; lipogranulomata	(36) (SEDA-6, 154)
Phenol	Face peeling; antipruritic	Milia; persistent erythema; skin pore prominence; telangiectasia; scarring; pigment alterations	(SEDA-7, 166)
Podophyllin	Treatment of condylomata acuminata	Carcinogen (?)	(37)
Polyethylene glycol	Vehicle constituent	Carcinogen (?)	(SEDA-6, 153)
Salicylic acid	Keratolytic drug	Thinning of the skin, telangiectasia, and (de)pigmentation after prolonged use	(SEDA-15, 151)
Selenium sulfide	Antiseborrheic drug	Reversible hair loss; structural hair defects (?); oiliness of the scalp	(38)
Tretinoin	Acne treatment	Ectropion	(SEDA-17, 185)
		Eruptive pyogenic granuloma	(SEDA-15, 151)

References

1. Ebihara T, Nakayama H. Pigmented contact dermatitis. Clin Dermatol 1997;15(4):593–9.
2. Bleiberg J, Brodkin RH, Abbey AA. Bleaching of hair after use of benzoyl peroxide acne lotions. Arch Dermatol 1973;108(4):583.
3. Bushkell LL. Letter: Bleaching by benzoyl peroxide. Arch Dermatol 1974;110(3):465.
4. Menter JM, Etemadi AA, Chapman W, Hollins TD, Willis I. In vivo depigmentation by hydroxybenzene derivatives. Melanoma Res 1993;3(6):443–9.
5. Lanigan RS, Yamarik TA. Final report on the safety assessment of BHT(1). Int J Toxicol 2002;21(Suppl 2):19–94.
6. Frost P, DeVita VT. Pigmentation due to a new antitumor agent. Effects of topical application of BCNU [1,3-bis(2-chloroethyl)-1-nitrosourea]. Arch Dermatol 1966; 94(3):265–8.
7. Sugai T, Takahashi Y, Takagi T. Pigmented cosmetic dermatitis and coal tar dyes. Contact Dermatitis 1977; 3(5):249–56.

8. Nguyen BC, Kochevar IE. Factors influencing sunless tanning with dihydroxyacetone. Br J Dermatol 2003; 149(2):332–40.
9. Rogers MJ, Whitefield M, Marks VJ. Yellow hair discoloration due to anthralin. J Am Acad Dermatol 1988;19 (2 Pt 1):370–1.
10. Muller R, Naumann E, Detmar M, Orfanos CE. Stabilitat von Cignolin (Dithranol) in teerhaltigen Salben mit und ohne Salicylsaurezusatz. Oxidation in Danthron und Dithranoldimer. [Stability of cignolin (dithranol) in ointments containing tar with and without the addition of salicylic acid. Oxidation to danthron and dithranol dimer.] Hautarzt 1987;38(2):107–11.
11. Stohs SJ, Ezzedeen FW, Anderson AK, Baldwin JN, Makoid MC. Percutaneous absorption of iodochlorhydroxyquin in humans. J Invest Dermatol 1984;82(2):195–8.
12. Gallardo MJ, Johnson DA. Cutaneous hypopigmentation following a posterior sub-tenon triamcinolone injection. Am J Ophthalmol 2004;137(4):779–80.
13. Coulson IH. "Fade out" photochromonychia. Clin Exp Dermatol 1993;18(1):87–8.

14. Camarasa JG, Serra-Baldrich E. Exogenous ochronosis with allergic contact dermatitis from hydroquinone. Contact Dermatitis 1994;31(1):57–8.

15. Clarys P, Barel A. Efficacy of topical treatment of pigmentation skin disorders with plant hydroquinone glucosides as assessed by quantitative color analysis. J Dermatol 1998;25(6):412–14.

16. Amazon K, Robinson MJ, Rywlin AM. Ferrugination caused by Monsel's solution. Clinical observations and experimentations. Am J Dermatopathol 1980;2(3): 197–205.

17. Wood C, Severin GL. Unusual histiocytic reaction to Monsel's solution. Am J Dermatopathol 1980; 2(3):261–4.

18. Bleehen SS. The treatment of hypermelanosis with 4-isopropylcatechol. Br J Dermatol 1976;94(6):687–94.

19. Goulden V, Layton AM, Cunliffe WJ. Long-term safety of isotretinoin as a treatment for acne vulgaris. Br J Dermatol 1994;131(3):360–3.

20. Adebajo SB. An epidemiological survey of the use of cosmetic skin lightening cosmetics among traders in Lagos, Nigeria. West Afr J Med 2002;21(1):51–5.

21. Larsen WG. Perfume dermatitis. J Am Acad Dermatol 1985;12(1 Pt 1):1–9.

22. Maibach H. Chronic dermatitis and hyperpigmentation from petrolatum. Contact Dermatitis 1978;4(1):62.

23. Loveman AB, Fliegelman MT. Discoloration of the nails; concomitant use of nail lacquer with resorcinol or resorcinol monoacetate (Euresol) as cause. AMA Arch Derm 1955;72(2):153–6.

24. Lee SM, Lee SH. Generalized argyria after habitual use of AgNO₃. J Dermatol 1994;21(1):50–3.

25. Halder RM, Richards GM. Management of dyschromias in ethnic skin. Dermatol Ther 2004;17(2):151–7.

26. Armijo Moreno M, Gutierrez Salmeron MT, Camacho Martinez F, Naranjo Sintes R, Armijo Lozano R, Garcia Mellado V, De Dulanto F. Necrosis de pene por dequalinium (dos observaciones). [Necrosis of the penis caused by dequalinium (2 cases).] Actas Dermosifiliogr 1976;67 (7–8):547–52.

27. Sankar NS, Donaldson D. Lessons to be learned: a case study approach. Finger discoloration due to silver nitrate exposure: review of uses and toxicity of silver in clinical practice. J R Soc Health 1998; 118(6):371–4.

28. Stransky L, Vasileva S, Mateev G. Contact bullous pemphigoid? Contact Dermatitis 1996;35(3):182.

29. Dawber RP, Calnan CD. Bird's nest hair. Matting of scalp hair due to shampooing. Clin Exp Dermatol 1976; 1(2):155–8.

30. Plantin P. [Question of the month: should coal-tar be forbidden?] Ann Dermatol Venereol 1997;124(2):205–7.

31. Pilkington T, Brogden RN. Acitretin. A review of its pharmacology and therapeutic use. Drugs 1992;43(4): 597–627.

32. de Groot AC, Nater JP, Bleumink E, de Jong MC. Does DNCB therapy potentiate epicutaneous sensitization to non-related contact allergens? Clin Exp Dermatol 1981; 6(2):139–44.

33. Yoshikura H, Zajdela F, Perin F, Perin-Roussel O, Jacquignon P, Latarjet R. Enhancement of 5-iododeoxyuridine-induced endogenous C-type virus activation by polycyclic hydrocarbons: apparent lack of parallelism between enhancement and carcinogenicity. J Natl Cancer Inst 1977;58(4):1035–40.

34. Pizer LI, Mitchell DH, Bentele B, Betz JL. A mammalian cell line designed to test the mutagenic activity of anti-herpes nucleosides. Int J Cancer 1987;40(1):114–21.

35. Itoi M, Ishii Y. [Teratogenicity of IDU ophthalmic.] Nippon Ganka Gakkai Zasshi 1972;76(1):52–4.

36. Cribier B, Welsch M, Heid E. Renal impairment probably induced by etretinate. Dermatology 1992; 185(4):266–8.

37. Baran R, Laugier P. Melanonychia induced by topical 5-fluorouracil. Br J Dermatol 1985;112(5):621–5.

38. Park YM, Kim TY, Kim HO, Kim CW. Reproducible elevation of liver transaminases by topical 8-methoxypsoralen. Photodermatol Photoimmunol Photomed 1994; 10(6):261–3.

Substances that affect the skin: Photocontact dermatitis

Photocontact dermatitis can be toxic or allergic in nature (1–4). Phototoxicity can occur in anybody if enough light energy and photosensitizer are present in the skin. Photoallergy is due to a cell-mediated hypersensitivity response, and therefore occurs in sensitized individuals only.

Compared with contact allergy, photocontact allergy is uncommon, although many chemicals have been responsible for photoallergic reactions.

The British Photodermatology Group has provided a summary of the methods and clinical use of photopatch-testing. The following potential photoallergens have been suggested as standard series for routine testing in all patients suspected of photosensitivity:

(a) benzophenone-3;
(b) butyl methoxydibenzoylmethane;
(c) 2-ethylhexyl-para-methoxycinnamate;
(d) musk ambrette;
(e) octyl dimethyl para-aminobenzoic acid;
(f) para-aminobenzoic acid (PABA).

Patients' own products, diluted as appropriate, should be tested as well (5). Currently, UV filters (and to a lesser extent fragrances) are the main photosensitizers, notably benzophenone-3. Sunscreen photosensitization occurs especially in patients with photodermatoses and photo-aggravated dermatoses (3). The UV filter isopropyl dibenzoylmethane caused so many cases of photosensitization that it was withdrawn.

In a review of photopatch-testing in 2390 patients with rashes that were confined to sun-exposed areas, about 70% of 4374 positive reactions were classified as photo-induced reactions, of which 222 (5%) were photoallergic reactions (6). NSAIDs, disinfectants, and phenothiazines were the main photoallergens. Photosensitive reactions to antimicrobial drugs, including topical agents, have been reviewed (7).

Topical photosensitizers are listed in Table 1 (1–4,8).

Table 1 Topical photosensitizers

Aceclofenac (9)	A
6-Acetoxy-2,4-dimethyl-m-dioxane (SEDA-10, 131)	T
Amyl dimethyl PABA (SEDA-10, 131)	T
Balsam of Peru (SEDA-19, 162)	T
Benoxaprofen (10)	A
Benzocaine (11)	A, T
Benzophenone-3 (oxybenzone) (SEDA-22, 170, 172)	A
Benzophenone-4 (sulizobenzone) (SEDA-19, 162)	A
Benzophenone-10 (mexenone) (SEDA-22, 170)	A
Benzydamine (SEDA-18, 164)	A
Bithionol (12)	A
Brilliant lake red	A, T
5-Bromo-4'-chlorsalicylanilide	A
Buclosamide (Jadit)	A, T
Butyl methoxydibenzoylmethane (SEDA-22, 170, 172)	A
Cadmium sulfide	A
Carbimazole (SEDA-10, 131)	A
β-Carotene (SEDA-5, 153)	A
Chloramphenicol (13)	T
Chlorhexidine (14)	A
Chlormercaptodicarboximide	A
Chloro-2-phenylphenol	A
Cinchocaine (dibucaine) (SEDA-5, 155) (SEDA-23, 167)	A
Cinnamates (15)	A
Cinnamic aldehyde (SEDA-8, 153)	A, T
Cinoxate (2-ethoxyethyl-para-methoxycinnamate)	A, T
Clarithromycin (16)	T
Clindamycin (13)	T
Coal tar derivatives (SEDA-8, 160)	A
Coumarin derivatives (SEDA-4, 106)	T
Desoximetasone (SEDA-14, 130)	T
Dibenzthione (sulbentine)	A
Dibromsalan	A
Dichlorophene	A, T
Diclofenac (17)	A
Digalloyl trioleate	A
Dimethoxane	A
Dimethoxydibenzoylmethane	A, T
Diphenhydramine hydrochloride (18,19)	A, T
Doxepin (SEDA-19, 159)	A
Dyes, for example methylthioninium chloride, fluorescein (SEDA-15, 150), rose Bengal, acridine orange, acriflavin, neutral red	A
Erythromycin (13)	T
Essential oils: bergamot oil, cedar oil, citron oil, lavender oil, lime oil, neroli oil, petitgrain oil, sandalwood oil (SEDA-10, 131) (SEDA-12, 134)	A
Fenofibrate (SEDA-22, 170)	A, T
Fenticlor (SEDA-14, 130)	A
Fepradinol (SEDA-23, 167)	T?
Fluorouracil	A
Formaldehyde (SEDA-19, 162)	T
Furocoumarins (20)	A
Glyceryl para-aminobenzoic acid (SEDA-10, 131)	A
Hexachlorophene (21)	A
Homosalate (homomenthyl salicylate) (22)	A
Hydrocortisone (23)	A
Isoamyl-para-methoxycimamate (SEDA-22, 172)	A
Isobutyl para-aminobenzoic acid	A, T
Isopropyl dibenzoylmethane (SEDA-22, 172)	A, T
Ketoprofen (SEDA-22, 170) (24)	A
Lithiol red-CA (D and C Red No. 11)	T
5-Methoxypsoralen (SEDA-23, 167)	A, T
8-Methoxypsoralen (methoxsalen) (SEDA-15, 150) (SEDA-17, 187)	A, T
4-Methylbenzylidene camphor (SEDA-22, 172)	A
6-Methylcoumarin (SEDA-17, 187)	A
Minoxidil (SEDA-11, 139)	A, T
Musk ambrette (SEDA-15, 150)	A
Musk moskene (25)	A
Musk xylene (26)	A
Mycanodin (27)	A
Octyl dimethyl PABA (SEDA-19, 161)	A
Octyl methoxycinnamate (SEDA-22, 172)	A
PABA (para-aminobenzoic acid and derivatives) (SEDA-22, 172)	A
Paraphenylenediamine (18)	A, T
Permanent orange (D and C Orange No. 17)	A
Phenothiazines (28)	A
Phenylbenzimidazole sulfonic acid (SEDA-22, 172)	A
2-Phenyl-5-methylbenzoxazole (Witisol)	A
Piroxicam (SEDA-15, 150) (24)	A
Procaine hydrochloride	A
Selenium disulfide (SEDA-16, 157)	?
Sulfanilamide (29)	A, T
Sulfisoxasole (30)	T
Suprofen (SEDA-18, 164) (24)	A
Tar (31)	T
Tetrachlorosalicylanilide (12)	A, T
Tetracyclines (13)	T
Tiaprofenic acid (SEDA-15, 150) (24)	A, T
Thiocolchicoside (32)	A
Toluidine red (D and C Red No. 35)	A
Tribromsalan (12)	A, T
Triclocarban (14)	A, T
Triclosan (12)	A, T
Zinc pyrithione	A?

A = photoallergy; T = phototoxicity

References

1. Rietschel RL, Fowler JF Jr, editors. Fisher's Contact Dermatitis. 4th ed. Baltimore: Williams and Wilkins, 1995.
2. De Groot AC, Weyland JW, Nater JP. Unwanted Effects of Cosmetics and Drugs used in Dermatology. 3rd ed. Amsterdam: Elsevier, 1994.
3. Schauder S, Ippen H. Contact and photocontact sensitivity to sunscreens. Review of a 15-year experience and of the literature. Contact Dermatitis 1997;37(5):221–32.
4. Dromgoole SH, Maibach HI. Sunscreening agent intolerance: contact and photocontact sensitization and contact urticaria. J Am Acad Dermatol 1990;22(6 Pt 1):1068–78.
5. British Photodermatology Group. Photopatch testing—methods and indications. Br J Dermatol 1997;136(3):371–6.
6. Neumann NJ, Holzle E, Plewig G, Schwarz T, Panizzon RG, Breit R, Ruzicka T, Lehmann P. Photopatch testing: the 12-year experience of the German, Austrian, and Swiss photopatch test group. J Am Acad Dermatol 2000;42(2 Pt 1):183–92.
7. Vassileva SG, Mateev G, Parish LC. Antimicrobial photosensitive reactions. Arch Intern Med 1998;158(18):1993–2000.
8. Rycroft RJG, Frosch PJ, Menne T, editors. Textbook of Contact Dermatitis. 3rd ed. Springer-Verlag, 1999.
9. Goday Bujan JJ, Garcia Alvarez-Eire GM, Martinez W, del Pozo J, Fonseca E. Photoallergic contact

dermatitis from aceclofenac. Contact Dermatitis 2001; 45(3):170.

10. Przybilla B, Schwab-Przybilla U, Ruzicka T, Ring J. Phototoxicity of non-steroidal anti-inflammatory drugs demonstrated in vitro by a photo-basophil-histamine-release test. Photodermatol 1987;4(2):73–8.

11. Allen JE. Drug-induced photosensitivity. Clin Pharm 1993;12(8):580–7.

12. Durbize E, Vigan M, Puzenat E, Girardin P, Adessi B, Desprez PH, Humbert PH, Laurent R, Aubin F. Spectrum of cross-photosensitization in 18 consecutive patients with contact photoallergy to ketoprofen: associated photoallergies to non-benzophenone-containing molecules. Contact Dermatitis 2003;48(3):144–9.

13. Smilack JD, Wilson WR, Cockerill FR 3rd. Tetracyclines, chloramphenicol, erythromycin, clindamycin, and metronidazole. Mayo Clin Proc 1991;66(12):1270–80.

14. Hasan T, Jansen CT. Photopatch test reactivity: effect of photoallergen concentration and UVA dosaging. Contact Dermatitis 1996;34(6):383–6.

15. Cook N, Freeman S. Photosensitive dermatitis due to sunscreen allergy in a child. Australas J Dermatol 2002; 43(2):133–5.

16. Parkash P, Gupta SK, Kumar S. Phototoxic reaction due to clarithromycin. J Assoc Physicians India 2002; 50:1192–3.

17. Montoro J, Rodriguez M, Diaz M, Bertomeu F. Photoallergic contact dermatitis due to diclofenac. Contact Dermatitis 2003;48(2):115.

18. Horio T. Allergic and photoallergic dermatitis from diphenhydramine. Arch Dermatol 1976;112(8):1124–6.

19. Lim HW, Young L, Hagan M, Gigli I. Delayed phase of hematoporphyrin-induced phototoxicity: modulation by complement, leukocytes, and antihistamines. J Invest Dermatol 1985;84(2):114–17.

20. Gregersen AB, Thestrup-Pedersen K, Paulsen E. Fytofotodermatit forarsaget af Moses' braendende busk. [Phytodermatitis caused by burning bush of Moses.] Ugeskr Laeger 2003;165(23):2400–1.

21. Tronnier H. Photoallergie und Photosensibilisierung durch Kosmetika. [Photoallergy and photosensitization due to cosmetics.] Med Klin 1971;65(11):510–14.

22. Gerberick GF, Ryan CA. Contact photoallergy testing of sunscreens in guinea pigs. Contact Dermatitis 1989;20(4):251–9.

23. Rietschel RL. Photocontact dermatitis to hydrocortisone. Contact Dermatitis 1978;4(6):334–7.

24. Warin RP, Smith RJ. Chronic urticaria. Investigations with patch and challenge tests. Contact Dermatitis 1982;8(2):117–21.

25. Parker RD, Buehler EV, Newmann EA. Phototoxicity, photoallergy, and contact sensitization of nitro musk perfume raw materials. Contact Dermatitis 1986; 14(2):103–9.

26. Bruze M, Gruvberger B. Contact allergy to photoproducts of musk ambrette. Photodermatol 1985; 2(5):310–14.

27. Burckhardt W, Mahler F, Schwarz-Speck M. Photoallergische Ekzeme durch Mycanodin. [Mycanodin induced eczematid photoallergy.] Dermatologica 1968; 137(4):208–15.

28. Neumann NJ, Lehmann P. The photopatch test procedure of the German, Austrian, and Swiss photopatch test group. Photodermatol Photoimmunol Photomed 2003; 19(1):8–10.

29. Jung EG, Schwarz K. Photoallergy to "jadit" with photo cross-reactions to derivative of sulfanilamide. Int Arch Allergy Appl Immunol 1965;27(5):313–17.

30. Chetty GN, Kamalam A, Thambiah AS. Acquired structural defects of the hair. Int J Dermatol 1981;20(2):119–21.

31. Plantin P. [Question of the month: should coal-tar be forbidden?] Ann Dermatol Venereol 1997;124(2):205–7.

32. Foti C, Vena GA, Angelini G. Photocontact allergy due to thiocolchicoside. Contact Dermatitis 1992;27(3):201–2.

Succimer

General Information

Succimer is the meso isomer of 2,3-dimethylmercapto-succinic acid (DMSA). It is used as a lead chelator for oral administration (1). Nausea, vomiting, diarrhea, and anorexia are common. Rashes, sometimes necessitating withdrawal, have been reported in up to 10% of adults and 5% of children, and mild transient rises in serum transaminase activity in 6–10% (mostly adults) (2,3). Life-threatening hyperthermia occurred on two occasions in one subject, but no details were given. Iron can be safely and effectively given to patients taking succimer, which (unlike dimercaprol) does not appear to deplete iron stores or to form a toxic chelate that would preclude the parenteral administration of iron (3).

The manufacturers have accumulated data on about 200 children treated with succimer, of whom about 10% had an adverse event (1). Gastrointestinal symptoms and raised serum transaminases were most frequently observed.

In a UK study, single oral doses of succimer or dimercaptopropane sulfonic acid in different combinations with or without acetylcysteine and potassium citrate were given to 191 patients considered to have mercury toxicity from amalgam dental fillings (4). After a single dose, about 5% of patients complained of mild gastrointestinal discomfort, fatigue, mental fuzziness, headache, and diuresis. These usually cleared within 6 hours of the dose and were considered to be due to heavy metal mobilization. There were no cases of hypersensitivity.

Organs and Systems

Hematologic

Mild to moderate neutropenia (5) and episodes of granulocytopenia, possibly related to succimer, have been reported (1,6).

In animals thrombocytopenia has occurred (7).

References

1. Glotzer DE. The current role of 2,3-dimercaptosuccinic acid (DMSA) in the management of childhood lead poisoning. Drug Saf 1993;9(2):85–92.

2. Mann KV, Travers JD. Succimer, an oral lead chelator. Clin Pharm 1991;10(12):914–22.

3. Anonymous. Drug reviews from the Formulary. Succimer Hosp Pharm 1991;26:974–6.
4. Hibberd AR, Howard MA, Hunnisett AG. Mercury from dental amalgam fillings: studies on oral chelating agents for assessing and reducing mercury burdens in humans. J Nutr Environ Med 1998;8:219–31.
5. Mann KV, Travers JD. Succimer, an oral lead chelator. Clin Pharm 1992;11:388.
6. Besunder JB, Anderson RL, Super DM. Short-term efficacy of oral dimercaptosuccinic acid in children with low to moderate lead intoxication. Pediatrics 1995; 96(4 Pt 1):683–7.
7. Marcus SM, Ruck B. Use of succimer. Clin Pharm 1992;11(5):387–8.

Sucralfate

General Information

Sucralfate, a basic aluminium salt of sucrose octasulfate, probably acts by binding to inflamed surfaces; it is possible, however, that its binding properties are more generalized, and it has been used as an intra-alimentary phosphate-binding agent in uremic patients.

Organs and Systems

Metal metabolism

Plasma aluminium concentrations rise in patients with renal insufficiency and one might expect aluminium to accumulate with long-term use of sucralfate (1); it is therefore unwise to use sucralfate in such patients (2).

Gastrointestinal

Bezoar formation has been recorded more than once in patients taking sucralfate, with esophageal obstruction by inspissated drug (SEDA-17, 421) (SEDA-18, 374) (3), and a gastric bezoar can be formed when tube feeds include sucralfate; the formation of bezoars reflects the binding of sucralfate to protein in the food. The French System of Pharmacovigilance on sucralfate has reported bezoars in 16 adults and five neonates (4). All the children were of low birth weights and developed bezoars in the stomach. The adults developed esophageal bezoars around nasogastric tubes. The risk factors for bezoar formation were severe illness, gut hypomotility, dehydration, overdosage with sucralfate, and nasogastric tube feeding. At a pH below 4, there is extensive polymerization of sucralfate, and a sticky viscid gel is formed, which may lead to the formation of a bezoar. In view of this, it has been recommended that sucralfate be used with caution in premature babies and in adults in intensive care who are being fed via a nasogastric tube.

Drug–Drug Interactions

Digoxin

Sucralfate may reduce the absorption of digoxin (5).

Fluoroquinolone antibiotics

The absorption of all fluoroquinolones is significantly impaired when they are co-administered with sucralfate (6).

In a man with prostatitis, co-administration of ciprofloxacin and sucralfate resulted in treatment failure, presumably because of impaired absorption of ciprofloxacin (7).

In an open, randomized, crossover study in 127 healthy volunteers, sucralfate 2 g reduced the AUC of a single oral dose of gemifloxacin 320 mg by 53% and the C_{max} by 69% (8). However, sucralfate had no effect when it was given 2 hours after gemifloxacin.

In two separate crossover studies in eight healthy volunteers sucralfate 1 g reduced the systemic availability of both norfloxacin 400 mg and ofloxacin 400 mg (9). However, sucralfate had no effect when it was given 2 hours after the antibiotics.

Phenytoin

In nine healthy subjects sucralfate reduced the AUC of a single oral dose of phenytoin 500 mg by 10% (10), and in another study it reduced the AUC of a single dose of phenytoin 300 mg by 20% (11). However, in six healthy volunteers sucralfate 1 g qds for 7 days had no effect on steady-state serum phenytoin concentrations (12).

Quinidine

Sucralfate may reduce the absorption of quinidine (5).

Warfarin

Concurrent sucralfate treatment has been claimed to reduce warfarin systemic availability (SEDA-12, 945) (5).

References

1. Leung AC, Henderson IS, Halls DJ. Dobbie JW. Aluminium hydroxide versus sucralfate as a phosphate binder in uraemia. BMJ 1989;286(6375):1379–81.
2. Marks IN. Sucralfate—safety and side effects. Scand J Gastroenterol Suppl 1991;185:36–42.
3. Anderson W, Weatherstone G, Veal C. Esophageal medication bezoar in a patient receiving enteral feedings and sucralfate. Am J Gastroenterol 1989;84(2):205–6.
4. Guy C, Ollagnier M. Sucralfate et bézoars: bilan de l'enquête officielle de pharmacovigilance et revue de la littérature. [Sucralfate and bezoars: data from the system of pharmacologic vigilance and review of the literature.] Therapie 1999;54(1):55–8.
5. Rey AM, Gums JG. Altered absorption of digoxin, sustained-release quinidine, and warfarin with sucralfate administration. DICP 1991;25(7–8):745–6.
6. Marchbanks CR. Drug–drug interactions with fluoroquinolones. Pharmacotherapy 1993;13(2 Pt 2):S23–8.

7. Spivey JM, Cummings DM, Pierson NR. Failure of prostatitis treatment secondary to probable ciprofloxacin–sucralfate drug interaction. Pharmacotherapy 1996;16(2):314–16.

8. Allen A, Bygate E, Faessel H, Isaac L, Lewis A. The effect of ferrous sulphate and sucralfate on the bioavailability of oral gemifloxacin in healthy volunteers. Int J Antimicrob Agents 2000;15(4):283–9.

9. Lehto P, Kivisto KT. Effect of sucralfate on absorption of norfloxacin and ofloxacin. Antimicrob Agents Chemother 1994;38(2):248–51.

10. Hall TG, Cuddy PG, Glass CJ, Melethil S. Effect of sucralfate on phenytoin bioavailability. Drug Intell Clin Pharm 1986;20(7–8):607–11.

11. Smart HL, Somerville KW, Williams J, Richens A, Langman MJ. The effects of sucralfate upon phenytoin absorption in man. Br J Clin Pharmacol 1985;20(3):238–40.

12. Malli R, Jones WN, Rindone JP, Labadie EL. The effect of sucralfate on the steady-state serum concentrations of phenytoin. Drug Metabol Drug Interact 1989;7(4):287–93.

Sufentanil

General Information

Sufentanil, a fentanyl analogue, is a highly lipid-soluble synthetic opioid with high affinity for OP_3 (μ) opioid receptors and a potency some 5–10 times that of fentanyl. It is a short-acting analgesic.

Its adverse effects include pruritus, sedation, nausea and vomiting, dizziness, urinary retention, light-headedness, miosis, and shivering (SEDA-16, 86). Respiratory depression also occurs (SEDA-21, 89). Motor neuron blockade, acute hypotension, and muscle weakness are rare, affecting under 1% of patients (SEDA-16, 86).

Drug studies

Placebo-controlled studies

In 41 patients undergoing abdominal hysterectomy randomly allocated in a double-blind, controlled study to sufentanil 50 micrograms for 8–16 hours via a lumbar epidural catheter before or at the end of surgery, the pre-emptive group ($n = 20$) used less sufentanil than the control group ($n = 21$) (1). The frequency of adverse effects was similar in the two groups; nine patients in the pre-emptive group and ten in the control group complained of nausea or vomiting and four patients in the pre-emptive group and five patients in the control group complained of mild pruritus.

Comparative studies

Bupivacaine

Intrathecal sufentanil and epidural bupivacaine were compared individually and in combination to establish dose-responsiveness for analgesia in labor in 100 women (2). There was no dose-responsiveness for doses of sufentanil between 2 and 10 micrograms. The ED_{50} for sufentanil was 2.3 micrograms alone (higher than that reported

above (3)) and 0.85 micrograms in combination with epidural bupivacaine. Adverse effects included pruritus (incidence 70–90%), nausea, and mild somnolence (10–30%). Transient fetal bradycardia was reported in two cases.

In a double-blind, randomized, placebo-controlled study in 80 patients of the analgesic efficacy of different subarachnoid applications of sufentanil and/or bupivacaine using a microcatheter for easy postoperative pain relief, sufentanil 10 micrograms, bupivacaine 5 mg, or a combination of sufentanil 2.5 micrograms and bupivacaine 2.5 mg provided immediate and adequate postoperative analgesia for 2–3 hours (4). The group who received only sufentanil had the highest incidence of pruritus and respiratory depression. The limitations of this study were highlighted in a letter, which questioned the value of the above procedure when other tried and tested perioperative pain management methods are available (5).

Clonidine

In a double-blind study of the effect of clonidine on intrathecal sufentanil, 53 nulliparous women received sufentanil 5 micrograms intrathecally either alone or with clonidine 30 micrograms (6). The addition of clonidine increased the incidence of hypotension (12% with sufentanil alone, 63% with clonidine) and sedation (23% with sufentanil alone and 46% with clonidine). There was no significant difference in the incidence of pruritus (88%). Again, no motor blockade was observed.

In another randomized, double-blind study in 40 primiparous women in labor at less than 5 cm cervical dilatation who requested epidural analgesia, the addition of clonidine 75 micrograms to epidural sufentanil 20 micrograms did not provide any advantages in analgesic efficacy or adverse effects (7).

Dextrose

The addition of 3.5% dextrose to sufentanil 10 micrograms given intrathecally in a randomized, double-blind study of 48 women in early labor produced a significant reduction in the incidence of clinically important pruritus (8). Dextrose did not compromise the quality and duration of analgesia.

Lidocaine

The analgesic efficacy of intrathecal sufentanil with or without lidocaine has been examined in two groups of outpatients undergoing lithotripsy or gynecological laparoscopy in order to determine optimal analgesia with rapid recovery and discharge (9,10). In a retrospective case-record study of 62 shock-wave lithotripsy procedures, the 25 cases performed using intrathecal sufentanil alone had better outcomes, significantly shorter post-anesthesia care unit time, and time for ambulation compared with 37 procedures performed with intrathecal lidocaine; pruritus was significantly more common with sufentanil (9). A double-blind, randomized study in 13 patients undergoing gynecological laparoscopy, who received either lidocaine 10 mg with sufentanil 10 micrograms or intrathecal sufentanil 20 micrograms, was terminated early owing to unacceptably frequent adverse effects and inferior analgesia in those given intrathecal sufentanil (10).

Piritramide

Sufentanil 1 microgram/ml plus 0.1% ropivacaine by epidural infusion has been compared with intravenous patient-controlled analgesia with piritramide in a double-blind, randomized study in 24 patients undergoing elective total hip replacement (11). The PCA group had significantly more adverse effects than the epidural group, including hypotension, nausea, and vomiting. There were no cases of respiratory depression, pruritus, hypertension, or dysrhythmias in either group. Epidural sufentanil was a better analgesic.

Combination studies

Adrenaline

In a randomized, double-blind, controlled study, the addition of adrenaline (100 micrograms/ml) significantly reduced the incidence of sedation and light-headedness after epidural sufentanil (40 micrograms) in 43 women who received epidural analgesia during early labor (12). However, adrenaline did not help in preventing maternal oxygen desaturation.

Bupivacaine

In a prospective dose-finding study, 170 women with cervical dilatation of 3–5 cm were randomized to receive intrathecal sufentanil 0, 2.5, 5.0, 7.5, or 10 micrograms combined with bupivacaine 5 mg (13). Bupivacaine combined with 2.5 micrograms sufentanil provided analgesia comparable to higher doses with a lower incidence of nausea and vomiting and less severe pruritus.

Bupivacaine and adrenaline

In a randomized, double-blind study in 243 parturients who received three doses of sufentanil (0.5, 0.75, and 1 microgram/ml) in combination with bupivacaine 0.625 mg/ml and adrenaline 1.25 micrograms/ml by continuous epidural infusion there were no differences in analgesic effects, but there was significantly more pruritus in those who received the highest dose of sufentanil (14). The authors suggested using the lowest dose of sufentanil (0.5 micrograms/ml) with bupivacaine solution to minimize the risk of adverse effects on the mother and neonate, with optimal analgesia.

Ropivacaine

In a randomized, double-blind study in 120 patients undergoing major abdominal surgery the combination of sufentanil 0.75 micrograms/ml with ropivacaine 0.2% provided optimal postoperative patient-controlled epidural analgesia with the fewest adverse effects of the regimens used (ropivacaine alone, ropivacaine and sufentanil 0.5, 0.75, or 1.00 microgram/ml) (15).

Organs and Systems

Cardiovascular

The incidence of hypotension with sufentanil is 7% and that of hypertension 3%. In a double-blind comparison of

morphine, pethidine, fentanyl, and sufentanil in balanced anesthesia, patients who received sufentanil had the least hemodynamic disturbances. In high doses, adverse effects such as bradycardia and hypotension can lead to complications in some patients (SEDA-16, 85). Sudden hypotension occurred on induction of anesthesia with sufentanil in four patients, in whom the dose was 8.4–22.7 micrograms/kg (16). Other workers noted similar findings at doses of 1 and 1.5 micrograms/kg.

Clinically significant bradycardia or asystole occurred on induction when sufentanil was used in conjunction with vecuronium (17,18).

The effect of sufentanil was examined in 10 healthy men to find out whether it has the same hemodynamic and sensory effects as when it is used in women in labor. Details of the method of recruitment of volunteers for this double-blind study were not provided, but they received either saline or sufentanil 10 micrograms intrathecally (19), and blood pressure, heart rates, oxyhemoglobin saturation, cold and pinprick sensation, motor block, and visual analogue scales for sedation pruritus and nausea were all measured. Pruritus and sensory changes to pinprick and cold occurred only in the sufentanil group and there were no significant hemodynamic changes in either group. In view of the frequency and severity of pruritus when sufentanil is used in labor, it is interesting that all five of the male volunteers experienced this symptom, three of them severely. These findings suggested that the hypotension observed with the use of intrathecal sufentanil during labor and the sensory changes may not be mediated by the same pathway. The authors proposed that the hypotension observed in such studies is a direct result of pain relief, which is not an issue in the pain-free men in this investigation.

Respiratory

Apneic episodes have been reported in patients given sufentanil (SEDA-20, 81) (SEDA-21, 89). Respiratory arrest occurred 55 minutes after epidural and intrathecal sufentanil and bupivacaine (SEDA-18, 82).

- A healthy 22-year-old woman at 41 weeks gestation presented for urgent cesarean section following fetal heart rate deceleration (20). She was given sufentanil 10 micrograms plus 0.1% bupivacaine 10 mg intrathecally and 8 minutes later became unrousable and apneic. After 3 minutes spontaneous ventilation resumed.

The authors suggested that giving the local anesthesia first and then the sufentanil later might have contributed to this presentation of spontaneous reversal of short-lived early-onset respiratory arrest.

When nasal sufentanil was used to induce anesthesia in children, ventilatory compliance was mildly or markedly reduced and one child required suxamethonium, oxygen, and positive pressure ventilation (SEDA-16, 86).

Respiratory depression has also been described after intrathecal sufentanil 5 micrograms (21).

- An 83-year-old woman scheduled for bilateral knee replacement surgery received midazolam 7.5 mg preoperatively. Continuous spinal anesthesia was planned, with combined general anesthesia.

Anesthesia was maintained with 0.3–0.5% of inspired isoflurane in 36% oxygen and 70% nitrous oxide while 5 mg of 0.5% bupivacaine was introduced into the subarachnoid space via an insertion at L3–4. Anesthesia extended to T11. During the procedure two top-up doses of bupivacaine 2.5 mg were administered. Postoperatively she was extubated immediately and was fully conscious on transfer to the recovery room, but 75 minutes later she had violent pain in both knees and received sufentanil 5 micrograms intrathecally. Analgesia was achieved in 10 minutes. At 15 minutes pruritus occurred and at 30 minutes she became unresponsive to verbal and painful stimuli and stopped breathing. Blood pressure was 120/60 mmHg, heart rate 72/minute, and oxygen saturation 97%. Ventilation with 100% oxygen via a facemask started immediately and naloxone 160 micrograms was injected intravenously, with full recovery of consciousness and respiration in 10 minutes.

This report is the first of respiratory depression after intrathecal sufentanil in a non-obstetric patient. Previous obstetric cases had occurred earlier and with larger doses of sufentanil. The site of action of sufentanil in this case is likely to have been supraspinal, by either direct cephalad migration in the CSF or through a systemic effect after vascular absorption.

Respiratory arrest has been reported in labor (22).

• A 20-year-old parturient received sufentanil 10 micrograms and bupivacaine 2.5 mg intrathecally as part of combined spinal-epidural analgesia and developed pruritus 15 minutes after the injection, followed by a sleepy feeling at 20 minutes. After 25 minutes she became unresponsive and apneic; her systolic blood pressure was 130 mmHg and her heart rate 60. The fetal heart rate was 86. She was ventilated manually with 100% oxygen and naloxone 0.4 mg was given with prompt recovery of consciousness and respiratory effort. Drowsiness persisted, and a naloxone infusion was initiated after top-up doses of naloxone had failed to relieve it. Subsequent analgesia was with bupivacaine alone. A vacuum-assisted vaginal delivery was performed after 3 hours. The infant's Apgar score was 8 at 1 minute and 9 at 5 minutes. The mother and baby were subsequently well.

This case highlights the low doses at which arrest may occur.

Violent coughing in young children and adolescents exposed to small doses of sufentanil (1 microgram/kg or less) has been reported (23). Specific cases were not alluded to and the literature remains divided on the significance and mechanism of this age-related effect.

Nervous system

An unexpected transient neurological deficit has been described in neurosurgical patients (SEDA-16, 85).

There have been three reports of neurological changes after the intrathecal administration of sufentanil plus bupivacaine (24,25).

• A 40-year-old pregnant woman developed acute confusion, aphasia, increased salivation, and difficulty in swallowing 15 minutes after intrathecal

administration of sufentanil 10 micrograms with bupivacaine 2.5 mg (25). There was spontaneous resolution 1 hour later with no need for pharmacological intervention.

• An 18-year-old nulliparous woman with an uncomplicated pregnancy developed difficulty in swallowing, respiratory abnormalities, and excessive tiredness 13 minutes after receiving sufentanil 5 micrograms with bupivacaine 1.25 mg as a spinal analgesic and disappearing over 20 minutes (24).

• A 36-year-old nulliparous woman complained of dyspnea and sensory block extending to the face 15 minutes after an intrathecal injection of sufentanil 5 micrograms with bupivacaine 1.25 mg (24).

In neither of the last two cases was there motor blockade or neonatal sequelae. Such adverse effects can be caused by sufentanil, bupivacaine, or both. Regardless of which drug caused these events, the intrathecal administration of a hypobaric solution to a patient in the sitting position might have contributed, since rostral spread of intrathecal drugs is accelerated in this setting. The use of smaller doses of sufentanil (2.5 or 5 micrograms) will also prevent such adverse effects.

Musculoskeletal

There have been isolated reports of chest wall rigidity after sufentanil (26).

Second-Generation Effects

Pregnancy

The effects of intrathecal and epidural sufentanil as an analgesic during labor have been described in 50 nulliparous patients in a randomized double-blind study, in which they received sufentanil 1–10 micrograms in preservative-free saline (27). The ED_{50} was 1.8 micrograms, based on those who requested further analgesia after 30 minutes. The incidence of adverse effects was similar in all groups (that is was not dose-related in this dosage range) and included pruritus of a similar intensity in all groups. There was no respiratory depression, but blood pressure and oxygen saturation fell. Other adverse effects included changes in temperature sensitivity at 30 minutes in 19 of the 50 subjects. One woman who received 5 micrograms of sufentanil had a fall in oxygen saturation to 90–92% with a respiratory rate of 16 breaths/minute 10–15 minutes after injection, but recovered spontaneously at 20 minutes. Fetal monitoring showed no significant bradycardia and there were no significant differences in 5-minute Apgar scores. It was suggested that hypotension was due to the effect of intrathecal opioid rather than to an effect on the autonomic nervous system and that the temperature sensitivity changes were due to a concentration-dependent local anesthetic effect of opioids. A drop in oxygen saturation in one subject indicated the need for observation for respiratory changes when sufentanil is given intrathecally.

Combined spinal epidural analgesia has been associated with reports of increased operative deliveries, possibly due to reduced perineal sensation and motor weakness. In a comparison of combined spinal epidural analgesia (intrathecal sufentanil 10 micrograms followed by epidural bupivacaine and fentanyl at their next request for analgesia) with intravenous pethidine analgesia (50 mg intravenously on demand up to a maximum of 200 mg in 4 hours) in 1223 randomly assigned healthy parturients there was no significant difference in the rates of cesarean delivery for dystocia (28). Maternal hypotension and pruritus requiring treatment occurred in 14% and 17% respectively of patients who received combined spinal epidural analgesia. Fetal heart rate deceleration occurred in 21% of patients who received pethidine compared with 18% of patients who received combined spinal epidural analgesia, and in each group most cases resolved spontaneously. However, profound fetal bradycardia (fetal heart rate of less than 60/minute, lasting 60 seconds or more), necessitating emergency cesarean section, occurred within 1 hour of administration of sufentanil in 8 of 400 mothers, while no such events occurred with pethidine. None of the cases responded to conservative management and none was associated with maternal hypotension. Immediate postnatal neonatal outcomes were similar between the two groups, as judged by Apgar scores and umbilical artery blood gases. These findings are significant, in that an increase in cesarean deliveries due to fetal bradycardia has not previously been reported, but findings in this study must be regarded with an element of caution, as fetal monitoring was more extensive in those given combined spinal epidural analgesia. The authors suggested that fetal bradycardia might have been due to uterine hyperstimulation, associated with intrathecal opioids (although they did not consistently monitor for this), and that fetal bradycardia resulted from reduced placental perfusion secondary to uterine tetany. Alternatively, since sufentanil is highly lipid soluble, it can be detectable in plasma within 39 minutes of intrathecal administration of 15 micrograms. Once in the plasma, transplacental transfer can occur and the drug can have a direct vagotonic effect on the fetus. However, they believed that the most probable explanation for the bradycardia was a direct consequence of hypoperfusion of the placenta secondary to maternal hypotension, although they pointed out that none of their cases was associated with this hemodynamic change in the mother.

In a double-blind, randomized study the analgesic efficacy of sufentanil 0.25 micrograms/ml with 0.125% bupivacaine was compared with fentanyl 2 micrograms/ml with 0.125% bupivacaine in 226 patients in labor with a patient-controlled epidural analgesic device (29). Overall analgesia was good, with no observed difference between the two groups. There was a significant difference in the occurrence of mild pruritus, with 10 cases in the fentanyl group ($n = 105$) and only two in the sufentanil group ($n = 101$). There were no gastrointestinal adverse effects. Sufentanil was deemed preferable owing to a lower incidence of adverse effects for equal analgesic potency.

An epidural mixture of sufentanil with ropivacaine has been used in a double-blind, randomized study in 100 women in the first stage of labor (30). They were randomized to receive 0.2% ropivacaine 12 mg either alone or with sufentanil 5, 10, or 15 micrograms. With combined sufentanil plus ropivacaine the duration of analgesia was about 40 minutes longer than with ropivacaine alone. There were no differences in analgesic efficacy or the incidence of opioid-related adverse effects in the three sufentanil groups. Sufentanil 5 micrograms plus ropivacaine 0.2% was therefore recommended.

Fetotoxicity

When epidural sufentanil is used for labor and delivery, the neonates can have subtle neurological signs of drug depression, including mild hypotonia, poor primary reflexes, and poor habituation to repeated stimuli at 1 and 4 hours of life (SEDA-16, 86).

The absence of motor block associated with combined spinal epidural analgesia using sufentanil has also been reported in an investigation in which intrathecal sufentanil 10 micrograms was compared with epidural lidocaine, adrenaline, and sufentanil 40 micrograms in early labor (31). Adverse effects were not significantly different between the groups, except for more frequent and severe pruritus in the intrathecal group. Although three subjects in each group had transient changes in fetal heart rate within 30 minutes of medication, no intervention was necessary.

Drug Administration

Drug dosage regimens

In a dose-finding, prospective, double-blind study, 60 men scheduled for unilateral extracorporeal shock-wave lithotripsy were randomized to receive 12.5, 15, 17.5, or 20 micrograms of intrathecal sufentanil (32). The results suggested that 15 micrograms of sufentanil may be the optimal intrathecal dose, since 20 micrograms produced significantly more pruritus than the lower doses and those who were given 12.5 micrograms needed significantly more supplementary analgesia.

Drug administration route

Serious consequences (respiratory arrest and hypotension) related to the use of intrathecal sufentanil have been described in parturients (SEDA-22, 101).

References

1. Akural EI, Salomaki TE, Tekay AH, Bloigu AH, Alahuhta SM. Pre-emptive effect of epidural sufentanil in abdominal hysterectomy. Br J Anaesth 2002; 88(6):803–8.
2. Camann W, Abouleish A, Eisenach J, Hood D, Datta S. Intrathecal sufentanil and epidural bupivacaine for labor analgesia: dose-response of individual agents and in combination. Reg Anesth Pain Med 1998; 23(5):457–62.
3. Duthie DJ. Remifentanil and tramadol. Br J Anaesth 1998;81(1):51–7.
4. Standl TG, Horn E, Luckmann M, Burmeister M, Wilhelm S, Schulte am Esch J. Subarachnoid sufentanil for early postoperative pain management in orthopedic patients: a placebo-controlled, double-blind study using spinal microcatheters. Anesthesiology 2001;94(2):230–8.

5. Gebhard RE, Fanelli G, Matuszczak M, Doehn M. Subarachnoid sufentanil for early postoperative pain management in orthopedic patients: more disadvantages than benefits? Anesthesiology 2001;95(6):1531–3.

6. Mercier FJ, Dounas M, Bouaziz H, Des Mesnards-Smaja V, Foiret C, Vestermann MN, Fischler M, Benhamou D. The effect of adding a minidose of clonidine to intrathecal sufentanil for labor analgesia. Anesthesiology 1998;89(3):594–601.

7. Connelly NR, Mainkar T, El-Mansouri M, Manikantan P, Venkata RR, Dunn S, Parker RK. Effect of epidural clonidine added to epidural sufentanil for labor pain management. Int J Obstet Anesth 2000;9(2):94–8.

8. Abouleish AE, Portnoy D, Abouleish EI. Addition of dextrose 3.5% to intrathecal sufentanil for labour analgesia reduces pruritis. Can J Anaesth 2000;47(12):1171–5.

9. Nelson CP, Francis TA, Wolf JS Jr. Comparison of shockwave lithotripsy outcomes in patients receiving sufentanil or lidocaine spinal anesthesia. J Endourol 2001;15(5):473–7.

10. Henderson CL, Schmid J, Vaghadia H, Fowler C, Mitchell GW. Selective spinal anesthesia for outpatient laparoscopy. III: sufentanil vs lidocaine–sufentanil. Can J Anaesth 2001;48(3):267–72.

11. Kampe S, Randebrock G, Kiencke P, Hunseler U, Cranfield K, Konig DP, Diefenbach C. Comparison of continuous epidural infusion of ropivacaine and sufentanil with intravenous patient-controlled analgesia after total hip replacement. Anaesthesia 2001;56(12):1189–93.

12. Armstrong KP, Kennedy B, Watson JT, Morley-Forster PK, Yee I, Butler R. Epinephrine reduces the sedative side effects of epidural sufentanil for labour analgesia. Can J Anaesth 2002;49(1):72–80.

13. Wong CA, Scavone BM, Loffredi M, Wang WY, Peaceman AM, Ganchiff JN. The dose-response of intrathecal sufentanil added to bupivacaine for labor analgesia. Anesthesiology 2000;92(6):1553–8.

14. Eriksson SL, Frykholm P, Stenlund PM, Olofsson C. A comparison of three doses of sufentanil in combination with bupivacaine–adrenaline in continuous epidural analgesia during labour. Acta Anaesthesiol Scand 2000;44(8):919–23.

15. Brodner G, Mertes N, Van Aken H, Mollhoff T, Zahl M, Wirtz S, Marcus MA, Buerkle H. What concentration of sufentanil should be combined with ropivacaine 0.2% wt/vol for postoperative patient-controlled epidural analgesia? Anesth Analg 2000;90(3):649–57.

16. Spiess BD, Sathoff RH, el-Ganzouri AR, Ivankovich AD. High-dose sufentanil: four cases of sudden hypotension on induction. Anesth Analg 1986;65(6):703–5.

17. Starr NJ, Sethna DH, Estafanous FG. Bradycardia and asystole following the rapid administration of sufentanil with vecuronium. Anesthesiology 1986;64(4):521–3.

18. Dobson JAR, Davies JM, Hodgson GH. Bradycardia after sufentanil and vecuronium. Can J Anaesth 1988;35:S121.

19. Riley ET, Hamilton CL, Cohen SE. Intrathecal sufentanil produces sensory changes without hypotension in male volunteers. Anesthesiology 1998;89(1):73–8.

20. Kehl F, Erfkamp S, Roewer N. Respiratory arrest during caesarean section after intrathecal administration of sufentanil in combination with 0.1% bupivacaine 10 ml. Anaesth Intensive Care 2002;30(5):698–9.

21. Fournier R, Gamulin Z, Van Gessel E. Respiratory depression after 5 micrograms of intrathecal sufentanil. Anesth Analg 1998;87(6):1377–8.

22. Katsiris S, Williams S, Leighton BL, Halpern S. Respiratory arrest following intrathecal injection of sufentanil and bupivacaine in a parturient. Can J Anaesth 1998;45(9):880–3.

23. Yemen TA, Bennet JA, Abrams J, Van Riper DF, Horrow JC. Small doses of sufentanil will produce violent coughing in young children. Anesthesiology 1998;89(1):271–2.

24. Abdou WA, Aveline C, Bonnet F. Two additional cases of excessive extension of sensory blockade after intrathecal sufentanil for labor analgesia. Int J Obstet Anesth 2000;9(1):48–50.

25. Fragneto RY, Fisher A. Mental status change and aphasia after labor analgesia with intrathecal sufentanil/bupivacaine. Anesth Analg 2000;90(5):1175–6.

26. Goldberg M, Ishak S, Garcia C, McKenna J. Postoperative rigidity following sufentanil administration. Anesthesiology 1985;63(2):199–201.

27. Arkoosh VA, Cooper M, Norris MC, Boxer L, Ferouz F, Silverman NS, Huffnagle HJ, Huffnagle S, Leighton BL. Intrathecal sufentanil dose response in nulliparous patients. Anesthesiology 1998;89(2):364–70.

28. Gambling DR, Sharma SK, Ramin SM, Lucas MJ, Leveno KJ, Wiley J, Sidawi JE. A randomized study of combined spinal-epidural analgesia versus intravenous meperidine during labor: impact on cesarean delivery rate. Anesthesiology 1998;89(6):1336–44.

29. Le Guen H, Roy D, Branger B, Ecoffey C. Comparison of fentanyl and sufentanil in combination with bupivacaine for patient-controlled epidural analgesia during labor. J Clin Anesth 2001;13(2):98–102.

30. Debon R, Allaouchiche B, Duflo F, Boselli E, Chassard D. The analgesic effect of sufentanil combined with ropivacaine 0.2% for labor analgesia: a comparison of three sufentanil doses. Anesth Analg 2001;92(1):180–3.

31. Dunn SM, Connelly NR, Steinberg RB, Lewis TJ, Bazzell CM, Klatt JL, Parker RK. Intrathecal sufentanil versus epidural lidocaine with epinephrine and sufentanil for early labor analgesia. Anesth Analg 1998;87(2):331–5.

32. Lau WC, Green CR, Faerber GJ, Tait AR, Golembiewski JA. Determination of the effective therapeutic dose of intrathecal sufentanil for extracorporeal shock wave lithotripsy. Anesth Analg 1999;89(4):889–92.

Sulfamazone

See also Non-steroidal anti-inflammatory drugs

General Information

Sulfamazone is a pyrazolone derivative. It causes benign intracranial hypertension in children (SEDA-5, 100) (1).

Reference

1. Laverda AM, Casara GL, Furlannt M, et al. Ipertensione endocranica acuta benigna da sulfafenazone. Riv Ital Pediatr 1981;7:83.

Sulfinpyrazone

General Information

Sulfinpyrazone, a pyrazolone derivative, is used both as a uricosuric agent and as an anti-platelet drug. It has similar adverse effects to those of phenylbutazone when taken for long term (SEDA-6, 104). In a large number of patients who took the drug for secondary prevention of myocardial infarction (an indication that was not subsequently accepted), the incidence of adverse effects was not high (1).

Organs and Systems

Respiratory

Sulfinpyrazone can precipitate bronchoconstriction in some aspirin-sensitive patients (2). There is no cross-sensitivity with dipyrone.

Hematologic

Prolonged treatment with sulfinpyrazone produces a high incidence of thrombocytopenia and granulocytopenia. After withdrawal, these effects are completely reversible (SED-9, 157) (3). Sulfinpyrazone also inhibits platelet aggregation (4).

Sulfinpyrazone has been implicated in the development of myelomonocytic leukemia and multiple myeloma when given with colchicine (3).

Urinary tract

Impairment of renal function and even acute renal insufficiency can follow sulfinpyrazone treatment, by various mechanisms: immunoallergic-induced acute interstitial nephritis, inhibition of renal prostaglandins, and precipitation of uric acid stones. These changes are probably reversible, since there have been cases in which renal impairment spontaneously normalized on withdrawal (5).

Susceptibility Factors

The antinatriuretic effects of sulfinpyrazone could be dangerous in patients with impaired cardiac function (6).

Drug–Drug Interactions

Aspirin

In low dosages (up to 2 g/day), aspirin reduces urate excretion and blocks the effects of sulfinpyrazone. In higher dosages (over 5 g/day), salicylates increase urate excretion.

Beta-blockers

Sulfinpyrazone interferes with the antihypertensive action of beta-blockers (7).

Phenylbutazone

Sulfinpyrazone has a biphasic interaction with phenylbutazone (enhancement followed by antagonism).

Warfarin

By reducing the metabolic clearance of warfarin, sulfinpyrazone enhances its hypoprothrombinemic effect, with life-threatening consequences (8).

References

1. Sherry S. The Anturan reinfarction trial. New Engl J Med 1980;303:50.
2. Szczeklik A, Czerniawska-Mysik G, Nizankowska E. Sulfinpyrazone and aspirin-induced asthma. N Engl J Med 1980;303(12):702–3.
3. Witwer MW, Schmid FR, Tesar JT. Acute myelomonocytic leukaemia and multiple myeloma after sulphinpyrazone and colchicine treatment of gout. BMJ 1976;2(6027):89.
4. Schwartz AD, Pearson HA. Aspirin, platelets, and bleeding. J Pediatr 1971;78(3):558–60.
5. Durham DS, Ibels LS. Sulphinpyrazone-induced acute renal failure. BMJ (Clin Res Ed) 1981;282(6264):609.
6. Hauselmann HJ, Studer H. Antinatriuretische Wirkung von Sulphinpyrazon. [Antinatriuretic effect of sulfinpyrazone.] Schweiz Med Wochenschr 1981;111(27–28):1030.
7. Brater DC. Drug–drug and drug–disease interactions with nonsteroidal anti-inflammatory drugs. Am J Med 1986;80(1A):62–77.
8. Bailey RR, Reddy J. Potentiation of warfarin action by sulphinpyrazone. Lancet 1980;1(8162):254.

Sulfites and bisulfites

See also Disinfectants and antiseptics

General Information

Sulfites and bisulfites have been used extensively as preservatives in the food industry and also in drugs and bronchodilator inhalant solutions (1,2) as preservatives. Sodium metabisulfite is used commonly as an antioxidant in foods and drugs. As an additive in various pharmaceutical products, metabisulfite can cause unpleasant adverse reactions.

Organs and Systems

Respiratory

Status asthmaticus and acute bronchospasm have been linked to the use of metabisulfites (3).

Hematologic

Preservatives in subconjunctival gentamicin were identified as the cause of conjunctival chemosis and capillary closure (4). Patients undergoing cataract surgery were divided into three groups: one was given a subconjunctival injection of a preservative-free solution of gentamicin at the end of the cataract procedure, another received a subconjunctival injection of gentamicin containing sodium metabisulfite and disodium edetate as preservatives, and the third was the control group not given a subconjunctival injection. There was a significant difference in the severity of conjunctival chemosis between patients who received gentamicin with and without preservatives (4).

Immunologic

The major symptoms of an adverse reaction to a sulfite are flushing, acute bronchospasm, and hypotension (SED-11, 492) (SEDA-10, 232) (SEDA-11, 221) (5). The incidence of sulfite sensitivity in an asthmatic population is estimated at about 10%. Sulfites have therefore been withdrawn from the composition of several medicines intended for asthmatic patients.

Metabisulfite-induced anaphylaxis through an IgE-mediated mechanism has been described in a patient who developed urticaria, angioedema, and nasal congestion following provocative challenge with sodium metabisulfite (6).

The presence of sodium metabisulfite as an antioxidant in commercial lidocaine with adrenaline significantly increased discomfort during injection (7).

Anaphylactic shock occurring during epidural anesthesia for cesarean section has been attributed to sodium metabisulfite (8).

Reports of contact allergy to topical medicaments containing sodium metabisulfite are rare (9). In two cases, a topical corticosteroid formulation that contained sodium metabisulfite (Trimovate cream) caused contact allergy; patch tests were positive with both sodium metabisulfite and Trimovate cream (10).

References

1. Gunnison AF, Jacobsen DW. Sulfite hypersensitivity. A critical review. CRC Crit Rev Toxicol 1987;17(3):185–214.
2. Monafo WW, West MA. Current treatment recommendations for topical burn therapy. Drugs 1990;40(3):364–73.
3. Maria Y, Vaillant P, Delorme N, Moneret-Vautrin DA. Les accidents graves liés aux metabisulfites. [Severe complications related to metabisulfites.] Rev Med Interne 1989;10(1):36–40.
4. Pande M, Ghanchi F. The role of preservatives in the conjunctival toxicity of subconjunctival gentamicin injection. Br J Ophthalmol 1992;76(4):235–7.
5. Chan TY, Critchley JA. Is chloroxylenol nephrotoxic like phenol? A study of patients with DETTOL poisoning. Vet Hum Toxicol 1994;36(3):250–1.
6. Sokol WN, Hydick IB. Nasal congestion, urticaria, and angioedema caused by an IgE-mediated reaction to sodium metabisulfite. Ann Allergy 1990;65(3):233–8.
7. Long CC, Motley RJ, Holt PJ. Taking the "sting" out of local anaesthetics. Br J Dermatol 1991;125(5):452–5.
8. Soulat JM, Bouju P, Oxeda C, Amiot JF. Choc anaphylactoide aux metabisulfites au cours d'une césarienne sous anesthésie péridurale. [Anaphylactoid shock due to metabisulfites during cesarean section under peridural anesthesia.] Cah Anesthesiol 1991;39(4):257–9.
9. Heshmati S, Maibach HI. Active sensitization to sodium metabisulfite in hydrocortisone cream. Contact Dermatitis 1999;41(3):166–7.
10. Tucker SC, Yell JA, Beck MH. Allergic contact dermatitis from sodium metabisulfite in Trimovate cream. Contact Dermatitis 1999;40(3):164.

Sulfonamides

General Information

The term "sulfonamide" is generic for derivatives of para-aminobenzenesulfonamide (sulfanilamide), which is similar in structure to para-aminobenzoic acid (PABA), a co-factor required by bacteria for folic acid synthesis. The sulfonamides act by competitive inhibition of the incorporation of PABA into tetrahydropteroic acid. Sulfonamides have a higher affinity for the microbial enzyme tetrahydropteroic acid synthetase than the natural substrate PABA. Sulfonamides have a wide range of antimicrobial activity against both Gram-positive and Gram-negative organisms (1). In therapeutic dosages they have only a bacteriostatic effect, and as single agents therefore have a limited role in drug therapy (1). Sulfonamides have been combined with trimethoprim or trimethoprim analogues, since such combinations result in a bactericidal effect (2). Adverse reactions during the administration of sulfamethoxazole + trimethoprim (co-trimoxazole, BAN) can be due to either compound. Although sulfonamides are thought to cause adverse reactions more often than trimethoprim, the culprit in the individual patient can only be determined by re-exposure to the individual agents.

Based on their pharmacological properties and clinical uses, sulfonamides can be classified into four groups (1):

1. short- or medium-acting sulfonamides;
2. long-acting sulfonamides;
3. topical sulfonamides;
4. sulfonamide derivatives used for inflammatory bowel disease.

Short- or medium-acting sulfonamides include the earliest varieties of azosulfonamides (Prontosil, Neoprontosil), sulfapyridine (Dagenan), sulfathiazole (Cibazol), sulfanilamide, and sulfadiazine. With the exception of sulfadiazine, these compounds are no longer used. Sulfadiazine and more recent compounds, including sulfafurazole (sulfisoxazole), sulfamethoxazole, sulfametrole, sulfacitine, and sulfamethizole, are rapidly absorbed and rapidly eliminated. Compared with the older generation they are more soluble, less toxic, and probably less allergenic. Sulfamethoxazole is a medium-acting sulfonamide that is often combined with trimethoprim (as co-trimoxazole). Long-acting sulfonamides include sulfametoxydiazine, sulfadimethoxine, and other compounds, of which many are no longer available, as they were associated with severe hypersensitivity reactions. Although these compounds have the advantage of long administration intervals, their long half-lives (over 100 hours) can be deleterious in case of adverse reactions. A long-acting drug that is still widely used is sulfadoxine (*N*-(5,6-dimethoxy-4-pyrimidinyl)-sulfanilamide). It is primarily used in combination with pyrimethamine (Fansidar) for the treatment and prophylaxis of malaria.

The topical use of sulfonamides has been discouraged, because of the high risk of sensitization. Nevertheless, sulfacetamide and sulfadicramide are still used topically for eye infections. Topical silver sulfadiazine (see monograph on Silver) is widely and successfully used in treating burns and leg ulcers (3,4). Since sulfonamides are easily absorbed through skin lesions, the same adverse reactions can occur as after systemic use.

A sulfonamide derivative with special use is sulfasalazine (salicylazosulfapyridine), which has been widely used to treat ulcerative colitis and regional ileitis (Crohn's disease). It is a compound of sulfapyridine and 5-aminosalicylate, linked by a diazo bond. Sulfasalazine is broken down in the large bowel to sulfapyridine, which is absorbed systemically, and 5-aminosalicylate, which reaches high concentrations in the feces (5). Sulfasalazine is not used for the antibacterial properties of the sulfapyridine, but for the local anti-inflammatory effect of 5-aminosalicylate in the gut. Because most of the adverse reactions are thought to be due to the absorbed sulfapyridine, the combination has largely been replaced in clinical practice by newer drugs that contain only 5-aminosalicylic acid (mesalazine), such as mesalazine itself and diazosalicylate (olsalazine) (5). The aminosalicylates are covered in a separate monograph.

Observational studies

In an open trial in 25 patients treated with sulfamethoxypyridazine (1 g/day) for mucous membrane pemphigoid unresponsive to topical steroid treatment, 12% of patients were withdrawn, 4% because of allergic reactions, the others because of significant hemolysis (6).

In children with acute uncomplicated *Plasmodium falciparum* malaria, pyrimethamine + sulfadoxine (25 mg + 500 mg) and artesunate (4 mg/kg) were well tolerated, and no adverse reactions attributable to treatment were recorded (7).

Comparative studies

In a randomized, open, multicenter study in 46 patients with sight-threatening ocular toxoplasmosis, those who took pyrimethamine + sulfadiazine had significantly more adverse events, especially malaise, than those who took pyrimethamine + azithromycin (8).

General adverse effects

The frequency and severity of the adverse effects of sulfonamides correspond to those seen with other antibacterial agents (2–5%). Dose-related effects, which tend to be more troublesome than serious, include gastrointestinal symptoms, headache, and drowsiness. Crystalluria can occur, but urinary obstruction is rare. Hematological adverse effects due to folic acid antagonism occur primarily in combination with trimethoprim. Hemolytic anemia occurs in patients with enzyme deficiencies and abnormal hemoglobins. Hypersensitivity

is thought to be the mechanism of many adverse effects of the sulfonamides. They can be life-threatening, and immediate withdrawal is recommended. The most important reactions include anaphylactic shock, a serum sickness-like syndrome, systemic vasculitis, severe skin reactions (Stevens–Johnson syndrome and toxic epidermal necrolysis), pneumonitis, hepatitis, and pancytopenia. Sulfonamides should not be used in the third trimester of pregnancy. In premature infants, they displace bilirubin from plasma albumin and can cause kernicterus. Carcinogenicity has not been reported with the use of sulfonamides.

Sulfanilamide and the history of adverse drug reactions

The first major drug catastrophe in the 20th century history of the public control of drugs occurred in 1937 in the USA. A pharmacist introduced Elixir Sulfanilamide, which consisted of sulfanilamide dissolved in diethylene glycol. It had been tested for flavor, appearance, and fragrance, but not for safety. After taking the drug, over 100 patients died in severe pain; many were children, who were given Elixir Sulfanilamide for sore throats and coughs. Public outrage created support for proposed legislation to reinforce the public control of drugs that was pending in the US Congress (9). This led to the US 1938 Food, Drug, and Cosmetic Act, which is still the country's legal foundation for the public control of drugs and devices intended for use in the diagnosis, cure, mitigation, treatment, or prevention of disease in humans or animals. It has been a model for similar legislation in many other countries.

The 1938 Food, Drug, and Cosmetic Act prohibited traffic in new drugs, unless they were safe for use under the conditions of use prescribed on their labels. The Act also explicitly required the labeling of drug products with adequate directions for use.

The burden of proof of harm of new drugs was laid on the Federal Food and Drug Agency (FDA). Companies that wanted to manufacture and sell new drugs in interstate commerce had to investigate their safety and report to the FDA. Unless the FDA, within a specified period of time, found that the safety of a drug had not been established, the company could proceed with its marketing. The FDA was also authorized to remove from the market any drug it could prove to be unsafe (10).

The US Supreme Court also established in 1941, in a legal case over drug adulteration, that responsible individuals in a company can be held personally accountable for the quality of the products manufactured by the company, and that distributors of pharmaceuticals are responsible for the quality of their products, even if they are manufactured elsewhere (11).

After World War II, the pharmaceuticals market changed radically, as many companies started industrial production of drugs that had previously been manufactured in pharmacies. Announcements of new industrially produced drugs were hailed as part of technological advancement, as significant a sign of progress as the launching of satellites and putting a man on the moon. However, public safeguards against the risks of drugs remained unchanged in most countries. Thus, control of the effects of drugs largely lay in the hands of the manufacturers, even though the responsibility for taking precautions rested with pharmacists and doctors.

Organs and Systems

Cardiovascular

Of 98 patients with drug-induced long QT interval, one taking sulfamethoxazole carried a single-nucleotide polymorphism (SNP; found in about 1.6% of the general population) in KCNE2, which encodes MinK-related peptide 1 (MiRP1), a subunit of the cardiac potassium channel I_{Kr} (12). Channels with the SNP were normal at baseline but were inhibited by sulfamethoxazole at therapeutic concentrations, which did not affect wild-type channels.

Cardiovascular reactions can be due to sulfonamide myocarditis or systemic vascular collapse, owing to severe adverse events such as widespread skin disease. Sulfonamide myocarditis has been described in relation to earlier sulfonamides and occurs in combination with other hypersensitivity reactions (13).

Respiratory

Respiratory reactions to sulfonamides include migratory pulmonary infiltrates, chronic pneumonia, asthma, and pulmonary angiitis. These reactions are thought to be mainly due to hypersensitivity, although the precise mechanisms are not well understood (14–16). The link to the drug has been proven in most cases by recurrence after re-exposure to the same sulfonamide or to co-trimoxazole.

Pulmonary reactions have been described with most sulfonamides. Pyrimethamine + sulfadoxine, used in malaria prophylaxis and treatment, also rarely causes pulmonary reactions (17–19). The sulfapyridine moiety of sulfasalazine, used in inflammatory bowel disease, can produce adverse pulmonary reactions (20).

The time between the last drug exposure and the first clinical symptoms varies from hours to a few days, and the lung pathology disappears in most patients within a few days after withdrawal. Most commonly, pulmonary involvement presents with fever, dyspnea, cough, and shortness of breath. Clinical examination reveals râles in the lungs, and there may be pulmonary infiltrates in the chest X-ray. Pulmonary function tests may show bronchial obstruction (18–21), and arterial blood gases show hypoxemia (19,20). Whereas bronchial obstruction is probably an immediate reaction (type I), pulmonary infiltrates may correspond to a type III reaction, similar to the mechanism responsible for extrinsic allergic alveolitis (20,21). Eosinophilia is present in 8–58% of cases (14,16,18,19,21,22). Histologically, the lung tissue is infiltrated by inflammatory cells, and in most cases the alveoli contain numerous macrophages and eosinophils in a protein-rich edema fluid.

Based on the predominant symptoms and their duration, four categories of sulfonamide-related pulmonary hypersensitivity reactions can be distinguished (23–25):

1. transient or migratory pulmonary infiltrations associated with eosinophilia (Loeffler's syndrome) (22,26–28)
2. chronic eosinophilic pneumonia (23,27)
3. asthma with pulmonary eosinophilia (14–16,21)
4. allergic angiitis with pulmonary involvement (25).

In the first three of these, the adverse reaction is limited to the lung, whereas in the fourth the lung involvement is part of a systemic reaction. Syndromes such as allergic granulomatosis and angiitis (Churg–Strauss syndrome) or Wegener's granulomatosis are not associated with the use of sulfonamides (25).

Nervous system

Neurological disturbances that have been attributed to sulfonamides include polyneuritis, neuritis, and optic neuritis (29,30). Tremor and ataxia have been described with co-trimoxazole (31,32). Aseptic meningitis can be separately caused by sulfonamides and trimethoprim. The occurrence of meningitis has been verified in most patients, with recurrence on re-exposure (33–42).

Sensory systems

Eyes

Drug induced uveitis is rare. Antibiotics that have been implicated include rifabutin and sulfonamides. Furthermore, nearly all antibiotics injected intracamerally have been reported to produce uveitis (43). Topical administration of a corticosteroid and a cycloplegic (such as atropine) is suitable as initial treatment. Withdrawal of causative drugs is not always necessary (44).

Transient myopia can be caused by topical or systematic sulfonamides (45–47).

Corneal ring formation has been described simultaneously with an erythematous skin rash in a patient known to have skin hypersensitivity (48).

Taste

In unmedicated young and elderly volunteers and HIV-infected patients, sulfamethoxazole applied to the tongue was described as sour by young subjects but bitter by elderly subjects (49).

Psychological, psychiatric

Headache, drowsiness, lowered mental acuity, and other psychiatric effects can be caused by sulfonamides (50). However, these adverse effects are rare, and the causative role of the drug is usually not clearly established.

Metabolism

Several sulfonamides, including co-trimoxazole in high doses, can produce hyperchloremic metabolic acidosis. This has even been seen in patients with extensive burns receiving topical mafenide (51). Mafenide (Sulfamylon) and its metabolite *para*-sulfamoylbenzoic acid inhibit carbonic acid anhydrase, resulting in reduced reabsorption of bicarbonate and thus bicarbonate wasting.

Electrolyte balance

Although co-trimoxazole in therapeutic doses can cause hyperkalemia (52), it is thought to be caused by the potassium-sparing effects of trimethoprim (53).

Hematologic

Sulfonamides have adverse effects on all bone marrow–derived cell lines. The resulting disturbances include hemolytic anemia, folate deficiency anemia, neutropenia, thrombocytopenia, and pancytopenia. While adverse effects on erythrocytes are rare, the rates of leukopenia, neutropenia, and thrombocytopenia are highly variable. In a hospital drug monitoring program, leukopenia or neutropenia occurred in 0.4% of 1809 patients treated with co-trimoxazole (54), and thrombocytopenia of mild-to-moderate degree in 0.1% (54,55), similar to figures recorded in other studies (56,57). Pancytopenia is an extremely rare form of adverse reaction to sulfonamides (58).

There were similar findings in children (59). It is generally believed that trimethoprim is primarily responsible for neutropenia due to co-trimoxazole.

Severe neutropenia often occurs in HIV-infected patients taking co-trimoxazole (60). It seems to be due to either folic acid deficiency or immunological mechanisms.

Erythrocytes

Sulfonamides rarely have adverse effects on erythrocytes. However, there are various mechanisms by which sulfonamide-induced hemolytic anemia can occur (61):

- abnormally high blood concentrations, due to large doses or reduced excretion of the drug in patients with renal disease (62)
- acquired hypersusceptibility, as reflected by the development of a positive Coombs' test (63,64)
- genetically determined abnormalities of erythrocyte metabolism, for example deficiency of glucose-6-phosphate dehydrogenase or of diaphorase (65,66)
- the presence of an abnormal, so-called "unstable", hemoglobin in the erythrocyte, for example hemoglobin Zürich (67,68), hemoglobin Torino (69), hemoglobin Hasharon (70), and hemoglobins H and M (66).

Simple and readily available in vitro methods have been used to demonstrate the pathogenetic mechanisms, including Coombs' test, Harris's test (71), a quantitative assay or screening for glucose-6-phosphate dehydrogenase activity after recovery (72,73), a test for Heinz bodies, the buffered isopropanol technique (74) to detect abnormal hemoglobins, and hemoglobin electrophoresis (61,66). The direct antiglobulin (Coombs') test can be negative in spite of an immune mechanism. If such a mechanism is suspected and the direct Coombs' test is negative, the indirect Coombs' test on the patient's serum with the addition of the suspected sensitizing agent can be of diagnostic value (75). Heinz bodies in the erythrocytes can be important for early differentiation of a sulfonamide-induced reaction, which could further progress to hemolytic anemia (76). This result can also be of help in distinguishing this from other kinds of anemia.

Sulfonamides are not directly associated with folate deficiency and megaloblastic anemias. Sulfasalazine can affect the absorption of folates, but inflammatory bowel disease can also be responsible for reduced folate absorption. Only in combination with trimethoprim are sulfonamides thought to deplete folate stores in patients with pre-existing deficiency of folate or vitamin B_{12} (77).

Leukocytes

Since the days when chloramphenicol was more commonly used, it has been recognized that many antimicrobial drug are associated with severe blood dyscrasias, such as aplastic anemia, neutropenia, agranulocytosis, thrombocytopenia, and hemolytic anemia. Information on this association has come predominantly from case series and hospital surveys (78–80). Some evidence can be extracted from population-based studies that have focused on aplastic anemia and agranulocytosis and their association with many drugs, including antimicrobial drugs (81,82). The incidence rates of blood dyscrasias in the general population have been estimated in a cohort study with a nested case-control analysis, using data from a General Practice Research Database in Spain (83). The study population consisted of 822 048 patients aged 5–69 years who received at least one prescription (in all 1 507 307 prescriptions) for an antimicrobial drug during January 1994 to September 1998. The main outcome measure was a diagnosis of neutropenia, agranulocytosis, hemolytic anemia, thrombocytopenia, pancytopenia, or aplastic anemia. The incidence was 3.3 per 100 000 person-years in the general population. Users of antimicrobial drugs had a relative risk (RR), adjusted for age and sex, of 4.4, and patients who took more than one class of antimicrobial drug had a relative risk of 29. Among individual antimicrobial drugs, the greatest risk was with cephalosporins (RR = 14), followed by the sulfonamides (RR = 7.6) and penicillins (RR = 3.1).

Agranulocytosis was not infrequent in the early sulfonamide era. The first cases were observed in association with sulfanilamide (84,85), Prontosil (84), sulfapyridine (85,86), sulfathiazole (87), sulfadiazine (87), and sulfasalazine (88). Even with topical silver sulfadiazine, agranulocytosis as a consequence of systemic absorption has been reported (89).

Special observations in patients with agranulocytosis favor an immunological/allergic mechanism rather than a toxic one. Several points justify this view:

1. the sulfonamide is well tolerated by most patients during the initial phase of treatment
2. sulfonamide concentrations in the serum, when determined, are not particularly high in patients with hematological complications
3. in some patients, skin rash, fever, and arthritis start concomitantly with or even before the appearance of leukopenia or agranulocytosis
4. re-exposure to a single dose can be followed by a second episode of severe agranulocytosis
5. an agglutinin for leukocytes has been identified in patients' serum shortly after withdrawal of the drug (86)
6. using in vitro techniques, positive reactions to the drug with the lymphocyte transformation test or inhibition of colony growth in bone marrow have been found (90,91); however, the results of lymphocyte transformation tests must be interpreted with caution—sometimes they are positive in patients who have been exposed to the drug without any evidence of a hypersensitivity reaction.

Platelets

Reports of drug-induced thrombocytopenia have been systematically reviewed (78). Among the 98 different drugs described in 561 articles the following antibiotics were found with level I (definite) evidence: co-trimoxazole, rifampicin, vancomycin, sulfisoxazole, cefalotin, piperacillin, methicillin, novobiocin. Drugs with level II (probable) evidence were oxytetracycline and ampicillin.

In another retrospective analysis of drug-induced thrombocytopenia reported to the Danish Committee on Adverse Drug Reactions, 192 cases caused by the most frequently reported drugs were included and analysed (92). There were pronounced drug-specific differences in the clinical appearance. Early thrombocytopenia was characteristic of cases caused by sulfonamides and co-trimoxazole. These drugs also often caused hemorrhage. Accompanying leukopenia was observed in some cases associated with co-trimoxazole. There were no patient-specific factors responsible for the heterogeneity of the clinical appearance, and factors related to the physician seemed to be of little significance.

Acute thrombocytopenia is rarely associated with the newer sulfonamides (4,93,94). The structurally related sulfonylureas and thiazide diuretics can also cause allergic thrombocytopenia (95). Although some in vitro tests have been reported to predict the occurrence of thrombocytopenia, none of these has been used routinely (96,97). Furthermore, a negative test result with a drug does not definitely exclude it as the responsible allergen.

Mouth

Salivary gland enlargement on repeated exposure to sulfafurazole (sulfisoxazole) has been described (98).

Gastrointestinal

Nausea, vomiting, and anorexia occur in a few patients taking sulfonamides (1). They are usually related to dosage, the disposition of the individual patient, and how the question concerning adverse effects is asked.

Liver

Increased activities of alanine transaminase and aspartate transaminase to over five times the upper limit of the reference range were reported in a randomized trial of sulfadiazine in toxoplasmic encephalitis (99).

Co-trimoxazole-induced hepatitis has been repeatedly reported. However, trimethoprim alone can also cause acute liver injury (100). Three forms of liver injury may be related to sulfonamides:

1. hepatitis of the hepatocellular type (101–105)
2. hepatitis of the mixed hepatocellular type accompanied by cholestatic features (106)
3. chronic active hepatitis, possibly leading to cirrhosis (107).

The number of cases of sulfonamide hepatitis published annually fell markedly after 1947, with the introduction of the newer short-acting derivatives (106).

Children can also be affected by drug-induced liver disease (108).

Hitherto, the connection with a sulfonamide has always been investigated by administering a test dose. Immunological in vitro methods that show sensitization to the drug, for example the lymphocyte transformation test, are of limited value. In some patients the hepatic injury develops in connection with a general reaction, such as serum sickness-like syndrome, generalized vasculitis, or rash (109,110). In patients with hypersensitivity, re-exposure can result in generalized malaise, nausea, back pain, and chills within one to several hours (103,107). However, symptoms can be delayed for as long as several days (106). Daily monitoring of liver function on re-exposure seems to be important, since subjective signs can be absent despite rising activities of serum transaminases and alkaline phosphatase (102).

Even in patients with chronic active hepatitis, the histopathology of the liver damage was indistinguishable from non-drug-induced pathology. The degree of piecemeal necrosis usually varies from one area to another. Antinuclear factor and lupus erythematosus factor were positive in some cases (107). Early recognition of drug-induced liver disease is of great importance, since liver injury can be completely reversible after withdrawal.

Pancreas

Pancreatitis has been attributed to sulfonamides. Sulfamethizole (34) and sulfasalazine (111) have been implicated by re-exposure. The 5-aminosalicylic acid moiety of sulfasalazine may also be responsible (112,113).

Urinary tract

Renal complications that occur in relation to sulfonamide administration include crystalluria, tubular necrosis, interstitial nephritis, and glomerular lesions as part of a vasculitis syndrome.

Sulfonamides and their metabolites are excreted in large amounts in the urine. They are relatively insoluble in the acid environment and tend to precipitate in the collecting tubules, calyces, and pelvis of the kidney, and possibly in the ureters. The course is typically benign but adequate hydration and alkalinization may be required (114). Nephrocalcinosis can cause hematuria, renal colic, or acute renal insufficiency (115). Urinary obstruction with anuria/oliguria was seen primarily with the earlier, less soluble sulfonamides. With the newer and more soluble sulfonamides crystal formation is rare, as is acute renal insufficiency due to other mechanisms. During recent years renal complications have been seen more often in patients with AIDS, because of the use of large doses of sulfonamides combined with trimethoprim against infection with *Pneumocystis jiroveci* (formerly *Pneumocystis carinii*) or *Toxoplasma* encephalitis. Reduced fluid intake and low urinary pH favor crystal formation, and so both adequate fluid intake (about 2 l/day for adults) and urine alkalinization are encouraged when larger doses of sulfonamides are used (60,115–120). For the diagnosis of sulfonamide crystalluria, the Lignin test is recommended. At room temperature crystals can even be found in the urine of patients taking sulfamethoxazole, which is readily soluble (121).

Other renal complications reported with sulfonamides are:

- acute tubular necrosis or tubulointerstitial nephritis (117,122);
- interstitial nephritis (123), in some cases combined with granulomatous lesions (124,125);
- acute vasculitis (126);
- acute renal insufficiency in association with a serum sickness-like syndrome, generalized vasculitis, or rashes in combination with hepatic damage (109).

Acute anuria or oliguria is often the first symptom, not only in patients with tubular necrosis or tubulointerstitial nephritis, but also in those with allergic vasculitis. Non-oliguric renal insufficiency can also occur. It is not yet clear whether tubular necrosis in association with sulfonamides is a toxic, collateral, or hypersusceptibility reaction. The unstable hydroxylamine metabolites of some sulfonamides can act as direct renal toxins.

In a French analysis of 22 510 urinary calculi performed by infrared spectroscopy, drug-induced urolithiasis was divided into two categories: first, stones with drugs physically embedded ($n = 238$; 1.0%), notably indinavir monohydrate ($n = 126$; 53%), followed by triamterene ($n = 43$; 18%), sulfonamides ($n = 29$; 12%), and amorphous silica ($n = 24$; 10%); secondly, metabolic nephrolithiasis induced by drugs ($n = 140$; 0.6%), involving mainly calcium/vitamin D supplementation ($n = 56$; 40%) and carbonic anhydrase inhibitors ($n = 33$; 24%) (127). Drug-induced stones are responsible for about 1.6% of all calculi in France. Physical analysis and a thorough drug history are important elements in the diagnosis.

Skin

Rashes are common during sulfonamide administration, and the rate increases with duration of therapy. Maculopapular reactions are most common and occur in about 1–3% of patients (128–132). In a survey of 5923 pediatric records, 3.46% of prescriptions for sulfonamides were followed by the development of a rash, although none was severe enough to require hospitalization (133).

Urticaria, fixed drug eruptions (131,134–137), erythema nodosum (138), photosensitivity reactions (139), and generalized skin reactions involving light-exposed areas (139–141) are less common. Topical silver sulfadiazine cause local reactions, consisting of rash, pruritus, or a burning sensation in 2.5% of patients (4,51).

- Fixed drug eruption has been described in a patient treated with the non-thiazide sulfonamide diuretic indapamide; an oral challenge test showed cross-reactivity to sulfamethoxazole and sulfadiazine (142).

Generalized cutaneous depigmentation after sulfamide therapy occurred in a 41-year-old man (143). Melanocytes were not seen on electron microscopy, but there were clear cells with the characteristics of Langerhans cells along the basal layer.

Other skin eruptions seen with sulfonamides include erythema multiforme, vesicular and bullous rashes, and exfoliative dermatitis (144). In erythema multiforme, linear depositions of IgA at the dermoepidermal junction have been suggested to play a pathogenic role (132).

- Linear IgA dermatosis with erythema multiforme-like clinical features has been reported in a 19-year-old man several days after completion of a 5-day-course treatment with sulfadimethoxine (500 mg bd) for a flu-like syndrome (134). Treatment with methylprednisolone (150 mg) with gradual dosage reduction was started. Slow improvement was followed by a flare-up after reduction to 80 mg/day. Therapy was changed to dapsone 100 mg/day, and there was a dramatic improvement.

The most severe skin reactions associated with sulfonamides are the severe forms of erythema multiforme, Stevens–Johnson syndrome, and toxic epidermal necrolysis (144–152). In a study from Cameroon, eight of ten patients with toxic epidermal necrolysis had taken sulfonamides (five sulfadoxine, three sulfamethoxazole); two patients died after taking sulfadoxine (153).

Mortality in drug-induced toxic epidermal necrolysis has been estimated to be about 20–30% (154,155), and in Stevens–Johnson syndrome 1–10% (33,146–148,151). Some severe skin reactions start with a maculopapular rash or generalized erythema. The culprit drug is often either a long-acting formulation or a short-acting drug that has been continued over a long period. In both toxic epidermal necrolysis and Stevens–Johnson syndrome immediate withdrawal of the sulfonamide and all other non-essential drugs is required, as well as adequate supportive therapy with fluids, proteins, and electrolytes, in order to prevent renal insufficiency and respiratory distress syndrome (154,155). Occasionally, toxic epidermal necrolysis must be distinguished from staphylococcal scalded skin syndrome (Lyell's syndrome) by histology. In toxic epidermal necrolysis, there is subepidermal cleavage of the skin at the level of the basal cells, resulting in full-thickness denudation, whereas in scalded skin syndrome the split occurs in the upper epidermis near the granular layer just beneath the stratum corneum (156).

The role of sulfonamides as an etiological factor in the Stevens–Johnson syndrome is extremely difficult to evaluate, except for patients with re-exposure or in situations where the drug was given prophylactically for meningitis (146) or pneumonia (147,148,151,152). In the first epidemiological study in 1968, 100 000 individuals were given prophylactic sulfadoxine (Fanasil) and 997 (1.0%) had skin reactions (146). Of these, about 100 had severe reactions, such as erythroderma with jaundice, Stevens–Johnson syndrome, or toxic epidermal necrolysis; 11 died from these complications, that is about one in 10 000 patients treated with the probably causative drug. It is not known how many would have had similar skin reactions unrelated to the drug. However, the benefit to risk balance of meningitis prophylaxis clearly favored the use of sulfonamides (146). A second report (147) showed an incidence of three cases of Stevens–Johnson syndrome in 480 healthy, newly recruited Bantu mineworkers treated prophylactically with sulfadimethoxine. In a third epidemiological study in Mozambique in 1981, 149 000 inhabitants in one town were given a single dose of sulfadoxine as mass prophylaxis in an attempt to stem an outbreak of cholera (148); 22 patients with typical Stevens–Johnson syndrome were admitted to hospital over 18 days; three died.

In one case toxic epidermal necrolysis caused by co-trimoxazole improved with high-dose methylprednisolone (157). However, previous studies of the use of glucocorticoids in toxic epidermal necrolysis have given contradictory results.

The combination of pyrimethamine and sulfadoxine, used for prophylaxis of chloroquine-resistant malaria (*Plasmodium falciparum*), causes severe skin reactions in one per 5000–8000 users, with fatal reactions in one per 11 000–25 000 users (158). Even at the stage of early rash or generalized erythema, this therapy should be withdrawn (129).

In an open prospective study in 95 HIV-infected patients with successfully treated *Pneumocystis jiroveci* pneumonia, pyrimethamine + sulfadoxine (25/500 mg) was given twice weekly to prevent relapse (159). There were allergic skin reactions in 16 patients, resulting in permanent withdrawal in six. Two patients developed serious adverse reactions (Stevens–Johnson syndrome), both of whom had continued to take prophylaxis despite progressive hypersensitivity reactions.

Most of the cutaneous adverse reactions to sulfonamides are associated with increased in vitro reactivity to sulfonamide metabolites, such as unstable hydroxylamines (160,161). In some cases glutathione deficiency has been proposed as a major mechanism. This seems to be important in patients with AIDS, in whom glutathione deficiency is frequent, and in whom skin rashes are much more common than in other patients (160,162). A predominance of slow acetylator phenotype has also been observed among patients with sulfonamide hypersensitivity reactions, and an association with the phenotypes HLA-A29, B-12, and DR-7 in patients with bullous cutaneous reactions (161,163–165).

A mechanism for generalized drug-induced delayed skin reactions to sulfamethoxazole may be perforin-mediated killing of keratinocytes by drug-specific CD4+ lymphocytes (166). The requirement of interferon gamma pretreatment of keratinocytes for efficient specific killing might explain the increased frequency of drug allergies in generalized viral infections such as HIV, when interferon gamma concentrations are raised.

Immunologic

Sulfa allergy refers to a specific hypersensitivity response to a group of chemicals containing a sulfonamide moiety covalently bound to a benzene ring; drugs structurally similar to sulfonamides may cross-react, for example sulfonylureas, thiazides, and furosemide (167). Sulfa allergy is most consistent with an immune-mediated reaction with delayed onset, 7–14 days after the start of therapy, characterized by fever, rash, and eosinophilia. IgG antibodies may be present and directed against proteins in the endoplasmic reticulum (about 80% of patients) or against the drug covalently bound to protein (about 5% of patients). High-dose methylprednisolone sodium succinate (250 mg every 6 hours for 48 hours) may not only alleviate the signs but also markedly attenuate the antibody response, as reported in a 19-year-old man (168).

Hypersusceptibility to sulfonamides has been proposed to be the mechanism for many adverse reactions, including anaphylactic shock, serum sickness-like syndrome,

systemic allergic vasculitis, drug fever (up to 1–2% in some series), lupus-like syndrome, myocarditis, pulmonary infiltrates, interstitial nephritis, aseptic meningitis, hepatotoxicity, blood dyscrasias (agranulocytosis, thrombocytopenia, eosinophilia, pancytopenia), and a wide variety of skin reactions (urticaria, erythema nodosum, erythema multiforme, erythroderma, toxic epidermal necrolysis, and photosensitivity).

Urticarial and maculopapular rashes are the most frequent adverse reactions to sulfonamides after gastrointestinal symptoms. Although hypersusceptibility is suspected to be the mechanism for these adverse effects, type I allergic reactions, which are induced by IgE antibodies, have been confirmed only rarely. It appears that with the older sulfonamides severe reactions were more frequent. In some patients who have immediate hypersensitivity reactions to sulfonamides, IgE has been found that can bind to an N4-sulfonamidoyl determinant (N4-SM) (169).

Prediction

It is desirable to predict hypersusceptibility reactions to sulfonamides. IgE-induced in vitro reactions to sulfonamides have mainly been studied in the last 15 years (169–171). A lymphocyte toxicity assay showed a positive result in about 70% of patients with a maculopapular rash, an urticarial reaction, or erythema multiforme (172). This biochemical test determines the percent of cell death due to toxic metabolites. The same in vitro reaction using the hydroxylamine metabolite of sulfamethoxazole gave significantly different results in six patients with fever and skin rash with or without hepatitis than in control patients (160). Unfortunately, in most adverse reactions it is not known whether the reaction is dose-related or allergic. Individual differences in metabolism predispose to idiosyncratic reactions, for example sulfonamides are metabolized by N-acetylation (mediated by a genetically determined polymorphic enzyme) and oxidation to potentially toxic metabolites (164,165). Fever and rash were observed significantly more often in slow than in fast acetylators (164,165). Systemic glutathione deficiency, with a consequently reduced capacity to scavenge such toxic metabolites, might contribute to these adverse reactions, particularly in patients with AIDS (173,174). In a child with dihydropteridine reductase deficiency, a variant of phenylketonuria, adverse drug reactions occurred to co-trimoxazole (175). Unfortunately, there are no reliable in vitro tests to predict idiosyncratic reactions in vivo (160,161,164,165,174).

Cross-reactivity

The immunogenicity of sulfonamide antimicrobials may be due to the presence of an arylamine group at the N4 position of the sulfonamide molecule. Thus, allergic cross-reactions between different sulfonamides can occur. Therefore, in cases of known hypersusceptibility to a specific sulfonamide exposure to other sulfonamides should be avoided. Cross-reactions can even occur with *para*-aminosalicylic acid and local anesthetics of the procaine type; however, the real frequency of these cross-sensitivities is not known and their significance is undetermined. It should be noted that as many as 50% of patients with rash have recovered in spite of continued treatment with the same drug (176), and even agranulocytosis did not occur after later re-exposures to the causative agent (162).

Susceptibility factors

In an in vitro study, plasma from HIV-positive patients was less able to detoxify nitrososulfamethoxazole than control plasma, suggesting that a disturbance in redox balance in HIV-positive patients may alter metabolic detoxification capacity, thereby predisposing to sulfamethoxazole hypersensitivity (177).

Types of reaction

Type I reactions

Anaphylactic shock occurs rarely with sulfonamides (160,169,170,178,179). Anaphylaxis to a central venous catheter (ARROWg+ard Blue Catheter) coated with chlorhexidine and sulfadiazine has been reported in a 50-year-old man (180).

Type III reactions

A serum sickness-like syndrome has been observed during sulfonamide administration. This diagnosis should be limited to patients with at least three of the symptoms of classical serum sickness, that is fever, rash, allergic arthritis, lymphadenopathy, and possibly leukopenia or neutropenia. Histologically, severe serum sickness-like syndrome seems to correspond to an allergic vasculitis (126,181). Most of the descriptions of serum sickness-like syndrome with histopathological documentation have been associated with older sulfonamides that are no longer used (182). In some severe forms of serum sickness-like syndrome, the reaction can be complicated by a number of unusual organ manifestations, including plasmacytosis, lymphocytosis, monoclonal gammopathy (183,184), interstitial myocarditis (13,33), allergic pneumonitis, nephropathy, liver damage, and nervous system disorders (126,181).

Lupus-like syndromes

Sulfonamides can cause three different clinical and biological syndromes similar or identical to systemic lupus erythematosus (185,186):

1. exacerbation of pre-existing lupus erythematosus
2. triggering of lupus erythematosus in a susceptible patient
3. serum sickness-like syndrome resembling lupus erythematosus clinically and serologically.

There may be positive LE cells and antinuclear factors. In exacerbation or triggering of lupus erythematosus, two pathogenetic mechanisms may be involved:

1. a reaction to the pharmacological properties of the drug, such as occurs with other drugs, such as hydralazine, diphenylhydantoin, procainamide, isoniazid, and practolol (185–190);
2. a hypersensitivity reaction (186,191,192).

In type I reactions, exposure time, and especially re-exposure time, are usually longer than 1–2 months. In type II reactions, exposure is more variable, lasting from hours to

days or up to 1–2 months (185–187). Some patients with ulcerative colitis have developed arthropathy, possibly polyserositis, hematological abnormalities, and even loss of consciousness with positive LE cell and antinuclear antibody tests during treatment with sulfasalazine (187,189).

Diagnosis

No diagnostic tests are available to confirm sulfonamide hypersensitivity, and while avoidance of the drug is generally appropriate when a previous hypersensitivity reaction is suspected, desensitization protocols are available for use in HIV patients in whom *Pneumocystis jiroveci* pneumonia prophylaxis or treatment is indicated (193).

Desensitization

Desensitization has been tried with sulfonamides and especially co-trimoxazole. Desensitization with the combination seems to be essential in patients with AIDS, since co-trimoxazole is the first choice against *Pneumocystis jiroveci* pneumonia and toxoplasmosis. Desensitization is successful in 75% of patients with AIDS (194–196). However, the procedure is not completely safe and even anaphylactic shock can occur (170).

Body temperature

Drug fever due to sulfonamides is usually accompanied by a skin reaction; however, fever without other manifestations can occur (164,165).

Long-Term Effects

Drug resistance

Salmonella typhimurium DT104 is usually resistant to ampicillin, chloramphenicol, streptomycin, sulfonamides, and tetracycline. An outbreak of 25 culture-confirmed cases of multidrug-resistant *S. typhimurium* DT104 has been identified in Denmark (197). The strain was resistant to the abovementioned antibiotics and nalidixic acid and had reduced susceptibility to fluoroquinolones. A swineherd was identified as the primary source (197). The DT104 strain was also found in cases of salmonellosis in Washington State, and soft cheese made with unpasteurized milk was identified as an important vehicle of its transmission (198).

Second-Generation Effects

Fertility

Male infertility with oligospermia has been reported during treatment with sulfasalazine (199,200). However, inflammatory bowel disease can also affect the maturation of spermatozoa (201).

Teratogenicity

The sulfonamides appear to have little if any effect on early human development. This is indicated by the absence of case reports or epidemiological survey data during pregnancy. In one study of 50 282 mother–child pairs, 1455 were exposed to sulfonamides during the first 4 months; there was no increase in the relative risk of any malformation (202,203).

Malaria during pregnancy is associated with an increased risk of severe anemia and babies of low birth weight. Effective intermittent therapy with pyrimethamine + sulfadoxine reduces parasitemia and severe anemia and improves birth weight in areas in which *Plasmodium falciparum* is sensitive to this combination. In an open, prospective trial in 287 pregnant women in the Gambia who were exposed to a single dose of a combination of artesunate and pyrimethamine + sulfadoxine there was no evidence of a teratogenic or otherwise harmful effect (204).

Fetotoxicity

Sulfonamides should not be given to pregnant women in the third trimester of pregnancy. They can displace bilirubin from plasma albumin and cause kernicterus (bilirubin encephalopathy) (205–208). For the same reason, the administration of sulfonamides to lactating women or premature infants should be avoided. Successful treatment of neonatal hyperbilirubinemia with higher bilirubin concentrations has been established using exchange transfusion and phototherapy.

Susceptibility Factors

Genetic factors

The acetylator phenotype of a patient can affect the frequency and severity of adverse reactions to drugs that are metabolized by acetylation (66,164,165).

In patients with porphyria, sulfonamides should not be used (209).

Other features of the patient

Although patients with HIV infection are more likely to develop generalized skin reactions to sulfonamides, they can be used for prophylaxis and therapy.

Relative contraindications to sulfonamides are systemic lupus erythematosus and a known predisposition to lupus-like reactions. Allergic reactions to antimicrobials are frequent in patients with Sjögren's syndrome. They are especially susceptible to reactions to penicillins, cephalosporins, and sulfonamides, but reactions to macrolides and tetracyclines also seem to be over-represented in these patients (210).

Drug Administration

Drug administration route

Sulfacetamide sodium (Albucid) in solutions stronger than 5% can cause burning and stinging when applied to the eyes, but this brief discomfort is usually tolerated without serious complaints. Sulfacetamide still compares favorably with newer antibiotics since it is effective against superficial ocular infections caused by a variety of microorganisms. However, serious allergic reactions can develop after ocular treatment (211).

The sulfonamides have a bacteriostatic rather than a bactericidal action. Many local anesthetics used in the eye are esters of *para*-aminobenzoic acid, and such drugs will interfere with the action of sulfonamides. Thus, to obtain the maximum effect from instillation of sulfonamide eye-drops, these drugs should not be used until the effect of the local anesthesia disappears.

Drug–Drug Interactions

Alkalis

Urine alkalinization increases the urinary excretion of sulfonamides (212,213).

Barbiturates

Sulfafurazole enhances the anesthetic effect of short-acting intravenous barbiturates, by competitive displacement from binding sites on plasma albumin (214).

CYP2C9

The inhibitory effect of sulfonamides on tolbutamide metabolism is mediated by CYP2C9, and therefore other drugs with narrow therapeutic ranges that are metabolized by CYP2C9, such as phenytoin and warfarin, deserve attention when certain sulfonamides (for example sulfaphenazole, sulfadiazine, sulfamethizole, and sulfafurazole) are co-administered (215).

Phenytoin

Attention is warranted when certain sulfonamides (for example sulfaphenazole, sulfadiazine, sulfamethizole, and sulfafurazole) are co-administered with CYP2C9 substrates with narrow therapeutic ranges, such as phenytoin.

Sulfonylureas

Hypoglycemia, often during the first hours of combining the two drugs, is the result of an important interaction between sulfonylureas and sulfonamides (216–219). For example, the half-life of tolbutamide was increased from 9.5 to 29 hours by chronic sulfaphenazole and from 9.2 to 26 hours by a single dose of sulfaphenazole (220). Interference by sulfonamides with the protein binding of sulfonylureas may contribute.

Most reports of this interaction have described hypoglycemia with tolbutamide in combination with sulfaphenazole (216,217,220,221), sulfafurazole (217), or co-trimoxazole (219,222). The inhibitory effect of sulfonamides on tolbutamide metabolism is mediated by CYP2C9 (215).

Chlorpropamide produces the same interaction (223).

The combination of gliclazide, fluconazole, and sulfamethoxazole can cause severe hypoglycemia (224).

Warfarin

Attention is warranted when certain sulfonamides (for example sulfaphenazole, sulfadiazine, sulfamethizole, and sulfafurazole) are co-administered with CYP2C9 substrates with narrow therapeutic ranges, such as warfarin (215).

Interference with Diagnostic Tests

Folate measurement

Sulfonamides, in contrast to trimethoprim, do not interfere with the microbiological assay of folate (77).

Theophylline

Sulfamethoxazole distorts the results of high performance liquid chromatography used for detection of theophylline plasma concentrations; the antibiotic should be withdrawn 24 hours before the procedure (SEDA-6, 7).

References

1. Zinner SH, Mayer KH. Basic principles in the diagnosis and management of infectious diseases: sulfonamides and trimethoprim. In: Mandell GL, Douglas RG, Bennett JE, editors. Principles and Practice of Infectious Diseases. 4th ed. Edinburgh: Churchill Livingstone, 1996:354.

2. Bushby SR, Hitchings GH. Trimethoprim, a sulphonamide potentiator. Br J Pharmacol Chemother 1968;33(1):72–90.

3. Ballin JC. Evaluation of a new topical agent for burn therapy. Silver sulfadiazine (silvadene). JAMA 1974;230(8):1184–5.

4. Lowbury EJ, Babb JR, Bridges K, Jackson DM. Topical chemoprophylaxis with silver sulphadiazine and silver nitrate chlorhexidine creams: emergence of sulphonamide-resistant Gram-negative bacilli. BMJ 1976;1(6008):493–6.

5. Sutherland LR, May GR, Shaffer EA. Sulfasalazine revisited: a meta-analysis of 5-aminosalicylic acid in the treatment of ulcerative colitis. Ann Intern Med 1993;118(7):540–9.

6. Thornhill M, Pemberton M, Buchanan J, Theaker E. An open clinical trial of sulphamethoxypyridazine in the treatment of mucous membrane pemphigoid. Br J Dermatol 2000;143(1):117–26.

7. von Seidlein L, Milligan P, Pinder M, Bojang K, Anyalebechi C, Gosling R, Coleman R, Ude JI, Sadiq A, Duraisingh M, Warhurst D, Alloueche A, Targett G, McAdam K, Greenwood B, Walraven G, Olliaro P, Doherty T. Efficacy of artesunate plus pyrimethamine-sulphadoxine for uncomplicated malaria in Gambian children: a double-blind, randomised, controlled trial. Lancet 2000;355(9201):352–7.

8. Bosch-Driessen LH, Verbraak FD, Suttorp-Schulten MS, van Ruyven RL, Klok AM, Hoyng CB, Rothova A. A prospective, randomized trial of pyrimethamine and azithromycin vs pyrimethamine and sulfadiazine for the treatment of ocular toxoplasmosis. Am J Ophthalmol 2002;134(1):34–40.

9. US Congress. House Committee on Interstate and Foreign Commerce and Its Subcommittee on Public Health and Environment, 1974. A Brief Legislative History of the Food, Drug, and Cosmetic Act. Committee Print No. 14. Washington DC: US Government Printing Offices, 1974:1–4.

10. USA, 52 Stat. 1040, 75th Congress, 3rd session, 25 June, 1938.

11. USA vs Dotterweich, 1941.

12. Sesti F, Abbott GW, Wei J, Murray KT, Saksena S, Schwartz PJ, Priori SG, Roden DM, George AL Jr, Goldstein SA. A common polymorphism associated with antibiotic-induced cardiac arrhythmia. Proc Natl Acad Sci USA 2000;97(19):10613–18.

13. French AJ, Weller CV. Interstitial myocarditis following the clinical and experimental use of sulfonamide drugs. Am J Pathol 1942;18:109.

14. Jones GR, Malone DN. Sulphasalazine induced lung disease. Thorax 1972;27(6):713–17.

15. Thomas P, Seaton A, Edwards J. Respiratory disease due to sulphasalazine. Clin Allergy 1974;4(1):41–7.

16. Scherpenisse J, van der Valk PD, van den Bosch JM, van Hees PA, Nadorp JH. Olsalazine as an alternative therapy in a patient with sulfasalazine-induced eosinophilic pneumonia. J Clin Gastroenterol 1988;10(2):218–20.

17. Svanbom M, Rombo L, Gustafsson L. Unusual pulmonary reaction during short term prophylaxis with pyrimethamine-sulfadoxine (Fansidar). BMJ (Clin Res Ed) 1984;288(6434):1876.

18. Berliner S, Neeman A, Shoenfeld Y, Eldar M, Rousso I, Kadish U, Pinkhas J. Salazopyrin-induced eosinophilic pneumonia. Respiration 1980;39(2):119–20.

19. Tydd TF. Sulphasalazine lung. Med J Aust 1976;1(16):570–3.

20. Wang KK, Bowyer BA, Fleming CR, Schroeder KW. Pulmonary infiltrates and eosinophilia associated with sulfasalazine. Mayo Clin Proc 1984;59(5):343–6.

21. Klinghoffer JF. Löffler's syndrome following use of a vaginal cream. Ann Intern Med 1954;40(2):343–50.

22. Fiegenberg DS, Weiss H, Kirshman H. Migratory pneumonia with eosinophilia associated with sulfonamide administration. Arch Intern Med 1967;120(1):85–9.

23. Crofton JW, Livingstone JL, Oswald NC, Roberts AT. Pulmonary eosinophilia. Thorax 1952;7(1):1–35.

24. Reeder WH, Goodrich BE. Pulmonary infiltration with eosinophilia (PIE syndrome). Ann Intern Med 1952;36(5):1217–40.

25. Chumbley LC, Harrison EG Jr, DeRemee RA. Allergic granulomatosis and angiitis (Churg–Strauss syndrome). Report and analysis of 30 cases. Mayo Clin Proc 1977;52(8):477–84.

26. Loeffler W. Ueber flüchtige Lungenilfiltrate (mit Eosinophilie). Beitr Klin Tuberk 1932;79:368.

27. Ellis RV, McKinlay CA. Allergic pneumonia. J Lab Clin Med 1941;26:1427.

28. Von Meyenburg H. Das eosinophile Lungenilfilträt: pathologische Anatomie und Pathogenese. Schweiz Med Wochenschr 1942;72:809.

29. Plogge H. Ueber zentrale und periphere nervöse Schäden nach Eubasinummedikation. Dtsch Z Nervenheilkd 1940;151:205.

30. Bucy PC. Toxic optic neuritis resulting from sulfanilamide. JAMA 1937;109:1007.

31. Borucki MJ, Matzke DS, Pollard RB. Tremor induced by trimethoprim-sulfamethoxazole in patients with the acquired immunodeficiency syndrome (AIDS). Ann Intern Med 1988;109(1):77–8.

32. Liu LX, Seward SJ, Crumpacker CS. Intravenous trimethoprim–sulfamethoxazole and ataxia. Ann Intern Med 1986;104(3):448.

33. Whalstrom B, Nystrom-Rosander C, Aberg H, Friman G. [Recurrent meningitis and perimyocarditis after trimethoprim.] Lakartidningen 1982;79(51):4854–5.

34. Barrett PV, Thier SO. Meningitis and pancreatitis associated with sulfamethizole. N Engl J Med 1963;268:36–7.

35. Haas EJ. Trimethoprim–sulfamethoxazole: another cause of recurrent meningitis. JAMA 1984;252(3):346.

36. Kremer I, Ritz R, Brunner F. Aseptic meningitis as an adverse effect of co-trimoxazole. N Engl J Med 1983;308(24):1481.

37. Auxier GG. Aseptic meningitis associated with administration of trimethoprim and sulfamethoxazole. Am J Dis Child 1990;144(1):144–5.

38. Biosca M, de la Figuera M, Garcia-Bragado F, Sampol G. Aseptic meningitis due to trimethoprim–sulfamethoxazole. J Neurol Neurosurg Psychiatry 1986;49(3):332–3.

39. Joffe AM, Farley JD, Linden D, Goldsand G. Trimethoprim–sulfamethoxazole-associated aseptic meningitis: case reports and review of the literature. Am J Med 1989;87(3):332–8.

40. Carlson J, Wiholm BE. Trimethoprim associated aseptic meningitis. Scand J Infect Dis 1987;19(6):687–91.

41. Gordon MF, Allon M, Coyle PK. Drug-induced meningitis. Neurology 1990;40(1):163–4.

42. Derbes SJ. Trimethoprim-induced aseptic meningitis. JAMA 1984;252(20):2865–6.

43. Moorthy RS, Valluri S, Jampol LM. Drug-induced uveitis. Surv Ophthalmol 1998;42(6):557–70.

44. Anonymous. Drug-induced uveitis can usually be easily managed. Drugs Ther Perspect 1998;11:11–14.

45. Bovino JA, Marcus DF. The mechanism of transient myopia induced by sulfonamide therapy. Am J Ophthalmol 1982;94(1):99–102.

46. Hook SR, Holladay JT, Prager TC, Goosey JD. Transient myopia induced by sulfonamides. Am J Ophthalmol 1986;101(4):495–6.

47. Carlberg O. Zur Genese der Sulfonamidmyopie. Acta Ophthalmol 1942;20:275.

48. Gutt L, Feder JM, Feder RS, Grammer LC, Shaughnessy MA, Patterson R. Corneal ring formation after exposure to sulfamethoxazole. Case reports. Arch Ophthalmol 1988;106(6):726–7.

49. Schiffman SS, Zervakis J, Westall HL, Graham BG, Metz A, Bennett JL, Heald AE. Effect of antimicrobial and anti-inflammatory medications on the sense of taste. Physiol Behav 2000;69(4–5):413–24.

50. Wade A, Reynolds JE. Sulfonamides. London: The Pharmaceutical Press, 1982:1457.

51. White MG, Asch MJ. Acid-base effects of topical mafenide acetate in the burned patient. N Engl J Med 1971;284(23):1281–6.

52. Alappan R, Buller GK, Perazella MA. Trimethoprim–sulfamethoxazole therapy in outpatients: is hyperkalemia a significant problem? Am J Nephrol 1999;19(3):389–94.

53. Marinella MA. Trimethoprim-induced hyperkalemia: An analysis of reported cases. Gerontology 1999;45(4):209–12.

54. Baumgartner A, Hoigné R, Müller U, et al. Medikamentöse Schäden des Blutbildes: Erfahrungen aus dem Komprehensiven Spital-Drug-Monitoring Bern, 1974–1979. Schweiz Med Wochenschr 1982;112:1530.

55. Muller U. Hämatologische Nebenwirkungen von Medikamenten. [Hematologic side effects of drugs.] Ther Umsch 1987;44(12):942–8.

56. Havas L, Fernex M, Lenox-Smith I. The clinical efficacy and tolerance of co-trimoxazole (Bactrim; Septrim). Clin Trials J 1973;3:81.

57. Hoigne R, Klein U, Muller U. Results of four-week course of therapy of urinary tract infections: a comparative study using trimethoprim with sulfamethoxazole (Bactrim; Roche) and trimethoprim alone In: Hejzlar M, Semonsky M, Masak S, editors. Advances in Antimicrobial and Antineoplastic Chemotherapy. Munchen-Berlin-Wien: Urban and Schwarzenberg, 1972:1283.

58. Scott JL, Cartwright GE, Wintrobe MM. Acquired aplastic anemia: an analysis of thirty-nine cases and review of the pertinent literature. Medicine (Baltimore) 1959;38(2):119–72.

59. Jick SS, Jick H, Habakangas JA, Dinan BJ. Co-trimoxazole toxicity in children. Lancet 1984;2(8403):631.

60. Malinverni R, Blatter M. Ambulante Therapie und Prophylaxe der haufigsten HIV-assoziierten opportunistischen Infektionen. [Ambulatory therapy and prevention of the most frequent HIV-associated opportunistic infections.] Schweiz Med Wochenschr 1991;121(34):1194–204.

61. Zinkham WH. Unstable hemoglobins and the selective hemolytic action of sulfonamides. Arch Intern Med 1977;137(10):1365–6.

62. de Leeuw N, Shapiro L, Lowenstein L. Drug-induced hemolytic anemia. Ann Intern Med 1963;58:592–607.

63. Worlledge SM. Immune drug-induced haemolytic anemias. Semin Hematol 1969;6(2):181–200.

64. Fishman FL, Baron JM, Orlina A. Non-oxidative hemolysis due to salicylazosulfapyridine: evidence for an immune mechanism. Gastroenterology 1973;64:727.

65. Cohen SM, Rosenthal DS, Karp PJ. Ulcerative colitis and erythrocyte G6PD deficiency. Salicylazosulfapyridine-provoked hemolysis. JAMA 1968;205(7):528–30.

66. Meyer UA. Drugs in special patient groups: Clinical importance of genetics in drug effects. In: Melmon KL, Morelli HF, Hoffman BB, Nierenberg DW editors. Nelmon and Morelli's Clinical Pharmacology, Basic Principles in Therapeutics. 3rd ed. New York-St Louis-San Francisco, etc: McGraw-Hill, 1992:875.

67. Frick PG, Hitzig WH, Stauffer U. Das Hämoglobin Zürich-Syndrom. [Hemoglobin-Zurich syndrome.] Schweiz Med Wochenschr 1961;91:1203–5.

68. Hitzig WH, Frick PG, Betke K, Huisman TH. Hämoglobin Zürich: eine neue Hämoglobinanomalie mit Sulfonamid-induzierter Innenkörperanämie. [Hemoglobin Zurich: a new hemoglobin anomaly with sulfonamide-induced inclusion body anemia.] Helv Paediatr Acta 1960;15:499–514.

69. Beretta A, Prato V, Gallo E, Lehmann H. Haemoglobin Torino—alpha-43 (CD1) phenylalanine replaced by valine. Nature 1968;217(133):1016–18.

70. Adams JG, Heller P, Abramson RK, Vaithianathan T. Sulfonamide-induced hemolytic anemia and hemoglobin Hasharon. Arch Intern Med 1977;137(10):1449–51.

71. Harris JW. Studies on the mechanism of a drug-induced hemolytic anemia. J Lab Clin Med 1956;47(5):760–75.

72. Beutler E. Red cell metabolism. Edinburgh/London: Churchill-Livingstone, 1986:16.

73. Gaetani GD, Mareni C, Ravazzolo R, Salvidio E. Haemolytic effect of two sulphonamides evaluated by a new method. Br J Haematol 1976;32(2):183–91.

74. Huisman TH. Hemoglobinopathies. Edinburgh/London: Churchill-Livingstone, 1986:15.

75. Shinton NK, Wilson C. Autoimmune haemolytic anaemia due to phenacetin and p-aminosalicylic acid. Lancet 1960;1:226.

76. Lyonnais J. Production de corps de Heinz associée à la prise de salicylazosulfapyridine. [Production of Heinz bodies after administration of salicylaszosulfapyridine.] Union Med Can 1976;105(2):203–5.

77. Streeter AM, Shum HY, O'Neill BJ. The effect of drugs on the microbiological assay of serum folic acid and vitamin B12 levels. Med J Aust 1970;1(18):900–1.

78. George JN, Raskob GE, Shah SR, Rizvi MA, Hamilton SA, Osborne S, Vondracek T. Drug-induced thrombocytopenia: a systematic review of published case reports. Ann Intern Med 1998;129(11):886–90.

79. Wright MS. Drug-induced hemolytic anemias: increasing complications to therapeutic interventions. Clin Lab Sci 1999;12(2):115–18.

80. Arneborn P, Palmblad J. Drug-induced neutropenia—a survey for Stockholm 1973–1978. Acta Med Scand 1982;212(5):289–92.

81. Baumelou E, Guiguet M, Mary JY. Epidemiology of aplastic anemia in France: a case-control study. I. Medical history and medication use. The French Cooperative Group for Epidemiological Study of Aplastic Anemia. Blood 1993;81(6):1471–8.

82. Anonymous. Anti-infective drug use in relation to the risk of agranulocytosis and aplastic anemia. A report from the International Agranulocytosis and Aplastic Anemia Study. Arch Intern Med 1989;149(5):1036–40.

83. Huerta C, Garcia Rodriguez LA. Risk of clinical blood dyscrasia in a cohort of antibiotic users. Pharmacotherapy 2002;22(5):630–6.

84. Johnston FD. Granulocytopenia following the administration of sulphanilamide compounds. Lancet 1938;2:1044.

85. Rinkoff SS, Spring M. Toxic depression of the myeloid elements following therapy with the sulfonamides: report of 8 cases. Ann Intern Med 1941;15:89.

86. Moeschlin S. Immunological granulocytopenia and agranulocytosis; clinical aspects. Sang 1955;26(1):32–51.

87. Rios Sanchez I, Duarte L, Sanchez Medal L. Agramulocitosis. Analisis de 29 episodes en 19 pacientes. [Agranulocytosis. Analysis of 29 episodes in 19 patients.] Rev Invest Clin 1971;23(1):29–42.

88. Ritz ND, Fisher MJ. Agranulocytosis due to administration of salicylazosulfapyridine (azulfidine). JAMA 1960;172:237.

89. Jarrett F, Ellerbe S, Demling R. Acute leukopenia during topical burn therapy with silver sulfadiazine. Am J Surg 1978;135(6):818–19.

90. Maurer LH, Andrews P, Rueckert F, McIntyre OR. Lymphocyte transformation observed in Sulfamylon agranulocytosis. Plast Reconstr Surg 1970;46(5):458–62.

91. Rhodes EG, Ball J, Franklin IM. Amodiaquine induced agranulocytosis: inhibition of colony growth in bone marrow by antimalarial agents. BMJ (Clin Res Ed) 1986;292(6522):717–18.

92. Pedersen-Bjergaard U, Andersen M, Hansen PB. Drug-specific characteristics of thrombocytopenia caused by non-cytotoxic drugs. Eur J Clin Pharmacol 1998;54(9–10):701–6.

93. Bottiger LE, Westerholm B. Thrombocytopenia. II. Drug-induced thrombocytopenia. Acta Med Scand 1972;191(6):541–8.

94. Gremse DA, Bancroft J, Moyer MS. Sulfasalazine hypersensitivity with hepatotoxicity, thrombocytopenia, and erythroid hypoplasia. J Pediatr Gastroenterol Nutr 1989;9(2):261–3.

95. Bottiger LE, Westerholm B. Thrombocytopenia. I. Incidence and aetiology. Acta Med Scand 1972;191(6):535–40.

96. Kelton JG, Meltzer D, Moore J, Giles AR, Wilson WE, Barr R, Hirsh J, Neame PB, Powers PJ, Walker I, Bianchi F, Carter CJ. Drug-induced thrombocytopenia is associated with increased binding of IgG to platelets both in vivo and in vitro. Blood 1981;58(3):524–9.

97. Kiefel V, Santoso S, Schmidt S, Salama A, Mueller-Eckhardt C. Metabolite-specific (IgG) and drug-specific antibodies (IgG, IgM) in two cases of trimethoprim–sulfamethoxazole-induced immune thrombocytopenia. Transfusion 1987;27(3):262–5.

98. Nidus BD, Field M, Rammelkamp CH Jr. Salivary gland enlargement caused by sulfisoxazole. Ann Intern Med 1965;63(4):663–5.

99. Chirgwin K, Hafner R, Leport C, Remington J, Andersen J, Bosler EM, Roque C, Rajicic N, McAuliffe V, Morlat P, Jayaweera DT, Vilde JL, Luft BJ. Randomized phase II trial of atovaquone with pyrimethamine or sulfadiazine for treatment of toxoplasmic encephalitis in patients with acquired immunodeficiency syndrome: ACTG 237/ANRS 039 Study. AIDS Clinical Trials Group 237/Agence Nationale de Recherche sur le SIDA, Essai 039. Clin Infect Dis 2002;34(9):1243–50.

100. Vial T, Biour M, Descotes J, Trepo C. Antibiotic-associated hepatitis: update from 1990. Ann Pharmacother 1997;31(2):204–20.

101. Fries J, Siragenian R. Sulfonamide hepatitis. Report of a case due to sulfamethoxazole and sulfisoxazole. N Engl J Med 1966;274(2):95–7.

102. Kaufman SF. A rare complication of sulfadimethoxine (Madribon) therapy. Calif Med 1967;107(4):344–5.

103. Konttinen A, Perasalo JO, Eisalo A. Sulfonamide hepatitis. Acta Med Scand 1972;191(5):389–91.

104. Konttinen A. Hepatotoxicity of sulphamethoxyridazine. BMJ 1972;2(806):168.

105. Sotolongo RP, Neefe LI, Rudzki C, Ishak KG. Hypersensitivity reaction to sulfasalazine with severe hepatotoxicity. Gastroenterology 1978;75(1):95–9.

106. Dujovne CA, Chan CH, Zimmerman HJ. Sulfonamide hepatic injury. Review of the literature and report of a case due to sulfamethoxazole. N Engl J Med 1967;277(15):785–8.

107. Tonder M, Nordoy A, Elgjo. Sulfonamide-induced chronic liver disease. Scand J Gastroenterol 1974;9(1):93–6.

108. Gutman LT. The use of trimethoprim–sulfamethoxazole in children: a review of adverse reactions and indications. Pediatr Infect Dis 1984;3(4):349–57.

109. Chester AC, Diamond LH, Schreiner GE. Hypersensitivity to salicylazosulfapyridine: renal and hepatic toxic reactions. Arch Intern Med 1978;138(7):1138–9.

110. Shaw DJ, Jacobs RP. Simultaneous occurrence of toxic hepatitis and Stevens–Johnson syndrome following therapy with sulfisoxazole and sulfamethoxazole. Johns Hopkins Med J 1970;126(3):130–3.

111. Block MB, Genant HK, Kirsner JB. Pancreatitis as an adverse reaction to salicylazosulfapyridine. N Engl J Med 1970;282(7):380–2.

112. Suryapranata H, De Vries H, et al. Pancreatitis associated with sulphasalazine. BMJ 1986;292:732.

113. Deprez P, Descamps C, Fiasse R. Pancreatitis induced by 5-aminosalicylic acid. Lancet 1989;2(8660):445–6.

114. Crespo M, Quereda C, Pascual J, Rivera M, Clemente L, Cano T. Patterns of sulfadiazine acute nephrotoxicity. Clin Nephrol 2000;54(1):68–72.

115. Perazella MA. Crystal-induced acute renal failure. Am J Med 1999;106(4):459–65.

116. Christin S, Baumelou A, Bahri S, Ben Hmida M, Deray G, Jacobs C. Acute renal failure due to sulfadiazine in patients with AIDS. Nephron 1990;55(2):233–4.

117. Miller MA, Gallicano K, Dascal A, Mendelson J. Sulfadiazine urolithiasis during antitoxoplasma therapy. Drug Invest 1993;5:334.

118. Simon DI, Brosius FC 3rd., Rothstein DM. Sulfadiazine crystalluria revisited. The treatment of *Toxoplasma* encephalitis in patients with acquired immunodeficiency syndrome. Arch Intern Med 1990;150(11):2379–84.

119. Furrer H, von Overbeck J, Jaeger P, Hess B. Sulfadiazin-Nephrolithiasis und Nephropathie. [Sulfadiazine nephrolithiasis and nephropathy.] Schweiz Med Wochenschr 1994;124(46):2100–5.

120. Craig WA, Kunin CM. Trimethoprim–sulfamethoxazole: pharmacodynamic effects of urinary pH and impaired renal function. Studies in humans. Ann Intern Med 1973;78(4):491–7.

121. Carbone LG, Bendixen B, Appel GB. Sulfadiazine-associated obstructive nephropathy occurring in a patient with the acquired immunodeficiency syndrome. Am J Kidney Dis 1988;12(1):72–5.

122. Robson M, Levi J, Dolberg L, Rosenfeld JB. Acute tubulo-interstitial nephritis following sulfadiazine therapy. Isr J Med Sci 1970;6(4):561–6.

123. Baker SB, Williams RT. Acute interstitial nephritis due to drug sensitivity. BMJ 1963;5346:1655–8.

124. Pusey CD, Saltissi D, Bloodworth L, Rainford DJ, Christie JL. Drug associated acute interstitial nephritis: clinical and pathological features and the response to high dose steroid therapy. Q J Med 1983;52(206):194–211.

125. Cryst C, Hammar SP. Acute granulomatous interstitial nephritis due to co-trimoxazole. Am J Nephrol 1988;8(6):483–8.

126. Van Rijssel TG, Meyler L. Necrotizing generalized arteritis due to the use of sulfonamide drugs. Acta Med Scand 1948;132:251.

127. Cohen-Solal F, Abdelmoula J, Hoarau MP, Jungers P, Lacour B, Daudon M. Les lithiases urinaires d'origine medicamenteuse. [Urinary lithiasis of medical origin.] Therapie 2001;56(6):743–50.

128. Bigby M, Jick S, Jick H, Arndt K. Drug-induced cutaneous reactions. A report from the Boston Collaborative Drug Surveillance Program on 15,438 consecutive inpatients, 1975 to 1982. JAMA 1986;256(24):3358–63.

129. Sonntag MR, Zoppi M, Fritschy D, Maibach R, Stocker F, Sollberger J, Buchli W, Hess T, Hoigne R. Exantheme unter häufig angewandten Antibiotika und anti-bakteriellen Chemotherapeutika (Penicilline, speziell Aminopenicilline, Cephalosporine und Cotrimoxazol) sowie Allopurinol. [Exanthema during frequent use of antibiotics and antibacterial drugs (penicillin, especially aminopenicillin, cephalosporin and cotrimoxazole) as well as allopurinol. Results of The Berne Comprehensive Hospital Drug Monitoring Program.] Schweiz Med Wochenschr 1986;116(5):142–5.

130. Hunziker T, Braunschweig S, Zehnder D, Hoigné R, Kunzi UP. Comprehensive Hospital Drug Monitoring (CHDM) adverse skin reactions, a 20-year survey. Allergy 1997;52(4):388–93.

131. Arndt KA, Jick H. Rates of cutaneous reactions to drugs. A report from the Boston Collaborative Drug Surveillance Program. JAMA 1976;235(9):918–23.

132. Gomez B, Sastre J, Azofra J, Sastre A. Fixed drug eruption. Allergol Immunopathol (Madr) 1985;13(2):87–91.

133. Ibia EO, Schwartz RH, Wiedermann BL. Antibiotic rashes in children: a survey in a private practice setting. Arch Dermatol 2000;136(7):849–54.

134. Tonev S, Vasileva S, Kadurina M. Depot sulfonamid associated linear IgA bullous dermatosis with erythema multiforme-like clinical features. J Eur Acad Dermatol Venereol 1998;11(2):165–8.

135. Kauppinen K, Stubb S. Fixed eruptions: causative drugs and challenge tests. Br J Dermatol 1985;112(5):575–8.

136. Pasricha JS. Drugs causing fixed eruptions. Br J Dermatol 1979;100(2):183–5.

137. Sehgal VN, Rege VL, Kharangate VN. Fixed drug eruptions caused by medications: a report from India. Int J Dermatol 1978;17(1):78–81.

138. Rollof SI. Erythema nodosum in association with sulphathiazole in children; a clinical investigation with special reference to primary tuberculosis. Acta Tuberc Scand Suppl 1950;24:1–215.

139. Kuokkanen K. Drug eruptions. A series of 464 cases in the Department of Dermatology, University of Turku, Finland, during 1966–1970. Acta Allergol 1972;27(5):407–38.

140. Epstein JH. Photoallergy. A review. Arch Dermatol 1972;106(5):741–8.

141. Harber LC, Bickers DR, Armstrong RB, et al. Drug photosensitivity: phototoxic and photoallergic mechanisms. Semin Dermatol 1982;1:183.

142. De Barrio M, Tornero P, Zubeldia JM, Sierra Z, Matheu V, Herrero T. Fixed drug eruption induced by indapamide. Cross-reactivity with sulfonamides. J Investig Allergol Clin Immunol 1998;8(4):253–5.

143. Martinez-Ruiz E, Ortega C, Calduch L, Molina I, Montesinos E, Revert A, Carda C, Navarro V, Jorda E. Generalized cutaneous depigmentation following sulfamide-induced drug eruption. Dermatology 2000;201(3):252–4.

144. Connor EE. Sulfonamide antibiotics. Prim Care Update Ob Gyns 1998;5:32–5.

145. Bottiger LE, Strandberg I, Westerholm B. Drug-induced febrile mucocutaneous syndrome with a survey of the literature. Acta Med Scand 1975;198(3):229–33.

146. Bergoend H, Loffler A, Amar R, Maleville J. Réactions cutanées survenues au cours de la prophylaxie de masse de la méningite cérébrospinale par un sulfamide long-rétard (à propos de 997 cas). [Cutaneous reactions appearing during the mass prophylaxis of cerebrospinal meningitis with a long-delayed action sulfonamide (apropos of 997 cases).] Ann Dermatol Syphiligr (Paris) 1968;95(5):481–90.

147. Taylor GM. Stevens–Johnson syndrome following the use of an ultra-long-acting sulphonamide. S Afr Med J 1968;42(20):501–3.

148. Hernborg A. Stevens–Johnson syndrome after mass prophylaxis with sulfadoxine for cholera in Mozambique. Lancet 1985;2(8463):1072–3.

149. Lyell A. A review of toxic epidermal necrolysis in Britain. Br J Dermatol 1967;79(12):662–71.

150. Bjornberg A. Fifteen cases of toxic epidermal necrolysis (Lyell). Acta Dermatol Venereol 1973;53(2):149–52.

151. Cohlan SQ. Erythema multiforme exudativum associated with use of sulfamethoxypyridazine. JAMA 1960;173:799–800.

152. Gottschalk HR, Stone OJ. Stevens–Johnson syndrome from ophthalmic sulfonamide. Arch Dermatol 1976;112(4):513–14.

153. Moussala M, Beharcohen F, Dighiero P, Renard G. Le syndrome de Lyell et ses manifestations ophtalmologiques en milieu camerounais. [Lyell's syndrome and its ophthalmologic manifestations in Cameroon.] J Fr Ophtalmol 2000;23(3):229–37.

154. Hoigne R. Interne Manifestationen und Labor-befunde beim Lyell-Syndrom. In: Braun-Falco O, Bandmann HJ, editors. Das Lyell-Syndrom. Bern-Stuttgart-Wien: Verlag H Huber, 1970:27.

155. Revuz J, Roujeau JC, Guillaume JC, Penso D, Touraine R. Treatment of toxic epidermal necrolysis. Creteil's experience. Arch Dermatol 1987;123(9):1156–8.

156. Amon RB, Dimond RL. Toxic epidermal necrolysis. Rapid differentiation between staphylococcal- and drug-induced disease. Arch Dermatol 1975;111(11):1433–7.

157. Soylu H, Akkol N, Erduran E, Aslan Y, Gunes Z, Yildiran A. Co-trimoxazole-induced toxic epidermal necrolysis treated with high dose methylprednisolone. Ann Med Sci 2000;9:38–40.

158. Miller KD, Lobel HO, Satriale RF, Kuritsky JN, Stern R, Campbell CC. Severe cutaneous reactions among American travelers using pyrimethamine–sulfadoxine (Fansidar) for malaria prophylaxis. Am J Trop Med Hyg 1986;35(3):451–8.

159. Schurmann D, Bergmann F, Albrecht H, Padberg J, Grunewald T, Behnsch M, Grobusch M, Vallee M, Wunsche T, Ruf B, Suttorp N. Twice-weekly pyrimethamine-sulfadoxine effectively prevents Pneumocystis carinii pneumonia relapse and toxoplasmic encephalitis in patients with AIDS. J Infect 2001;42(1):8–15.

160. Shear NH, Rieder MJ, Spielberg SP, et al. Hypersensitivity reactions to sulfonamide antibiotics are mediated by a hydroxylamine metabolite. Clin Res 1987;35:717.

161. Shear NH, Spielberg SP. In vitro evaluation of a toxic metabolite of sulfadiazine. Can J Physiol Pharmacol 1985;63(11):1370–2.

162. Nixon N, Eckert JF, Holmesk B. The treatment of agranulocytosis with sulfadiazine. Am J Med Sci 1943;206:713.

163. Roujeau JC, Bracq C, Huyn NT, Chaussalet E, Raffin C, Duedari N. HLA phenotypes and bullous cutaneous reactions to drugs. Tissue Antigens 1986;28(4):251–4.

164. Shear NH, Spielberg SP, Grant DM, Tang BK, Kalow W. Differences in metabolism of sulfonamides predisposing to idiosyncratic toxicity. Ann Intern Med 1986;105(2):179–84.

165. Rieder MJ, Shear NH, Kanee A, Tang BK, Spielberg SP. Prominence of slow acetylator phenotype among patients with sulfonamide hypersensitivity reactions. Clin Pharmacol Ther 1991;49(1):13–17.

166. Schnyder B, Frutig K, Mauri-Hellweg D, Limat A, Yawalkar N, Pichler WJ. T cell-mediated cytotoxicity against keratinocytes in sulfamethoxazol-induced skin reaction. Clin Exp Allergy 1998;28(11):1412–17.

167. Dwenger CS. 'Sulpha' hypersensitivity. Anaesthesia 2000;55(2):200–1.

168. Bedard K, Smith S, Cribb A. Sequential assessment of an antidrug antibody response in a patient with a systemic delayed-onset sulphonamide hypersensitivity syndrome reaction. Br J Dermatol 2000;142(2):253–8.

169. Carrington DM, Earl HS, Sullivan TJ. Studies of human IgE to a sulfonamide determinant. J Allergy Clin Immunol 1987;79(3):442–7.

170. Sher MR, Suchar C, Lockey RF. Anaphylactic shock induced by oral desensitization to trimethoprim/sulfmethoxazole. J Allergy Immunol 1986;77:133.

171. Gruchalla RS, Sullivan TJ. Detection of human IgE to sulfamethoxazole by skin testing with sulfamethoxazoyl-poly-L-tyrosine. J Allergy Clin Immunol 1991;88(5):784–92.

172. Ghajar BM, Naranjo CA, Shear NH, Lanctot KL. Improving the accuracy of the differential diagnosis of idiosyncratic adverse drug reactions (IADRs): skin eruptions and sulfonamides. Clin Pharmacol Ther 1990;47(2):127.

173. Delomenie C, Mathelier-Fusade P, Longuemaux S, Rozenbaum W, Leynadier F, Krishnamoorthy R, Dupret JM. Glutathione S-transferase (GSTM1) null genotype and sulphonamide intolerance in acquired immunodeficiency syndrome. Pharmacogenetics 1997;7(6):519–20.

174. Coopman SA, Johnson RA, Platt R, Stern RS. Cutaneous disease and drug reactions in HIV infection. N Engl J Med 1993;328(23):1670–4.

175. Woody RC, Brewster MA. Adverse effects of trimethoprim–sulfamethoxazole in a child with dihydropteridine reductase deficiency. Dev Med Child Neurol 1990;32(7):639–42.

176. Kreuz W, Gungor T, Lotz C, Funk M, Kornhuber B. "Treating through" hypersensitivity to cotrimoxazole in children with HIV infection. Lancet 1990;336(8713):508–9.

177. Naisbitt DJ, Vilar FJ, Stalford AC, Wilkins EG, Pirmohamed M, Park BK. Plasma cysteine deficiency and decreased reduction of nitrososulfamethoxazole with HIV infection. AIDS Res Hum Retroviruses 2000;16(18):1929–38.

178. Binns PM. Anaphylaxis after oral sulphadiazine; two reactions in the same patient within eight days. Lancet 1958;1(7013):194–5.

179. Reichmann J. Anaphylaktischer Schock durch intravenöse Sulfonamidapplikation mit letalem Ausgang. [Anaphylactic shock caused by intravenous sulfonamide application with fatal outcome.] Dtsch Gesundheitsw 1960;15:1139–41.

180. Stephens R, Mythen M, Kallis P, Davies DW, Egner W, Rickards A. Two episodes of life-threatening anaphylaxis in the same patient to a chlorhexidine–sulphadiazine-coated central venous catheter. Br J Anaesth 2001;87(2):306–8.

181. Rich AR. Additional evidence of the role of hypersensitivity in the etiology of periarteritis nodosa. Bull Johns Hopkins Hosp 1942;71:375.

182. Zeek PM, Smith CC, Weeter JC. Studies on periarteritis nodosa. III. Differentiation between vascular lesions of periarteritis nodosa and of hypersensitivity. Am J Pathol 1948;24:889.

183. Delage C, Lagace R. Maladie sérique avec hyperplasie ganglionnaire pseudo-lymphomateuse secondaire à la prise de salicylazosulfapyridine. [Serum sickness with pseudolymphomatous lymph node hyperplasia caused by salicylazosulfapyridine.] Union Med Can 1975;104(4):579–84.

184. Han T, Chawla PL, Sokal JE. Sulfapyridine-induced serum-sickness-like syndrome associated with plasmacytosis, lymphocytosis and multiclonal gamma-globulinopathy. N Engl J Med 1969;280(10):547–8.

185. Lee SL, Rivero I, Siegel M. Activation of systemic lupus erythematosus by drugs. Arch Intern Med 1966;117(5):620–6.

186. Hoigne R, Biedermann HP, Naegeli HR. INH-induzierter systemischer Lupus erythematodes: 2. Beobachtungen mit Reexposition. Schweiz Med Wochenschr 1975;105:1726.

187. Clementz GL, Dolin BJ. Sulfasalazine-induced lupus erythematosus. Am J Med 1988;84(3 Pt 1):535–8.

188. Alarcon-Segovia D. Drug-induced lupus syndromes. Mayo Clin Proc 1969;44(9):664–81.

189. Griffiths ID, Kane SP. Sulphasalazine-induced lupus syndrome in ulcerative colitis. BMJ 1977;2(6096):1188–9.

190. Hess E. Drug-related lupus. N Engl J Med 1988;318(22):1460–2.

191. Cohen P, Gardner FH. Sulfonamide reactions in systemic lupus erythematosus. JAMA 1966;197(10):817–19.

192. Honey M. Systemic lupus erythematosus presenting with sulphonamide hypersensitivity reaction. BMJ 1956;(4978):1272–5.

193. Tilles SA. Practical issues in the management of hypersensitivity reactions: sulfonamides. South Med J 2001;94(8):817–24.

194. Torgovnick J, Arsura E. Desensitization to sulfonamides in patients with HIV infection. Am J Med 1990;88(5):548–9.

195. Finegold I. Oral desensitization to trimethoprim–sulfamethoxazole in a patient with acquired immunodeficiency syndrome. J Allergy Clin Immunol 1986;78(5 Pt 1):905–8.

196. Papakonstantinou G, Fuessl H, Hehlmann R. Trimethoprim-sulfamethoxazole desensitization in AIDS. Klin Wochenschr 1988;66(8):351–3.

197. Villar RG, Macek MD, Simons S, Hayes PS, Goldoft MJ, Lewis JH, Rowan LL, Hursh D, Patnode M, Mead PS. Investigation of multidrug-resistant *Salmonella* serotype typhimurium DT104 infections linked to raw-milk cheese in Washington State. JAMA 1999;281(19):1811–16.

198. Molbak K, Baggesen DL, Aarestrup FM, Ebbesen JM, Engberg J, Frydendahl K, Gerner-Smidt P, Petersen AM, Wegener HC. An outbreak of multidrug-resistant, quinolone-resistant *Salmonella enterica* serotype typhimurium DT104. N Engl J Med 1999;341(19):1420–5.

199. Levi AJ, Toovey S, Hudson E. Male infertility due to sulphasalazine. Gastroenterology 1981;80:1208.

200. Tobias R, Sapire KE, Coetzee T, Marks IN. Male infertility due to sulphasalazine. Postgrad Med J 1982;58(676):102–3.

201. Karbach U, Ewe K, Schramm P. Samenqualität bei Patienten mit Morbus Crohn. [Quality of semen in patients with Crohn's disease.] Z Gastroenterol 1982;20(6):314–20.

202. Heinonen OP, Slone D, Shapiro S. Antimicrobial and antiparasitic agents. In: Heinonen OP, Slone D, Shapiro S,

editors. Birth Defects and Drugs in Pregnancy. 4th ed. Boston-Bristol-London: John Wright PSG Inc, 1982:296.

203. Karkinen-Jaaskelainen, Saxen L. Maternal influenza, drug consumption, and congenital defects of the central nervous system. Am J Obstet Gynecol 1974;118(6):815–18.

204. Deen JL, von Seidlein L, Pinder M, Walraven GE, Greenwood BM. The safety of the combination artesunate and pyrimethamine–sulfadoxine given during pregnancy. Trans R Soc Trop Med Hyg 2001;95(4):424–8.

205. Brodersen R. Prevention of kernicterus, based on recent progress in bilirubin chemistry. Acta Paediatr Scand 1977;66(5):625–34.

206. Diamond I, Schmid R. Experimental bilirubin encephalopathy. The mode of entry of bilirubin-14C into the central nervous system. J Clin Invest 1966;45(5):678–89.

207. Andersen DH, Blanc WA, Crozier DN, Silverman WA. A difference in mortality rate and incidence of kernicterus among premature infants allotted to two prophylactic antibacterial regimens. Pediatrics 1956;18(4):614–25.

208. Wadsworth SJ, Suh B. In vitro displacement of bilirubin by antibiotics and 2-hydroxybenzoylglycine in newborns. Antimicrob Agents Chemother 1988;32(10):1571–5.

209. Peterkin GA, Khan SA. Iatrogenic skin disease. Practitioner 1969;202(207):117–26.

210. Antonen JA, Markula KP, Pertovaara MI, Pasternack AI. Adverse drug reactions in Sjögren's syndrome. Frequent allergic reaction and a specific trimethoption associated systemic reaction. Scand J Pheumatol 1999;28(3):157–9.

211. Hugues FC, Le Jeunne C. Systemic and local tolerability of ophthalmic drug formulations. An update. Drug Saf 1993;8(5):365–80.

212. Hartshorn EA. Drug interaction. Drug Intell 1968;2:174.

213. Kabins SA. Interactions among antibiotics and other drugs. JAMA 1972;219(2):206–12.

214. Csogor SI, Kerek SF. Enhancement of thiopentone anaesthesia by sulphafurazole. Br J Anaesth 1970;42(11):988–90.

215. Komatsu K, Ito K, Nakajima Y, Kanamitsu S, Imaoka S, Funae Y, Green CE, Tyson CA, Shimada N, Sugiyama Y. Prediction of in vivo drug–drug interactions between tolbutamide and various sulfonamides in humans based on in vitro experiments. Drug Metab Dispos 2000;28(4):475–81.

216. Christensen LK, Hansen JM, Kristensen M. Sulphaphenazole-induced hypoglycaemic attacks in tolbutamide-treated diabetic. Lancet 1963;41:1298–301.

217. Soeldner JS, Steinke J. Hypoglycemia in tolbutamide-treated diabetes; Report of two casses with measurement of serum insulin. JAMA 1965;193:398–9.

218. Dubach UC, Bückert A, Raaflaub J. Einfluss von Sulfonamiden auf die blutzuckersenkende Wirkung oraler Antidiabetica. Schweiz Med Wochenschr 1966;44:1483.

219. Wing LM, Miners JO. Cotrimoxazole as an inhibitor of oxidative drug metabolism: effects of trimethoprim and sulphamethoxazole separately and combined on tolbutamide disposition. Br J Clin Pharmacol 1985;20(5):482–5.

220. Pond SM, Birkett DJ, Wade DN. Mechanisms of inhibition of tolbutamide metabolism: phenylbutazone, oxyphenbutazone, sulfaphenazole. Clin Pharmacol Ther 1977;22(5 Pt 1):573–9.

221. Hansen JM, Christensen LK. Drug interactions with oral sulphonylurea hypoglycaemic drugs. Drugs 1977;13(1):24–34.

222. Schattner A, Rimon E, Green L, Coslovsky R, Bentwich Z. Hypoglycemia induced by co-trimoxazole in AIDS. BMJ 1988;297(6650):742.

223. Baciewicz AM, Swafford WB Jr. Hypoglycemia induced by the interaction of chlorpropamide and co-trimoxazole. Drug Intell Clin Pharm 1984;18(4):309–10.

224. Abad S, Moachon L, Blanche P, Bavoux F, Sicard D, Salmon-Ceron D. Possible interaction between gliclazide,

fluconazole and sulfamethoxazole resulting in severe hypoglycaemia. Br J Clin Pharmacol 2001;52(4):456–7.

Sulfonylureas

General Information

Sulfonylureas act by inhibiting ATP-sensitive potassium channels (K_{ATP} channels) in pancreatic beta cells, increasing the amount of insulin released. The beta cells of patients taking these drugs are chronically stimulated. Changes in the pattern of insulin secretion and increased peripheral resistance to insulin both result in increased output of glucose from the liver. A rise in the number of insulin receptors, amelioration of the postbinding defect, and inhibition of the increased glucose output from the liver have been described (SEDA-5, 391), mostly in in vitro or animal experiments of short duration. The K_{ATP} channels in the beta cells and other tissues have been reviewed, including a discussion of the effects of various sulfonylureas (1). Enhanced action on beta cells by the addition of ADP suggests that the action of sulfonylureas varies with the metabolic state of the islet. Chlorpropamide and glibenclamide have high islet-binding specificity, while glibenclamide also binds with high affinity to extra-pancreatic binding sites.

Increased insulin release reduces blood glucose and glycosuria and contributes to a reduction in energy loss. This leads to increased storage of body fat when more is eaten than is necessary to meet daily energy needs and provokes feelings of hunger. Traditionally therefore, the sulfonylureas have been regarded as being unsuitable for overweight diabetics, who primarily need to lose weight. However, the results of the Diabetes Control and Complications Trial (DCCT) (2) and the UK Prospective Diabetes Study (UKPDS) (3) have shown that a sustained increase in the blood glucose concentration accelerates the development of secondary complications of diabetes mellitus. Being overweight may therefore be the price to be paid for normalization of blood glucose. However, not all secondary changes, such as macroangiopathy, seem to depend directly on the blood glucose concentration.

The potencies and the durations of action of oral hypoglycemic drugs vary (see Table 1). Oral drugs may make the cell more sensitive to insulin, and it is difficult to predict how long the hypoglycemic effect will last. The blood concentration does not always determine the duration of action. When the concentration is falling, stimulation of insulin secretion can continue for some time.

There have been reviews of oral hypoglycemic drugs (4–8).

Maturity-onset diabetes of the young (MODY) is characterized by type 2 diabetes at or before adolescence. It is a genetically heterogeneous disease, for which at least five different genes have been identified. MODY3, one of the most common forms, is characterized by a mutation in the hepatocyte nuclear factor (HNF)-1α gene. MODY3 can be very sensitive to sulfonylureas (SEDA-22, 475) (9,10).

Table 1 Doses, durations of action, and half-lives of sulfonylureas

RINN	Dose (mg)		Duration of action (hours)	Half-life (hours)	
				Renal function	
	Mean/day	Maximum/day		Normal	Anuric
Acetohexamide	250–1000	1500	12–24	16	48
Carbutamide[a]	500–1500	2500			
Chlorpropamide	100–500	1000	20–60	35	200
Glibenclamide (glyburide)	2.5–10	20	12–18	5–8	11
Glibornuride	12.5–100		10–15		
Gliclazide	40–240	240	12–18	8–11	
Glimepiride	1–4	6	12–20	5–8	
Glipizide	2.5–20	30	6–12	3–5	Unchanged[b]
Gliquidone	15–90	120	6–12	6–10	Unchanged[b]
Glisoxepide	2–12	15	5–10		
Glymidine (glycodiazine)	500–1500	3000	6–12		
Tolazamide	100–500	1000	12–16	8–10	
Tolbutamide	500–2000	3000	6–12	3–5	48

[a] Obsolete
[b] Hypoglycemia occurs despite the unchanged half-life

Three new cases have been presented, all with a mutation in the HNF-1α gene; low-dose glibenclamide was the best treatment in all cases (11).

The UK Prospective Diabetes Study (3) has shown that timely treatment, by reducing blood glucose concentrations before subjective complaints develop, reduces secondary complications in type 2 diabetes mellitus.

Combinations of oral hypoglycemic drugs

The different mechanisms of action of the various classes of hypoglycemic drugs makes combined therapy feasible: the sulfonylureas and meglitinides stimulate insulin production by different mechanisms, the biguanides reduce glucose production by the liver and excretion from the liver, acarbose reduces the absorption of glucose from the gut, and the thiazolidinediones reduce insulin resistance in fat. It is not necessary to wait until the maximal dose of one drug has been reached before starting another. However, sulfonylureas and meglitinides should no longer be used when endogenous insulin production is minimal. Combinations of insulin with sulfonylureas or meglitinides should only be used while the patient is changing to insulin, except when long-acting insulin is given at night in order to give the islets a rest and to stimulate daytime insulin secretion.

Large studies of the effects of lifestyle changes, the effects of drugs in preventing or postponing the complications of diabetes, or the usefulness of various combinations are regularly published. The different mechanisms of action of the various classes give different metabolic effects and different adverse effects profiles (12). Comparative costs of the various therapies in the USA have been presented (13).

This subject has been reviewed in relation to combined oral therapy. In a systematic review of 63 studies with a duration of at least 3 months and involving at least 10 patients at the end of the study, and in which HbA$_{1c}$ was reported, five different classes of oral drugs were almost equally effective in lowering blood glucose concentrations (14). HbA$_{1c}$ was reduced by about 1–2% in all cases.

Combination therapy gave additive effects. However, long-term vascular risk reduction was demonstrated only with sulfonylureas and metformin.

The adverse effects of combined drug therapy are attributable to adverse effects of the individual drugs. Increased adverse effects or new adverse effects in patients taking combinations have not been reported.

Sulfonylureas + meglitinides

Glipizide, nateglinide, and their combination have been compared in a double-blind, randomized, placebo-controlled study in 20 patients with type 2 diabetes not requiring insulin (15). Before a standardized breakfast they took glipizide 10 mg, nateglinide 120 mg, both, or placebo; 4 hours after the meal blood glucose concentrations were significantly higher after nateglinide, but peak and integrated glucose concentrations did not differ. Integrated insulin concentrations were higher with glipizide. There were three episodes of hypoglycemia in the glipizide alone group and three in the combined group; three required treatment with glucose.

Sulfonylureas + thiazolidinediones

Troglitazone 100 or 200 mg/day or placebo was given for 16 weeks to 259 patients already taking sulfonylurea therapy (16). HbA$_{1c}$ was 0.4 and 0.7% lower and blood glucose concentrations fell. The most common event was hypoglycemia, but this did not occur more often when troglitazone was added. Liver enzymes increased to the same extent in the three groups and never rose above normal. No patients withdrew because of drug-related effects.

Organs and Systems

Cardiovascular

Early studies suggested that tolbutamide caused excessive cardiovascular deaths (17) as reported in the University Group Diabetes Program (UGDP) (SEDA-4, 301), but the UK Prospective Diabetes Study did not find different mortality in patients treated with insulin, glibenclamide, or chlorpropamide (3).

This effect of tolbutamide has been attributed to prevention of ischemic preconditioning, a protective manoeuvre that reduces myocardial damage after temporary stoppage of coronary blood flow (18). Transient myocardial ischemia augments post-ischemic myocardial function and prevents dysrhythmias. K_{ATP} channels play a role in this so-called ischemic preconditioning. In 48 atrial trabeculae, obtained during catheterization, the recovery of the developed muscle force in patients treated with a sulfonylurea was only half of what was found in nondiabetics or diabetics treated with insulin. This suggests that inhibition of K_{ATP} channels by oral sulfonylureas might contribute to increased cardiovascular mortality (19). The question of whether the findings obtained mainly with glibenclamide can be generalized to all sulfonylureas has been discussed, since sulfonylureas differ greatly in their ability to interfere with vascular or cardiac K_{ATP} channels (20). Both glimepiride and glibenclamide (21) improved glycemia in 29 patients in a randomized, double-blind, placebo-controlled, crossover study of a number of susceptibility factors for ischemic heart disease (plasminogen activator inhibitor activity, plasminogen activator inhibitor antigen, LDL cholesterol, C peptide, proinsulin, des-31,32 proinsulin, etc.), but K_{ATP} channels were not investigated.

Glibenclamide prevented the increase in tolerance to myocardial ischemia normally observed during the second of two sequential exercise tests (22).

Respiratory

- A 76-year-old man who had taken glibenclamide for 2 weeks, having switched from voglibose, developed pneumonitis; a lymphocyte stimulation test was positive for glibenclamide (23).

Sensory systems

A change in taste sensation has been reported with glipizide (24).

Metabolism

In 36 Japanese patients who were relatively lean but had excess abdominal fat, glibenclamide and voglibose caused loss of weight and abdominal fat (25). The loss of abdominal fat was related to glycemic control. The ratio of subcutaneous to abdominal fat shifted toward subcutaneous fat only in those who took voglibose. Both voglibose and glibenclamide improved insulin sensitivity and the acute response to insulin.

Hypoglycemia
DoTS classification (BMJ 2003;327:1222–5)
Adverse effect: Hypoglycemia due to sulfonylureas
Dose-relation: toxic effect
Time-course: time-independent
Susceptibility factors: disease (impaired liver or kidney function, alcoholism); drug interactions; reduced food intake; exercise

Hypoglycemia is the most frequent complication in patients with diabetes taking oral hypoglycemic drugs (26–28).

Presentation
In general, hypoglycemia caused by oral hypoglycemic drugs is more dangerous and of longer duration than hypoglycemia caused by insulin (29), and the most dangerous hypoglycemic attacks are those that result from long-acting drugs, such as chlorpropamide, and later sulfonylureas, such as glibenclamide (SEDA-4, 303). Sulfonylureas are mostly used by elderly people, and the characteristic warning symptoms of hypoglycemia (dizziness, breathlessness, sweating, and a feeling of hunger) are often absent or not well-interpreted.

Neurological symptoms are common and hypoglycemia can cause hemiplegia, which can be confused with neurological symptoms of other origin (transient ischemic attack, stroke, etc.). A bilateral case has been reported (30).

- A 68-year-old man started to take glibenclamide and 1 week later developed a blurred voice and right-sided hemiplegia with a blood glucose of 1.4 mmol/l. Ten minutes after intravenous glucose 50 g his motor function returned to normal. Six hours later he developed slurred speech and left-sided hemiplegia; his blood glucose was 1.9 mmol/l. During glucose administration his deficit resolved.

- A 75-year-old man taking gliclazide 80 mg bd and metformin 850 mg tds became hypoglycemic and was treated successfully (31). All hypoglycemic drugs were withdrawn, but he received more through his doctor's prescription computer and again became hypoglycemic on two occasions. On the second he became unconscious for 4.5 hours and his plasma glucose was 1.2 mmol/l. After resuscitation his abbreviated mental test was 5/10 and did not improve. He later became very aggressive and died of bronchopneumonia.

Three patients became comatose due to hypoglycemia (32):

- an 83-year-old woman who took two times 5 mg glibenclamide bd;
- a 61-year-old man who took 2 mg glimepiride bd and 500 mg metformin bd;
- a 79-year-old woman who took 5 mg glibenclamide tds and metformin 850 mg bd.

All of these patients had general malaise, reduced food intake, and vomiting; glucose had to be given for a long time and one patient died with pneumonia.

Frequent attacks of hypoglycemia can result in encephalopathy, and after withdrawal of the hypoglycemic drug cerebral injury can persist. It is not exceptional for prolonged hypoglycemic coma to end fatally (33,34). In 494 cases of severe hypoglycemia, 10% of the patients died and 9% had permanent sequelae (35).

Factitious hypoglycemia can take a long time to diagnose.

- A 20-year-old woman with unexplained hypoglycemia had an exploratory laparotomy with pancreatic biopsy, which showed a histological picture compatible with hyperplasia (36). Glipizide was detected in the blood at a concentration of 0.72 (usual target range 0.1–0.49) µg/ml. The diagnosis was factitious hypoglycemia.

- A 33-year-old nurse with unexplained hypoglycemia had only small increases in insulin and C-peptide, and glibenclamide was found in her serum (37). However, she denied using it and did not want psychiatric therapy.

Reported cases again illustrate that hypoglycemia induced by tablets tends to relapse and that long-term observation after normalizing the blood glucose concentration is necessary.

Hypoglycemia has been reported in a worker, not wearing a mask, working with a machine preparing ultrafine sulfonylurea powder (38).

Incidence

In 13 963 sulfonylurea users over 65 years of age, there were 255 severe attacks of hypoglycemia during 20 715 patient-years of use (39).

In an open comparative study in 57 patients acarbose and gliclazide had the same effects on HbA_{1c}, blood glucose, and lipids, although the ratio of HDL:LDL cholesterol increased during acarbose therapy (40). Of those who took gliclazide 10% reported at least one mild hypoglycemic reaction.

In an 8-week, non-interventional cohort study in 22 045 patients with type 2 diabetes, of whom 4.9% discontinued therapy, adverse advents occurred in 2.3% (41). There were attacks of hypoglycemia in 0.3%. Of the 6547 patients taking glimepiride, 2.5% had adverse reactions and 0.4% had hypoglycemic reactions.

In an open, multicenter study, 849 patients with poorly controlled diabetes were treated with glimepiride monotherapy for 6 months in doses that were titrated from 1 to 6 mg (42). The authors tried to identify factors that could predict the response to glimepiride. Patients who achieved a fasting blood glucose below 7.7 mmol/l and HbA_{1c} below 7.5% or a reduction in fasting blood glucose of over 20% and/or in HbA_{1c} of at least 10% were defined as responders (57% of the 849 patients). Earlier treatment with other oral hypoglycemic drugs or long-standing diabetes increased the rate of non-responders. In 9.2% of the patients there were episodes of hypoglycemia, 1.4 per patient, and third-party or medical assistance was required five times as often. A family history of type 2 diabetes doubled the risk; a high HbA_{1c} reduced the risk.

In a retrospective study in Hong Kong, drug-induced hypoglycemia accounted for 0.5% of admissions; 50% of the episodes were related to sulfonylureas (43). These patients were older, predominantly female, in poorer general health, and needing assistance in daily activities, including feeding. Co-morbidities, such as macrovascular complications, renal insufficiency, and concurrent infections, were common. Low plasma albumin concentrations probably reflected poor nutritional status. Of those who had recurrent admissions, 67% lived in old peoples' homes, compared with 22% in those without previous admissions. The prognosis in this group was poor: 23% died within 1 year. Patients taking gliclazide ($n = 13$) or glipizide ($n = 10$) accounted for 37% of the episodes. They had more vascular complications than patients who used glibenclamide or chlorpropamide. They had a higher frequency of previous admissions (47 versus 19%) and a higher mortality rate (1 year, 47 versus 10%; 5 years, 72 versus 34%).

In a period of 12 months 23 episodes of severe hypoglycemia were recorded in those taking a sulfonylurea in a district with a population of 367 051 (8655 with diabetes) (44). The total cost of emergency treatment was estimated to be up to \$92 078/year.

Causes and susceptibility factors

Most sulfonylureas are at least partly metabolized in the liver (SEDA-9, 709) (45), and hence liver insufficiency, liver disease, and liver enzyme inhibition (alcohol) or induction (drugs) can alter the half-life of the drug and its duration of action.

Renal dysfunction is another cause of hypoglycemia (46). Some sulfonylureas, such as chlorpropamide (30%) and tolbutamide (50%), are excreted by the kidney. Other drugs, such as acetohexamide, glibenclamide (glyburide), glibornuride, and glymidine, are mainly metabolized, but some of their metabolites also have a hypoglycemic effect and are excreted by the kidneys, so that renal insufficiency can prolong their hypoglycemic actions. The reduction in insulin metabolism in diseased kidneys (nephropathy) can contribute to hypoglycemia, since it increases the half-life of insulin.

Hypoglycemia can also result from drug interactions, with the simultaneous use of drugs that have glucose-lowering effects or that inhibit the clearance of oral hypoglycemic drugs.

The conclusion (SEDA-22, 475) (47) that fasting is well tolerated and that old age is no contraindication to sulfonylurea therapy has not been accepted by others (48,49), as the previous study included only a small number of relatively healthy patients with type 2 diabetes.

Hypoglycemia can result from overdosage of sulfonylureas (50,51). Factitious hypoglycemia induced by tablets is difficult to diagnose, since C peptide concentrations will be high and not suppressed. Reduced intake of food or alcohol can also play a role (52).

Severe hypoglycemia induced by long-acting and short-acting sulfonylureas in Basel, Switzerland (200 000 inhabitants), has been analysed in a retrospective study in 28 patients (median age 73 years) (53); 11 men and 5 women (2.24 per 1000 person-years) were taking long-acting sulfonylureas (15 glibenclamide, 1 chlorpropamide) and 2 men and 10 women (0.75 per 1000 person-years) short-acting sulfonylureas (10 glibornuride, 2 gliclazide). Metformin was only involved when combined with a sulfonylurea. There were no deaths. Reduced food intake ($n = 9$), increased activity ($n = 2$), impaired renal function ($n = 2$), alcohol ($n = 2$), too many tablets ($n = 3$), and no obvious factor ($n = 10$) were the causes.

Drug-induced hypoglycemia in 102 non-alcoholic, non-epileptic patients has been reviewed (54). There were susceptibility factors for hypoglycemia in 94; 84 were over 60 years old, of whom 70 were over 70 years; 66 had renal impairment, of whom 28 also had reduced energy intake, 10 had reduced energy intake, 30 had infections, 5 had liver cirrhosis, and 10 had malignant neoplasia; 14 had used hypoglycemia-potentiating drugs, such as beta-blockers ($n = 8$), cimetidine ($n = 2$), co-trimoxazole ($n = 2$), and aspirin ($n = 2$). Forty patients had protracted hypoglycemia lasting 12–72 hours. Head trauma ($n = 4$), skeletal injury ($n = 3$), seizures ($n = 8$), transient asymptomatic myocardial ischemia ($n = 2$), and transient right hemiplegia ($n = 1$) were seen. Five patients died. Ten used glibenclamide + metformin, 14 used glibenclamide + insulin, and 53 used only glibenclamide.

To study the impact of Munchausen's syndrome, 129 patients with unexplained hypoglycemia in France had blood tests for sulfonylureas, which were found in 22 cases—glibenclamide in 19 patients and gliclazide in 3 (55). The concentrations were usually higher than the usual target concentration: in seven cases they were five times higher and the highest value was 18 times higher. In most cases an insulinoma was suggested and pancreatectomy was planned.

Management

Treatment of sulfonylurea-induced hypoglycemia and of overdose with sulfonylureas has been reviewed (56). If intravenous dextrose is insufficient, octreotide is recommended (57) but not diazoxide. In patients with insulin reserve, dextrose can stimulate insulin secretion and paradoxically worsen the condition. Patients with drug-induced hypoglycemia should not be given glucagon, since it will stimulate insulin secretion. Hypoglycemia can last for up to 5 days. Continued observation is important, because recurrence after temporary recovery is common.

Nutrition

In patients taking maximal doses of sulfonylureas, plasma homocysteine concentrations were raised during secondary failure with poor metabolic control, which may indicate increased vascular risk (58). The concentrations correlated inversely with endogenous insulin concentrations.

Electrolyte balance

Mild hyponatremia has been reported with sulfonylureas, most commonly with chlorpropamide (59,60). The mechanism with chlorpropamide is secretion of ADH (61).

In 70 non-insulin-dependent patients with diabetes, taking one of five different oral hypoglycemic drugs, 21% of prescriptions were associated with a low plasma sodium concentration, but it was lower than 129 mmol/l in only 8% (62). Every oral hypoglycemic agent was associated with a low plasma sodium concentration, which normalized on withdrawal. Extreme hyponatremia was only seen with chlorpropamide and, in one case, with glibenclamide.

Fluid balance

Water retention with oliguria, uremia, and edema has been reported with gliclazide (63). Resistance to diuretics can be caused by chlorpropamide (64) or, to a lesser extent, tolbutamide. Changing to a sulfonylurea without an antidiuretic effect (glibenclamide) or to one that enhances water excretion (acetohexamide, glipizide, or tolazamide) (65) may be advisable.

Hematologic

The most dangerous adverse reaction of sulfonylureas is agranulocytosis. Aplastic anemia (66), red cell aplasia (67), pure white cell aplasia (68), bone marrow aplasia, and hemolytic anemia have been described during treatment with chlorpropamide (69), glibenclamide (70), or tolbutamide (71).

Thrombocytopenia has been described with chlorpropamide (72), tolbutamide (73), glibenclamide (74), and glimepiride (75).

- A 68-year-old man, who had taken pipotiazine and trihexyphenidyl for 12 years for chronic psychosis, took glimepiride for hyperglycemia. No platelet counts were performed before or during this. He had no symptoms of bleeding. He developed a petechial rash and hematomas on his trunk, legs, and face, hemorrhagic bullae in his mouth, and gingival bleeding. There was thrombocytopenia (1×10^9/l), with no malignant cells in a bone marrow aspirate and no serological evidence of recent viral infection. All medications were withdrawn and he was given prednisone and human immunoglobulin. After 7 days the hemorrhagic syndrome abated, although his platelet count was still 2×10^9/l. After four weeks the platelet count was 23×10^9/l and the prednisone was gradually withdrawn. After 6 months the platelet count was normal (346×10^9/l).

Glibenclamide can cause hemolysis by a non-immune mechanism (76).

- A 68-year-old man with a long history of type 2 diabetes and a slowly progressive myelodysplastic syndrome for 2 years took glibenclamide 5 mg/day for more than a year, buformin 150 mg/day, and voglibose 0.6 mg/day. His hemoglobin was 8.4 g/dl. No other cause of hemolysis was found and glibenclamide was withdrawn. His hemoglobin rose to 11.1 g/dl.

Eosinophilic infiltrations have been described with tolbutamide (SEDA-8, 917) (77), and chronic eosinophilic pneumonia has been described with chlorpropamide (78) and tolazamide (79).

Gastrointestinal

Gastrointestinal tract disturbances are frequent with sulfonylureas. They comprise nausea, vomiting, heartburn, dyspepsia, a metallic taste, and abdominal pain (80). They are less troublesome when the drug is taken after meals.

Liver

The risk of hepatotoxicity with the sulfonylureas varies with both the drug and the dosage. It has been described with chlorpropamide (81), tolazamide (82), tolbutamide (83), glipizide (84), and glibenclamide (85). Anicteric, cytolytic hepatitis has been described after glibenclamide (86).

Hepatic granulomas have been reported as a hypersensitivity reaction to chlorpropamide (87). Cholestatic jaundice from sulfonylureas is also probably of allergic origin; it is rare and has been described with glibenclamide (88), also in combination with hepatorenal syndrome (89), acetohexamide (90), chlorpropamide (91), gliclazide (92), and tolazamide (93).

- A 64-year-old man who had taken glibenclamide 10 mg/day for 4 years developed cholestasis (94). There was no extrahepatic obstruction on ERCP and serological tests for hepatitis A, B, and C, *Helicobacter pylori*, and antimitochondrial or antinuclear antibodies were all negative. Liver biopsy showed portal and periportal inflammation, edema, and prominent centrilobular hepatocanalicular cholestasis. When glibenclamide was withdrawn and insulin given, the laboratory values normalized within 8 weeks. Rechallenge was considered unethical.

Hepatitis has been described with glibenclamide (95) and gliclazide (96).

- A 60-year-old woman with normal liver function tests developed acute hepatitis 6 weeks after starting to take gliclazide. No viruses, autoimmune factors, or metabolic factors that could have caused hepatitis could be found. A lymphocyte transformation test was not performed. A liver biopsy was compatible with drug-related acute hepatitis. When gliclazide was withdrawn she improved. She took glibenclamide and recovered fully within 6 weeks.
- A 64-year-old man who took gliclazide 160 mg bd for 3 months developed hepatitis (97). No other cause could be detected. Gliclazide was withdrawn. A liver biopsy after 2 weeks showed resolving acute hepatitis, consistent with a drug reaction, and 3 months later the liver profile was normal.
- A 42-year-old woman with newly diagnosed diabetes and no other known diseases developed a slightly abnormal liver profile (98). Good glycemic control was obtained with metformin 850 mg bd and gliclazide 80 mg bd. After 4 weeks she developed a pruritic skin rash, which resolved after 4 days of treatment with fexofenadine. A liver profile 2 weeks later was abnormal. Metformin was withdrawn, but 3 days later she was icteric and gliclazide was withdrawn. A liver biopsy was consistent with cirrhosis and there were moderate inflammatory infiltrates. The liver function tests improved and after 3 weeks she was rechallenged with metformin without exacerbation.

In the last case cirrhosis may have contributed to the adverse effect of gliclazide.

Pancreas

A possible relation between 2 years of treatment with a sulfonylurea and damage to the islets of Langerhans has been reported (99). A fatal case of pancreatitis has been attributed to glibenclamide (100).

In a case-control study in 1.4 million people in Sweden, 462 who were hospitalized for pancreatitis without gallbladder disease were compared with 1781 randomly selected controls; 6% of the cases and 3% of the controls had diabetes (101). Diet and insulin therapy were not associated with an increased risk, but the risk of pancreatitis with glibenclamide had a crude odds ratio of 3.2 and was higher in people aged over 70 years and in those taking beta-blockers.

Urinary tract

Nephrotic syndrome and immune complex glomerulonephritis have been attributed to chlorpropamide (102).

Skin

Photosensitization has been described with carbutamide (103), tolbutamide (104), chlorpropamide (105), and glibenclamide (106), sometimes combined with porphyrinuria.

Allergic skin reactions have been described with all sulfonylureas. They include pruritic rashes, erythema nodosum, urticaria, blisters (86), erythema multiforme, exfoliative dermatitis, Quincke's edema, erythroderma, and itching, while lichenoid drug reactions with ulceration have occurred after chlorpropamide and tolazamide (107). More generalized hypersensitivity reactions may prove fatal, but rarely.

Erythema multiforme has been attributed to glibenclamide (108).

- A 69-year-old woman, who had taken gliclazide 40 mg/day for 3 months, was switched to glibenclamide 2.5 mg/day. She had malaise for 2 days, followed by anorexia, fever, and 2 days later erythema multiforme over her whole body. She also had liver dysfunction, renal impairment, and rhabdomyolysis. A lymphocyte stimulation test was positive for glibenclamide, which was withdrawn; the rash improved and the laboratory tests normalized within 4 days.

Pigmented purpuric dermatosis has been attributed to glipizide (109).

- A 66-year-old man took glipizide for 4 weeks and developed brownish, non-pruritic, purpuric, scaling patches on his upper legs and buttocks. Biopsy showed dilated capillaries with surrounding extravasated erythrocytes, perivascular lymphocytic infiltrates, and areas of hemosiderin deposition. After withdrawal of glipizide the rash cleared.

Immunologic

Hypersensitivity vasculitis has been described with glibenclamide (110). Glibenclamide contains a sulfa moiety and can cause allergic reactions in someone who is allergic to sulfonamides.

- A 57-year-old man with a previously undocumented sulfa allergy used atenolol 100 mg/day, hydrochlorothiazide 25 mg/day, docusate sodium 100 mg/day, and ranitidine 300 mg bd for several months (111). He started to take celecoxib 200 mg/day, and 1 month later developed erythema multiforme and difficulty in breathing caused by swelling of the throat. He improved after withdrawal of his drugs and further treatment. He was then instructed to reintroduce his previous drugs one a day. One day later, after taking glibenclamide 5 mg, he developed new lesions and dyspnea. After 3 weeks he had another relapse when he reintroduced hydrochlorothiazide. He omitted glibenclamide, celecoxib, and hydrochlorothiazide, but continued to use insulin, metformin, ranitidine, and psyllium. The urticarial lesions disappeared.

Celecoxib and hydrochlorothiazide also have sulfa moieties and could have contributed in this case.

Death

Of 2275 diabetic patients aged 45–74 years with proven coronary artery disease, followed for 7.7 years, 990 were treated with diet alone, 79 with metformin, 953 with glibenclamide, and 253 with a combination of metformin and glibenclamide (112). They were compared with 9047 non-diabetics. Mortality was lowest in the non-diabetics; death rates in the others were: diet alone 26%, metformin 32%, glibenclamide 34%, and combined therapy 44%.

Second-Generation Effects

Pregnancy

Sulfonylureas ($n = 68$) and metformin ($n = 50$) have been compared retrospectively with insulin ($n = 42$) in pregnancy (113). There were no severe attacks of hypoglycemia, no jaundice, and no differences in neonatal morbidity. However, in those who took metformin, pre-eclampsia and perinatal deaths were more common. Since metformin was given to obese women, and since obesity contributes to pre-eclampsia and perinatal mortality, this may have been an effect of obesity.

In 404 pregnant women at 11–33 weeks of gestation, with a fasting blood glucose of 5.3–7.8 mmol/l, randomly assigned to insulin or glibenclamide, there were no differences in perinatal outcome (114). Glibenclamide was not found in cord blood. The data were analysed separately for women with mean glucose concentrations at home above and below 5.8 mmol/l. In the high blood glucose group there were large children for gestational age in 19% (insulin) and 17% (glibenclamide), compared with 10% (insulin) and 11% (glibenclamide) in the low glucose group; it is not clear whether these differences were significant. There were no other differences (for example macrosomia, insulin in cord blood) between the groups.

Teratogenicity

There is anecdotal evidence of a risk of teratogenicity of sulfonylureas, and on theoretical grounds it is inadvisable to give sulfonylureas to women of fertile age. In women using self-administered hypoglycemic drugs during pregnancy, chlorpropamide, glibenclamide, and tolbutamide were associated with serious malformations, such as microtia, deafness, facial deformities, ventricular septal defect (with or without aortic rotation), atrial septal defect, and a single umbilical artery (115). Of 332 children of women using a sulfonylurea during the first week of pregnancy, 12% had major and 5% had minor abnormalities, related to the increase in HbA$_{1c}$ (116). An effect of high blood glucose could not be excluded. Chromosomal damage is described with chlorpropamide (117), which may have contributed to the development of a cleft palate in another case (118). The choice for pregnant women with diabetes is between insulin given frequently in a short-acting form to avoid overdosage, or a continuous insulin infusion system, since overdosage of insulin can harm the developing fetus.

Fetotoxicity

Hypoglycemia has been reported in a neonate whose mother had taken tolbutamide (119).

- A woman with pre-existing hypertension took labetalol 600 mg/day and tolbutamide for gestational diabetes

and had long-standing hypoglycemia. She had started to take tolbutamide 500 mg/day in week 23 and increased the dosage to 1500 mg/day in week 29. Her HbA$_{1c}$ concentration was 5.0–5.8%. She felt no intrauterine movements during week 34 and an emergency cesarean section was performed. The baby had diabetic fetopathy (details not specified) and a blood glucose concentration of 0.8 mmol/l. Despite the administration of 20% glucose 10 ml as a bolus and then 8 ml/hour, the blood glucose remained below 1 mmol/l, and 10 hours after birth octreotide, a somatostatin analogue, was given. Intravenous glucose was discontinued after 3 days and octreotide on day 9. There were no signs of encephalopathy. C peptide, proinsulin, and insulin concentrations in the child were inappropriately high. Serum tolbutamide in the child was 141 µmol/l at 3 hours and the half-life was 46 hours.

The half-life of tolbutamide in this case was much longer than the reported half-life in adults of 7 hours, but the normal half-life in neonates is not known. The activity of CYP2C9, which metabolizes tolbutamide, may be reduced in the first 2 days of life.

Transient diabetes insipidus was seen in a child born to a mother who took chlorpropamide during pregnancy (120).

Neonatal thrombocytopenia and congenital malformations have been associated with administration of tolbutamide to the mother (121).

Susceptibility Factors

Age

Old age increases sensitivity to sulfonylureas and the frail elderly are at greatest risk (122).

Renal disease

Glimepiride (6), which is metabolized in the liver, was given for 3 months to two groups of diabetic patients with renal impairment: those with creatinine clearances of 30–60 ml and 10–30 ml (123). The goal was to reach a fasting blood glucose concentration below 10 mmol/l. There was recurrent hypoglycemia in one patient who did not need further drug therapy. There was one "silent" myocardial infarct. There were no other adverse effects. Serum insulin and C peptide concentrations did not change. There was increased clearance of glimepiride in the group with low creatinine clearances, probably caused by altered protein binding, increasing the unbound fraction available for hepatic metabolism.

Other features of the patient

Hypopituitarism, hypoadrenalism, and hypothyroidism all increase sensitivity to sulfonylureas because of reduced secretion of counter-regulatory hormones.

In insuloma, sensitivity to sulfonylureas is increased because insulin secretion from the tumor cells is greater than from normal islet cells.

Exercise training can force a reduction in the dose of various drugs in the treatment of diabetes (124). The hypoglycemic action of exercise in combination with sulfonylurea on postabsorptive glucose concentration is mainly caused by greater inhibition of glucose production in the liver (125).

Prolonged hypoglycemia in patients with end-stage renal disease prompted a search for predisposing factors in such patients with type 2 diabetes taking oral therapy only (126). Seven patients with and 31 without prolonged attacks of hypoglycemia, all on hemodialysis, were studied. All were using glibenclamide, except for three controls who took tolbutamide. The hypoglycemic episodes lasted 28–256 hours and glucose 83–2000 g was given for each episode. A recent fall in food intake, previous hypoglycemic episodes, longer duration of episodes, and a history of cerebrovascular disease were associated with prolonged hypoglycemia. There were no relations to age, sex, beta-blockers, ACE inhibitors, or drug doses. There were no cases of liver disease or alcohol abuse. Glibenclamide is seven times more highly concentrated in the pancreatic islets than other sulfonylureas, it has a long half-life, and its degradation products have hypoglycemic activity (SEDA-14, 1510).

Drug Administration

Drug formulations

New formulations of some sulfonylureas offer the possibility of once-daily therapy. They include gliclazide MR (SEDA-25, 511) and glipizide GITS (SEDA-22, 444) (SEDA-23, 475).

Gliclazide is available in various formulations with different kinetics in vivo and in vitro (127). Gliclazide MR is a modified-release formulation that allows once-a-day dosing. In a double-blind study 800 patients were randomized to gliclazide or gliclazide MR; there were no differences in adverse reactions or hypoglycemia (128). When comparing identical doses of Diamicron™ and Diabrezide™ in an open, crossover study, Diabrezide had a larger acute and mid-term hypoglycemic effect than Diamicron (129).

In a small study, gliclazide MR 30–120 mg/day had similar efficacy to 80–320 mg/day of the immediate-release formulation. The most commonly observed adverse events were arthralgia, arthritis, back pain, and bronchitis, which may not all have been directly related to the drug, as they also occurred with placebo. There was symptomatic hypoglycemia in about 5%.

Glipizide GITS was also studied in 19 patients with type 2 diabetes in an open, randomized, two-way, crossover study for 5 days, comparing 20 mg/day and 10 mg bd (130). Despite lower serum concentrations with glipizide GITS, the effects on serum concentrations of glucose, insulin, and C-peptide were the same. This may explain the low overall rate of hypoglycemia and lack of weight gain with glipizide GITS.

From time to time, drug names are confused and the wrong drug is prescribed or dispensed instead of the one intended. Of all the errors that occur, sulfonylureas are often implicated (131). Examples include chlorpropamide instead of chlorpromazine, chloroquine or etodolac instead of chlorpropamide, glyburide instead of thyroxine, and oxybutynin hydrochloride or acetohexamide

instead of acetazolamide (SEDA-16, 490) (SEDA-17, 495) (SEDA-18, 414) (SEDA-19, 395) (SEDA-21, 443).

Drug dosage regimens

There were no differences in episodes of hypoglycemia, concentrations of glucose, insulin, HbA1c, or lipids, or body weight when glibenclamide was given in one daily dose instead of divided doses (132).

Drug overdose

A suicide attempt with chlorpropamide has been reported (50).

- A 23-year-old woman took chlorpropamide 5–10 g. She needed assisted respiration and cardiac pacing for bradycardia (probably due to blockade of potassium channels), fluid infusion, and forced diuresis for 3 days. Notwithstanding continuous glucose infusion and glucose boluses she relapsed into severe hypoglycemia with convulsions. Only on day 27 was her urine free of chlorpropamide and her blood glucose normal.

Chlorpropamide is the longest-acting sulfonylurea. The high doses of glucose this patient was given may have stimulated further insulin secretion, thus contributing to the long period of fluctuating hypoglycemia. In the preceding 5 years 12 fatal cases of chlorpropamide poisoning with 3–15 g were seen in the same institution.

- Glibenclamide self-poisoning has been reported in a 48-year-old man with von Willebrand disease, Prinzmetal angina, hepatitis C, and depression (51). He had frequent hypoglycemic attacks, which were not reduced by reducing the dose of glibenclamide. Laparotomy for an insulinoma was considered until a glibenclamide concentration of 0.32 µg/ml was found, although glibenclamide was supposed to have been withdrawn.

Permanent right-sided hemiplegia, dysphasia, and hepatitis occurred after a suicide attempt with gliclazide (133).

- A 14-year-old non-diabetic girl took 15 tablets of gliclazide (1200 mg) and had gastric lavage 6 hours later. She developed lethargy, vomiting, and generalized tonic-clonic convulsions. Her blood glucose concentration was 0.8 mmol/l, aspartate transaminase 147 U/l (2.45 µkat/l), alanine transaminase 102 U/l (1.07 µkat/l), bilirubin 78 µmol/l (direct 31 µmol/l), and alkaline phosphatase 63 U/l. Electroencephalography showed voltage suppression in the left hemisphere and generalized slow-wave activity. A CT scan showed cerebral edema. Hypoglycemia was controlled within 24 hours with intravenous glucose. The convulsions could not be controlled with phenytoin, dexamethasone, or mannitol, given for cerebral edema, but they stopped on day 9. After 3.5 months of follow-up she could perceive words but could not speak and was severely hemiplegic.

Drug–Drug Interactions

General

Drug mechanisms that result in potentiation of the hypoglycemic effects of the sulfonylureas include:

- prolongation of the half-life by inhibition of metabolism or excretion (phenylbutazone, coumarins, chloramphenicol, doxycycline, bezafibrate, probenecid, sulfaphenazole, naproxen, fenyramidol);
- competition with plasma protein binding sites (NSAIDs, salicylates, and sulfonamides);
- potentiation of their hypoglycemic action by inhibition of gluconeogenesis, enhancement of oxidation of glucose, or stimulation of insulin secretion (beta-adrenoceptor antagonists, monoamine oxidase inhibitors, salicylates).

Examples are given in Table 2.

ACE inhibitors

In a retrospective case-control study, a primary diagnosis of hypoglycemia was identified in 413 patients registered as diabetic in 1993 (134). Five controls of the same age and sex, without hypoglycemia, were selected for each case from the same cohort. The relative risks of

Table 2 Drug interactions with oral hypoglycemic drugs

Interactions	Mechanisms
Enhanced hypoglycemia	
ACE inhibitors	7
Alcohol	3
Allopurinol	1 or 6
Azapropazone	2
Beta-adrenoceptor antagonists	3
Bezafibrate	7
Chloramphenicol	1
Cimetidine	7
Coumarin anticoagulants	7
Isoniazid	7
Levodopa	3
Naproxen	2
Perhexiline	3
Probenecid	1, 2, or 6
Pyrazolones	1, 2, or 6
Salicylates	2 or 6
Sulfonamides	1, 2 or 6
Reduced hypoglycemia	
Acetazolamide	7
Furosemide	7
Glucocorticoids	5
Oral contraceptives	5
Phenothiazines	7
Rifampicin	4
Sulfamethoxydiazine	7
Thiazide diuretics	5

Key to mechanisms:
[1]—Inhibition of drug-metabolizing enzymes
[2]—Displacement of drug from protein-binding sites
[3]—Impairment of glucose homeostatic mechanism
[4]—Induction of metabolizing enzymes
[5]—Increased insulin resistance
[6]—Reduced renal secretion
[7]—Unknown

hypoglycemia with ACE inhibitors, beta-blockers, calcium antagonists, and salicylates were determined. There was an association between enalapril and sulfonylureas. However, other ACE inhibitors could not be identified as a risk factor. There was no interaction with beta-blockers, calcium channel blockers, or salicylates.

The interaction of ACE inhibitors with sulfonylureas has also been illustrated in case reports (135,136).

- A 67-year-old man using glucocorticoids for asthma, ranitidine 300 mg/day, and enalapril 5 mg/day developed a low blood glucose (1.2 mmol/l) within 48 hours of starting to take glibenclamide 5–10 mg/day.
- A 64-year-old man, who used, amongst other drugs, glibenclamide 2.5 mg/day and metformin 850 mg bd, lost consciousness after a week of dwindling appetite and loose stools. His blood glucose was 2.2 mmol/l. He had renal impairment (creatinine 362 µmol/l). He also used ranitidine and ramipril 2.5 mg/day, which could have contributed to both the hypoglycemic effect and renal insufficiency.

In the second case, renal insufficiency could have reduced the clearance of the active metabolites of glibenclamide.

Alcohol

A disulfiram-like effect after use of alcohol has been described with chlorpropamide, but also with gliclazide, glipizide, and acetohexamide. However, the hepatic effects of sulfonylureas include inhibition of the enzymatic degradation of ethanol, an effect that is only partly comparable with the action of disulfiram, which blocks the degradation of aldehyde but not that of ethanol itself. This interaction results in a vasomotor reaction, with giddiness, tachycardia, headache, angina pectoris, and skin reactions. The most prominent drug to elicit these effects is chlorpropamide, but tolbutamide and other drugs can also do it. The specific effect of alcohol and chlorpropamide has been propagated to be of use as a genetic marker, but this has not been confirmed (SEDA-7, 407).

Excessive use of alcohol, sometimes found in older persons living alone, may also contribute to changes in sensitivity to oral hypoglycemic drugs. Low doses of alcohol (4.35 mmol/l/kg, comparable to one or two drinks) in fasting diabetics taking glibenclamide 20 mg/day in a randomized, double-blind, placebo-controlled study caused a greater fall in blood glucose concentrations than saline and increased counter-regulatory hormone concentrations (137).

Clarithromycin

Two men aged 82 and 72 years with impaired renal function and taking glibenclamide 5 mg/day and glipizide 15 mg/day, respectively, became comatose due to hypoglycemia within 48 hours of starting to take clarithromycin (138). Clarithromycin inhibits cytochrome CYP3A4. It should be used carefully in patients with diabetes and reduced renal function taking oral drugs.

Diltiazem

The interaction of tolbutamide with diltiazem has been studied in eight healthy men (139). Tolbutamide had no effect on diltiazem, but diltiazem increased the AUC of tolbutamide by 10% without an effect on blood glucose concentrations.

Hydroxychloroquine

The addition of hydroxychloroquine to sulfonylureas has been investigated in a placebo-controlled study in 125 adipose patients whose diabetes was not well enough controlled with a sulfonylurea alone (140). During the first six months HbA$_{1c}$ was significantly reduced by 1.02%. There were no significant differences in adverse effects, but those who took hydroxychloroquine had a greater incidence of minor corneal changes.

Rifampicin

Reduced efficacy of gliclazide has been attributed to induction of CYP2C9 by rifampicin (141).

- A 65-year-old man who had taken gliclazide 80 mg/day for 2 years took rifampicin for an infection with *Mycobacterium gordonae*, after which the dose of gliclazide had to be increased to 120 mg/day and later to 160 mg/day. After 75 days of combined therapy, gliclazide 80 mg/day gave a plasma concentration of 1.4 µg/ml; 7 months after stopping rifampicin it increased to 4.7 µg/ml. Gliclazide was then reduced to 80 mg/day.

It is important to check the blood glucose concentration if rifampicin is given in combination with oral hypoglycemic drugs.

Sulfonamides

Tolbutamide is mainly metabolized by CYP2C9, which also has a role in the metabolism of sulfonamides. Of various sulfonamides, sulfaphenazole had the largest inhibitory effect on the metabolism of tolbutamide in vitro (142). This gives a theoretical basis for being careful when tolbutamide and sulfonamides are co-administered.

References

1. Ashcroft FM, Gribble FM. ATP-sensitive K+ channels and insulin secretion: their role in health and disease. Diabetologia 1999;42(8):903–19.
2. The Diabetes Control and Complications Trial Research Group. The effect of intensive treatment of diabetes on the development and progression of long-term complications in insulin-dependent diabetes mellitus. N Engl J Med 1993;329(14):977–86.
3. Turner RC, Holman RR, Cull CA, Stratton IM, Matthews DR, Frighi V, Manley E, Neil A, McElroy H, Wright D, Kohner E, Fox C, Hadden D. Intensive blood-glucose control with sulphonylureas or insulin compared with conventional treatment and risk of complications in patients with type 2 diabetes (UKPDS 33). UK Prospective Diabetes Study (UKPDS) Group. Lancet 1998;352(9131):837–53.
4. DeWitt DE, Evans TC. Perioperative management of oral antihyperglycemic agents: special consideration for metformin. Semin Anesth 1998;17:267–72.
5. Anonymous. New oral antihyperglycaemic agents expand armamentarium in the battle against type 2 diabetes mellitus. Drugs Ther Perspect 1998;12:6–9.
6. Parulkar AA, Fonseca VA. Recent advances in pharmacological treatment of type 2 diabetes mellitus. Compr Ther 1999;25(8–10):418–26.
7. DeFronzo RA. Pharmacologic therapy for type 2 diabetes mellitus. Ann Intern Med 1999;131(4):281–303.
8. Lebovitz HE. Insulin secretagogues: old and new. Diabetes Rev 1999;7:139–53.
9. Hathout EH, Cockburn BN, Mace JW, Sharkey J, Chen-Daniel J, Bell GI. A case of hepatocyte nuclear factor-1 alpha diabetes/MODY3 masquerading as type 1 diabetes in a Mexican–American adolescent and responsive to a low dose of sulfonylurea. Diabetes Care 1999;22(5):867–8.
10. Hansen T, Eiberg H, Rouard M, Vaxillaire M, Moller AM, Rasmussen SK, Fridberg M, Urhammer SA, Holst JJ, Almind K, Echwald SM, Hansen L, Bell GI, Pedersen O. Novel MODY3 mutations in the hepatocyte nuclear factor-1alpha gene: evidence for a hyperexcitability of pancreatic beta-cells to intravenous secretagogues in a glucose-tolerant carrier of a P447L mutation. Diabetes 1997;46(4):726–30.
11. Pearson ER, Liddell WG, Shepherd M, Corrall RJ, Hattersley AT. Sensitivity to sulphonylureas in patients with hepatocyte nuclear factor-1alpha gene mutations: evidence for pharmacogenetics in diabetes. Diabet Med 2000;17(7):543–5.
12. Inzucchi SE. Oral antihyperglycemic therapy for type 2 diabetes: scientific review. JAMA 2002;287(3):360–72.
13. Holmboe ES. Oral antihyperglycemic therapy for type 2 diabetes: clinical applications. JAMA 2002;287(3):373–6.
14. Van Gaal LF, De Leeuw IH. Rationale and options for combination therapy in the treatment of type 2 diabetes. Diabetologia 2003;46(Suppl 1):M44–50.
15. Carroll MF, Izard A, Riboni K, Burge MR, Schade DS. Control of postprandial hyperglycemia: optimal use of short-acting insulin secretagogues. Diabetes Care 2002;25(12):2147–52.
16. Buysschaert M, Bobbioni E, Starkie M, Frith L. Troglitazone in combination with sulphonylurea improves glycaemic control in Type 2 diabetic patients inadequately controlled by sulphonylurea therapy alone. Troglitazone Study Group. Diabet Med 1999;16(2):147–53.
17. Leibowitz G, Cerasi E. Sulphonylurea treatment of NIDDM patients with cardiovascular disease: a mixed blessing? Diabetologia 1996;39(5):503–14.
18. Schwartz TB, Meinert CL. The UGDP controversy: thirty-four years of contentious ambiguity laid to rest. Perspect Biol Med 2004;47(4):564–74.
19. Cleveland JC Jr, Meldrum DR, Cain BS, Banerjee A, Harken AH. Oral sulfonylurea hypoglycemic agents prevent ischemic preconditioning in human myocardium. Two paradoxes revisited. Circulation 1997;96(1):29–32.
20. Wascher TC. Sulfonylureas and cardiovascular mortality in diabetes: a class effect? Circulation 1998;97(14):1427–8.
21. Britton ME, Denver AE, Mohamed-Ali V, Yudkin JS. Effects of glimepiride vs glibenclamide on ischaemic heart disease risk factors and glycaemic control in patients with type 2 diabetes mellitus. Clin Drug Invest 1998;16:303–17.
22. Tomai F, Danesi A, Ghini AS, Crea F, Perino M, Gaspardone A, Ruggeri G, Chiariello L, Gioffre PA. Effects of K(ATP) channel blockade by glibenclamide on the warm-up phenomenon. Eur Heart J 1999;20(3):196–202.
23. Ishibashi R, Takagi Y, Ozaki S. [A case with glibenclamide induced pneumonitis.] Jpn J Chest Dis 1999;58:758–62.
24. Feinglos MN, Lebovitz HE. Long-term safety and efficacy of glipizide. Am J Med 1983;75(5B):60–6.
25. Takami K, Takeda N, Nakashima K, Takami R, Hayashi M, Ozeki S, Yamada A, Kokubo Y, Sato M, Kawachi S, Sasaki A, Yasuda K. Effects of dietary

treatment alone or diet with voglibose or glyburide on abdominal adipose tissue and metabolic abnormalities in patients with newly diagnosed type 2 diabetes. Diabetes Care 2002;25(4):658–62.

26. Sulfonylurea drugs: basic and clinical considerations. A symposium presented before the 13th International Diabetes Federation Congress. Sydney, Australia, 20 November 1988. Proceedings. Diabetes Care 1990;13(Suppl 3):1–58.

27. Berger W, Caduff F, Pasquel M, Rump A. Die relative Haufigkeit der schweren Sulfonylharnstoff-Hypoglykämie in den letzten 25 Jahren in der Schweiz. Resultät von zwei gesamtschweizerischen Umfragen in den Jahren 1969 und 1984. [The relatively frequent incidence of severe sulfonylurea-induced hypoglycemia in the last 25 years in Switzerland. Results of 2 surveys in Switzerland in 1969 and 1984.] Schweiz Med Wochenschr 1986;116(5):145–51.

28. Ohsawa K, Koike N, Takamura T, Nagai Y, Kobayashi K. Hypoglycemic attacks after administration of bezafibrate in three cases of non-insulin dependent diabetes mellitus. J Jpn Diabetes Soc 1994;37:295–300.

29. Colagiuri S, Miller JJ, Petocz P. Double-blind crossover comparison of human and porcine insulins in patients reporting lack of hypoglycaemia awareness. Lancet 1992;339(8807):1432–5.

30. Wattoo MA, Liu HH. Alternating transient dense hemiplegia due to episodes of hypoglycemia. West J Med 1999;170(3):170–1.

31. Croxson SC, McConvey R, Molodynski L. Profound hypoglycaemia and cognitive impairment. Pract Diabetes Int 2001;18:315–16.

32. van Vonderen MG, Thijs A. Hypoglykemie bij orale bloed glucoseverlagende middelen: kans oprecidief na herstel van de glucosespiegel. [Hypoglycemia caused by oral hypoglycemic agents: risk of relapse after normalisation of blood glucose.] Ned Tijdschr Geneeskd 2002;146(7):289–92.

33. Auzepy P, Caquet R. Hypoglycémies gravesdues a l'insuline. Risques et accidents des médicaments antidiabétiques. [Severe hypoglycemia due to insulin. Risks and adverse effects of antidiabetic drugs.] Sem Hop 1983;59(10):697–705.

34. Asplund K, Wiholm BE, Lithner F. Glibenclamide-associated hypoglycaemia: a report on 57 cases. Diabetologia 1983;24(6):412–17.

35. Kennedy TD, Keat AC, Chester M, et al. Predisposing factors in fatal glibenclamide induced hypoglycaemia. Pract Diabetes 1988;5:217.

36. Gorgojo GG, Cancer E, Andreu M, Camblor M, Lajo T, Alvarez V, Moreno B. Hipoglucemia factitia induca por glipizida en una paciente con síndrome de Münchhausen. Endocrinologia 1998;45:38–42.

37. Meier JJ, Hucking K, Gruneklee D, Schmiegel W, Nauck MA. Unterschiede im Insulin-Sekretionsverhalten erleichtern die Differentialdiagnose von Insulinom und Hypoglycaemia factitia. [Differences in insulin secretion facilitate the differential diagnosis of insulinoma and factitious hypoglycaemia.] Dtsch Med Wochenschr 2002;127(8):375–8.

38. Ludwig A. Akzidentelle Hypoglykämie durch Inhalation von Sulfonylharnstoffstaub. Arbeitsmed Sozialmed Praventivmed 1991;26:31–2.

39. Anonymous. Sulfonylureas and hypoglycemia in the elderly. Hosp Practice 1996;31:28:167.

40. Salman S, Salman F, Satman I, Yilmaz Y, Ozer E, Sengul A, Demirel HO, Karsidag K, Dinccag N, Yilmaz MT. Comparison of acarbose and gliclazide as first-line agents in patients with type 2 diabetes. Curr Med Res Opin 2001;16(4):296–306.

41. Scholz GH, Schneider K, Knirsch W, Becker G. Effect and tolerability of glimepiride in daily practice: a non-interventional observational cohort study Clin Drug Invest 2001;21:597–604.

42. Charpentier G, Vaur L, Halimi S, Fleury F, Derobert E, Grimaldi A, Oriol V, Etienne S, Altman JJ; DIAMETRE. Predictors of response to glimepiride in patients with type 2 diabetes mellitus. Diabetes Metab 2001;27(5 Pt 1):563–71.

43. So WY, Chan JC, Yeung VT, Chow CC, Ko GT, Li JK, Cockram CS. Sulphonylurea-induced hypoglycaemia in institutionalized elderly in Hong Kong. Diabet Med 2002;19(11):966–8.

44. Leese GP, Wang J, Broomhall J, Kelly P, Marsden A, Morrison W, Frier BM, Morris AD; DARTS/MEMO Collaboration. Frequency of severe hypoglycemia requiring emergency treatment in type 1 and type 2 diabetes: a population-based study of health service resource use. Diabetes Care 2003;26(4):1176–80.

45. Tomizawa HH. Properties of glutathione insulin transhydrogenase from beef liver. J Biol Chem 1962;237:3393–6.

46. Pettipierre B, Fabre J. Effet de l'insuffisance rénale sur l'action hypoglycémiante des sylfonylurées. Cinétique de la chlorpropamide en cas de néphropathie. [The effect of renal insufficiency on the hypoglycemic action of sulfonylureas. Kinetics of chlorpropamide in a case of nephropathy.] Schweiz Med Wochenschr 1972;102(16):570–8.

47. Burge MR, Schmitz-Fiorentino K, Fischette C, Qualls CR, Schade DS. A prospective trial of risk factors for sulfonylurea-induced hypoglycemia in type 2 diabetes mellitus. JAMA 1998;279(2):137–43.

48. Shorr RI. Hypoglycemia from glipizide and glyburide. JAMA 1998;279(18):1441–2.

49. Gambassi G, Carbonin P, Bernabei R. Hypoglycemia from glipizide and glyburide. JAMA 1998;279(18):1442–3.

50. Ciechanowski K, Borowiak KS, Potocka BA, Nowacka M, Dutkiewicz G. Chlorpropamide toxicity with survival despite 27-day hypoglycemia. J Toxicol Clin Toxicol 1999;37(7):869–71.

51. Torello AL, Canonge RS, Pascual CH, Manteca JM. Occult ingestion of sulfonylureas: a diagnostic challenge. Endocrinol Nutr 2000;47:174–5.

52. Seltzer HS. Severe drug-induced hypoglycemia: a review. Compr Ther 1979;5(4):21–9.

53. Stahl M, Berger W. Higher incidence of severe hypoglycaemia leading to hospital admission in type 2 diabetic patients treated with long-acting versus short-acting sulphonylureas. Diabet Med 1999;16(7):586–90.

54. Ben-Ami H, Nagachandran P, Mendelson A, Edoute Y. Drug-induced hypoglycemic coma in 102 diabetic patients. Arch Intern Med 1999;159(3):281–4.

55. Trenque T, Hoizey G, Lamiable D. Serious hypoglycemia: Munchausen's syndrome? Diabetes Care 2001;24(4):792–3.

56. Moore DF, Wood DF, Volans GN. Features, prevention and management of acute overdose due to antidiabetic drugs. Drug Saf 1993;9(3):218–29.

57. Boyle PJ, Justice K, Krentz AJ, Nagy RJ, Schade DS. Octreotide reverses hyperinsulinemia and prevents hypoglycemia induced by sulfonylurea overdoses. J Clin Endocrinol Metab 1993;76(3):752–6.

58. Drzewoski J, Czupryniak L, Chwatko G, Bald E. Total plasma homocysteine and insulin levels in type 2 diabetic patients with secondary failure to oral agents. Diabetes Care 1999;22(12):2097–9.

59. Hirokawa CA, Gray DR. Chlorpropamide-induced hyponatremia in the veteran population. Ann Pharmacother 1992;26(10):1243–4.

60. Kadowaki T, Hagura R, Kajinuma H, Kuzuya N, Yoshida S. Chlorpropamide-induced hyponatremia: incidence and risk factors. Diabetes Care 1983;6(5):468–71.

61. Chan TY. Drug-induced syndrome of inappropriate antidiuretic hormone secretion. Causes, diagnosis and management. Drugs Aging 1997;11(1):27–44.

62. Gin H, Lars I, Morlat P, Beauvieux JM, Aubertin J. Hyponatrémie induite par les sulfamides hypoglycémiants. [Hyponatremia induced by hypoglycemic sulfonamides: a study of 70 patients.] Ann Med Interne (Paris) 1988;139(7):455–9.

63. Tsumura K. Clinical evaluation of glimepiride (HOE490) in NIDDM, including a double blind comparative study versus gliclazide. Diabetes Res Clin Pract 1995;28(Suppl):S147–9.

64. Ravina A. Antidiuretic action of chlorpropamide. Lancet 1973;2(7822):203.

65. Moses AM, Howanitz J, Miller M. Diuretic action of three sulfonylurea drugs. Ann Intern Med 1973;78(4):541–4.

66. Traumann KJ, Grom E, Schwarzkopf H. Panzytopenie bei Diabetes-mellitus-Therapie mit Tolbutamid? [Pancytopenia in diabetes mellitus treatment with tolbutamide?] Dtsch Med Wochenschr 1975;100(6):250–1.

67. Gill MJ, Ratliff DA, Harding LK. Hypoglycemic coma, jaundice, and pure RBC aplasia following chlorpropamide therapy. Arch Intern Med 1980;140(5):714–15.

68. Levitt LJ. Chlorpropamide-induced pure white cell aplasia. Blood 1987;69(2):394–400.

69. Saffouri B, Cho JH, Felber N. Chlorpropamide-induced haemolytic anaemia. Postgrad Med J 1981;57(663):44–5.

70. Nataas OB, Nesthus I. Immune haemolytic anaemia induced by glibenclamide in selective IgA deficiency. BMJ (Clin Res Ed) 1987;295(6594):366–7.

71. Malacarne P, Castaldi G, Bertusi M, Zavagli G. Tolbutamide-induced hemolytic anemia. Diabetes 1977;26(2):156–8.

72. Cunliffe DJ, Gorst DW, Palmer HM. Chlorpropamide-induced thrombocytopenia. Postgrad Med J 1977;53(616):87–8.

73. Sauer H, Fischer K, Landbeck G. [Allergic thrombocytopenia in tolbutamide therapy of diabetes mellitus.] Med Welt 1962;36:1899–903.

74. Vaatainen N, Fraki JE, Hyvonen M, Neittaanmaki H. Purpura with a linear epidermo-dermal deposition of IgA. Acta Derm Venereol 1983;63(2):169–70.

75. Cartron G, Jonville-Bera AP, Autret-Leca E, Colombat P. Glimepiride-induced thrombocytopenic purpura. Ann Pharmacother 2000;34(1):120.

76. Noto H, Tsukamoto K, Kimura S. Glyburide-induced hemolysis in myelodysplastic syndrome. Diabetes Care 2000;23(1):129.

77. Bernhard H. Long-term observations on oral hypoglycemic agents in diabetes; The effect of carbutamide and tolbutamide. Diabetes 1965;14:59–70.

78. Bell RJ. Pulmonary infiltration with eosinophils caused by chlorpropamide. Lancet 1964;42:1249–50.

79. Bondi E, Slater S. Tolazamide-induced chronic eosinophilic pneumonia. Chest 1981;80(5):652.

80. Berger W, Constam GR, Siegenthaler W. Die Behandlungsmoglichkeiten des Diabetes mellitus mit Biguaniden. Klinische Erfahrungen bei 122 Diabetikern mit Dimethylbiguanid (Glucophage). [Therapeutic possibilities in diabetes mellitus with biguanides. Clinical experiences in 122 diabetics with dimethylbiguanide (Glucophage).] Schweiz Med Wochenschr 1966;96(40):1335–42.

81. Schneider HL, Hornbach KD, Kniaz JL, Efrusy ME. Chlorpropamide hepatotoxicity: report of a case and review of the literature. Am J Gastroenterol 1984;79(9):721–4.

82. Nakao NL, Gelb AM, Stenger RJ, Siegel JH. A case of chronic liver disease due to tolazamide. Gastroenterology 1985;89(1):192–5.

83. Rumboldt Z, Bota B. Favorable effects of glibenclamide in a patient exhibiting idiosyncratic hepatotoxic reactions to both chlorpropamide and tolbutamide. Acta Diabetol Lat 1984;21(4):387–91.

84. Clementsen P, Hansen CL, Hoegholm A. Glipizidinduceret toksisk hepatitis. [Glipizide induced toxic hepatitis.] Ugeskr Laeger 1986;148(13):771–2.

85. De Rosa G, Corsello SM, Pizzi C, et al. Epatopatia citolitica amitterica da glibenclamide. Epatologia 1980;26:73.

86. Wongpaitoon V, Mills PR, Russell RI, Patrick RS. Intrahepatic cholestasis and cutaneous bullae associated with glibenclamide therapy. Postgrad Med J 1981;57(666):244–6.

87. Rigberg LA, Robinson MJ, Espiritu CR. Chlorpropamide-induced granulomas. A probable hypersensitivity reaction in liver and bone marrow. JAMA 1976;235(4):409–10.

88. Lambert M, Geubel A, Rahier J, Branquinho F. Cholestatic hepatitis associated with glibenclamide therapy. Eur J Gastroenterol Hepatol 1990;2:389–91.

89. Krivoy N, Zaher A, Yaacov B, Alroy G. Fatal toxic intrahepatic cholestasis secondary to glibenclamide. Diabetes Care 1996;19(4):385–6.

90. Rank JM, Olson RC. Reversible cholestatic hepatitis caused by acetohexamide. Gastroenterology 1989;96(6):1607–8.

91. Gupta R, Sachar DB. Chlorpropamide-induced cholestatic jaundice and pseudomembranous colitis. Am J Gastroenterol 1985;80(5):381–3.

92. Dourakis SP, Tzemanakis E, Sinani C, Kafiri G, Hadziyannis SJ. Gliclazide-induced acute hepatitis. Arch Hell Med 1998;15:87–9.

93. Bridges ME, Pittman FE. Tolazamide-induced cholestasis. South Med J 1980;73(8):1072–4.

94. Tholakanahalli VN, Potti A, Heyworth MF. Glibenclamide-induced cholestasis. West J Med 1998;168(4):274–7.

95. Goodman RC, Dean PJ, Radparvar A, Kitabchi AE. Glyburide-induced hepatitis. Ann Intern Med 1987;106(6):837–9.

96. Dourakis SP, Tzemanakis E, Sinani C, Kafiri G, Hadziyannis SJ. Gliclazide-induced acute hepatitis. Eur J Gastroenterol Hepatol 2000;12(1):119–21.

97. Subramanian G, Walmsley D, Blewitt RW. Gliclazide-induced hepatitis. Pract Diabetes Int 2003;20:18–20.

98. Chitturi S, Le V, Kench J, Loh C, George J. Gliclazide-induced acute hepatitis with hypersensitivity features. Dig Dis Sci 2002;47(5):1107–10.

99. Tavani E, Giardini R. Alterazioni istopatologiche delle isole di Langerhans in un caso di diabete mellito trattato con sulfaniluree. [Histopathological changes in the islands of Langerhans in a case of diabetes mellitus treated with sulfonylurea.] Pathologica 1978;70(999–1000):105–8.

100. Roblin X, Abinader Y, Baziz A. Pancréatite aiguë sous gliclazide. [Acute pancreatitis induced by gliclazide.] Gastroenterol Clin Biol 1992;16(1):96.

101. Blomgren KB, Sundstrom A, Steineck G, Wiholm BE. Obesity and treatment of diabetes with glyburide may both be risk factors for acute pancreatitis. Diabetes Care 2002;25(2):298–302.

102. Appel GB, D'Agati V, Bergman M, Pirani CL. Nephrotic syndrome and immune complex glomerulonephritis associated with chlorpropamide therapy. Am J Med 1983;74(2):337–42.

103. Temime P, Oddoze L, Privat Y, Costes A, Maurin J. [Erythrodermia secondary to an intense photosenitization caused by carbutamide (BZ 55).] Bull Soc Fr Dermatol Syphiligr 1962;69:124–5.

104. Kar PK, Das Gupta SK, Das KD. Tolbutamide photosensitivity. J Indian Med Assoc 1984;82(8):289–91.

105. Feuerman E, Frumkin A. Photodermatitis induced by chlorpropamide. A report of five cases. Dermatologica 1973;146(1):25–9.

106. Fujii S, Nakashima T, Kaneko T. Glibenclamide-induced photosensitivity in a diabetic patient with erythropoietic protoporphyria. Am J Hematol 1995;50(3):223.

107. Barnett JH, Barnett SM. Lichenoid drug reactions to chlorpropamide and tolazamide. Cutis 1984;34(6):542–4.

108. Aoki T, Sobajima H, Suzuki Y, Sassa H. [A case of erythema multiforme and rhabdomyolysis induced by Daonil (glibenclamide) 2.5 mg tablet.] J Jpn Diabetes Soc 1999;42:759–63.

109. Adams BB, Gadenne AS. Glipizide-induced pigmented purpuric dermatosis. J Am Acad Dermatol 1999;41(5 Pt 2):827–9.

110. Clarke BF, Campbell IW, Ewing DJ, Beveridge GW, MacDonald MK. Generalized hypersensitivity reaction and visceral arteritis with fatal outcome during glibenclamide therapy. Diabetes 1974;23(9):739–42.

111. Ernst EJ, Egge JA. Celecoxib-induced erythema multiforme with glyburide cross-reactivity. Pharmacotherapy 2002;22(5):637–40.

112. Fisman EZ, Tenenbaum A, Boyko V, Benderly M, Adler Y, Friedensohn A, Kohanovski M, Rotzak R, Schneider H, Behar S, Motro M. Oral antidiabetic treatment in patients with coronary disease: time-related increased mortality on combined glyburide/metformin therapy over a 7.7-year follow-up. Clin Cardiol 2001;24(2):151–8.

113. Hellmuth E, Damm P, Molsted-Pedersen L. Oral hypoglycaemic agents in 118 diabetic pregnancies. Diabet Med 2000;17(7):507–11.

114. Langer O, Conway DL, Berkus MD, Xenakis EM, Gonzales O. A comparison of glyburide and insulin in women with gestational diabetes mellitus. N Engl J Med 2000;343(16):1134–8.

115. Piacquadio K, Hollingsworth DR, Murphy H. Effects of in-utero exposure to oral hypoglycaemic drugs. Lancet 1991;338(8771):866–9.

116. Towner D, Kjos SL, Leung B, Montoro MM, Xiang A, Mestman JH, Buchanan TA. Congenital malformations in pregnancies complicated by NIDDM. Diabetes Care 1995;18(11):1446–51.

117. Berger W. Orale Antidiabetika 1977. [Oral antidiabetics 1977.] ZFA (Stuttgart) 1978;54(9):513–24.

118. Ansaldi E, Gilardi GB. Chlorpropamide and cleft palate. J Foetal Med 1984;4:50.

119. Christesen HB, Melander A. Prolonged elimination of tolbutamide in a premature newborn with hyperinsulinaemic hypoglycaemia. Eur J Endocrinol 1998;138(6):698–701.

120. Uhrig JD, Hurley RM. Chlorpropamide in pregnancy and transient neonatal diabetes insipidus. Can Med Assoc J 1983;128(4):368,370–1.

121. Schiff D, Aranda JV, Stern L. Neonatal thrombocytopenia and congenital malformations associated with administration of tolbutamide to the mother. J Pediatr 1970;77(3):457–8.

122. Shorr RI, Ray WA, Daugherty JR, Griffin MR. Incidence and risk factors for serious hypoglycemia in older persons using insulin or sulfonylureas. Arch Intern Med 1997;157(15):1681–6.

123. Profozic V, Mrzljac V, Nazar I, Metelko Z, Rosenkranz B, Lange C, Malerczyk V. Safety, efficacy, and pharmacokinetics of glimepiride in diabetic patients with renal impairment over a 3-month period. Diabetol Croat 1999;28:25–32.

124. Valenta LJ, Elias AN. Insulin-induced lipodystrophy in diabetic patients resolved by treatment with human insulin. Ann Intern Med 1985;102(6):790–1.

125. Cusi K, DeFronzo RA. Treatment of NIDDM IDDM, and other insulin-resistant states with IGF-I. Diabetes Rev 1995;3:206–36.

126. Krepinsky J, Ingram AJ, Clase CM. Prolonged sulfonylurea-induced hypoglycemia in diabetic patients with end-stage renal disease. Am J Kidney Dis 2000;35(3):500–5.

127. McGavin JK, Perry CM, Goa KL. Gliclazide modified release. Drugs 2002;62(9):1357–64.

128. Drouin P. Diamicron MR once daily is effective and well tolerated in type 2 diabetes: a double-blind, randomized, multinational study. J Diabetes Complications 2000;14(4):185–91.

129. Galeone F, Fiore G, Mannucci E. Medium-term hypoglycaemic effects of two different oral formulations of gliclazide. Diabet Med 1999;16(7):618–19.

130. Chung M, Kourides I, Canovatchel W, Sutfin T, Messig M, Chaiken RL. Pharmacokinetics and pharmacodynamics of extended-release glipizide GITS compared with immediate-release glipizide in patients with type II diabetes mellitus. J Clin Pharmacol 2002;42(6):651–7.

131. Aronson JK. Confusion over similar drug names. Problems and solutions. Drug Saf 1995;12(3):155–60.

132. Wan Mohamad WB, Tun Fizi A, Ismail RB, Mafauzy M. Efficacy and safety of single versus multiple daily doses of glibenclamide in type 2 diabetes mellitus. Diabetes Res Clin Pract 2000;49(2–3):93–9.

133. Caksen H, Kendirci M, Tutus A, Uzum K, Kurtoglu S. Gliclazide-induced hepatitis, hemiplegia and dysphasia in a suicide attempt. J Pediatr Endocrinol Metab 2001;14(8):1157–9.

134. Thamer M, Ray NF, Taylor T. Association between antihypertensive drug use and hypoglycemia: a case-control study of diabetic users of insulin or sulfonylureas. Clin Ther 1999;21(8):1387–400.

135. Parlapiano C, Paoletti V, Campana E, Giovanniello T, Pantone P. Increased risk of hypoglycemia from enalapril plus ranitidine with glibenclamide: a clinical case. Adv Ther 1999;16:130–2.

136. Collin M, Mucklow JC. Drug interactions, renal impairment and hypoglycaemia in a patient with type II diabetes. Br J Clin Pharmacol 1999;48(2):134–7.

137. Burge MR, Zeise TM, Sobhy TA, Rassam AG, Schade DS. Low-dose ethanol predisposes elderly fasted patients with type 2 diabetes to sulfonylurea-induced low blood glucose. Diabetes Care 1999;22(12):2037–43.

138. Bussing R, Gende A. Severe hypoglycemia from clarithromycin–sulfonylurea drug interaction. Diabetes Care 2002;25(9):1659–61.

139. Dixit AA, Rao YM. Pharmacokinetic interaction between diltiazem and tolbutamide. Drug Metabol Drug Interact 1999;15(4):269–77.

140. Gerstein HC, Thorpe KE, Taylor DW, Haynes RB. The effectiveness of hydroxychloroquine in patients with type 2 diabetes mellitus who are refractory to sulfonylureas—a randomized trial. Diabetes Res Clin Pract 2002;55(3):209–19.

141. Kihara Y, Otsuki M. Interaction of gliclazide and rifampicin. Diabetes Care 2000;23(8):1204–5.

142. Dische FE, Wernstedt C, Westermark GT, Westermark P, Pepys MB, Rennie JA, Gilbey SG, Watkins PJ. Insulin as an amyloid-fibril protein at sites of repeated insulin injections in a diabetic patient. Diabetologia 1988;31(3):158–61.

Sulindac

See also Non-steroidal anti-inflammatory drugs

General Information

There is still no firm evidence that by acting through an active metabolite, sulindac has any distinct advantage over other members of the group of NSAIDs that are related to indometacin. However, its good tolerance in elderly patients has been stressed (1). Its pattern of adverse effects is similar to that of indometacin (2), with an incidence ranging from 17 (3) to 50% (4). Sulindac causes fewer gastrointestinal adverse effects than aspirin, but in some studies the incidence equalled that of ibuprofen (5), fenoprofen (6), and indometacin (7).

Organs and Systems

Cardiovascular

Several cardiac abnormalities have been reported, including congestive heart failure, dysrhythmias, and palpitation (8).

Respiratory

Pulmonary infiltrates were described in a woman with osteoarthritis who had been taking sulindac for 6 months (9).

Nervous system

Adverse effects on the nervous system were found in 2.5–6.5% of patients in one study (4). Dizziness, drowsiness and headache, somnolence, vertigo, insomnia, and blurred vision, that is all adverse effects described with indometacin, have been observed. Acute reversible encephalopathy with rash and fever has been described.

Like other NSAIDs, sulindac can cause aseptic meningitis in patients with systemic lupus erythematosus (SEDA-7, 109). Recurrent aseptic meningitis, described in a patient with no underlying connective tissue disease who had tolerated other NSAIDs, suggested immunological hypersensitivity to sulindac (10).

Psychological, psychiatric

Psychiatric symptoms, bizarre behavior, and paranoia have been attributed to sulindac (11).

Electrolyte balance

The risk of severe hyperkalemia with sulindac has been documented in a series of four cases (12).

Hematologic

Agranulocytosis (probably due to toxicity rather than hypersusceptibility) can be caused by sulindac (13), as can bone marrow aplasia (14) and severe thrombocytopenia (15,16), which may be the consequence of autoimmune platelet destruction in the presence of sulindac or its metabolite (SEDA-7, 109). Immune-mediated hemolytic anemia with a positive direct antiglobulin test has been reported (SEDA-18, 103).

Aplastic anemia in a woman with osteoarthritis taking sulindac relapsed 3 years later during therapy with fenbufen, suggesting that extreme caution should be exercised before giving NSAIDs to a patient with a history of NSAID-related aplastic anemia (17).

Gastrointestinal

Sulindac can cause all of the gastrointestinal adverse effects that are associated with indometacin, from dyspepsia to peptic ulcer. Nausea and abdominal pain are the most frequent, followed by constipation (18). Surprisingly, a study in healthy volunteers showed no gastroscopic mucosal damage after 7 days (19). This recalls past papers showing a lack of mucosal damage in short-term therapy, even with NSAIDs known to be gastrotoxic. A giant esophageal ulcer has been described (20). A preterm neonate developed fatal hemorrhagic gastritis with oral sulindac (21).

Ulcers in an ileal pouch with chronic bleeding have been described (22).

Sulindac reduces the number and size of rectal and colon polyps (23) and colon-mucosal synthesis of prostaglandin E_2 and 6-keto-prostaglandin $F_{1\alpha}$ is markedly reduced in patients taking sulindac. As this occurs concomitantly with the regression of polyps, it supports the hypothesis that prostaglandins are implicated in the regulation of colonic polyp growth (24). These observations have been confirmed in two other studies. Low-dose rectal sulindac produced complete adenoma remission in 87% of 15 colectomized patients with familial adenomatous polyposis. Polyp number and size fell significantly in 22 patients who took sulindac 150 mg bd for 3 months (25). After rectal administration of sulindac two patients had histologically proven mild gastritis (26).

Liver

Sulindac can cause toxic hepatitis, and several cases, some with positive rechallenge, have been described (27,28). A retrospective cohort study with secondary case-control analysis suggested that sulindac has a higher incidence of acute liver damage than all other NSAIDs, although the calculated risk is very low (27 per 100 000 prescriptions) (29). Liver function impairment is generally mild and reversible. Analysis of spontaneous reports to the FDA and the Danish Committee on ADRs (SEDA-18, 103) has confirmed these data.

Abdominal pain, nausea, high fever with chills, icterus, high liver enzyme activities, and hepatomegaly are characteristic and are probably caused by hypersensitivity. The occurrence of fever, rash, and/or eosinophilia in 35–55% of patients seems to confirm a hypersensitivity mechanism (SEDA-18, 103).

Cholestatic jaundice (30) and acute cholangitis in combination with acute pancreatitis (SEDA-13, 79) have been described.

Pancreas

There are several reports of pancreatitis associated with sulindac (SEDA-4, 66) (SEDA-7, 109). Symptoms resembling acute pancreatitis appeared after 3–90 days. Rechallenge was positive in one case (31). Acute cholangitis in combination with acute pancreatitis has been described (SEDA-13, 79).

Urinary tract

Sulindac may be less likely to cause renal toxicity than other NSAIDs (32), at least when it is used in low dosages, but there is some disagreement on this point (33–35), and five cases of nephrotic syndrome and renal insufficiency have been described (36,37).

Analysis of small renal and biliary stones has shown that sulindac or its metabolite was present in the material (SEDA-15, 99), and the labeling of sulindac was revised in 1989 to warn physicians of this phenomenon. However, despite the presence of sulindac or its metabolites in some renal stones, patients taking long-term sulindac are not at risk of an increased incidence of renal stone formation compared with those taking other NSAIDs (38).

Skin

The Stevens–Johnson syndrome has been reported in women who all recovered after the drug was withdrawn and corticosteroids given (SEDA-6, 95). Toxic epidermal necrolysis has also been reported (39–41).

A reaction like lupus pernio, with purple discoloration, swelling, red papules, and desquamation of the distal parts of several toes, which resolved after drug suspension and recurred after resumption, has been observed (42), as have subcutaneous fat necrosis (SEDA-11, 92), and fixed drug reaction (SEDA-12, 84).

Immunologic

Several types of proven or suspected hypersensitivity have already been mentioned, for example in connection with the liver, but the exact mechanism of a particular adverse effect has not always been clear. One case of fever, pharyngitis, cervical lymphadenopathy, leukopenia, liver abnormalities, proteinuria, pulmonary infiltrates, and abdominal pain has been described. Another patient who previously took sulindac without problems developed pruritus, dyspnea, perioral edema, and lethargy after taking a single dose of sulindac 150 mg.

Pneumonitis is probably part of a general hypersensitivity reaction (SEDA-6, 94) (9,43).

An anaphylactic reaction has been described (44). Sulindac is also thought to have been responsible for a severe multisystem reaction (possibly again anaphylactic) involving the cardiovascular, hepatic, pulmonary, and hematological systems in a patient with quiescent systemic lupus erythematosus (45).

Second-Generation Effects

Fetotoxicity

The use of oral sulindac for closure of patent ductus arteriosus has been evaluated in a prospective comparison with intravenous indometacin. Sulindac promoted ductal constriction without compromising renal function in preterm infants, but its use was associated with severe gastrointestinal complications (46).

Susceptibility Factors

Patients with sodium depletion are at risk of developing hyponatremia with all NSAIDs. Sulindac also provoked hyponatremia in an elderly patient taking a salt-restricted diet (47).

Drug Administration

Drug overdose

Agranulocytosis of short duration was described after an overdose of sulindac 12 g (48). Eight cases of sulindac overdose have been reported to the UK National Poisons Information Service; all the patients remained asymptomatic (SEDA-9, 89).

Drug–Drug Interactions

Furosemide

Data on sulindac inhibition of the diuretic effect of furosemide are contradictory (49).

Lithium

Unlike other NSAIDs, sulindac does not seem to interact with lithium (SEDA-10, 82). However, in one case it may have increased serum lithium concentrations (50).

Propranolol

Like indometacin, sulindac interacted with propranolol and a thiazide diuretic in a hypertensive patient (SEDA-6, 95).

Thiazide diuretics

Like indometacin, sulindac interacted with propranolol and a thiazide diuretic in a hypertensive patient (SEDA-6, 95).

Topical dimethylsulfoxide

Two cases of peripheral neuropathy attributed to a combination of oral sulindac and topical dimethylsulfoxide have been reported (SEDA-9, 89).

Warfarin

Potentiation of warfarin effects by sulindac has been reported (51).

References

1. Davis P. Comparative efficacy and tolerance of sulindac (Clinoril) in geriatric and nongeriatric patients. Curr Ther Res 1985;37:945.
2. Anonymous. Clinoril adverse reactions. FDA Drug Bull 1979;9(5):29.
3. Delcambre B. The sulindac profile—use of sulindac in hospital and private practice: multicentre study in general practice. Eur J Rheumatol Inflamm 1978;1:47.
4. Bordier P, Knutz DD. Sulindac: clinical results of treatment of osteoarthritis. Eur J Rheumatol Inflamm 1978;1:27.
5. Andrade L, Fernandez A. Sulindac in the treatment of osteoarthritis: a double blind 8 week study comparing sulindac with ibuprofen and 96 weeks of long term therapy. Eur J Rheumatol Inflamm 1978;1:36.
6. Durance RA, Jacobi RK, Thompson M, Whittington JR. A multicentre comparative analgesic study of fenoprofen and sulindac in rheumatoid arthritis. Curr Ther Res 1979;26:79.

7. Calin A, Britton M. Sulindac in ankylosing spondylitis. Double-blind evaluation of sulindac and indomethacin. JAMA 1979;242(17):1885–6.

8. Anonymous. Clinoril sulindac: cardiac abnormalities. ADR Highlights 1979;July 3.

9. Takimoto CH, Lynch D, Stulbarg MS. Pulmonary infiltrates associated with sulindac therapy. Chest 1990;97(1):230–2.

10. Greenberg GN. Recurrent sulindac-induced aseptic meningitis in a patient tolerant to other nonsteroidal anti-inflammatory drugs. South Med J 1988;81(11):1463–4.

11. Kruis R, Barger R. Paranoid psychosis with sulindac. JAMA 1980;243(14):1420.

12. Nesher G, Zimran A, Hershko C. Hyperkalemia associated with sulindac therapy. J Rheumatol 1986;13(6):1084–5.

13. Romeril KR, Duke DS, Hollings PE. Sulindac induced agranulocytosis and bone marrow culture. Lancet 1981;2(8245):523.

14. Miller JL. Marrow aplasia and sulindac. Ann Intern Med 1980;92(1):129.

15. Stambaugh JE Jr, Gordon RL, Geller R. Leukopenia and thrombocytopenia secondary to clinoril therapy. Lancet 1980;2(8194):594.

16. Rosenbaum JT. Thrombocytopenia associated with sulindac. Arthritis Rheum 1981;24(5):753–4.

17. Andrews R, Russell N. Aplastic anaemia associated with a non-steroidal anti-inflammatory drug: relapse after exposure to another such drug. BMJ 1990;301(6742):38.

18. Anonymous. Sulindac (Clinoril)—a new drug for arthritis. Med Lett Drugs Ther 1979;21(1):1–2.

19. Graham DY, Smith JL, Holmes GI, Davies RO. Nonsteroidal anti-inflammatory effect of sulindac sulfoxide and sulfide on gastric mucosa. Clin Pharmacol Ther 1985;38(1):65–70.

20. Levine MS, Rothstein RD, Laufer I. Giant esophageal ulcer due to Clinoril. Am J Roentgenol 1991;156(5):955–6.

21. Ng PC, So KW, Fok TF, To KF, Wong W, Liu K. Fatal haemorrhagic gastritis associated with oral sulindac treatment for patent ductus arteriosus. Acta Paediatr 1996;85(7):884–6.

22. Bertoni G, Sassatelli R, Bedogni G, Nigrisoli E. Sulindac-associated ulcerative pouchitis in familial adenomatous polyposis. Am J Gastroenterol 1996;91(11):2431–2.

23. Rigau J, Pique JM, Rubio E, Planas R, Tarrech JM, Bordas JM. Effects of long-term sulindac therapy on colonic polyposis. Ann Intern Med 1991;115(12):952–4.

24. Smalley WE, DuBois RN. Colorectal cancer and nonsteroidal anti-inflammatory drugs. Adv Pharmacol 1997;39:1–20.

25. Giardiello FM, Offerhaus JA, Tersmette AC, Hylind LM, Krush AJ, Brensinger JD, Booker SV, Hamilton SR. Sulindac induced regression of colorectal adenomas in familial adenomatous polyposis: evaluation of predictive factors. Gut 1996;38(4):578–81.

26. Winde G, Schmid KW, Schlegel W, Fischer R, Osswald H, Bunte H. Complete reversion and prevention of rectal adenomas in colectomized patients with familial adenomatous polyposis by rectal low-dose sulindac maintenance treatment. Advantages of a low-dose nonsteroidal anti-inflammatory drug regimen in reversing adenomas exceeding 33 months. Dis Colon Rectum 1995;38(8):813–30.

27. Kaul A, Reddy JC, Fagman E, Smith GF. Hepatitis associated with use of sulindac in a child. J Pediatr 1981;99(4):650–1.

28. Smith FE, Lindberg PJ. Life-threatening hypersensitivity to sulindac. JAMA 1980;244(3):269–70.

29. Garcia Rodriguez LA, Williams R, Derby LE, Dean AD, Jick H. Acute liver injury associated with nonsteroidal anti-inflammatory drugs and the role of risk factors. Arch Intern Med 1994;154(3):311–16.

30. Giroux Y, Moreau M, Kass TG. Cholestatic jaundice caused by sulindac. Can J Surg 1982;25(3):334–5.

31. Lilly EL. Pancreatitis after administration of sulindac. JAMA 1981;246(23):2680.

32. Bunning RD, Barth WF. Sulindac. A potentially renal-sparing nonsteroidal anti-inflammatory drug. JAMA 1982;248(21):2864–7.

33. Dunn MJ, Simonson M, Davidson EW, Scharschmidt LA, Sedor JR. Nonsteroidal anti-inflammatory drugs and renal function. J Clin Pharmacol 1988;28(6):524–9.

34. Stillman MT, Schlesinger PA. Nonsteroidal anti-inflammatory drug nephrotoxicity. Should we be concerned? Arch Intern Med 1990;150(2):268–70.

35. Whelton A, Stout RL, Spilman PS, Klassen DK. Renal effects of ibuprofen, piroxicam, and sulindac in patients with asymptomatic renal failure. A prospective, randomized, crossover comparison. Ann Intern Med 1990;112(8):568–76.

36. Champion de Crespigny PJ, Becker GJ, Ihle BU, Walter NM, Wright CA, Kincaid-Smith P. Renal failure and nephrotic syndrome associated with sulindac. Clin Nephrol 1988;30(1):52–5.

37. Pagniez D, Gosset D, Hardouin P, Noel C, Delvallez L, Dequiedt P. Evolution vers la hyalinose segmentaire et focale d'un syndrome néphrotique à lésions glomérulaires minimes chez une patiente traitée par le sulindac. [Development toward segmental and focal hyalinosis of a nephrotic syndrome with minimal glomerular lesions in a patient treated with sulindac.] Nephrologie 1988;9(2):90–1.

38. Ito S, Hasegawa H, Nozawa S, Murasawa A, Nakano M, Arakawa M. Sulindac usage may not be associated with an increased incidence of renal stone formation in patients with rheumatoid arthritis. J Rheumatol 1999;9:119–21.

39. Breton JC, Pibouin M, Allain H, et al. Toxic epidermal necrolysis induced by sulindac. Therapie 1985;40:67.

40. Small RE, Garnett WR. Sulindac-induced toxic epidermal necrolysis. Clin Pharm 1988;7(10):766–71.

41. Hovde O. Sulindakindusert toksisk epidermal nekrolyse. [Sulindac-induced toxic epidermal necrolysis.] Tidsskr Nor Laegeforen 1990;110(19):2537–8.

42. Reinertsen JL. Unusual pernio-like reaction to sulindac. Arthritis Rheum 1981;24(9):1215.

43. Fein M. Sulindac and pneumonitis. Ann Intern Med 1981;95(2):245.

44. Burrish GF, Kaatz BL. Sulindac-induced anaphylaxis. Ann Emerg Med 1981;10(3):154–5.

45. Hyson CP, Kazakoff MA. A severe multisystem reaction to sulindac. Arch Intern Med 1991;151(2):387–8.

46. Ng PC, So KW, Fok TF, Yam MC, Wong MY, Wong W. Comparing sulindac with indomethacin for closure of ductus arteriosus in preterm infants. J Paediatr Child Health 1997;33(4):324–8.

47. Chamontin B, Fille A, Salva P, Salvador M. L'inhibition sélective des prostaglandines existe-t-elle? A propos d'une hyponatrémie sous sulindac. [Does selective inhibition of prostaglandins exist? Apropos of hyponatrémia with sulindac.] Presse Méd 1988;17(40):2140–1.

48. Gross GE. Granulocytosis and a sulindac overdose. Ann Intern Med 1982;96(6 Pt 1):793–4.

49. Brater DC, Anderson S, Baird B, Campbell WB. Effects of ibuprofen, naproxen, and sulindac on prostaglandins in men. Kidney Int. 1985;27(1):66–73.

50. Jones MT, Stoner SC. Increased lithium concentrations reported in patients treated with sulindac. J Clin Psychiatry 2000;61(7):527–8.

51. Ross JR, Beeley L. Sulindac, prothrombin time, and anticoagulants. Lancet 1979;2(8151):1075.

Sulmazole

See also Phosphodiesterase type III, selective inhibitors of

General Information

Sulmazole is an inhibitor of phosphodiesterase type III.

Sulmazole commonly causes adverse gastrointestinal effects; dose-related anorexia, nausea, and vomiting have been reported in about 50% of patients given an intravenous infusion (1,2) and also after single oral doses (3). Cardiac dysrhythmias, mostly ventricular, have been reported occasionally with sulmazole (4). Other reported adverse effects in small numbers of patients include headache (1), temporary visual disturbances (2,5), discoloration of the urine (attributed to a metabolite) (2,6), and a small reduction in platelet count (1).

References

1. Renard M, Jacobs P, Dechamps P, Dresse A, Bernard R. Hemodynamic and clinical response to three-day infusion of sulmazol (AR-L 115 BS) in severe congestive heart failure. Chest 1983;84(4):408–13.
2. Renard M, Jacobs P, Melot C, Dresse A, Bernard R. Le sulmazol: un nouvel agent inotrope positif. [Sulmazole: a new positive inotropic agent.] Ann Cardiol Angeiol 1984;33(4):219–22.
3. Berkenboom GM, Sobolski JC, Depelchin PE, Contu E, Dieudonne PM, Degre SG. Clinical and hemodynamic observations on orally administered sulmazol (ARL115BS) in refractory heart failure. Cardiology 1984;71(6):323–30.
4. Hagemeijer F, Segers A, Schelling A. Cardiovascular effects of sulmazol administered intravenously to patients with severe heart failure. Eur Heart J 1984;5(2):158–67.
5. Thormann J, Schlepper M, Kramer W, Gottwik M, Kindler M. Effects of AR-L 115 BS (Sulmazol), a new cardiotonic agent, in coronary artery disease: improved ventricular wall motion, increased pump function and abolition of pacing-induced ischemia. J Am Coll Cardiol 1983;2(2):332–7.
6. Timmis AD, Smyth P, Jewitt DE. Milrinone in heart failure. Effects on exercise haemodynamics during short term treatment. Br Heart J 1985;54(1):42–7.

Sulpiride and levosulpiride

General Information

Sulpiride and its levorotatory isomer levosulpiride are dopamine receptor antagonists. The pharmacology, efficacy, and tolerability of levosulpiride for dyspepsia and emesis have been reviewed (1).

Levosulpiride has been evaluated in 15 double-blind, randomized trials in patients with dyspepsia (1818 patients in all, of whom 676 were treated with levosulpiride) and in 11 trials in patients with emesis (718 patients in all, of whom 383 were treated with levosulpiride) (1). Levosulpiride was effective in the treatment of dyspepsia and emesis. The incidence of adverse effects was 11% in 840 patients with dyspepsia. Most of them were mild and resulted in treatment withdrawal in only 0.9% of cases. The common adverse effects were drowsiness, breast tenderness, and hoarseness.

Reference

1. Corazza GR, Tonini M. Levosulpiride for dyspepsia and emesis. A review of its pharmacology, efficacy and tolerability. Clin Drug Invest 2000;19:151–62.

Sulprostone

See also Prostaglandins

General Information

Sulprostone is a synthetic prostaglandin analogue of PGE_2 used for inducing uterine contraction.

In large series, sulprostone has had good tolerability with a very low complication rate. The most severe complication is myocardial infarction secondary to coronary spasm, with a frequency of one in 20 000, usually in smokers and women over 35 years of age with cardiovascular disease (SEDA-23, 436).

Organs and Systems

Cardiovascular

Several experimental studies have provided support for the hypothesis that coronary spasm plays a major role in the pathophysiology of myocardial infarction during the administration of sulprostone. However, the possibility of myocardial infarction is not mentioned in the product information.

- Two cases of myocardial infarction (one fatal) have been reported in patients receiving sulprostone with mifepristone (1,2).
- Myocardial infarction has been reported in a woman aged 35 years with normal coronary arteries and good left ventricular function (3).
- A 30-year-old woman developed uterine atony and bleeding after induced abortion because of fetal death at 17 weeks of gestation (4). Sulprostone was given intravenously at a rate of 500 micrograms/hour. When additional sulprostone was injected into the uterine cervix, the patient sustained a myocardial infarction, with ventricular fibrillation and cardiocirculatory arrest, most probably due to coronary artery spasm. She was resuscitated and recovered completely.

Sulprostone should be used with care, particularly in patients with cardiac risk factors, and only in settings equipped to manage complications.

Cardiac dysrhythmias have been reported after the administration of misoprostol.

- A 38-year-old woman developed complete heart block, ventricular fibrillation, and subsequent asystole about 7 minutes after intravenous sulprostone 30 micrograms over 5 minutes, after she had previously been given a total dose of intramyometrial sulprostone 500 micrograms at seven different points for postpartum hemorrhage after cesarean section (5).

The time-course suggested that the most likely cause of the arrest was the intravenous sulprostone. Contributory causes may have been hemorrhagic shock, electrolyte abnormalities, and hypothermia (from massive blood transfusion).

- Cardiac arrest occurred in a 39-year-old woman 3.5 hours after the administration of sulprostone 250 micrograms directly into the uterine wall for postpartum hemorrhage after manual removal of the placenta (6). She had specific contraindications to sulprostone, as formulated by the French authorities: age over 35 years, heavy cigarette smoking, and cardiovascular risk factors.

In the Netherlands, sulprostone is registered for intravenous administration only. The authors strongly advised against administration directly into the uterine wall.

Nervous system

Seizures have been described during pregnancy termination induced by sulprostone (7).

Liver

Sulprostone has been associated with minor abnormalities of liver function (8).

Urinary tract

Sulprostone has been associated with minor abnormalities of kidney function (8).

Reproductive system

Sulprostone can cause rupture of the uterine cervix (9).

- A 43-year-old woman, who had previously had a first trimester miscarriage that required evacuation of the uterus and a normal vaginal delivery at term 4 years before, was admitted for an abortion at 16 weeks. Ripening of the cervix was started with a pessary of gemeprost 1 mg. After 3 hours, when the cervix was 1 cm dilated, an intramuscular injection of sulprostone 500 mg was given. After 30 minutes she developed persistent abdominal pain, which became a continuous cramping and then a shooting pain; a male fetus of 170 g was aborted. There was a 3 cm longitudinal cervical rupture located posteriorly that reached the posterior fornix.

References

1. Anonymous. A death associated with mifeprostone/sulprostone. Lancet 1991;337:969–70.
2. Ulmann A, Silvestre L, Chemama L, Rezvani Y, Renault M, Aguillaume CJ, Baulieu EE. Medical termination of early pregnancy with mifepristone (RU 486) followed by a prostaglandin analogue. Study in 16,369 women. Acta Obstet Gynecol Scand 1992;71(4):278–83.
3. Feenstra J, Borst F, Huige MC, Oei SG, Stricker BH. Acuut myocardinfarct na toediening van sulproston. [Acute myocardial infarct following sulprostone administration.] Ned Tijdschr Geneeskd 1998;142(4):192–5.
4. Kulka PJ, Quent P, Wiebalck A, Jager D, Strumpf M. Myocardial infarction after sulprostone therapy for uterine atony and bleeding: a case report. Geburtshilfe Frauenheilk 1999;59:634–7.
5. Chen FG, Koh KF, Chong YS. Cardiac arrest associated with sulprostone use during caesarean section. Anaesth Intensive Care 1998;26(3):298–301.
6. Beerendonk CC, Massuger LF, Lucassen AM, Lerou JG, van den Berg PP. Circulatiestilstand na gebruik van sulproston bij fluxus post partum. [Circulatory arrest following sulprostone administration in postpartum hemorrhage.] Ned Tijdschr Geneeskd 1998;142(4):195–7.
7. Brandenburg H, Jahoda MG, Wladimiroff JW, Los FJ, Lindhout D. Convulsions in epileptic women after administration of prostaglandin E2 derivative. Lancet 1990;336(8723):1138.
8. Ranjan V, Hingorani V, Kinra G, Agarwal N, Pande Y. Evaluation of sulprostone for second trimester abortions and its effects on liver and kidney function. Contraception 1982;25(2):175–84.
9. Corrado F, D'Anna R, Cannata ML. Rupture of the cervix in a sulprostone induced abortion in the second trimester. Arch Gynecol Obstet 2000;264(3):162–3.

Sultiame

See also Antiepileptic drugs

General Information

Sultiame is a carbonic anhydrase inhibitor that has been used as an antiepileptic agent in most forms of epilepsy except absence seizures.

In 86 patients there was a good correlation between the weight-related dose of sultiame and the sultiame serum concentration (1). The half-life was 8.7 hours. In children the half-life was shorter and the clearance higher than in adults, and sultiame concentrations in children were lower than in adults, dose for dose.

Sultiame as monotherapy has been studied in a double-blind, placebo-controlled trial for 6 months in 66 children with benign childhood epilepsy with centrotemporal spikes (2). The number of adverse events per day of exposure was similar with sultiame and placebo, and no patient withdrew because of adverse effects.

The most common adverse effects of sultiame are gastrointestinal disturbances, ataxia, dizziness, headache, paresthesia, anorexia, weight loss, sedation, behavioral disorders, and metabolic acidosis (SEDA-21, 74) (3). There have been rare reports of neuropathy and acute tubular necrosis (3).

Organs and Systems

Psychological, psychiatric

- A 9-year-old boy with rolandic epilepsy developed impaired vigilance, depressed mood, fatigue, loss of drive, and listlessness when given sultiame 5 mg/kg/day

(4). All his symptoms disappeared within a few days of withdrawal.

References

1. May TW, Korn-Merker E, Rambeck B, Boenigk HE. Pharmacokinetics of sulthiame in epileptic patients. Ther Drug Monit 1994;16(3):251–7.
2. Rating D, Wolf C, Bast T. Sulthiame as monotherapy in children with benign childhood epilepsy with centrotemporal spikes: a 6-month randomized, double-blind, placebo-controlled study. Sulthiame Study Group. Epilepsia 2000;41(10):1284–8.
3. Perucca E. Sulthiame. In: Dam M, Gram L, editors. Comprehensive Epileptology. New York: Raven Press, 1990:617–20.
4. Weglage J, Pietsch M, Sprinz A, Feldmann R, Denecke J, Kurlemann G. A previously unpublished side effect of sulthiame in a patient with Rolandic epilepsy. Neuropediatrics 1999;30(1):50.

Sunscreens, substances used in

General Information

Solar UV rays are classified into three groups: UVA rays have the longest wavelength and account for 90% of the total; UVB rays have higher energy and are the most damaging; UVC rays are filtered out by the ozone layer.

Topical sunscreens

Topical sunscreens are made up of constituents that either absorb or reflect incident radiation; absorbents are organic chemicals, reflectants are inorganic chemicals.

The commonest absorbents are *para*-aminobenzoic acid (PABA) and its derivatives, cinnamates, benzophenones, and salicylates, none of which offers significant protection against UVA. Dibenzoylmethane derivatives and anthranilates, which also work by absorbing radiation, are more effective UVA filters.

Reflectant inorganic components, such as zinc oxide and titanium dioxide, provide significant UVA protection, as well as good UVB protection. However, they are opaque and can leave a visible white film, despite the use of "microfined" particles in most products, and some users find them cosmetically less acceptable.

The Sun Protection Factor (SPF) is the ratio of the amount of UVB radiation that is just enough to produce sunburn on protected skin to the amount that will produce the same effect on unprotected skin. For example, skin protected by a sunscreen with an SPF of 10 should be able to withstand a given intensity of UVB rays for 10 times as long as unprotected skin before burning. As no assessment of UVA protection is included, the SPF should not be used as the basis for recommending a sunscreen to a patient who is sensitive to UVA.

Some products also carry a star rating system to indicate UVA protection, four stars representing the greatest; this rating is not an absolute measure, but indicates UVA protection relative to UVB, and its usefulness is controversial. Objective testing of widely available sunscreen agents has shown UVA protection to be significantly less than for UVB.

People vary in their susceptibility to sunburn, as follows:

I— Always burns, never tans
II— Burns easily, sometimes tans
III— Tans easily, burns rarely
IV— Always tans, never burns

Those who burn easily (types I and II) should be advised to choose a preparation with a high SPF (15 or more) that will provide good protection against UVB and adequate protection against UVA. Darker subjects (skin types III and IV) can safely use sunscreens with a lower SPF (around 10).

General adverse effects

Ultraviolet-absorbent organic sun filters, particularly derivatives of PABA, dibenzoylmethane, and anthranilates, can cause both allergic and photoallergic contact dermatitis. PABA-containing formulations can stain clothing yellow and cause stinging or drying of the skin.

Organs and Systems

Immunologic

Photopatch-testing with sunscreens in Sweden has been reviewed (1). Between 1990 and 1996, 355 patients with suspected photosensitivity were photopatch-tested with seven sunscreens (benzophenone-3 (Eusolex 4360), isopropyldibenzoylmethane (Eusolex 8020), butylmethoydibenzoylmethane (Parsol 1789), octylmethoxycinnamate (Parsol MCX), PABA, phenylbenzimidazole sulfonic acid (Eusolex 232), 4-methylbenzylidene camphor (Eusolex 6300); 2% petrolatum). There were 42 allergic reactions in 28 patients. The most common allergen was benzophenone-3 (Eusolex 4360), with 15 photocontact and one contact allergic reaction, followed by eight photocontact and four allergic contact reactions to isopropyl dibenzoylmethane (Eusolex 8020). In six cases, photocontact reactions were due to butylmethoxydibenzoylmethane (Parsol 1789). Phenylbenzimidazole sulfonic acid (Eusolex 232) caused two cases of photocontact allergy, and benzophenone-3 caused contact urticaria in one patient (1). There was a similar frequency of photocontact dermatitis to Eusolex 4360, Eusolex 8020, and Parsol 1789 in an Italian study, in which nine of 36 patients had positive reactions when photopatch-tested with sunscreens (UVA 10 J/m^2) (2).

In 19 patients with positive photopatch tests to sunscreens among all the patients that were photopatch-tested between 1992 and 1999 (total not stated) there were 21 positive photopatch tests to sunscreen agents (3). Nine patients reacted to oxybenzone, eight to butylmethoxydibenzoylmethane, three to methoxycinnamate, and one to benzophenone. There were no reactions to *para*-aminobenzoic acid (PABA), reflecting the increased use of PABA-free sunscreens. Six patients also had positive patch tests to components of the sunscreen base, such as fragrances, which can complicate the diagnosis.

Oxybenzone is the most frequently used benzophenone in sunscreens, estimated to be present in 20–30% of commercial products. Phototoxicity and allergic contact dermatitis have been described, but reports of immediate-type hypersensitivity are scarce.

- A 22-year-old woman with a history of atopy had anaphylaxis 10 minutes after widespread application of an oxybenzone-containing sunscreen (4). Blinded patch tests with the sunscreen and its ingredients yielded wheal and flare reactions after 15 minutes to the sunscreen and to oxybenzone. Some days before skin testing the woman had had contact urticaria on the face after kissing a friend who had applied the same sunscreen.

A positive patch test to polyvinylpyrrolidone/eicosene (10% in petrolatum on days 2 and 4) was found in a patient who had used a sun block (5).

Photo-induced contact urticaria to benzophenone-3 and benzophenone-10, possibly in combination with delayed hypersensitivity, has been described (6). Urticaria occurred within minutes of UVA irradiation (10 J), 24 hours after the application of the benzophenones.

Octyl triazone is a UVB absorber structurally unrelated to the benzophenones. Photocontact allergy to this agent in a sunscreen has been described (7).

References

1. Berne B, Ros AM. 7 years experience of photopatch testing with sunscreen allergens in Sweden. Contact Dermatitis 1998;38(2):61–4.
2. Ricci C, Pazzaglia M, Tosti A. Photocontact dermatitis from UV filters. Contact Dermatitis 1998;38(6):343–4.
3. Cook N, Freeman S. Report of 19 cases of photoallergic contact dermatitis to sunscreens seen at the Skin and Cancer Foundation. Australas J Dermatol 2001;42(4):257–9.
4. Emonet S, Pasche-Koo F, Perin-Minisini MJ, Hauser C. Anaphylaxis to oxybenzone, a frequent constituent of sunscreens. J Allergy Clin Immunol 2001;107(3):556–7.
5. Smith HR, Armstrong K, Wakelin SH, White IR. Contact allergy to PVP/eicosene copolymer. Contact Dermatitis 1999;40(5):283.
6. Bourrain JL, Amblard P, Beani JC. Contact urticaria photoinduced by benzophenones. Contact Dermatitis 2003;48(1):45–6.
7. Sommer S, Wilkinson SM, English JS, Ferguson J. Photoallergic contact dermatitis from the sunscreen octyl triazone. Contact Dermatitis 2002;46(5):304–5.

Suprofen

See also Non-steroidal anti-inflammatory drugs

General Information

Suprofen, alpha-methyl-4-(2-thienylcarbonyl)-phenyl-acetic acid, was specifically promoted as a non-narcotic analgesic for many painful conditions, and was withdrawn from the market worldwide in 1987. It caused an unusual clinical syndrome of acute flank pain and nephrotoxicity (SEDA-12, 89). It is still available as a 1% ointment in some countries.

Organs and Systems

Urinary tract

The pathogenesis of suprofen nephrotoxicity in young healthy volunteers involved a transient reduction in renal plasma flow and glomerular filtration rate, possibly due to intratubular precipitation of uric acid (1).

Skin

Suprofen ointment can cause photodermatitis (SEDA-17, 113).

Susceptibility Factors

A case-control study identified as susceptibility factors for adverse effects of suprofen male sex, hay fever and asthma, exercise, and alcohol consumption (2).

References

1. Abraham PA, Halstenson CE, Opsahl JA, Matzke GR, Keane WF. Suprofen-induced uricosuria. A potential mechanism for acute nephropathy and flank pain. Am J Nephrol 1988;8(2):90–5.
2. Strom BL, West SL, Sim E, Carson JL. The epidemiology of the acute flank pain syndrome from suprofen. Clin Pharmacol Ther 1989;46(6):693–9.

Suramin

General Information

Suramin is a trypanocide that has been used in the treatment of African trypanosomiasis and onchocerciasis, and has been studied in AIDS (SEDA-10, 277) (SEDA-15, 335). However, the high doses that are required for a worthwhile effect are extraordinarily toxic. It is particularly likely to cause adverse effects in the malnourished and has therefore largely been abandoned for the treatment of trypanosomiasis and onchocerciasis, but it still seems uniquely capable of killing the adult onchocerciasis worm, although results are sometimes incomplete even in that respect (SEDA-20, 283).

Suramin is mainly used now in the treatment of hormone-refractory prostate cancer, in which it has shown some antitumor effect, although accompanied by extensive and sometimes severe adverse effects (1), and in the treatment of high-grade glioma. Since it suppresses adrenocortical function it is usually given in conjunction with glucocorticoids. The concomitant use of glucocorticoids and anti-androgen withdrawal usually makes it difficult to establish the true response to suramin.

Observational studies

AIDS

For a time, unsuccessful attempts were made to treat AIDS with suramin (2), because of its proven ability to impair the in vitro infectivity (and inhibit the cytopathic effect) of human T cell lymphotropic virus type III (HTLV-III) or lymphadenopathy-associated virus (LAV). However, it is no longer used for this indication. Its adverse effects were more severe and numerous than in its traditional field of use: two-thirds of patients had malaise, fever, and raised transaminases, and a quarter had adrenal insufficiency. Erythematous drug eruptions (particularly on sun-exposed surfaces) were common; some patients had a burning sensation of the skin, particularly on the limbs. The most common laboratory abnormalities were proteinuria, microscopic pyuria, trace hemoglobinuria, and occasional granular casts. There were rises in hepatic transaminase activities in some patients, usually during the second and third weeks, and others had eosinophilia (maximum 14%) during a drug eruption. There was a high incidence of keratopathy (SEDA-14, 263).

Hormone-refractory prostate cancer

Much work relating to the use of suramin in prostatic cancer involves drug combinations, including amino-glutethimide, epirubicin, and hydrocortisone, with or without androgen deprivation, and in these studies it is hardly possible to determine which drug was responsible for a given adverse effect.

The adverse effects of suramin that were reported in a group of 69 patients with hormone-refractory prostate cancer were anorexia (19%), malaise and fatigue (40%), paresthesia (10%), weakness (9%), and skin rash (6%). In another group of patients there were higher frequencies of adverse effects: fatigue occurred in 70% and neuropathy in 16%. Hematological abnormalities occurred often, but were mostly mild and consisted of neutropenia (30%), anemia (74%), thrombocytopenia (26%), and coagulopathy (30%). Other common adverse effects have included uremia (21%), increased serum transaminase activities (19%), nausea and vomiting (30%), constipation (9%), edema (33%), dysrhythmias (7%), mild hyperglycemia (86%), and rash (60%) (SEDA-20, 283).

In 81 patients intravenous suramin (peak plasma concentration 300 μg/ml trough concentration 175 μg/ml) combined with aminoglutethimide 250 mg qds in patients with progressive androgen-refractory prostate cancer after antiandrogen treatment had been withdrawn, effectiveness was limited, whereas most adverse effects were attributed to suramin (3). There were 38 episodes of grade 3 and 4 toxic effects in 29 patients. Severe thrombocytopenia occurred in four patients. There were four episodes of atrial fibrillation. One patient developed uremia which required dialysis. One patient developed grade 3 neurosensory changes, but none had neuromotor changes. There was one episode of grade 4 rash, which was probably attributable to aminoglutethimide, consisting of diffuse erythematous exfoliating papules over the chest, back, arms, and face. All adverse effects were reversible.

The efficacy and adverse effects of treatment with suramin for hormone-refractory prostate cancer have been evaluated in 27 patients (4). The treatment regimen consisted of a loading phase, targeted to reach suramin serum concentrations of 180–250 μg/ml using a dose of 1.4 g/m² at 3-day intervals. Constant suramin concentrations were obtained with a dose of 0.5–1 g/m² every 7–10 days. Six patients did not complete the suramin loading phase because of adverse effects and were withdrawn. About one-third of the assessable patients had a more than 50% reduction in prostate specific antigen and/or serum alkaline phosphatase. Two of these also had a reduction in metastases on bone scan. Another 48% of the patients had unchanged prostate specific antigen or serum alkaline phosphatase during treatment with suramin, suggesting stable disease. The mean survival time was 41 weeks. Responders had a survival of 70 weeks compared with 12 weeks among non-responders. However, the adverse effects were substantial. The most common adverse effects were renal impairment (18 patients), 10 of whom had a mild increase in serum creatinine and seven had a moderate increase. One patient died of multiorgan failure, including renal shutdown. Suramin treatment was interrupted for 7–14 days when the creatinine clearance was under 40 ml/minute, which resulted in improvement in renal function. A sensimotor polyneuropathy occurred in 18 patients and typically presented as paresthesia involving the limbs, combined with reduced nerve conducting velocity. Mild and moderate sensorimotor polyneuropathy occurred in 14 patients. Severe polyneuropathy occurred in two cases and led to the withdrawal of suramin. These effects were only partially reversible. Eleven patients had no neurotoxic symptoms. Allergic rashes occurred in 30% of patients and consisted of a moderate, diffuse, morbilliform rash during the loading phase of suramin treatment, usually disappearing within a few days without further therapy. Two patients with more severe and prolonged rashes were treated with high-dose corticosteroids with a beneficial effect. Hematological toxicity consisted of anemia in 22% of the patients, who all needed blood transfusions, leukopenia in 15%, of whom one with a severe leukopenia was successfully treated by granulocyte-macrophage colony stimulating factor, and thrombocytopenia, which occurred in 15% of patients and led to spontaneous bleeding in two. The platelet count returned to normal in both cases after the withdrawal of suramin. Vortex keratopathy occurred in 15% of the patients. Corneal changes were always minimal and vision was not affected. One patient had a retinal bleed, which led to withdrawal. Severe infections occurred in 26% of the patients, and also led to the withdrawal of suramin and required intravenous antibiotics. These results have further confirmed that suramin has a limited but statistically significant effect in the treatment of hormone-refractory prostate cancer. Although the severity of adverse effects were somewhat less than in previous studies they were still substantial. The toxicity of suramin seems to be closely related to the cumulative dose, peak concentration, and treatment regimen, and toxicity may be reduced by reducing daily doses and giving additional treatment-free intervals.

Suramin has been combined with epirubicin in 26 patients with hormone-refractory prostate cancer (5). No additional therapeutic effect was found compared with suramin or epirubicin alone. Suramin was given in an initial daily dose of 350 mg/m^2, with weekly infusions thereafter, targeted to maintain suramin plasma concentrations at 200–250 μg/ml for a maximum of 6 months. Cortisone acetate was added after 4 weeks in order to prevent adrenal insufficiency. Epirubicin was given as a weekly intravenous bolus from the start, also for a maximum of 6 months. The median duration of therapy with suramin and epirubicin was 9 (2–29) weeks. The toxic effects of this combined treatment included grade 1–2 nausea and vomiting (54%), fatigue (54%), anorexia (58%), stomatitis (52%), diarrhea (8%), mild rash (11%), neutropenia, usually mild (65%), low-grade fever (26%), mild increases in serum creatinine concentrations (27%), proteinuria (58%), and peripheral neurotoxicity (mild 23%, severe 4%); alopecia was caused by the epirubicin in 58%.

The use of suramin plus hydrocortisone and androgen deprivation and the use of multiple courses of suramin have been assessed in 59 patients with newly diagnosed metastatic prostate cancer (6). Suramin (doses aimed at plasma concentrations between a trough of 150 μg/ml and a peak of 250 μg/ml) was given in a 78-day fixed dosage schedule (one cycle) and suramin treatment cycles were repeated every 6 months to a total of four cycles. There was significant broad-spectrum toxicity throughout the study, leading to withdrawal of treatment in 33 patients. Cardiovascular events (dysrhythmias, hypotension, and congestive heart failure), neurotoxic effects, and respiratory effects were more frequent than expected. In consequence, repeated courses of suramin could be given in a minority of cases only. The authors felt that in the light of the relatively non-toxic palliation achieved with standard hormonal therapy, suramin in this dosage schedule has only limited use in patients with newly diagnosed metastatic prostate cancer.

The effects of fixed-dose suramin plus hydrocortisone have been studied in 50 patients with hormone-refractory prostate cancer (7). Suramin was initially given as a 30-minute test infusion of 200 mg. In the absence of allergic reactions, additional 24-hour intravenous infusions of 500 mg/m^2 were given daily for the next 5 days. Thereafter, 2-hour intravenous infusions (350 mg/m^2) were given weekly on an outpatient basis for 12 weeks or until disease progression. The median duration of response was 16 weeks and the median time to disease progression 13 weeks. Fatigue and lymphopenia were the most commonly reported adverse effects, in 27 patients (54%) and 39 patients (78%) respectively. Skin rash occurred in 12 patients (24%). Suramin was withdrawn in three patients because of acute renal insufficiency ($n = 2$) and Stevens–Johnson syndrome ($n = 1$).

In a randomized study in 390 patients suramin has been given in a fixed low dose (3.192 g/m^2), intermediate dose (5.320 g/m^2), or high dose (7.661 g/m^2) to determine whether its efficacy and toxicity in the treatment of patients with hormone-refractory prostate cancer is dose-dependent (8). There was no clear dose–response relation for survival or progression-free survival, but toxicity increased especially with the higher dose. There were neurological adverse effects in 40% of the patients and cardiac adverse effects in 15%. This raises questions about the usefulness of suramin, particularly in high doses, in advanced prostate cancer. However, in another phase I study of suramin with once- or twice-monthly dosing in patients with advanced cancer, suramin was relatively safely administered without using plasma concentrations to guide dosing (9). Dose-limiting toxic effects included fatigue, neuropathy, anorexia, and renal toxicity. Diffuse colitis, erythema multiforme, and hemolytic anemia were reported as unusual effects.

High-grade glioma

The efficacy, toxicity, and pharmacology of suramin have been studied in 12 patients with recurrent or progressive recurrent high-grade gliomas aged 26–67 years (10). Suramin was given in doses similar to those used in patients with hormone-refractory prostate cancer. Treatment-related adverse effects were usually mild and reversible. Three patients developed transient grade 3–4 toxicity (leukopenia, a rise in serum creatinine, and diarrhea). There was no coagulopathy or central nervous system bleeding. All patients reached target suramin concentrations. The pharmacology of suramin was not affected by anticonvulsant therapy. Median time to progression was 55 days (range 17–242) and median survival was 191 days (range 42–811). There were no partial or complete remissions at 12 weeks. However, the clinical outcome in three patients suggested that effect of suramin may be delayed. One patient who progressed after 12 weeks had a subsequent marked reduction in tumor size and maintained an excellent partial response for over 2 years without other therapy. The two others had disease stabilization and lived for 16 and 27 months respectively. Based on these observations, suramin and radiotherapy are now being used concurrently in patients with newly diagnosed glioblastoma multiforme to study survival as the primary outcome.

Renal cell carcinoma

Suramin was not effective in one phase II study in advanced renal cell carcinoma, in which it was given in a fixed dose plus hydrocortisone to 22 patients (19 men, three women, aged 30–74 years) (11). Three patients had grade 4 toxicity (hypersensitivity, urethral obstruction, hypotension, and neutropenic sepsis). Eleven developed grade 3 toxicity, mainly abdominal pain, anemia, diarrhea, erythema, dyspnea, fatigue, and fever.

Placebo-controlled studies

The antitumor effect of suramin has been evaluated in a prospective randomized trial in 458 patients with hormone-refractory prostate cancer and significant opioid analgesic-dependent pain (12). Reduction of pain and opioid requirements served as surrogates for tumor responsiveness. The patients were given either suramin (aiming at sustained plasma concentrations of 100–300 μg/ml) plus hydrocortisone (40 mg/day) or placebo plus hydrocortisone. Patients treated with suramin plus hydrocortisone had greater reductions in combined pain and opioid analgesic intake. Suramin did not reduce the quality of life or performance status. However, overall survival was similar. Most of the adverse events were mild or moderate and were easily managed medically.

Frequent adverse effects of suramin were rash, chills, fever, and taste disturbance. In contrast to the results of earlier studies, in which different suramin dosage regimens were used, neurological, renal, hepatic, and coagulation abnormalities were rare.

Organs and Systems

Nervous system

The neurological adverse effects of suramin have been reviewed in the context of a broad review of neuropathies associated with malignancy and chemotherapy (13).

Neurotoxicity is a dose-limiting adverse effect of suramin and there are two distinct types of neuropathy: a mild, length-dependent, axonal polyneuropathy, and a more serious subacute demyelinating, Guillain–Barré-like polyneuropathy. The reported incidence of neuropathy is 25–90% with a mean of about 50%. Various neuropathies were noted in four of 38 patients infused with suramin for various malignancies (14).

The milder axonal polyneuropathy is the most common neurological adverse effect of suramin and causes distal paresthesia, reduced pain and vibration sensation in the feet, weak toe extensors, and absent ankle jerks; this neuropathy is largely reversible. Milder neuropathies occurred in 50–70% of patients with plasma concentrations below 300 µg/ml, and severe motor neuropathy was rare in this category of patients.

The more severe demyelinating neuropathies appear to be dose-related and occur when peak suramin plasma concentrations are maintained above 350 µg/ml; the effective serum concentration in cancers is about 250 µg/ml (SEDA-20, 283) (15,16). A Guillain–Barré-like polyradiculoneuropathy occurs in 10–20% of patients after 1–5 months of treatment, with a maximum at 2–9 weeks after the start of treatment. The first symptoms are distal limb and or facial paresthesia, followed by diffuse, symmetrical, proximal weakness and areflexia. About 25% of these patients eventually require ventilation. The CSF protein content may be raised.

In 24 patients with hormone-refractory prostate cancer given suramin twice weekly intravenously targeted to reach plasma concentrations of 50–100, 101–150, 151–200, or 201–250 µg/ml plus doxorubicin, fatigue occurred in 18 and was dose-limiting in two (17). Eight developed neurological symptoms, of whom three, all receiving the highest dose, developed grade 3 toxicity. There were five cases of neuropathies. Two patients had evidence of a demyelinating neuropathy, one of whom developed a Guillain–Barré-like syndrome and inflammatory myopathy. A further patient had a mixed axonal and demyelinating peripheral neuropathy. Two patients developed a motor neuropathy that exacerbated pre-existing neurological defects. Other frequent adverse events were proteinuria, leukopenia, and alopecia. However, the respective roles of suramin and doxorubicin in causing these adverse effects were uncertain.

Evidence of an underlying distal axonal polyneuropathy can be detected by electromyelography (18). Electroencephalography shows slow motor conduction velocities and electromyography shows reduced recruitment in both proximal and distal muscles. In the more severe cases denervation emerges. Sural nerve biopsies have shown a reduced density of the large and small myelinated fibers, occasional axonal degeneration, and demyelination. Epineural and endoneural mononuclear inflammatory cell infiltrates are sometimes seen. After withdrawal of treatment symptoms may deteriorate further for several weeks with recovery, sometimes incomplete, after 1–2 months.

The precise mechanism of the neurotoxicity of suramin is unknown, although both inhibition of the effects of nerve growth factors and a possible immune-mediated effect, consistent with the many immunomodulating effects, have been suggested. In a recent experimental study in dorsal root ganglion cell cultures suramin disrupted the transport and metabolism of glycolipids, with accumulation of the GM1 ganglioside and ceramide, leading to cell death (19).

Sensory systems

Photophobia, lacrimation, and palpebral edema are recognized late effects of suramin, and there is evidence of a late optic atrophy of suramin (20).

High-dose treatments for cancers seem to produce changes in most patients consistent with a vortex keratopathy (SEDA-21, 320), although it can be entirely symptomless. Other cases have a hyperoptic refractory shift leading to blurred vision. Of 114 patients, 19 developed ocular symptoms and signs while taking suramin sodium for metastatic cancer of the prostate (21). Of these, 13 developed bilateral corneal epithelial whorl-like deposits, in 10 cases associated with a foreign body sensation and lacrimation. Symptoms in all cases resolved with topical lubricants. Three patients developed asymptomatic corneal deposits. Seven had blurred vision and had a mean hyperopic shift in refractive error of 1.13 (range 0.75–2.00) diopters, which persisted throughout treatment. None of these patients had a reduction in best-corrected visual acuity. At the very least, ophthalmological surveillance is necessary when suramin is used.

Suramin has been used in the treatment of AIDS and adrenal carcinoma, in both of which there was a high incidence of keratopathy (SED-13, 836).

Endocrine

The adrenal glands are sensitive to the toxic effects of suramin; both glucocorticoid and mineralocorticoid functions can be impaired at doses normally used, necessitating replacement therapy (22).

Hematologic

Occasional cases of hemolytic anemia and agranulocytosis have been reported in patients taking suramin (SED-13, 836). Severe neutropenia has been attributed to suramin in six cases (23). Plasma concentrations of platelet-derived growth factor-AB (PDGF-AB) and fibroblast growth factor basic correlated with the time-course of the neutropenia, which was unpredictable and occurred both during and after withdrawal of suramin. Plasma concentrations of suramin and G-CSF did not correlate with the neutropenia, but there was a rapid response to G-CSF.

Blood coagulation can be altered by suramin, which causes accumulation of glycosaminoglycans, which have heparin-like properties (24). In patients who had received suramin intravenously for 2 weeks there was inhibition of factors V, VIII, IX, X, XI, and XII, while thrombin, prothrombin, and factor VII were unaffected (25). The inhibition of factor V was virtually irreversible, although the effect of suramin on the other factors is readily reversed by dilution.

In one patient with cancer, immunological complement-mediated destruction of circulating platelets was induced by suramin, demanding urgent treatment (26).

Gastrointestinal

Suramin can cause vomiting (27).

Liver

In three men with severe chronic active hepatitis, suramin treatment prolonged the prothrombin time in all three, caused a rise in bilirubin in two, and may have led to hemorrhage from esophageal varices in one patient and to hepatic encephalopathy in another (28).

Urinary tract

Suramin can cause acute renal failure (29,30).

Skin

Skin effects were prominent in patients treated with the high doses needed in malignancies, including morbilliform rashes in 67%, UV recall in 35%, urticaria in 18%, and keratotic papules in 12% (31). Late reactions include various skin eruptions, hyperesthesia and paresthesia (particularly affecting the palms and soles of the feet); erythema multiforme as part of a generalized skin reaction has been well documented in some individual cases (32) and toxic epidermal necrolysis has been reported (33).

A single dose of intravenous hydrocortisone 200 mg was protective against skin complications in another small group of patients.

Second-Generation Effects

Teratogenicity

Suramin has generally been avoided in pregnancy because its safety is uncertain; it is teratogenic in experimental animals (34–36).

Drug–Drug Interactions

Furosemide

In 26 patients treated with suramin for hormone-refractory prostate cancer, furosemide reduced the total body clearance of suramin by 36% (37). In view of the increased risk of severe adverse effects after treatment with higher plasma concentrations of suramin, it would be prudent to alter dosage schemes in patients treated with both suramin and furosemide.

Warfarin

In 13 men with advanced hormone-refractory prostate cancer the interaction between suramin and warfarin was studied because of potential worries that suramin may affect blood coagulation (38). After initial stabilization to an International Normalized Ratio (INR) of about 2.0 suramin plus hydrocortisone was started, after which warfarin requirements fell by 0.50–0.78 mg/day. The difference did not reach statistical significance. There were no bleeding problems. These results suggest that suramin and warfarin can be safely co-administered, provided that coagulation status is monitored.

References

1. Knox JJ, Moore MJ. Treatment of hormone refractory prostate cancer. Semin Urol Oncol 2001;19(3):202–11.
2. Broder S, Yarchoan R, Collins JM, Lane HC, Markham PD, Klecker RW, Redfield RR, Mitsuya H, Hoth DF, Gelmann E, et al. Effects of suramin on HTLV-III/LAV infection presenting as Kaposi's sarcoma or AIDS-related complex: clinical pharmacology and suppression of virus replication in vivo. Lancet 1985;2(8456):627–30.
3. Dawson N, Figg WD, Brawley OW, Bergan R, Cooper MR, Senderowicz A, Headlee D, Steinberg SM, Sutherland M, Patronas N, Sausville E, Linehan WM, Reed E, Sartor O. Phase II study of suramin plus aminoglutethimide in two cohorts of patients with androgen-independent prostate cancer: simultaneous antiandrogen withdrawal and prior antiandrogen withdrawal. Clin Cancer Res 1998;4(1):37–44.
4. Garcia-Schurmann JM, Schulze H, Haupt G, Pastor J, Allolio B, Senge T. Suramin treatment in hormone- and chemotherapy-refractory prostate cancer. Urology 1999;53(3):535–41.
5. Falcone A, Antonuzzo A, Danesi R, Allegrini G, Monica L, Pfanner E, Masi G, Ricci S, Del Tacca M, Conte P. Suramin in combination with weekly epirubicin for patients with advanced hormone-refractory prostate carcinoma. Cancer 1999;86(3):470–6.
6. Hussain M, Fisher EI, Petrylak DP, O'Connor J, Wood DP, Small EJ, Eisenberger MA, Crawford ED. Androgen deprivation and four courses of fixed-schedule suramin treatment in patients with newly diagnosed metastatic prostate cancer: a Southwest Oncology Group Study. J Clin Oncol 2000;18(5):1043–9.
7. Calvo E, Cortes J, Rodriguez J, Sureda M, Beltran C, Rebollo J, Martinez-Monge R, Berian JM, de Irala J, Brugarolas A. Fixed higher dose schedule of suramin plus hydrocortisone in patients with hormone refractory prostate carcinoma a multicenter Phase II study. Cancer 2001;92(9):2435–43.
8. Small EJ, Halabi S, Ratain MJ, Rosner G, Stadler W, Palchak D, Marshall E, Rago R, Hars V, Wilding G, Petrylak D, Vogelzang NJ. Randomized study of three different doses of suramin administered with a fixed dosing schedule in patients with advanced prostate cancer: results of intergroup 0159, cancer and leukemia group B 9480. J Clin Oncol 2002;20(16):3369–75.
9. Ryan CW, Vokes EE, Vogelzang NJ, Janisch L, Kobayashi K, Ratain MJ. A phase I study of suramin with once- or twice-monthly dosing in patients with advanced cancer. Cancer Chemother Pharmacol 2002;50(1):1–5.

10. Grossman SA, Phuphanich S, Lesser G, Rozental J, Grochow LB, Fisher J, Piantadosi S; New Approaches to Brain Tumor Therapy CNS Consortium. Toxicity, efficacy, and pharmacology of suramin in adults with recurrent high-grade gliomas. J Clin Oncol 2001;19(13):3260–6.

11. Schroder LE, Lew D, Flanigan RC, Eisenberger MA, Seay TE, Hammond N, Needles BM, Crawford ED. Phase II evaluation of suramin in advanced renal cell carcinoma. A Southwest Oncology Group study. Urol Oncol 2001;6(4):145–8.

12. Small EJ, Meyer M, Marshall ME, Reyno LM, Meyers FJ, Natale RB, Lenehan PF, Chen L, Slichenmyer WJ, Eisenberger M. Suramin therapy for patients with symptomatic hormone-refractory prostate cancer: results of a randomized phase III trial comparing suramin plus hydrocortisone to placebo plus hydrocortisone. J Clin Oncol 2000;18(7):1440–50.

13. Amato AA, Collins MP. Neuropathies associated with malignancy. Semin Neurol 1998;18(1):125–44.

14. La Rocca RV, Meer J, Gilliatt RW, Stein CA, Cassidy J, Myers CE, Dalakas MC. Suramin-induced polyneuropathy. Neurology 1990;40(6):954–60.

15. Chaudhry V, Eisenberger MA, Sinibaldi VJ, Sheikh K, Griffin JW, Cornblath DR. A prospective study of suramin-induced peripheral neuropathy. Brain 1996;119(Pt 6):2039–52.

16. Soliven B, Dhand UK, Kobayashi K, Arora R, Martin B, Petersen MV, Janisch L, Vogelzang NJ, Vokes EE, Ratain MJ. Evaluation of neuropathy in patients on suramin treatment. Muscle Nerve 1997;20(1):83–91.

17. Tu SM, Pagliaro LC, Banks ME, Amato RJ, Millikan RE, Bugazia NA, Madden T, Newman RA, Logothetis CJ. Phase I study of suramin combined with doxorubicin in the treatment of androgen-independent prostate cancer. Clin Cancer Res 1998;4(5):1193–201.

18. Rosen PJ, Mendoza EF, Landaw EM, Mondino B, Graves MC, McBride JH, Turcillo P, deKernion J, Belldegrun A. Suramin in hormone-refractory metastatic prostate cancer: a drug with limited efficacy. J Clin Oncol 1996;14(5):1626–36.

19. Gill JS, Windebank AJ. Suramin induced ceramide accumulation leads to apoptotic cell death in dorsal root ganglion neurons. Cell Death Differ 1998;5(10):876–83.

20. Thylefors B, Rolland A. The risk of optic atrophy following suramin treatment of ocular onchocerciasis. Bull World Health Organ 1979;57(3):479–80.

21. Hemady RK, Sinibaldi VJ, Eisenberger MA. Ocular symptoms and signs associated with suramin sodium treatment for metastatic cancer of the prostate. Am J Ophthalmol 1996;121(3):291–6.

22. Kobayashi K, Weiss RE, Vogelzang NJ, Vokes EE, Janisch L, Ratain MJ. Mineralocorticoid insufficiency due to suramin therapy. Cancer 1996;78(11):2411–20.

23. Dawson NA, Lush RM, Steinberg SM, Tompkins AC, Headlee DJ, Figg WD. Suramin-induced neutropenia. Eur J Cancer 1996;32A(9):1534–9.

24. Horne MK 3rd, Stein CA, LaRocca RV, Myers CE. Circulating glycosaminoglycan anticoagulants associated with suramin treatment. Blood 1988;71(2):273–9.

25. Horne MK 3rd, Wilson OJ, Cooper M, Gralnick HR, Myers CE. The effect of suramin on laboratory tests of coagulation. Thromb Haemost 1992;67(4):434–9.

26. Seidman AD, Schwartz M, Reich L, Scher HI. Immune-mediated thrombocytopenia secondary to suramin. Cancer 1993;71(3):851–4.

27. Cheson BD, Levine AM, Mildvan D, Kaplan LD, Wolfe P, Rios A, Groopman JE, Gill P, Volberding PA, Poiesz BJ, et al. Suramin therapy in AIDS and related disorders.

28. Loke RH, Anderson MG, Coleman JC, Tsiquaye KN, Zuckerman AJ, Murray-Lyon IM. Suramin treatment for chronic active hepatitis B—toxic and ineffective. J Med Virol 1987;21(1):97–9.

29. Figg WD, Cooper MR, Thibault A, Headlee D, Humphrey J, Bergan RC, Reed E, Sartor O. Acute renal toxicity associated with suramin in the treatment of prostate cancer. Cancer 1994;74(5):1612–14.

30. Smith A, Harbour D, Liebmann J. Acute renal failure in a patient receiving treatment with suramin. Am J Clin Oncol 1997;20(4):433–4.

31. Lowitt MH, Eisenberger M, Sina B, Kao GF. Cutaneous eruptions from suramin. A clinical and histopathologic study of 60 patients. Arch Dermatol 1995;131(10):1147–53.

32. Katz SK, Medenica MM, Kobayashi K, Vogelzang NJ, Soltani K. Erythema multiforme induced by suramin. J Am Acad Dermatol 1995;32(2 Pt 1):292–3.

33. Falkson G, Rapoport BL. Lethal toxic epidermal necrolysis during suramin treatment. Eur J Cancer 1992;28A(6–7):1294.

34. Mercier-Parot L, Tuchmann-Duplessis H. Action abortive et tératogène d'un trypanocide, la suramine. [Abortifacient and teratogenic effect of suramin, a trypanocide.] C R Seances Soc Biol Fil 1973;167(11):1518–22.

35. Freeman SJ, Lloyd JB. Evidence that suramin and aurothiomalate are teratogenic in rat by disturbing yolk sac-mediated embryonic protein nutrition. Chem Biol Interact 1986;58(2):149–60.

36. Manner J, Seidl W, Heinicke F, Hesse H. Teratogenic effects of suramin on the chick embryo. Anat Embryol (Berl) 2003;206(3):229–37.

37. Piscitelli SC, Forrest A, Lush RM, Ryan N, Whitfield LR, Figg WD. Pharmacometric analysis of the effect of furosemide on suramin pharmacokinetics. Pharmacotherapy 1997;17(3):431–7.

38. Meyer M, Jeong E, Bolinger B, Chen L, Lenehan P, Slichenmyer W, Natale RB. Phase 1 drug interaction study of suramin and warfarin in patients with prostate cancer. Am J Clin Oncol 2001;24(2):167–71.

Suriclone

General Information

Suriclone, a cyclopyrrolone analogue of zopiclone, has similar pharmacology to the benzodiazepines, binding close to the same site of the GABA receptor–chloride channel complex. It is effective as an anxiolytic and has the notable advantages of minimal sedation and cognitive toxicity, and milder withdrawal effects than those of diazepam or lorazepam (1). Its withdrawal from further development is a mystery.

Reference

1. Lader M. Clin pharmacology of anxiolytic drugs: Past, present and future. In: Biggio G, Sanna E, Costa E, editors. GABA-A Receptors and Anxiety. From Neurobiology to Treatment. New York: Raven Press, 1995:135.

Suxamethonium

See also Neuromuscular blocking drugs

General Information

Suxamethonium consists of two acetylcholine molecules linked together. Initially, it acts like acetylcholine by depolarizing the motor end-plate. However, unlike acetylcholine, which on dissociation from the receptor is immediately destroyed by acetylcholinesterase present in the neuromuscular junction, suxamethonium is hydrolysed by a (pseudo)cholinesterase present in the plasma but not at the neuromuscular junction. Most of an injected dose of suxamethonium is normally destroyed before it reaches the neuromuscular junction. If the activity of plasma cholinesterase in a particular patient is reduced, more of the suxamethonium reaches the neuromuscular junction and its action is proportionately prolonged. The molecules of suxamethonium that reach the acetylcholine receptor sites interact repeatedly with them, producing prolonged depolarization of the motor end-plate, which becomes surrounded by an electrically inactive zone. The end-result is flaccid paralysis. The action of suxamethonium is terminated by diffusion away from the neuromuscular junction. Hydrolysis results in choline and succinylmonocholine, which has a very weak competitive blocking action and is further slowly hydrolysed by plasma cholinesterase to choline and succinic acid.

About 10% of an intravenous dose of suxamethonium is excreted unchanged in the urine with a half-life of 1–2 minutes (1). The half-life is prolonged in patients with pseudocholinesterase deficiency or an abnormal pseudocholinesterase.

The usual adult dose of suxamethonium chloride is 0.5–1.5 mg/kg, which provides clinical relaxation for some 4–9 minutes. However, the normal response is highly variable and relaxation for up to 15 minutes can result from normal doses. Suxamethonium iodide has about two-thirds the potency of the chloride.

General adverse effects

Suxamethonium has several unwanted and potentially dangerous adverse effects. Generalized muscle fasciculations are associated, to a varying degree, with muscle pain, an acute rise in serum potassium, which under certain conditions can result in dysrhythmias and cardiac arrest, raised intraocular and intragastric pressures, and rhabdomyolysis and myoglobinuria with a rare risk of renal insufficiency. Bradycardia and junctional rhythms are relatively common. Normal doses can cause prolonged paralysis (on rare occasions for several hours) in patients with congenital or acquired plasma cholinesterase abnormality or deficiency.

Anaphylactoid reactions have been documented, and signs suggestive of histamine release are not uncommon. These are mostly mild such as flushing of the skin. Occasionally bronchospasm and/or hypotension can lead to circulatory arrest. Suxamethonium is the relaxant most commonly associated with the syndrome of malignant hyperthermia.

Tumor-inducing effects have not been reported.

Tachyphylaxis and resistance

Tachyphylaxis to the neuromuscular blocking effects of suxamethonium is associated with repeated doses. Prolonged exposure of the neuromuscular junction to suxamethonium (resulting from repeated bolus injections or during an infusion of the drug, or as a consequence of delayed hydrolysis subsequent to genetic or acquired plasma cholinesterase deficiency) is accompanied by the development of a phase II block, with non-depolarizing characteristics and a variably prolonged recovery. This depends on both the dose and the duration of exposure to suxamethonium. A cumulative dose of 3–4 mg/kg and an exposure time of 20–30 minutes can be sufficient during halothane anesthesia (2). However, there is wide variation between patients (3), and monitoring of neuromuscular transmission (train-of-four or post-tetanic count) is advisable with cumulative doses greater than 3 mg/kg.

Resistance to suxamethonium has been seen in von Recklinghausen's disease (4) and nemaline myopathy (5).

Organs and Systems

Cardiovascular

Bradycardia and other dysrhythmias are common (80% in some series) and occur after the first and subsequent injections of suxamethonium in infants and children. In adults, these effects are seen more commonly after second or later injections, particularly when the interval between the doses is 2–5 minutes. However, it has been suggested that bradycardia and asystole may now be more frequently seen than previously in adults after a single injection of suxamethonium, as a result of the increased use of fentanyl or the omission of atropine beforehand (6). Nodal rhythm and wandering pacemaker are frequent. The bradycardia is sometimes extreme (asystolic periods of 15–30 seconds duration have been reported). Usually these minor dysrhythmias revert to normal after a few minutes. Halothane can prolong their presence. The incidence of bradycardic asystole is not known, as atropine (the effective therapy) is usually quickly given.

Over the years cardiac arrest in apparently healthy children has occurred unexpectedly, most cases having been attributed to suxamethonium-induced hyperkalemia in patients with previously undetected myopathies (7–17). Several children have died of this complication. A diagnosis of Duchenne dystrophy or another unspecified progressive myopathy was made in 80% of the patients reported to the American Malignant Hyperthermia Registry who were subsequently tested for myopathies (18). Pointing out that hyperkalemia was detected in 72% of the patients from whom blood samples were taken, the authors suggested that calcium, sodium bicarbonate, hyperventilation, and glucose and insulin should be considered for the treatment of anesthesia-related cardiac arrest in children. This is certainly good advice. Standard resuscitative efforts in such cases are often ineffective, as severe hyperkalemia prevents the restoration of a stable cardiac rhythm. It should be stressed that resuscitative efforts should not be stopped until hyperkalemia has been aggressively treated. Excessive doses of adrenaline, calcium, sodium bicarbonate, and glucose/

insulin may be required. Peritoneal dialysis (19), hemodialysis (20), and cardiopulmonary bypass (21) have been used successfully to treat suxamethonium-induced hyperkalemic cardiac arrest.

Regarding the risk of this rare but life-threatening complication in children with undetected myopathy or muscular dystrophy, it has been suggested that the routine use of suxamethonium in pediatric anesthesia be abandoned. It should be reserved for emergency intubation or when immediate securing of the airway is necessary.

Tachycardia and a rise in blood pressure are occasionally seen. Other supraventricular and ventricular dysrhythmias are much less common. Ventricular fibrillation associated with suxamethonium is usually the result of hyperkalemia, but has also been reported in hypercalcemia (22) and is often seen in the course of malignant hyperthermia. Atropine, especially when given intravenously just before suxamethonium, is the most effective agent for the prevention of dysrhythmias. Hexafluorenium, D-tubocurarine, pancuronium, and other non-depolarizer blockers have also been reported as being effective in prevention. Severe hypotension can occur in patients with anaphylactoid reactions.

On theoretical grounds, suxamethonium, being akin to acetylcholine, should produce effects not only at the neuromuscular junction, but also at autonomic ganglia, at muscarinic receptors, and at postganglionic parasympathetic receptors. However, these other types of cholinoceptors are not so sensitive to its action. Nevertheless, stimulation of sympathetic ganglia has been invoked as being possibly responsible for the tachycardia and rise in blood pressure that sometimes occur transiently after its use. Likewise, stimulation of parasympathetic ganglia or direct stimulation of cardiac muscarinic receptors may be responsible for bradycardia. Differences in resting sympathetic and vagal tone have been said to account for the more frequent occurrence of tachycardia in "vagotonic" adults and bradycardia in "sympathotonic" children. The transient mild rise in blood pressure is possibly the result of the initial fasciculation, inducing an increase in venous return, which may also reflexly result in a slowing of the heart rate. Stimulation of afferent receptors in the carotid sinus has also been claimed to cause reflex bradycardia. Small doses (20–25 mg) are said to convert nodal to sinus rhythm, and larger doses to depress the sinoatrial node and so to cause bradycardia and nodal rhythm. Fasciculation probably produces an increase in afferent discharge from muscle spindles, which may account for the reported arousal pattern on the electroencephalogram; this in turn is postulated as a cause of tachycardia and a rise in blood pressure.

It has been hypothesized that suxamethonium modulates noradrenaline release from postganglionic sympathetic nerve terminals by presynaptic nicotine (+) and muscarinic (−) receptors on these nerve terminals (23). The refractory period of these presynaptic nicotinic receptors is postulated as being longer than that of the muscarinic receptors, which results in a net muscarinic effect (bradycardia) after a second injection of suxamethonium within 4–5 minutes of the first. To explain the occurrence of bradycardia after an initial injection of suxamethonium in young children, it is postulated that sympathetic nerve terminals mature later, so that muscarinic (bradycardic) effects are unopposed by noradrenaline secretion in younger patients.

Some controversial correspondence has followed the report of four cases of fatal cardiac arrest among 150 patients who were given suxamethonium by paramedics in out-of-hospital emergencies (24). The authors suggested that this might militate against suxamethonium-facilitated endotracheal intubation in this setting. Others, however, have argued that there was no evidence for a causal role of suxamethonium in those cases (25). Patients with critical conditions, such as respiratory failure requiring endotracheal intubation, may have a cardiac arrest without being given suxamethonium. Furthermore, undetected esophageal intubation was considered to be an alternative explanation of cardiac arrest. Indeed, when endotracheal intubation is attempted in these often dramatic and stressful circumstances by health-care providers who have no routine experience in this, there may be a high rate of esophageal intubation. In one study 18 of 108 patients who had been intubated by paramedics were found to have the tube in their esophagus (26). So the role of suxamethonium in the above report is questionable. On the other hand, suxamethonium is part of the protocol for emergency intubation in many centers worldwide and suxamethonium-associated cardiac arrest, apart from anecdotal instances, has not been reported to be a relevant problem (27). Suxamethonium may increase the success rate of emergency intubations while reducing the incidence of traumatic intubations (28). Therefore, rapid-sequence intubation with an induction agent such as etomidate and suxamethonium is probably still the technique of choice for airway management in emergencies. Whoever uses this technique must be aware of contraindications to suxamethonium and must have frequent practice in endotracheal intubation.

Respiratory

Apnea of variable duration results from muscle paralysis. The return of spontaneous respiration is normally rapid, but it may be delayed if phase II block develops. This will only be of consequence if it is not detected and spontaneous respiration is permitted before it is adequate. Exacerbation of muscle weakness in Duchenne muscular dystrophy after injection of suxamethonium can lead to delayed respiratory failure postoperatively (29).

Bronchospasm is a feature of about one-third of anaphylactoid reactions to suxamethonium and laryngeal edema can also occur, producing intubation problems (30) or respiratory distress and cyanosis after extubation (31).

Nervous system

An arousal pattern can occur on the electroencephalogram, possibly as a result of increased afferent traffic from muscle spindles. This has been speculated as the cause of perioperative dreaming in children in whom an intermittent-suxamethonium technique has been used during light anesthesia (SEDA-13, 102) (32). Suxamethonium must be used with caution in neurological disease and is better avoided altogether when there is a risk of a dangerous rise in serum potassium. A transient rise in intracranial pressure has been observed after injection of suxamethonium, probably as a result of increased cerebral blood volume (33,34). This might be regarded as noxious in patients with intracranial lesions. However, when suxamethonium was given to patients with markedly raised intracranial pressure who received artificial ventilation on the intensive care unit, no adverse effects were observed (35).

Patients with severe head injuries require endotracheal intubation and controlled ventilation. Rapid-sequence intubation using an intravenous anesthetic plus suxamethonium is the standard technique for this, as the patient may have a full stomach. However, suxamethonium has been suggested by some to have a negative effect by causing increased intracranial pressure. The literature on this has been reviewed (36). The authors found only two studies that specifically addressed the effects of suxamethonium on intracranial pressure in patients with head injuries (35,37). In both studies suxamethonium was given to patients who were already being ventilated in the intensive care unit. There were no adverse effects of suxamethonium on intracranial pressure or cerebral perfusion pressure. However, when suxamethonium was given to lightly anesthetized patients undergoing resection of intracranial tumors, there were significant increases in intracranial pressure (38,39). These could be prevented by pretreatment with a small dose of a non-depolarizing muscle relaxant (39). The importance of an adequate level of anesthesia for intubating patients at risk of intracranial hypertension should be stressed. A lightly anesthetized patient will have large increases in intracranial pressure during intubation, no matter which muscle relaxant is used, because of a stress response that includes venous vasoconstriction and a massive increase in central venous pressure, resulting in impaired venous outflow from the cranium and thereby increased intracranial blood volume.

Neuromuscular function

Muscle pain

The depolarization of the motor end-plate receptors produced by suxamethonium (either directly or via repetitive discharge generation by the motor nerve terminals) (40) results in generalized and desynchronized contraction of skeletal muscle fibers. These fasciculations result in aching muscle pain (in up to 90% of patients), most commonly in the neck, pectoral region, shoulders, and back. The pain is most often experienced the day after operation and is worse in ambulatory patients. It is more common in women than in men. Children, elderly patients, athletes, and pregnant women (41) complain less often. Africans also seem to be less susceptible (42).

Mechanism

The cause of the pain is unknown, although there are many hypotheses such as damage to muscle (43,44) resulting from asynchronous contractions of adjacent muscle fibers (45), irreversible damage to muscle spindles (46), potassium flux (47), lactic acid (48), serotonin (49), calcium influx-associated damage to muscle spindles (50), and prostaglandins (51,52). The pain appears not to be related to the extent or intensity of the observed fasciculations.

Prevention

Various preventive measures have been recommended, but none is effective in all cases. One reliable method is the injection of a small non-paralysing dose of a non-depolarizing neuromuscular blocker 2–3 minutes before the injection of suxamethonium (53–57) in preventing fasciculations, but the patient must be carefully observed, since an unexpected degree of paralysis occasionally ensues (SEDA-6, 130).

Other measures, much disputed, include the prior injection of diazepam (58,59), procaine or lidocaine (57), vitamin C, suxamethonium itself (10 mg), and aspirin (51,52). The combined use of atracurium 0.05 mg/kg and lidocaine 1.5 mg/kg reduced the incidence of postoperative myalgia to 5% compared with 75% in controls (57). Thiopental, injected immediately beforehand, is also said to have some effect, as is giving the suxamethonium slowly.

Myotonic reactions

Rarely, on injecting suxamethonium, contracture, instead of the usual relaxation, of skeletal muscles ensues. In denervated muscles the postulated mechanism is direct activation of the contractile mechanism by suxamethonium because of the widespread chemosensitivity of the muscle fiber membranes.

Paradoxical contracture is most often associated with myotonia dystrophica and myotonia congenita. A myotonic reaction has also been reported in a patient with hyperkalemic periodic paralysis (60). Suxamethonium is therefore contraindicated in these conditions, even though normal responses are sometimes seen. Contracture has also been reported as a result of denervation in Pancoast's syndrome and after plexus injuries and, rarely, in patients with amyotrophic lateral sclerosis or multiple sclerosis (61–63).

Failure of relaxation and generalized muscular rigidity after suxamethonium is sometimes also seen in patients who develop the syndrome of malignant hyperthermia. Isolated masseter muscle rigidity can occur after the administration of suxamethonium, being reported particularly in children given both suxamethonium and halothane. Most experts define masseter muscle rigidity as a major increase in masseter muscle tone severe enough to make mouth opening impossible and to prevent laryngoscopy and endotracheal intubation. Referring to the high incidence of positive results with halothane-caffeine contracture testing, some believe that up to 50% of patients with masseter muscle rigidity are susceptible to malignant hyperthermia (64–67). Others are not convinced of such a high degree of correlation (68) and hold that divers other factors are responsible for the majority of cases (69–71). While severe masseter muscle rigidity is rare (72), smaller increases in jaw tension of about 60 seconds duration occur almost invariably after suxamethonium administration (73,74). Such increases in masseter muscle tone can be attenuated by using propofol as an induction agent and by precurarization, that is pretreatment with a small dose of a non-depolarizing muscle relaxant (74) This might be important during rapid sequence induction of anesthesia.

A hypothesis has been offered to explain muscle hyperexcitability in response to suxamethonium (75). Voltage clamp experiments on alpha subunits of human muscle sodium channels, heterologously expressed in HEK 293 cells, showed that succinic acid, a metabolite of suxamethonium, shifted steady-state activation in the direction of more negative membrane potentials. The EC_{50} for this effect was 0.39 mmol/l. This might lead to muscle hyperexcitability in vivo. Clearly, it is not currently possible to claim any direct clinical implications of this study, but two facts should be considered. After the administration of a routine dose of suxamethonium, blood concentrations of 0.17 mmol/l have been reported (76) Thus, equimolar concentrations of succinic acid are to be expected, given that cholinesterase activity is not impaired. Moreover, succinic acid is a citric acid cycle intermediate, ubiquitous in body tissues. In conditions of ischemia and hypoxia, tissue and serum concentrations of succinic acid increase up to 0.2 mmol/l (77,78). Thus, the administration of suxamethonium to a hypoxic patient may well lead to succinic acid concentrations that affect muscle sodium channel excitability in vitro.

Rhabdomyolysis

Myoglobinuria (79) and raised serum creatine kinase activity (44) have been reported after suxamethonium and appear to be evidence of muscle damage, probably resulting from fasciculation. Repeated bolus doses of suxamethonium result in higher plasma myoglobin concentrations (80) and creatine kinase activities (44). Myoglobinemia seems to be much more common in children than in adults (SEDA-10, 107) (SEDA-11, 121) (81) and is more marked when halothane is used (82). On occasion, myoglobinuria results in renal insufficiency (83–88).

There is an association between (latent) muscular dystrophy (usually of the Duchenne or Becker type) and the production of rhabdomyolysis by suxamethonium (84,85,89,90). Suxamethonium can cause excessive muscle damage in these patients, as manifested not only by severe myoglobinemia and raised serum creatine kinase activity but also by acute exacerbation of muscle weakness postoperatively (SEDA-11, 121) (7,29,84,91,92). Massive potassium release can result in hyperkalemic cardiac arrest. Such patients may also develop features suggestive of the syndrome of malignant hyperthermia (93,94). Suxamethonium should not be used in patients with Duchenne muscular dystrophy or who have a family history suspect for the condition.

Prolonged paralysis

Prolonged paralysis can result from idiosyncrasy, overdose, or reduced or abnormal plasma cholinesterase activity. There are geographical and racial differences in sensitivity to suxamethonium (SEDA-6, 129) (95,96); some of these differences arise from dietary and other environmental factors and others result from variations in plasma cholinesterase genotypes. Genotypically normal patients may be paralysed by a usual (1 mg/kg) dose of suxamethonium for as short a time as 2 minutes or (rarely) as long as 20 minutes, and the duration in general inversely reflects plasma cholinesterase activity (97).

Prolonged paralysis after suxamethonium has also been reported in von Recklinghausen's disease (98), but resistance to suxamethonium has also been seen (4).

Sensory systems

Shortly after the introduction of suxamethonium it was noted that it can increase intraocular pressure (99), an observation that has subsequently been confirmed in several other studies (100–114). The increase in intraocular pressure occurs promptly after intravenous injection of suxamethonium, peaks at 1–2 minutes, and returns to baseline after 6–10 minutes (102,109). The mean increase is about 4–8 mmHg, with a range of 5–15 mmHg.

Mechanism

Several mechanisms have been suggested to explain the effect of suxamethonium on intraocular pressure. One of the first ideas was to blame fasciculation and contraction of the extraocular muscles of the eye (115). However, a study in humans undergoing enucleation showed that suxamethonium produces an increase in intraocular pressure even after detachment of the extraocular muscles (116). So activity of the extraocular muscles may increase intraocular pressure, but there must be other factors. Observing that suxamethonium administration was almost invariably followed by retraction of the eyeball, some investigators suggested increased tone of intraorbital smooth muscles as a mechanism (117), but in fact there is very little intraorbital extraocular smooth muscle in humans. This idea has therefore not been widely accepted. There appears to be some effect of suxamethonium on the intraocular smooth muscles, as indicated by the observation that there is a rapid rise in anterior chamber thickness and a diminution of lens thickness after suxamethonium administration (118). These changes could be explained by a relaxing effect of suxamethonium on the ciliary muscle, which would in turn result in increased aqueous humor outflow resistance and a consequent increase in intraocular pressure (116). However, this mechanism would not be expected to produce pressure increases of the magnitude observed after suxamethonium injection. A vasodilatory effect on conjunctival vessels has been observed (119), and this has been interpreted as indirect evidence of choroidal vasodilatation (120). On the other hand, an increase in ocular blood flow has not been detected after suxamethonium administration but after subsequent endotracheal intubation (121). In conclusion, there is no satisfactory explanation for the suxamethonium-associated increase in intraocular pressure, but increased tone of extraocular muscles, increased aqueous humor outflow resistance, and increased choroidal blood volume are probably important elements.

Prevention

Many efforts have been made to find a technique to prevent the suxamethonium-associated increase in intraocular pressure. Some attenuation of the pressure response has been demonstrated with defasciculation doses of non-depolarizing muscle relaxants (122), but this could not be reproduced in subsequent studies (100–102,123). The same is true for self-taming, that is pretreatment with a small dose of suxamethonium (124,125). Other drugs that have been used with some effect are diazepam (105,126,127), lidocaine (107,114,121,128,129), glyceryl trinitrate (130), nifedipine (131), and beta-blockers (132), but none of these completely prevented increases in intraocular pressure.

The most effective method of attenuating the intraocular pressure response to suxamethonium plus endotracheal intubation is to provide a deep level of anesthesia by using intravenous anesthetics and opiates (133–137). In 60 patients who received thiopental/suxamethonium, propofol/suxamethonium, or propofol/alfentanil/suxamethonium for anesthesia induction, the increase in intraocular pressure after suxamethonium plus endotracheal intubation was completely blocked by propofol plus alfentanil (137). Combining an intravenous anesthetic with a rapid-onset opioid, such as alfentanil, prevents increases in intraocular pressure (137). When the ultra-short-acting opioid remifentanil (1 microgram/kg) was given in combination with propofol (2 mg/kg) and suxamethonium (1 mg/kg) for endotracheal intubation during induction of anesthesia the highest intraocular pressure recorded was 18 mmHg, whereas peak values up to 35 mmHg occurred in the control group without remifentanil (138).

Implications for surgery

A particular problem is the clinical impact of a rise in intraocular pressure during operation in cases of penetrating eye injury, which is usually performed as an emergency, when it is often not clear whether the patient has eaten recently. While it is commonly accepted that anesthesia in these patients should be induced in a rapid-sequence technique, that is by giving an hypnotic and suxamethonium followed rapidly by endotracheal intubation, in order to reduce the risk of pulmonary aspiration of gastric contents, there is considerable controversy about what to do in the case of penetrating eye injuries. As suxamethonium provokes an increase in intraocular pressure in intact eyes, there is concern that its use could result in loss of intraocular contents and damage to the eye if the eyeball is opened. This, however, has not hitherto been observed, either in clinical studies or in animal experiments (139–141). Several experts regard suxamethonium as being appropriate for rapid-sequence intubation in patients with penetrating eye injuries (142–146).

Similarly, there are difficulties in strabismus surgery, which is commonly performed in children, with the goal of correcting the optical axes of the eyes by shortening certain extraocular muscles. The "forced duction test" can be used to differentiate between a paretic muscle and a restrictive force that prevents ocular movement. Suxamethonium, by increasing the tone of the extraocular muscles, can produce considerable alterations in the results of that test, sometimes lasting as long as 20 minutes (147). Suxamethonium should therefore be avoided in strabismus surgery. Furthermore, in a retrospective study there was an increased incidence of masseter muscle rigidity in patients with strabismus (148). A positive halothane-caffeine contracture test was subsequently found in 25% of the adults and 50% of the children in whom masseter rigidity had occurred (64–67). In line with that, there were more patients with strabismus in a group of patients who had experienced an episode of malignant hyperthermia than in the general surgical population in the USA (149). Based on these observations, it has been assumed that patients with strabismus might have an increased risk of malignant hyperthermia (146,150), which has been regarded as another reason for avoiding suxamethonium in strabismus surgery (151). On the other hand, the incidence of strabismus was not different in two groups of patients, with or without a positive halothane–caffeine contracture test (152). In conclusion, there are some indirect clues to an increased risk of malignant hyperthermia in patients with strabismus, but for the time being there is not enough evidence to contraindicate suxamethonium. However, there are reasons for reserving its use for special circumstances, such as rapid-sequence induction in patients with an increased risk of pulmonary aspiration. First, the surgical procedure can be impaired by increased tone in the extraocular muscles. Secondly, patients with strabismus may have a higher risk of suxamethonium-associated masseter muscle rigidity. Thirdly, most patients with strabismus are children, in whom the suxamethonium is best avoided (SEDA-19, 139).

Electrolyte balance

An immediate rise in serum potassium occurs after the administration of suxamethonium. The rise is normally small, 0.5 mmol/l or less (4). However, in some cases it can be larger, and cases of cardiac arrest associated with hyperkalemia have been reported in critically ill patients after prolonged immobilization (153–161). Cardiac arrest also occurred in a patient with wound botulism (162).

- A 28-year-old previously healthy man was admitted with a 4-week history of progressive symmetrical muscle weakness that had started in his neck and descended to both arms and legs. He also complained of diplopia, dysphonia, and dysphagia. On the day of admission, he noted difficulty in breathing. He had a history of intermittent diamorphine abuse, and had been injecting "black tar" heroin subcutaneously for the past month. Several hours after admission he had to be intubated, and was given etomidate 20 mg plus suxamethonium 80 mg. Within 60 seconds he developed a wide complex tachycardia, which degenerated into ventricular fibrillation refractory to electrical countershock and standard resuscitative measures. His serum potassium concentration 10–12 minutes after the onset of cardiocirculatory arrest was 6.8 mmol/l, having been 4.7 mmol/l several hours before. Calcium chloride, sodium bicarbonate, and glucose/insulin were given, and 25 minutes after the arrest began the heart rhythm converted to sinus tachycardia. The electrocardiogram subsequently showed no structural abnormalities. A serological test taken on the day of admission was positive for botulinum toxin type A. He eventually survived without any residual deficits and was discharged from hospital after 63 days.

The authors suggested that suxamethonium should be avoided in patients with suspected botulism and in patients with muscle weakness of unknown origin. Wound botulism had been observed before in drug users who have injected black tar heroin (163). Botulinum toxin inhibits presynaptic acetylcholine release, resulting in muscle weakness. In animals chronic administration of botulinum toxin caused an increase in the number of postsynaptic acetylcholine receptors with distribution across the muscle surface (164) and postsynaptic acetylcholine receptors converted into the immature type with prolonged channel opening times (165). With huge numbers of muscle fibers altered in that way, suxamethonium may cause hyperkalemic cardiac arrest by producing massive potassium efflux.

One major concern for anesthetists is suxamethonium-associated hyperkalemia in apparently fit patients without obvious risk factors. Life-threatening hyperkalemia occurred in three Japanese women who underwent cesarean section (166).

- Cardiac arrest occurred in a 34-year-old woman who was given suxamethonium 120 mg. She had been immobilized and treated with high-dose magnesium sulfate and ritodrine for 5 weeks before the event because of preterm uterine contractions. Her preoperative creatine kinase activity was 4050 IU/l. After rapid-sequence induction of anesthesia and injection of suxamethonium she became cyanotic and pulseless and the electrocardiogram showed ventricular fibrillation. The serum potassium concentration after 25 minutes of cardiopulmonary resuscitation, which included the administration of adrenaline, sodium bicarbonate, and calcium chloride, was 5.7 mmol/l. During resuscitation vaginal vacuum delivery was performed. Finally, she was defibrillated successfully and made a full recovery.
- Two other patients had been immobilized and treated with magnesium and ritodrine for several weeks. Preoperative creatine kinase activities were 2120 IU/l and 630 IU/l. In both cases, serum potassium increased by 2.3 mmol/l within 2–3 minutes after suxamethonium injection (from 4.0 to 6.3 mmol/l and from 4.9 to 7.2 mmol/l). This was accompanied by tall peaked T waves and a short period of ventricular tachycardia in one case and by tall peaked T waves and widened QRS complexes in the other.

The authors suggested that the combined effects of immobilization and prolonged magnesium administration might have resulted in a denervation-like state of large groups of skeletal muscles. The drawback of that explanation is that an awake and healthy person will always move normally even when confined to bed. As long as muscle cells receive physiological stimulation via the neuromuscular junction in patients without muscle weakness, denervation-like changes should not occur to a significant extent. In addition, denervation alone is not known to be associated with an increase in plasma creatine kinase activity, a strong indicator of muscle cell damage, which was found in all the patients reported here. Unfortunately, the authors did not document creatine kinase activities or myoglobin concentrations after suxamethonium, which might have given some idea about additional suxamethonium-induced rhabdomyolysis.

It can be assumed that these three patients had some form of myopathy, either acquired during their previous course or pre-existing. It would have been interesting to know if they had any clinical symptoms, such as muscle pain or weakness. Pre-existing myopathy would be unlikely if plasma creatine kinase activities had been normal before. However, this information was not given in the paper. On the other hand, myopathy could have been acquired during the course of pregnancy and hospital treatment. Various drugs and toxins have been associated with myopathies (167). Hypermagnesemia can produce muscle weakness but magnesium sulfate has not so far been reported to cause myopathy. Therefore, the role of ritodrine in these cases should be questioned. This selective beta$_2$-adrenoceptor agonist has previously been linked to myopathic changes in a patient treated for preterm labor (168). In addition, glucocorticoid treatment, probably used to promote fetal lung development, might be a contributory factor. Long-term glucocorticoid treatment is associated with myopathic changes (167).

In the end, the exact mechanism of suxamethonium-associated hyperkalemia in these cases cannot be determined. Given the huge numbers of patients who receive suxamethonium during rapid-sequence induction of anesthesia for cesarean section, even after some time of treatment for preterm labor without adverse effects, it would be overzealous to call for a restricted use of suxamethonium in these patients. Rather, this report is in support of preoperative screening of plasma creatine kinase activity. Probably suxamethonium should not be used in patients with raised plasma creatine kinase activity. It is a good idea to check creatine kinase activity preoperatively in women due to undergo cesarean section after prolonged immobilization and pretreatment with magnesium sulfate and a beta$_2$-adrenoceptor agonist such as ritodrine.

Mechanism

The underlying mechanisms of and mortality from suxamethonium-associated hyperkalemic cardiac arrest have been reviewed (169). The rise in serum potassium probably results from repetitive opening of receptor-linked ion channels and suxamethonium-induced fasciculation, although it can occur in the absence of visible fasciculation. Muscle injury with excessive leakage of potassium is postulated as a cause of the hyperkalemia. Reuptake of potassium into muscle cells may also be hindered. It has been shown that denervation results in a spread of the normally small receptor area of the motor end-plate over the entire muscle fiber membrane, so that eventually the whole membrane surface is directly excitable by depolarizing agents such as acetylcholine or suxamethonium (170). The immature extrajunctional receptor-linked ion channels so formed remain open for a longer time than those at normal motor end-plates. Depolarization by suxamethonium thereby results in an excessive efflux of potassium from ion channels spread over the entire muscle fiber membrane and not just, as normally occurs, from the circumscribed motor end-plate region (171–173). Prolonged immobilization can also result in extrajunctional receptor spread (174) and a greater increase in serum potassium than usual after suxamethonium.

Rhabdomyolysis is also a mechanism for hyperkalemia, and it has been said that almost all reported cases of hyperkalemic cardiac arrest considered to have resulted from rhabdomyolysis occurred in children and adolescents with underlying muscular dystrophies (169). Hyperkalemia during rapid acute rhabdomyolysis is more likely to result in unsuccessful resuscitation than hyperkalemia due to the potassium efflux that results from upregulation of acetylcholine receptors.

Susceptibility factors

The rise in serum potassium can be prolonged (SEDA-11, 122) (175) and exaggerated (SEDA-10, 108) (176) in patients taking beta-blockers. In renal insufficiency the rise after suxamethonium is similar to that in healthy patients (177) and is only dangerous if the serum potassium is already high (above 5.5 mmol/l). However, several conditions can lead to a massive rise in serum potassium, resulting in ventricular fibrillation and cardiac arrest. These include burns (178,179), massive trauma (180,181), and neurological diseases or injuries, especially when denervation is a feature, such as spinal cord injury (182), hemiplegia, multiple sclerosis, or muscular dystrophy (183), peripheral nerve injuries (62,184) and polyneuropathy (185,186). Hyperkalemia has also been reported after suxamethonium in patients with tetanus (187), encephalitis (188), Parkinson's disease (SEDA-6, 129) (189), muscle wasting secondary to chronic arterial insufficiency (190), metastatic embryonal rhabdomyosarcoma (SEDA-14, 114) (191), ruptured cerebral aneurysms (SEDA-5, 134) (192), hyperparathyroidism (22), and in patients with severe and long-lasting sepsis (193,194).

There are times when patients are most susceptible to hyperkalemia. In patients with burns or trauma this is generally between 10 and 60 days after the injury, or longer if there is persistent infection and delayed healing. In neurological diseases or injuries the danger period is usually from 3 weeks to 6 months after onset. However, in some cases, such as patients with transverse spinal lesions and tetraplegia, dangerous hyperkalemia has been reported as early as 24–48 hours after the injury, and likewise severe potassium rises have been reported more than 6 months after injury or onset of disease, particularly in patients with progressive lesions (SEDA-6, 128) (183).

Extrajunctional spread of acetylcholine receptors and expression of the immature type of these receptors with prolonged channel opening times have been shown after burns, which may be why there can be massive potassium release after suxamethonium administration. As the increase in acetylcholine receptor density on the muscle surface takes some time to develop, there should be an interval after the accident during which suxamethonium can be safely given. However, the length of this interval is controversial. Referring to a lack of reports of hyperkalemic complications during the first week after the injury, it has been suggested that suxamethonium can be given safely during the first 6–7 days after major thermal injury (195). However, based on the results of animal experiments, suxamethonium might be safe for up to 48 hours after the injury only (195).

The use of suxamethonium in intensive care units has been critically reviewed (196). Several cases of hyperkalemic cardiac arrest after suxamethonium have occurred in intensive care patients (153,155–157,159,160). Of particular concern is the risk of hyperkalemic cardiac arrest when suxamethonium is given to critically ill patients

after a period of immobilization (154). The exact mechanism is not known, but extrajunctional spread of acetylcholine receptors is believed to play a major role. It is strongly recommended that suxamethonium should not be given to patients who have been immobilized in the intensive care unit for more than a few days.

In yet another report of suxamethonium-induced fatal hyperkalemic cardiac arrest in an intensive care unit it was assumed that severe mucositis after cancer chemotherapy might have contributed to the hyperkalemic response (197).

- A 37-year-old woman with acute myelogenous leukemia was admitted to an intensive care unit (ICU) with mental status changes and progressive dyspnea due to pneumonia. Intubation was performed before ICU admission using a sedative without neuromuscular blockade. She had received chemotherapy with cytarabine, daunorubicin, and intrathecal methotrexate for brain metastases. After chemotherapy and before ICU admission her course was complicated by continuous neutropenic fevers and by painful mucositis causing dysphagia and bleeding. After 10 days of ventilator treatment in the ICU and treatment with ceftazidime, gentamicin, metronidazole, vancomycin, amphotericin, and aciclovir, her condition improved, allowing withdrawal of ventilator support and extubation. A few hours later, however, she gradually developed severe respiratory distress and required re-intubation. The serum potassium concentration before intubation was 4.3 mmol/l. For endotracheal intubation she received intravenous etomidate 14 mg and suxamethonium 100 mg. Immediately after intubation she developed a broad-complex tachycardia and her blood pressure could not be measured. Chest compression and advanced cardiac life support were started. Her serum potassium concentration was 13.1 mmol/l. Intravenous calcium chloride, sodium bicarbonate, and insulin/glucose were therefore given. The serum potassium fell to 6.5 mmol/l but rose to 7.4 mmol/l 15 minutes later, despite additional antihyperkalemic treatment. She finally died.

Despite this having been a case of suxamethonium-induced hyperkalemic cardiac arrest after several days of ventilator treatment on the intensive care unit, the authors did not believe that upregulation and extrajunctional spread of acetylcholine receptors were the underlying mechanisms. They implied that mobilization and daily physiotherapy would have both prevented these typical denervation-like changes and ruled out a neuromuscular disorder. Rather they suggested that severe generalized mucositis had resulted in a state that they compared to an "internal burns injury." However, these speculations were not substantiated by additional data. In particular, they gave no information on the presuxamethonium neuromuscular state of the patient. Some form of polyneuropathy and/or myopathy could have been present, and this was not ruled out by the fact that the patient could breathe spontaneously and sit in a chair. While it is true that severe mucositis represents a state of widespread cellular damage similar to severe burn injuries, it is not clear why this itself should result in hyperkalemia after suxamethonium. To our knowledge suxamethonium only has effects on excitable cells. Even in patients with severe thermal injuries, no case of hyperkalemia after suxamethonium has been reported within the first 48 hours after the accident, and suxamethonium-induced hyperkalemia in burned patients is believed to result from upregulation of acetylcholine receptors, owing to thermal damage of nerve fibers (structural denervation) and immobilization (functional denervation) (170). Apart from immobilization due to the severity of the illness it is very unlikely that mucositis should have similar effects. Mucositis itself should therefore not be regarded as a risk factor for suxamethonium-associated hyperkalemia.

In a survey of intensive care units in the UK, more than two-thirds of the respondents would have chosen suxamethonium in a clinical scenario requiring re-intubation in a patient with abdominal sepsis and weaning failure after 20 days of ICU stay (198). The authors concluded that there is a lack of appreciation of the dangers of suxamethonium in critically ill patients in intensive care units.

The use of suxamethonium in patients with renal insufficiency was controversial in the 1970s, after some cases of hyperkalemic cardiac arrest in such patients. As several studies did not show exaggerated potassium release, suxamethonium is now considered safe for patients with renal insufficiency, if preoperative hyperkalemia is excluded. The observation of some cases of postoperative hyperkalemia recently prompted a review of the literature (199). The authors found sufficient evidence to support the current consensus: suxamethonium can be used in patients with renal insufficiency, but it should not be given if there is pre-existing hyperkalemia; doses of suxamethonium should not be given repeatedly, as this can result in sinus bradycardia.

Suxamethonium is said to be contraindicated in patients with hyperkalemia (that is a serum potassium concentration over 5.5 mmol/l). This, however, has been questioned (200). In an analysis of their anesthetic database, the authors identified 38 patients with a preoperative serum potassium concentration over 5.5 mmol/l who subsequently received suxamethonium. In no case were dysrhythmias or any complications documented and there were no deaths. While they admitted that minor complications might not have found their way into the database, the authors felt that major problems caused by suxamethonium in these patients were unlikely. They suggested that the use of suxamethonium in patients with serum potassium concentrations above 5.5 mmol/l may be acceptable when other muscle relaxants have inappropriate profiles. As their analysis included only a few patients with serum potassium concentrations above 6.0 mmol/l they recommended the use of antihyperkalemic treatment before suxamethonium in these patients.

Prevention

It has been claimed that non-depolarizing drugs given before suxamethonium attenuate the rise in potassium, but this has been repeatedly shown to be unreliable. It seems advisable to avoid the use of suxamethonium completely in such patients. This subject has been extensively reviewed (201,202).

Gastrointestinal

Suxamethonium can increase intragastric pressure. This is probably a result of fasciculation of the abdominal muscles (203), although a vagal effect can also contribute. The rise is highly variable, ranging from zero to more than 85 cm H_2O according to many different investigations (204–207). The intragastric pressure at which the lower esophageal sphincter opens is also variable, with a mean of about 28 cm H_2O, depending partly on the angle between the esophagus and the cardia of the stomach (208,209). There is therefore a danger that the suxamethonium-induced rise in intragastric pressure may produce incompetence of the lower esophageal sphincter and result in regurgitation. This risk is likely to be increased in patients with hiatus hernia, gastric and intestinal dilatation, ascites, and intra-abdominal tumors. Pregnant patients are especially susceptible, as the tonus of the lower esophageal sphincter can also be reduced in pregnancy. It has been suggested, however, that suxamethonium causes, either by a direct action on the lower esophageal sphincter or indirectly through a pinch action of the diaphragm, increased resistance to opening of the lower esophagus, which counteracts the increased intragastric pressure (210). Attenuating fasciculation by giving small doses of non-depolarizing blockers reduces the rise in gastric pressure (203,206,211).

Urinary tract

In severe renal disease, suxamethonium should only be given if the serum potassium is below 5.5 mmol/l. The excretion of neostigmine and pyridostigmine can be impaired in renal insufficiency, and this has been reported to have resulted in prolongation of the action of suxamethonium given some hours later (212).

Myoglobinuria resulting from suxamethonium administration can cause acute renal insufficiency (83,84,213).

Musculoskeletal

The problem of suxamethonium-associated postoperative myalgia has been reviewed (214). Key statements are:

- there is no correlation between the severity of muscle fasciculation, changes in serum creatine phosphokinase or serum potassium, and postoperative myalgia;
- although not proven, mechanical muscle damage is still assumed to be an underlying mechanism;
- several classes of pretreatment drugs reduce the incidence and severity of myalgia; combining two agents may be the most useful method;
- so far, the lowest incidence of post-suxamethonium myalgia has been reported when a small dose of a non-depolarizing neuromuscular blocking agent was given together with lidocaine as pretreatment.

In addition, there was a reduced incidence and intensity of post-suxamethonium myalgia when anesthesia had been maintained by propofol infusion compared with isoflurane (215).

Immunologic

From the results of intradermal injections, suxamethonium has only 1% of the histamine-releasing activity of D-tubocurarine (216). However, through the years there have been many reports of reactions, varying from flushing and urticaria to bronchospasm (217,218) and severe shock (219–222). That suxamethonium was responsible was suggested in some cases by the fact that the patients reacted on different occasions with raised plasma histamine and catecholamine concentrations (223–225). The association was confirmed in other cases by repeatedly injecting the drug, thereby producing bronchospasm several times in the course of the one anesthetic (226,227). Skin testing has also yielded confirmation, although this can be dangerous (220). Analysis of large series of patients (228–233) who have had severe anaphylactoid reactions during anesthesia, using more sophisticated laboratory and immunological investigations in addition to intradermal skin tests, suggests that suxamethonium may be much more commonly associated with such reactions than was previously believed. In 18 cases (234) cardiovascular collapse was the predominant feature in 72% and bronchospasm in 33%; cardiac arrest occurred in five patients. In addition, two reports (235,236) of anaphylactic reactions involving both thiopental and suxamethonium have raised the question of "aggregate"-induced reactions (235) occurring when drugs are given in such a way that they can interact in the injection system.

Body temperature

The syndrome of malignant hyperthermia can be triggered by suxamethonium. Mortality is more than 60% in untreated patients. This syndrome is reported as occurring once in every 15 000–150 000 anesthetics. It may be more common in the Japanese. However, there are also abortive forms of malignant hyperthermia, and many of the typical signs may be produced by other conditions, so that it is difficult to ascertain the precise incidence. Autosomal dominant inheritance, with reduced penetrance and variable expressivity, is the proposed genetic basis. The cause is unknown, but it is thought to be associated with a rise in free ionized myoplasmic calcium, possibly owing to a failure of the sarcoplasmic reticulum to bind calcium. As a result, aerobic and anaerobic metabolism are increased, resulting in the typical features of the syndrome. Halothane and suxamethonium are the most frequent triggers, although almost all of the inhalational anesthetic agents have been incriminated. While other muscle relaxants (pancuronium, D-tubocurarine) have been suggested as triggers in a few cases, and many other drugs used in anesthetized patients also, convincing evidence is lacking. It has been suggested that stress plays a role in the development of malignant hyperthermia (237).

Dantrolene (238,239) is the agent of choice for treatment of malignant hyperthermia and greatly reduces the mortality to under 10% if given in time (240) together with general supportive measures. Dantrolene itself has adverse effects that are mostly minor in nature, such as nausea and vomiting, when it is used acutely. However, a report has suggested that it may have contributed to uterine atony, with resulting excessive hemorrhage when given prophylactically after a cesarean section (241), and muscle weakness associated with its oral prophylactic use in a patient with compromised respiratory function is reported to have exacerbated postoperative respiratory depression to such an extent that artificial ventilation

was required (SEDA-14, 114) (242). The combination with calcium channel blockers, such as verapamil, may result in severe cardiovascular depression and hyperkalemia (SEDA-12, 113) (243,244), so that extreme care is required.

Second-Generation Effects

Pregnancy

Maternal doses of suxamethonium up to 200 mg have been reported as not resulting in detectable concentrations in neonates. Very large bolus doses (300–500 mg) have produced umbilical vein concentrations up to 2 micrograms/ml, but the neonates showed no adverse effects (245,246). Extreme reduction in plasma cholinesterase activity, either caused by organophosphorus poisoning (247) or genetically determined (SEDA-15, 123) (248,249), has resulted in weakness and respiratory depression in neonates after normal or small (247) maternal doses.

Susceptibility Factors

Genetic factors

Plasma cholinesterase deficiency can be hereditary or acquired. The hereditary form is believed to account for two-thirds of suxamethonium-sensitive patients. Genetically determined plasma cholinesterase variants hydrolyse suxamethonium much more slowly. About 96% of the population are homozygotes for the normal "typical" gene, one in 25 are heterozygotes ("typical"/ "atypical") and have a slightly prolonged (about 2–4 times normal) response to suxamethonium, and one in 2000–3000 are homozygotes for the "atypical" gene and have a markedly prolonged response (2–3 hours). The "silent" gene is much rarer and homozygotes (about 0.0006% of the population) have virtually no plasma cholinesterase activity; in them complete paralysis after suxamethonium lasts many hours.

Acquired plasma cholinesterase deficiency is clinically less important, since paralysis from suxamethonium seldom lasts for more than 20–30 minutes. However, this can be avoided by not using suxamethonium in patients known to be at risk. Clinically important prolongation of suxamethonium-paralysis is only to be expected, with the exception of some drug-induced effects, in patients with more than one cause for a reduction in pseudocholinesterase activity. In malnutrition and liver disease (250,251) the synthesis of plasma cholinesterase in the liver is reduced. Neonates have about 50% of normal adult plasma cholinesterase activity. In pregnancy there is a rapid fall in plasma cholinesterase activity of about 25% in the first trimester, which only returns to normal some 6–8 weeks postpartum (252–254). Occasionally much larger falls occur. The lowest average values have been reported during the first week of the puerperium (SEDA-5, 135) (255,256). Similar changes have been reported in gestational trophoblastic disease (hydatidiform mole) (257). Cancer is sometimes associated with lower plasma cholinesterase activity (SEDA-5, 136) (258). There is also a report of multiple esterase deficiencies in Hodgkin's disease (259). Plasma cholinesterase activity has also been reported to be reduced by up to 70–80% in patients with renal disease and burns. Plasmapheresis (SEDA-5, 135) (260,261) removes cholinesterase, along with other proteins, from the plasma.

Numerous drugs also reduce plasma cholinesterase synthesis or activity, for example estrogens, glucocorticoids, phenelzine, organophosphorus compounds (such as ecothiopate eye-drops, insecticides), carbamates (insecticides, bambuterol), cytotoxic drugs, metoclopramide, the ester-type local anesthetic drugs, and pancuronium. Anticholinesterases also prolong the action of suxamethonium. Several reviews are recommended for detailed information about plasma cholinesterase and its relevance in anesthetic practice (96,262–264).

Hepatic disease

In severe liver dysfunction the synthesis of plasma cholinesterase may be reduced to such an extent that the action of suxamethonium can be prolonged (SED-8, 282). This is usually not more than 2 or 3 times the normal duration.

Other features of the patient

Suxamethonium-induced fasciculation or increased muscle tone can be dangerous in patients with fractures or dislocations (especially vertebral, when the drug is relatively contraindicated), in patients with open-eye injuries or after the eyeball is opened surgically, when an increase in abdominal pressure must be avoided (pheochromocytoma, aortic aneurysm, full stomach, ileus), and in patients in whom a rise in arterial pressure may be catastrophic (cerebral aneurysm, raised intracranial pressure). Prolonged paralysis, occasionally lasting hours, is a risk if the patient is, or has been, taking certain drugs.

Pregnancy

In pregnancy the risk of regurgitation has to be weighed against the advantage of rapid intubation. The use of "precurarization" with small doses of non-depolarizing drugs may reduce the intensity of the fasciculation, but is by no means reliable. If possible, relaxation is better achieved by using a non-depolarizing agent alone.

Muscle disorders

Patients with muscle disorders (dystrophia myotonica, myotonia congenita, myasthenia gravis, and hyperkalemic periodic paralysis) tend to react unpredictably to suxamethonium. In myasthenia gravis, small doses of suxamethonium may be tried and the resulting effect monitored. In the other diseases listed non-depolarizers, cautiously used, are preferable. Cardiac arrest has been reported in patients with pseudohypertrophic muscular dystrophy (Duchenne type) and excessive muscle damage may be produced by suxamethonium in this condition.

Myasthenic syndromes

In myasthenia gravis responses to suxamethonium are unpredictable (265–268). Resistance has been reported and the development of a phase II block can occur more readily, occasionally leading to prolonged paralysis. The measures used to treat the condition, for example plasmapheresis or anticholinesterases, further complicate the picture. Patients with the Eaton–Lambert syndrome are very sensitive to all relaxants.

Asthma or allergic reactions

In patients with asthma or a history of previous allergy, suxamethonium should be used with caution, in view of its potential for causing allergic reactions and bronchospasm. When a patient or a relative has had a previous adverse reaction to an anesthetic, the possibilities of an atypical cholinesterase genotype or malignant hyperthermia should also be considered. Patients with certain musculoskeletal and developmental abnormalities, such as a tendency to joint dislocations, squint, ptosis, hernias, some forms of cryptorchidism, pectus excavatum, kyphosis, foot deformities, and myopathic features, and also those who have reacted to a previous injection of suxamethonium with generalized muscle rigidity or masseter spasm, may be more prone to malignant hyperthermia. Dantrolene should be available to every area where anesthetic agents are used.

Patients at risk of aspiration

The choice of muscle relaxants for rapid sequence induction of anesthesia in patients at risk of aspiration has been controversial for many years. Suxamethonium has been used for decades, because it has a fast onset and a short duration of action, although it can have severe adverse effects. Alternatives have been suggested, all of which have their own pros and cons, but suxamethonium has withstood the test of time and is still widely used. On this background, the use of rocuronium versus suxamethonium has been subjected to a Cochrane review, in which 40 studies addressing the issue were identified, 26 of which were combined for analysis (269). For rocuronium, the relative risk of excellent intubating conditions was 0.87 (95% CI = 0.81, 0.94) compared with suxamethonium. In a subgroup of patients who had been given propofol as an induction agent, there was no difference between rocuronium and suxamethonium. The reviewers concluded that overall suxamethonium creates excellent intubation conditions more reliably than rocuronium and should still be used as a first-line muscle relaxant for rapid sequence intubation. Rocuronium, when used with propofol, reliably created excellent intubation conditions and was consequently suggested as a second-line alternative to suxamethonium. In addition, some have suggested that intubating under deep anesthesia without a neuromuscular blocker is an acceptable third-line alternative if neither suxamethonium nor rocuronium is considered appropriate. To allow rapid-sequence intubation of the trachea without a muscle relaxant, adequate doses of propofol (2.0–2.5 mg/kg) or etomidate (0.3 mg/kg) and a fast-onset opioid, such as alfentanil (50 micrograms/kg) or remifentanil (4 micrograms/kg) are required (270–275).

Drug–Drug Interactions

Antidysrhythmic drugs

Quinidine potentiates not only non-depolarizing muscle relaxants but also depolarizing drugs (276).

Verapamil can potentiate the block produced by both types of neuromuscular blocking agent (277).

Beta-blockers can prolong and possibly exaggerate the rise in serum potassium resulting from the injection of suxamethonium (SEDA-10, 108) (SEDA-11, 122) (175,176).

Aprotinin (Trasylol)

Aprotinin (Trasylol) slightly reduces plasma cholinesterase activity and would only be expected to prolong the action of suxamethonium in combination with other factors. However, re-paralysis has been reported when this agent was used after operations during which suxamethonium had been given alone or in combination with normal doses of D-tubocurarine (278).

Bambuterol

Bambuterol, a beta$_2$-adrenoceptor agonist that is used to relieve bronchospasm, approximately doubles the duration of action of suxamethonium (SEDA-14, 114) (279). Plasma cholinesterase activity was reduced significantly even 10–12.5 hours after a single dose of 30 mg had been given to patients. The interaction is due to the binding of carbamate groups to plasma cholinesterase.

Cardiac glycosides

Cardiac glycosides and suxamethonium can interact, resulting in an increased risk of dysrhythmias (280), perhaps through alterations in intracellular calcium (22). In 24 patients with ischemic heart disease taking digoxin who underwent abdominal surgery ventricular extra beats with bigemini or severe bradycardia were recorded in two patients and episodes of torsade de pointes occurred in two others during endotracheal intubation (281). The authors suggested that endotracheal intubation in digitalized patients should be performed without suxamethonium. However, considering the frequency with which digitalized patients receive suxamethonium and the paucity of reports of clinical problems, this interaction is probably of minor importance.

Cytotoxic and immunosuppressive drugs

Nitrogen mustard and related alkylating agents, such as cyclophosphamide, chlorambucil, triethylmelamine, and thiophosphoramide, prolong the action of suxamethonium (282,283). Plasma cholinesterase activity is reduced, possibly by alkylation of the enzyme. It has been suggested that azathioprine may potentiate suxamethonium by inhibition of phosphodiesterase activity (SEDA-4, 87) (284).

Donepezil

Donepezil acts primarily as a reversible inhibitor of acetylcholinesterase with a half-life of over 70 hours. Prolonged paralysis lasting several hours and requiring postoperative mechanical ventilation in the intensive care unit has been reported after the use of suxamethonium in a patient taking long-term donepezil (285).

- An 85-year-old woman with a history of mild Alzheimer's disease and hypertension underwent abdominal hysterectomy. Anesthesia was induced with suxamethonium 100 mg and 40 minutes later pancuronium 2 mg. After 2 hours, when surgery was finished, train-of-four stimulation elicited three twitches, and neostigmine 5 mg plus glycopyrrolate 1 mg was given to reverse neuromuscular block. She was subsequently able to follow commands and was breathing adequately; four twitches were observed during train-of-four stimulation. Several minutes after extubation she became apneic and had to be reintubated. Further neostigmine 1 mg was given, but neuromuscular block persisted without any response to peripheral nerve stimulation. In a blood sample taken 60 minutes after the second dose of neostigmine plasma cholinesterase activity was 2.1 (reference range 7.1–19) U/ml. The dibucaine number was 45 (reference range 81–87)%, and the fluoride number was 84 (44–54)%.

The authors of this report subsequently tested the effect of donepezil on plasma cholinesterase activity in vitro. Supratherapeutic concentrations (0.02 mg/ml) reduced plasma cholinesterase activity to 53% of baseline. Dibucaine and fluoride numbers were not affected by neostigmine or donepezil. Others have shown previously that therapeutic doses of donepezil inhibit acetylcholinesterase by 64% (286). Prolonged paralysis in this case may have been due to the combined effects of atypical plasma cholinesterase and additional inhibition of plasma cholinesterase activity by donepezil. Unfortunately, preoperative plasma cholinesterase activity was not known and low cholinesterase activity was detected under the influence of neostigmine, which inhibits both plasma cholinesterase and acetylcholinesterase. Because a very high dose of neostigmine resulted in intensification rather than reversal of neuromuscular block, overdose of neostigmine may have caused paradoxical neuromuscular block (287). Hypothetically, paradoxical block is a combination of desensitization and open channel block (SED-13, 298). So the additional dose of neostigmine should have been omitted. In addition, an excess of acetylcholine at the end-plate might have been the result of combined inhibition of acetylcholinesterase by both donepezil and neostigmine. Until more is known, neostigmine and other cholinesterase inhibitors should be used with caution in patients taking donepezil.

- A 72-year-old woman with a symptomatic hiatus hernia, osteoarthritis, and Alzheimer's disease was taking fluoxetine 20 mg/day, donepezil hydrochloride 10 mg/day, nimesulide 12.5 mg/day, and omeprazole 20 mg/day (288). There still was no twitch response to peripheral nerve stimulation 20 minutes after rapid-sequence induction of anesthesia with propofol 2.5 mg/kg and suxamethonium 1 mg/kg. She then gradually developed a weak twitch response, and 50 minutes after induction of anesthesia four twitches with a fade were elicited by train-of-four stimulation. No additional medication was given and after the end of the procedure 10 minutes later she was extubated uneventfully. She refused further blood testing and so her plasma cholinesterase activity at that time is not known. However, her anesthetic notes from a previous operation did not reveal any problems with prolonged paralysis after suxamethonium.

It is not proven that donepezil was the cause of the prolonged duration of action of suxamethonium in this case. However, a case with some similarities has been reported before (285). In addition, there has been another report linking donepezil therapy to both prolonged duration of action of suxamethonium and reduced sensitivity to atracurium (289). Recovery of neuromuscular function should therefore be monitored when suxamethonium is given to patients taking donepezil. The withdrawal of donepezil 2–3 weeks before an operation cannot be supported, because this might have adverse effects on cognitive function. The issue has been highlighted in a recent letter, and the author concluded that "a brief prolongation of muscle relaxation is very rarely a problem (although its mismanagement may be)" (290).

Ecothiopate

Ecothiopate eye-drops, used in the treatment of glaucoma, prolong the action of suxamethonium considerably (291,292). Ecothiopate is a long-acting anticholinesterase that inhibits the activity of both acetylcholinesterase and plasma cholinesterase. Plasma cholinesterase activity may be reduced to 5% or less and on withdrawal requires 1–2 months for recovery to normal values (293,294). The prolonged anticholinesterase effect is due to conversion of the enzyme to its stable phosphoryl derivative. If a patient has used ecothiopate eye-drops in the previous 2 months or so, suxamethonium should not be given, unless normal plasma cholinesterase activity can be demonstrated. Various organophosphorus insecticides, such as parathion and malathion, may also result in prolonged paralysis after suxamethonium due to reduced free cholinesterase activity (247,295), produced in a similar manner to that in the case of ecothiopate.

Estrogens and estrogen-containing contraceptives

Estrogens and estrogen-containing contraceptives prolong the action of suxamethonium. Plasma cholinesterase activity is reduced, possibly by estrogenic inhibition of the hepatic synthesis of plasma cholinesterase, and its isozymes are modified (262,296,297). Diethylstilbestrol, included in this group, is reported to have caused paralysis for 3 hours in a patient with other aggravating factors (SEDA-4, 89) (298). One would, however, expect little prolongation of suxamethonium paralysis since the decrease in plasma cholinesterase activity (after contraceptives, at least) averages only about 20%. Prednisone, cortisol, and dexamethasone also reduce plasma cholinesterase activity to a mild or moderate degree (SEDA-15, 122) (299–301).

General anesthetics

When mixed in solution, thiopental will hydrolyse suxamethonium, owing to a pH effect. Ketamine may prolong the action of suxamethonium slightly (302,303); a phase II block might be prolonged more significantly (303), although there is no clinical experience reported. Decreased presynaptic acetylcholine synthesis or release has been postulated as the mechanism (304). In another study there was no significant shift in the dose–response curve for suxamethonium with ketamine (305).

Inhalational agents potentiate muscle relaxants, which is of more clinical importance with regard to non-depolarizing agents. Tachyphylaxis and phase II block develop earlier and after smaller total doses of suxamethonium when volatile agents such as halothane, enflurane, or isoflurane (306,307) are used instead of balanced anesthesia. Halothane can increase the incidence of cardiac dysrhythmias, especially bradycardia and nodal rhythm, after suxamethonium. Atropine and glycopyrrolate, particularly when given intravenously just before, afford some protection (SEDA-5, 136) (308).

Lithium carbonate

Lithium carbonate delays the onset and prolongs the action of depolarizing relaxants (309,310). The principal mechanism of action is disputed. Factors suggested have been the development of dual block, reduced sensitivity of the end-plate for suxamethonium, diminished synthesis or release of acetylcholine, and plasma cholinesterase inhibition (310–312). The clinical importance is also disputed.

Local anesthetics

Procaine and cocaine are esters that are hydrolysed by plasma cholinesterase and can therefore competitively enhance the action of suxamethonium (313). Chloroprocaine may have a similar action. Lidocaine also interacts, although the mechanism is not clear unless very high doses are used (314).

Magnesium sulfate

Magnesium sulfate is used mostly in the treatment of toxemia of pregnancy. Serum magnesium concentrations may be raised and, as magnesium inhibits the release of acetylcholine and reduces the sensitivity of the postjunctional membrane, the action of non-depolarizing agents will be prolonged. It is not so clear, however, why the action of suxamethonium is also prolonged (315–318). Suxamethonium-induced fasciculation are reportedly prevented (SEDA-5, 135) (319). It has been suggested that the administration of intravenous magnesium sulfate should be stopped 20–30 minutes before muscle relaxants are given. Monitoring with a nerve stimulator is advisable.

Metoclopramide

Metoclopramide inhibits the activity of plasma cholinesterase and can prolong the action of suxamethonium (SEDA-14, 115) (320–322).

Neostigmine

Neostigmine inhibits both plasma cholinesterase and acetylcholinesterase, so that if any suxamethonium is still circulating, its action will be prolonged (by about a factor of two). This may present problems when neostigmine is administered to antagonize phase II block (323) (in which hypothetical desensitization block and open channel block elements may also be intensified) or shortly after suxamethonium is given. In renal insufficiency both neostigmine and pyridostigmine can cause prolongation (by 1–2 hours) of the action of suxamethonium given several hours after renal transplant operations.

Non-depolarizing muscle relaxants

Non-depolarizing muscle relaxants and suxamethonium are mutually antagonistic. These agents are often given in small non-paralysing doses before suxamethonium to reduce fasciculation and other adverse effects. Gallamine is slightly more effective than D-tubocurarine, and both are more effective than pancuronium. This precurarization tends to prolong the onset of action of (probably by direct antagonism) and to shorten (D-tubocurarine) or lengthen (pancuronium) its duration of action (324). The latter effect may well be due to inhibition of plasma cholinesterase by pancuronium. When compared with pancuronium, pretreatment with either atracurium or vecuronium was associated with a significantly shorter time to 90% twitch recovery after a standard dose of suxamethonium (325). When non-depolarizing agents are given after suxamethonium, even more than 30 minutes later, their action is considerably potentiated and prolonged (89,326,327). This effect (and also the production of a phase II block when suxamethonium is used alone in high or frequently repeated doses) may be the result of inhibition of transmitter release through a prejunctional action of suxamethonium (328). Suxamethonium given some time after a paralysing dose of a non-depolarizing agent (for example for peritoneal closure) produces varying effects depending on the depth of residual curarization and on the dosage of suxamethonium (SEDA-21, 141) (329–331). As it is uncertain what type of block results, this practice cannot be recommended, although few problems with subsequent reversal have been reported.

Phenelzine

Phenelzine, a monoamine oxidase inhibitor, has been reported to cause significant prolongation of suxamethonium paralysis due to depressed plasma cholinesterase levels (to about 10% of normal). Recovery of plasma cholinesterase activity took 2 weeks (332).

Tacrine (tetrahydroaminoacridine) and hexafluorenium

Tacrine (tetrahydroaminoacridine) and hexafluorenium, used sometimes to potentiate and prolong the action of suxamethonium (333,334), inhibit plasma cholinesterase. Hexafluorenium also inhibits acetylcholinesterase and has a weak neuromuscular blocking action of the non-depolarizing type; a phase II block develops fairly rapidly when repeated injections of even small doses (0.2–0.3 mg/kg) of suxamethonium are given in combination with hexafluorenium (335). Fasciculation is reportedly reduced and hyperkalemia prevented (336), as is the increase in intraocular pressure (337), when hexafluorenium is given before suxamethonium. Because of a lack of consistency of successful results from various investigators, this method is not recommended for patients who are especially at risk from hyperkalemia or increased intraocular pressure. Simultaneous injection of hexafluorenium and suxamethonium can cause severe bronchospasm.

Trimetaphan

Trimetaphan can double the duration of suxamethonium block (338–340). The mechanism is not clear, but may be a competitive effect at the neuromuscular junction. Blockade of end-plate ionic channels has also been suggested (341).

References

1. Dal Santo G. Kinetics of distribution of radioactive labeled muscle relaxants. 3. Investigations with ^{14}C-succinyldicholine and ^{14}C-succinylmonocholine during controlled conditions Anesthesiology 1968;29(3):435–43.
2. DeCook TH, Goudsouzian NG. Tachyphylaxis and phase II block development during infusion of succinylcholine in children. Anesth Analg 1980;59(9):639–43.
3. Ramsey FM, Lebowitz PW, Savarese JJ, Ali HH. Clinical characteristics of long-term succinylcholine neuromuscular blockade during balanced anesthesia. Anesth Analg 1980;59(2):110–16.
4. Baraka A. Myasthenic response to muscle relaxants in von Recklinghausen's disease. Br J Anaesth 1974;46(9):701–3.
5. Heard SO, Kaplan RF. Neuromuscular blockade in a patient with nemaline myopathy. Anesthesiology 1983;59(6):588–90.
6. Sorensen M, Engbaek J, Viby-Mogensen J, Guldager H, Molke Jensen F. Bradycardia and cardiac asystole following a single injection of suxamethonium. Acta Anaesthesiol Scand 1984;28(2):232–5.
7. Linter SP, Thomas PR, Withington PS, Hall MG. Suxamethonium associated hypertonicity and cardiac arrest in unsuspected pseudohypertrophic muscular dystrophy. Br J Anaesth 1982;54(12):1331–2.
8. Genever EE. Suxamethonium-induced cardiac arrest in unsuspected pseudohypertrophic muscular dystrophy. Case report. Br J Anaesth 1971;43(10):984–6.
9. Henderson WA. Succinylcholine-induced cardiac arrest in unsuspected Duchenne muscular dystrophy. Can Anaesth Soc J 1984;31(4):444–6.
10. Solares G, Herranz JL, Sanz MD. Suxamethonium-induced cardiac arrest as an initial manifestation of Duchenne muscular dystrophy. Br J Anaesth 1986;58(5):576.
11. Sullivan M, Thompson WK, Hill GD. Succinylcholine-induced cardiac arrest in children with undiagnosed myopathy. Can J Anaesth 1994;41(6):497–501.
12. Bush GH. Suxamethonium-associated hypertonicity and cardiac arrest in unsuspected pseudohypertrophic muscular dystrophy. Br J Anaesth 1983;55(9):923.
13. Schaer H, Steinmann B, Jerusalem S, Maier C. Rhabdomyolysis induced by anaesthesia with intraoperative cardiac arrest. Br J Anaesth 1977;49(5):495–9.
14. Seay AR, Ziter FA, Thompson JA. Cardiac arrest during induction of anesthesia in Duchenne muscular dystrophy. J Pediatr 1978;93(1):88–90.
15. Parker SF, Bailey A, Drake AF. Infant hyperkalemic arrest after succinylcholine. Anesth Analg 1995;80(1):206–7.
16. Schulte-Sasse U, Eberlein HJ, Schmucker I, Underwood D, Wolbert R. Sollte die verwendung von succinylcholin in der kinderanästhesie neu uberdacht werden? [Should the use of succinylcholine in pediatric anesthesia be re-evaluated?] Anaesthesiol Reanim 1993;18(1):13–19.
17. Farrell PT. Anaesthesia-induced rhabdomyolysis causing cardiac arrest: case report and review of anaesthesia and the dystrophinopathies. Anaesth Intensive Care 1994;22(5):597–601.

18. Larach MG, Rosenberg H, Gronert GA, Allen GC. Hyperkalemic cardiac arrest during anesthesia in infants and children with occult myopathies. Clin Pediatr (Phila) 1997;36(1):9–16.

19. Jackson MA, Lodwick R, Hutchinson SG. Hyperkalaemic cardiac arrest successfully treated with peritoneal dialysis. BMJ 1996;312(7041):1289–90.

20. Lin JL, Huang CC. Successful initiation of hemodialysis during cardiopulmonary resuscitation due to lethal hyperkalemia. Crit Care Med 1990;18(3):342–3.

21. Lee G, Antognini JF, Gronert GA. Complete recovery after prolonged resuscitation and cardiopulmonary bypass for hyperkalemic cardiac arrest. Anesth Analg 1994;79(1):172–4.

22. Smith RB, Petruscak J. Succinylcholine, digitalis, and hypercalcemia: a case report. Anesth Analg 1972;51(2):202–5.

23. Nigrovic V. Succinylcholine, cholinoceptors and catecholamines: proposed mechanism of early adverse haemodynamic reactions. Can Anaesth Soc J 1984;31(4):382–94.

24. Pace SA, Fuller FP. Out-of-hospital succinylcholine-assisted endotracheal intubation by paramedics. Ann Emerg Med 2000;35(6):568–72.

25. Menegazzi JJ, Wayne MA. Succinylcholine-assisted endotracheal intubation by paramedics. Ann Emerg Med 2001;37(3):360–1.

26. Katz SH, Falk JL. Misplaced endotracheal tubes by paramedics in an urban emergency medical services system. Ann Emerg Med 2001;37(1):32–7.

27. Zink BJ, Snyder HS, Raccio-Robak N. Lack of a hyperkalemic response in emergency department patients receiving succinylcholine. Acad Emerg Med 1995;2(11):974–8.

28. Dronen SC, Merigian KS, Hedges JR, Hoekstra JW, Borron SW. A comparison of blind nasotracheal and succinylcholine-assisted intubation in the poisoned patient. Ann Emerg Med 1987;16(6):650–2.

29. Smith CL, Bush GH. Anaesthesia and progressive muscular dystrophy. Br J Anaesth 1985;57(11):1113–18.

30. Ravindran RS, Klemm JE. Anaphylaxis to succinylcholine in a patient allergic to penicillin. Anesth Analg 1980;59(12):944–5.

31. Cohen S, Liu KH, Marx GF. Upper airway edema — an anaphylactoid reaction to succinylcholine? Anesthesiology 1982;56(6):467–8.

32. O'Sullivan EP, Childs D, Bush GH. Peri-operative dreaming in paediatric patients who receive suxamethonium. Anaesthesia 1988;43(2):104–6.

33. Halldin M, Wahlin A. Effect of succinylcholine on the intraspinal fluid pressure. Acta Anaesthesiol Scand 1959;3:155–61.

34. Marsh ML, Dunlop BJ, Shapiro HM, Gagnon RL, Rockoff MA. Succinylcholine-intracranial pressure effects in neurosurgical patients. Anesth Analg 1980;59:550–1.

35. Kovarik WD, Mayberg TS, Lam AM, Mathisen TL, Winn HR. Succinylcholine does not change intracranial pressure, cerebral blood flow velocity, or the electroencephalogram in patients with neurologic injury. Anesth Analg 1994;78(3):469–73.

36. Clancy M, Halford S, Walls R, Murphy M. In patients with head injuries who undergo rapid sequence intubation using succinylcholine, does pretreatment with a competitive neuromuscular blocking agent improve outcome? A literature review. Emerg Med J 2001;18(5):373–5.

37. Brown MM, Parr MJ, Manara AR. The effect of suxamethonium on intracranial pressure and cerebral perfusion pressure in patients with severe head injuries following blunt trauma. Eur J Anaesthesiol 1996;13(5):474–7.

38. Minton MD, Grosslight K, Stirt JA, Bedford RF. Increases in intracranial pressure from succinylcholine: prevention by prior nondepolarizing blockade. Anesthesiology 1986;65(2):165–9.

39. Stirt JA, Grosslight KR, Bedford RF, Vollmer D. "Defasciculation" with metocurine prevents succinylcholine-induced increases in intracranial pressure. Anesthesiology 1987;67(1):50–3.

40. Standaert FG, Adams JE. The actions of succinylcholine on the mammalian motor nerve terminal. J Pharmacol Exp Ther 1965;149:113–23.

41. Thind GS, Bryson TH. Single dose suxamethonium and muscle pain in pregnancy. Br J Anaesth 1983;55(8):743–5.

42. Coxon JD. Muscle pain after suxamethonium. Br Anaesth 1962;34:750.

43. Paton WD. The effects of muscle relaxants other than muscular relaxation. Anesthesiology 1959;20(4):453–63.

44. Tammisto T, Airaksinen M. Increase of creatine kinase activity in serum as sign of muscular injury caused by intermittently administred suxamethonium during halothane anaesthesia. Br J Anaesth 1966;38(7):510–15.

45. Waters DJ, Mapleson WW. Suxamethonium pains: hypothesis and observation. Anaesthesia 1971;26(2):127–41.

46. Rack PM, Westbury DR. The effects of suxamethonium and acetylcholine on the behaviour of cat muscle spindles during dynamics stretching, and during fusimotor stimulation. J Physiol 1966;186(3):698–713.

47. Mayrhofer O. Die Wirksamkeit von d-Tubocurarin zur Verhütung der Muskelschmerzen nach Succinylcholin. [The efficacy of d-tubocurarine in the prevention of muscle pain after succinylcholine.] Anaesthesist 1959;8:313.

48. Konig W. Über Beschwerden nach Anwendung von Succinylcholin. Anaesthesist 1956;5:50.

49. Kaniaris P, Galanopoulou T, Varonos D. Effects of succinylcholine on plasma 5-HT levels. Anesth Analg 1973;52(3):425–7.

50. Collier CB. Suxamethonium pains and early electrolyte changes. Anaesthesia 1978;33(5):454–61.

51. Naguib M, Farag H, Magbagbeola JA. Effect of pre-treatment with lysine acetyl salicylate on suxamethonium-induced myalgia. Br J Anaesth 1987;59(5):606–10.

52. McLoughlin C, Nesbitt GA, Howe JP. Suxamethonium induced myalgia and the effect of pre-operative administration of oral aspirin. A comparison with a standard treatment and an untreated group. Anaesthesia 1988;43(7):565–7.

53. Cullen DJ. The effect of pretreatment with nondepolarizing muscle relaxants on the neuromuscular blocking action of succinylcholine. Anesthesiology 1971;35(6):572–8.

54. Jansen EC, Hansen PH. Objective measurement of succinylcholine-induced fasciculations and the effect of pretreatment with pancuronium or gallamine. Anesthesiology 1979;51(2):159–60.

55. Blitt CD, Carlson GL, Rolling GD, Hameroff SR, Otto CW. A comparative evaluation of pretreatment with nondepolarizing neuromuscular blockers prior to the administration of succinylcholine. Anesthesiology 1981;55(6):687–9.

56. Erkola O, Salmenpera A, Kuoppamaki R. Five nondepolarizing muscle relaxants in precurarization. Acta Anaesthesiol Scand 1983;27(6):427–32.

57. Raman SK, San WM. Fasciculations, myalgia and biochemical changes following succinylcholine with atracurium and lidocaine pretreatment. Can J Anaesth 1997;44(5 Pt 1):498–502.

58. Fahmy NR, Malek NS, Lappas DG. Diazepam prevents some adverse effects of succinylcholine. Clin Pharmacol Ther 1979;26(3):395–8.

59. Manchikanti L. Diazepam does not prevent succinylcholine-induced fasciculations and myalgia. A

comparative evaluation of the effect of diazepam and D-tubocurarine pretreatments. Acta Anaesthesiol Scand 1984;28(5):523–8.

60. Flewellen EH, Bodensteiner JB. Anesthetic experience in a patient with hyperkalemic periodic paralysis. Anesthesiol Rev 1980;7:44.

61. Brim VD. Denervation supersensitivity: the response to depolarizing muscle relaxants. Br J Anaesth 1973;45(2):222–6.

62. Kelly EP. A rise in serum potassium after suxamethonium following brachial plexus injury. Anaesthesia 1982;37(6):694–5.

63. Orndahl G, Stenberg K. Myotonic human musculature: stimulation with depolarizing agents. Mechanical registration of the effects of succinyldicholine, succinylmonocholine and decamethonium. Acta Med Scand 1962;172(Suppl 389):3–29.

64. Allen GC, Rosenberg H. Malignant hyperthermia susceptibility in adult patients with masseter muscle rigidity. Can J Anaesth 1990;37(1):31–5.

65. Flewellen EH, Nelson TE. Halothane-succinylcholine induced masseter spasm: indicative of malignant hyperthermia susceptibility? Anesth Analg 1984;63(7):693–7.

66. O'Flynn RP, Shutack JG, Rosenberg H, Fletcher JE. Masseter muscle rigidity and malignant hyperthermia susceptibility in pediatric patients. An update on management and diagnosis. Anesthesiology 1994;80(6):1228–33.

67. Rosenberg H, Fletcher JE. Masseter muscle rigidity and malignant hyperthermia susceptibility. Anesth Analg 1986;65(2):161–4.

68. Gronert GA. Management of patients in whom trismus occurs following succinylcholine. Anesthesiology 1988;68(4):653–5.

69. Van der Spek AF, Fang WB, Ashton-Miller JA, Stohler CS, Carlson DS, Schork MA. The effects of succinylcholine on mouth opening. Anesthesiology 1987;67(4):459–65.

70. Meakin G, Walker RW, Dearlove OR. Myotonic and neuromuscular blocking effects of increased doses of suxamethonium in infants and children. Br J Anaesth 1990;65(6):816–18.

71. Littleford JA, Patel LR, Bose D, Cameron CB, McKillop C. Masseter muscle spasm in children: implications of continuing the triggering anesthetic. Anesth Analg 1991;72(2):151–60.

72. Lazzell VA, Carr AS, Lerman J, Burrows FA, Creighton RE. The incidence of masseter muscle rigidity after succinylcholine in infants and children. Can J Anaesth 1994;41(6):475–9.

73. Leary NP, Ellis FR. Masseteric muscle spasm as a normal response to suxamethonium. Br J Anaesth 1990;64(4):488–92.

74. Ummenhofer WC, Kindler C, Tschaler G, Hampl KF, Drewe J, Urwyler A. Propofol reduces succinylcholine induced increase of masseter muscle tone. Can J Anaesth 1998;45(5 Pt 1):417–23.

75. Jenkins JG. Masseter muscle rigidity after vecuronium. Eur J Anaesthesiol 1999;16(2):137–9.

76. Polta TA, Hanisch EC Jr, Nasser JG, Ramsborg GC, Roelofs RI. Masseter spasm after pancuronium. Anesth Analg 1980;59(7):509–11.

77. Albrecht A, Wedel DJ, Gronert GA. Masseter muscle rigidity and nondepolarizing neuromuscular blocking agents. Mayo Clin Proc 1997;72(4):329–32.

78. Cheung PY, Tyebkhan JM, Peliowski A, Ainsworth W, Robertson CM. Prolonged use of pancuronium bromide and sensorineural hearing loss in childhood survivors of congenital diaphragmatic hernia. J Pediatr 1999;135(2 Pt 1):233–9.

79. Airaksinen MM, Tammisto T. Myoglobinuria after intermittent administration of succinylcholine during halothane anesthesia. Clin Pharmacol Ther 1966;7(5):583–7.

80. Plotz J, Braun J. Serummyoglobin nach Wiederholungsgaben von Succinylcholin und der Einfluss von Dantrolen. [Serum myoglobin following intermittent administration of succinylcholine and the effect of dantrolene. Clinical studies of children in halothane anesthesia.] Anaesthesist 1985;34(10):513–15.

81. Plotz J. Nebenwirkungen von Succinylcholin auf die Skelettmuskulatur in Halothannarkose bei Kindern: Prophylaxe mit Diallylnortoxiferin, 'self-taming' und Dantrolen. Therapiewoche 1984;34:3168.

82. Harrington JF, Ford DJ, Striker TW. Myoglobinemia after succinylcholine in children undergoing halothane and non-halothane anesthesia. Anesthesiology 1984;61:A431.

83. Hool GJ, Lawrence PJ, Sivaneswaran N. Acute rhabdomyolytic renal failure due to suxamethonium. Anaesth Intensive Care 1984;12(4):360–4.

84. McKishnie JD, Muir JM, Girvan DP. Anaesthesia-induced rhabdomyolysis—a case report. Can Anaesth Soc J 1983;30(3 Pt 1):295–8.

85. Pedrozzi NE, Ramelli GP, Tomasetti R, Nobile-Buetti L, Bianchetti MG. Rhabdomyolysis and anesthesia: a report of two cases and review of the literature. Pediatr Neurol 1996;15(3):254–7.

86. Bhave CG, Gadre KC, Gharpure BS. Myoglobinuria following the use of succinylcholine. J Postgrad Med 1993;39(3):157–9.

87. Gokhale YA, Marathe P, Patil RD, Prasar S, Kamble P, Hase NK, Agrawal MB, Deshmukh SN, Menon PS. Rhabdomyolysis and acute renal failure following a single dose of succinylcholine. J Assoc Physicians India 1991;39(12):968–70.

88. Lee SC, Abe T, Sato T. Rhabdomyolysis and acute renal failure following use of succinylcholine and enflurane: report of a case. J Oral Maxillofac Surg 1987;45(9):789–92.

89. Ryan JF, Kagen LJ, Hyman AI. Myoglobinemia after a single dose of succinylcholine. N Engl J Med 1971;285(15):824–7.

90. Gibbs JM. A case of rhabdomyolysis associated with suxamethonium. Anaesth Intensive Care 1978;6(2):141–5.

91. Miyamoto K, Sasaki M, Okudo T, et al. Four cases suspected of malignant hyperthermia induced by halothane and succinylcholine. Hiroshima J Anesth 1983;18:157.

92. Lewandowski KB. Strabismus as a possible sign of subclinical muscular dystrophy predisposing to rhabdomyolysis and myoglobinuria: a study of an affected family. Can Anaesth Soc J 1982;29(4):372–6.

93. Larsen UT, Juhl B, Hein-Sorensen O, de Fine Olivarius B. Complications during anaesthesia in patients with Duchenne's muscular dystrophy (a retrospective study) Can J Anaesth 1989;36(4):418–22.

94. Wang JM, Stanley TH. Duchenne muscular dystrophy and malignant hyperthermia—two case reports. Can Anaesth Soc J 1986;33(4):492–7.

95. Steegmuller H. On the geographical distribution of pseudo-cholinesterase variants. Humangenetik 1975;26(3):167–85.

96. Pantuck EJ, Pantuck CB. Cholinesterases and anticholinesterases. In: Katz RL, editor. Muscle Relaxants. Amsterdam: Excerpta Medica, 1975:155.

97. Viby-Mogensen J. Correlation of succinylcholine duration of action with plasma cholinesterase activity in subjects with the genotypically normal enzyme. Anesthesiology 1980;53(6):517–20.

98. Yamashita M, Matsuki A, Oyama T. Anaesthetic considerations on von Recklinghausen's disease (multiple neurofibromatosis). Abnormal response to muscle relaxants. Anaesthesist 1977;26(6):317–18.

99. Hofmann H, Holzer H. Die Wirkung von Muskelrelaxanzien auf den intraokularen Druck. [Effect

of muscle relaxants on the intraocular pressure.] Klin Monatsbl Augenheilkd 1953;123(1):1–16.

100. Bowen DJ, McGrand JC, Palmer RJ. Intraocular pressures after suxamethonium and endotracheal intubation in patients pretreated with pancuronium. Br J Anaesth 1976;48(12):1201–5.

101. Bowen DJ, McGrand JC, Hamilton AG. Intraocular pressure after suxamethonium and endotracheal intubation. The effect of pre-treatment with tubocurarine or gallamine. Anaesthesia 1978;33(6):518–22.

102. Cook JH. The effect of suxamethonium on intraocular pressure. Anaesthesia 1981;36(4):359–65.

103. Craythorne NW, Rottenstein HS, Dripps RD. The effect of succinylcholine on intraocular pressure in adults, infants and children during general anesthesia. Anesthesiology 1960;21:59–63.

104. Dear GD, Hammerton M, Hatch DJ, Taylor D. Anaesthesia and intra-ocular pressure in young children. A study of three different techniques of anaesthesia. Anaesthesia 1987;42(3):259–65.

105. Feneck RO, Cook JH. Failure of diazepam to prevent the suxamethonium-induced rise in intra-ocular pressure. Anaesthesia 1983;38(2):120–7.

106. Goldsmith E. An evaluation of succinylcholine and gallamine as muscle relaxants in relation to intraocular tension. Anesth Analg 1967;46(5):557–61.

107. Grover VK, Lata K, Sharma S, Kaushik S, Gupta A. Efficacy of lignocaine in the suppression of the intra-ocular pressure response to suxamethonium and tracheal intubation. Anaesthesia 1989;44(1):22–5.

108. Lincoff HA, Ellis CH, DeVoe AG, DeBeer EJ, Impastato DJ, Berg S, Orkin L, Magda H. The effect of succinylcholine on intraocular pressure. Am J Ophthalmol 1955;40(4):501–10.

109. Pandey K, Badola RP, Kumar S. Time course of intra-ocular hypertension produced by suxamethonium. Br J Anaesth 1972;44(2):191–6.

110. Robertson GS, Gibson PF. Suxamethonium and intra-ocular pressure. Anaesthesia 1968;23(3):342–9.

111. Sarmany BJ. Über die Wirkung von verschiedenen Narkotica auf den intraoculären Druck. [On the effect of various narcotics on intraocular pressure.] Anaesthesist 1967;16(10):296–8.

112. Schwartz H, DeRoetth A. Effect of succinylcholine on intraocular pressure in human. Anesthesiology 1958;19:112–13.

113. Taylor TH, Mulcahy M, Nightingale DA. Suxamethonium chloride in intraocular surgery. Br J Anaesth 1968;40(2):113–18.

114. Warner LO, Bremer DL, Davidson PJ, Rogers GL, Beach TP. Effects of lidocaine, succinylcholine, and tracheal intubation on intraocular pressure in children anesthetized with halothane–nitrous oxide. Anesth Analg 1989;69(5):687–90.

115. Kornblueth W, Jampolsky A, Tamler E, Marg E. Contraction of the oculorotary muscles and intraocular pressure. A tonographic and electromyographic study of the effect of edrophonium chloride (Tensilon) and succinylcholine (Anectine) on the intraocular pressure. Am J Ophthalmol 1960;49:1381–7.

116. Kelly RE, Dinner M, Turner LS, Haik B, Abramson DH, Daines P. Succinylcholine increases intraocular pressure in the human eye with the extraocular muscles detached. Anesthesiology 1993;79(5):948–52.

117. Bjork A, Halldin M, Wahlin A. Enophthalmus elicited by succinylcholine; some observations on the effect of succinylcholine and noradrenaline on the intraorbital muscles studied on man experimental animals. Acta Anaesthesiol Scand 1957;1(1–2):41–53.

118. Abramson DH. Anterior chamber and lens thickness changes induced by succinylcholine. Arch Ophthalmol 1971;86(6):643–7.

119. Halldin M, Wahlin A, Koch T. Observations of the conjunctival vessels under the influence of succinylcholine with intravenous anaesthesia. Acta Anaesthesiol Scand 1959;3:163–71.

120. Adams AK, Barnett KC. Anaesthesia and intraocular pressure. Anaesthesia 1966;21(2):202–10.

121. Robinson R, White M, McCann P, Magner J, Eustace P. Effect of anaesthesia on intraocular blood flow. Br J Ophthalmol 1991;75(2):92–3.

122. Miller RD, Way WL, Hickey RF. Inhibition of succinylcholine-induced increased intraocular pressure by nondepolarizing muscle relaxants. Anesthesiology 1968;29(1):123–6.

123. Meyers EF, Krupin T, Johnson M, Zink H. Failure of nondepolarizing neuromuscular blockers to inhibit succinylcholine-induced increased intraocular pressure, a controlled study. Anesthesiology 1978;48(2):149–51.

124. Verma RS. "Self-taming" of succinylcholine-induced fasciculations and intraocular pressure. Anesthesiology 1979;50(3):245–7.

125. Meyers EF, Singer P, Otto A. A controlled study of the effect of succinylcholine self-taming on intraocular pressure. Anesthesiology 1980;53(1):72–4.

126. Cunningham AJ, Albert O, Cameron J, Watson AG. The effect of intravenous diazepam on rise of intraocular pressure following succinylcholine. Can Anaesth Soc J 1981;28(6):591–6.

127. Fjeldborg P, Hecht PS, Busted N, Nissen AB. The effect of diazepam pretreatment on the succinylcholine-induced rise in intraocular pressure. Acta Anaesthesiol Scand 1985;29(4):415–17.

128. Mahajan RP, Grover VK, Munjal VP, Singh H. Double-blind comparison of lidocaine, tubocurarine and diazepam pretreatment in modifying intraocular pressure increases. Can J Anaesth 1987;34(1):41–5.

129. Murphy DF, Eustace P, Unwin A, Magner JB. Intravenous lignocaine pretreatment to prevent intraocular pressure rise following suxamethonium and tracheal intubation. Br J Ophthalmol 1986;70(8):596–8.

130. Mahajan RP, Grover VK, Sharma SL, Singh H. Intranasal nitroglycerin and intraocular pressure during general anesthesia. Anesth Analg 1988;67(7):631–6.

131. Indu B, Batra YK, Puri GD, Singh H. Nifedipine attenuates the intraocular pressure response to intubation following succinylcholine. Can J Anaesth 1989;36(3 Pt 1):269–72.

132. Grover VK, Kakkar RK, Grewal S, Sharma S, Gupta A. Efficacy of topical timolol to prevent intraocular pressor response to suxamethonium and tracheal intubation. J Anaesth Clin Pharmacol 1996;12:107–11.

133. Edmondson L, Lindsay SL, Lanigan LP, Woods M, Chew HE. Intra-ocular pressure changes during rapid sequence induction of anaesthesia. A comparison between thiopentone and suxamethonium and thiopentone and atracurium. Anaesthesia 1988;43(12):1005–10.

134. Mirakhur RK, Shepherd WF, Darrah WC. Propofol or thiopentone: effects on intraocular pressure associated with induction of anaesthesia and tracheal intubation (facilitated with suxamethonium). Br J Anaesth 1987;59(4):431–6.

135. Polarz H, Bohrer H, Fleischer F, Huster T, Bauer H, Wolfrum J. Effects of thiopentone/suxamethonium on intraocular pressure after pretreatment with alfentanil. Eur J Clin Pharmacol 1992;43(3):311–13.

136. Sweeney J, Underhill S, Dowd T, Mostafa SM. Modification by fentanyl and alfentanil of the intraocular

pressure response to suxamethonium and tracheal intubation. Br J Anaesth 1989;63(6):688–91.

137. Zimmerman AA, Funk KJ, Tidwell JL. Propofol and alfentanil prevent the increase in intraocular pressure caused by succinylcholine and endotracheal intubation during a rapid sequence induction of anesthesia. Anesth Analg 1996;83(4):814–17.

138. Alexander R, Hill R, Lipham WJ, Weatherwax KJ, el-Moalem HE. Remifentanil prevents an increase in intraocular pressure after succinylcholine and tracheal intubation. Br J Anaesth 1998;81(4):606–7.

139. Donlon JV. Succinylcholine and open eye injury. Anesthesiology 1986;64:525–6.

140. Wang ML, Seiff SR, Drasner K. A comparison of visual outcome in open-globe repair: succinylcholine with D-tubocurarine vs nondepolarizing agents. Ophthalmic Surg 1992;23(11):746–51.

141. Moreno RJ, Kloess P, Carlson DW. Effect of succinylcholine on the intraocular contents of open globes. Ophthalmology 1991;98(5):636–8.

142. Cunningham AJ, Barry P. Intraocular pressure—physiology and implications for anaesthetic management. Can Anaesth Soc J 1986;33(2):195–208.

143. Donlon JV. Anesthesia and eye, ear, nose, and throat surgery. In: Miller RD, editor. Anesthesia. 4th ed. New York: Churchill Livingstone, 1994:2175–96.

144. Hunter JM. Anaesthetic drugs and the eye. In: Mostafa SM, editor. Anaesthesia for Ophthalmic Surgery. Oxford: Oxford University Press, 1991:32–44.

145. McGoldrick KE. The open globe: is an alternative to succinylcholine necessary? J Clin Anesth 1993;5(1):1–4.

146. McGoldrick KE. Anesthesia and the eye. In: Barash PG, Cullen BF, Stoelting RK, editors. Clinical Anesthesia. 3rd ed. Philadelphia: Lippincott-Raven, 1996:911–28.

147. France NK, France TD, Woodburn JD Jr, Burbank DP. Succinylcholine alteration of the forced duction test. Ophthalmology 1980;87(12):1282–7.

148. Carroll JB. Increased incidence of masseter spasm in children with strabismus anesthetized with halothane and succinylcholine. Anesthesiology 1987;67(4):559–61.

149. Strazis KP, Fox AW. Malignant hyperthermia: a review of published cases. Anesth Analg 1993;77(2):297–304.

150. Dodd MJ, Phattiyakul P, Silpasuvan S. Suspected malignant hyperthermia in a strabismus patient. A case report. Arch Ophthalmol 1981;99(7):1247–50.

151. Schwartz N, Eisenkraft JB, Raab EL. Masseter muscle spasm, succinylcholine, and strabismus surgery. Anesthesiology 1988;69(4):635–6.

152. Ranklev E, Henriksson KG, Fletcher R, Germundsson K, Oldfors A, Kalimo H. Clinical and muscle biopsy findings in malignant hyperthermia susceptibility. Acta Neurol Scand 1986;74(6):452–9.

153. Berkahn JM, Sleigh JW. Hyperkalaemic cardiac arrest following succinylcholine in a longterm intensive care patient. Anaesth Intensive Care 1997;25(5):588–9.

154. Biccard BM, Grant IS, Wright DJ, Nimmo SR, Hughes M. Suxamethonium and critical illness polyneuropathy. Anaesth Intensive Care 1998;26(5):590–1.

155. Dornan RI, Royston D. Suxamethonium-related hyperkalaemic cardiac arrest in intensive care. Anaesthesia 1995;50(11):1006.

156. Hansen D. Suxamethonium-induced cardiac arrest and death following 5 days of immobilization. Eur J. Anaesthesiol 1998;15(2):240–1.

157. Hemming AE, Charlton S, Kelly P. Hyperkalaemia, cardiac arrest, suxamethonium and intensive care. Anaesthesia 1990;45(11):990–1.

158. Horton WA, Fergusson NV. Hyperkalaemia and cardiac arrest after the use of suxamethonium in intensive care. Anaesthesia 1988;43(10):890–1.

159. Lee YM, Fountain SW. Suxamethonium and cardiac arrest. Singapore Med J 1997;38(7):300–1.

160. Markewitz BA, Elstad MR. Succinylcholine-induced hyperkalemia following prolonged pharmacologic neuromuscular blockade. Chest 1997;111(1):248–50.

161. Matthews JM. Succinylcholine-induced hyperkalemia and rhabdomyolysis in a patient with necrotizing pancreatitis. Anesth Analg 2000;91(6):1552–4.

162. Chakravarty EF, Kirsch CM, Jensen WA, Kagawa FT. Cardiac arrest due to succinylcholine-induced hyperkalemia in a patient with wound botulism. J Clin Anesth 2000;12(1):80–2.

163. Passaro DJ, Werner SB, McGee J, Mac Kenzie WR, Vugia DJ. Wound botulism associated with black tar heroin among injecting drug users JAMA 1998;279(11):859–63.

164. Simpson LL. The effects of acute and chronic botulinum toxin treatment on receptor number, receptor distribution and tissue sensitivity in rat diaphragm. J Pharmacol Exp Ther 1977;200(2):343–51.

165. Koltgen D, Ceballos-Baumann AO, Franke C. Botulinum toxin converts muscle acetylcholine receptors from adult to embryonic type. Muscle Nerve 1994;17(7):779–84.

166. Sato K, Nishiwaki K, Kuno N, Kumagai K, Kitamura H, Yano K, Okamoto S, Ishikawa K, Shimada Y. Unexpected hyperkalemia following succinylcholine administration in prolonged immobilized parturients treated with magnesium and ritodrine. Anesthesiology 2000;93(6):1539–41.

167. Pascuzzi RM. Drugs and toxins associated with myopathies. Curr Opin Rheumatol 1998;10(6):511–20.

168. Sholl JS, Hughey MJ, Hirschmann RA. Myotonic muscular dystrophy associated with ritodrine tocolysis. Am J Obstet Gynecol 1985;151(1):83–6.

169. Gronert GA. Cardiac arrest after succinylcholine: mortality greater with rhabdomyolysis than receptor upregulation. Anesthesiology 2001;94(3):523–9.

170. Martyn JA, White DA, Gronert GA, Jaffe RS, Ward JM. Up-and-down regulation of skeletal muscle acetylcholine receptors. Effects on neuromuscular blockers. Anesthesiology 1992;76(5):822–43.

171. Axelsson J, Thesleff S. A study of supersensitivity in denervated mammalian skeletal muscle. J Physiol 1959;147(1):178–93.

172. Kendig JJ, Bunker JP, Endow S. Succinylcholine-induced hyperkalemia: effects of succinylcholine on resting potentials and electrolyte distributions in normal and denervated muscle. Anesthesiology 1972;36(2):132–7.

173. Gronert GA, Lambert EH, Theye RA. The response of denervated skeletal muscle to succinylcholine. Anesthesiology 1973;39(1):13–22.

174. Fischbach GD, Robbins N. Effect of chronic disuse of rat soleus neuromuscular junctions on postsynaptic membrane. J Neurophysiol 1971;34(4):562–9.

175. O'Brien DJ, Moriarty DC, Hope CE. The effect of pre-existing beta blockade on potassium flux in patients receiving succinylcholine. Can Anaesth Soc J 1986;3:S89.

176. McCammon RL, Stoelting RK. Exaggerated increase in serum potassium following succinylcholine in dogs with beta blockade. Anesthesiology 1984;61(6):723–5.

177. Koide M, Waud BE. Serum potassium concentrations after succinylcholine in patients with renal failure. Anesthesiology 1972;36(2):142–5.

178. Schaner PJ, Brown RL, Kirksey TD, Gunther RC, Ritchey CR, Gronert GA. Succinylcholine-induced

hyperkalemia in burned patients. 1. Anesth Analg 1969;48(5):764–70.

179. Tolmie JD, Joyce TH, Mitchell GD. Succinylcholine danger in the burned patient. Anesthesiology 1967;28(2):467–70.

180. Mazze RI, Escue HM, Houston JB. Hyperkalemia and cardiovascular collapse following administration of succinylcholine to the traumatized patient. Anesthesiology 1969;31(6):540–7.

181. Birch AA Jr, Mitchell GD, Playford GA, Lang CA. Changes in serum potassium response to succinylcholine following trauma. JAMA 1969;210(3):490–3.

182. Stone WA, Beach TP, Hamelberg W. Succinylcholine — danger in the spinal-cord-injured patient. Anesthesiology 1970;32(2):168–9.

183. Cooperman LH. Succinylcholine-induced hyperkalemia in neuromuscular disease. JAMA 1970;213(11):1867–71.

184. Tobey RE, Jacobsen PM, Kahle CT, Clubb RJ, Dean MA. The serum potassium response to muscle relaxants in neural injury. Anesthesiology 1972;37(3):332–7.

185. Beach TP, Stone WA, Hamelberg W. Circulatory collapse following succinylcholine: report of a patient with diffuse lower motor neuron disease. Anesth Analg 1971;50(3):431–7.

186. Fergusson RJ, Wright DJ, Willey RF, Crompton GK, Grant IW. Suxamethonium is dangerous in polyneuropathy. BMJ (Clin Res Ed) 1981;282(6260):298–9.

187. Roth F, Wuthrich H. The clinical importance of hyperkalaemia following suxamethonium administration. Br J Anaesth 1969;41(4):311–16.

188. Cowgill DB, Mostello LA, Shapiro HM. Encephalitis and a hyperkalemic response to succinycholine. Anesthesiology 1974;40(4):409–11.

189. Gravlee GP. Succinylcholine-induced hyperkalemia in a patient with Parkinson's disease. Anesth Analg 1980;59(6):444–6.

190. Rao TL, Shanmugam M. Succinylcholine administration — another contraindication? Anesth Analg 1979;58(1):61–2.

191. Krikken-Hogenberk LG, de Jong JR, Bovill JG. Succinylcholine-induced hyperkalemia in a patient with metastatic rhabdomyosarcoma. Anesthesiology 1989;70(3):553–5.

192. Iwatsuki N, Kuroda N, Amaha K, Iwatsuki K. Succinylcholine-induced hyperkalemia in patients with ruptured cerebral aneurysms. Anesthesiology 1980;53(1):64–7.

193. Kohlschutter B, Baur H, Roth F. Suxamethonium-induced hyperkalaemia in patients with severe intra-abdominal infections. Br J Anaesth 1976;48(6):557–62.

194. Khan TZ, Khan RM. Changes in serum potassium following succinylcholine in patients with infections. Anesth Analg 1983;62(3):327–31.

195. Gronert GA. Succinylcholine hyperkalemia after burns. Anesthesiology 1999;91(1):320–2.

196. Booij LH. Is succinylcholine appropriate or obsolete in the intensive care unit? Crit Care 2001;5(5):245–6.

197. Al-Khafaji AH, Dewhirst WE, Cornell CJ Jr, Quill TJ. Succinylcholine-induced hyperkalemia in a patient with mucositis secondary to chemotherapy. Crit Care Med 2001;29(6):1274–6.

198. Soliman IE, Park TS, Berkelhamer MC. Transient paralysis after intrathecal bolus of baclofen for the treatment of post-selective dorsal rhizotomy pain in children. Anesth Analg 1999;89(5):1233–5.

199. Yaksh TL. A drug has to do what a drug has to do. Anesth Analg 1999;89(5):1075–7.

200. Schow AJ, Lubarsky DA, Olson RP, Gan TJ. Can succinylcholine be used safely in hyperkalemic patients? Anesth Analg 2002;95(1):119–22.

201. Gronert GA, Theye RA. Pathophysiology of hyperkalemia induced by succinylcholine. Anesthesiology 1975;43(1):89–99.

202. Yentis SM. Suxamethonium and hyperkalaemia. Anaesth Intensive Care 1990;18(1):92–101.

203. Muravchick S, Burkett L, Gold MI. Succinylcholine-induce fasciculations and intragastric pressure during induction of anesthesia. Anesthesiology 1981;55(2):180–3.

204. Salem MR, Wong AY, Lin YH. The effect of suxamethonium on the intragastric pressure in infants and children. Br J Anaesth 1972;44(2):166–70.

205. Roe RB. The effect of suxamethonium on intragastric pressure. Anaesthesia 1962;17:179–81.

206. Miller RD, Way WL. Inhibition of succinylcholine-induced increased intragastric pressure by nondepolarizing muscle relaxants and lidocaine. Anesthesiology 1971;34(2):185–8.

207. La Cour D. Rise in intragastric pressure caused by suxamethonium fasciculations. Acta Anaesthesiol Scand 1969;13(4):255–61.

208. Marchand P. The gastro-oesophageal sphincter and the mechanism of regurgitation. Br J Surg 1955;42(175):504–13.

209. Greenan J. The cardio-oesophageal junction. Br J Anaesth 1961;33:432–9.

210. Smith G, Dalling R, Williams TI. Gastro-oesophageal pressure gradient changes produced by induction of anaesthesia and suxamethonium. Br J Anaesth 1978;50(11):1137–43.

211. La Cour D. Prevention of rise in intragastric pressure due to suxamethonium fasciculations by prior dose of D-tubocurarine. Acta Anaesthesiol Scand 1970;14(1):5–15.

212. Bishop MJ, Hornbein TF. Prolonged effect of succinylcholine after neostigmine and pyridostigmine administration in patients with renal failure. Anesthesiology 1983;58(4):384–6.

213. Bennike KA, Jarnum S. Myoglobinuria with acute renal failure possibly induced by suxamethonium. A case report. Br J Anaesth 1964;36:730–6.

214. Wong SF, Chung F. Succinylcholine-associated postoperative myalgia. Anaesthesia 2000;55(2):144–52.

215. Manataki AD, Arnaoutoglou HM, Tefa LK, Glatzounis GK, Papadopoulos GS. Continuous propofol administration for suxamethonium-induced postoperative myalgia. Anaesthesia 1999;54(5):419–22.

216. Bourne JG, Collier HO, Somers GF. Succinylcholine (succinoylcholine), muscle-relaxant of short action Lancet 1952;1(25):1225–9.

217. Smith NL. Histamine release by suxamethonium. Anaesthesia 1957;12(3):293–8.

218. Bele-Binda N, Valeri F. A case of bronchospasm induced by succinylcholine. Can Anaesth Soc J 1971;18(1):116–19.

219. Redderson C, Perkins HM, Adler WH, Gravenstein JS. Systemic reaction to succinylcholine: a case report. Anesth Analg 1971;50(1):49–52.

220. Sitarz L. Anaphylactic shock following injection of suxamethonium. Anaesth Resusc Intensive Ther 1974;2(1):83–6.

221. Mandappa JM, Chandrasekhara PM, Nelvigi RG. Anaphylaxis to suxamethonium. Two case reports. Br J Anaesth 1975;47(4):523–5.

222. James OF, Aseervatham SD, Fortunaso B, Clancy R. Anaphylactoid reaction to suxamethonium. Anaesth Intensive Care 1979;7(3):288.

223. Kepes ER, Haimovici H. Allergic reaction to succinylcholine. JAMA 1959;171:548–9.

224. Jerums G, Whittingham S, Wilson P. Anaphylaxis to suxamethonium. A case report. Br J Anaesth 1967;39(1):73–7.

225. Moss J, Fahmy NR, Sunder N, Beaven MA. Hormonal and hemodynamic profile of an anaphylactic reaction in man. Circulation 1981;63(1):210–13.

226. Fellini AA, Bernstein RL, Zauder HL. Bronchospasm due to suxamethonium; report of a case. Br J Anaesth 1963;35:657–9.

227. Katz AM, Mulligan PG. Bronchospasm induced by suxamethonium. A case report. Br J Anaesth 1972;44(10):1097–9.

228. Fisher MM, Munro I. Life-threatening anaphylactoid reactions to muscle relaxants. Anesth Analg 1983;62(6):559–64.

229. Laxenaire MC, Moneret-Vautrin DA, Vervloet D, Alazia M, Francois G. Accidents anaphylactoïdes graves peranesthésiques. [Severe peranesthetic anaphylactic accident.] Ann Fr Anesth Reanim 1985;4(1):30–46.

230. Laxenaire MC, Moneret-Vautrin DA, Vervloet D. The French experience of anaphylactoid reactions. Int Anesthesiol Clin 1985;23(3):145–60.

231. Galletly DC, Treuren BC. Anaphylactoid reactions during anaesthesia. Seven years' experience of intradermal testing. Anaesthesia 1985;40(4):329–33.

232. Youngman PR, Taylor KM, Wilson JD. Anaphylactoid reactions to neuromuscular blocking agents: a commonly undiagnosed condition? Lancet 1983;2(8350):597–9.

233. Vuitton D, Neidhardt-Audion M, Girardin P, Racadot E, Geissmann C, Laurent R, Barale F. Caractéristiques épidemiologiques de 21 accidents anaphylactoïdes peranesthésiques observés dans une population de 12,855 sujets opérés. [Epidemiologic characteristics of 21 peranesthetic anaphylactoid accidents observed in a population of 12,855 surgically treated patients.] Ann Fr Anesth Reanim 1985;4(2):167–72.

234. Laxenaire MC, Moneret-Vautrin DA, Boileau S. Choc anaphylactique au suxaméthonium: à propos de 18 cas. [Anaphylactic shock induced by suxamethonium.] Ann Fr Anesth Reanim 1982;1(1):29–36.

235. Wright PJ, Shortland JR, Stevens JD, Parsons MA, Watkins J. Fatal haemopathological consequences of general anaesthesia. Br J Anaesth 1989;62(1):104–7.

236. Moneret-Vautrin DA, Widmer S, Gueant JL, Kamel L, Laxenaire MC, Mouton C, Gerard H. Simultaneous anaphylaxis to thiopentone and a neuromuscular blocker: a study of two cases. Br J Anaesth 1990;64(6):743–5.

237. Gronert GA, Thompson RL, Onofrio BM. Human malignant hyperthermia: awake episodes and correction by dantrolene. Anesth Analg 1980;59(5):377–8.

238. Britt BA. Dantrolene. Can Anaesth Soc J 1984;31(1):61–75.

239. Ward A, Chaffman MO, Sorkin EM. Dantrolene. A review of its pharmacodynamic and pharmacokinetic properties and therapeutic use in malignant hyperthermia, the neuroleptic malignant syndrome and an update of its use in muscle spasticity. Drugs 1986;32(2):130–68.

240. Kolb ME, Horne ML, Martz R. Dantrolene in human malignant hyperthermia. Anesthesiology 1982;56(4):254–62.

241. Weingarten AE, Korsh JI, Neuman GG, Stern SB. Postpartum uterine atony after intravenous dantrolene. Anesth Analg 1987;66(3):269–70.

242. Hara Y, Kato A, Horikawa H, Kato Y, Ichiyanagi K. [Postoperative respiratory depression thought to be due to oral dantrolene pretreatment in a malignant hyperthermia-susceptible patient.] Masui 1988;37(4):483–7.

243. Saltzman LS, Kates RA, Corke BC, Norfleet EA, Heath KR. Hyperkalemia and cardiovascular collapse after verapamil and dantrolene administration in swine. Anesth Analg 1984;63(5):473–8.

244. Rubin AS, Zablocki AD. Hyperkalemia, verapamil, and dantrolene. Anesthesiology 1987;66(2):246–9.

245. Moya F, Kvisselgaard N. The placental transmission of succinylcholine. Anesthesiology 1961;22:1–6.

246. Kvisselgaard N, Moya F. Investigation of placental thresholds to succinylcholine. Anesthesiology 1961;22:7–10.

247. Weis OF, Muller FO, Lyell H, Badenhorst CH, van Niekerk P. Materno-fetal cholinesterase inhibitor poisoning. Anesth Analg 1983;62(2):233–5.

248. Hoefnagel D, Harris NA, Kim TH. Transient respiratory depression of the newborn. Its occurrence after succinylcholine administration to the mother. Am J Dis Child 1979;133(8):825–6.

249. Cherala SR, Eddie DN, Sechzer PH. Placental transfer of succinylcholine causing transient respiratory depression in the newborn. Anaesth Intensive Care 1989;17(2):202–4.

250. Hodges RJ, Harkness J. Suxamethonium sensitivity in health and disease; a clinical evaluation of pseudocholinesterase levels. BMJ 1954;4878:18–22.

251. Birch JH, Foldes FF, Rendell-Baker L. Causes and prevention of prolonged apnea with succinylcholine. Curr Res Anesth Analg 1956;35(6):609–33.

252. Shnider SM. Serum chlonesterase activity during pregnancy, labor and the puerperium. Anesthesiology 1965;26:335–9.

253. Robertson GS. Serum cholinesterase deficiency. II. Pregnancy. Br J Anaesth 1966;38(5):361–9.

254. Hazel B, Monier D. Human serum cholinesterase: variations during pregnancy and post-partum. Can Anaesth Soc J 1971;18(3):272–7.

255. Evans RT, Wroe JM. Plasma cholinesterase changes during pregnancy. Their interpretation as a cause of suxamethonium-induced apnoea. Anaesthesia 1980;35(7):651–4.

256. Robson N, Robertson I, Whittaker M. Plasma cholinesterase changes during the puerperium. Anaesthesia 1986;41(3):243–9.

257. Davies JM, Carmichael D, Dymond C. Plasma cholinesterase and trophoblastic disease. Gestational trophoblastic disease and reduced activity of plasma cholinesterase. Anaesthesia 1983;38(11):1071–4.

258. Kaniaris P, Fassoulaki A, Liarmakopoulou K, Dermitzakis E. Serum cholinesterase levels in patients with cancer. Anesth Analg 1979;58(2):82–4.

259. Goertz B, Spieckermann B, Leven B, et al. Succinylunverträglichkeit mit achtwöchiger Atemlähmung. Intensivmedizin 1977;14:88.

260. Evans RT, MacDonald R, Robinson A. Suxamethonium apnoea associated with plasmaphoresis. Anaesthesia 1980;35(2):198–201.

261. Paterson JL, Walsh ES, Hall GM. Progressive depletion of plasma cholinesterase during daily plasma exchange. BMJ 1979;2(6190):580.

262. Whittaker M. Plasma cholinesterase variants and the anaesthetist. Anaesthesia 1980;35(2):174–97.

263. Jensen FS, Viby-Mogensen J, Ostergaard D. Significance of plasma cholinesterase for the anaesthetist. Curr Anaesth Crit Care 1991;2:232.

264. Davis L, Britten JJ, Morgan M. Cholinesterase. Its significance in anaesthetic practice. Anaesthesia 1997;52(3):244–60.

265. Foldes FF. Myasthenia gravis. In: Katz RL, editor. Muscle Relaxants. Amsterdam: Excerpta Medica, 1975:345.

266. Azar I. The response of patients with neuromuscular disorders to muscle relaxants: a review. Anesthesiology 1984;61(2):173–87.

267. Martz DG, Schreibman DL, Matjasko MJ. Neurological diseases. In: Katz RL, Benumof JL, Kadis LB, editors. Anesthesia and Uncommon Diseases. 3rd ed. Philadelphia: W.B. Saunders, 1990:560.

268. Miller JD, Lee C. Muscle diseases. In: Katz RL, Benumof JL, Kadis LB, editors. Anesthesia and Uncommon Diseases. 3rd ed. Philadelphia: W.B. Saunders, 1990:590.

269. Perry J, Lee J, Wells G. Rocuronium versus succinylcholine for rapid sequence induction intubation (Cochrane Review). The Cochrane Library. Oxford: Update Software, 2003:1.

270. Beck GN, Masterson GR, Richards J, Bunting P. Comparison of intubation following propofol and

alfentanil with intubation following thiopentone and suxamethonium. Anaesthesia 1993;48(10):876–80.

271. Scheller MS, Zornow MH, Saidman LJ. Tracheal intubation without the use of muscle relaxants: a technique using propofol and varying doses of alfentanil. Anesth Analg 1992;75(5):788–93.

272. Wong AK, Teoh GS. Intubation without muscle relaxant: an alternative technique for rapid tracheal intubation. Anaesth Intensive Care 1996;24(2):224–30.

273. Stevens JB, Vescovo MV, Harris KC, Walker SC, Hickey R. Tracheal intubation using alfentanil and no muscle relaxant: is the choice of hypnotic important? Anesth Analg 1997;84(6):1222–6.

274. Klemola UM, Mennander S, Saarnivaara L. Tracheal intubation without the use of muscle relaxants: remifentanil or alfentanil in combination with propofol. Acta Anaesthesiol Scand 2000;44(4):465–9.

275. Erhan E, Ugur G, Alper I, Gunusen I, Ozyar B. Tracheal intubation without muscle relaxants: remifentanil or alfentanil in combination with propofol. Eur J Anaesthesiol 2003;20(1):37–43.

276. Miller RD, Way WL, Katzung BG. The potentiation of neuromuscular blocking agents by quinidine. Anesthesiology 1967;28(6):1036–41.

277. Durant NN, Nguyen N, Katz RL. Potentiation of neuromuscular blockade by verapamil. Anesthesiology 1984;60(4):298–303.

278. Chasapakis G, Dimas C. Possible interaction between muscle relaxants and the kallikrein-trypsin inactivator "Trasylol". Report of three cases. Br J Anaesth 1966;38(10):838–9.

279. Fisher DM, Caldwell JE, Sharma M, Wiren JE. The influence of bambuterol (carbamylated terbutaline) on the duration of action of succinylcholine-induced paralysis in humans. Anesthesiology 1988;69(5):757–9.

280. Avery GS. Check-list to potential clinically important interactions. Drugs 1973;5(3):187–211.

281. Blanloeil Y, Pinaud M, Nicolas F. Arythmies per-operatoires chez le coronarien digitalise. Vingt-quatre cas. [Perioperative cardiac arrhythmias in digitalized patients with ischemic heart disease.] Anesth Analg (Paris) 1980;37(11–12):669–74.

282. Zsigmond EK, Robins G. The effect of a series of anti-cancer drugs on plasma cholinesterase activity. Can Anaesth Soc J 1972;19(1):75–82.

283. Gurman GM. Prolonged apnea after succinylcholine in a case treated with cytostatics for cancer. Anesth Analg 1972;51(5):761–5.

284. Dretchen KL, Morgenroth VH 3rd, Standaert FG, Walts LF. Azathioprine: effects on neuromuscular transmission. Anesthesiology 1976;45(6):604–9.

285. Sprung J, Castellani WJ, Srinivasan V, Udayashankar S. The effects of donepezil and neostigmine in a patient with unusual pseudocholinesterase activity. Anesth Analg 1998;87(5):1203–5.

286. Friedhoff LT, Rogers SL. Correlation between the clinical efficacy of donepezil HCl (E2020) and red-blood cell (RBC) acetylcholinesterase (ACHE) inhibition in patients with Alzheimer's disease. Clin Pharmacol Ther 1997;61:177.

287. Bevan DR, Donati F, Kopman AF. Reversal of neuromuscular blockade. Anesthesiology 1992;77(4):785–805.

288. Crowe S, Collins L. Suxamethonium and donepezil: a cause of prolonged paralysis. Anesthesiology 2003;98(2):574–5.

289. Sanchez Morillo J, Demartini Ferrari A, Roca de Togores Lopez A. Interacción entre donepezilo y bloqueantes musculares en la enfermedad de Alzheimer. [Interaction of donepezil and muscular blockers in Alzheimer's disease.] Rev Esp Anestesiol Reanim 2003;50(2):97–100.

290. Heath ML. Donepezil and succinylcholine. Anaesthesia 2003;58(2):202.

291. Gesztes T. Prolonged apnoea after suxamethonium injection associated with eye drops containing an anticholinesterase agent. Br J Anaesth 1966;38(5):408–9.

292. Pantuck EJ. Ecothiopate iodide eye drops and prolonged response to suxamethonium. Br J Anaesth 1966;38(5):406–7.

293. Deroetth A Jr, Dettbarn WD, Rosenberg P, Wilensky JG, Wong A. Effect of phospholine iodide on blood cholinesterase levels of normal and glaucoma subjects. Am J Ophthalmol 1965;59:586–92.

294. McGavi DD. Depressed levels of serum-pseudocholinesterase with ecothiophate–iodide eyedrops. Lancet 1965;19:272–3.

295. Barnes JM, Davies DR. Blood cholinesterase levels in workers exposed to organo-phosphorus insecticides. BMJ 1951;4735:816–9.

296. Robertson GS. Serum protein and cholinesterase changes in association with contraceptive pills. Lancet 1967;1(7484):232–5.

297. Whittaker M, Charlier AR, Ramaswamy S. Changes in plasma cholinesterase isoenzymes due to oral contraceptives. J Reprod Fertil 1971;26(3):373–5.

298. Archer TL, Janowsky EC. Plasma pseudocholinesterase deficiency associated with diethylstilbestrol therapy. Anesth Analg 1978;57(6):726–32.

299. Foldes FF, Arai T, Gentsch HH, Zarday Z. The influence of glucocorticoids on plasma cholinesterase. Proc Soc Exp Biol Med 1974;146(3):918–20.

300. Verjee ZH, Behal R, Ayim EM. Effect of glucocorticoids on liver and blood cholinesterases. Clin Chim Acta 1977;81(1):41–6.

301. Bradamante V, Kunec-Vajic E, Lisic M, Dobric I, Beus I. Plasma cholinesterase activity in patients during therapy with dexamethasone or prednisone. Eur J Clin Pharmacol 1989;36(3):253–7.

302. Bovill JG, Coppel DL, Dundee JW, Moore J. Current status of ketamine anaesthesia. Lancet 1971;1(7712):1285–8.

303. Tsai SK, Lee CM, Tran B. Ketamine enhances phase I and phase II neuromuscular block of succinylcholine. Can J Anaesth 1989;36(2):120–3.

304. Amaki Y, Nagashima H, Radnay PA, Foldes FF. Ketamine interaction with neuromuscular blocking agents in the phrenic nerve-hemidiaphragm preparation of the rat. Anesth Analg 1978;57(2):238–43.

305. Johnston RR, Miller RD, Way WL. The interaction of ketamine with D-tubocurarine, pancuronium, and succinylcholine in man. Anesth Analg 1974;53(4):496–501.

306. Hilgenberg JC, Stoelting RK. Characteristics of succinylcholine-produced phase II neuromuscular block during enflurane, halothane, and fentanyl anesthesia. Anesth Analg 1981;60(4):192–6.

307. Donati F, Bevan DR. Long-term succinylcholine infusion during isoflurane anesthesia. Anesthesiology 1983;58(1):6–10.

308. Cozanitis DA, Dundee JW, Khan MM. Comparative study of atropine and glycopyrrolate on suxamethonium-induced changes in cardiac rate and rhythm. Br J Anaesth 1980;52(3):291–3.

309. Hill GE, Wong KC, Hodges MR. Potentiation of succinylcholine neuromuscular blockade by lithium carbonate. Anesthesiology 1976;44(5):439–42.

310. Hill GE, Wong KC, Hodges MR. Lithium carbonate and neuromuscular blocking agents. Anesthesiology 1977;46(2):122–6.

311. Schou M. Possible mechanisms of action of lithium salts: approaches and perspectives. Biochem Soc Trans 1973;1:81.

312. Whittaker M, Spencer R. Plasma cholinesterase variants in patients having lithium therapy. Clin Chim Acta 1977;75(3):421–5.

313. Matsuo S, Rao DB, Chaudry I, Foldes FF. Interaction of muscle relaxants and local anesthetics at the neuromuscular junction. Anesth Analg 1978;57(5):580–7.

314. Usubiaga JE, Wikinski JA, Morales RL, Usubiaga LE. Interaction of intravenously administered procaine, lidocaine and succinylcholine in anesthetized subjects. Anesth Analg 1967;46(1):39–45.

315. Morris R, Ciesecke A. Potentiation of muscle relaxants by magnesium sulfate therapy in toxemia in pregnancy. South Med J 1968;61:25.

316. Skaredoff MN, Roaf ER, Datta S. Hypermagnesaemia and anaesthetic management. Can Anaesth Soc J 1982;29(1):35–41.

317. Ghoneim MM, Long JP. The interaction between magnesium and other neuromuscular blocking agents. Anesthesiology 1970;32(1):23–7.

318. Giesecke AH Jr, Morris RE, Dalton MD, Stephen CR. Of magnesium, muscle relaxants, toxemic parturients, and cats. Anesth Analg 1968;47(6):689–95.

319. De Vore JS, Asrani R. Magnesium sulfate prevents succinylcholine-induced fasciculations in toxemic parturients. Anesthesiology 1980;52(1):76–7.

320. Kambam JR, Parris WC, Franks JJ, Sastry BV. The inhibitory effect of metoclopramide on plasma cholinesterase activity. Anesth Analg 1988;67:S107.

321. Kao YJ, Turner DR. Prolongation of succinylcholine block by metoclopramide. Anesthesiology 1989;70(6):905–8.

322. Kao YJ, Tellez J, Turner DR. Dose-dependent effect of metoclopramide on cholinesterases and suxamethonium metabolism. Br J Anaesth 1990;65(2):220–4.

323. Gissen AJ, Katz RL, Karis JH, Papper EM. Neuromuscular block in man during prolonged arterial infusion with succinylcholine. Anesthesiology 1966;27(3):242–9.

324. Ivankovich AD, Sidell N, Cairoli VJ, Dietz AA, Albrecht RF. Dual action of pancuronium on succinylcholine block. Can Anaesth Soc J 1977;24(2):228–42.

325. Ebeling BJ, Keienburg T, Hausmann D, Apffelstaedt C. Das Wirkungsprofil von Succinylcholin nach Präcurarisierung mit Atracurium, Vecuronium oder Pancuronium. [Profile of the effect of succinylcholine after pre-curarization with atracurium, vecuronium or pancuronium.] Anästhesiol Intensivmed Notfallmed Schmerzther 1996;31(5):304–8.

326. d'Hollander AA, Agoston S, De Ville A, Cuvelier F. Clinical and pharmacological actions of a bolus injection of suxamethonium: two phenomena of distinct duration. Br J Anaesth 1983;55(2):131–4.

327. Katz RL. Modification of the action of pancuronium by succinylcholine and halothane. Anesthesiology 1971;35(6):602–6.

328. Bowman WC. Non-relaxant properties of neuromuscular blocking drugs. Br J Anaesth 1982;54(2):147–60.

329. Walts LF, Dillon JB. Clinical studies of the interaction between D-tubocurarine and succinylcholine. Anesthesiology 1969;31(1):35–8.

330. Scott RP, Norman J. Effect of suxamethonium given during recovery from atracurium. Br J Anaesth 1988;61(3):292–6.

331. Kim KS, Na DJ, Chon SU. Interactions between suxamethonium and mivacurium or atracurium. Br J Anaesth 1996;77(5):612–16.

332. Bodley PO, Halwax K, Potts L. Low serum pseudocholinesterase levels complicating treatment with phenelzine. BMJ 1969;3(669):510–12.

333. Foldes FF, Hillmer NR, Molloy RE, Monte AP. Potentiation of the neuromuscular effect of succinylcholine by hexafluorenium. Anesthesiology 1960;21:50–8.

334. Gordh T, Wahlin A. Potentiation of the neuromuscular effect of succinylcholine by tetrahydro-amino-acridine. Acta Anaesthesiol Scand 1961;5:55–61.

335. Walts LF, DeAngelis J, Dillon JB. Clinical studies of the interaction of hexafluorenium and succinylcholine in man. Anesthesiology 1970;33(5):503–7.

336. Radnay PA, El-Gaweet ES, Novakovic M, Badola R, Cizmar S, Duncalf D. Prevention of succinylcholine induced hyperkalemia by neuroleptanesthesia and hexafluorenium in anephric patients. Anaesthesist 1981;30(7):334–7.

337. Katz RL, Eakins KE, Lord CO. The effects of hexafluorenium in preventing the increase in intraocular pressure produced by succinylcholine. Anesthesiology 1968;29(1):70–8.

338. Tewfik GI. Trimetaphan; its effect on the pseudo-cholinesterase level of man. Anaesthesia 1957;12(3):326–9.

339. Sklar GS, Lanks KW. Effects of trimethaphan and sodium nitroprusside on hydrolysis of succinylcholine in vitro. Anesthesiology 1977;47(1):31–3.

340. Poulton TJ, James FM 3rd, Lockridge O. Prolonged apnea following trimethaphan and succinylcholine. Anesthesiology 1979;50(1):54–6.

341. Nakamura K, Hatano Y, Mori K. The site of action of trimethaphan-induced neuromuscular blockade in isolated rat and frog muscle. Acta Anaesthesiol Scand 1988;32(2):125–30.

Suxibuzone

See also Non-steroidal anti-inflammatory drugs

General Information

Suxibuzone, a derivative of phenylbutazone, is an NSAID that has been used topically. Skin reactions, gastrotoxicity, nephrotoxicity, headache, and vertigo have been noted. The carcinogenic potential of suxibuzone in animals has attracted attention (1) and put an end to sales in some countries.

Reference

1. Anonymous. Other action on suxibuzone. Scrip 1982;669:14.